PRINCIPLES OF
Neurosurgery

PRINCIPLES OF
Neurosurgery

Edited by

Setti S. Rengachary, MD
Professor of Neurosurgery
University of Minnesota Medical School
Minneapolis, Minnesota

Robert H. Wilkins, MD
Professor and Chief
Division of Neurosurgery
Duke University Medical Center
Durham, North Carolina

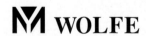 **WOLFE**

LONDON ST. LOUIS BALTIMORE BOSTON CHICAGO PHILADELPHIA SYDNEY TORONTO

Editors: Elizabeth Greenspan, David Yoon
Art Director: Kathryn Greenslade
Designers: Anne Kenney (interior), Talar Agasyan, Jennifer Bergamini (cover, chapter opener), Carol Drozdyk, Ric Sevilla
Illustration Supervisor: Patricia Holtz
Illustrators: Alan Landau, Gary Welch, SueAnn Fung-Ho, Nicholas Guarracino, Scott Bodell (Ch. 11), M.B. Mackay (Ch. 37), Jon Coulter (Ch. 40), Patricia Gast (line drawings), Ruth Soffer (inking)

10 9 8 7 6 5 4 3 2 1

Originated in Singapore by Colourscan Overseas Co., PTE, Ltd.

Produced in Hong Kong by Mandarin Offset

Printed and bound in Hong Kong, 1994

Library of Congress Cataloging-in-Publication Data
Principles of neurosurgery / edited by Setti S. Rengachary, Robert H. Wilkins
    p. cm.
    Includes bibliographical references and index.
    ISBN 1-56375-022-8
    1. Nervous system—Surgery. I. Rengachary, Setti S. II. Wilkins, Robert H.
    [DNLM: 1. Neurosurgery. WL 368P9571 1993]
RD593.P752 1993
617.4'8—dc20
DNLM/DLC
                                                                    93-10153

British Library Cataloguing in Publication Data
A catalogue record for this book is available from the British Library.

DEDICATION

This book is dedicated to house officers in clinical neurosciences throughout the world.

S.S.R.
R.H.W.

In memory of Alan Landau—gifted artist, kind friend.

The Publishers

FOREWORD

Fifty years ago, few textbooks dealing with neurosurgery were available. In the last two or three decades there has been an explosive increase in the number of published monographs, texts, and atlases of neurosurgical interest. There have been several brief introductory texts targeted for medical students, several operative atlases, a number of detailed comprehensive texts covering the entire field of neurosurgery, and a large number of subject-specific monographs. However, little has been written primarily for the neurosurgical resident.

Setti S. Rengachary and Robert H. Wilkins, the editors of this volume, have also edited a number of other successful and popular texts, and both of the editors have trained neurosurgical residents for many years. Neurosurgical residents, especially the junior and mid-level residents, are often overwhelmed by the literature available. This book is uniquely planned for their educational needs as well as for medical students with an interest in neurosurgery.

An excellent cast of experienced and knowledgeable experts were recruited to write the 51 chapters in this comprehensive text. The format and style emphasize illustrations, with high-quality color drawings and with many tables and algorithms, which help to simplify the understanding of the concepts and subjects discussed. The style of presentation makes this book most appealing and easy to read. The text is well organized and well subdivided so it can be used as a quick reference. The references in most chapters are well selected and not excessive. The unique format makes it easy to review material previously studied.

I am sure most neurosurgical trainees join me in congratulating the editors for this most instructive educational text, and I am sure most neurosurgical residents will have it on their desks.

Hugo V. Rizzoli, MD
Professor Emeritus of Neurological Surgery
George Washington University Medical Center
Washington, DC

PREFACE

The proverb "a little picture is worth a thousand words" is especially true when core textbooks are designed for beginners trying to understand a complex subject. *Principles of Neurosurgery* applies this proverb to neurologic surgery. It is intended to give a broad overview of the subject to medical students and junior house officers in the clinical neurosciences. The chapter topics chosen cover core areas of neurosurgery; the text is comprehensive without being encyclopedic. What differentiates *Principles of Neurosurgery* from other neurosurgery texts is the extraordinary visual appeal it provides to the subject matter. A large number of color illustrations, tables, algorithms, photographs, and flow charts are incorporated in every chapter. The illustrations provide the major fabric, with appropriate text material interwoven. This enables a beginning student to grasp the subject more easily; attractive visual input makes the learning of sophisticated concepts an easy and enjoyable process. Virtually all of the illustrations have been prepared by dedicated and highly skilled artists specifically for this text, using state-of-the-art technology. In attempting to present the subject in an attractive manner, rigor and accuracy have not been overlooked. All of the contributing authors have worked in close collaboration with the artists to ensure imaginative original style and accuracy. We hope that *Principles of Neurosurgery* will be a landmark publication among introductory texts in neurosurgery.

We thank Elizabeth Greenspan of Mosby for her initiative, extraordinary diligence, and dedication in overseeing and coordinating all phases of production of this book; we also thank Jane Hunter for her continued support.

Setti S. Rengachary, MD
Robert H. Wilkins, MD

CONTENTS

CONTENTS

CONTRIBUTORS

Chad D. Abernathey, MD, PC
Department of Neurosurgery
Mercy Medical Center
Cedar Rapids, Iowa

A. Leland Albright, MD
Associate Professor of Neurosurgery
University of Pittsburgh
Chief of Pediatric Neurosurgery
Children's Hospital of Pittsburgh
Pittsburgh, Pennsylvania

Mitchell S. Anscher, MD
Assistant Professor of Radiation Oncology
Duke University Medical Center
Durham, North Carolina

James I. Ausman, MD, PhD
Professor and Head
Department of Neurosurgery
University of Illinois College of Medicine at Chicago
Chicago, Illinois

Issam A. Awad, MD, MSc, FACS
Director, Neurovascular Surgery Program
and Yale Cerebrovascular Center
Yale University School of Medicine
New Haven, Connecticut

H. Hunt Batjer, MD
Associate Professor of Neurological Surgery
University of Texas Southwestern Medical Center
Dallas, Texas

Allan J. Belzberg, MD
Assistant Professor of Neurosurgery
Johns Hopkins School of Medicine
Co-Director, Peripheral Nerve Injury Unit
Johns Hopkins Hospital
Baltimore, Maryland

Mark Bernstein, MD
Associate Professor of Surgery
University of Toronto
Head, Division of Neurosurgery
The Toronto Hospital
Toronto, Ontario

José Biller, MD, FACP
Professor of Neurology
Northwestern University Medical School
Director, Stroke Program
Northwestern Memorial Hospital
Searle Family Center for Neurological
Disorders
Chicago, Illinois

Peter McL. Black, MD, PhD
Franc D. Ingraham Professor of Neurosurgery
Harvard Medical School
Neurosurgeon-in-Chief
Brigham and Women's Hospital
The Children's Hospital
Boston, Massachusetts

Bennett Blumenkopf, MD
Associate Professor of Neurological Surgery
Vanderbilt University Medical Center
Nashville, Tennessee

Michael F. Brothers, MD, FRCP(C)
Assistant Professor of Radiology
and Neurosurgery
Duke University Medical Center
Durham, North Carolina

Arturo Camacho, MD
Resident in Neurological Surgery
Mayo Clinic and Mayo Graduate School
of Medicine
Rochester, Minnesota

James N. Campbell, MD
Professor of Neurosurgery
Johns Hopkins School of Medicine
Co-Director, Peripheral Nerve Injury Unit
Johns Hopkins Hospital
Baltimore, Maryland

Samuel F. Ciricillo, MD
Clinical Instructor
Department of Neurological Surgery
School of Medicine
University of California, San Francisco
San Francisco, California

Robert J. Coffey, MD
Assistant Professor of Neurosurgery
Mayo Medical School
Senior Associate Consultant
Mayo Clinic
Rochester, Minnesota

Derek A. Duke, MD
Resident, Department of Neurosurgery
Mayo Clinic
Rochester, Minnesota

Michael S. B. Edwards, MD
Professor in Residence
Departments of Pediatrics and
    Neurological Surgery
Vice-Chairman, Department of
    Neurological Surgery
School of Medicine
University of California, San Francisco
San Francisco, California

Mark B. Eisenberg, MD
Chief Resident
Department of Neurosurgery
Mount Sinai Medical Center
New York, New York

Allan H. Friedman, MD
Associate Professor of Neurosurgery
Duke University Medical Center
Durham, North Carolina

Fred H. Geisler, MD, PhD
Director, Comprehensive Spine
    Care Center
Chicago Institute of Neurosurgery
    and Neuroresearch
Chicago, Illinois

James Tait Goodrich, MD, PhD
Associate Professor of Neurosurgery,
    Pediatrics, Plastic and Reconstructive Surgery
Albert Einstein College of Medicine
Bronx, New York

Mark N. Hadley, MD
Assistant Professor of Neurological Surgery
University of Alabama at Birmingham
Birmingham, Alabama

Edward C. Halperin, MD
Associate Professor of Radiation Oncology
Department of Radiation Oncology
Duke University Medical Center
Durham, North Carolina

Griffith R. Harsh IV, MD
Associate Professor of Surgery
Harvard Medical School
Associate Visiting Neurosurgeon
Massachusetts General Hospital
Boston, Massachusetts

Martin C. Holland, MD
Senior Resident, Division of Neurosurgery
School of Medicine
University of California, Los Angeles
Los Angeles, California

John A. Jane, MD
Chairman
Department of Neurological Surgery
University of Virginia Health Sciences Center
Charlottesville, Virgnia

Patrick J. Kelly, MD
Professor of Neurological Surgery
Mayo Medical School
Rochester, Minnesota

Douglas W. Laske, MD
Senior Staff Fellow, Surgical Neurology Branch
National Institute of Neurological Disorders and Stroke
National Institutes of Health
Bethesda, Maryland

Christopher M. Loftus, MD, FACS
Associate Professor of Surgery (Neurosurgery)
University of Iowa College of Medicine
Iowa City, Iowa

CONTRIBUTORS

Paul N. Manson, MD
Professor of Plastic Surgery
Johns Hopkins University
Chairman, Division of Plastic Surgery
R. Adams Cowley Shock Trauma Center
Maryland Institute for Emergency Medical
    Services Systems
Baltimore, Maryland

Neil A. Martin, MD
Associate Professor of Neurosurgery
School of Medicine
University of California, Los Angeles
Los Angeles, California

Mitsunori Matsumae, MD
Department of Neurosurgery
Tokai University School of Medicine
Kanagawa, Japan

Robert J. McBroom, MD
Assistant Professor
University of Toronto
Division of Orthopaedics
The Wellesley Hospital & St. Michael's Hospital
Toronto, Ontario

Jeffrey D. McDonald, MD
Resident, Department of Neurological Surgery
School of Medicine
University of California, San Francisco
San Francisco, California

Ossama Al-Mefty, MD, FACS
Professor of Neurological Surgery
Stritch School of Medicine
Loyola University of Chicago
Maywood, Illinois

Raj K. Narayan, MD
Associate Professor of Neurosurgery
Baylor College of Medicine
Chief of Neurosurgery
Ben Taub General Hospital
The Methodist Hospital
Houston, Texas

Paul B. Nelson, MD
Director and Professor of Neurological Surgery
Indiana University Medical Center
Indianapolis, Indiana

Eric S. Nussbaum, MD
Resident, Department of Neurosurgery
University of Minnesota Medical School
Minneapolis, Minnesota

W. Jerry Oakes, MD
Professor of Surgery (Neurosurgery)
University of Alabama at Birmingham
Birmingham, Alabama

Edward Oldfield, MD, FACS
Chief, Surgical Neurology Branch
National Institute of Neurological
    Disorders and Stroke
National Institutes of Health
Bethesda, Maryland

Steven Onesti, MD
Attending Neurosurgeon
New England Baptist Hospital
Boston, Massachusetts

T.C. Origitano, MD, PhD
Assistant Professor of Neurological Surgery
    and Physiology
Loyola University Medical Center
Maywood, Illinois

Dachling Pang, MD, FRCS(C), FACS
Professor of Neurological Surgery
Chief, Pediatric Neurosurgery
School of Medicine
University of California, Davis
Sacramento, California

Roy A. Patchell, MD
Associate Professor of Neurology and
    Neurosurgery
Chief, Neuro-Oncology
University of Kentucky College of Medicine
Lexington, Kentucky

Richard G. Perrin, MD
Associate Professor
University of Toronto
Chief, Division of Neurosurgery
The Wellesley Hospital
Toronto, Ontario

John A. Persing, MD
Professor and Chief
Plastic and Reconstructive Surgery
Yale University School of Medicine
New Haven, Connecticut

Joseph A. Petronio, MD
Fellow, Pediatric Neurosurgery
University of Utah
Primary Children's Medical Center
Salt Lake City, Utah

Kalmon D. Post, MD
Professor and Chairman
Department of Neurosurgery
Mount Sinai Medical Center
New York, New York

Setti S. Rengachary, MD
Professor of Neurosurgery
University of Minnesota Medical School
Minneapolis, Minnesota

Mark L. Rosenblum, MD
Chairman, Department of Neurological Surgery
Henry Ford Hospital
Detroit, Michigan

S. Clifford Schold, Jr., MD
Professor and Chairman
Department of Neurology
University of Texas Southwestern Medical Center
Dallas, Texas

Chandranath Sen, MD
Associate Professor of Neurological Surgery
Mount Sinai School of Medicine
Associate Attending Surgeon
Mount Sinai Medical Center
New York, New York

Christopher I. Shaffrey, MD
Chief Resident
Department of Neurological Surgery
University of Virginia Health Sciences Center
Charlottesville, Virginia

Mark E. Shaffrey, MD
Chief Resident
Department of Neurological Surgery
University of Virginia Health Sciences
    Center
Charlottesville, Virginia

Konstantin V. Slavin, MD
Research Fellow, Department of Neurosurgery
The Neuropsychiatric Institute
University of Illinois College of Medicine
    at Chicago
Chicago, Illinois

Robert A. Solomon, MD
Associate Professor of Neurological Surgery
College of Physicians and Surgeons
Columbia University
New York, New York

Leslie N. Sutton, MD
Associate Professor of Neurosurgery
    and Pediatrics
University of Pennsylvania School
    of Medicine
Associate Neurosurgeon
Children's Hospital of Philadelphia
Philadelphia, Pennsylvania

Ronald R. Tasker, MD
Professor of Surgery
University of Toronto
Senior Neurosurgeon
The Toronto Hospital
Toronto, Ontario

Dennis A. Turner, MD
Assistant Professor of Neurosurgery and
    Neurobiology
Duke University Medical Center
Durham, North Carolina

CONTRIBUTORS

Marion L. Walker, MD
Professor of Neurosurgery and Pediatrics
University of Utah
Primary Children's Medical Center
Salt Lake City, Utah

Philip R. Weinstein, MD
Professor and Vice-Chairman
Department of Neurological Surgery
School of Medicine
University of California, San Francisco
San Francisco, California

Jack E. Wilberger, MD, FACS
Associate Professor of Surgery
Medical College of Pennsylvania
Vice-Chairman, Department of Neurosurgery
Director, Neurotrauma
Co-Director, AGH Comprehensive Epilepsy Services
Allegheny General Hospital
Pittsburgh, Pennsylvania

Robert H. Wilkins, MD
Professor and Chief
Division of Neurosurgery
Duke University Medical Center
Durham, North Carolina

Allen R. Wyler, MD
Medical Director, Epilepsy Center
Swedish Medical Center
Seattle, Washington

Byron Young, MD
Chief, Division of Neurosurgery
Johnston-Wright Chair of Surgery
University of Kentucky College of
    Medicine
Lexington, Kentucky

Chapter 1

Landmarks in the History
of Neurosurgery

James Tait Goodrich

If a physician makes a wound and cures a free-man, he shall receive ten pieces of silver, but only five if the patient is the son of a plebeian or two if he is a slave. However it is decreed that if a physician treats a patient with a metal knife for a severe wound and has caused the man to die—his hands shall be cut off.—Code of Hammurabi

Landmarks in the history of neurologic surgery are the focus of this chapter. After reading it, perhaps the neurosurgeon will explore more carefully the subsequent chapters in this volume to avoid having his or her "hands cut off."

In order to identify major trends in neurosurgery I have organized its history into six periods. In each era the key themes, personalities, and neurosurgical techniques developed and used will be discussed. This review focuses on concepts and ideas in the hope of stimulating further reading in the subject.

GREEK AND EARLY BYZANTINE PERIOD: THE ORIGINS OF NEUROSURGERY

The intellectual development of neurosurgery begins in the golden age of Greece. The use of trephination in head injury dates back to much earlier periods, but little is known about how it was used in wound management. In fact, much early trephination appears to have been done for religious or psychologic purposes. During the ancient period there were no surgeons who restricted themselves *in stricto sensu* to "neurosurgery." Head injuries, however, appear to have been plentiful, the result of wars and internecine conflicts, as recorded by Herodotus and Thucydides as well as Homer. War was then, as now, the principal source of material for the study and treatment of head injury.

The earliest medical writings from this period are generally thought to be those attributed to Hippocrates (460–370 BC), that most celebrated of the Asclepiadae (Fig. 1.1).[1] Hippocrates was the first to describe a number of neurologic conditions, many of them resulting from battlefield injuries. He understood that the location of the injury to the skull was important. The vulnerability of the brain to injury was categorized from lesser to greater by location, with injury to the bregma representing a greater risk than injury to the temporal region, which in turn was more dangerous than injury to the occipital region.[2]

One of the most interesting observations from this school comes from the *Aphorisms*, which include one of the earliest descriptions of subarachnoid hemorrhage: "When persons in good health are suddenly seized with pains in the head, and straightway are laid down speechless, and breathe with stertor, they die in seven days, unless fever comes on."[3]

Hippocrates described the use of the trephine. He argued for trephination in brain contusions but not in depressed skull fractures (the prognosis was too grave) and cautioned that it should never be done over a skull suture due to the risk of injury to the underlying dura. In the same spirit he recommended "watering" the trephine bit well to prevent overheating and injury to the dura.

In the section on "Wounds of the Head," Hippocrates warned against incising the brain, as convulsions can occur on the opposite side. He also warned against making a skin incision over the temporal artery, as this could lead to contralateral convulsions (or perhaps severe hemorrhage from skin?). He understood simple concepts of cerebral localization and appreciated the serious prognosis in head injury.

From the region of the Bosporus to the crowded schools of Alexandria came Herophilus of Chalcedon (fl. ca. 300 BC), the great early anatomist. Unlike his predecessors, Herophilus dissected human bodies in addition to animals—more than 100, by his own account. Herophilus engaged in the arduous task of developing an anatomic nomenclature and forming a language of anatomy. He traced the origin of nerves to the spinal cord and divided them into motor and sensory tracts. He made the important differentiation of nerves from tendons, which were often confused at that time. He was among the first to describe in detail the ventricles and venous sinuses of the brain, in particular the confluens sinuum or *torcular Herophili*. He described for the first time the choroid plexus, so named by him for its resemblance to the vascular membrane of the fetus. Herophilus described in detail the fourth ventricle and noted the peculiar arrangement at its base, which he called the "calamus scriptorius" because it "resembles the groove of a pen for writing." Among his many other contributions was his recognition of the brain as the central organ of the nervous system and the seat of intelligence.[4]

Herophilus is also remembered for introducing one of the longest-standing errors in anatomic physiology:

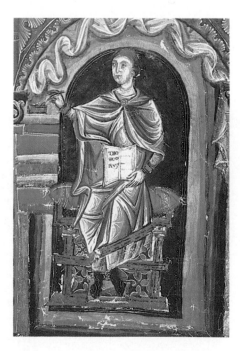

Figure 1.1
A depiction of Hippocrates in an early eighth century manuscript.

Principles of Neurosurgery

the rete mirabile, a structure present in artiodactyls but not in humans, which acts as an anastomotic network at the base of the brain. This structure was to become important in early physiologic theories of human brain function. The rete mirabile was later described in detail by Galen of Pergamus and canonized by Arabic and medieval scholars. Not until the sixteenth century, with the authoritative accounts of Vesalius and Berengario da Carpi, was its absence in humans recognized.

Rufus of Ephesus (fl. ca. AD 98–117) lived during the reign of Trajan in the beautiful city of Ephesus. Because so many of Rufus's manuscripts survived, they heavily influenced the medieval compilers. Due to his great skill as a surgeon, many of his surgical writings were transcribed through the sixteenth century.[5] Rufus's description of the membranes covering the brain is classic. He distinguished between the cerebrum and cerebellum and described the corpus callosum. He understood the anatomy of the ventricular system and gave details of the lateral ventricle; he also described the third and fourth ventricles, as well as the aqueduct of Sylvius. Rufus also provided anatomic descriptions of the pineal gland and hypophysis, and his accounts of the fornix and the quadrigeminal plate are accurate and elegant. Rufus also described the optic chiasm and recognized that it is related to vision. The singular accuracy of Rufus's studies must be credited to his use of dissection (mostly monkeys) in an era during which most Greeks abhorred anatomic dissection.

Though Aulus Cornelius Celsus (25 BC–AD 50) was not a surgeon, as a medical encyclopedist he had an important influence on surgery. He reviewed the rival medical schools of his time—dogmatic, methodic, and empiric—fairly and with moderation. As counsel to the emperors Tiberius and Gaius (Caligula), he was held in great esteem. His book, *De re medicina*,[6] is one of the earliest extant medical documents after the Hippocratic writings. It is elegantly written and has therefore had a large influence on medical history. In fact, when printing was introduced in the fifteenth century, Celsus's works were printed before those of Hippocrates and Galen.

In the field of neurosurgery Celsus made a number of interesting observations. *De re medicina* 8.4 contains an early description of an epidural hematoma resulting from a bleeding middle meningeal artery.[6] He recommended that the surgeon always operate on the side of greater pain and place the trephine where the pain is best localized. Considering the innervation of the dura and its sensitivity to pressure, this has proved to be a good clinical suggestion. He also provided accurate descriptions of hydrocephalus and facial neuralgia. He knew that a fracture of the cervical spine can cause vomiting and difficulty in breathing, whereas injury of the lower spine can cause weakness or paralysis of the leg, as well as urinary retention or incontinence.

Galen of Pergamus (Claudius Galenus, AD 129–200) needs little introduction to a medical audience. He was an original investigator, compiler, and codifier, as well as a leading advocate of the doctrines of Hippocrates and the Alexandrian school. As physician to the gladiators of Pergamus he had access to many human subjects, particularly with traumatic injuries.

His experience as a physician and his scientific studies enabled Galen to make a variety of contributions to neuroanatomy. He differentiated between the pia mater and the dura mater. He described the corpus callosum, the ventricular system, the pineal and pituitary glands, and the infundibulum. He predated Monro in describing the structure later called the foramen of Monro. He also gave an accurate description of the aqueduct of Sylvius. He performed such anatomic experiments as transection of the spinal cord, which led him to describe loss of function below the level of the lesion. In the dog he sectioned the recurrent laryngeal nerve and recognized that hoarseness was a consequence (Fig. 1.2). Moreover, Galen made the first recorded attempt at identifying and numbering the cranial nerves. He actually demonstrated 11 of the 12 nerves, but he combined several, thus arriving at a total of only seven. He regarded the olfactory nerve as merely a prolongation of the brain and hence did not count it.[7]

Galen held original views concerning brain functions. He believed the brain controlled intelligence, fantasy, memory, and judgment. This was an important departure from the teaching of earlier schools, Aristotle's for example. Galen discarded Hippocrates' notion that the brain is only a gland and attributed to it the powers of voluntary action and sensation.

In neurology, Galen made a number of important observations. He recognized that cervical injury can cause disturbance in arm function. In a study of spinal cord injury, Galen detailed a classic case of what is today known as Brown-Séquard syndrome—that is, a hemiplegia with contralateral sensory loss in a subject with a hemisection of the cord.[8] Galen's description of the symptoms and signs of hydrocephalus is classic—it enabled him to predict which patients has a poor prog-

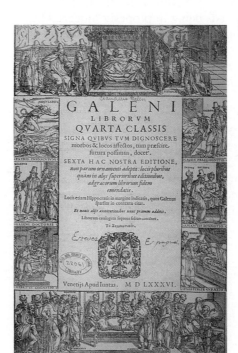

Figure 1.2
Title page from Galen's *Opera omnia*, Juntine edition, Venice. The border contains a number of allegorical scenes showing the early practice of medicine. The lower panel shows Galen performing his classic study on the recurrent larygneal nerve.

nosis. Galen was much more liberal about head injury than Hippocrates, arguing for elevation of depressed skull fractures, fractures with hematomas, and comminuted fractures. Galen recommended removing the bone fragments, particularly those pressing into the brain. Galen was more optimistic than Hippocrates about brain injuries, commenting "we have seen a severely wounded brain healed." He provided an extensive description of the safe use of the trephine, pointing out that the dura should not be violated.

Paul of Aegina (AD 625–690), trained in the Alexandrian school, was the last great Byzantine physician. He was a compiler of works in both the Latin and Greek schools, and his writings were consulted well into the seventeenth century. More importantly, he was a skilled surgeon to whom patients came from far and wide. He venerated the teachings of the ancients as tradition required, but he introduced his own techniques with good results. His classic work, *The Seven Books of Paul of Aegina,* contains an excellent section on head injury and the use of the trephine.[9,10] Paul classified skull fractures in several categories: fissure, incision, expression, depression, arched fracture, and, in infants, dent. In dealing with fractures he used an interesting skin incision: two incisions intersecting one another at right angles, giving the Greek letter X, with one leg of the incision incorporating the scalp wound. The patient's ear was to be stuffed with wool so that the noise of the trephine would not cause distress. The wound was dressed with a broad bandage soaked in oil of roses and wine, with care taken to avoid compressing the brain (Paulus Aeginetes 6.90).[10]

In discussing hydrocephalus Paul of Aegina introduced the concept of the man-handling midwife. He was the first to suggest the possibility that an intraventricular hemorrhage might cause hydrocephalus:

> The hydrocephalic affection...occurs in infants, owing to their heads being improperly squeezed by midwives during parturition, or from some other obscure cause; or from the rupture of a vessel or vessels, and the extravasated blood being converted into an inert fluid....(Paulus Aeginetes 6.3)[10]

Several of the instruments that Paul designed for neurosurgical procedures can be seen in his earlier manuscripts. Elevators, raspatories, bone biters, all came from this period, and trephine bits with conical styles and different biting edges were introduced by Paul. His wound management was also quite sophisticated—he used wine (helpful in antisepsis, though this concept was then unknown) and stressed that dressings should be applied with no compression to the brain. Paul's influence on Arabic medicine, in particular on Albucasis, who is discussed below, was enormous.

ARABIC AND MEDIEVAL MEDICINE: SCHOLARSHIP AND SOMNOLENCE

From approximately AD 750 to 1200 the major intellectual centers of medicine were the Arabic and Byzantine cultures. As Western Europe revived after AD 1000, the study of surgery and medicine returned there as well.

ARABIC SCHOLARSHIP

Arabic schools translated and systematized the surviving Greek and Roman texts. Thanks to their incredible zeal, the best of Greek medicine was made available to Arabic readers by the end of the ninth century. Unfortunately, a rigid scholastic dogmatism became characteristic. Also, the translators too frequently rendered their favorite view instead of the author's.

Arabic medicine flourished from the tenth century through the twelfth century. Among the most illustrious scholars were Avicenna, Rhazes, Avenzoar, Albucasis, and Averroes. In the writings of these great physicians one sees an extraordinary effort to canonize the writings of their Greek and Roman predecessors. Arab scholars and physicians served as guardians and academics of what now became Hippocratic and Galenic dogma, while the wonderful advances in surgery and anatomy developed by the Alexandrians, among others, were lost or ignored.

Physicians rarely did surgery in this era. It was expected that the physician would write learnedly and speak ex cathedra, but assign the menial task of surgery to an individual of a lower class, that is, to a surgeon.

Arabic medicine did introduce a great medical tradition—bedside medicine and teaching. But the lack of dissection and the practice of surgery by individuals of substantially less status than physicians reduced interest in surgery. The only major contribution to surgery was the reintroduction of the Egyptian technique of using the hot cautery to control bleeding (Fig. 1.3). Regrettably, the hot cautery was often used instead of the scalpel to create surgical incisions—a rather destructive way to proceed.

The writings of Rhazes (Abu Bakr Muhammad ibn Zakariya' al-Razi, 865–925) indicate that he was a scholarly physician, loyal to Hippocratic teachings and learned in diagnosis. Although primarily a court physician and not a surgeon, his writings on surgical topics remained influential through the eighteenth century.[11] Rhazes was one of the first to introduce the concept of concussion. Head injury, he wrote, is among the most devastating of all injuries. He advocated surgery only for penetrating injuries of the skull; the outcome was almost always fatal. Rhazes understood that a skull fracture, because it causes compression of the brain, requires elevation to prevent lasting injury.

Avicenna (Abu 'Ali al-Husayn ibn 'Abdallah ibn

Sina, 980–1037), the famous physician and philosopher of Baghdad, was known as the "second doctor" (the first being Aristotle). His works were translated into Latin and were a dominant force in the major European universities well into the eighteenth century. He disseminated the Greek teachings so persuasively that their influence is felt to this day. In his major work, *Canon medicinae*, an encyclopedic effort founded on the writings of Galen and Hippocrates, the observations reported are mostly clinical, bearing primarily on materia medica (Fig. 1.4).[12] Within Avicenna's *Canon* are a number of interesting neurologic findings, such as the first accurate clinical explication of epilepsy, for which treatment consisted of various medicants and herbals. It appears that Avicenna conducted anatomic studies inasmuch as he gives a correct anatomic discussion of the vermis of the cerebellum and the "tailed nucleus," now known as the caudate nucleus. His greatest contribution may be his translation of Galen's collected works.

In the Arab tradition Albucasis (Abu 'l-Qasim ibn 'Abbas al-Zahrawi, 936–1013) was a great compiler as well as a serious scholar, whose writings (some thirty volumes!) were focused mainly on surgery, dietetics, and materia medica. In the introduction to his *Compendium* there is an interesting discussion of why the Arabs had made so little progress in surgery: He attributed it to a lack of anatomic study and inadequate knowledge of the classics. He popularized the frequent use of emetics as prophylaxis against disease, a practice that survived, as "purging," into the nineteenth century.

The final section of the *Compendium* is a lengthy summary of surgical practice at that time.[13–15] This work was used extensively in the schools of Salerno and Montpellier and hence was an important influence in medieval Europe. Illustrations of surgical instruments to accompany the text describing their use were a unique feature. Many of the instruments were designed by Albucasis, and some were based on those described by Paul of Aegina. His design of a "nonsinking" trephine is classic (he placed a collar on the trephine to prevent plunging), the basis of many later instrument designs.

Albucasis' treatise on surgery is an extraordinary work—a rational, comprehensive, and well-illustrated text designed to teach the surgeon the details of each treatment, including the types of wound dressings to be used. Yet one can only wonder how patients tolerated some of Albucasis' techniques. For chronic headache he applied a hot cautery to the occiput, burning through the skin but not the bone. Another headache treatment he described required hooking the temporal artery, twisting it, placing ligatures, and then in essence ripping it out! Albucasis recognized the diagnosis of spinal injury, particularly dislocation of the vertebrae: In total subluxation, with the patient showing involuntary activity (passing urine and stool) and flaccid limbs, he appreciated that death was almost certain. Some of the methods he advocated for reduction of lesser spinal injuries, depending on combinations of spars and winches, were rather dangerous. He held that bone fragments in the spinal canal should be removed.

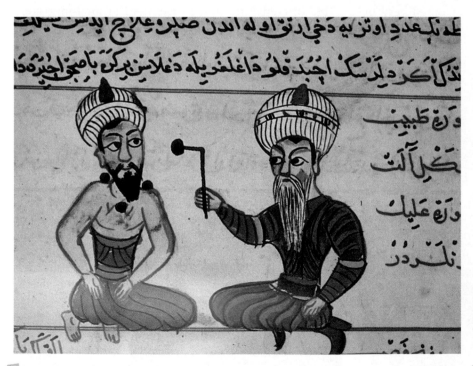

Figure 1.3 Arabic physician applying cautery—source unknown.

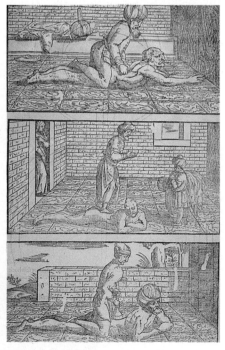

Figure 1.4 Engraved leaf from Avicenna's *Canon medicinae* showing an Arabic physician manipulating a spinal injury. (From Avicenna, 1556)

For hydrocephalus (which he, like Paul of Aegina, associated with the midwife grasping the head too roughly) Albucasis recommended drainage, although he noted that the outcome was almost always fatal. He attributed these poor results to "paralysis" of the brain from relaxation. With regard to the site for drainage, Albucasis noted that the surgeon must never cut over an artery, as hemorrhage could lead to death. In the child with hydrocephalus he would "bind" the head with a wrap and then put the child on a "dry diet" with little fluid—a progressive treatment plan for hydrocephalus.[13,14]

MEDIEVAL EUROPE

Constantinus Africanus (1020–1087) introduced Arabic medicine to the school of Salerno and thus to Europe (Fig. 1.5). He had studied in Baghdad, where he came under the influence of the Arabists. Later, he retired to the monastery at Monte Cassino and there translated Arabic manuscripts into Latin, albeit rather inaccurately. Thus began a new wave of translation of medical texts, this time into Latin.[16] His work allows one to gauge how much medical and surgical knowledge was lost or distorted by multiple translations, particularly of anatomic works. It is also notable that Constantinus reintroduced anatomic dissection with the annual dissection of a pig. Unfortunately the anatomic observations that did not match those recorded in the Greek classics were ignored! Surgical education and practice continued to slumber (Fig. 1.6).

Roger of Salerno (fl. 1170) was a surgical leader in the Salernitan tradition, the first writer on surgery in Italy. His work on surgery was to have a tremendous influence on the medieval period. His *Practica chirurgiae* offered some interesting surgical techniques.[17] Roger introduced an unusual technique of checking for a tear of the dura or CSF leakage in a patient with a skull fracture by having the patient hold his or her breath (Valsalva maneuver) and watching for a CSF leak or air bubbles. A pioneer in the techniques of managing nerve injury, he argued for reanastomosis of severed nerves, and he paid particular attention to alignment. Several chapters of his text are devoted to the treatment of skull fractures.

When a fracture occurs it is accompanied by various wounds and contusions. If the contusion of the flesh is small but that of the bone great, the flesh should be divided by a cruciate incision down to the bone and everywhere elevated from the bone. Then a piece of light, old cloth is inserted for a day, and if there are fragments of the bone present, they are to be thoroughly removed. If the bone is unbroken on one side, it is left in place, and if necessary elevated with a flat sound (spatumile) and the bone is perforated by chipping with the spatumile so that clotted blood may be soaked up with a wad of wool and feathers. When it has consolidated, we apply lint and then, if it is necessary (but not until after the whole wound has become level with the skin), the patient may be bathed. After he leaves the bath, we apply a thin cooling plaster made of wormwood with rose water and egg.[17]

He offered little new in the field of anatomy, contenting himself with recapitulating earlier treatises, in

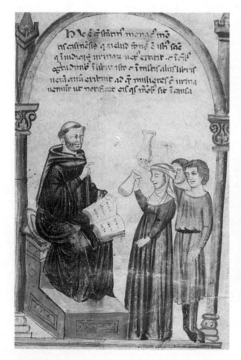

Figure 1.5 Constantinus Africanus making a diagnosis using both a text reference and uroscopy (from a medieval manuscript).

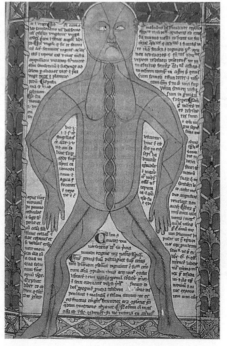

Figure 1.6 One of the "five-figure series," showing a medieval understanding of the nervous system.

Principles of Neurosurgery

particular those of Albucasis and Paul of Aegina. He strongly favored therapeutic plasters and salves; fortunately he was not a strong advocate of the application of grease to dural injuries. Citing the writings of the "Bamberg Surgery,"[18] he advocated trephination in the treatment of epilepsy.

An unusually inventive medieval surgeon, Theodoric Borgognoni of Cervia (1205–1298) is remembered as a pioneer in the use of aseptic technique—not the "clean" aseptic technique of today but rather a method based on avoidance of "laudable pus." He attempted to discover the ideal conditions for good wound healing; he concluded that they comprised control of bleeding, removal of contaminated or necrotic material, avoidance of dead space, and careful application of a wound dressing bathed in wine (Fig. 1.7).

His surgical work, written in 1267, provides one of the best views of medieval surgery.[19] He argued for meticulous (almost Halstedian!) surgical techniques. The aspiring surgeon was to train under competent surgeons and be well read in the field of head injury. Interestingly, he argued that parts of the brain could be removed through a wound with little effect on the patient. He appreciated the importance of skull fractures, especially depressed ones, recognizing that they should be elevated. Punctures of the dura, he believed, could cause abscess and convulsions. To assist the patient in tolerating surgery, he developed his own "soporific sponge," which contained opium, mandragora, hemlock, and other ingredients. It was applied to the nostrils until the patient fell asleep. This may well have been better, for both patient and surgeon, than no medication (Figs. 1.8, 1.9).

The ablest Italian surgeon of the thirteenth century,

professor at the University of Bologna, William of Saliceto (1210–1277) wrote a *Chirurgia*[20] which was highly original, though it does show the influence of Galen and Avicenna. William replaced the Arabic technique of incision by cautery with the surgical knife. He also devised techniques for nerve suture. In neurology, he recognized that the cerebrum governs voluntary motion and the cerebellum involuntary function.

Leonard of Bertapalia (1380?–1460) was a prominent figure in fifteenth century surgery. He came from a small town near Padua and established an extensive, lucrative practice there and in nearby Venice. He was among the earliest proponents of anatomic research—in fact, he gave a course of surgery in 1429 that included the dissection of an executed criminal (Fig. 1.10). Leonard appears to have had a strong interest in injuries of the head—he devoted a third of his book to surgery of the nervous system.[21,22] He considered the brain the most precious organ, regarding it as the source of voluntary and involuntary functions. His insights into skull fractures were remarkable: Always avoid materials that might cause pus, never use a compressive dressing that might drive bone into the brain, and if a piece of bone pierces the brain, remove it.

Lanfranchi of Milan (d. 1306), a pupil of William of Saliceto, continued his teacher's practice of using a knife instead of cautery. In his *Cyrurgia parva* he pioneered the use of suture for repairs.[23] He offered classic guidelines for performing trephination in skull fractures and "release of irritation" of dura. He even developed a technique of esophageal intubation for surgery, a technique not commonly practiced until the twentieth century.

Guy de Chauliac (1300–1386) was the most influential surgeon of the fourteenth and fifteenth centuries

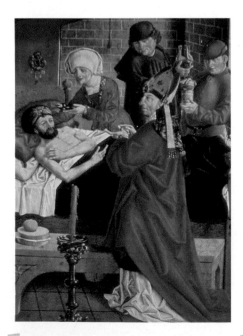

Figure 1.7 A medieval physician attending to a patient.

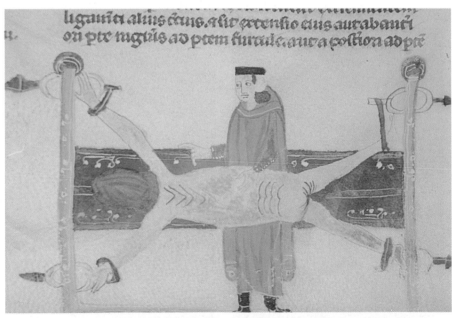

Figure 1.8 Medieval scene with a surgeon about to operate on a patient who has all four limbs tied down and head bagged to muffle the screams.

and a writer of rare learning and fine historical sense. Guy de Chauliac's *Ars chirurgica* was copied and translated into the seventeenth century; in fact it was the principal didactic surgical text up to that time.[24,25]

The discussion of head injuries in his *Ars chirurgica* reveals the breadth of his knowledge and intellect. He noted that the head should be shaved prior to surgery to prevent hair from getting into the wound and interfering with primary healing. When dealing with depressed skull fractures he advocated putting wine into the depression to assist healing—an interesting early form of antisepsis. He categorized head wounds into seven types and described the management of each in detail. A scalp wound requires only cleaning and debridement, whereas a compound depressed skull fracture must be treated by trephination and elevation. He advocated repair by primary suture and claimed good results. He used egg albumin to provide adequate hemostasis, always a difficult problem for surgeons.

SIXTEENTH CENTURY: ANATOMIC EXPLORATION

In the sixteenth century a whole range of new surgical concepts were developed. Physicians and surgeons rediscovered basic investigative techniques. The introduction of anatomic dissection of humans had the most profound influence—great figures like Leonardo da Vinci, Berengario da Carpi, Nicholas Massa, Andreas Vesalius, and others re-explored the human body. Anatomic errors, many ensconced since the Greco-Roman era, were corrected, and great interest in surgery developed. The radically inventive research of the Renaissance laid the foundations of modern neurosurgery.

Leonardo da Vinci (1452–1519) was the quintessential Renaissance man. Multitalented, recognized as an artist, an anatomist, and a scientist, Leonardo went to the dissection table so as better to understand surface anatomy and its bearing on his artistic creations. On the basis of these studies he founded iconographic and physiologic anatomy (Fig. 1.11).[26–28] A well-read man, familiar with writings of Galen, Avicenna, Mondino, and others, he also appreciated their errors.

In his anatomic studies Leonardo provided the first crude diagrams of the cranial nerves, the optic chiasm, and the brachial and lumbar plexuses. Leonardo made the first wax casting of the ventricular system and in so doing obtained the earliest accurate view. His casting technique involved removing the brain from the calvarium and injecting melted wax through the fourth ventricle. Tubes were placed in the lateral ventricles to allow air to escape. When the wax hardened he removed the brain, leaving a cast behind—simple but elegant.

In connection with his artistic studies he developed the concept of "antagonism" in muscle control. His experimental studies included sectioning a digital nerve and noting that the affected finger no longer had sensation, even when placed in a fire. Unfortunately, Leonardo's great opus on anatomy, which was to be published in some 20 volumes, never appeared.[29] From 1519, the year of Leonardo's death, until the middle of the sixteenth century, his anatomic manuscripts circulated among Italian artists through the guidance of Francesco da Melzi, Leonardo's associate. Later they were lost, and were rediscovered only in the eighteenth century, by William Hunter.

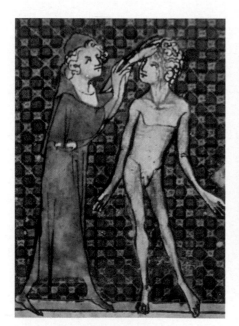

Figure 1.9 Medieval surgeon performing a craniotomy.

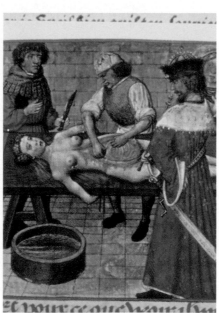

Figure 1.10 Medieval dissection scene.

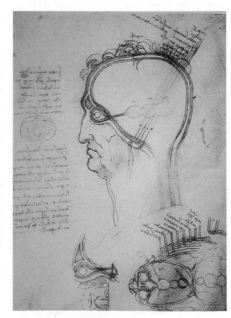

Figure 1.11 From Leonardo's anatomic codices: a classic early view of the cell theory, localizing function to the ventricles. (From da Vinci L, 1911–1916).

Principles of Neurosurgery

Ambroise Paré (1510–1590), a poorly educated and humble Huguenot, became one of the greatest figures in surgery; indeed, he is considered the father of modern surgery. As a result of long military experience he was able to incorporate a great deal of practical knowledge into his works. He published in the vernacular rather than Latin, thus allowing wider dissemination of his work. Paré was a popular surgeon with the royalty. The fatal injury sustained by Henri II of France was an important case, from which some insight into Paré's understanding of head injury can be obtained. Paré attended the king and was present at the autopsy. The patient developed a subdural hematoma. Paré's clinical observations included headache, blurred vision, vomiting, lethargy, and decreased respiration. Using the clinical observations and the history, Paré postulated that the injury was due to a tear in one of the bridging cortical veins. An autopsy confirmed the findings.

Among Paré's surgical works,[30,31] the part on the brain best reflects contemporary practice. Book X is devoted to skull fractures. Paré advanced an interesting technique of elevating a depressed skull fracture using the Valsalva maneuver: "…for a breath driven forth of the chest and prohibited passage forth, swells and lifts the substance of the brain and meninges where upon the frothing humidity and sanies sweat forth."[31] This maneuver enabled the expulsion of blood and pus.

His surgical techniques also demonstrate a remarkable advance over previous writers. Paré provided an extensive discussion on the use of trephines, shavers, and scrapers (Fig. 1.12). He described the removal of osteomyelitic bone, incising the dura and evacuating blood clots and pus, procedures previously carried out

with great trepidation. He advocated debridement, emphasizing that all foreign bodies must be removed. Paré's most useful advance in surgery was the discovery that boiling oil should not be used in gunshot wounds. Rather, he made a dressing of egg yolk, rose oil, and turpentine, which he found greatly improved wound healing and dramatically reduced morbidity and mortality. He also discarded the use of hot cautery to control bleeding, substituting the use of ligatures, which enhanced healing and reduced blood loss, particularly in amputations.

In 1518 a remarkable book by Giacopo Berengario da Carpi (1470–1550) appeared.[32] This book came about because of Berengario's success in treating Lorenzo de' Medici, Duke of Urbino, who had received a serious cranial injury and survived. In a dream shortly after this episode Berengario was visited by the god Hermes Trismegistus (Thrice-Great Mercury), who encouraged him to a write a treatise on head injuries. As a result his marvelous *Tractatus* appeared, the first printed work devoted solely to treating injuries of the head. Not only are original surgical techniques discussed but also illustrations of the cranial instruments for dealing with skull fractures (Fig. 1.13). Berengario introduced the use of interchangeable cranial drill bits for trephination. Included in the text are a number of case histories with descriptions of the patients, methods of treatment, and clinical outcomes. This work remains our best sixteenth century account of brain surgery.

Berengario, like Leonardo da Vinci, was an excellent anatomist who gave one of the earliest and most complete discussions of the ventricular system. He provided early descriptions of the pineal gland, choroid plexus,

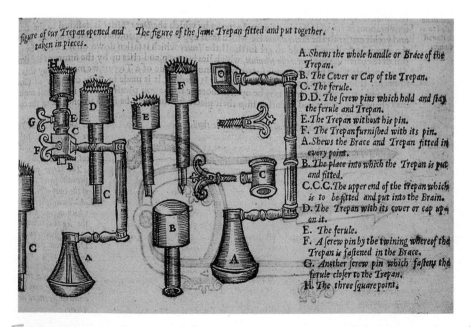

Figure 1.12 A page from the English translation of Paré, showing some early neurosurgical instruments. (From Paré A, 1649).

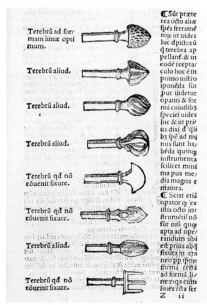

Figure 1.13 Woodcut from Berengario da Carpi's *Tractatus de Fractura Calvae* showing early neurosurgical instruments—the trephines show a sophisticated design to avoid plunging. (From Berengario da Carpi J, 1518).

and lateral ventricles. His anatomic illustrations are believed to be the first published from actual anatomic dissections. In addition his anatomic writings were among the first to challenge dogmatic belief in the writings of Galen and others.

A striking and beautifully illustrated work appeared in 1536 (with an expanded version in 1537) written by a professor of medicine from Marburg, Johannes Dryander (Johann Eichmann, 1500–1560).[33,34] This work contains 16 plates showing successive Galenic dissections of the brain (Fig. 1.14). The dura mater, cortex, and posterior fossa are illustrated in detail. Dryander performed public dissections of the skull, dura, and brain, the results of which he published in this little monograph. Despite inaccuracies in the work, reflecting medieval scholasticism, it can be considered the first textbook of neuroanatomy.

Volcher Coiter (1534–1576) was an army surgeon and city physician at Nuremberg who had the good fortune to study under Fallopius, Eustachius, and Aldrovandi. These scholars provided the impetus for Coiter's original anatomic and physiologic investigations. He described the anterior and posterior spinal roots and distinguished gray from white matter in the spinal cord. His interest in the spine led him to conduct anatomic and pathologic studies of the spinal cord, including a study on the decerebrate model. He did a number of experiments on living subjects. He trephined the skulls of birds, lambs, goats, and dogs. He was the first to associate the pulsation of the brain with the arterial pulse. He even opened the brain and removed parts of it, reporting no ill effects—an early, surprising attempt at cerebral localization.[35]

Using a combination of surgical skill and a Renaissance flair for design, Giovanni Andrea della Croce (1509?–1580)[36] produced some beautifully engraved scenes of neurosurgical operations, performed in family homes, especially in the bedrooms; most were simple trephinations. Croce also designed a number of trephination instruments, some of which improved on their predecessors. His trephine drill was rotated by means of an attached bow, in the manner of a carpenter's drill. Various trephine bits with conical designs are proposed and illustrated. The illustrations of surgical instruments include elevators for lifting depressed bone.

Croce's writing is mainly a compilation of important authorities from Hippocrates to Albucasis, but his recommendations for treatment and his instrumentation are surprisingly modern.

A discussion of surgery in the sixteenth century would not be complete without mention of the great anatomist, Andreas Vesalius (1514–1564). Rejecting the views of his Galenic teachers, Vesalius provided a new and dramatic approach to anatomic dissection. Following on the theme of earlier sixteenth century anatomists like Berengario da Carpi, Vesalius argued that dissection should be done by teachers, not by prosectors. His anatomic descriptions are his own observations rather than an interpretation of the Galenic writings.

Vesalius' magnum opus, *De Humani Corporis Fabrica*,[37] has a section on the anatomy of the brain that presents detailed anatomic discussions with excellent illustrations (Fig. 1.15). Vesalius noted that "heads of beheaded men are the most suitable [for study] since they can be obtained immediately after execution with the friendly help of judges and prefects."[38]

Vesalius was primarily a surgeon and the section of text on the brain and the dural coverings discusses mechanisms of injury and how the various membranes and bone have been designed to protect the brain. Interestingly, close examination of several of the illustrated initial letters in the text shows little cherubs performing trephinations!

A remarkable work on anatomy by Charles Estienne

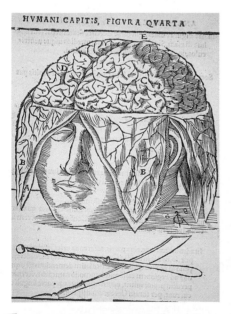

Figure 1.14 Illustration from Dryander's *Anatomie* showing a dissection of the skull and brain. (From Dryander J, 1537).

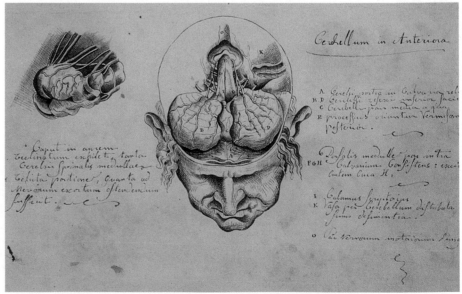

Figure 1.15 An original drawing of the brain from the school of Titian, done for Vesalius's book. (See Vesalius A, 1543).

(1504–1564) appeared in Paris in 1546.[39] Although published 3 years after Andreas Vesalius' work, the book had actually been completed in 1539, but legal problems delayed publication. This work contains a wealth of beautiful anatomic plates with the subjects posed against sumptuous, imaginative Renaissance backgrounds (Fig. 1.16). The anatomic detail is not as good as Vesalius' and repeats many of the errors of Galen, but the plates on the nervous system are quite graphic. Despite some errors, they detail the anatomy of the skull and brain more accurately than previous works.

SEVENTEENTH CENTURY: ORIGINS OF NEUROLOGY

The seventeenth century, like the Renaissance, was a period of spectacular growth in science and medicine. Isaac Newton, Francis Bacon, William Harvey, and Robert Boyle made important contributions in physics, experimental design, the discovery of the circulation of blood, and physiologic chemistry. Open public communication of scientific ideas came with the advent of the scientific society (e.g., the Royal Society of London, the Académie des Sciences in Paris, and the Gesellschaft Naturforschenden Aerzte in Germany), which elevated scientific education and improved the exchange of scientific information.

The figure most remembered for his original investigation of the brain is Thomas Willis (1621–1675), after whom the circle of Willis is named (Fig. 1.17). A fashionable London practitioner, educated at Oxford, Willis published his *Cerebri Anatome* in London in 1664 (Fig. 1.18).[40] This book was the most accurate anatomic study of the brain up to that time. He was assisted in this work by Richard Lower (1631–1691), who showed that when parts of the "circle" were tied off, the anastomotic network still provided blood to the brain. The engravings were done by the prominent London personality, Sir Christopher Wren (1632–1723).

Willis introduced the concept of "neurology," or the doctrine of neurons, using the term in a purely anatomic sense. The word did not enter general use until Samuel Johnson defined it in his dictionary of 1765, according to which neurology encompassed the entire field of anatomy, function, and physiology. The circle of Willis was also detailed in other anatomic works of this period by Vesling,[41] Casserius,[42] Fallopius,[43] and Humphrey Ridley.[44]

Humphrey Ridley (1653–1708) produced an important anatomic work on the brain, written in the vernacular and widely circulated.[44] Ridley was educated at Merton College, Oxford, and at the University of Leiden, where he received his doctorate in medicine in 1679. At the time his work on the brain appeared, many ancient theories of the brain remained prevalent. Shifting away from the earlier cell theory, however, seventeenth century anatomists recognized the brain as a distinct anatomic entity. Instead of residing within the ventricles, cerebral function was thought to be a property of the brain parenchyma.

Ridley recorded a number of original observations in his volume on brain anatomy. He conducted his anatomic studies on freshly executed criminals, most of whom had been hanged, causing vascular engorgement of the brain and hence allowing easier identification of the anatomy. His description of the circle of Willis was

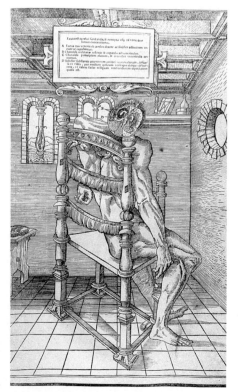

Figure 1.16
A plate from Estienne's *De Dissectione* showing a neurologic dissection of the brain. (From Estienne C, 1546).

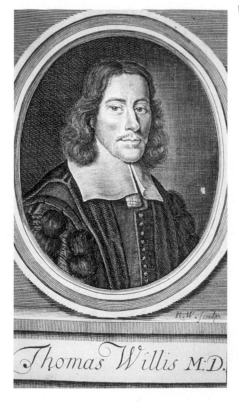

Figure 1.17
Thomas Willis (1621–1675).

even more accurate than Willis's and included a complete account of both the posterior cerebral artery and the superior cerebellar artery. The anastomotic principle of this network was even further elucidated. His understanding of the deep nuclei and in particular the anatomy of the posterior fossa was superior to that of Willis. In addition, Ridley gave a thorough description of the arachnoid membrane. Of interest is Ridley's argument in favor of the belief that the rete mirabile exists. The first accurate description of the fornix and its pathways appears in this monograph.

Although Wilhelm Fabricius von Hilden (1560–1634) had received a classical education in his youth, family misfortune did not allow him a formal medical education. Following the apprenticeship system then prevalent, he studied the lesser field of surgery. Fortunately, the teachers he selected were among the finest wound surgeons of the day. With this education, he had a distinguished career in surgery, during which he made a number of advances.

His large work, *Observationum et Curationum,* included over 600 surgical cases and a number of important and original observations on the brain.[45] Congenital malformations, skull fractures, techniques for bullet extraction, and field instruments were described. He performed operations for intracranial hemorrhage (with cure of insanity), vertebral displacement, congenital hydrocephalus, and occipital tumor of the newborn; he also carried out trephinations for abscess and a cure of an old aphasia. He even removed a splinter of metal from the eye using a magnet, a cure that enhanced his reputation.

Johann Schultes (Scultetus) of Ulm (1595–1645) provided in his *Armamentarium Chirurgicum XLIII* the first descriptive details of neurosurgical instruments to appear since those published by Berengario in 1518.[46] This work was translated into many languages, influencing surgery throughout Europe. Its importance lies in the exact detail of surgical instrument design and in the presentation of tools from antiquity to the present. Many of the instruments illustrated are still in use today. In addition, Scultetus gave details of operations for dealing with injuries of the skull and brain.

James Yonge (1646–1721) was among the first since Galen to argue emphatically that "wounds of the brain are curable." Appropriately enough, Yonge's remarkable little monograph was entitled *Wounds of the Brain Proved Curable.*[47] Yonge was a Plymouth naval surgeon, remembered mostly for his flap amputation technique. In his monograph Yonge gives a detailed account of a brain operation on a child aged 4 years with extensive compound fractures of the skull from which brain tissue issued forth. The surgery was a success and the child lived. Yonge also included reports on more than 60 cases of brain wounds that he found in the literature, beginning with Galen, which had been cured.

EIGHTEENTH CENTURY: ADVENTUROUS SURGEONS

The eighteenth century was a period of intense activity in the medical and scientific world. Chemistry as a true science was propelled forward in the works of Priestley, Lavoisier, Volta, Watt, and many others. Clinical bedside medicine, essentially lost since the Byzantine era, was reintroduced by Thomas Sydenham, William Cullen, and Herman Boerhaave. Diagnostic examination of the patient advanced in this period; especially notable is Auenbrugger's introduction of percussion of the chest. Withering introduced the use of digitalis for cardiac problems. William Jenner provided the world with cowpox inoculation for smallpox, reducing the terror of this scourge.

Perceival Pott (1714–1788) was the greatest English surgeon of the eighteenth century. His list of contributions, several of which apply to neurosurgery, is enor-

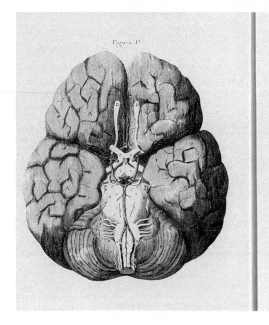

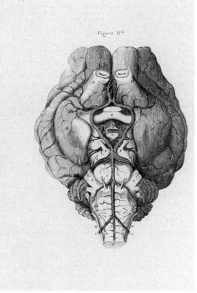

Figure 1.18 A depiction in Willis's *Cerebri Anatome* of what is now called the circle of Willis. (From Willis T, 1664).

mous. His work *Remarks on That Kind of Palsy of the Lower Limbs Found to Accompany a Curvature of the Spine* describes the condition now known as Pott's disease.[48] His clinical descriptions are excellent, with the gibbous and tuberculous condition of the spine well outlined. Interestingly, he failed to associate the spinal deformity with the paralysis. He also described an osteomyelitic condition of the skull with a collection of pus under the pericranium, now called Pott's puffy tumor. Pott felt strongly that these lesions should be trephined to remove the pus and decompress the brain.

In the ongoing argument over whether to trephine, Pott was a strong proponent of intervention (Fig. 1.19). In his classic work on head injury,[49] Pott appreciated that symptoms of head injury were due to injury of the brain and not of the skull. He made an attempt to differentiate between "compression" and "concussion" injury of the brain.

The reasons for trepanning in these cases are, first, the immediate relief of present symptoms arising from pressure of extravasated fluid; or second, the discharge of matter formed between the skull and dura mater, in consequence of inflammation; or third, the prevention of such mischief, as experience has shown may most probably be expected from such kind of violence offered to the last mentioned membrane....

In the...mere fracture without depression of bone, or the appearance of such symptoms as indicate commotion, extravasation, or inflammation, it is used as a preventative, and therefore is a matter of choice, more than immediate necessity.[49]

Pott's astute clinical observations, bedside treatment, and aggressive management of head injuries made him the first modern neurosurgeon. His caveats, presented in the preface to his work on head injury, still hold today.

John Hunter (1728–1793) was one of the most remarkable and talented figures in English medicine. His knowledge and skills in anatomy, pathology, and surgery and his dedication to his work allowed him to make a number of important contributions. He had minimal formal education, though Perceival Pott was an early teacher. In his book *A Treatise on the Blood, Inflammation, and Gun-Shot Wounds*,[50] Hunter drew on his years of military experience (he served as a surgeon with the English forces during the Spanish campaign of 1761–1763). Unfortunately, the section on skull fractures took up only one paragraph and offered nothing original. However, his discussion of vascular disorders was quite advanced, with an appreciation of the concept of collateral circulation. His views on this subject grew out of his observations on a buck whose carotid artery he tied off; the response was, of course, development of collateral circulation.

Benjamin Bell (1749–1806) was among the most prominent and successful surgeons in Edinburgh. He was one of the first to emphasize the importance of reducing pain during surgery. His text, *A System of Surgery*,[51] is written with extraordinary clarity and precision, qualities that made it one of the most popular surgical texts in the eighteenth and nineteenth centuries. In the section on head injury there is an interesting and important discussion of the differences between concussion, compression, and inflammation of the brain—each requiring different modes of treatment.[51] Bell stressed the importance of relieving compression of the brain, whether it be caused by a depressed skull fracture or pressure caused by pus or blood—a remarkably aggressive approach for this period (Fig. 1.20). Bell was among the first to note that hydrocephalus is often associated with spina bifida. His treatment of a

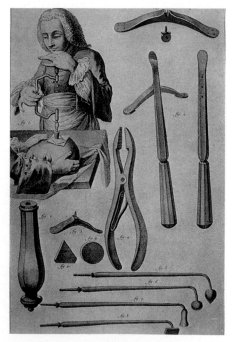

Figure 1.19
An eighteenth-century trephination in Diderot's *Encyclopédie.*

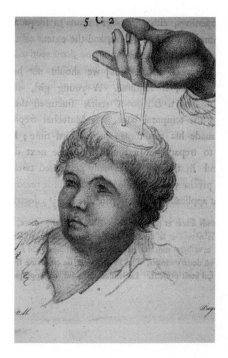

Figure 1.20
Bell's depiction of how to elevate a depressed skull fracture. (From Bell B, 1783–1788).

myelomeningocele involved placing a ligature around the base of the myelomeningocele sac. The concept of an epidural hematoma and its symptoms were appreciated by Bell: He argued for a rapid and prompt evacuation. His discussion of the symptoms of brain compression due to external trauma is classic.

A great variety of symptoms...indicating a compressed state of the brain [among which]...the most frequent, as well as the most remarkable, are the following: Giddiness; dimness of sight; stupefaction; lots of voluntary motion; vomiting; an apoplectic stertor in the breathing; convulsive tremors in different muscles; a dilated state of the pupils, even when the eyes are exposed to a clear light; paralysis of different parts, especially of the side of the body opposite to the injured part of the head; involuntary evacuation of the urine and faeces; an oppressed, and in many case an irregular pulse.... (volume 3, chapter 10, section 3)[51]

Lorenz Heister (1683–1758) produced another of the most popular surgical textbooks of the eighteenth century. A German surgeon and anatomist (a common combination at the time), he published his *Chirurgie* in 1718. It was subsequently translated into a number of languages and circulated widely.[52] The wide range of surgical knowledge it communicated and its many illustrations made it popular. In the treatment of head injury Heister remained conservative with regard to trephination (Fig. 1.21). In wounds involving only concussion and contusion, he felt trephination to be too dangerous. Considering the risk of infection and injury to the brain, this was not too far off the mark.

XXVII. But when the Cranium is so depressed, whether in Adults or Infants, as to suffer a Fracture, or Division of its Parts, it must instantly be relieved: the Part depressed, which adheres, after cleaning the Wound, must be restored to its

Place, what is separated must be removed, and the extravasated Blood be drawn off through the Aperture.... (p. 100)[52]

Heister introduced a number of techniques that proved most useful. To control scalp hemorrhage he used a "crooked needle and thread" that when placed and drawn tight reduced bleeding. He also pointed out that when the assistant applied pressure to the skin, edge bleeding could be reduced. In spinal injuries Heister argued for exposing the fractured vertebrae and removing fragments that damaged the spinal marrow, even though he recognized that grave outcomes of such attempts were not uncommon.

Francois-Sauveur Morand (1697–1773) published a monograph that describes one of the earliest operations for abscess of the brain. Morand had a patient, a monk, who developed an otitis and subsequently mastoiditis with temporal abscess.[53] He trephined over the carious bone and discovered pus. He placed a catgut wick within the wound, but it continued to drain. He reopened the wound and this time opened the dura (a very adventurous maneuver for this period) with a cross-shaped incision and found a brain abscess. He explored the abscess with his finger, removing as much of the contents as he could, and then instilled balsam and turpentine into the cavity. He placed a silver tube for drainage, and as the wound healed he slowly withdrew the tube. The abscess healed, and the patient survived.

Domenico Cotugno (1736–1822) was a Neapolitan physician who offered a small monograph in which he gave the classic descriptions of cerebrospinal fluid and sciatica.[54] He performed a number of experiments on the bodies of some 20 adults. Using the technique of lumbar puncture, he was able to demonstrate the characteristics of CSF. In *De Ischiade Nervosa Commentarius* he demonstrated the "nervous" origin of sciatica, differentiating it from arthritis, with which it was generally equated at that time. Cotugno discovered the pathways of CSF, showing that it circulates in the pia-arachnoid interstices and flows

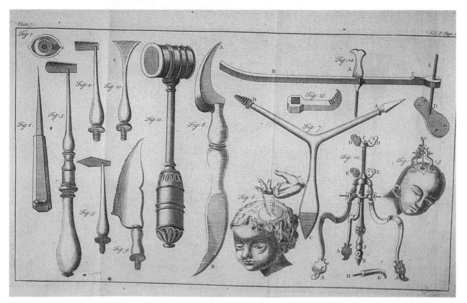

Figure 1.21 Heister's trephination equipment and techniques. (From Heister L,1743).

Principles of Neurosurgery

through the brain and spinal cord via the aqueduct and convexities. He also described the hydrocephalus ex vacuo seen in cerebral atrophy.

In 1709, a small and now very rare monograph by Daniel Turner (1667–1741) appeared.[55] The book was entitled *A Remarkable Case in Surgery: Wherein an Account is given of an uncommon Fracture and Depression of the Skull, in a Child about Six Years old; accompanied with a large Abscess or Aposteme upon the Brain...*(Fig. 1.22). This rather poignant piece of writing is perhaps our best view of the treatment of brain injuries in the early eighteenth century.

The case is most disturbing to read, written in the frank and somewhat verbose style of this period. Turner was "...called in much hast, to a Child about the Age of Six Years...wounded by a Catstick.... He was taken up for dead and continued speechless for some time." Turner examined the head, found a considerable depression, and arrived at the prognosis that the child was in great danger. He sent for the barber to shave the head; while waiting for the barber he opened a vein in the arm to bleed the child, taking about 6 ounces. The patient regained consciousness, vomiting and complaining of a headache. Turner chose to delay surgery. But finding the child the next day still vomiting, restless, and hot, he decided on an exploration. Through a typical X incision he found "the Bones were beat thro' both meninges into the substance of the brain." He elevated the bone and found "...a cavity sufficient to contain near two Ounces of Liquor." Postoperatively the patient was awake with "...a quick pulse, thirst and headache...but no vomiting. He was very sensible." He visited the child the next day and found him still feverish but without other symptoms. He removed the dressings and realized the extent of the fracture, which had been only partially elevated. He now took a trephine, removed what bone he thought it was safe to remove, and applied a clyster.

A careful report of the operation follows, including a description of a piece of bone that flew across the room upon elevation. Four pieces of bone were removed. The dura now pulsated nicely. The wound was cleaned out with soft sponges soaked in claret. The patient was carried to bed and refreshed with "two or three Spoonfulls of his Cephalic Julep." Despite all this effort and although the patient was doing well, upon removing the dressings "an offensive smell" and fetid matter were noted. A consultant's advice was to redress the wound. Instead, Turner opened the right jugular vein and bled 6 ounces. A vesicatory was also applied to the neck and an emollient clyster given in the evening. The next day Turner was still not satisfied with what was happening, and so he re-explored the wound, venting a great deal of purulent matter.

This patient was to have several additional explorations for removal and drainage of pus. Cannulas were placed for drainage and the wound carefully tended, but despite all this the patient died after 12 weeks.

Louis Sebastian (also listed as Nicolas) Saucerotte (1741–1814) was first surgeon to the King of Poland and later a surgeon in the French Army. As has often been the case in the history of neurosurgery, war provided Saucerotte with training and the opportunity for insight into the management of head injury. He reintroduced the concept of the contre-coup injury. In a review of head injury, he described in detail a series of intracranial injuries and their symptoms, including compression of the brain due to blood clot.[56] Saucerotte described a classic case of incoordination, including opisthotonos and rolling of the eyes, due to a cerebellar lesion. He divided the brain into "areas" of injury, pointing out that areas of severe injury are at the base of the brain, while injuries of the forebrain are the best tolerated.

During the eighteenth century there was a remarkable change in approaches to surgery of the brain. Surgeons became much more aggressive in their management of head injuries and the clinical symptoms associated with brain injury were better recognized.

NINETEENTH AND TWENTIETH CENTURIES: ANESTHESIA, ANTISEPSIS, AND CEREBRAL LOCALIZATION

Three major innovations made possible the great advances in neurosurgery during the nineteenth century. Anesthesia allowed patients freedom from pain during surgery, antisepsis and aseptic technique enabled the surgeon to operate with a greatly reduced risk of postoperative complications due to infection, and the concept of cerebral localization helped the surgeon make the diagnosis and plan the operative approach.

In the first half of the century, improvements in surgical technique and neuropathology helped prepare the way for these innovations. John Abernethy (1764–1831) succeeded John Hunter at St. Bartholomew's Hospital and followed his tradition of experimentation and observation. Abernethy's surgical technique did not differ from that of his predecessors; what is remarkable in his

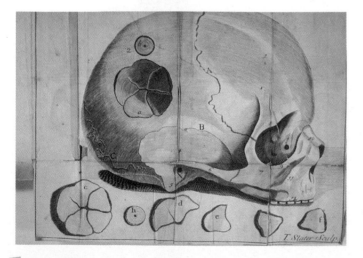

Figure 1.22 A child with a severe skull fracture. (From Turner D, 1709).

Surgical Observations[57] is the thoughtful, very thorough discussion of all the mechanisms of injury to the brain and spinal cord. He performed one of the earliest known procedures for removal of a painful neuroma. The neuroma was resected and the nerve reanastomosed; the pain resolved and sensation returned, proving the efficacy of the anastomosis.

Sir Charles Bell (1774–1842), a Scottish surgeon and anatomist, was a prolific writer. He was educated at the University of Edinburgh and spent most of his professional career in London. He is remembered for many contributions to the neurosciences, including the differentiation of the motor and sensory components of the spinal root. He wrote a number of works on surgery, many of which were beautifully illustrated with his own drawings. These hand-colored illustrations were unrivaled at the time in detail, accuracy, and beauty (Fig. 1.23). This is one of the earliest works with detailed illustrations to assist the surgeon in mastering neurosurgical techniques.

In describing a trephination Bell gave a view of the technique as practiced in 1821:

> Let the bed or couch on which the patient is lying be turned to the light—have the head shaved—put a wax-cloth on the pillow—let the pillow be firm, to support the patient's head. Put tow or sponge by the side of the head—let there be a stout assistant to hold the patient's head firmly, and let others put their hands on his arms and knees.

> The surgeon will expect the instruments to be handed to him in this succession—the scalpel; the rasparatory; the trephine; the brush, the quill, and probe, from time to time; the elevator, the forceps, the lenticular (p. 6).[58]

Also in the first half of the nineteenth century, a number of industrious individuals provided the basis for study of neuropathologic lesions. Several excellent atlases appeared, beautifully colored and pathologically correct. Among the best known are those of Robert Hooper, Jean Cruveilhier, Robert Carswell, and Richard Bright. Cruveilhier's is the most dramatic in appearance.

Jean Cruveilhier (1791–1874) was the first occupant of a new chair of pathology at the University of Paris. He had at his disposal an enormous collection of autopsy material provided by the deadhouse at the Salpêtrière and the Musée Dupuytren, on the basis of which he made a number of original descriptions of pathologies of the nervous system, including spina bifida (Fig. 1.24), spinal cord pathology, cerebellopontine angle tumor, disseminated sclerosis, muscular atrophy, and perhaps the best early description of meningioma (Fig. 1.25). This work was published in a series of fascicles issued over 13 years.[59] The detailed descriptions of Cruveilhier and others provided the basis for the later cerebral localization studies. An understanding of tumors and their clinical-pathologic effects on the brain was critical for the later development of neurosurgery and neurologic examination. Harvey Cushing was the first to call attention to Cruveilhier's accuracy in pathology and clinical correlation. He used portions of Cruveilhier's works in his treatise on acoustic neuromas and his classic meningioma work.[60,61]

ANESTHESIA

Various methods of reducing sensibility to pain were tried by surgeons over the centuries. Mandrake, *Cannabis,* opium and other narcotics, the "soporific sponge" (saturated with opium), and alcohol had all been tried. In 1844, Horace Wells, a dentist in Hartford, Connecticut, introduced the use of nitrous oxide

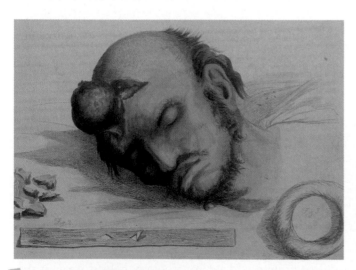

Figure 1.23 Charles Bell's illustrations of a large tumor. (From Bell C, 1821).

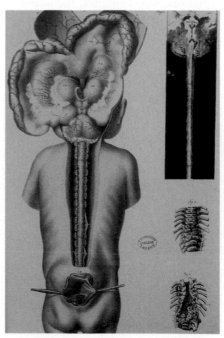

Figure 1.24 Plate showing a child with spina bifida and hydrcephalus: an excellent example of the quality of pathologic illustrations in the first half of the nineteenth century. (From Cruveilhier J, 1829–1842).

in dental procedures; however, the death of one of his patients stopped him from investigating further. At the urging of W.T.O. Morton, J.C. Warren used ether on October 16, 1846, to induce a state of insensibility in a patient, during which a vascular tumor of the submaxillary region was removed. Similar efforts were undertaken in the United Kingdom by J.Y. Simpson, who preferred chloroform, introduced in 1847, as an anesthetic agent. There were many arguments about which was the best agent. However, the end result was that the surgeon did not need to restrain the patient or operate at breakneck speed, and patients were free of pain during the procedure.

ANTISEPSIS

Even with the best surgical technique, three-minute (!) trephinations, the patient might well die postoperatively of suppuration and infection. Fever, purulent material, brain abscess, draining wounds, all defeated the best surgeons. No surgeon could open the dura mater without inviting disaster until the risk of infection could be reduced.

Surgery was revolutionized when, using concepts developed by Louis Pasteur, Joseph Lister introduced antisepsis in the operating room (Fig. 1.26). For the first time a surgeon, using aseptic technique and a clean operating theater, could operate on the brain with a reasonably small likelihood of infection. The steam sterilizer, the scrub brush, and Halsted's rubber gloves truly heralded a revolution in surgery.

CEREBRAL LOCALIZATION

To make a diagnosis of a brain lesion or brain injury was not meaningful until the concept of localization was formulated (Fig. 1.27). Before the 1860s, the brain was thought to act as a single unit. Then during the 1860s several investigators, including G.T. Fritsch and E. Hitzig[62] as well as Paul Broca (Fig. 1.28), introduced the concept that each part of the brain corresponds to a particular function.

Paul Broca (1824–1880) conceived the idea of speech localization in 1861. His studies were based on the work by Ernest Auburtin (1825–1893?), who had as a patient a gentleman who attempted suicide by shooting himself through the frontal region. He survived, but was left with a defect in the left frontal bone. Through this defect Auburtin was able to apply a spatula to the anterior frontal lobe and with pressure abolish speech, which returned when the spatula was removed. The clinical implications were immediately recognized by Auburtin. Broca further localized speech in an epileptic patient who was aphasic and could only emit the utterance "tan," for which the patient became named. At the autopsy of Tan, Broca found softening of the third left frontal convolution, and from this he postulated the cerebral localization of speech.[63,64] Later, Karl Wernicke (1848–1904) identified a different area of the brain where speech was associated with conduction defects.[65]

These studies led to an explosion of research on the localization of brain function, such as the use of ablation by David Ferrier (1843–1928).[66] John Hughlings

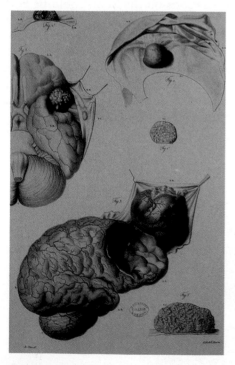

Figure 1.25 Examples of meningiomas. (From Cruveilhier J, 1829–1842).

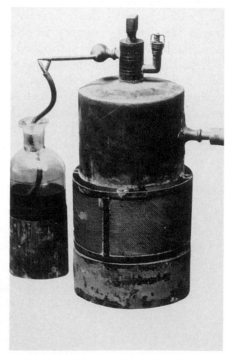

Figure 1.26 Early Lister carbolic acid sprayer.

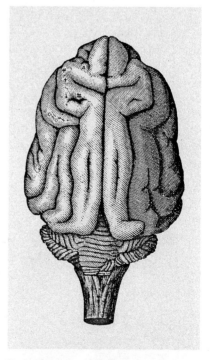

Figure 1.27 Illustration of the exposed cortex of a dog's brain showing sites of stimulation. (From Fritsch GT, Hitzig E, 1870).

Jackson (1835–1911), the founder of modern neurology, demonstrated important areas of function by means of electrical studies and developed the concept of epilepsy.[67] Robert Bartholow (1831–1904), working in Ohio, published a series of three cases of brain tumors in which he correlated the clinical observations with the anatomic findings.

Bartholow later performed an amazing clinical study correlating these types of pathologic findings. In 1874 he took under his care a lady named Mary Rafferty who had developed a large cranial defect, which had in turn exposed portions of each cerebral hemisphere. Through these defects he electrically stimulated the brain; unfortunately she subsequently died of meningitis. Bartholow records that "two needles insulated were introduced into left side until their points were well engaged in the dura mater. When the circuit was closed, distinct muscular contractions occurred in the right arm and leg."[69] Bartholow stimulated a number of different areas, carefully recording his observations. These clinical observations supported his postulated functional localizations in the brain. The ethics of his studies, though, might be called into question today!

_____ ADVANCES IN SURGICAL TECHNIQUES

The surgical personalities of the nineteenth century were quite varied and in most cases very talented. Until the end of the nineteenth century, neurosurgery was not specialized; brain operations were performed by general surgeons, top-hatted, bewhiskered, and always pontifical!

Sir Rickman Godlee (1859–1925) (Fig. 1.29) removed one of the most celebrated brain tumors, the first to be successfully diagnosed by cerebral localization, in 1884.[70] The patient, a man by the name of Henderson, had suffered for 3 years from focal motor seizures. They started as focal seizures of the face and proceeded to involve the arm and then the leg. In the 3 months prior to surgery the patient also developed weakness and eventually had to give up his work. A neurologist, A. H. Bennett, basing his conclusions on the findings of a neurologic examination, localized a brain tumor and recom-

mended removal to the surgeon. Godlee made an incision over the Rolandic area and removed the tumor through a small cortical incision. The patient survived the surgery with some mild weakness and did well, only to die a month later from infection. The operation was observed by Hughes Bennett, the physician who made the diagnosis and localization, and J. Hughlings Jackson and David Ferrier, two local neurologists, all of whom were extremely interested in whether the cerebral localization studies would provide results in the operating theatre. The results were good; this operation was a landmark in the progress of neurosurgery.

William Gowers (1845–1915) was one of an extraordinary group of English neurologists. Using some of the recently developed techniques in physiology and pathology, he made great strides in refining the concept of cerebral localization. Gowers was noted for the clarity and organization of his writing; his works remain classics.[71–73] Such studies allowed surgeons to consider operating on the CNS for other than desperate conditions.

Sir Victor Alexander Haden Horsley (1857–1916) was another English general surgeon who furthered the development of neurosurgery during this period. Horsley began his experimental studies on the brain in the early 1880s, during the height of the cerebral localization controversies. He worked with Sharpey-Schäfer in using faradic stimulation to analyze and localize motor functions in the cerebral cortex, internal capsule, and spinal cord of primates.[74] In a classic study with Gotch (1891), using a string galvanometer, he showed that electrical currents originate in the brain.[75] These experimental studies showed Horsley that localization was possible and that operations on the brain could be conducted safely using techniques adapted from general surgery. In 1887, working with William Gowers, Horsley performed a laminectomy on Gowers' patient, Captain Golby, a 45-year-old army officer. Golby was slowly losing function in his legs from a spinal cord tumor. Gowers localized the tumor by examination and suggested to Horsley where to operate; the tumor, a benign "fibromyxoma" of the fourth thoracic root, was successfully removed.[76]

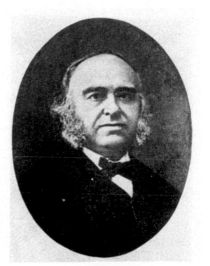

Figure 1.28
Paul Broca
(1824–1880): a
pioneer in cerebral
localization studies.

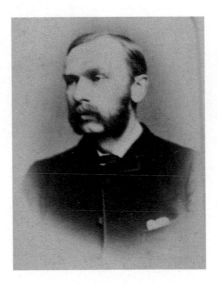

Figure 1.29
Rickman J. Godlee
(1849–1925).

Principles of Neurosurgery

Horsley made a number of technical contributions to neurosurgery, including the use of beeswax to stop bone bleeding. He performed one of the earliest operations for craniostenosis and relief of increased intracranial pressure. For patients with inoperable tumors, he developed the decompressive craniectomy. He also developed the technique of sectioning the posterior root of the trigeminal nerve for pain relief, the first effective treatment for trigeminal neuralgia. Using his technical gifts he helped Clarke design the first useful stereotactic unit for brain surgery. The Horsley-Clarke stereotactic frame is the source by which all subsequent designs have been inspired.[77]

During World War I, Horsley was sent to Mesopotamia to help develop hygienic procedures in a desert outpost. Ironically, he died within 2 days of arrival after contracting a severe desert fever.

William Macewen (1848–1924), a Scottish surgeon and pioneer in the field of neurosurgery, successfully accomplished on July 29, 1879, a brain operation for tumor (Fig. 1.30). Using meticulous technique and the recently developed neurologic examination, he localized and removed a periosteal tumor over the right eye from a 14-year-old. The patient went on to live 8 more years, only to die of Bright's disease; at autopsy no tumor was detected. By 1888, Macewen had operated on 21 neurosurgical cases with only 3 deaths and 18 successful recoveries—a remarkable turnabout from earlier studies. He considered his success to be due to excellent cerebral localization and good aseptic techniques. Macewen's monograph on pyogenic infections of the brain and their surgical treatment, published in 1893,[78] was the earliest to deal with the successful treatment of brain abscess. His morbidity and mortality statistics are as good as those in any series reported today. Without good results, the neurologist of that era was hesitant to recommend surgery; Macewen helped immensely to make the case for performing operations on the brain that had previously been considered too dangerous.

Fedor Krause (1857–1937) was a general surgeon

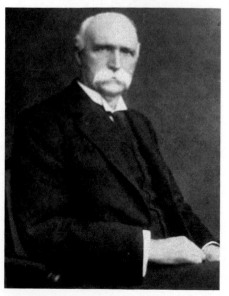

Figure 1.30
William Macewen (1848–1924).

whose keen interest in neurosurgery made him the father of German neurologic surgery. His three-volume atlas on neurosurgery, published in 1909–1912, was one of the first to detail the techniques of good neurosurgery; it has since been through some 60 editions.[79] Krause, like William Macewen, was a major proponent of aseptic technique in neurosurgery. His atlas describes a number of interesting techniques. The "digital" extirpation of a meningioma is graphically illustrated. A number of original neurosurgical techniques are reviewed, including resection of scar tissue for treatment of epilepsy. Krause was a pioneer in the extradural approach to the gasserian ganglion for treatment of trigeminal neuralgia. To deal with tumors of the pineal region he pioneered the supracerebellar-infratentorial approach. Krause was the first to suggest that tumors of the cerebellopontine angle (e.g., acoustic neuromas) could be operated on safely.

William W. Keen (1837–1924), professor of surgery at Jefferson Medical College in Philadelphia, was one of the strongest American advocates for the use of listerian techniques in surgery, advancing the concepts of surgical bacteriology, asepsis, and antisepsis. A description of Keen's surgical set up provides a contemporary view of this innovative surgeon's approach to antisepsis:

All carpets and unnecessary furniture were removed from the patient's room. The walls and ceiling were carefully cleaned the day before operation, and the woodwork, floors, and remaining furniture were scrubbed with carbolic solution. This solution was also sprayed in the room on the morning preceding but not during the operation. On the day before operation, the patient's head was shaved, scrubbed with soap, water, and ether, and covered with wet corrosive sublimate dressing until operation, then ether and mercuric chloride washings were repeated. The surgical instruments were boiled in water for 2 hours, and new deep-sea sponges (elephant ears) were treated with carbolic and sublimate solutions before usage. The surgeon's hands were cleaned and disinfected by soap and water, alcohol, and sublimate solution (pp. 1001–1002).[80]

One of the earliest American monographs on neurosurgery, *Linear Craniotomy*, was prepared by Keen.[81] He described the difficult differentiation between microcephalus and craniosynostosis. He then performed, in 1890, one of the first operations for craniostenosis in America. He developed a technique for treatment of spastic torticollis by division of the spinal accessory nerve and the posterior roots of the first, second, and third spinal nerves.[82] He was also responsible for introducing the Gigli saw, first described in Europe in 1897, into American surgery in 1898.[83,84]

The first American monograph devoted to brain surgery was written not by a neurosurgeon but by the New York neurologist Allen Starr (1854–1932) (Fig. 1.31).[85] Starr was Professor of Nervous Diseases at

Columbia and an American leader in neurology. He trained in Europe, working in the laboratories of Erb, Schultze, Meynert, and Nothnagle, experiences that gave him a strong foundation in neurologic diagnosis. Working closely with Charles McBurney (1845–1913), a general surgeon, he came to the realization that brain surgery not only could be done safely but was necessary in the treatment of certain neurologic problems (Fig. 1.32).[86,87] He summarized his views in the preface:

> Brain surgery is at present a subject both novel and interesting. It is within the past five years only that operations for the relief of epilepsy and of imbecility, for the removal of clots from the brain, for the opening of abscesses, for the excision of tumors, and the relief of intra-cranial pressure have been generally attempted.... It is the object of this book to state clearly those facts regarding the essential features of brain disease which will enable the reader to determine in any case both the nature and situation of the pathological process in progress, to settle the question whether the disease can be removed by surgical interference, and to estimate the safety and probability of success by operation.[85]

Starr was highly regarded by surgeons. In 1923 Harvey Cushing, reviewing one of his own cases, commented about Allen Starr:

> I am confident that if Allen Starr, in view of his position in neurology and his interest in surgical matters, had taken to the scalpel rather than the pen we would now be thirty years ahead in these matters, and I am sure his fingers must many times have itched when he stood alongside an operating table and saw the operator he was coaching hopelessly fumble with the brain.[88]

Harvey William Cushing (1869–1939) is considered the founder of American neurosurgery (Fig. 1.33). Educated at Johns Hopkins under one of the premier general surgeons, William Halsted (1852–1922), Cushing learned meticulous surgical technique from his mentor. As was standard then, Cushing spent time in Europe; he worked in the laboratories of Theodore Kocher in Bern, investigating the physiology of CSF. These studies led to his important monograph in 1926 on the third circulation.[89] It was during this period of experimentation that the cerebral phenomenon of increased intracranial pressure in association with hypertension and bradycardia was defined; it is now called the "Cushing phenomenon." While traveling through Europe, he met several important surgical personalities like Macewen and Horsley. They provided the impetus to consider neurosurgery as a full-time endeavor.

Cushing's contributions to the literature of neurosurgery are too extensive to be listed in this brief chapter. Among his most significant is a monograph on pituitary surgery published in 1912.[90] This monograph inaugurated a career in pituitary studies. Cushing's syndrome was defined in his final monograph on the pituitary, dated 1932.[91] In a classic monograph written with Perceival Bailey in 1926, Cushing brought a rational approach to the classification of brain tumors.[92] His monograph on meningioma, written with Louise Eisenhardt in 1938, still remains the standard for the profession.[93]

Cushing retired as Moseley Professor of Surgery at Harvard in 1932. By the time he completed his 2000th brain tumor operation,[94] he had unquestionably made

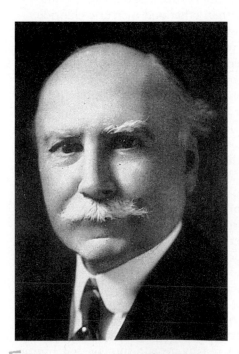

Figure 1.31 Allen Starr (1854–1932).

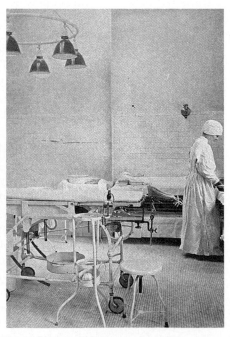

Figure 1.32 Operating room at the New York Neurological Institute, ca. 1910.

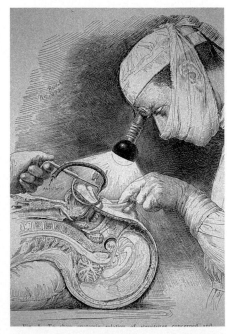

Figure 1.33 Harvey Cushing operating transsphenoidally—from his S. Weir Mitchell lecture.

some preeminent contributions to neurosurgery, based on meticulous, innovative surgical techniques and the effort to understand brain function from physiologic and pathologic points of view. An ardent bibliophile, Cushing spent his final years in retirement as Stirling Professor of Neurology at Yale, where he put together his extraordinary monograph on Andreas Vesalius.[95] Cushing's life has been faithfully recorded by his close friend and colleague John F. Fulton.[96]

Walter Dandy (1886–1946), who trained under Cushing at Johns Hopkins, made a number of important contributions to neurosurgery. Based on Luckett's serendipitous finding of air in the ventricles after a skull fracture,[97] Dandy developed the technique of pneumoencephalography (Fig. 1.34).[98,99] This technique provided the neurosurgeon the opportunity to localize a tumor by analyzing the displacement of air in the ventricles.[100] A Philadelphia neurosurgeon, Charles Frazier, commented in 1935 on the importance of pneumoencephalography and the difference it made in the practice of neurosurgery:

> Only too often, after the most careful evaluation of the available neurologic evidence, no tumor would be revealed by exploration, the extreme intracranial tension would result in cerebral herniation to such an extent that sacrifice of the bone flap became necessary, and subsequently the skin sutures would give way before the persistent pressure, with cerebral fungus and meningitis as inevitable consequences. But injection of air has done away with all these horrors. The neurologist has been forced to recognize its important place in correct intracranial localization and frequently demands its use by the neurosurgeon.[101]

Dandy was an innovative neurosurgeon, far more aggressive in style and technique than Cushing. He was the first to show that acoustic neuromas could be totally removed.[102,103] He devoted a great deal of effort to the treatment of hydrocephalus.[104,105] He introduced the technique of removing the choroid plexus to reduce the production of CSF.[106] He was among the first to attack cerebral aneurysms by obliterating them using snare ligatures or metal clips.[107] His monograph on the third ventricle and its anatomy remains a standard to this day, with illustrations that are among the best ever produced.[108]

In the field of spinal surgery, two important American figures appeared in the first quarter of the twentieth century: Charles Elsberg (1871–1948), Professor of Neurosurgery at the New York Neurological Institute, and Charles Frazier (1870–1936), Professor of Surgery at the University of Pennsylvania. Work in the nineteenth century by J.L. Corning had shown that lumbar puncture can be performed safely.[109] H. Quincke popularized this procedure, and from there spinal surgery developed.[110,111]

Charles Frazier's book on spinal surgery, published in 1918, was the most comprehensive work on the subject available[112]; he summarized much of the existing literature and established that spinal surgery could be done safely. His experience in World War I led him to devote his career to neurosurgery.

Charles Elsberg was another pioneer in spinal surgery. His techniques were impeccable and led to excellent results. By 1912 he had reported on a series of 43 laminectomies and by 1916 he had published the first of what were to be three monographs on surgery of the spine.[113,114] He introduced the technique of myelotomy, allowing a intramedullary tumor to deliver itself, so the tumor could be removed later, at a second-stage procedure (Fig. 1.35). He worked with a fierce intensity and was always looking for new techniques. Working with Cornelius Dyke, a neuroradiologist at the New York Neurological Institute, he treated spinal glioblastomas with directed radiation in the operating room

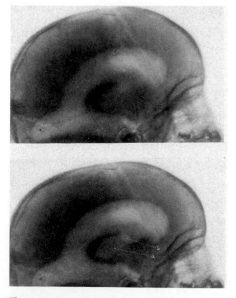

Figure 1.34 Radiograph showing pneumoencephalography. (From Dandy WE, 1918).

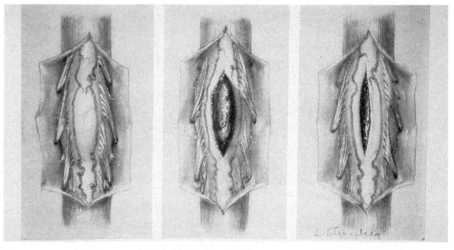

Figure 1.35 Elsberg's two-stage procedure for removing an intramedullary tumor. A myelotomy is made at the first operation over the tumor. The pressure of the tumor causes its extrusion; then in a later operation the surgeon can remove the extruded tumor safely. (From Elsberg CA. *Tumors of the Spinal Cord.* New York: Hoeber; 1925:381.)

after the tumor had been exposed! These procedures were performed with the patients receiving only local anesthesia. During the half hour therapy, while the radiation was being delivered, the surgeon and assistants stood off in the distance behind a glass shield.[115]

Besides the pioneering techniques of Dandy, Cushing, and others, a number of diagnostic techniques were introduced whereby the neurosurgeon could localize lesions less haphazardly, thereby shifting the emphasis from the neurologist to the neurosurgeon. One such technique, myelography using opaque substances, was brought forward by Jean Athanase Sicard (1872–1929).[116] Using a radiopaque iodized oil, the spinal cord and its elements could be outlined on x-ray. Antonio Caetano de Egas Moniz (1874–1955), Professor of Neurology at Lisbon, perfected arterial catheterization techniques and the cerebral angiogram in animal studies. To do this required that a number of iodine compounds be studied, many of which caused convulsions and paralysis in laboratory animals. But his ideas were sound and by 1927 angiography, used in combination with pneumoencephalography, offered the neurosurgeon the first detailed view of the intracranial contents.[117,118]

In 1929, Alexander Fleming published a report on the first observation of a substance that appeared to block the growth of a bacterium. This substance, identified as penicillin, heralded a new era of medicine and surgery.[119] With World War II, antibiotics were perfected in the treatment of bacterial infection, reducing even further the risk of infection during craniotomy.

CONCLUSION

The first half of the twentieth century brought the formalization of the field of neurosurgery. In the 1920s, Elsberg, Cushing, and Frazier persuaded the American College of Surgeons to designate neurosurgery as a separate specialty. It has taken some 5000 years of constant study and the experience of generations to make neurosurgery what it is today.

In the 1990s the neurosurgery patient can have a painless operation with minimal risk of infection, and surgery will rarely be in the wrong location. Thanks to MRI and CT, the localization of neurologic problems is hardly an issue. This is a far cry from our Asclepiad fathers, who could only whisper secret incantations and provide herbal medicaments that rarely worked.

REFERENCES

1. Hippocrates; Foesio A, trans-ed. Του μεγαλου Ιπποκρατους παντων των ιατρων κορυφαιου τα ευρισκομενα: *Magni Hippocratis Medicorum Omnium Facile Principis, Opera Omnia Quae Extant.* Geneva: Samuel Chouet; 1657–1662.

2. Hippocrates; Leonicenus N, Laurentianus L, trans. *Aphorismi, cum Galeni Commentariis; Praedictiones, cum Galeni Commentariis.* Paris: Simon Sylvius; 1527.

3. Clarke E. Apoplexy in the Hippocratic writings. *Bull Hist Med.* 1963;37:301.

4. Marx KFH. *Herophilus: ein Beitrag zur Geschichte der Medicin.* Carlsruhe und Baden; 1838.

5. *Medicae Artis Principes post Hippocratem et Galenum.* Geneva: Henri Estienne; 1567.

6. Celsus. *Medicinae Libri VIII.* Venice: Aedes Aldi et Andreae Asulani Soceri; 1528.

7. Galen. *Omnia Quae Extant Opera in Latinum Sermonem Conversa.* 5th ed. Venice: Juntas; 1576–1577.

8. Galen. Experimental section and hemisection of the spinal cord (taken from *De locis affectibus*). *Ann Med Hist.* 1917;1:367.

9. Paulus Aeginetes. *Opus de Re Medica Nunc Primum Integrum.* Köln: Joannes Soter; 1534.

10. Paulus Aeginetes; Adams F, trans. *The Seven Books of Paulus Aegineta.* London: Sydenham Society; 1844–1847.

11. Rhazes. *Opera Parva.* Lyons: Gilbertus de Villiers, Johannis de Ferris; 1511.

12. Avicenna. *Liber canonis, de medicinis cordialibus, et cantica.* Basel: Joannes Heruagios; 1556.

13. Albucasis. *Liber Theoricae Necnon Practicae Alsaharavii.* Augsburg: Sigismundus Grimm & Marcus Vuirsung; 1519.

14. Albucasis; Spink MS, Lewis GL, trans-ed. *Albucasis on Surgery and Instruments.* Berkeley, Calif: University of California Press; 1973.

15. Al-Rodhan NRF, Fox JL. Al-Zahrawi and Arabian neurosurgery, 936–1013 AD. *Surg Neurol.* 1986;25:92–95.

16. Constantinus Africanus. *Constantini Africani Post Hippocratem et Galenum.* Basel: Henricus Petrus; 1536.

17. Roger of Salerno. *Practica chirurgiae.* In: *Guy de Chauliac Cyrurgia...et Cyrurgia Bruni, Teodorici, Rolandi, Lanfranci, Rogerii, Bertapalie.* Venice: Bernardinus Venetus de Vitalibus; 1519.

18. Corner G, trans. The Bamberg Surgery. *Bull Inst Hist Med* 1937; 5:1–32.

19. Theodoric Bishop of Cervia; Campbell E, Colton J, trans. *The Surgery of Theodoric, ca. A.D. 1267.* New York, NY: Appleton-Century-Crofts; 1955–1966.

20. William of Saliceto. *Chirurgia.* Venice: F di Pietro; 1474.

21. Leonard of Bertapalia. *Chirurgia.* In: *Guy de Chauliac Cyrurgia...et Cyrurgia Bruni, Teodorici, Rolandi, Lanfranci, Rogerii, Bertapalie.* Venice: Bernardinus Venetus de Vitalibus; 1519.

22. Leonard of Bertapalia; Ladenheim JC, trans. *On Nerve Injuries and Skull Fractures.* Mount Kisco, NY: Futura Publishing; 1989.

23. Lanfranchi of Milan. *Chirurgia.* In: *Guy de Chau-*

liac *Cyrurgia...et Cyrurgia Bruni, Teodorici, Rolandi, Lanfranci, Rogerii, Bertapalie.* Venice: Bernardinus Venetus de Vitalibus; 1519.

24. Guy de Chauliac. *Chirurgia magna.* In: *Guy de Chauliac Cyrurgia...et Cyrurgia Bruni, Teodorici, Rolandi, Lanfranci, Rogerii, Bertapali.* Venice: Bernardinus Venetus de Vitalibus; 1519.

25. Guy de Chauliac. *Guy de Chauliac (A.D. 1363) on Wounds and Fractures.* Chicago, Ill: Published by translator; 1923.

26. Leonardo da Vinci. *Quaderni d'Anatomia.* Christiania: Jacob Dybwad; 1911–1916.

27. Hopstock H. Leonardo as an anatomist. In: Singer C, ed. *Studies in the History of Medicine.* Oxford: Clarendon Press; 1921.

28. Leonardo da Vinci; Keele KD, Pedretti C, eds. *Corpus of the Anatomical Studies in the Collection of Her Majesty the Queen at Windsor Castle.* New York, NY: Harcourt Brace Jovanovich; 1979.

29. Goodrich JT. Sixteenth century Renaissance art and anatomy: Andreas Vesalius and his great book—a new view. *Medical Heritage.* 1985;1:280–288.

30. Paré A; Guillemeau J, trans. *Opera.* Paris: Jacobus Du Puys; 1582.

31. Paré A; Johnson T, trans. *The Workes of That Famous Chirurgion Ambroise Parey.* London: Richard Coates; 1649.

32. Berengario da Carpi J. *Tractatus de Fractura Calvae Sive Cranei.* Bologna: Hieronymus de Benedictus; 1518.

33. Dryander J. *Anatomiae.* Marburg: Eucharius Ceruicornus; 1537.

34. Hanigan WC, Ragen W, Foster R. Dryander of Marburg and the first textbook of neuroanatomy. *Neurosurgery.* 1990;26:489–498.

35. Coiter V. *Externarum et Internarum Principalium Humani Corporis Partium Tabulae Atque Anatomicae Exercitationes Observationesque Variae.* Nürnberg: Theodoricus Gerlatzenus; 1573.

36. Croce GA della. *Chirurgiae Libri Septem.* Venice: Jordanus Zilettus; 1573.

37. Vesalius A. *De Humani Corporis Fabrica Libri Septem.* Basel: Joannes Oporinus; 1543.

38. Vesalius A; Singer C, trans-ed. *Vesalius on the Human Brain.* London: Oxford University Press; 1952.

39. Estienne C. *De Dissectione Partium Corporis Humani Libri Tres.* Paris: Simon Colinaeus; 1546.

40. Willis T. *Cerebri Anatome: Cui Accessit Nervorum Descriptio et Usus.* London: J Flesher; 1664.

41. Vesling J. *Syntagma Anatomicum.* 2nd ed. Padua: Paulus Frambottus; 1651.

42. Spiegal A van de, Casserius G. *De Humani Corporis Fabrica Libri Decem, Tabulis XCIIX Aeri Incisis Elegantissimis.* Venice: Evangelista Deuchinus; 1627.

43. Fallopius G. *Observationes Anatomicae.* Venice: Marcus Antonius Ulmus; 1561.

44. Ridley H. *The Anatomy of the Brain, Containing Its Mechanisms and Physiology: Together With Some New Discoveries and Corrections of Ancient and Modern Authors Upon That Subject.* London: Samuel Smith; 1695.

45. Fabry W. *Observationum et Curationum Chirurgicarum Centuriae.* Lyons: JA Huguetan, 1641.

46. Scultetus J. Χειροπλοθηκη...*Armamentarium Chirurgicum XLIII.* Ulm: Balthasar Kühnen; 1655.

47. Yonge J. *Wounds of the Brain Proved Curable, Not Only by the Opinion and Experience of Many (the Best) Authors, but the Remarkable History of a Child Four Years Old Cured of Two Very Large Depressions, With the Loss of a Great Part of the Skull, a Portion of the Brain Also Issuing Thorough a Penetrating Wound of the Dura and Pia Mater.* London: Henry Faithorn and John Kersey; 1682.

48. Pott P. *Remarks on That Kind of Palsy of the Lower Limbs, Which is Frequently Found to Accompany a Curvature of the Spine.* London: J Johnson; 1779.

49. Pott P. *Observations on the Nature and Consequences of Wounds and Contusions of the Head, Fractures of the Skull, Concussions of the Brain.* London: C Hitch and L Hawes; 1760.

50. Hunter J. *A Treatise on the Blood, Inflammation, and Gun-Shot Wounds.* London: J Richardson; 1794.

51. Bell B. *A System of Surgery.* Edinburgh: C Elliot; 1783–1788.

52. Heister L. *A General System of Surgery in Three Parts.* London: W Innys; 1743.

53. Morand F-S. *Opuscules de chirurgie.* Paris: Guillaume Desprez; 1768–1772.

54. Cotugno D. *De Ischiade Nervosa Commentarius.* Napoli: Fratres Simonii; 1764.

55. Turner D. *A Remarkable Case in Surgery: Wherein an Account is Given of an Uncommon Fracture and Depression of the Skull, in a Child About Six Years Old; Accompanied With a Large Abscess or Aposteme Upon the Brain. With Other Practical Observations and Useful Reflections Thereupon. Also an Exact Draught of the Case, Annex'd. And for the Entertainment of the Senior, but Instruction of the Junior Practitioners, Communicated.* London: R Parker; 1709.

56. Saucerotte N. *Mélanges de chirurgie.* Paris: Gay; 1801.

57. Abernethy J. *Surgical Observations.* London: Longman et al.; 1809–1810.

58. Bell C. *Illustrations of the Great Operations of Surgery.* London: Longman et al.; 1821.

59. Cruveilhier J. *Anatomie pathologique du corps humain.* Paris: J-B Baillière; 1829–1842.

60. Flamm ES. The neurology of Jean Cruveilhier. *Med Hist.* 1973;17:343–353.

61. Bakay L. Historical vignette: Cruveilhier on meningiomas (1829–1842). *Surg Neurol.* 1989;32:159–164.

62. Fritsch GT, Hitzig E. Über die elektrische Erregbarkeit des Grosshirns. *Arch Anat Physiol Wiss Med.* 1870:300–332.

63. Broca P. Remarques sur le siège de la faculté du language articulé suivie d'une observation d'aphémie

(perte de la parole). *Bull Soc Anat Paris.* 1861;36: 330–357.

64. Broca P. Perte de la parole: ramollissement chronique et destruction partielle du lobe antérieur gauche du cerveau. *Bull Soc Anthropol Paris.* 1861;2:235–238.

65. Wernicke C. *Der aphasische Symptomenkomplex.* Breslau: M Cohn & Weigert; 1874.

66. Ferrier D. *The Functions of the Brain.* London: Smith, Elder and Co; 1876.

67. Jackson JH. In: Taylor J, ed. *Selected Writings of John Hughlings Jackson.* New York, NY: Basic Books; 1958.

68. Bartholow R. Tumours of the brain: clinical history and comments. *Am J Med Sci.* 1868;110(ns):339–359.

69. Bartholow R. Experimental investigations into the functions of the human brain. *Am J Med Sci.* 1874;67:305–313.

70. Bennett AH, Godlee RJ. Excision of a tumour from the brain. *Lancet.* 1884;2:1090–1091.

71. Gowers WR. *The Diagnosis of Diseases of the Spinal Cord.* London: J and A Churchill; 1880.

72. Gowers WR. *Epilepsy and Other Chronic Convulsive Diseases.* London: J and A Churchill; 1881.

73. Gowers WR. *Lectures on the Diagnosis of Diseases of the Brain.* London: J and A Churchill; 1886–1888.

74. Horsley VAH, Sharpey-Schäfer EA. A record of experiments upon the functions of the cerebral cortex. *Philos Trans R Soc Lond Biol.* 1889;179:1–45.

75. Gotch F, Horsley VAH. On the mammalian nervous system, its functions, and their localisation determined by an electrical method. *Philos Trans R Soc Lond Biol.* 1891;182:267–526.

76. Gowers WR, Horsley VAH. A case of tumour of the spinal cord: removal; recovery. *Med Chir Trans.* 1888; 71:377–430.

77. Horsley VAH, Clarke RH. The structure and functions of the cerebellum examined by a new method. *Brain.* 1908;31:45–124.

78. Macewen W. *Pyogenic Infective Diseases of the Brain and Spinal Cord.* Glasgow: J Maclehose & Sons; 1893.

79. Krause F; Haubold H, Thorek M, trans. *Surgery of the Brain and Spinal Cord Based on Personal Experiences.* New York, NY: Rebman Co; 1909–1912.

80. Stone JL. W.W. Keen: America's pioneer neurological surgeon. *Neurosurgery.* 1985;17:997–1110.

81. Keen WW. *Linear Craniotomy.* Philadelphia, Pa: Lea Bros and Co; 1891.

82. Keen WW. A new operation for spasmodic wry neck, namely, division or exsection of the nerves supplying the posterior rotator muscles of the head. *Ann Surg.* 1891; 13:44–47

83. Keen WW. On the use of the Gigli wire saw to obtain access to the brain. *Phila Med J.* 1898;1:32–33.

84. Bingham WF. W.W. Keen and the dawn of American neurosurgery. *J Neurosurg.* 1986;64:705–717.

85. Starr MA. *Brain Surgery.* New York: William Wood & Co; 1893.

86. Starr MA. Discussion on the present status of the surgery of the brain, 2: a contribution to brain surgery, with special reference to brain tumors. *Trans Med Soc NY.* 1896;119–134.

87. McBurney C, Starr MA. A contribution to cerebral surgery: diagnosis, localization and operation for removal of three tumors of the brain, with some comments upon the surgical treatments of brain tumors. *Am J Med Sci.* 1893;105(ns):361–387.

88. Cushing H. Neurological surgeons, with the report of one case. *Arch Neurol Psychiatr.* 1923;10:381–390.

89. Cushing H. *The Third Circulation: Studies in Intracranial Physiology and Surgery.* London: Oxford University Press; 1926.

90. Cushing H. *The Pituitary Body and Its Disorders: Clinical States Produced by Disorders of the Hypophysis Cerebri.* Philadelphia, Pa: JB Lippincott Co; 1912.

91. Cushing H. *Papers Relating to the Pituitary Body, Hypothalamus, and Parasympathetic Nervous System.* Springfield, Ill: Charles C Thomas Publisher; 1932.

92. Bailey P, Cushing H. *A Classification of the Tumors of the Glioma Group on a Histogenetic Basis With a Correlated Study of Prognosis.* Philadelphia, Pa: JB Lippincott Co; 1926.

93. Cushing H, Eisenhardt L. *Meningiomas: Their Classification, Regional Behavior, Life History and Surgical End Results.* Springfield, Ill: Charles C Thomas Publisher; 1938.

94. Cushing H. *Intracranial Tumors: Notes Upon a Series of Two Thousand Verified Cases With Surgical Mortality Percentages Pertaining Thereto.* Springfield, Ill: Charles C Thomas Publisher; 1932.

95. Cushing H. *A Bio-Bibliography of Andreas Vesalius.* New York, NY: Schuman; 1943.

96. Fulton JF. *Harvey Cushing: A Biography.* Springfield, Ill: Charles C Thomas Publisher; 1946.

97. Luckett WH. Air in the ventricles following a fracture of the skull. *Surg Gynecol Obstet.* 1913; 17:237–240.

98. Dandy WE. Ventriculography following the injection of air into the cerebral ventricles. *Ann Surg.* 1918;68:5–11.

99. Dandy WE. Röntgenography of the brain after the injection of air into the spinal canal. *Ann Surg.* 1919;70:397–403.

100. Dandy WE. Localization or elimination of cerebral tumors by ventriculography. *Surg Gynecol Obstet.* 1920;30:329–342.

101. Frazier CH. Fifty years of neurosurgery. *Arch Neurol Psychiatr.* 1935;34:907–922.

102. Dandy WE. An operation for the total extirpation of tumors in the cerebellopontine angle: a preliminary report. *Bull Johns Hopkins Hosp.* 1922; 33:344–345.

103. Dandy WE. An operation for the total removal of cerebello-pontine (acoustic) tumors. *Surg Gynecol Obstet.* 1925;41:129–148.

104. Dandy WE, Blackfan DD. An experimental and clinical study of internal hydrocephalus. *JAMA.* 1913;61:2216–2217.

105. Dandy WE, Blackfan DD. Internal hydrocephalus: an experimental, clinical and pathologic study. *Am J Dis Child.* 1914;8:406–482.

106. Dandy WE. An operative procedure for hydrocephalus. *Bull Johns Hopkins Hosp.* 1922;33:189–190.

107. Dandy WE. Intracranial aneurysm of the internal carotid artery cured by operation. *Ann Surg.* 1938;107:654–659.

108. Dandy WE. *Benign Tumors of the Third Ventricles.* Springfield, Ill: Charles C Thomas Publisher; 1933.

109. Corning JL. Spinal anesthesia and local medication of the cord. *N Y Med J.* 1885;42:483–485.

110. Quincke HI. Die Lumbalpunction des Hydrocephalus. *Berl Klin Wochenschr.* 1891;28:929–933, 965–968.

111. Quincke HI. Die diagnostische und therapeutische Bedeutung der Lumbalpunction: klinischer Vortrag. *Dtsch Med Wochenschr.* 1905;31:1825–1828, 1869–1872.

112. Frazier C. *Surgery of the Spine and Spinal Cord.* New York, NY: Appleton; 1918.

113. Elsberg CA. Surgery of intramedullary affections of the spinal cord: anatomic basis and technic with report of cases. *JAMA.* 1912;59:1532–1536.

114. Elsberg CA. *Diagnosis and Treatment of Surgical Diseases of the Spinal Cord and Its Membranes.* Philadelphia, Pa: WB Saunders Co; 1916.

115. Pool L. *The Neurological Institute of New York, 1909–1974, With Personal Anecdotes.* Lakeville, Conn: Pocket Knife Press; 1975:59.

116. Sicard JA, Forestier J. Méthode radiographique d'exploration de la cavité épidurale par le lipiodol. *Rev Neurol.* 1921;37:1264–1266.

117. Moniz CE. L'encéphalographie artérielle: son importance dans la localisation des tumeurs cérébrales. *Rev Neurol.* 1927;2:72–90.

118. Moniz CE. *Diagnostic des tumeurs cérébrales et épreuve de l'encéphalographie artérielle.* Paris: Masson & Cie; 1931.

119. Fleming A. On the antibacterial action of cultures of a *Penicillium,* with special reference to their use in the isolation of *B. influenzae. Br J Exp Pathol.* 1929;10:226–236.

ADDITIONAL READINGS

Bakay L. *An Early History of Craniotomy From Antiquity to the Napoleonic Era.* Springfeld, Ill: Charles C Thomas Publisher; 1985.

Ballance CA. *A Glimpse Into the History of the Surgery of the Brain.* London: Macmillan and Co; 1922.

Bucy PC, ed. *Neurosurgical Giants: Feet of Clay and Iron.* New York, NY: Elsevier; 1985.

Clarke E, Dewhurst K. *An Illustrated History of Brain Function.* Oxford: Sandforn; 1972.

Clarke E, O'Malley CD. *The Human Brain and Spinal Cord: A Historical Study Illustrated by Writings from Antiquity to the Twentieth Century.* Berkeley, Calif: University of California Press; 1968.

Gurdjian ES. *Head Injury from Antiquity to the Present, With Special Reference to Penetrating Head Wounds.* Springfield, Ill: Charles C Thomas Publisher; 1973

Haymaker W, Schiller F. *The Founders of Neurology.* 2nd ed. Springfield, Ill: Charles C Thomas Publisher; 1970.

Horrax G. *Neurosurgery: An Historical Sketch.* Springfield, Ill: Charles C Thomas Publisher; 1952.

Leonardo RA. *History of Surgery.* New York, NY: Froben Press; 1943.

McHenry LC. *Garrison's History of Neurology, Revised and Enlarged, With a Bibliography of Classical, Original and Standard Works in Neurology.* Springfield, Ill: Charles C Thomas Publisher; 1969.

Meyer A. *Historical Aspects of Cerebral Anatomy.* London: Oxford University Press; 1971.

Poynter FNL, ed. *The History and Philosophy of Knowledge of the Brain and Its Functions.* Springfield, Ill: Charles C Thomas Publisher; 1958.

Rose FC, Bynum WF. *Historical Aspects of the Neurosciences: A Festschrift for Macdonald Critchley.* New York, NY: Raven Press; 1982.

Spillane JD. *The Doctrine of the Nerves: Chapters in the History of Neurology.* Oxford: Oxford University Press; 1981.

Sachs E. *The History and Development of Neurological Surgery.* New York, NY: Hoeber; 1952.

Soury J. *Le système nerveux central: structure et fonctions, histoire, critiques des théories et des doctrines.* Paris: Georges Carré; 1899.

Walker AE. *A History of Neurological Surgery.* Baltimore, Md: Williams & Wilkins; 1951.

Wilkins RH, Brody IA. *Neurological Classics.* New York, NY: Johnson Reprint Co; 1973.

Chapter 2

Increased Intracranial Pressure, Cerebral Edema, and Brain Herniation

Setti S. Rengachary, Derek A. Duke

The vertebrate cranium is a rigid structure. The major intracranial contents are the *brain* (including the neuroglial elements and interstitial fluid), *blood* (arterial and venous), and *cerebrospinal fluid* (Fig. 2.1). Because the intracranial volume is constant, when an intracranial mass is introduced, compensation must occur through a reciprocal decrease in the volume of venous blood and CSF. This is the Monro-Kellie-Burrows doctrine (Fig. 2.2), which has been confirmed by many experimental and clinical observations. Only in children whose sutures have not yet fused can the cranium itself expand to accommodate extra volume.

Figure 2.1 Intracranial Contents and Their Respective Volumes

Content	Volume	Percentage of Total Volume
Brain (70%) and interstitial fluid (10%)	1400 mL	80%
Blood	150 mL	10%
CSF	150 mL	10%
Total	1700 mL	100%

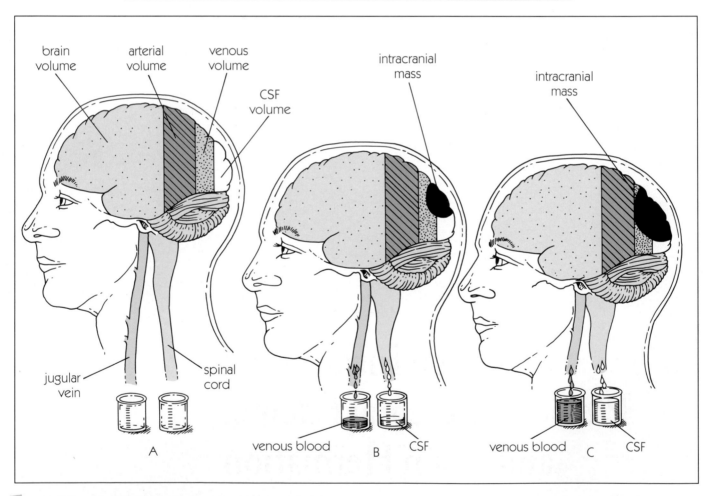

Figure 2.2 Monro-Kellie-Burrows doctrine. **(A)** Physiologic state with normal intracranial pressure (ICP). The major intracranial components are brain (80%), arterial and venous blood (10%), and CSF (10%). The cranium is a rigid container, the intracranial volume is constant, and the normal intracranial contents are shown with ICP within physiologic range (10 to 15 mm Hg). **(B)** Intracranial mass with compensation (normal ICP). This patient has an intracranial mass (space-occupying lesion) of moderate size. Because intracranial volume is constant, the increasing volume caused by the mass is compensated by a decrease in the intracranial content. Venous volume decreases through egress of venous blood from the intracranial cavity into the jugular veins. CSF volume decreases because of egress of CSF through the foramen magnum into the spinal canal. The brain itself is nearly incompressible, and thus no significant change in its volume occurs; neither is there change in arterial volume. Intracranial volume is constant and there is no net rise in ICP (pressure buffering). **(C)** Intracranial mass with decompensation and elevated ICP. The intracranial mass is much larger, beyond the pressure-buffering capacity of venous blood and CSF; there is a net rise in ICP.

Principles of Neurosurgery

To maintain pressure within the physiologic range the venous system collapses easily, squeezing venous blood out through the jugular veins or through the emissary and scalp veins. CSF, likewise, can be displaced through the foramen magnum into the spinal subarachnoid space. When these compensatory mechanisms have been exhausted, minute changes in volume produce precipitous increases in pressure.[1] This can be demonstrated in an experimental model by inserting a Foley catheter in the epidural space and inflating the balloon gradually. The curve produced by plotting intracranial pressure against volume (Fig. 2.3) is initially flat, due to the pressure-buffering capacity offered by displacement of CSF and venous blood; later, there is a precipitous increase in pressure because compensatory mechanisms have been exceeded.[1] Brain parenchyma and arterial blood do not participate to any significant extent in the intracranial pressure-buffering mechanism.

Compliance (dV/dP) is the change in volume observed for a given change in pressure. This represents the accommodative potential of the intracranial space. Compliance is high when cranial cavity will permit the accommodation of a large mass with very little change in pressure. In clinical practice, however, what is measured is *elastance (dP/dV)*, the inverse of compliance; that is, the change in pressure observed for a given change in volume. It represents the resistance to outward expansion of an intracranial mass. Elastance can be measured at the bedside by injecting 1 mL of sterile saline through the ventricular catheter in 1 second and observing the change in pressure—an increase of less than 2 mm Hg implies low elastance and high compliance. The high risk of infection associated with this maneuver precludes its performance.

THE BLOOD-BRAIN BARRIER

Not all substances that are carried in the blood reach neural tissue—a barrier blocks entry of many substances into the brain.[2] This barrier resides in the cerebral capillaries. Its function is to regulate the flow of biologically active substances into the brain and to protect the sensitive neural tissue from toxic materials.

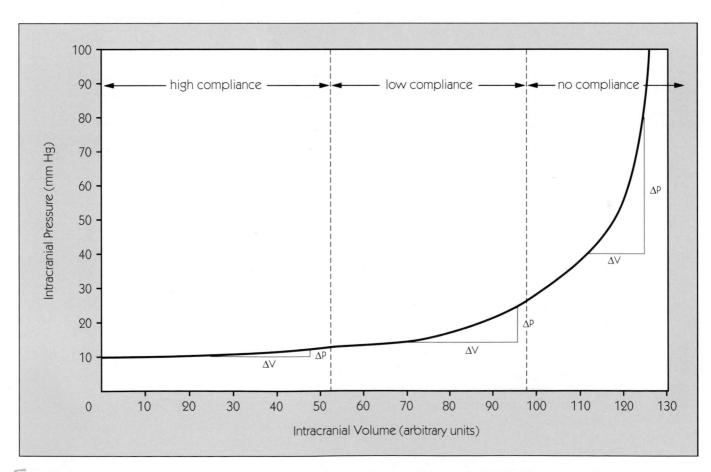

Figure 2.3 Pressure-volume curve. If an intracranial balloon is expanded slowly in a laboratory animal and the ICP and the balloon's volume are plotted, an exponential curve results. In the initial phase there is virtually no increase in ICP because of the compensatory decrease in CSF and venous volumes. The compliance is high (elastance low). With further expansion of the balloon, the ICP begins to rise. Compliance is low (elastance high). In the terminal stages, when the compensatory mechanisms are exhausted, there is a steep rise in pressure (no compliance, highest elastance).

Comparison of the structural differences between somatic capillaries and brain capillaries helps us to understand the anatomic basis of the blood-brain barrier (Fig. 2.4). In the somatic capillary, blood components pass freely through the fenestrae between endothelial cells. Also, certain materials are transported directly across the capillary cell wall through bulk transport via pinocytotic vesicles. The endothelial cells of brain capillaries, on the other hand, are connected by tight junctions. These junctions act as a barrier to the passive movement of many substances across the endothelium. There are two mechanisms by which material may be transported across the endothelial cells. Lipid-soluble substances can usually penetrate all capillary endothelial cell membranes in a passive manner. Amino acids and sugars are transported across the capillary endothelium by specific carrier-mediated mechanisms.

The physiology of the blood-brain barrier is especially important in certain clinical settings. First, when there is a disruption of the blood-brain barrier by any cause, plasma components easily cross the barrier into neural tissue, causing *vasogenic edema*. Second, tight junctions can be transiently opened artificially by the intraarterial injection of a bolus of an osmotic agent,

such as mannitol, which dehydrates the endothelial cells. During this brief interval, which lasts for a few hours, certain chemotherapeutic or other agents can be administered that would not otherwise cross the barrier. Third, when mannitol is given intravenously, the concentration in the cerebral capillary is quite low; however, it is sufficient to create an osmotic gradient between the cerebral tissue and the capillary, allowing withdrawal of interstitial fluid into the capillary lumen. An intact tight junction is necessary for this to occur. If the tight junctions are not intact, mannitol will permeate the neural tissue, preventing the formation of an osmotic gradient.

CEREBRAL EDEMA

Cerebral edema may be defined as a state of increased brain volume due to an increase in water content.[3,4] There are three types of cerebral edema (Fig. 2.5).

Vasogenic edema is the most common form of brain edema encountered in clinical practice (Fig. 2.6). It results from increased permeability of capillaries. The tight junctions between the endothelial cells become incompetent, allowing escape of plasma filtrate into the

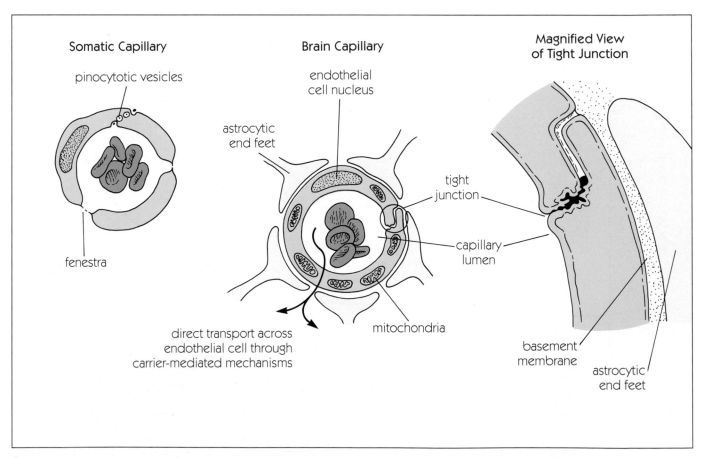

Figure 2.4 Differences between somatic and brain capillaries. In the somatic capillary, fenestrations between endothelial cells allow free flow of plasma components into the tissues. In addition, there is bulk flow of plasma components across endothelial cells via pinocytotic vesicles. In the brain capillary, the endothelial cells are attached to each other by tight junctions. There are no intervening fenestrae. Certain selected plasma components cross the endothelial membrane if they are lipid-soluble; others, such as amino acids and sugars, are transported across the endothelial cells through carrier-mediated mechanisms. The large number of mitochondria in the brain endothelial cells generate energy for active transport.

Figure 2.5 Types and Characteristics of Cerebral Edema

	Vasogenic Edema (extracellular edema)	Cytotoxic Edema (intracellular edema)	Interstitial Edema
Pathogenesis	increased capillary permeability	cellular swelling (neuronal, glial, and endothelial cells)	increased brain water due to impairment of absorption of cerebrospinal fluid
Location of edema	mainly white matter	gray and white matter	transpendymal flow of CSF and interstitial edema in the periventricular white matter in hydrocephalus
Composition of edema fluid	plasma filtrate containing plasma proteins	increased intracellular water and sodium due to failure of membrane transport	cerebrospinal fluid
Extracellular fluid volume	increased	decreased	increased
Pathologic lesion causing edema	primary or metastatic tumor, abscess, late stages of infarction, trauma	early stages of infarction, water intoxication	obstructive or communicating hydrocephalus
Effect of steroids	effective	not effective	not effective
Effect of mannitol	effective	effective	questionable

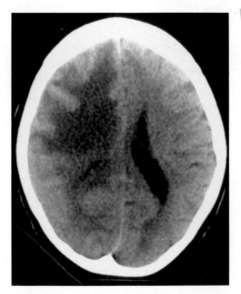

Figure 2.6 CT scan of a patient with vasogenic edema caused by metastatic tumor. Note that the edema involves predominantly the white matter.

intercellular space (Fig. 2.7). The phenomenon of contrast enhancement in CT and MRI scans is, in part, due to breakdown of the blood-brain barrier and resultant vasogenic edema. Vasogenic edema is most commonly seen with trauma, tumor, and abscess. The edema is more marked in white matter than in gray matter.

Cytotoxic edema most commonly results from hypoxia of the neural tissue. The hypoxia affects the ATP-dependent sodium pump mechanism in the cell membrane, promoting an accumulation of intracellular sodium and the subsequent flow of water into the cell to maintain osmotic equilibrium. Thus, the edema is primarily intracellular and affects virtually all cells, including the endothelial cells, astrocytes, and neurons. Because of the swelling of these cells, the interstitial space is considerably narrowed (see Fig. 2.7). The two most common causes of cytotoxic edema are tissue hypoxia and water intoxication. The CT scan commonly shows only subtle or no changes indicative of cytotoxic edema in the early phases of ischemic stroke.

Interstitial edema results from transudation of CSF in obstructive hydrocephalus. This is best observed on CT or MRI scans as periventricular low density due to retrograde transependymal flow of CSF into the interstitial space of the white matter (Fig. 2.8). This is most commonly observed in the frontal region. This finding indicates active hydrocephalus requiring surgical therapy.

CEREBRAL BLOOD FLOW

Normal cerebral blood flow averages 55 to 60 mL/100 g brain tissue/min. In the gray matter the blood flow is 75 mL/100 g/min, whereas in the white matter it is only 45 mL/100 g/min. This flow is sufficient to meet the metabolic needs of the brain. The most significant factor that determines cerebral blood flow at any given time is the cerebral perfusion pressure, which is the effective blood pressure gradient across the brain. It is the difference between the incoming mean arterial pressure and the opposing intracranial pressure. The mean arterial pressure is the diastolic pressure plus one third of the pulse pressure. With increased intracranial pressure there is a tendency for the cerebral perfusion pressure to decrease.

Three major factors regulate cerebral blood flow under physiologic conditions (Fig. 2.9): systemic blood pressure, CO_2 and hydrogen ion concentration in the arterial blood, and oxygen concentration. The ability to maintain blood flow to the brain at a constant level over a wide range of

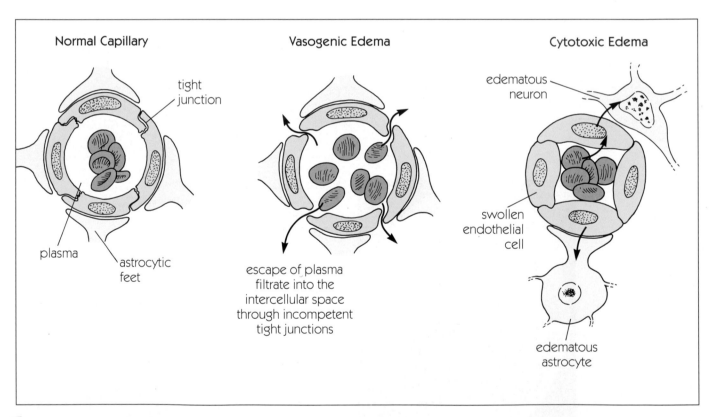

Figure 2.7 Normal appearance of a cerebral capillary contrasted with the changes that occur in vasogenic or cytotoxic edema. Under normal conditions, the intercellular tight junctions are intact. In vasogenic edema, the tight junctions are not competent, allowing leakage of plasma into the interstitial space. In cytotoxic edema, there is a primary failure of ATP-dependent sodium pump mechanism resulting in intracellular accumulation of sodium and secondarily water.

Principles of Neurosurgery

mean arterial pressures (50 to 160 mm Hg) is called autoregulation. When the mean arterial pressure is low, the cerebral arterioles dilate to allow adequate flow at the decreased pressure. Conversely, an increase in systemic blood pressure causes the arterioles to constrict and maintain the flow within physiologic range.

Cerebral blood flow cannot always be regulated. When the mean arterial blood pressure falls below 50 mm Hg, such as in hypovolemic shock, there is inadequate perfusion of the brain. When the mean arterial pressure exceeds 150 mm Hg the autoregulatory system fails. There is a passive increase in blood flow proportionate to the increase in systemic pressure, causing, in extreme cases, exudation of fluid from the vascular system with resultant vasogenic edema. This cascade results in hypertensive encephalopathy. Carbon dioxide tension is the most potent stimulus for cerebrovascular dilatation. There is a graded increase in cerebral blood flow with increase from 15 to 80 mm Hg Pco_2. Hyperventilation, by decreasing the CO_2 tension in the blood, decreases cerebral blood flow and cerebral blood volume in the brain. Hypoxia causes cerebrovascular dilation, which becomes apparent when the oxygen tension in the blood drops down to 50 mm Hg, and becomes maximal around 20 mm Hg.

PATHOLOGIC EFFECTS OF INCREASED INTRACRANIAL PRESSURE

Normal intracranial pressure (ICP) ranges from 10 to 15 mm Hg (136 to 204 mm H_2O). This is primarily con-

tributed by arterial pulsations transmitted to the brain directly and through the choroid plexus. An increase in ICP always occurs when there is a disparity between intracranial volume and the intracranial contents. Common causes of raised ICP are listed in Figure 2.10.

An increase in ICP can cause deleterious effects on the brain in two ways. First, brain ischemia may occur when the cerebral perfusion pressure is reduced to critical levels. Second, focal masses can cause distortion and herniation of the brain, resulting in compression of critical brain stem structures. The presence of herniation syndromes with occlusion of the tentorial incisura or the aqueduct further elevates the ICP by blocking CSF pathways. As a general rule, an increase in ICP without shift of brain structures is better tolerated than an increase secondary to focal mass. Examples of generalized increased pressure without brain shift include pseudotumor cerebri and chronic hydrocephalus. In these disorders, the patient may or may not have a headache.

TYPES OF BRAIN HERNIATION

The brain is supported by dural folds that prevent undue movements of the brain within the cranial cavity (Fig. 2.11). There are two major dural folds—the *falx cerebri* and the *tentorium cerebelli*. The falx cerebri is a sickle-shaped dural fold in the midline that separates the two cerebral hemispheres. The tentorium cerebelli is a tent-shaped dural fold that separates the occipital lobes from the posterior fossa structures. The tentorial incisura, or hiatus, is the dural opening that surrounds the rostral brain stem.

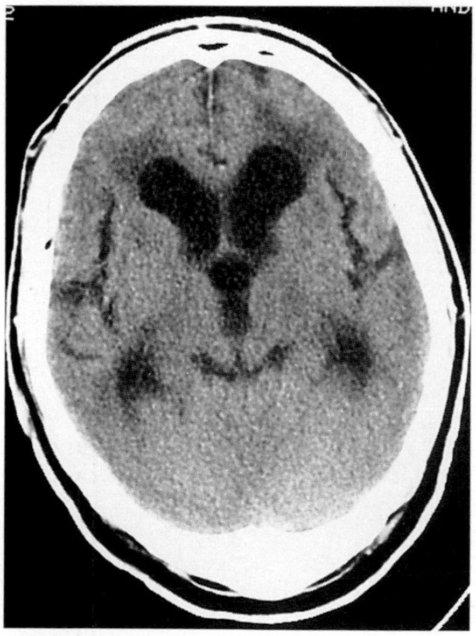

Figure 2.8 CT scan of a patient with active hydrocephalus showing periventricular low density representing transependymal flow of CSF (interstitial edema).

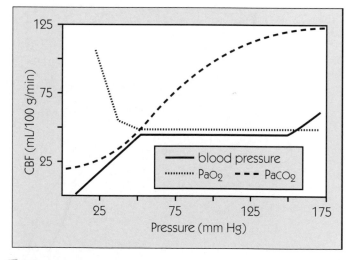

Figure 2.9 Effects of arterial blood pressure, $Paco_2$, and Pao_2 on cerebral blood flow (CBF).

Figure 2.10 Common Causes of Increased Intracranial Pressure

Pathologic Process	Representative Examples
Localized masses	Hematomas: epidural, subdural, intracerebral Neoplasms: gliomas, meningiomas, metastases Abscesses Focal edema due to trauma, infarction, tumor
Obstruction to CSF pathways	Obstructive hydrocephalus Communicating hydrocephalus
Obstruction to major venous sinuses	Depressed skull fracture over major venous sinuses, thromboembolic disease from contraceptive pills
Diffuse brain edema or swelling	Encephalitis, meningitis, diffuse head injury, subarachnoid hemorrhage, Reye's syndrome, lead encephalopathy, water intoxication from fluid overload, near-drowning
Idiopathic	Pseudotumor cerebri

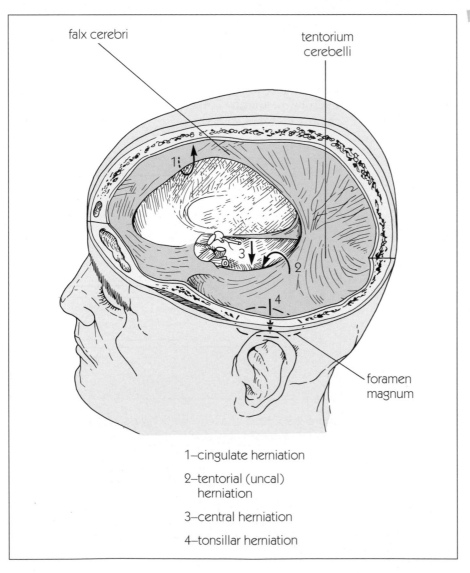

Figure 2.11 Dural folds within the cranial cavity and associated herniation sites.

1—cingulate herniation

2—tentorial (uncal) herniation

3—central herniation

4—tonsillar herniation

Cingulate Herniation

A focal mass lesion in the supratentorial compartment exerts progressive pressure locally on the ipsilateral hemisphere. The increase in ICP may not be uniform; it is greatest close to the mass, thus creating a pressure gradient. A supratentorial mass lesion may displace the cingulate gyrus, which is next to the free edge of the falx cerebri, and cause it to herniate under the falx to the opposite side. There is usually displacement of the ventricular system as well (Fig. 2.12). The anterior cerebral artery may be compromised by the tight, sharp edge of the falx cerebri. There are no clinical signs and symptoms specific to a cingulate herniation.

Uncal Herniation

Uncal herniation is the most dramatic and most common herniation syndrome observed clinically. Uncal herniation is often seen with lesions of the middle cranial fossa, such as acute epidural hematoma, subdural hematoma, temporal lobe contusions, or temporal lobe neoplasms. An expansile mass of the middle fossa causes the uncus, the inferomedial-most structure of the temporal lobe, to herniate between the rostral brain stem and the tentorial edge into the posterior fossa (see Fig. 2.12). In postmortem studies, a deep groove may be noticed at the lateral margin of the uncus as a manifestation of the herniation. In some instances, the medial displacement of the brain stem may cause compression of the brain stem against the opposite tentorial edge, producing a notch called Kernohan's notch.

With uncal herniation, the clinical syndrome consists of progressively impaired consciousness, dilated ipsilateral pupil, and contralateral hemiplegia. The impaired consciousness results from compression of the reticular activating system in the rostral brain stem. The dilated pupil is due to compression of the third nerve, which carries the parasympathetic pupilloconstrictor fibers. Contralateral hemiplegia results from direct compression of the cerebral peduncle, which carries corticospinal fibers to the opposite side. When a Kernohan's notch is present, the hemiplegia will be on the ipsilateral side. In some patients with uncal herniation, the posterior cerebral artery may be compromised, causing secondary infarction of the occipital lobe on one or both sides.

Central Transtentorial Herniation

In contrast to uncal herniation, which occurs from mass lesions located close to the tentorial hiatus, central transtentorial herniation occurs with mass lesions far removed from the tentorial hiatus, such as in frontal,

Figure 2.12 Types of brain herniation.

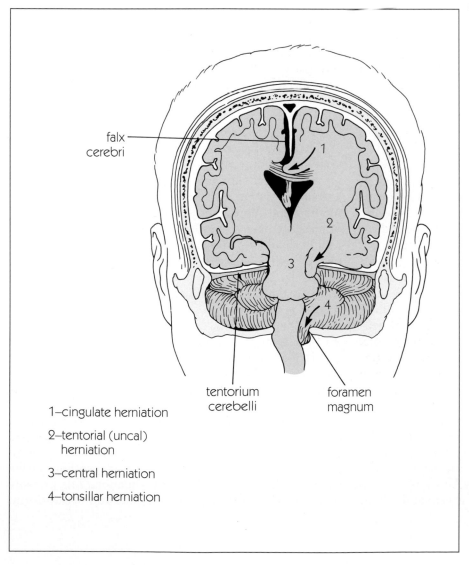

falx cerebri

tentorium cerebelli

foramen magnum

1–cingulate herniation

2–tentorial (uncal) herniation

3–central herniation

4–tonsillar herniation

parietal, or occipital areas. Bilateral mass lesions, such as bilateral subdural hematomas, can also cause central herniation. There is a downward displacement of the diencephalon and midbrain centrally through the tentorial incisura (see Fig. 2.12). The clinical syndrome in central herniation is not as easily recognizable as that of uncal herniation. The patient with central transtentorial herniation tends to have bilaterally small reactive pupils, exhibits Cheyne-Stokes respirations, is quite obtunded, and may show loss of vertical gaze.

Tonsillar Herniation

Acute tonsillar herniation generally results from acute expansion of posterior fossa lesions. It may result from an ill-advised lumbar puncture in a patient with a mass lesion within the cranial cavity. The tonsil of the cerebellum herniates through the foramen magnum into the upper spinal canal, compressing the medulla (see Fig. 2.12). The manifestations of acute medullary compression are cardiorespiratory impairment, hypertension, high pulse pressure, Cheyne-Stokes respirations, neurogenic hyperventilation, and impaired consciousness. The patient may have a stiff neck or be in an opisthotonic position. Decorticate or decerebrate posturing may be present as well.

SYMPTOMS AND SIGNS

The most common symptom of increased ICP is headache. It is generalized in nature and is worse at night or when the patient is recumbent, presumably due to the increase in CO_2 tension and increased venous pressure. The pain-sensitive structures within the cranial cavity are the dura and the blood vessels. Focal mass lesions that distort the dura and stretch the vessels tend to cause headache more frequently than diffuse generalized increase in ICP without focal mass effect, such as in pseudotumor cerebri or hydrocephalus. The headache, if present, may be associated with nausea and vomiting. Projectile vomiting is thought to be indicative of intracranial mass and increased pressure, but clinical experience has shown that all vomiting, regardless of the cause, is projectile and one cannot assign intracranial etiology from the nature of vomiting. The vomiting associated with increased ICP is usually not associated with nausea. Vomiting associated with neurologic signs such as ataxia, papilledema, and cranial nerve paralysis is most likely associated with an intracranial lesion. Papilledema is another cardinal sign of increased ICP.

The symptoms of increased ICP vary depending on whether the increased pressure is of a chronic, slowly progressive nature or results from an acute, rapidly evolving lesion, such as a clot that follows trauma. When there is an acute and rapid rise in ICP the patient generally becomes obtunded and there may be signs of brain stem compression from herniation. This is manifested by

irregular breathing patterns, decorticate or decerebrate rigidity, hemiplegia, and pupillary inequality.

MONITORING INTRACRANIAL PRESSURE

The most significant factor determining morbidity and mortality in patients with neurosurgical disorders is increased intracranial pressure. Continuous ICP monitoring is very useful for assessing intracranial dynamics in patients with suspected increased pressure. There are no clinical indicators that can be used at an early stage of rising ICP to forestall a further rise. The classic clinical indicators described in the literature occur in the end stage and they are not sensitive enough to show subtle changes in pressure. Equally important is the role of ICP monitoring in assessing treatment regimens for increased pressure. The two most common indications for ICP monitoring are closed head injury and subarachnoid hemorrhage. Although significant neurologic impairment can occur in neurosurgical disorders without elevation of pressure (head injury), the vast majority have significant elevation of ICP.

TECHNIQUES OF MONITORING ICP

Intracranial pressure is best measured directly and continuously from the cranial cavity. Although lumbar puncture can indirectly indicate ICP, it is neither safe nor accurate. It is not safe because it might precipitate tonsillar or uncal herniation. It may not be accurate if the subarachnoid pathways in the vicinity of the tentorial incisura are blocked, for then the spinal subarachnoid compartment is isolated from the supratentorial subarachnoid compartment.

There are two commonly used pressure-monitoring systems in contemporary neurosurgical practice. An intraventricular catheter connected to a manometer and a drainage system is the simplest and most economical method and represents the standard against which all other systems are compared. The ventricular catheter ideally should be tunneled under the skin and brought out through a separate stab wound, well away from the ventricular entry site, to minimize the risk of infection, which is the most significant complication of intraventricular pressure monitoring. Using an electronic transducer, the waveform can be monitored as well (Fig. 2.13). The major advantage of this method is that the ventricular catheter is used not only to measure the pressure, but also as a treatment modality allowing continuous drainage of CSF when the pressure exceeds physiologic limits.

A second method is the use of a fiberoptic transducer-tipped catheter system.[5] The transducer-tipped catheter can be placed within the ventricle or brain parenchyma or in the subdural space, depending on the surgeon's choice and the clinical situation. The pressure monitor gives both a digital readout and a waveform.

The advantages of this system are: 1) the zero point does not have to be reset with changes in head position because the pressure-sensing transducer is within the cranial cavity, and 2) it is not susceptible to blockage by debris and air bubbles because it is not a fluid-coupled system. The disadvantages of this system are: 1) higher cost; 2) inability to tunnel—the fiberoptic cables tend to break at acute angles, so that extended monitoring using the same port carries a higher risk of infection; 3) baseline drift—with prolonged monitoring the indicated pressures become less reliable; and 4) possible inaccuracy of intraparenchymal pressure readings—there is some concern about whether they truly reflect intracranial pressure.

ICP WAVEFORMS

The waveform of normal ICP typically shows three arterial components superimposed on the respiratory rhythm (Fig. 2.14). The first arterial wave is the percussion wave, followed by the tidal wave, which ends in the dicrotic notch. This notch is followed by the dicrotic wave. Under physiologic conditions, the percussion wave is the tallest, with the tidal and dicrotic waves having progressively smaller amplitudes (Fig. 2.15A). When the ICP rises even to a modest degree (20 mm Hg) the waveform may change, with the peaks of the tidal or dicrotic waves exceeding that of the percussion wave

(Fig. 2.15B). Such alterations in the morphology of the pressure tracing indicate decreasing compliance and increasing ICP.

When the ICP waveforms are registered over a period of time, certain trends may become apparent (Fig. 2.16). Plateau waves, or type A waves, are characterized by an abrupt elevation in ICP for 5 to 20 minutes followed by a rapid fall in the pressure to the resting level.[6] The amplitude may reach as high as 50 to 100 mm Hg. Plateau waves may be clinically marked by a decreasing level of conciousness, restlessness, increased tone in the extremities, and tonic-clonic movements. Plateau waves may represent transient surges in ICP secondary to increased cerebral blood volume, possibly related to CO_2 retention. B waves, which have a frequency of 0.5 to 2 per minute, are related to rhythmic variations in breathing. The C waves are rhythmic variations related to Traub-Meyer-Hering waves of systemic blood pressure and have a smaller amplitude, with a frequency of about 6 per minute. B and C waves have questionable clinical significance.

TREATMENT

The most direct way to normalize raised ICP to the physiologic range is to eliminate the cause. If the increased pressure is due to a mass effect, such as a

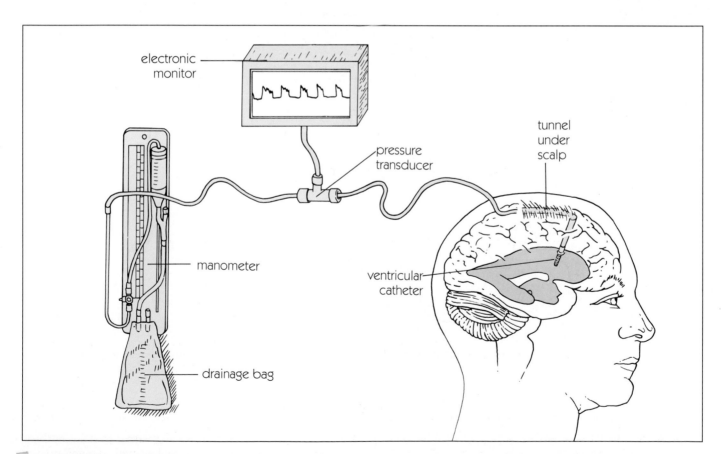

Figure 2.13 ICP monitoring system using ventricular catheter, pressure transducer, manometer, and drainage bag.

blood clot, prompt evacuation of the offending lesion will restore ICP to normal more effectively than any other measure.

VENTRICULAR DRAINAGE

Drainage of CSF from the ventricular system is the simplest, most effective, and quickest method of decreasing ICP. This modality is particularly effective in patients with cerebral edema. Experimental work has shown that the vasogenic edema fluid that has extravasated into the interstitial space is cleared by diffusion into either the ventricular system or the subarachnoid space.[7,8] Draining the ventricular fluid and decreasing the intraventricular pressure promotes rapid diffusion of edema fluid from the site of pathology.[9] This experimental observation

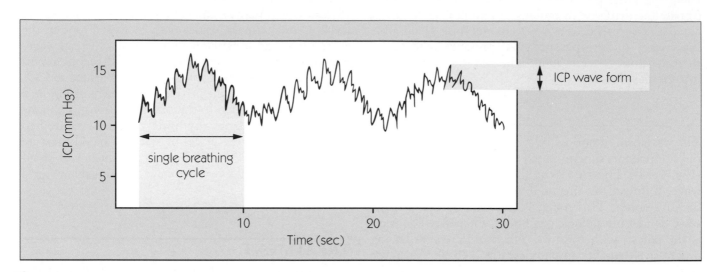

Figure 2.14 Normal ICP waveform superimposed on respiratory rhythm.

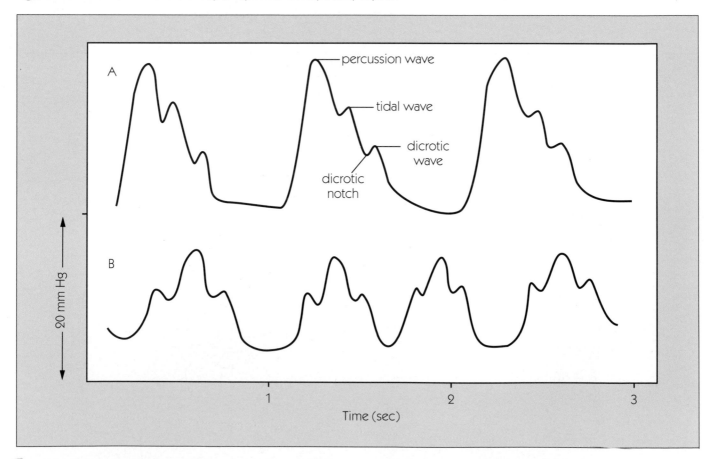

Figure 2.15 (A) ICP waveform under physiologic conditions. Three peaks are generally recognizable. The first, and usually tallest, is the percussion wave, followed by the tidal wave, the dicrotic notch, and the dicrotic wave. Note that the tidal and dicrotic waves have progressively lesser amplitudes than the percussion wave. (B) Abnormal intracranial waveform with high ICP. The amplitude of the tidal wave exceeds the amplitude of the percussion wave.

Principles of Neurosurgery

provides a logical foundation for the use of ventricular drainage in the management of vasogenic edema. Ventriculostomy is also highly effective in patients who have acute subarachnoid hemorrhage with acute communicating hydrocephalus. In patients with critically increased ICP, a ventricular catheter system can be used not only to monitor pressure continuously, but to drain the ventricular system automatically when the pressure exceeds the upper limits of the physiologic range. In ventilator-dependent patients ventricular drainage may be particularly effective at preventing sharp rises in ICP during suctioning or turning.

MANNITOL

Mannitol is the universally used osmotic agent to treat cerebral edema (other osmotic agents such as urea and glycerol are no longer used in contemporary neurosurgical practice). It has many pharmacologic effects, but the most significant one is its osmotic effect. It is not metabolized and it does not cross the blood-brain barrier. It increases serum osmolality and thus helps to draw fluid from the brain parenchyma into the vascular space. The normal serum osmolality is 275 to 290 mOsm/kg. An increase in serum osmolality of as little as 10 mOsm/kg is enough to have a significant effect on cerebral edema. Mannitol is generally given in small boluses rather than as a continuous drip. The usual dose is 0.25 g/kg at 4 to 6 hour intervals. In addition to the osmotic effect, mannitol decreases CSF production, increases cerebral blood flow and cerebral oxygen consumption, and decreases blood viscosity, thereby improving perfusion. Mannitol is generally effective for 48 to 72 hours. Its use beyond 72 hours is ineffective because mannitol slowly leaks out of the blood vessel, especially in areas of blood-brain barrier breakdown, with loss of osmotic gradient. Serum osmolality and electrolytes should be carefully monitored during mannitol therapy.

HYPERVENTILATION

Hyperventilation causes a fall in ICP by reducing intracranial blood flow and blood volume through vasoconstriction. Hyperventilation is generally initiated for acute management of increased ICP, but sustained hyperventilation as a mode of therapy has not been found to be beneficial because of compensatory mechanisms that come into play.[10] Also, recent studies show that some patients with increased ICP, such as patients with acute head trauma, may have low blood flow to begin with. Hyperventilation in such individuals may worsen the clinical condition.[11] Hyperventilation, if undertaken, should be moderate, bringing the P_{CO_2} down to 28 to 32 mm Hg. Reducing the P_{CO_2} much further will decrease blood flow to critically low levels, compounding the ischemia produced by increased ICP.

LOOP DIURETICS

Furosemide has been used as an adjunct to mannitol because they seem to have synergistic effect. Furosemide alone, however, cannot be depended on to reduce ICP. Because its primary action is on the kidney, it is not dependent on the intact blood-brain barrier for its effect. It is thought to reduce CSF production as well.

STEROIDS

Dexamethasone is used for treating chronic increases in ICP, especially those related to vasogenic edema caused by primary or metastatic neoplasms. It is ineffective in the management of vasogenic edema related to head trauma or cerebral infarction. It is thought to stabilize the cell membrane and restore the normal permeability of endothelial cells. This is brought about by inhibition of lysosomal activity, suppression of polyunsaturated fatty acid production that causes edema, and decrease of free radical production. The usual loading dose is 10 mg given

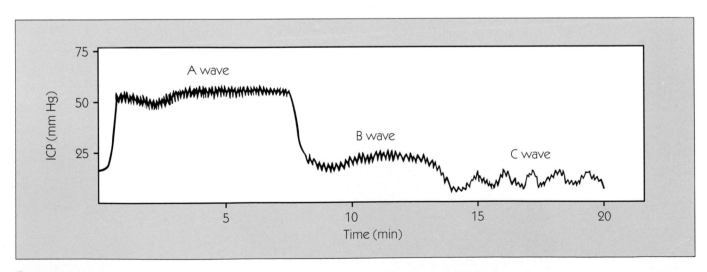

Figure 2.16 Examples of abnormal ICP waveforms with trend recording. Plateau waves, or A waves, are characterized by abrupt elevation in ICP for 5 to 20 minutes followed by a rapid fall in pressure to the resting level. Plateau waves herald neurologic worsening. B and C waves have questionable clinical significance.

intravenously followed by 4 mg every 6 hours. When the appropriate therapeutic goal has been achieved, the dose should be slowly tapered over a period of 3 to 4 days.

BARBITURATE COMA

Induction of coma with short-acting barbiturates is the last resort in the management of raised ICP when all other measures fail. Its clinical use is controversial. Barbiturates decrease the ICP by several mechanisms. They inhibit the release of fatty-acid peroxidation products by scavenging free radicals from the mitochondrial respiratory chain. They also inhibit cerebral metabolism and reduce cerebral blood flow. The most commonly used drug is thiopental, which is given in a loading dose of 3 to 10 mg/kg over a 10 minute period and a maintenance dose of 1 to 2 mg/kg/h. The serum level should be maintained at 3 to 4 mg/L. Patients in barbiturate coma require intensive monitoring of hemodynamic function, ICP, and blood gases. Vasopressors may have to be administered if hypotension results. Barbiturate therapy is usually withdrawn when the ICP normalizes and there is a good intracranial compliance; no clinical indicators are available to dictate termination of therapy.

REFERENCES

1. Langfitt TW, Weinstein JD, Kassell NF. Cerebral vasomotor paralysis produced by intracranial hypertension. *Neurology.* 1965;15:622–641.
2. Pollay M, Roberts PA. Blood-brain barrier: a definition of normal and altered function. *Neurosurgery.* 1980;6:675–685.
3. Ignelzi RJ. Cerebral edema: present perspectives. *Neurosurgery.* 1979;4:338–342.
4. Fishman RA. Brain edema. *N Engl J Med.* 1975; 293:706–711.
5. Kanter MJ, Narayan RK. Intracranial pressure monitoring. *Neurosurg Clin North Am.* 1991;2:257–265.
6. Lundberg N. Continuous recording and control of ventricular fluid pressure in neurosurgical practice. *Acta Psychiatr Neurol Scand Suppl.* 1960;149:1.
7. Reulen HJ, Grahm R, Spatz M, Klatzo I. Role of pressure gradients and bulk flow in dynamics of vasogenic brain edema. *J Neurosurg.* 1977;46:24–35.
8. Ohata K, Marmarou A. Clearance of brain edema and macromolecules through the cortical extracellular space. *J Neurosurg.* 1992;77:387–396.
9. Reulen HJ, Tsuyumu M, Tack A, Fenske AR, Prioleau GR. Clearance of edema fluid into cerebrospinal fluid. *J Neurosurg.* 1978;48:754–764.
10. Raichle ME, Plum F. Hyperventilation and cerebral blood flow. *Stroke.* 1972;3:566–575.
11. Bouma GJ, Muizelaar P, Choi SC, Newlon PG, Young HF. Cerebral circulation and metabolism after severe traumatic brain injury: the elusive role of ischemia. *J Neurosurg.* 1991;75:685–693.

Impaired Consciousness

Setti S. Rengachary, Derek A. Duke

Coma, or loss of consciousness, may be defined as a loss of awareness of one's self or environment (Fig. 3.1). Comatose state constitutes an acute neurosurgical emergency and is one of the most frequent reasons for a neurosurgical consultation in the emergency room.[1] Evaluation of the patient, history-taking, clinical assessment, basic resuscitation efforts, laboratory investigations, and radiologic assessment should occur in rapid sequence or concurrently, if possible; there is no justification for a sequential and leisurely evaluation. The comatose patient poses a chal-

Figure 3.1 Terms Used to Describe Altered States of Consciousness

Coma
Unawareness of self and environment.

Alpha Coma
An apparently comatose state in which the patient exhibits EEG rhythms within the alpha-frequency range, paradoxically resembling an awake EEG pattern.[13,14] Alpha coma is generally observed in the following groups of patients: 1) those who survive cardiopulmonary arrest with global ischemic changes in the brain, 2) those with a focal brain stem lesion at or just caudal to the pontomesencephalic junction, and 3) those with metabolic or toxic encephalopathies.

Persistent Vegetative State
(Syn.: akinetic mutism, coma vigile, neocortical death, apallic syndrome, cerebral death) A state of wakefulness without the ability to appreciate or respond to external stimuli.

Brain Death
A comatose state with an irreversible total loss of cerebral and brain stem functions preceding cessation of cardiac activity.

Locked-in State
(Syn.: pseudocoma, ventral pontine syndrome, deefferented state, cerebro-medullospinal disconnection) A state of unimpaired consciousness with tetraplegia and pseudobulbar paralysis. Patients generally have preserved vertical but absent horizontal eye movements. They respond to verbal stimuli with coded lid movements.

Lethargy
A mild decrease in the level of alertness; patient responds when spoken to but clearly lacks concentration and the attention span is short.

Obtundation
A moderate decrease in the level of alertness; patients generally tend to sleep when undisturbed but can be aroused to answer simple questions appropriately.

Stupor
A severe decrease in the level of alertness; patients respond to continuous vigorous stimulation (shaking or shouting) with unintelligible sounds, if any. Verbal responses are absent.

Confusion
Clouded, slow thinking.

Delirium
A hyperactive, agitated, confused state with hallucinations, paranoid ideations, and signs of autonomic overactivity.

Syncope (Fainting)
Transient loss of consciousness from a reversible, temporary impairment of blood flow to the brain.

Sleep
Cyclic loss of consciousness reversible with stimulation.

Principles of Neurosurgery

lenge to the diagnostic acumen of the physician and the treatment resources available.

A unique feature in the clinical assessment of the comatose patient is the inability to obtain a history from the patient, unless the patient is known to the physician from previous admissions. The history must be obtained from previous medical records, relatives, friends, law enforcement officials, or anyone else available. The circumstances in which the patient was found by the paramedics may be valuable. Knowing about a history of trauma from a fall, assault, penetrating wound, or auto accident is helpful. The patient should be searched for empty pill containers. A history of psychiatric illness, suicide attempt, epilepsy, illicit drug use, endocrine or other metabolic disorder, cardiac ir-regularity, hypertension, vascular disease, or coagulo-pathy may be helpful in determining the etiology of impaired consciousness.

EMERGENCY MANAGEMENT

First, the airway is inspected. If the patient vomits, the head should be turned to one side to prevent aspiration. Depending on the circumstances, an oral airway, nasal airway, endotracheal tube, or cricothyrotomy may be necessary. Whether to place the patient on a ventilator depends on the blood gases, tidal volume, rate of respirations, oxygen saturation, and level of consciousness. Vital signs, including temperature, pulse, respiratory rate, and blood pressure, should be recorded. The head, neck, trunk, and extremities are checked for signs of external trauma. Periorbital ecchymosis (raccoon eyes) (Fig. 3.2), drainage of clear fluid or blood from the nose, and Battle's sign are all indicative of trauma. The odor of alcohol in inebriation, ammoniacal odor in uremia, musty odor in hepatic coma, and spoiled fruit odor in diabetic coma should be noted, if present. An intravenous line should be started and the appropriate electrolyte solution administered. If the

patient is hypotensive, other sources of bleeding should be sought (for example, in the abdominal and pelvic areas). After cervical spine films have been taken to rule out cervical spine trauma, the patient is checked for meningeal signs such as neck stiffness, Kernig's sign, and Brudzinski's sign.

CLINICAL ASSESSMENT

LEVEL OF CONSCIOUSNESS

Assessing the level of consciousness is of foremost importance.[2] Level of consciousness varies from the patient who is fully alert and responsive to verbal comands to one who is totally incognizant of the environment and of herself or himself. To assess the level of consciousness, the Glasgow coma scale, which is particularly helpful in patients with head injury, has been devised (see Chapter 16).[3] The three parameters taken into consideration are eye opening response, verbal response, and motor response.

EYELIDS

Comatose patients have their eyes closed due to the tonic contraction of the orbicularis oculi muscles (Fig. 3.3). If one opens the eyelids they gradually and smoothly close. Hysterical patients cannot mimic this gradual closure, but keep their eyes closed forcibly, resisting opening by the examiner.

RESTING POSITION OF THE EYES

A quick inspection of the eyes at rest may give an idea of the general location of the pathologic lesion (Fig. 3.4). Patients with large destructive lesions in the *frontal lobe*, such as an acute intracerebral hematoma, will have conjugate deviation of the eyes away from the side of paral-

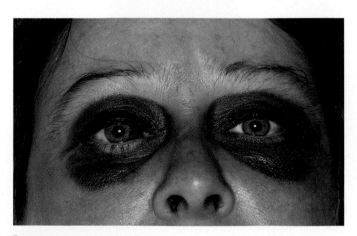

Figure 3.2 Bilateral periorbital ecchymosis (raccoon eyes) indicative of a fracture of the floor of the anterior cranial fossa.

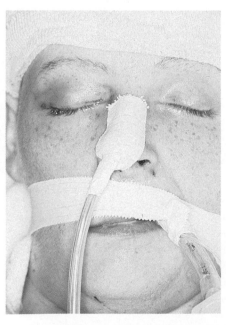

Figure 3.3 Deeply comatose patient with the eyes closed.

ysis, looking toward the lesion. In *deep-seated thalamic lesions* there may be "wrong-way" gaze paresis, that is, the conjugate deviation may be toward the paralysis and away from the lesion. In *unilateral pontine lesions* the conjugate deviation is toward the side of paralysis. A disconjugate gaze may imply an internuclear opthalmoplegia, paresis of individual muscles, or preexisting tropia or phoria. Spontaneous slow horizontal roving eye movements may indicate a good prognosis in that they usually imply an intact brain stem. They have essentially the same clinical significance as a positive response to the doll's eye maneuver, which is discussed below. It is to be emphasized that *in a deeply comatose patient with a structural lesion in the brain, true nystagmus with fast and slow components is never observed.*

--- PUPILS

Examination of pupillary size, equality, and response to light (both direct and consensual) gives valuable information regarding the integrity of the brain stem, especially the midbrain area (Fig. 3.5).

Pupillary abnormality is one of the cardinal features differentiating surgical disorders from medical disorders; pupillary abnormalities in a comatose patient generally herald structural changes in the brain, especially the brain stem, whereas in metabolic coma such abnormalities are not observed. In patients who are on a ventilator and who have received paralyzing agents, pupillary examination may be the only objective neurologic test possible. Resting pupillary size is determined under ambient light. In the critical care setting, the pupils should not be pharmacologically dilated to observe the fundus because this eliminates one of the prime objective means to assess brain stem integrity. One should check for orbital trauma, including injury to the iris that could cause pupillary dilation; this dilatation has no value for neurologic localization. Previous cataract surgery will impair mobility of the iris and thus the pupillary reaction.

A significant pupillary abnormality that one encounters in neurosurgical practice is the unilaterally dilated and fixed pupil (see Fig. 3.5A, left). This generally indicates uncal herniation with compression of the third cranial nerve at the tentorial edge, resulting in impairment of the parasympathetic pupilloconstrictor fibers within the nerve. Pupillary dilation can also occur with sudden expansion or rupture of an internal carotid

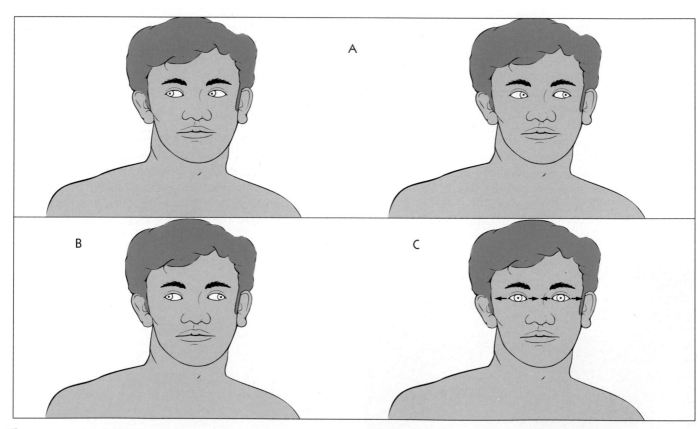

Figure 3.4 Resting position of the eyes. (**A**) *Left* Patient with a large right frontal destructive lesion. There is tonic conjugate deviation of the eyes toward the lesion away from the paralysis. *Right* With deep-seated thalamic lesions on the right side, there is "wrong-way" gaze deviation; there is tonic deviation of the eyes away from the lesion and toward paralysis. With a right pontine lesion there is conjugate deviation of the eyes toward the side of paralysis (not shown). (**B**) A disconjugate gaze may imply an internuclear opthalmoplegia, paresis of individual muscles, or preexisting tropia or phoria. (**C**) Spontaneous slow horizontal roving eye movements have a good prognostic value in that they usually imply an intact brain stem.

artery aneurysm or because of an intrinsic lesion of the midbrain (for example, acute hematoma). In extreme midbrain compression both pupils become fixed and dilated (Fig. 3.6). Fixed and dilated pupils also characterize the terminal stages of brain death, whatever the etiology. *Pontine tegmental lesions* produce small pinpoint pupils with a flicker of reaction to light, which sometimes can be appreciated only with a magnifying lens. *Medullary lesions* may cause a unilateral Horner's syndrome, which is characterized by miosis, ptosis, enophthalmos, and reduced sweating on the face homolateral to the lesion in the brain stem. *Hypothalamic lesions* may also produce Horner's syndrome. It is to be emphasized

that afferent optic abnormalities, such as an optic nerve transection, do not cause pupillary inequality. In such a situation, the direct response to light may be absent, but the consensual response is intact.

EYE MOVEMENTS

Forced downward deviation of the eyes occurs in lesions of the thalamus or the tectum of the midbrain. This would be associated with nonreactive pupils (Parinaud's syndrome). *Skew deviation*, or vertical divergence, follows lesions of the cerebellum or brain stem. *Ocular bobbing*, or conjugate downward movement from the

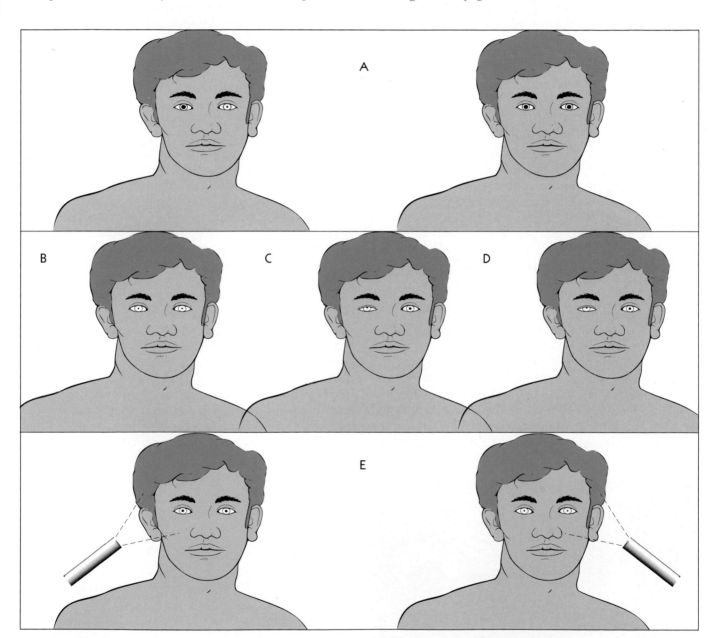

Figure 3.5 (A) Midbrain lesions. *Left* Third nerve paresis or a unilateral midbrain lesion produces an ipsilaterally dilated pupil. This is generally indicative of uncal herniation. *Right* Bilaterally fixed and dilated pupils in bilateral midbrain lesions, anoxic encephalopathy, and brain death. (B) Pontine lesion: bilaterally small pinpoint pupils. (C) Medullary lesions: unilateral Horner's syndrome with miosis, ptosis, enophthalmos. (D) Hypothalamic lesion producing Horner's syndrome. (E) Optic nerve injury on the right with no reaction to direct light but with consensual response.

primary position through a very small arc, usually follows lesions in the pontine tegmentum.[4] In such a situation there is usually lateral gaze paralysis.

Disconjugate movements may be seen in cranial nerve paralysis. The two most commonly paralyzed nerves are the sixth nerve due to a generalized increased intracranial pressure or the third nerve due to uncal herniation.

Oculocephalic Reflex (Doll's Eye Movement)

Elicitation of the oculocephalic reflex is a quick bedside test to determine the integrity of the brain stem (Fig. 3.7). This brain stem reflex has an afferent limb, a central relay, and an efferent arc. The afferent response is from the vestibular end organs through the vestibular nerve terminating in the vestibular nuclei. The efferent arc is the medial longitudinal fasciculus connecting the nuclei of the third, fourth, and sixth cranial nerves on the ipsilateral and opposite sides. In deeply comatose patients with absence of brain stem function, the doll's eye' movement is completely abolished (see Fig. 3.7D). The whole reflex is inhibited by the cerebral cortex. This reflex cannot be demonstrated in an alert, conscious individual because of the intact inhibitory influences from the cerebral hemispheres. In an unconscious patient, however, the presence or absence of this reflex gives an indication of the integrity of the brain stem. If the brain stem is intact, the eyes lag behind and roll towards the opposite side if the head is briskly turned to one side (see Fig. 3.7C). Before eliciting the doll's eye movement, one should be certain that there is no cervical spine injury.

Oculovestibular Reflex (Ice Water Caloric Test)

Elicitation of the oculovestibular reflex gives the same information as the doll's eye maneuver. This test is particularly useful in patients who have a head injury and possibly an associated spine injury. Before doing the test, one inspects the ear canal to make certain that the tympanic membranes are intact. The head is kept flexed 30° from the horizontal. Approximately 30 mL of ice cold water is injected into the external auditory canal. In normal awake individuals stimulation from the cold water induces nystagmus, with the fast component away from the stimulated side. In comatose patients the fast component is lost. Thus, cold caloric stimulation causes slow deviation of the eyes towards the irrigated side (Fig. 3.8A) lasting for 2 to 3 minutes before the eye returns to the neutral position. Patients with brain stem damage exhibit no response to cold caloric stimulation; the eyes assume a fixed forward gaze (Fig. 3.8B). The caloric test is also helpful for differentiating organic coma from hysterical coma. Hysterical patients will develop nystagmus from caloric testing. Caloric testing may also reveal gaze paralysis, individual muscle paresis, or internuclear opthalmoplegia. It is to be noted that *in metabolic encephalopathy, at least in the early stages, the oculocephalic reflexes are intact.*

RESPIRATIONS

Using bedside observations, clinical neurologists have described several classic patterns of respiration that correlate with various levels of anatomic involvement of the CNS. These patterns of respiration have been useful for years in the clinical evaluation of patients.[5] Most comatose patients with neurosurgical disorders and a Glasgow coma score less than 9 are intubated soon after arrival to insure adequate oxygenation of the brain. Because these patients are intubated, paralyzed, and ventilated, the classic respiratory patterns cannot be observed. However, the standard descriptions of various classic patterns are given for completeness of discussion of the subject.

Cheyne-Stokes respirations are generally seen in patients with diffuse forebrain lesions (Fig. 3.9A). Patients with diffuse forebrain lesions are thought to be hypersensitive to normal levels of CO_2. This results in a hyperventilatory phase, which blows off CO_2 and results in apnea for a brief period. CO_2 accumulates to normal levels during the apneic interval; thus, cycles of hyperventilation and apnea alternate. Cheyne-Stokes breathing can be seen occasionally for brief periods in a normal individual during sleep. In Cheyne-Stokes respirations

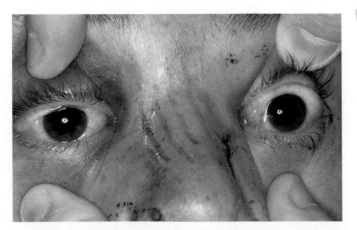

Figure 3.6 Bilaterally fixed and dilated pupils in a deeply comatose patient.

the hyperventilation phase is longer than the apnea phase. As a result, the patients are generally alkalotic.

Central neurogenic hyperventilation is a rare phenomenon seen in the head-injured patient with a severe midbrain lesion (Fig. 3.9B). In true neurogenic hyperventilation the partial pressure of oxygen (P_{O_2}) is high and that of carbon dioxide (P_{CO_2}) is low. Many episodes of hyperventilation seen in comatose individuals are not true neurogenic hyperventilation, but rather the result of pulmonary edema and aspiration pneumonitis. In such individuals, the P_{O_2} is below normal in spite of the tachypnea.

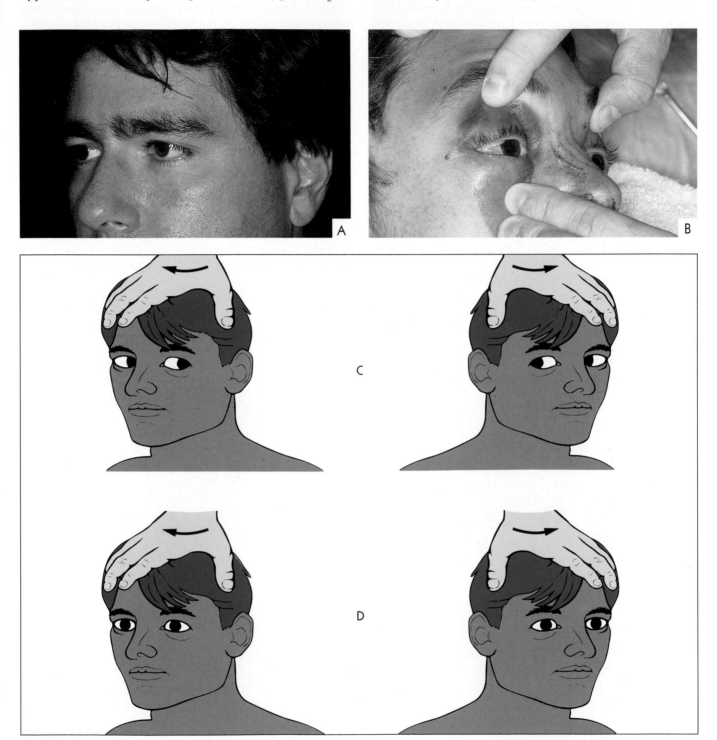

Figure 3.7 Oculocephalic reflex (doll's eye movements). **(A)** In a fully conscious individual, doll's eye movements are absent. The eyes point in the direction in which the head points. **(B)** In an unconscious patient with intact brain stem function, doll's eye movements can be elicited. As one briskly turns the head to one side, the eyes lag behind and roll toward the opposite side **(C)**. In a deeply comatose patient with absent brain stem function the doll's eye movements are absent **(D)**. The eyes have a fixed forward stare and move with the head.

Apneustic breathing is characterized by a prolonged pause at full inspiration (Fig. 3.9C). This phenomenon is quite rare. It usually reflects a lesion of the mid to caudal pons. Usually it is seen in patients with brain stem stroke from basilar artery occlusion.

Ataxic breathing occurs in patients with medullary lesions where the respiratory center is located (Fig. 3.9D). The breathing is very irregular with deep and shallow breaths occurring randomly. It represents impairment of the orderly cyclic respiratory rhythm. Lesions in the posterior cranial fossa may produce this pattern in the terminal stages.

Cluster pattern is also seen in lower medullary lesions (Fig. 3.9E). Clusters of breath occur in an irregular sequence with varying pauses between clusters. Clustered breathing and gasping respirations occur in end-stage medullary failure.

_____ MOTOR FUNCTION

A quick assessment of motor function helps to localize lesions in the nervous system. The patient who can obey orders and perform simple motor tasks on command obviously has intact corticospinal tracts and the related integrative pathways. When asking a patient to squeeze a hand on command, one should make sure that the grasp reflex is not mistaken for volitional contraction. This can be done by asking the patient to release the hand on command. Patients with reflex grasp but without volitional contraction will not be able to release the hand on command. A better test is to ask the patient to hold up two fingers. If a patient does not respond to vocal stimuli, a painful stimulus, such as pressure on the supraorbital notch, sternum, or nailbed, should be applied. Usually, the patient moves the extremities defensively to ward off the painful stimulus (Fig. 3.10A). At a lesser level of response, the patient may slightly withdraw the limb from the painful source without any complicated purposeful defensive movements. *Decorticate posturing* (Fig. 3.10B), either spontaneously or in response to stimuli, is characterized by flexion of the arms and wrists and extension of the lower extremities. The lesion is generally thought to be in cerebral white matter, internal capsule, and the thalamus. In *decerebrate rigidity* (Fig. 3.10C) the patient has the upper and lower extremities in complete extension. In extreme cases the patient may assume an opisthotonic position. In decerebrate posturing, the lesion is slightly more caudal in the upper brain stem. *Flaccidity* of the extremities with no response to any noxious stimuli is seen in moribund patients with medullary failure (Fig. 3.10D).

_____ OTHER BRAIN STEM FUNCTIONS

Other brain stem reflexes that are commonly tested include corneal, gag, and cough reflexes. The corneal

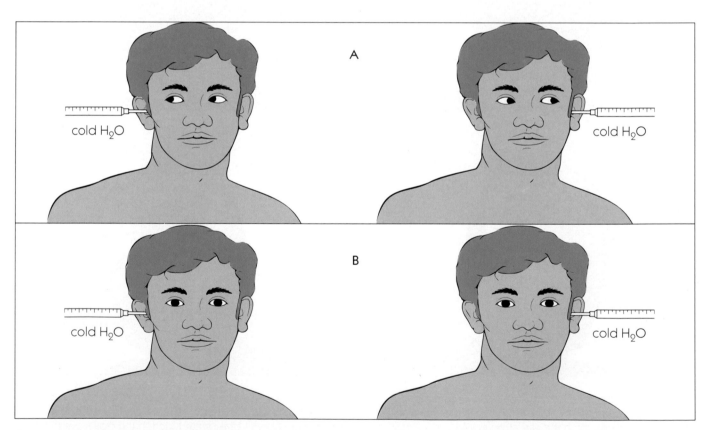

Figure 3.8 Oculovestibular reflex (ice water caloric test). **(A)** Cold caloric stimulation in a comatose patient causes slow tonic deviation of the eyes toward the stimulated side, if the brain stem is intact. **(B)** With a damaged brain stem, the eyes are immobile despite cold caloric stimulation.

reflex is tested by lightly touching the edge of the cornea with a wisp of cotton. There is usually prompt eye closure. Intact corneal reflex implies that the facial nerve and the pathway from the first division of the trigeminal nerve to the facial nerve nucleus are intact. The gag reflex is tested by touching the pharynx with a cotton swab. The cough reflex is tested by suctioning the patient or manipulating the endotracheal tube.

DIAGNOSTIC TESTS

Admission laboratory studies include complete blood count, electrolytes, liver function tests, renal function tests, serum alcohol level, and toxic drug screen of both blood and urine. If poisoning is suspected, gastric lavage is instituted and gastric contents are sent for analysis. A fingerstick test for glucose is taken, and if the glucose level is low, 50% glucose is administered. The rationale for using 50% glucose blindly in comatose individuals is now being questioned because there is some evidence that high glucose concentrations may increase the infarct size in patients with impending stroke.[6,7]

After initial clinical assessment and drawing of blood samples, a CT scan is done without contrast administration. The CT scan has considerable value in patients in coma. A negative CT scan in a coma patient implies a metabolic process such as uremic, diabetic, or anoxic encephalopathy. A structural lesion (for example, intracerebral hematoma, brain tumor, abscess) will be clearly visible on the scan. If the CT scan is normal and the patient has meningeal signs and fever, a lumbar puncture should be performed to rule out meningitis or subarachnoid hemorrhage.

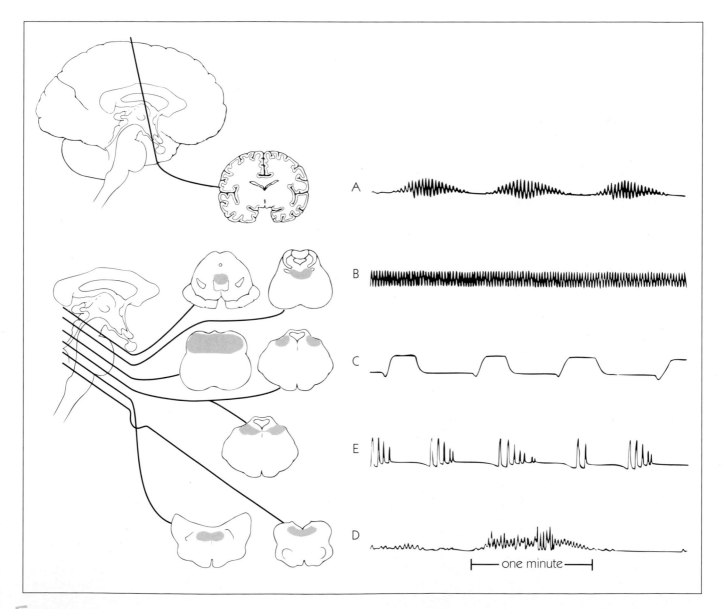

Figure 3.9 (A) Cheyne-Stokes respiration. Periods of hyperventilation alternate with apneic intervals. (B) Central neurogenic hyperventilation. (C) Apneustic breathing. (D) Ataxic breathing. (E) Cluster pattern.

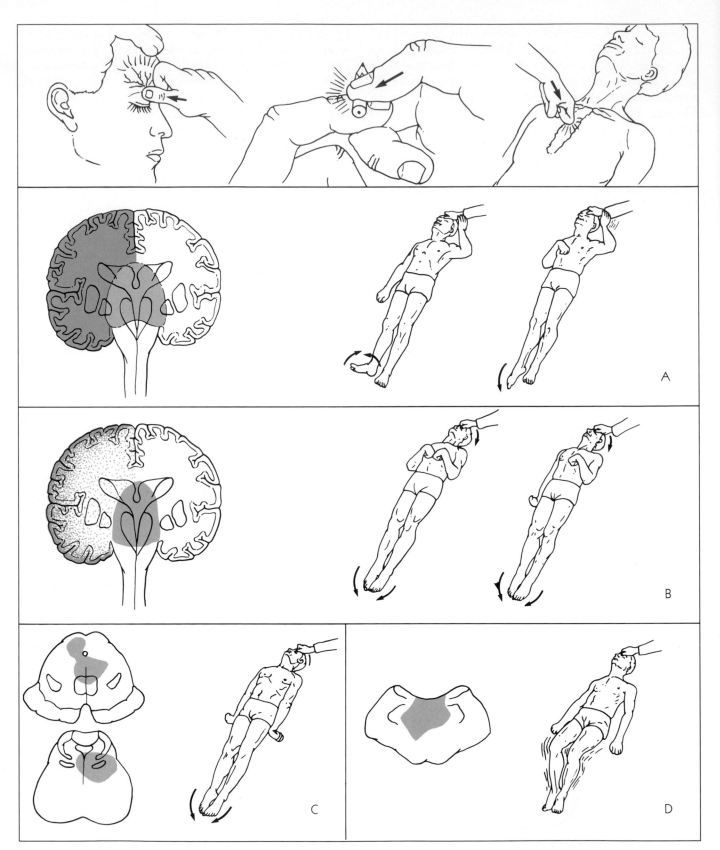

Figure 3.10 Various motor responses to painful stimuli in a comatose patient. Three methods of inducing pain are illustrated: supraorbital pressure, pressure on the finger nailbed with a pencil, and sternal rub. (A) With a hemispheric lesion the patient is hemiplegic on the opposite side. The patient has purposeful defensive movements on the nonparalyzed side.

(B) With a bilateral lesion in the deep white matter and thalamus there is decorticate posturing characterized by flexion of the arms and wrists and extension of the legs. (C) With upper brain stem lesions there is decerebrate rigidity—the patient has both upper and lower extremities in extreme extension. (D) Medullary lesions produce generalized flaccidity.

PATHOGENESIS OF COMA

The conscious state depends on the integrity of the reticular activating system in the rostral pons, midbrain, and thalamus (Fig. 3.11). This system receives collateral input from all the incoming sensory pathways (specific sensory systems). Projections from the rostral end of the reticular activating system from the thalamic nuclei radiate diffusely to the entire cerebral cortex. The thalamocortical connection is bidirectional in that regulatory input to the reticular activating system is directed from the cortex and the input to the cortex is derived from the reticular nuclei. Impairment of consciousness can occur in two types of lesions: focal destruction in the reticular core of the rostral brain stem or a diffuse lesion in both cerebral hemispheres. Therefore, the causes of impaired consciousness can be broadly classified into four major categories. *Diffuse cortical lesions* can result from hypoxia, hypoglycemia, hyperosmolar coma, acid-base imbalance, uremia, hepatic coma, etc. In this situation the neurons of the cerebral cortex are diffusely affected. *Supratentorial mass lesions,* either extrinsic or intrinsic, in the cerebral hemispheres may cause compression and uncal herniation, which results in compression of the rostral brain stem and thus impairment of the reticular activating system. This is a common mechanism of coma in a neurosurgical setting. *Direct lesions* in the rostral brain stem itself, for example, acute

hemorrhage or trauma, may result in coma. *Infratentorial lesions* with secondary compression on the brain stem caused by large cerebellar tumors, large cerebellar hemorrhage, or infarction may impair consciousness.

RELATED STATES

PERSISTENT VEGETATIVE STATE

This state is also called akinetic mutism, coma vigile, neocortical death, apallic syndrome, or cerebral death.[8,9] The term *vegetative* is used because only vegetative or autonomic functions are preserved. In this state patients appear wakeful, but there is no cognitive function. Although they may open their eyes, they do not track and explore the surroundings. Purposeful movements of the eyes in response to commands are absent. These patients do not vocalize or verbalize, their faces are expressionless, and they generally assume a fetal position with the limbs flexed. They do not have any purposeful motion of the extremities in response to noxious stimuli. They continue to have normal spontaneous respirations and normal cardiac and gastrointestinal activity. They are totally dependent for all activities of daily living, including eating, drinking, and attention to personal hygiene. Sleep-wake cycles may

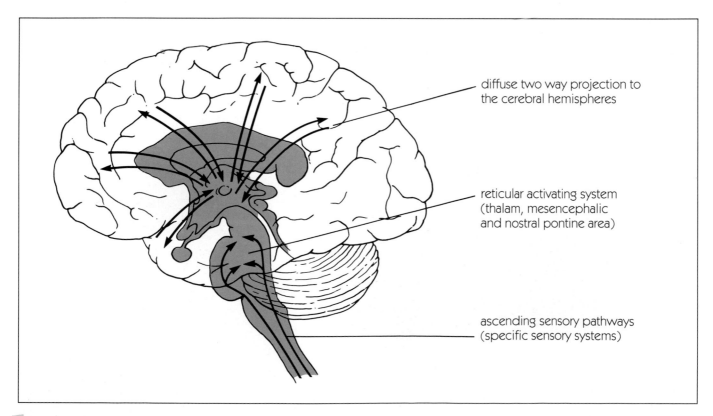

diffuse two way projection to the cerebral hemispheres

reticular activating system (thalam, mesencephalic and nostral pontine area)

ascending sensory pathways (specific sensory systems)

Figure 3.11 Anatomic substrate of consciousness. The anatomy of the reticular activating system is depicted in this illustration. This system receives collateral input from all incoming sensory pathways (specific sensory systems). There is a two-way projection (afferent and efferent) from the reticular core to the cerebral cortex.

remain intact. A positron emission tomographic (PET) scan will show low cerebral metabolic rate for glucose.

Patients may get into a persistent vegetative state in one of two ways. A patient may start with a chronic nervous disorder that has a continuous downhill course, such as Alzheimer's disease. Or the patient may suffer an acute insult to the brain that causes coma and may partially recover from the coma only to go into a persistent vegetative state. Most patients in a persistent vegetative state were first comatose.

LOCKED-IN SYNDROME

The so-called locked-in syndrome, also called pseudocoma, ventral pontine syndrome, deefferent state or cerebromedullospinal disconnection,[10,11] occurs due to a lesion in the pons affecting both corticospinal and corticobulbar tracts bilaterally. The distal part of the reticular formation in the pons and tegmentum may be involved but does not appear to be critical in maintaining consciousness. Thus the patient is tetra-plegic and has pseudobulbar paralysis and is unable to communicate except by coded blinking motions. Horizontal eye motions are affected as well. The patient is fully conscious because the reticular activating system in the rostral brain stem is intact. This is a very unique neurologic

syndrome and one should be cognizant of it to avoid mistaking this for coma.

Blood flow studies of the cerebral hemispheres in patients with locked-in syndrome and in patients with chronic vegetative state have shown that blood flow is nearly normal in the former and considerably decreased in the latter. Figure 3.12 illustrates the location of the lesion in locked-in syndrome.

BRAIN DEATH

Brain death is defined as total and irreversible loss of function of the cerebral hemispheres and the brain stem. Some institutions, however, have made minor modifications to this definition. The patient may continue to have some spinal reflex activity, which does not preclude declaring the patient brain dead.

As a general rule, a brain-dead patient lacks the clinical attributes of a functioning brain stem and cerebral hemispheres. This is manifested by coma and unresponsiveness to deep painful stimuli. Reflexes mediated by the brain stem are all absent. The pupils are fixed and maximally dilated. The corneal, cough, and gag reflexes are absent. The doll's eye testing and cold caloric stimulation do not induce any response. There are no spontaneous respirations. Apnea can be

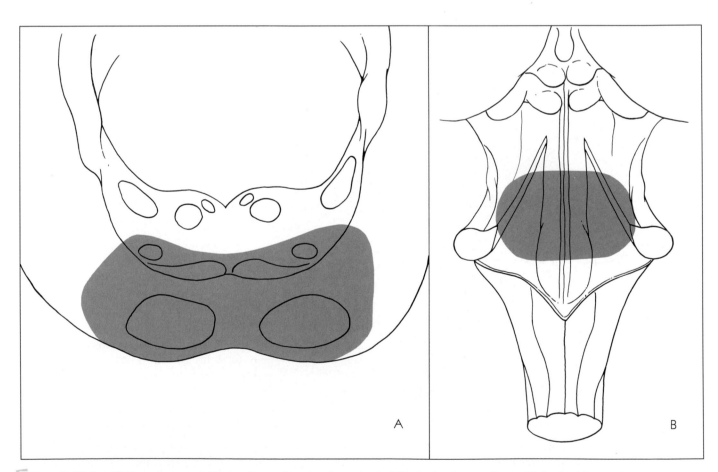

A

B

Figure 3.12 Axial (A) and coronal (B) sections, showing the extent of the lesion in a patient with locked-in syndrome.

Principles of Neurosurgery

further tested by disconnecting the patient from the respirator to allow the Pco_2 to rise to 60 mm Hg of mercury. At this stage the patient who does not initiate breathing is assumed to have no spontaneous respiratory effort. Generally, all of the extremities are flaccid with no response to painful stimuli. The deep tendon reflexes are generally absent, but their presence does not preclude declaration of brain death. Similarly, a withdrawal response in the feet may be present. An EEG will show isoelectric tracing in spite of high-gain setting. Before brain death is declared, it must be ascertained that the patient is not intoxicated with sedative or hypnotic drugs and is not hypothermic. Objective criteria seldom used in clinical practice are radionuclide brain scan and arteriogram, both of which can confirm a total lack of cerebral blood flow.[2]

It is customary when declaring brain death to examine the patient twice, 6 hours apart, to make certain the state is irreversible. After a patient meets the criteria for brain death, within minutes to a few days cardiac activity invariably ceases. Because there is no exception to this rule, it has become customary to declare patients legally dead if they meet the brain-death criteria. Brain-dead patients who continue to have good cardiac function and perfusion are potential organ donors. When the criteria are met and the patient is declared brain-dead, the family should be approached for potential organ donation.

REFERENCES

1. Posner JB. The comatose patient. *JAMA*. 1975; 232:1313.
2. Fisher CM. The neurological examination of the comatose patient. *Acta Neurol Scand Suppl*. 1969; 36:273–290.
3. Teasdale G, Jennet B. Assessment of coma and impaired consciousness—a practical scale. *Lancet*. 1974;2:81.
4. Fisher CM. Ocular bobbing. *Arch Neurol*. 1964; 11:543–546.
5. North JB, Jennet S. Abnormal breathing patterns associated with acute brain damage. *Arch Neurol*. 1974;32:338.
6. Couten-Meyers G, Myers RE, Schoolfield L. Hyperglycemia enlarges infarct size in cerebrovascular occlusion in cats. *Stroke*. 1988;19:623–630.
7. Vazquez-Curz J, Vilalta JL, Ferer I, Perez-Gallofre A, Folch J. Progressing cerebral infarction in relation to plasma glucose in gerbils. *Stroke*. 1990;21: 1621–1624.
8. Feldman MH. Physiologic observations in a chronic case of "locked-in" syndrome. *Neurology*. 1971;21:459–478.
9. Nordgren RE, Markesbery WR, Fukuda K, Reeves AG. Seven cases of cerebromedullospinal disconnection: the "locked-in" syndrome. *Neurology*. 1971; 21:1140–1148.
10. Munsat TL, Stuart WH, Cranford RE. Guidelines on the vegetative state: commentary on the American Academy of Neurology statement. *Neurology*. 1989;39:123–124.
11. American Academy of Neurology. Position of the American Academy of Neurology on certain aspects of the care and management of the persistent vegetative state patient. *Neurology*. 1989;39: 125–126.
12. Levy DE, Sidtis JJ, Rottenberg DA, et al. Differences in cerebral blood flow and glucose utilization in vegetation versus locked-in patients. *Ann Neurol*. 1987;22:673–682.
13. Iragui VJ, McCuthen CB. Physiologic and prognostic significance of "alpha coma." *J Neurol Neurosurg Psychiatry*. 1983;46:632.
14. Westmoreland BF, Klass DW, Shargbough FW, Reagan TJ. Alpha-coma: electroencephalographic, clinical, pathologic and etiologic correlations. *Arch Neurol*. 1975;32:713–718.

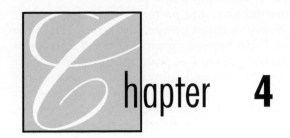

Perioperative Care
of the Neurosurgical Patient

Dennis A. Turner

This chapter discusses the major principles of the preoperative, intraoperative, and postoperative care of neurosurgical patients. Accurate preoperative assessment of the patient's condition improves preoperative and intraoperative management, minimizes problems in the immediate postoperative course and substantially decreases the overall surgical risks. The neurosurgeon follows generally accepted guidelines for patient care and management, which must be adhered to strictly in order to decrease the average surgical risk for a cohort of patients. The informed consent should include an enumeration of risks associated with the procedure in addition to rationale and expected outcome.

PREOPERATIVE CARE

Once the decision to perform a procedure is finalized, the general goal of preoperative care is to minimize the surgical risks, taking into account specific patient characteristics and the particular technique.[1–5] The more information one has regarding the region of interest, the shorter and less problematic the surgery and recovery will be.[6] Surgery of the nervous system must be planned in the context of the patient's general medical condition. Medical problems and risk factors, such as hypertension and diabetes, should be treated prior to surgical intervention, if possible. A scheme of perioperative risks devised for carotid endarterectomy by Sundt and coworkers[7,8] classifies risk factors neurologically, medically, angiographically, and according to their stability or instability prior to surgery. This system can be applied to a wide range of neurosurgical procedures.

Preparation for a nervous system operation includes three stages: 1) preventing problems related to the specific nervous system approach being taken, 2) evaluating and treating systemic medical risks and general risks associated with any surgical procedure, and 3) discussing and obtaining an informed consent from the patient and family.[6] The extent of this preparation is dictated by how urgent it is to alleviate the nervous system abnormalities.

SPECIFIC NERVOUS SYSTEM PREPARATION

The primary goal of preparation is to stabilize abnormalities of the nervous system as much as possible. Even in emergencies, the wait for the operating suite may be 15 to 30 minutes, during which time an emergent lesion may cause considerable secondary damage. Figure 4.1 lists some of the ways in which the nervous system can be temporarily protected, obviating secondary damage. For example, performing CSF drainage preoperatively may help stabilize the patient, protecting against damage caused by increased intracranial pressure; performing a temporizing procedure such as a ventriculostomy may help if there is hydrocephalus, as with an obstructive tumor in the posterior fossa; and stabilizing intracranial edema and pressure can lessen the risks of general anesthesia induction, which may raise intracranial pressure considerably.

Conditions that increase risk need to be recognized and treatment plans instituted preoperatively to prevent surprising perioperative complications. To stabilize comatose patients before a procedure the airway must be controlled and seizures treated. Many neurological disorders, such as Parkinson's disease and multiple sclero-

Figure 4.1 Neurologic Preoperative Risks and Management

Nervous System Risk Factors	Management Scheme to Decrease Risk
Increased ICP	CSF drainage via ventricular or lumbar catheter Steroids: dexamethasone, prednisone, or hydrocortisone Controlled anesthesia induction: hyperventilation, narcotics
Coma	Early intubation, assessment, and systemic stabilization ICP management: CSF drainage, mannitol as needed Treatment of urinary retention: bladder catheter
Seizures	Control of seizures: parenteral medication, with loading of phenytoin (20 mg/kg) or phenobarbital (15 mg/kg) Treatment of status with additional agents as required
Contaminated or open wound	Antibiotics to cover skin contaminants and prompt debridement and secondary closure

sis, require maximal medical treatment before and during surgery to minimize temporary worsening of the neurological state or morbidity. Parkinson's patients continue their medications (particularly the Sinemet or L-dopa) to avoid pulmonary and bradykinesia-related complications, while multiple sclerosis patients may benefit from a steroid boost in the perioperative period. The measures instituted preoperatively to prevent further secondary damage to the nervous system or clinical worsening postoperatively depend on the nature and urgency of the operative procedure.

EVALUATION AND TREATMENT OF SYSTEMIC ABNORMALITIES

Figure 4.2 lists a number of common systemic risk factors that require evaluation and treatment to insure optimal safety during anesthetic delivery and the procedure. Some of these abnormalities may require significant treatment and may even preclude either anesthesia or the procedure until corrected (e.g., severe arrythmia or coagulation disorder), while others (e.g., metabolic imbalance or inadequate nutritional status) do not increase the intraoperative risks and can be managed intraoperatively if necessary. For example, hyperglycemia should be treated with sufficient insulin to lower the blood sugar to less than 300 mg/100 mL; intraoperatively the patient should receive an insulin drip and frequent blood sugar measurements should be taken. Hypertension should be treated until blood pressure is in the range of 160/90 mm Hg or less, if possible, and preparations should be made for uncontrolled pressure spikes during both the anesthesia induction and, particularly, the period following anesthesia and extubation. These pressure elevations can be treated with either nitroprusside intravenously or a continuous drip of nitroglycerin. Platelets may need to be supplemented, if there are abnormalities in platelet number (50,000/mm³) or function that cannot be rapidly corrected. Pulmonary function tests, cardiology consultation as needed for cardiovascular risk assessment, and endocrine evaluation may be required in addition to the standard ECG and serum tests for electrolytes, renal function, blood count, and coagulation factors. The urgency of the procedure must be weighed against the risk of postponement (with the attendant risk of neurological worsening) or inadequately treating the systemic complicating factor.

INFORMED CONSENT

The patient and family must be realistically and constructively informed of the potential risks and likely

Figure 4.2 Systemic Preoperative Risks and Management

Systemic Risk Factors	Management Scheme
Cardiovascular	Control of hypertension, hypotension, and arrhythmias
Respiratory	Pulmonary function tests and chest x-ray to assess complicating lesions and need for bronchodilation
Endocrine	Diabetes management, pituitary assessment, steroid coverage for stress management
Hematologic	Coagulation disorders and platelets; anemia evaluation
Gastrointestinal	Risk of aspiration; general nutrition for healing
Genitourinary	Management of urinary infections and drainage
Renal	Need for dialysis in patient with renal compromise
Fluids and electrolytes	Metabolic balance, control of electrolytes
Infection	Identification of source, treatment with antibiotics

outcome of the proposed procedure, and this discussion must be thoroughly documented (Fig. 4.3). Informed consent is crucial in high risk patients and when the benefits of the procedure may only marginally outweigh the risks. The surgeon must compare the benefits and risks of the proposed treatment to alternative treatments, including nonoperative approaches. The reasons for recommending the proposed treatment should be clearly presented to the patient and/or the family representatives. The patient's and family's awareness of the advantages and disadvantages of the treatment plan will enhance their cooperation during the recovery following surgical intervention as well as increase their understanding of (though not necessarily their sympathy towards) complications that occur.

PREOPERATIVE MEDICATIONS

During the preoperative evaluation, the surgeon should determine if additional medications are required to facilitate the intraoperative course and enhance the patient's recovery (Fig. 4.4). For example, perioperative steroid management may be necessary for cerebral edema or for a prophylactic effect on the CNS. The suggested dose of dexamethasone for this effect (such as on brain tumors) is 10 to 20 mg for a loading dose and 4 to 6 mg every 6 hours before, during, and after the procedure. If the risk of seizures from a primary cortical abnormality is thought to be greater than 5% to 10%, management with anticonvulsants should be considered, particularly to minimize neighborhood seizures commonly associated with CNS procedures. Perioperative antibiotics, such as cephalosporins, vancomycin, or nafcillin for staph coverage, can decrease the risk of infection in clean procedures but are more advantageous for treating contaminated and overtly infected cases. Pre- and postoperative antibiotic use has also undergone considerable scrutiny, particularly in clean cases where the risk is substantially lower than in contaminated cases.[9] Several studies indicate that if the

antibiotics are in the tissues during the operation, they may prevent the usual mild tissue contamination that occurs during an open procedure from developing into an overt infection. However, gentleness with tissues, good operating technique in closing tissue layers, and attention to blood supply are fundamental; the surgeon cannot rely on antibiotics to treat infections caused by inadequacies in these areas. The current trend is to administer antibiotics directly before and during procedures only, in order to treat contamination from the skin surface and potential seeding, while avoiding the selection for antibiotic-resistant organisms caused by lengthy regimens.[9,10] In many cases, such as contaminated or infected wounds, a full course of antibiotics both during and after the procedure may prevent more severe infections and aid in healing.

INTRAOPERATIVE CONSIDERATIONS

MEDICATIONS AND ANESTHETICS

The patient should undergo routine preoperative preparation; the patient should have an empty stomach (to avoid aspiration) and, if indicated, should be sedated prior to intubation.[6] The risk of increased intracranial pressure (ICP) can be minimized at the time of induction, for example, by spraying lidocaine on the patient's vocal cords or hyperventilating the patient to a P_{CO_2} near 25 to 27 mm Hg (Fig. 4.5). Muscle paralysis may be contraindicated for certain procedures, particularly those where either a twitch or EMG response is required to document the status or location of peripheral nerves. Examples of the latter include procedures for nerve root decompression, where a muscle twitch may indicate potential root damage, and surgery for acoustic neuroma, where the facial nerve may be located using an EMG recording prior to direct visualization with the microscope. Medications that protect neural structures

---

Figure 4.3 Preoperative Preparation and Informed Consent

1. Nature of the condition	Clinical history, exam, diagnostic tests
2. Proposed treatment and associated possible complications	Possible benefit when balanced against known and/or unexpected risks
3. Alternative forms of treatment	Benefits and risks compared to natural history and proposed treatment, including nonoperative management
4. Customary and usual treatment schemes	Recommended standard of care
5. Expected benefit of proposed treatment is not guaranteed	

Principles of Neurosurgery

from damage, such as steroid protocols, and prophylactic antibiotics should also be continued intraoperatively.

The recommended anesthesia for most neurosurgical procedures is the balanced type, which includes a mixture of intravenous narcotics, inhalation agents, and nitrous oxide as needed for adequate analgesia. Agents that raise ICP (including most inhalation agents, such as halothane and isofluorane) should be avoided in circumstances where this would be harmful, although a high ICP may be partially overcome with hyperventilation and additional balanced agents (such as narcotics and neuroleptics) that prevent vascular engorgement. Of course, the particular circumstances and neurological status of the patient should be considered (e.g., a comatose patient needs only light anesthesia during surgery).

Figure 4.4 Perioperative Medication Management

Type of Medication	Rationale and Duration of Treatment
Perioperative antibiotics	First dose prior to anesthesia; continue throughout surgery until skin closed, unless infection demonstrated or wound contaminated
Perioperative steroids	Useful for spinal cord injury, brain tumor edema, and increased ICP; dexamethasone 10 to 20 mg loading, 4 to 6 mg every 6 hours
Hypertonic solutions	Mannitol 1 g/kg for increased ICP and to help retraction; 3% saline for persistent hyponatremia
Antihypertensives	To prevent immediate postoperative bleeding and for management of subarachnoid hemorrhage
Anticonvulsants	Full preoperative load when risk of seizures exceeds 5% to 10% or after seizure occurs

Figure 4.5 Intraoperative Medications

Type of Medication	Rationale and Medication-Related Problems
Intravenous narcotics	Postoperative sedation may be pronounced
Inhalation agents	Increased ICP due to venous vasodilation
Hyperventilation	Maintain low P_{CO_2} and vasoconstriction
Nitrous oxide	Only as a supplement to other anesthetics
Muscle paralysis agents	For induction and intubation but not when stimulating excitable structures (nerves and brain) for locating muscle or EMG response
Local anesthetics	On vocal cords during induction to decrease ICP and in skin incisions to decrease overall need for general anesthetic
Hypertensives (pressors)	Persistent hypotension intraoperatively

Physiological variables should be assessed during induction and intubation, including ECG, arterial pressure, and, if critical, ICP using a ventriculostomy to allow venting of CSF (Fig. 4.6). End-tidal CO_2 measurements also allow assessment of ventilation adequacy. Other types of physiological monitoring include evoked potentials to evaluate axonal conduction along pertinent pathways, EMG recording of end-organs associated with the operative field (such as EMG recording of the facial nerve during surgery for acoustic neurinoma), and monitoring of bladder and anal sphincter function during procedures involving sacral nerve roots or the conus and swallowing during sectioning of the upper cervical nerves and accessory nerves for torticollis. Physiological monitoring may substantially decrease the risk of damage to critical neurological structures in close proximity to the exposure.

Procedures performed on patients in the sitting position, particularly those involving the posterior fossa, require constant vigilance because of the increased risk related to veins unable to collapse under negative pressure. The veins in this category include those embedded in bone (e.g., the mastoid emissary vein), large muscular structures, and, particularly, the dural venous sinuses. These veins may remain open regardless of the intraluminal venous pressure, enabling the vein to pull room gas directly into the circulation, which causes air embolism. The patient must be monitored constantly. Specific methods to detect air embolism have been developed, including Doppler monitoring of the heart for abnormal mixing of air within its chambers, and end-tidal CO_2 measurement. Air embolism is treated by withdrawing the air through a right atrial catheter in addition to identifying and stopping the source in the surgical field.

Intraoperative management includes determining the proper surgical position, the types of perioperative monitoring required, and how to minimize complications such as infection, bleeding, and peripheral nerve palsies due to pressure. Each position has its own risks and attention must be directed towards secondary problems. For instance, the ulnar nerves should always be carefully padded and the axilla should be well protected during surgery in the lateral position. Figure 4.7 illustrates standard positions; other positions include those that provide extensile exposure for peripheral nerve problems in the upper and lower extremities, the lateral thoracotomy position for exposure of T2-L1 in complex spine procedures, and the lateral retroperitoneal position for lumbar spine procedures. Positioning should be discussed with the anesthesiologist either before or at the time of surgery.

Air embolism is one of the more severe complications associated with the sitting position.[2-4] The larger the difference in elevation between the surgical site and the right atrium, the more likely it is that air embolism will occur, particularly if the central venous pressure is low. Another risk factor is operative manipulation of venous sinuses and large emissary veins within bones. Since these venous structures cannot collapse under negative pressure, they pull air into the venous system at a rapid rate. Effective surveillance includes a precordial Doppler for early detection and monitoring the end-tidal CO_2 for a decreased CO_2 value caused by the room air quickly filling up alveoli. Immediate measures to halt the air flow include raising the venous pressure, tamponading the wound with wet sponges, and lowering the patient so blood egresses from the venous channels. If unchecked, air embolism can severely raise the right heart pressure due to pulmonary embolism, open the fo-

Figure 4.6 Intraoperative Monitoring

Risk or Structure	Type of Monitoring Performed
Cardiovascular system	Pulse, ECG, pulmonary artery catheter for cardiac output
Blood pressure	Indwelling arterial cannula or external automatic self-inflating cuff
Respiration	End-tidal expired CO_2
Air embolism	End-tidal expired CO_2 precordial Doppler
Specific structure monitoring	Facial nerve stimulation and EMG recording; spinal cord evoked potentials during decompression or fixation; peripheral nerve monitoring during repair; EMG recording during selective rhizotomy

ramen ovale, and lead to severe arterial embolism. There is even a risk of air embolism in the supine and prone positions, depending on the location of the operative site and the right atrium and central venous pressures. However, the sitting or lounge position, compared to the prone position, causes considerably less venous oozing throughout the procedure.

CONTINUOUS SURGICAL MANAGEMENT

Additional management during surgery should be directed towards maintaining the preoperative evaluation and treatment paradigms (e.g., blood clotting factors should be continued as needed for an abnormal coagulopathy). Intraoperative antibiotics, steroids, and anticonvulsants should be maintained. Induced hypo- or

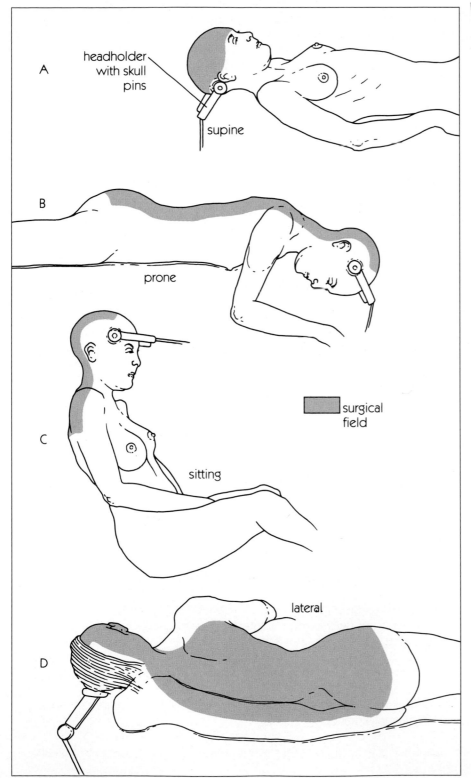

Figure 4.7 Typical positions for patients undergoing neurosurgical procedures, and the regions of access for each particular position (shaded areas). Note that for all craniotomy procedures (apart from those performed supine with a head roll), a headholder with skull pins is used to clamp the patient to the operating room bed securely and prevent damage to the eyes and face. Each position has a number of variations and precautions, discussed more fully in the text. **(A)** Supine position—frontal craniotomies, carotid endarterectomy procedures, anterior cervical discectomy procedures, and transsphenoidal adenomectomy. **(B)** Prone position—posterior occipital and suboccipital craniotomy and craniectomy procedures and cervical, thoracic, and lumbar laminectomy procedures. **(C)** Sitting or lounge position—posterior fossa and cervical spine procedures. **(D)** Lateral or park bench position—posterior fossa and retromastoid craniectomy procedures, lateral thoracotomy and anterolateral lumbar spine approaches, lateral cervical, thoracic and lumbar spine procedures, and lumboperitoneal shunt placement.

hypertension for complex vessel exposure and direct replacement of blood loss to insure stability may be required. Adequate monitoring can indicate neurological changes during surgery that require the surgeon to make changes in surgical technique. Monitoring techniques that help confirm the level of surgery, the field of exposure, and delineate the pathologic abnormalities include regular x-ray film, fluoroscopy, intraoperative ultrasound, and angiography.

Instances occur in which the operation may be significantly altered or terminated (e.g., due to severe bleeding, hypotension, impending cardiac or respiratory instability, or severe air embolism). Contingency plans and alternative routes of treatment, such as unplanned ICU observation, are sometimes necessary.

POSTOPERATIVE CARE

Postoperative care of the patient should include knowledge of complications related to the procedure as well as general complications, as discussed in detail by Horwitz and Rizzoli.[3,4] Familiarity with rare complications can be helpful. A thorough understanding of how the CNS reacts to stress and anesthesia can help predict an individual patient's response to a situation. For instance,

Figure 4.8 Early Postoperative Problems

Event or Disease	Management
Subarachnoid/intraventricular blood	CSF drainage from subarachnoid space
Vasospasm following SAH	Maintain blood volume and pressure
CSF leak from operative site	CSF drainage, proper positioning
Respiratory insufficiency	Treat atelectasis, intubation if severe
Seizures	Remove source of cortical irritation and hemorrhage, if possible
Postoperative clot formation	May require direct evacuation of clot
Infection	Early or late: antibiotics, drainage, debridement
Inappropriate serum dilution	Fluid restriction, hypertonic saline

Figure 4.9 Phases and Risks of Wound Healing

1. Risks for poor healing	Prior radiation, diabetes, small vessel disease, previous infection
2. Suture type for closure	Absorbable versus permanent (incision location, use of suture site, likelihood of heavy work dictate type of suture and density of suturing)
3. First 4 days	Inflammatory healing only with no tissue crossbridges
4. Intermediate period	Proliferative changes, cell and collagen turnover, cell migration, and capillary formation
5. Reorganization phase	Continued remodeling and strengthening of wound for up to 2 years

patients with significant pre-existing CNS disease often recover slowly from the anesthesia and exhibit a prolonged deficit for the first 6 to 12 postoperative hours.[11]

ACUTE POSTOPERATIVE RECOVERY AND EARLY PROBLEMS

The patient's recovery following complex procedures involves either a specialized neurosurgical ICU or a general surgical ICU.[13] Management of cardiac or respiratory instability, CSF drainage (such as with ventriculostomy), ICP management, and care of patients with altered mental status can be facilitated by a knowledgeable ICU staff. In the early postoperative period (particularly the first 48 hours), close observation may help detect early problems, such as postoperative bleeding or hematomas, or local CNS problems that may or may not be directly related to the surgical procedure, including dural sinus thrombosis, acute seizures, inappropriate serum dilution, and early assessment for infection (Fig. 4.8). This stabilization period allows complete recovery from the anesthetics and evaluation for new postoperative deficits or systemic instabilities (e.g., cardiac or respiratory).

WOUND HEALING AND ACTIVITY

Figure 4.9 briefly describes the phases of wound healing. The type of sutures used depends on the expected rate of healing and anticipated problems, for example, prior radiation to an incision site may considerably inhibit healing, necessitating several layers of permanent sutures to insure wound closure. The presence of associated medical diseases, particularly diabetes, will slow the healing process, as will vessel diseases such as arteriosclerosis. However, good operative technique and clear apposition of important layers (such as the fascia and subcutaneous tissues) without overlap or infolding will decrease the chances of wound dehiscence or infection. For many incisions (such as those for a lumbar laminectomy), avoiding significant stress on the incision may be critical to wound healing for up to 2 to 3 months after the procedure.

The surgeon must decide when to mobilize the patient following surgery and what level of activity should be achieved. Ambulation is beneficial and prevents deep venous thrombosis, aspiration, and atelectasis. The advantages of early ambulation, however, have to be countered with contravening factors such as the need to prevent CSF leak through a dural incision in some cases and the maintenance of cervical traction for an unstable spine and postoperative comfort.

The objective of early postoperative care and observation is the management of immediate complications. Later in the postoperative course, the goal is to gradually bring the patient up to the level of functioning that the postoperative neurologic status allows. Subsequent rehabilitation or long-term nursing care is necessary for patients who will not return to their preoperative level of independent functioning or who require additional recovery time.

LATE POSTOPERATIVE PROBLEMS

Late postoperative complications include slow but progressive neurological conditions such as hydrocephalus, deep venous thrombosis and pulmonary embolism, delayed hemorrhage within operative sites, and infection (Fig. 4.10). Constant vigilance is required to recognize and assess problems before they become serious. The surgeon must be aware of the potential problems following the procedure and the time frame in which they occur to improve proper diagnosis and treatment. Thus hydrocephalus several months following a sub-

Figure 4.10 Late Postoperative Complications

Class of Complication	Examples of Complications
Late infections	Discitis, CSF shunt infections, cranioplasty infections
Late hemorrhage	Hemosiderosis after hemispherectomy
CSF leak	Meningitis following surgery or trauma
Late hydrocephalus	Subarachnoid hemorrhage, posterior fossa surgery
Deep venous thrombosis	Pulmonary embolism and risk of death
Pituitary insufficiency	Thyroid, gonadal, and steroid hormone insufficiency
Late seizures	Late development of epileptic focus due to scar or irritation

arachnoid hemorrhage, unexpected thyroid deficiency following a transsphenoidal adenomectomy for a nonsecreting adenoma, or lumbar discitis presenting several weeks after a discectomy procedure will not be unexpected. These complications may seem so remote from the surgery that they are not considered, delaying diagnosis until there is secondary damage or instability (e.g., late hormone insufficiency).

CONCLUSION

Many postoperative difficulties can be anticipated and their impact eliminated or ameliorated. Anticipated complications and difficulties can often be circumvented if preoperative and intraoperative planning is sufficient. The goal is to decrease the risks associated with the procedure and facilitate recovery, maximizing the patient's independent functional capabilities.

The author was supported by a NINDS grant, a Merit Review Award from the Durham VAMC, and grants from the B.S. Turner Foundation and the ADRDA.

REFERENCES

1. Keller TS. Preoperative evaluation of a neurosurgical patient. In: Wilkins RH, Rengachary SS, eds. *Neurosurgery.* New York, NY: McGraw-Hill; 1985: 366–368.
2. Wise BL. *Preoperative and Postoperative Care in Neurological Surgery.* Springfield, Ill: Charles C Thomas Publisher; 1978.
3. Horwitz NH, Rizzoli HV. *Postoperative Complications of Intracranial Neurological Surgery.* Baltimore, Md: Williams & Wilkins; 1982.
4. Horwitz NH, Rizzoli HV. *Postoperative Complications of Extracranial Neurological Surgery.* Baltimore, Md: Williams & Wilkins; 1987.
5. Stern WE. Preoperative evaluation; complications, their prevention and treatment. In: Youmans JR, ed. *Neurological Surgery.* Philadelphia, Pa: WB Saunders Co; 1985:1051–1116.
6. Wilkins RH, Odom GL. General operative technique. In: Youmans JR, ed. *Neurological Surgery.* Philadelphia, Pa: WB Saunders Co; 1985:1136–1159.
7. Sundt TM Jr, Sandok BA, Whisnant JP. Carotid endarterectomy: complications and preoperative assessment of risk. *Mayo Clin Proc.* 1975;50:301–306.
8. Turner DA, Tracy J, Haines SJ. Risk of late stroke and survival following carotid endarterectomy procedures for symptomatic patients. *J Neurosurg.* 1990; 73:193–200.
9. Haines SJ. Prophylactic antibiotics. In: Wilkins RH, Rengachary SS, eds. *Neurosurgery.* New York, NY: McGraw-Hill; 1985:448–452.
10. Friedman AH, Wilkins RH. *Neurosurgical Management for the House Officer.* Baltimore, Md: Williams & Wilkins; 1984.
11. Albin MS. Neuroanesthesia. In: Wilkins RH, Rengachary SS, eds. *Neurosurgery.* New York, NY: McGraw-Hill; 1985:384–395.
12. Mollman HD, Haines SJ. Risk factors for postoperative neurosurgical wound infections. *J Neurosurg.* 1986;64:902–906.
13. Wirth FP, Ratcheson RA. *Neurosurgical Critical Care.* Baltimore, Md: Williams & Wilkins; 1987.

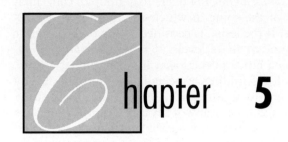

Chapter **5**

Spinal Dysraphism

Leslie N. Sutton

The term *spinal dysraphism* refers to a group of congenital anomalies of the spine in which the midline structures fail to fuse. If the lesion is confined to the bony posterior arches at one or more levels, it is termed *spina bifida*. Simple spina bifida of the lower lumbar spine is a common radiologic finding, especially in children, and by itself carries no significance; in contrast, bony spina bifida may accompany any of several complex anomalies involving the spinal cord, nerve roots, dura, and even the pelvic visceral structures. In these cases, spinal dysraphism constitutes a major source of disability among children and adults.

There are two distinct syndromes of spinal dysraphism: 1) *spina bifida cystica*, which includes the familiar myelomeningocele, is characterized by herniation of elements through the skin as well as the bony defect and is obvious at birth, and 2) *spina bifida occulta*, in which the underlying neural defect is masked by intact overlying skin. The external signs are often subtle; symptoms may not develop until late childhood, or even adulthood, as the result of spinal cord tethering. Included in the latter group are diastematomyelia, lipomyelomeningocele, hypertrophied filum terminale, and anterior sacral meningocele. The early recognition of these entities is important, since neurologic function may be preserved only by early and appropriate surgical intervention.

MYELOMENINGOCELE

Myelomeningocele is the most common significant birth defect involving the spine. The incidence of the condition ranges from one case per 1000 live births in the United States to almost 9 cases per 1000 in areas of Ireland.[1] The etiology is unknown, but evidence exists for both environmental and genetic influences. The risk of having additional children with myelomeningocele increases markedly after the birth of an affected child.[2]

Embryologically, the abnormality manifests between 3 and 4 weeks of gestation. At this point in development, the neural plate folds into the neural tube, a process termed *neurulation*. Neurulation begins in the dorsal midline, and progresses cephalad and caudad simultaneously. The last portion of the tube to close is the posterior end (neuropore) at 28 days. Myelomeningocele presumably occurs when the posterior neuropore fails to close, or if it reopens as the result of distention of the spinal cord's central canal with cerebrospinal fluid. The spinal abnormality is only a portion of a more widespread complex of central nervous system abnormalities, which also include hydrocephalus, gyral anomalies, and the Chiari malformation of the hindbrain.

Recent developments in prenatal diagnosis of fetal anomalies have made antenatal recognition of myelomeningocele commonplace. Families at risk are routinely

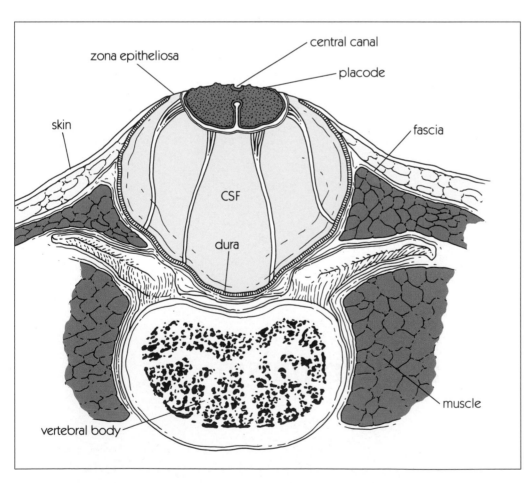

Figure 5.1 Cross sectional anatomy of a myelomeningocele. The neural placode is visible on the back, usually at the center of the sac. It is separated from the full-thickness skin by a fringe of pearly tissue, the "zone epitheliosa." The neural tissue herniates through a defect in the skin, fascia, muscle, and bone. The dorsal dura and zona epitheliosa converge to attach laterally to the placode, forming the roof of the sac.

zona epitheliosa
central canal
placode
skin
fascia
CSF
dura
muscle
vertebral body

offered amniocentesis and ultrasound screening, which have a combined accuracy of more than 90%.[3,4] Families can be professionally counseled regarding the expected prognosis and decisions about abortion.

The initial step in managing the newborn with myelomeningocele is a careful physical examination by a pediatrician. A thorough evaluation should reveal associated anomalies, including cardiac and renal defects, that might contraindicate surgical closure of the spine defect. A large head or bulging fontanelle suggests active hydrocephalus and heralds the need for a head ultrasound. Stridor, apnea, or bradycardia in the absence of overt intracranial hypertension suggests a symptomatic Chiari malformation, which carries a poor prognosis.[5] The myelomeningocele is inspected; the red, granular neural placode is surrounded by the pearly "zona epitheliosa," which must be entirely excised to prevent the appearance of a dermoid inclusion cyst. Most myelomeningoceles are slightly oval with the long axis oriented vertically. If the lesion is oriented more horizontally, a horizontal skin closure is often preferable. The neurological examination is difficult in the newborn infant, and it is hard to separate voluntary leg motion from reflex movement. It must be assumed that any leg movement in response to a painful stimulus to that limb is reflexive. Contractures and foot deformity usually denote paralysis at that segmental level. Virtually all affected neonates have abnormal bladder function, but this is difficult to assess in the newborn. A patulous anus lacking in sensation confirms sacral denervation.

Recent data suggest that if broad spectrum antibiotics are administered, closure of the myelomeningocele can be safely delayed for up to a week to allow time for discussion with the parents.[6] The parents should be told the infant's prognosis based on the functional spinal level, and it should be emphasized that closure of the defect is a lifesaving measure but will not alter the pre-existing neurologic deficits. Pending plans for definitive care, the infant is nursed in the prone position with a sterile, saline-soaked gauze dressing loosely applied to the sac or placode.

Generally the back is closed first, and a CSF shunting procedure, if needed, is deferred. In cases with massive hydrocephalus, the back closure and the shunt can be done at the same time to protect the back closure from CSF leakage. The goal of back closure is to seal the spinal cord with multiple tissue layers to inhibit the entrance of bacteria from the skin and to prevent CSF leakage while preserving neurologic function and preventing tethering of the spinal cord. Accomplishing this goal requires a thorough understanding of the three-dimensional anatomy of the tissue layers involved (Fig. 5.1).

Surgical Technique

General anesthesia is used, and the patient is placed in the prone position, with rolls under the chest and hips to allow the abdomen to hang freely (Fig. 5.2). If the sac remains intact, fluid is aspirated and sent for culture. The surgeon gently attempts to approximate the base of the sac or defect vertically, then horizontally, to deter-

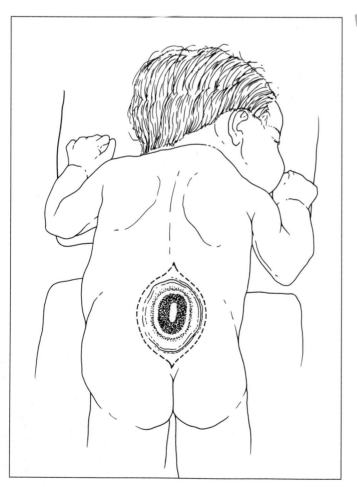

Figure 5.2 Positioning the patient for myelomeningocele closure. The infant is placed in the prone position, with rolls beneath the chest and iliac crests to minimize epidural bleeding. The skin incision is outlined circumferentially on the outside of the zona epitheliosa. A vertical orientation of the elliptical incision is appropriate for most closures.

mine which direction of closure will produce the smallest skin defect. An elliptical incision is made, oriented along that axis, just outside the junction of the normal, full-thickness skin and the thin, pearly zona epitheliosa. Full-thickness skin forming the base of the sac is viable and should not be excised. The incision is carried through the subcutaneous tissue until the glistening layer of everted dura or fascia is encountered. The base of the sac is mobilized medially until it is seen to enter the fascial defect (Fig. 5.3A). The sac is entered by radially incising the cuff of skin surrounding the placode. This skin is sharply excised circumferentially around the placode with iris scissors and discarded (Fig. 5.3B). It is important to excise all of the zona epitheliosa to prevent later formation of an epidermoid cyst. At this point, the placode is lying freely above the everted dura (Fig. 5.4).

In some instances it is appropriate to "reconstruct" the placode so that it fits better within the dural canal and a pial surface is in contact with the dural closure to prevent tethering. Interrupted 6-0 sutures approximate the pia-arachnoid-neural junction of one side of the placode with the other, folding the placode into a tube. The central canal is closed along its entire length.

Attention is then directed to the dura, which is everted and loosely attached to the underlying fascia. The dura is undermined bluntly and reflected medially on each side until enough has been mobilized to enable a closure (see Fig. 5.4). The dura is closed in a watertight fashion using a running suture of 4-0 neurilon. If possible, the fascia is closed as a separate layer by incising it laterally in a semicircle on both sides, elevating it from the underlying muscle, and reflecting it medially. Like the dura, the fascia is closed with a continuous stitch of 4-0 suture material (Fig. 5.5). The fascia is poor at the caudal end of a lumbar myelomeningocele as well as with most sacral lesions, thus closure at this level may be incomplete.

The skin is mobilized by blunt dissection with large scissors or a finger. It may be necessary to free up the skin anteriorly all the way to the abdomen (see Fig. 5.5). In most instances, midsagittal (vertical) plane closure is easiest, but occasionally horizontal closure results in less tension. A two-layer closure using vertical interrupted mattress skin sutures is preferred.

Very large lesions require special techniques. Various types of Z-plasties and relaxation incisions have been

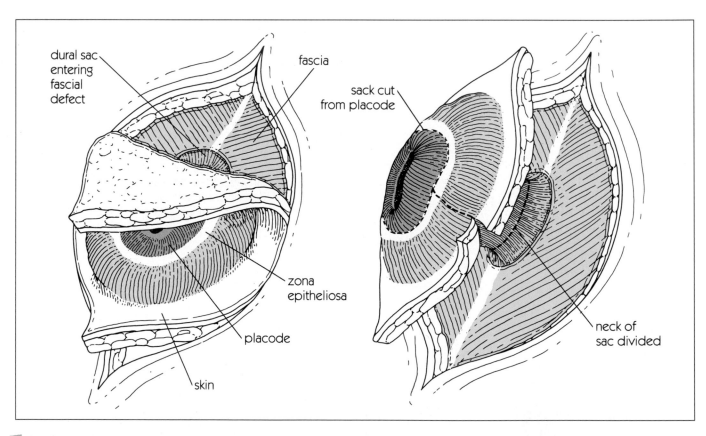

Figure 5.3 (A) Mobilizing the sac. The skin is undermined medially until the dural sac is seen to enter the fascial defect. **(B)** Excising the fringe of skin surrounding the placode.

A radial cut is used to enter the sac, and it is continued around the placode to excise the skin. A separate circumferential cut amputates the base of the sac.

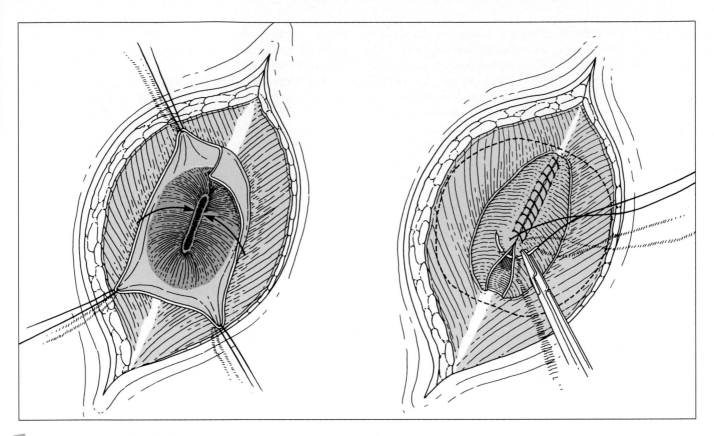

Figure 5.4 Mobilizing and closing the dura. The dura is undermined and closed using a continuous 4-0 nonabsorbable suture.

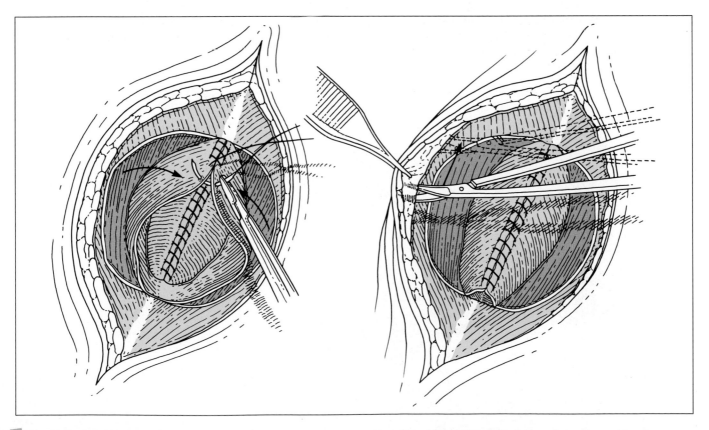

Figure 5.5 The fascial closure. The fascia is closed with a continuous stitch. The caudal end of the repair may be incomplete. Skin is mobilized by blunt dissection with scissors or a finger.

described but are rarely necessary. Large circular defects can be easily closed using a simple rotation flap (Fig. 5.6).

Care of the child with a myelomeningocele is life-long; it only begins with the surgical closure. Any deterioration in neurologic function signals a progressive process such as shunt malfunction, hydromyelia, tethered cord, or symptomatic Chiari malformation. Significant advancements have been made in the treatment of these children over the past two decades, particularly in the widespread use of multidisciplinary teams of specialists to manage their urologic, orthopedic, and other needs. Among those who undergo early back closure, 92% will survive infancy[7] and 86% will be alive 5 years later.[8] Death is due to problems associated with the Chiari II malformation, restrictive lung disease secondary to chest deformity, shunt malfunction, or urinary sepsis. Approximately 75% of children with myelomeningocele are ambulatory, although most require braces and crutches.[7] Approximately 75% of surviving infants will have normal intelligence (defined as IQ>80),[7] although only 59% to 60% of those requiring shunts for hydrocephalus will have normal intelligence.

OCCULT SPINA BIFIDA AND THE TETHERED CORD SYNDROME

Developmental anomalies involving the caudal portion of the neural tube are increasingly important in clinical practice, largely due to advances in diagnostic techniques and a consequent change in the philosophy of treatment. Greater awareness of these conditions by pediatricians, orthopedists, and urologists, and the development of MRI have lead to earlier recognition of these relatively rare problems.

The term *occult spinal dysraphism* actually encompasses several separate, possibly coexisting, entities (Fig. 5.7). Most of these entities are localized to the lower spine segments and hidden by full-thickness skin. Embryologically, they arise from abnormal retrogressive differentiation of the caudal cell mass, a process by which the previously formed tail structures undergo a precise, ordered necrosis, leaving only the filum terminale, the coccygeal ligament, and the terminal ventricle of the conus as remnants by 11 weeks of gestation. Failure of regression presumably gives rise to the hypertrophied filum terminale; abnormal and incomplete regression results in lipomyelomeningocele. The embryology of diastematomyelia remains poorly understood, but it may involve persistence of the fetal neurenteric canal between the yolk sac and the amniotic cavity, allowing herniation of endodermal elements through a split notochord, and causing migrating mesenchymal elements to form the bony "spike."

Symptoms may have several causes. Abnormal formation of the spinal cord and roots during embryogenesis can result in permanent neurologic deficits, as seen in myelomeningocele. Local masses growing within the spinal canal (lipomas or neurenteric cysts) can cause compression. Tethered cord syndrome, the result of traction on the spinal cord, occurs with any of the entities associated with occult spinal dysraphism. It can also occur in the adult in whom the conus has already completed its ascent.

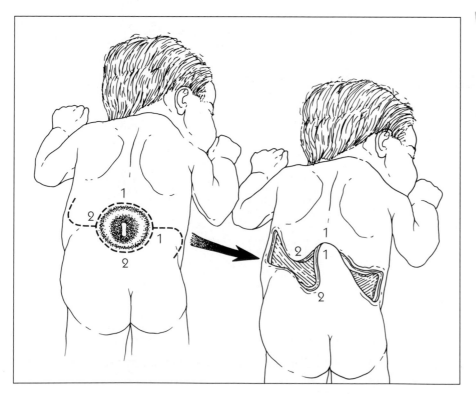

Figure 5.6 Simple rotation flap. **(A)** An S-shaped horizontal incision is made, encompassing the circular defect. **(B)** The points are approximated to the hollows, relieving tension both vertically and horizontally. The resulting skin closure has a W-shape.

To recognize occult dysraphic states one must appreciate the significance of the various syndromes that occur in association with the various entities. The *cutaneous syndrome* refers to any midline skin anomaly overlying the lower spine. This anomaly often signals a dysraphic state, and its recognition is especially important in the infant, in whom urologic or orthopedic complaints are not yet manifest. The cutaneous abnormality may include the striking "faun's tail" of hair (Fig. 5.8), dermal sinus tract, hemangioma (Fig. 5.9), or skin-covered fatty mass (Fig. 5.10). The *orthopedic syndrome* is apparent at birth or develops progressively in childhood. Common components include high arched feet, clawtoes, unequal leg length, and scoliosis. The *urologic syndrome* should be considered in any infant or small child who has an abnormal voiding pattern, new onset of incontinence after toilet-training, or with urinary tract infection in a child of any age. The *neurologic syndrome*

Figure 5.7 Occult Spinal Dysraphism
The number of patients seen over 7 years at Children's Hospital of Philadelphia

Myelomeningocele	132
Occult spinal dysraphism	60
Lipomyelomeningocele	34
Diastematomyelia	7
Anterior meningocele	2
Congenital dermal sinus	14
Hypertrophied filum	3

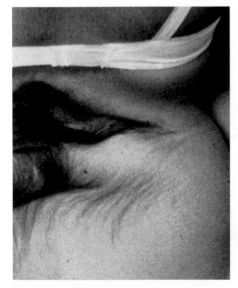

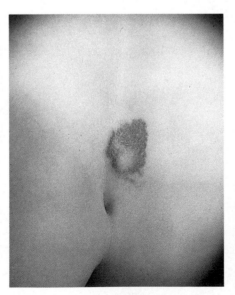

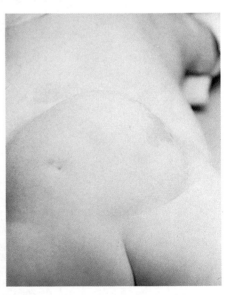

Figure 5.8 Faun's tail. This patch of hair in the midlline overlying the lower spine is highly suggestive of a dysraphic state. It is not associated with any particular entity, and it may occur in lipomyelomeningocele, diastematomyelia, or hypertrophied filum terminale. (Reprinted with permission from Rothman RH, Simeone FA. *The Spine*. 3rd ed. Philadelphia, Pa: WB Saunders Co; 1992)

Figure 5.9 Hemangioma and dermal sinus. Dermal sinus tracts overlying the distal sacrum or coccyx are common in normal infants and do not generally represent dysraphic states. Any midline hemangioma or sinus tract over the lumbar spine warrants an investigation. (Reprinted with permission from Rothman RH, Simeone FA. *The Spine*. 3rd ed. Philadelphia, Pa: WB Saunders Co; 1992)

Figure 5.10 Lipomyelomeningocele in an infant. The skin-covered fatty mass in the lumbosacral region is typical.

Figure 5.11 Presenting Symptoms and Signs of Occult Spinal Dysraphism

Foot deformity	39%
Scoliosis	14%
Gait abnormality	16%
Leg weakness	48%
Sensory abnormality	32%
Urinary incontinence	36%
Recurrent UTI	20%
Fecal incontinence	32%
Cutaneous abnormality	48%

Adapted from James HE, Walsh JW, 1981

presents as leg muscle atrophy or weakness, numbness of the feet, or radicular lower extremity pain and can occur at any age. In summary, patients may present with any of the above syndromes, but, in general, infants primarily present with skin manifestations, older children present with urologic, neurologic, or orthopedic syndromes, and adults often complain of pain (Fig. 5.11).[9]

The current study of choice for a suspected occult spinal dysraphic lesion is MRI scanning, which is usually definitive. In newborn infants the image quality can be suboptimal because of their small size, and if the clinical suspicion is high, a repeat study at 6 months is indicated. The study is examined for the level of the conus, which should not be below L-2, the presence of fatty masses, a split cord, and a thickened filum. A large distended urinary bladder suggests sacral root dysfunction. In some cases of hypertrophied filum terminale the MRI scan may be equivocal, and if the clinical suspicion is high, surgical exploration may be warranted.[10]

LIPOMYELOMENINGOCELE

Lipomyelomeningocele is one of the more common forms of occult spinal dysraphism seen in pediatric neurosurgical practice. The term is actually a misnomer, because it

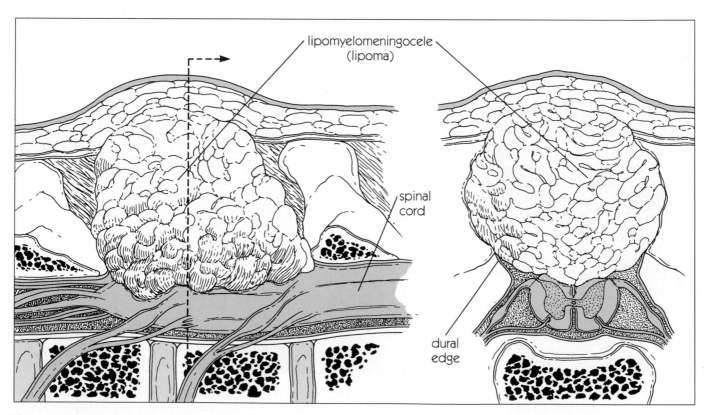

Figure 5.12 (A) Dorsally inserting lipomyelomeningocele. The mass of the lipoma, attaches broadly on the dorsal surface of the conus, extending through a dural and bony defect to be continuous with the subcutaneous mass. The nerve roots are ventral to the lipoma. **(B)** Cross-sectional view of a dorsal lipoma. The lateral lines of attachment are formed by the lipoma and the dural edge, and must be divided to release the tether. Note that the nerve roots are ventral to this line.

suggests herniation of neural elements through a spina bifida defect into a meningeal sac, which is not the case. In fact, the lipomatous tissue inserts into the conus, and it is fat that herniates through the bony defect dorsally to attach to a subcutaneous mass. Nonetheless, the term has gained wide acceptance and is likely to stay. Chapman's[11] distinction between lipomyelomeningoceles that insert caudally into the conus and those that attach to the dorsal surface of the spinal cord is of considerable value in planning the operative approach. If the lipoma inserts into the dorsal surface of the conus, there is usually a substantial subcutaneous mass (Fig. 5.12). Along the lateral interface of the attachment of the lipoma to the spinal cord, the dura and pia are also fused. Sensory roots emerge just anterior to this "lateral line of fusion," and, as a result, neither the sensory nor motor roots lie within the actual substance of the lipoma. Alternatively, the lipoma joins the conus at its caudal end, almost as a continuation of the cord itself. The remaining lipomatous mass then lies entirely within the spinal canal or extends dorsally through a spina bifida defect. The fatty tumor either replaces the filum terminale, or a separate filum lies anteriorly. The nerve roots usually lie anterior to the lipoma, although they can lie within the fibrous anterior portion of the mass itself (Fig. 5.13). Transitional forms of these two types may occur, but this schema is extremely useful in planning surgery.

The surgical indications for lipomyelomeningocele have undergone an evolution over the past 20 years. Although early neurosurgeons advised against prophylactic surgery, virtually all modern authorities strongly favor it.[10-13] The goals of surgery are to untether the spinal cord, remove as much of the lipomatous mass as possible, and reconstruct the dura to avoid leakage of

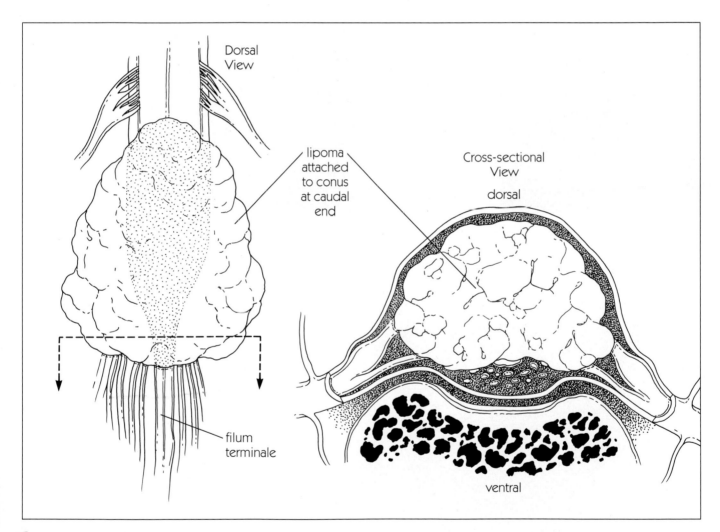

Figure 5.13 Cross-sectional view of a caudal lipoma. The roots run anteriorly and may attach to the ventral wall of the lipoma.

CSF and discourage retethering. Surgical planning begins with review of the MRI scan. The lipoma can usually be determined to fit either the dorsal group (Fig. 5.14) or the caudal group (Fig. 5.15).

Surgical Technique

General anesthesia is used, and the patient is positioned prone so the abdomen hangs free. An elliptical skin incision surrounding the subcutaneous mass is made along a vertical axis. The subcutaneous tissue is then incised circumferentially down to the lumbodorsal fascia (Fig. 5.16). The lipoma is undermined and separated bluntly from the underlying fascia, until it can be seen to enter the fascial defect medially. A self-retaining

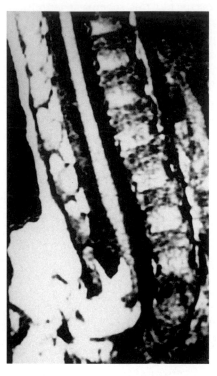

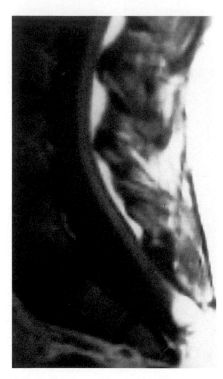

Figure 5.14 MRI of a dorsally inserting lipoma. The mass inserts dorsally within the conus. It extends through a spina bifida defect to be continuous with the subcutaneous mass. (Reprinted with permission from Rothman RH, Simeone FA. *The Spine.* 3rd ed. Philadelphia, Pa: WB Saunders Co; 1992)

Figure 5.15 MRI of caudal lipoma. The lipoma is entirely within the caudal spinal canal, and the cord is tethered to the caudal portion of the thecal sac. (Reprinted with permission from Rothman RH, Simeone FA. *The Spine.* 3rd ed. Philadelphia, Pa: WB Saunders Co; 1992)

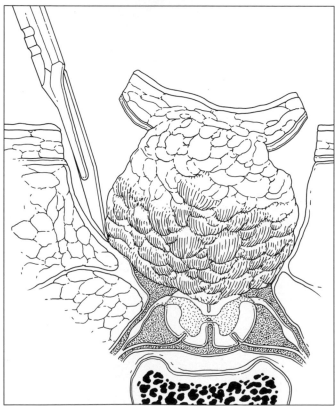

Figure 5.16 Initial exposure of a spinal lipoma. The skin has been elliptically incised around the subcutaneous mass and the incision carried to the lumbodorsal fascia. Dissection has proceeded medially, until the stalk of the lipoma is seen entering the spinal canal through the spinal bifida and the dural defect.

retractor is inserted, and the lowest intact laminar arch is palpated. The fascia overlying this spinous process and lamina is opened in the midline, and a laminectomy of this segment is performed, exposing the underlying normal dura. At this point it can help to amputate the large fatty mass with its island of skin attached at the level of its stalk.

Starting at the level of normal dura cephalad to the mass, the epidural fat is melted with a bipolar cautery until the dural defect with fatty tissue extruding through it is encountered. A midline dural opening is made above the defect, exposing the spinal cord. As the dural opening is carried inferiorly toward the defect, a transverse band of thick, fibrous tissue, which kinks the spinal cord, is noted at the rostral end of the lipoma stalk. This is opened widely along with the dura. The dural opening is extended caudally on either side of the exiting lipoma circumferentially (Fig. 5.17).

At this point, the lipoma will usually be found to correspond to one of the two types previously described. Lipomas that insert into the conus dorsally can be removed from the dorsal aspect of the cord in a plane superficial to the lateral lines of fusion, with the nerve roots emerging anteriorly (Fig. 5.18). These lines of fusion are divided laterally, first on one side and then the other, with a bipolar cautery and microscissors or a knife blade over a dissector. The operating microscope and laser help shave down the mass of the lipoma. The

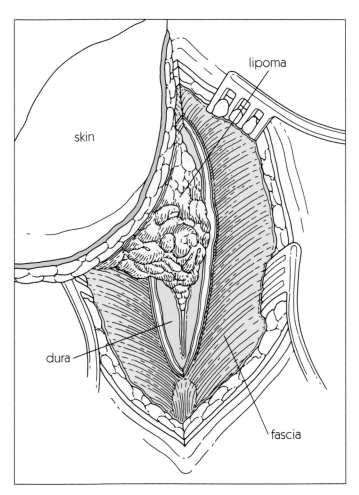

Figure 5.17 Surgery for spinal lipoma (continued). A laminectomy of the lowest intact neural arch has been performed and the dura opened at this level. The dural incision is extended caudally until the lipoma is encountered.

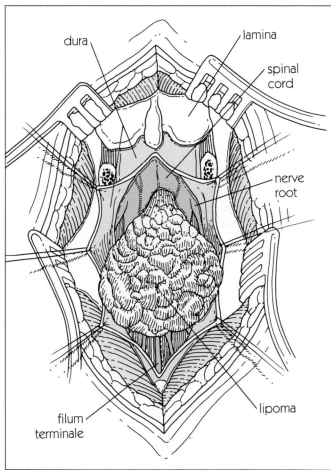

Figure 5.18 Lateral dissection of the lines of fusion. The lateral lines of fusion are sharply incised on either side of the lipoma. A tunnel can usually be formed between the lateral lines of fusion and the nerve roots beneath.

filum is identified and divided. After the lipoma has been largely removed from the spinal cord, it is sometimes possible to reapproximate the pial edges of the cord to reconstitute the normal tubular configuration (Fig. 5.19), which discourages retethering.

Lipomas that insert caudally into the conus must be sectioned distally to the take-off of any functional roots. It is unnecessary to remove all of the gross lipoma; attempting this can cause damage to the conus and roots. Simple sectioning of the lipoma releases the point of tethering and fulfills the goal of the operation.

When the cord is free of adhesions, the dura is closed. In some cases, the dura is approximated and closed with a running suture directly. In most cases, however, a graft is required to prevent stricture of the canal. The muscle and fascia are closed as much as possible, and the skin is closed in the usual fashion.

Surgery is relatively safe. The major problems are postoperative CSF leaks and pseudomeningoceles, which require re-exploration. Most series report a small number of patients whose condition is made worse by the procedure; however, when the procedure is compared with untreated cases, which are characterized by progressive worsening and disability, the benefits outweigh the risks.

DIASTEMATOMYELIA

The term *diastematomyelia*, which derives from the Greek word *diastema*, meaning cleft, refers to a congenital splitting of the spinal cord. The term is used to describe the split, not the bony spike that often accompanies the abnormality. Clinically, it presents as tethered cord syndrome. It occurs predominantly in females and most often in the lower thoracic or upper lumbar spine. Most patients have a midline cutaneous abnormality, but it does not necessarily correspond to the level of the cleft. The most common finding is a hairy patch, but a variety of other cutaneous abnormalities are seen. Spinal deformity (kyphoscoliosis), which eventually develops in virtually all patients, is thought to be due primarily to the bony structure abnormalities, rather than neurologic involvement.

Neurologic symptoms are due to spinal cord tethering and may not occur until adulthood, if at all. Symptoms can include back pain, gait disturbance, muscular atrophy, spasticity, or urologic complaints. These abnormalities are not specific, and other conditions, such as spinal cord tumor, Friedrich's ataxia, and syringomyelia, must be considered in the differential diagnosis. Neurologic deterioration can occur following corrective surgery for scoliosis, if spinal cord tethering is not recognized beforehand.

The classic appearance of diastematomyelia on plain spine roentgenograph is a fusiform interpedicular widening of the spinal canal on the AP view with a midline oval bony mass projecting posteriorly from the vertebral body. The spur is usually not visible on lateral views. Myelography will confirm the diagnosis, but MRI is currently the primary diagnostic test.[14] The coronal study shows

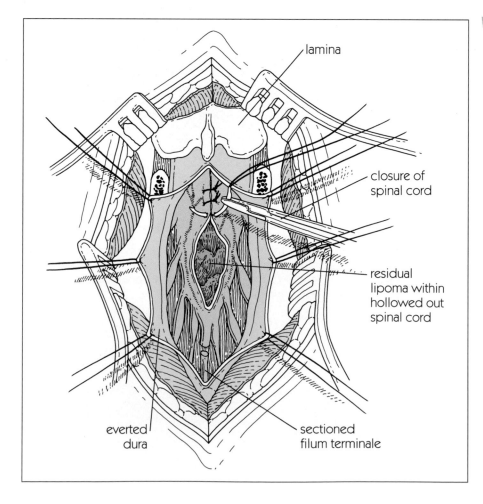

lamina

closure of spinal cord

residual lipoma within hollowed out spinal cord

everted dura

sectioned filum terminale

Figure 5.19 Reconstruction of the spinal cord. The lipoma has been largely removed with a CO_2 laser, creating a cavity within the conus. This may be closed with interrupted sutures to prevent retethering.

the split nicely, but severe kyphoscoliosis can make the study difficult to interpret. Newer imaging sequences, in which the scan is obtained along the curve of the spine, will likely solve this problem. It is important to evaluate the entire spine so secondary lesions such as lipomas or hypertrophied fila are not missed.

Clear indications for surgery include progressive neurologic deficit and scoliosis. When performing surgery to untether the cord for scoliosis, it is usually advisable to operate on the diastematomyelia first as a separate procedure; removal of the bony spike most often results in the temporary loss of evoked potential signals, which can reduce the safety of the orthopedic procedure.[15] The management of the asymptomatic patient remains controversial. Some authors favor prophylactic surgery within the first 2 years in asymptomatic children.[16–18] Others favor a more conservative approach because of the potential risks of surgery and the significant number of patients who remain asymptomatic (or with stable deficits) throughout growth.[19,20]

Surgical Technique

If surgery is to be undertaken, the technique described by Matson and by Meacham is generally employed. The patient is positioned as for a standard laminectomy. The paraspinal muscles on either side of the midline are freed and retracted laterally as in any standard laminectomy, but vigorous blunt dissection with a periosteal elevator and sponges is avoided, since spina bifida can coexist with the bony septum. The laminectomy is initiated at least one full segment above and below the septum, and it is carried out around the bony spike itself, exposing the dural cleft (Fig. 5.20A). The cleft will usually extend cephalad to the spur but hug it tightly caudally, which indicates tethering. A septal elevator frees the septum from the surrounding dura. The superficial portion of the septum is removed by a rongeur or a high-speed drill that has a diamond burr within the investing dural sheath, which protects the spinal cord. Once the cleft is decompressed, the dura is opened around the cleft, and all intradural adhesions at the cleft are divided (Fig. 5.20B). The dural cuff and the deeper portions of the septum are removed to the level of the anterior spinal canal. It is not necessary or appropriate to close the anterior dura. The posterior dura is closed in a watertight fashion, using a graft if necessary. If an associated hypertrophied filum is suspected, it is divided, using a separate laminectomy if needed.

The procedure should be considered largely prophylactic, although some patients may show neurologic

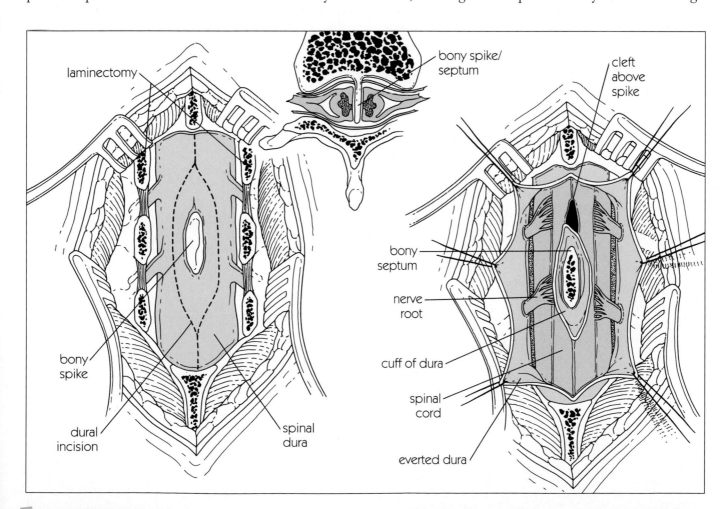

Figure 5.20 (A) Diastematomyelia. Full laminectomy has been performed above and below the bony septum and the bone has been removed laterally to expose the dural cleft. The proposed dural incision is shown. (B) Diastematomyelia, dura open. The cuff of dura is used to protect the spinal cord as the bony septum is drilled to the level of the vertebral body below. Note that the caudal end of the split cord tightly hugs the inferior surface of the bony spike, suggesting tethering.

improvement. Complications include worsening of neurologic status and CSF leak. Late deterioration after surgery can be due to failure to remove the spike completely, failure to address associated lesions or, rarely, to regrowth of the septum.

ANTERIOR SACRAL MENINGOCELE

Anterior sacral meningocele is a relatively rare condition in which there is herniation of the dural sac through a defect in the anterior surface of the spine, usually in the sacrum. The sac is composed of an outer dural membrane and an inner arachnoid membrane. It contains CSF and, occasionally, neural elements. If the sac is large, it may present as a pelvic mass. Most anterior meningoceles are congenital, as evidenced by their appearance in children. Unlike the typical posterior myelomeningocele, there is no association with hydrocephalus or Chiari malformation. The embryology of these lesions is incompletely understood; most likely, the primary problem is a defect in dural development, resulting in a defect through which the arachnoid herniates, resulting in pulsations that erode the bone.

The lesion is more commonly detected in women, but this most likely reflects the gynecologic presentation of a pelvic mass. Symptoms are usually produced by pressure of the presacral mass on adjacent pelvic structures, causing constipation, urinary urgency, dysparunia, or low back pain. Headache with defecation is occasionally described by children. The cardinal sign is a smooth, cystic mass detected on rectal or pelvic examination.

MRI scanning is the imaging study of choice. When communication between the pelvic cyst and the spinal subarachnoid space is not evident, a metrizamide CT-myelographic study may be indicated.

Surgical treatment of symptomatic lesions is advised since there is no possibility of spontaneous regression, and untreated female patients have a significant risk of pelvic obstruction at the time of labor.[21] Asymptomatic lesions may be followed without operation, if there is no possibility of pregnancy and the lesion does not enlarge on repeated rectal examinations.

Aspiration of the cyst through the rectum or vagina may result in meningitis and should not be performed. If the meningocele is discovered at laparotomy for other reasons, the operation should be terminated and further workup carried out. Surgical treatment via laparotomy has been described,[21] but the sacral laminectomy approach is preferable[22] because it allows visualization of the intraspinal contents of the cyst, resection of adhesions, and sectioning of the filum terminale. The goal of surgery is to untether the spinal cord, decompress the pelvic mass, and obliterate the CSF fistula.

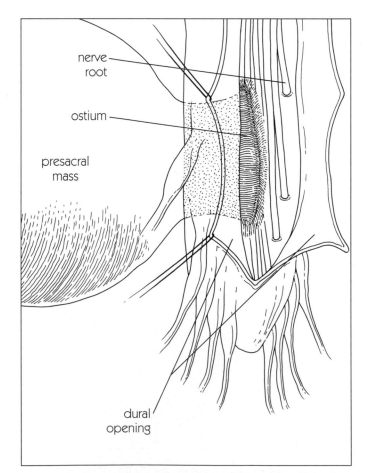

Figure 5.21 Approach to anterior sacral meningocele by sacral laminectomy. The posterior dura is opened longitudinally, exposing the sacral nerve roots and the ostium to the pelvic mass.

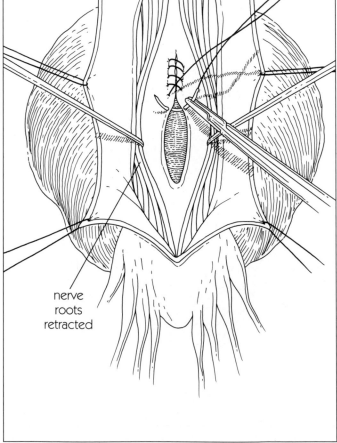

Figure 5.22 Anterior sacral meningocele. The nerve roots are retracted, and the ostium is oversewn using a continuous suture. No attempt is made to resect the pelvic mass.

Principles of Neurosurgery

Surgical Technique

The surgical technique has been reviewed by several authors.[23–25] Antibiotic coverage and a bowel prep are begun 48 hours prior to surgery in case bowel perforation occurs. Under general anesthesia the patient is positioned for laminectomy. A lumbosacral laminectomy is performed from L5-S4, and the posterior dura is opened longitudinally (Fig. 5.21). Nerve roots within the dural canal are carefully retracted, and the filum terminale is divided to expose the dural ostium leading to the pelvic sac. If no roots enter the sac and the neck is narrow, the anterior dura is simply oversewn (Fig. 5.22). If the sac arises as a caudal extension of the dural sac, and the sacral roots have exited above, the dural sleeve may simply be ligated. If the anterior defect is wide and cannot be mobilized into the field sufficiently for primary closure, digital collapse of the sac through the rectum can be helpful or a fascial graft can be sewn to the edges of the defect. If roots exit through the defect, the dura or graft will have to be plicated around the roots as they exit. The posterior dura is closed. Postoperatively, stool softeners are given to prevent straining. In difficult cases, a second pelvic procedure is required.[21]

The results of surgery described in the literature have generally been good. Complications have included meningitis, CSF leak, and neurologic problems when roots have entered the meningocele sac.

CONGENITAL DERMAL SINUS AND HYPERTROPHIED FILUM TERMINALE

The term *congenital dermal sinus* refers to a group of congenital malformations in which a tubular tract lined with squamous epithelium extends from the skin overlying the spine inward to varying depths. The sinus terminates in the subcutaneous tissue, bone, dura, subarachnoid space, filum terminale, or within an intradural dermoid cyst or neuroglial mass within the spinal cord itself. They occur at all levels within the spine but are most commonly seen in the lower lumbosacral area, where they are frequently confused with simple pilonidal sinuses. Pilonidal sinuses are acquired lesions in adults, believed to be secondary to trauma or chronic inflammation, that have no connection with the subarachnoid space or neural elements. In contrast, congenital dermal sinus is a significant lesion because it enables skin flora to enter the spinal fluid pathways, resulting in repeated bouts of meningitis, and it causes spinal cord tethering, which leads to progressive neurologic problems. The hallmark of the lesion is a midline cutaneous dimple overlying the spine. There can be other associated cutaneous abnormalities (see Fig. 5.12), such as hemangiomas or hairy patches. Shallow dimples located at the tip of the coccyx in infants are normal variants that do not have neurologic significance.

Prophylactic surgery is performed as early as possible, even in newborns, to excise the entire tract. When there is clinical evidence of spinal cord compression, MRI scanning is indicated to determine the extent of abscesses or dermoid cysts. In asymptomatic cases, the lesions can simply be explored and the tract followed to its termination. The surgeon undertaking such an operation must be prepared to carry out an extensive intradural dissection, since the tract can extend for a considerable distance. In typical cases, the sinus tract begins at the skin dimple and proceeds cephalad through the soft tissues overlying the spine to traverse the dorsal dura. Once intradural, the tract often becomes continuous with the filum terminale, which is thickened and may contain dermoid elements (Fig. 5.23).

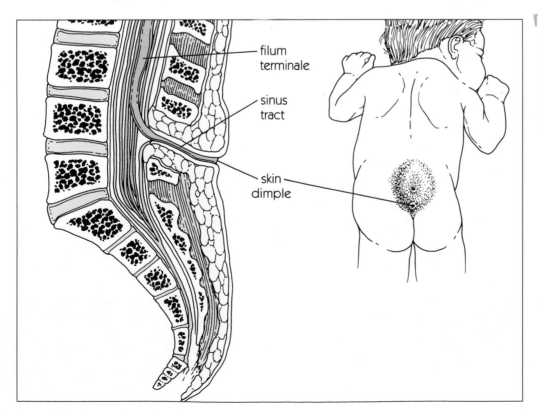

filum terminale

sinus tract

skin dimple

Figure 5.23 Cross-sectional anatomy of typical congenital dermal sinus tract. The tract may extend to any depth, but it often continues in a cephalad direction, enters the dura, and becomes continuous with the filum terminale.

Surgical Technique

The operation begins with an elliptical skin incision that surrounds the sinus opening and encompasses any abnormal skin surrounding it. The tract is sharply dissected and followed through the defect in the fascia. If the tract appears to continue through the dura, a laminectomy is performed above the level of the tract. If the tract attaches to the dura, the dura is opened above the attachment in the midline and incised inferiorly around the point of entry. Any intradural tract must be followed to its termination, even if this involves an extensive laminectomy, since remaining tissue has the capacity to grow into a dermoid inclusion cyst. Intradural dermoids are completely removed, if possible without violating the capsule. If the cyst has ruptured or has been infected, a dense arachnoiditis with scarred nerve roots will prevent complete excision. In this case, judicious intracapsular removal of purulent material and dermoid material is performed, and no attempt is made to remove the scarred capsular wall from the nerve roots. A watertight dural closure is accomplished, except when closure would compress residual infected dermoid cyst material, in which case the dura is left open and the muscle and fascia are closed.

The syndrome of the hypertrophied filum terminale may occur without a cutaneous dimple or sinus tract. If a patient presents with the typical picture of the tethered cord syndrome, an MRI scan is indicated. The scan will demonstrate the low-lying conus, but it may not demonstrate the thickened filum. In these cases, a metrizamide CT-myelogram can demonstrate the pathology, although surgical exploration may be more expeditious.

REFERENCES

1. Elwood JH, Nevin NC. Factors associated with anencephalus and spina bifida in Belfast. *Br Prev Med.* 1973;27:73–86.
2. Holmes LB, Driscoll SG, Atkins L. Etiologic heterogeneity of neural tube defects. *N Engl J Med.* 1976;294:365–369.
3. Globus MS, Loughman WD, Epstein CJ, et al. Prenatal genetic diagnosis in 3000 amniocentesis. *N Engl J Med.* 1979;300:157–173.
4. Powledge TM, Fletcher J. Guidelines for the ethical, social and legal issues in prenatal diagnosis. *N Engl J Med.* 1979;300:168–172.
5. Charney EB, Rorke LB, Sutton LN, et al. Management of Chiari II complications in infants with myelomeningocele. *J Pediatr.* 1987;111: 364–371.
6. Charney EB, Weller SC, Sutton LN, et al. Management of the newborn with myelomeningocele: time for a decision-making process. *Pediatrics.* 1985;75:58–64.
7. Sutton LN, Charney EB, Bruce DA, et al. Myelomeningocele–the question of selection. *Clin Neurosurg.* 1986;33:371–382.
8. McLone DG. Results of treatment of children born with a myelomeningocele. *Clin Neurosurg.* 1983; 30:407–412.
9. James HE, Walsh JW. *Current Problems in Pediatrics. Spinal Dysraphism.* Chicago, Ill: Yearbook Medical Publisher;1981; XI:8.
10. Brophy JD, Sutton LN, Zimmerman RA, et al. Magnetic resonance imaging of lipomyelomeningocele and tethered cord. *Neurosurgery.* 1989;25: 336–340.
11. Chapman PH.Congenital intraspinal lipomas: anatomic considerations and surgical treatment. *Childs Brain.* 1982;9:37–47.
12. Bruce DA, Schut L. Spinal lipomas in infancy and childhood. *Childs Brain.* 1979;5:192.
13. Hoffman HJ, Taechorlarn C, Hendrick B, et al. Lipomyelomeningoceles and their management. In: Humphreys RP, ed. *Concepts in Pediatric Neurosurgery.* Basel: Karger; 1985:5:107–117.
14. Riegel DH. Sacral agenesis and diastematomyelia. McLaurin R, ed. *Pediatric Neurosurgery. Surgery of the Developing Nervous System.* New York, NY: Grune and Stratton; 1982:79–94.
15. Pang D. Tethered cord syndrome: newer concepts. In: *Neurosurgery Update II.* Chicago Ill: McGraw Hill Book Co; 1991:336–344.
16. Matson DD, Woods RP, Campbell JR, et al. Diastematomyelia (congenital clefts of the spinal cord): diagnosis and surgical treatment. *Pediatrics.* 1950; 6:98-112.
17. Guthkelch AN. Diastematomyelia with median septum. *Brain.* 1974;97:729–742.
18. Meacham WF. Surgical treatment of diastematomyelia. *J Neurosurg.* 1967;27:78–85.
19. Cohen J, Sledge CB. Diastematomyelia: an embryological interpretation with report of a case. *Am J Dis Child.* 1960;100:257–263.
20. Eid K, Hochberg J, Saunders DE. Skin abnormalities of the back in diastematomyelia. *Plast Reconstr Surg.* 1979;63:534–539.
21. Amacher AL, Drake CG, McLaughlin AD. Anterior sacral meningocele. *Surg Gynecol Obstet.* 1968; 126:986-994.
22. Adson AW. Spina bifida cystica of the pelvis: diagnosis and surgical treatment. *Minn Med.* 1938;21: 468–475.
23. Mapstone TB, White RJ, Takacka Y. Anterior sacral meningocele. *Surg Neurol.* 1981;16:44–47.
24. Smith HP, Davis CH. Anterior sacral meningocele: two case reports and discussion of surgical approach. *Neurosurgery.* 1980;7:61–67.
25. Villarejo F, Scavone C, Blazquez MG, et al. Anterior sacral meningocele: review of the literature. *Surg Neurol.* 1983;19:57–71.

Chapter 6

Hydrocephalus in Children

A. Leland Albright

CEREBROSPINAL FLUID

PHYSIOLOGY

CSF is a clear, colorless fluid that fills both the ventricles within the brain and the subarachnoid spaces around the brain and spinal cord. CSF is produced continuously, predominantly by choroid plexus within the lateral, third, and fourth ventricles (Fig. 6.1). Choroid plexus consists of numerous villi, each composed of single-layer cuboidal epithelial cells around a core of highly vascularized connective tissue. An ultrafiltrate from the capillaries is processed by the epithelial cells and diffuses into the ventricles as CSF at a rate of 0.30 to 0.35 mL/min, or approximately 500 mL/d, in children and adults.[1] CSF production rates can be decreased by sclerosis of the choroid plexus (secondary to ventriculitis) and can be increased by choroid plexus papillomas. The total CSF volume in children is 65 to 140 mL. CSF secretion is partially regulated by the enzymes sodium-potassium ATPase and carbonic anhydrase, and it is affected by medications that inhibit these enzymes.

CSF normally flows through the pathways shown in Figure 6.1 and is absorbed by arachnoid villi, diverticula of arachnoid that invaginate the sagittal sinus, and the major cortical veins along that sinus. Clusters of arachnoid villi, called arachnoid granulations, are visible to the naked eye. A layer of endothelial cells separates arachnoid villi from the systemic circulation. Water and electrolytes pass freely through the membranes; proteins are actively transported out by pinocytosis.

The mechanism by which CSF exits via the arachnoid villi is unclear, although some resistance must be overcome, since there is no CSF absorption if the CSF pressure is less than 6.8 mm H_2O.[1] CSF production and absorption are normally in equilibrium. Equal production and absorption generate a CSF pressure of approximately 11 cm H_2O.

PATHOPHYSIOLOGY

Hydrocephalus is the abnormal accumulation of CSF within the ventricles and/or subarachnoid spaces. It is typ-

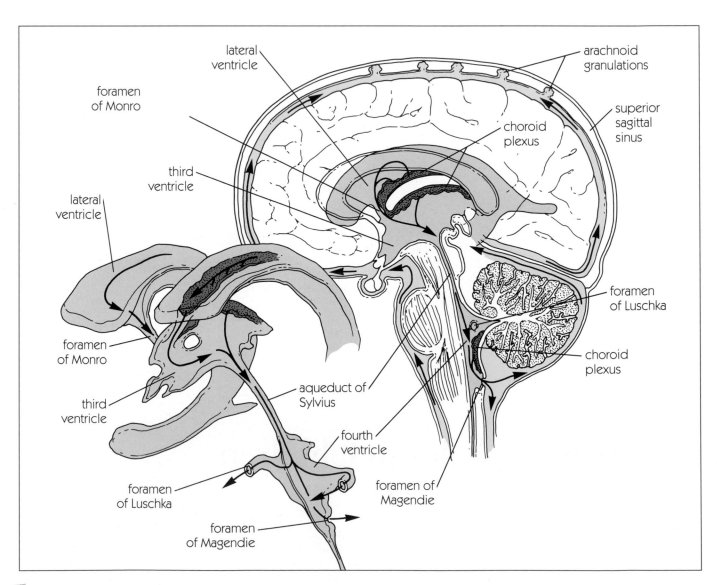

Figure 6.1 Normal CSF pathways.

ically associated with dilatation of the ventricles and increased intracranial pressure. The incidence of hydrocephalus in children is not well known, since it occurs both as an isolated disorder and in association with numerous other conditions. Hydrocephalus occurs as an isolated congenital disorder in approximately 1/1000 live births and in association with spina bifida in 1/1000 births in the United States. Hydrocephalus almost always results from an obstruction in the CSF pathways and only rarely from overproduction of CSF. Common sites and causes of obstruction are shown in Figure 6.2. As intracranial pressure rises, CSF absorption via the arachnoid villi increases somewhat, but CSF production remains constant.[2] If progressive ventriculomegaly separates ependymal cells lining the ventricles, some CSF exits transependymally via bulk flow through the white matter.

CLASSIFICATION

Hydrocephalus has been classified as obstructive or nonobstructive, a poor classification since all hydrocephalus except hydrocephalus ex vacuo (associated with brain atrophy) involves some impediment to CSF flow. A more commonly used classification is communicating or noncommunicating, a distinction based traditionally (but no longer in practice) on whether dye injected into the lateral ventricles could be detected in CSF withdrawn by lumbar puncture. With the former definition, noncom-

munication resulted from obstruction of the aqueduct or basal foramina. Currently the term noncommunicating hydrocephalus refers to hydrocephalus that results from lesions that obstruct the ventricular system, either at the aqueduct or basal foramina, and communicating refers to hydrocephalus that results from lesions that obstruct the subarachnoid space. A third classification describes hydrocephalus as physiologic, i.e., secondary to CSF overproduction by choroid plexus papillomas, or nonphysiological; however, this classification is of little relevance because such papillomas are rare. A fourth classification describes hydrocephalus as internal or external, depending on whether the site of obstruction is proximal or distal to the basal foramina. Lastly, hydrocephalus can be classified by etiology and site of obstruction (see Fig. 6.2). Hydrocephalus may also be secondary to increased intracranial venous pressure due to sinus thrombosis or to stenosis of the jugular foramina in achondroplasia.

PATHOLOGY—PROXIMAL TO DISTAL

LATERAL VENTRICLES

Two abnormalities within the lateral ventricles cause hydrocephalus. *Choroid plexus papilloma* (CPP) causes hydrocephalus, usually in the first three years of life, by oversecretion of CSF. CSF production rates of 1.0 to 1.4

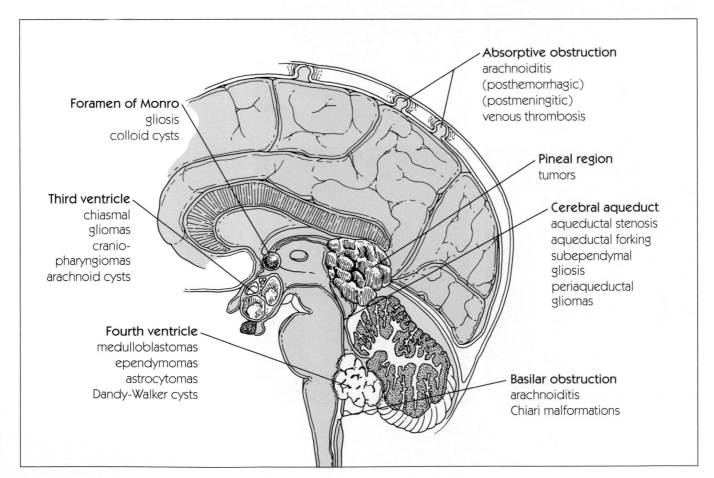

Figure 6.2 Common sites of and causes of CSF obstruction.

Labels in figure:

Foramen of Monro
gliosis
colloid cysts

Third ventricle
chiasmal
gliomas
cranio-
pharyngiomas
arachnoid cysts

Fourth ventricle
medulloblastomas
ependymomas
astrocytomas
Dandy-Walker cysts

Absorptive obstruction
arachnoiditis
(posthemorrhagic)
(postmeningitic)
venous thrombosis

Pineal region
tumors

Cerebral aqueduct
aqueductal stenosis
aqueductal forking
subependymal
gliosis
periaqueductal
gliomas

Basilar obstruction
arachnoiditis
Chiari malformations

mL/min, i.e., 3 to 4 times the normal rate, have been documented in children with CPP.[3,4] After removal of the papilloma, hydrocephalus resolves in approximately two thirds of the cases. It persists in the remaining third—probably because of microhemorrhages that obstruct the aqueduct or the basal meninges—and is treated with a shunt. The second disorder, *choroid plexus (villous) hypertrophy*, is rare. It is usually associated with considerable ventriculomegaly and is difficult to treat with shunts.[5,6] CSF overproduction has not been documented yet in this disorder. Scans demonstrate substantial enlargement of choroid plexus in the trigones of the lateral ventricles.

FORAMINA OF MONRO

Congenital atresia of both foramina of Monro is rare. Occasionally, occlusion of one foramen, by atresia, a congenital membrane, or gliosis after intraventricular hemorrhage (IVH) or ventriculitis, causes unilateral ventriculomegaly, which is often occult until after age 5 and may enlarge the hemicalvarium above the dilated ventricle (Fig. 6.3). In children with spina bifida whose hydrocephalus has been treated by a shunt, the nonshunted ventricle occasionally expands; decompression of one ventricle by the shunt apparently deforms the contralateral foramen of Monro and causes a functional stenosis.[7] If the nonshunted ventricle enlarges progressively, it is usually treated by inserting a ventricular catheter that is connected into the shunt system.

THIRD VENTRICLE

Cysts and neoplasms within the third ventricle commonly cause hydrocephalus. *Colloid* cysts occur superiorly and anteriorly within the third ventricle, usually obstruct both foramina of Monro, and cause either inter-

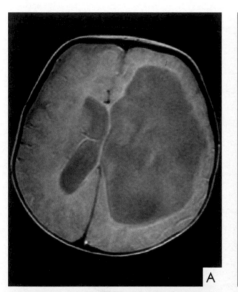
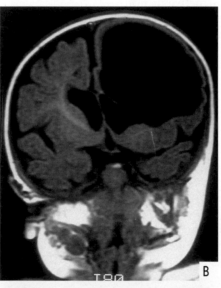
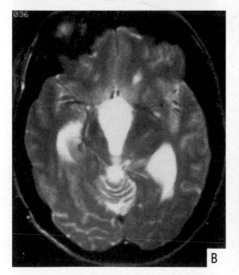
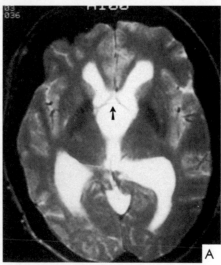

Figure 6.3 (A,B) Unilateral hydrocephalus secondary to posthemorrhagic gliosis of the foramen of Monro.

Figure 6.4 (A,B) Arachnoid cyst within the third ventricle. The cyst wall is evident (arrow) at the foramina of Monro (B).

Principles of Neurosurgery

mittent, acute, life-threatening hydrocephalus or chronic hydrocephalus. The treatment is customarily stereotactic aspiration of the cyst or removal via craniotomy, rather than CSF shunts.[8,9]

Ependymal/arachnoid cysts within the third ventricle (Fig. 6.4) usually cause hydrocephalus later in childhood. Patients may present with the bobble-head doll syndrome, a rhythmic head nodding two to three times per second similar to the bobbing wooden heads on antique dolls with wire spring necks. These cysts have been treated by fenestration,[10] but they are probably best treated by a shunt with a ventricular catheter fenestrated to drain both the lateral ventricles and the cyst.[11,12]

Dermoid cysts rarely occur in the third ventricle. When they do, the resultant hydrocephalus is treated by removing the cyst.

The two common pediatric neoplasms that obstruct the third ventricle are craniopharyngiomas and chiasmal-hypothalamic astrocytomas. Hydrocephalus secondary to craniopharyngiomas usually resolves after removal of the tumor. Most third ventricular gliomas cannot be surgically removed adequately to restore CSF pathways, so hydrocephalus is treated by a shunt.

AQUEDUCT OF SYLVIUS

The normal aqueduct in a newborn is 12 to 13 mm long and only 0.2 to 0.5 mm in diameter,[13] and is thus prone to obstruction. Lesions that obstruct the pediatric aqueduct include congenital aqueductal malformations (stenosis, forking, septum, or subependymal gliosis) (Fig. 6.5), pineal region neoplasms or arteriovenous malformations, and periaqueductal neoplasms.

Aqueductal stenosis, i.e., true luminal narrowing, is unusual, occurring in only 4% to 8% of infants with obstruction of the aqueduct.[14] Two much commoner abnormalities are subependymal gliosis, secondary either to in utero infections (e.g., toxoplasmosis), intraventricular hemorrhage, or mumps encephalitis in early childhood, and aqueductal forking, a malformation. Congenital hydrocephalus secondary to aqueductal occlusion is generally severe. Hydrocephalus at or distal to the aqueduct

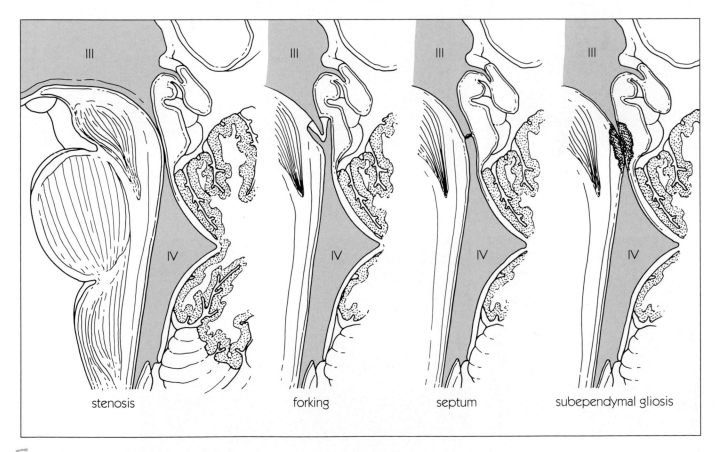

Figure 6.5 Left to right: stenosis, forking, septum, subependymal gliosis.

causes distention of the third ventricle and separation of the thalami, thinning or perforation of the septum pellucidum, thinning of the corpus callosum, and compression of the cerebral hemispheres (Fig. 6.6). Less than 2% of cases of congenital aqueductal stenosis are due to the recessively-inherited X-linked Bickers-Adams-Edwards syndrome, which is associated with flexion-adduction of the thumbs ("cortical" thumbs) in 25% of cases.[15]

Any pineal region mass can obstruct the inlet to the aqueduct and produce hydrocephalus, which is often treated perioperatively with an external ventricular drain (EVD). Many pineal region tumors are highly radiosensitive; thus tumor irradiation, as well as surgical removal, may obviate the need for a shunt.

Low-grade astrocytomas are the most common periaqueductal neoplasms that cause hydrocephalus. Children with neurofibromatosis have been diagnosed as having "late-onset aqueductal stenosis" on the basis of CT scans that revealed no neoplasms. Recently, however, MR scans in many of these children reveal periaqueductal hyperintense signals on T2-weighted images, indicative of low-grade astrocytomas (Fig. 6.7).[16]

FOURTH VENTRICLE

The fourth ventricle outlets in infants are obstructed commonly by Dandy-Walker cysts or by obliteration of the basal foramina, and in older children by neoplasms.

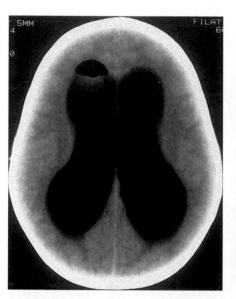
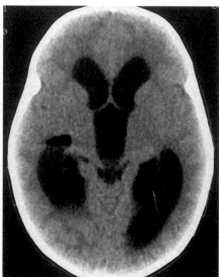
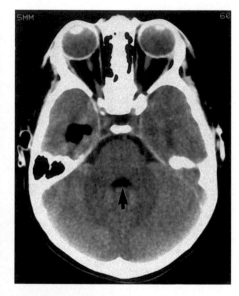

Figure 6.6 CT scan of an infant with aqueductal stenosis, demonstrating lateral and third ventricular distention, separation of the thalami, and compression of the cerebral hemispheres. The fourth ventricle (arrow) is normal.

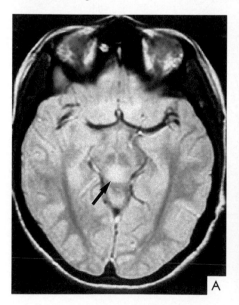
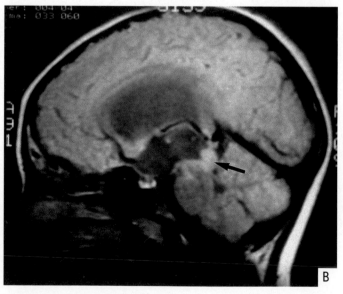

Figure 6.7 Axial (A) and sagittal (B) T2-weighted MR images demonstrating hydrocephalus secondary to a periaqueductal astrocytoma (arrow). The lesion was not visible on CT scans.

Dandy-Walker cysts are developmental anomalies characterized by a cyst—lined by pia-arachnoid and ependyma—within the fourth ventricle, hypoplasia of the vermis, and "atrophy" of the cerebellar hemispheres (Fig. 6.8). Over 85% of children with Dandy-Walker cysts have hydrocephalus, because the cyst obstructs either the aqueduct or the basal foramina or both.[17] The lateral and third ventricles communicate with the cyst in approximately 50% of cases in my experience.

Medulloblastomas typically occur within the fourth ventricle and are associated with the hydrocephalus in 85% of cases at the time of diagnosis. Hydrocephalus occurs in association with approximately 65% of posterior fossa astrocytomas, 75% of ependymomas, and 25% of brain stem gliomas.

The basal foramina of Lushka and Magendie are occluded by meningitis and subarachnoid hemorrhage, processes that cause arachnoiditis. The lateral, third, and fourth ventricles enlarge above the obstruction. Chiari II malformations in infants with myelomeningoceles cause hydrocephalus by preventing CSF, which exits through the basal foramina into the cervical subarachnoid spaces, from ascending into the intracranial subarachnoid spaces (Fig. 6.9).[18]

ARACHNOID GRANULATIONS

Sclerosis of the arachnoid granulations, after meningitis, subarachnoid hemorrhage, or trauma, impedes CSF outflow. The subarachnoid spaces over the cerebral con-

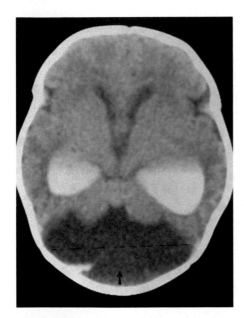

Figure 6.8 Axial CT scan on an infant with a Dandy-Walker cyst (arrow). Iohexal (white) injected into the lateral ventricles did not enter the cyst.

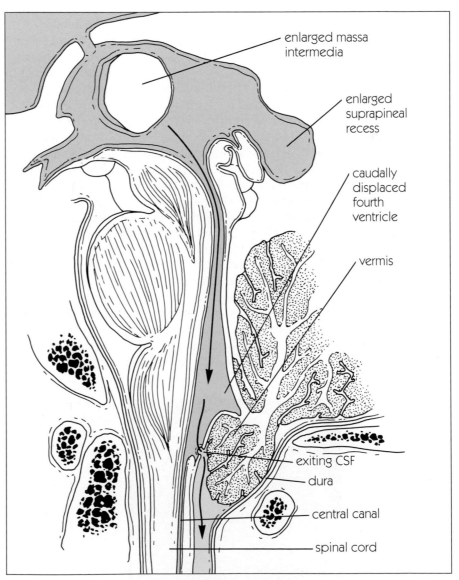

enlarged massa intermedia

enlarged suprapineal recess

caudally displaced fourth ventricle

vermis

exiting CSF

dura

central canal

spinal cord

Figure 6.9 CSF flow in Chiari II malformation associated with myelomeningocele. CSF exits the basal foramina but is prevented from ascending into the cranial subarachnoid spaces by the Chiari malformation.

vexities enlarge (Fig. 6.10), producing so-called external hydrocephalus, and the ventricles may dilate. This disorder is confused with subdural effusions, which are typically bifrontal, and with cerebral atrophy, which is rarely, if ever, present in children with macrocephaly.

ETIOLOGY, SYMPTOMS, AND SIGNS

PREMATURE INFANTS

Hydrocephalus in premature infants is caused predominantly by intraventricular hemorrhage (IVH), which causes 1) subependymal gliosis that occludes the cerebral aqueduct, 2) basal arachnoiditis that occludes the basal foramina, or 3) fibrosis that obstructs the arachnoid villi. Premature infants can develop considerable ventriculomegaly before their heads enlarge; the poorly myelinated premature brain is so easily compressed that the ventricles can enlarge substantially without enlarging the skull proportionately.

Posthemorrhagic hydrocephalus (PHH) usually develops within 4 weeks after IVH. There is a general correlation between the amount of intraventricular hemorrhage and the likelihood of PHH. Infants with PHH may have no symptoms, or may have only increasing spells of apnea and bradycardia (Fig 6.11). Poor feeding and vomiting are uncommon signs of hydrocephalus in premature infants. If moderate ventriculomegaly and pressure develop, the anterior fontanelle becomes convex, mildly tense, and nonpulsatile, and the scalp veins distend. Premature infants rarely develop lateral rectus palsies or the setting-sun sign common in older infants; because of the plasticity of the premature brain and skull, the intracranial pressure does not increase to levels sufficient to cause these signs. As ventriculomegaly increases and persists, the infant's head develops a globoid shape and the circumference of the head increases at an abnormal rate: Circumference increases 0.5 cm/wk in sick premature infants and 1 cm per week in healthy premature infants, but in infants with PHH, the circumference often increases 2 cm/wk. Seizures are not a sign of hydrocephalus in premature infants or older children.

FULL-TERM INFANTS

The common causes of hydrocephalus in full-term infants are listed in Figure 6.12. The symptoms include irritability, vomiting, and drowsiness. Signs of hydrocephalus include macrocephaly; a convex, tense, nonpulsatile anterior fontanelle; distended scalp veins; separated cranial sutures (especially the sagittal and coronal); frontal bossing; an excessively resonant cranial percussion note (positive Macewen's sign); poor head control; lateral rectus paresis; and the setting-sun sign, in which the eyes are inferiorly deviated. Paralysis of upgaze usually heralds dilatation of the suprapineal recess.

Normal head circumference at birth is 33 to 36 cm. During the first year, head circumference increases 2 cm/mo during the first 3 months, 1 cm/mo from 4 to 6 months, and 0.5 cm/mo from 7 to 12 months. A diagnosis of hydrocephalus is indicated more strongly by circumference increases across centile curves than by circumferences that are above but parallel to the 95% centile. Papilledema is rare in infants, although retinal hemorrhages can be seen in rapidly increasing, severe intracranial pressure. Chorioretinitis in a child with hydrocephalus indicates an in utero infection with cytomegalovirus, toxoplasmosis, or lues.

OLDER CHILDREN

Hydrocephalus that develops after infancy is usually caused by neoplasms. The predominant symptom of hydrocephalus in older children is headache, which typically occurs on awakening, is dull and steady, may be associated with lethargy and vomiting, and often improves after vomiting. Headaches secondary to neo-

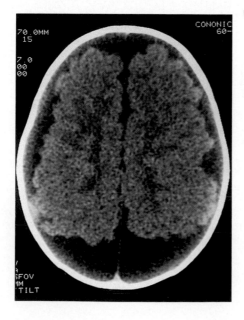

Figure 6.10 Enlarged subarachnoid spaces over the cerebral hemispheres, secondary to impaired CSF absorption.

Principles of Neurosurgery

plasms slowly increase in frequency and severity over days or weeks. Children often complain of blurred vision or double vision.

Children with headaches, vomiting, and drowsiness but no fever are, unfortunately, often misdiagnosed as having early meningitis; a CT or MR scan should be obtained in these children to rule out hydrocephalus or a tumor before a lumbar puncture is performed. Decreased school performance and behavioral disturbances are occasional signs of hydrocephalus in older children, as are endocrinopathies (precocious puberty, short stature, hypothyroidism).

Common signs of hydrocephalus in older children include papilledema and unilateral or bilateral lateral rectus palsies. Hyperreflexia and clonus are also common. The traditional "cracked-pot" sound of hydrocephalus in older children is of diagnostic value only for those who know what a cracked pot sounds like. Rarely, children with hydrocephalus develop transient or permanent blindness if the posterior cerebral arteries are compressed against the tentorium. Treatment is urgent if the child has become lethargic. If the hydrocephalus is extreme, heart rate and respiration slow, posturing develops, and blood pressure increases.

DIAGNOSTIC STUDIES

Skull radiographs demonstrate separation of the cranial sutures in infants, and in older children they demonstrate a beaten-copper appearance or enlargement of the sella. These findings are nonspecific and should be supplemented by scans. Periventricular punctate calcifications in infants with hydrocephalus indicate in utero cytomegalovirus infection. Disseminated calcifications indicate toxoplasmosis.

Before the advent of CT in 1976, three procedures were commonly used in the evaluation of children suspected of having hydrocephalus: transillumination, ventriculography, and angiography. These procedures did not demonstrate the brain directly and have been superseded. Cerebral angiography is currently used only in children whose hydrocephalus has a vascular cause, e.g., vein of Galen arteriovenous malformations or stenosis of the jugular foramina, which is seen in infants with achondroplasia.

Cranial ultrasonography can be performed in infants via the anterior fontanelle and is particularly useful for serial evaluations of ventricular size after IVH. Ultrasonography demonstrates lateral and third ventricle morphology, intraventricular masses, and periventricular leukomalacia

Figure 6.11 Symptoms and Signs of Hydrocephalus in Children

Premature Infants	Infants	Toddlers and Older
Apnea	Irritability	Headache
Bradycardia	Vomiting	Vomiting
Tense fontanelle	Drowsiness	Lethargy
Distended scalp veins	Macrocephaly	Diplopia
	Tense fontanelle	Blurred vision
Globoid head shape	Distended scalp veins	Papilledema
Rapid head growth	Frontal bossing	Lateral rectus palsy
	Abnormal percussion note	Hyperreflexia/clonus
	Poor head control	
	Lateral rectus palsy	
	"Setting-sun" sign	

Figure 6.12 Causes of Hydrocephalus in Infants

Aqueductal occlusion

Chiari type II malformation

Dandy-Walker syndrome

Cerebral malformations
    encephalocoele
    holoprosencephaly
    hydranencephaly

Arachnoid cysts

Neoplasms

Vein of Galen malformations

well, but it does not evaluate the fourth ventricle nor the subarachnoid spaces well. Ultrasonography is often used to detect and monitor fetal hydrocephalus.

From 1976 to 1986, CT was the definitive method of diagnosing hydrocephalus in children of all ages. Scans performed without intravenous contrast material demonstrate ventricular size and shape as well as the presence of blood or abnormal calcium deposits. Increased intracranial pressure from hydrocephalus is indicated by compression of sulci, obliteration of subarachnoid spaces over the convexity, and transependymal absorption of CSF into white matter anterior to the frontal horns (Fig. 6.13). CT scans after intravenous contrast injections reveal abnormalities such as tumors and abscesses. CT scans are still adequate for evaluating the extent of ventriculomegaly but their use is limited because they are performed predominantly in only the axial plane, require irradiation, and have considerably less sensitivity than MRI.

Since 1986, CT has been augmented by MRI, which demonstrates the brain and ventricles in the axial, coronal, and sagittal projections, transependymal absorption more clearly than CT, and low-grade gliomas that may not be apparent on CT scans, and provides information about CSF flow in the aqueduct. MRI does not demonstrate either calcium deposits or the skull well.

In patients with hydrocephalus secondary to Dandy-Walker cysts or other arachnoid cysts, there is often the question as to whether the cyst communicates with the lateral ventricles. This question cannot be definitively answered by either CT or MRI and requires the intraventricular instillation of iohexal, 3 to 5 mL (180 mg/mL), usually instilled into the lateral ventricles. A CT scan obtained 1 to 4 hours later will evaluate communication between the two (Fig. 6.14).

TREATMENT

MEDICAL

No medications treat hydrocephalus effectively. If CSF production were reduced 33%, ICP would decrease by only 1.5 cm H_2O; thus, although acetazolamide and furosemide decrease CSF production for a few days, they do not cause ventriculomegaly to resolve. Acetazolamide is needed in large doses, 100 mg/kg/d in three doses per day. It causes metabolic acidosis, which requires treatment with a systemic alkalizer. The combined use of acetazolamide and furosemide for 6 months was reported to "successfully avoid" a shunt in 22 of 49 infants older than 2 weeks with hydrocephalus of various causes, but neither the likelihood of normal ventricular size nor the intellectual outcome were reported.[19]

SURGICAL

The surgical treatment of hydrocephalus has been summarized by Pudenz.[20] Whenever possible, the obstructing lesion that causes hydrocephalus should be removed. Unfortunately, this is impossible in most cases of congenital hydrocephalus. When CSF flow is obstructed at the aqueduct or distal to it, a ventriculostomy, a surgically created opening in the third ventricle to alleviate hydrocephalus without a shunt, theoretically has considerable appeal. Neurosurgeons have created openings both in the anterior third ventricle via open craniotomies and in the floor of the third ventricle, either stereotactically or endoscopically. Several studies have found success rates of 40% to 60% following percutaneous third ventriculostomies. Kelly recently used stereotactic endoscopic third ventriculostomy to successfully treat 15 of 16 patients with nontumoral adolescent/adult onset hydrocephalus secondary

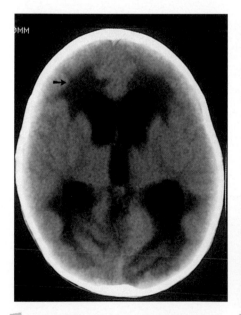

Figure 6.13 Axial CT scan demonstrating transependymal absorption of CSF (arrow) into frontal white matter.

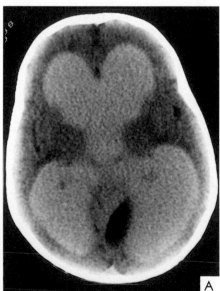
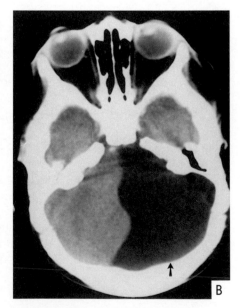

Figure 6.14 Axial CT scans of an infant with hydrocephalus (**A**) secondary to a posterior fossa arachnoid cyst (**B**). Iohexal injected into the ventricles did not communicate into the cyst (arrow).

to aqueductal stenosis. Ventriculostomies are most successful in treating hydrocephalus secondary to acquired aqueductal stenosis, but they are of intermediate value in those with congenital aqueductal stenosis and myelomeningocele; they are not indicated in patients with communicating hydrocephalus.[22,23] The ventriculostomy does not always remain patent and, even if it does, the subarachnoid spaces may not expand adequately to transmit CSF to the arachnoid villi. Currently, there are no known techniques to predict whether a ventriculostomy will effectively treat the hydrocephalus.

Choroid plexectomies, removing choroid plexus from the lateral ventricles, have been done in the past but do not reliably treat hydrocephalus, probably because of CSF production by residual choroid plexus in the third and fourth ventricles. Endoscopic choroid plexus coagulation is effective in treating hydrocephalus in only 50% of cases, for the same reason.

SHUNTS

CSF shunts are silastic tubes that divert CSF from the ventricles into other body cavities. All shunts have ventricular catheters, a valve that permits flow in one direction, and distal tubing. Many shunts have reservoirs that can be percutaneously aspirated of CSF. Shunt valves are of three main configurations: spring-ball, diaphragm, and slit (Fig. 6.15), and are designed to open in various pressure ranges: ultra low (2 to 4 cm H_2O), low (4 to 7 cm H_2O), medium (8 to 12 cm H_2O) and high (13 to 15 cm H_2O); medium pressure valves are used most often. Currently designed valves open at the designated pressure and remain open as long as the pressure differential across the valve is greater than the opening pressure, a differential that is altered by patient position (i.e., decreased when supine and increased when erect).

Ventricular catheters can be inserted through three routes: frontal, parietal, and occipital (Fig. 6.16). A recent study demonstrated that the likelihood of long-term shunt function is significantly higher for frontally inserted shunts than for others (Fig. 6.17), although short-term duration of function is similar in frontal and parietal shunts.[24,25] Frontal shunts lie anterior to the choroid plexus, whereas those inserted parietally or occipitally often lie in proximity to the choroid plexus, which attaches to the catheter, obstructing its foramina. Most ventricular catheters are inserted in the right, (usually) nondominant, hemisphere. Catheter placement

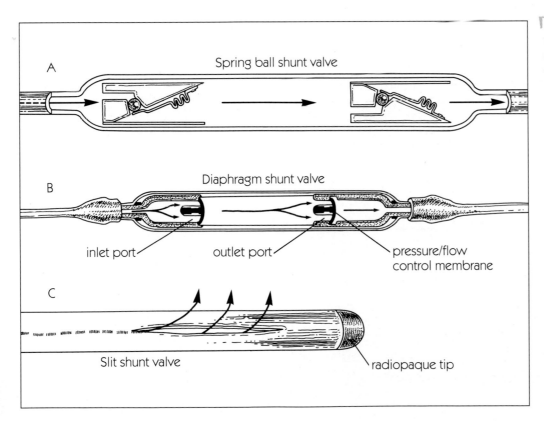

Figure 6.15 Diagram of three shunt valve mechanisms: spring-ball (**A**), diaphragm (**B**), slit valve (**C**).

A — Spring ball shunt valve

B — Diaphragm shunt valve

inlet port   outlet port   pressure/flow control membrane

C — Slit shunt valve   radiopaque tip

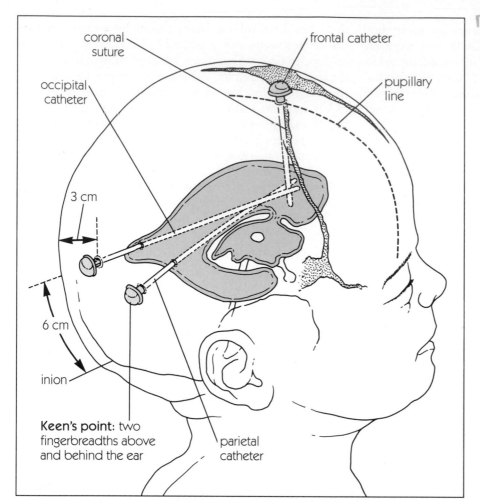

coronal suture

occipital catheter

3 cm

6 cm

inion

Keen's point: two fingerbreadths above and behind the ear

frontal catheter

pupillary line

parietal catheter

Figure 6.16 Three routes for insertion of ventricular shunt catheters: frontal, parietal, and occipital.

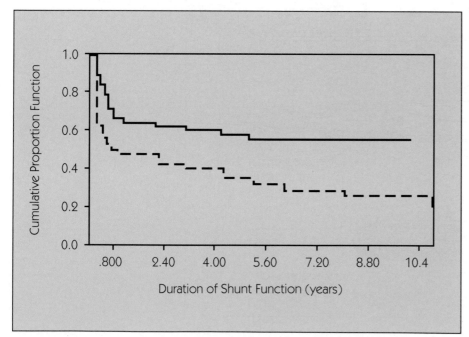

Figure 6.17 Function of frontal (solid line) and parietal (broken line) shunts. (Reprinted from Albright AL, Haines SJ, Taylor FH, 1988)

Principles of Neurosurgery

may be aided by intraoperative ultrasound or endoscopy. Ventricular catheter length, from the cerebral cortex to the floor of the frontal horn, is approximately 4.5 cm in a full-term infant and in an adult approximately 6.5 cm. The infant-length ventricular catheter is usually outgrown between 6 and 10 years of age and replaced with a longer catheter. If a child has loculated ventricles, either the septations need to be fenestrated, via endoscopy or craniotomy, or multiple ventricular catheters must be inserted.

Shunts are passed distally through subcutaneous removable tubes or trocars and into the peritoneal cavity via either a small incision and open dissection or a percutaneous trocar (Fig. 6.18). Common sites of peritoneal catheter insertion are in the epigastric midline immediately below the xiphoid process and at the lateral edge of the lateral rectus abdominis muscle. In full-term infants and throughout childhood, the entire shunt tubing, i.e., 40 to 50 cm, can be left within the peritoneal cavity so that the child does not outgrow the distal end of the shunt. The peritoneum is the preferred site for the distal end of the shunt because it easily contains enough tubing to allow for growth, and if a shunt infection occurs, the morbidity of peritoneal infection is low.

If the peritoneal cavity is not an appropriate site for the distal end of the shunt because of recent or pending operations, recent peritonitis, or multiple abdominal adhesions, the second preferred site is usually the atrium.

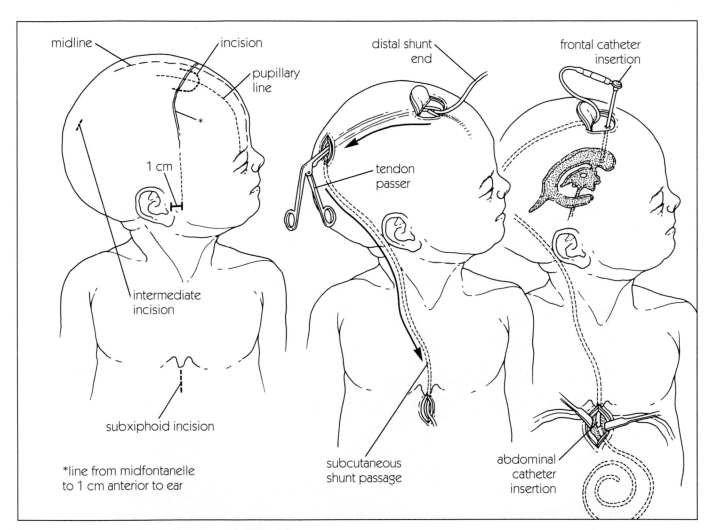

Figure 6.18 Placement of a frontal VP shunt. Patient positioned and coordinates marked; subcutaneous shunt passage; ventricular catheter insertion; peritoneal catheter insertion.

In the past, atrial catheters were inserted via a cutdown on the common facial vein and threaded through the external jugular vein into the right atrium. They are now inserted most easily with techniques used by pediatric surgeons to insert central venous catheters, that is, inserting a guidewire and peelaway catheter into the right atrium under fluoroscopic guidance, then inserting the shunt tubing through the peel away sheath. The right atrium lies at approximately T6-T7.

In children older than 4 to 5 years, the pleural cavity is a third possible site for distal shunt catheter placement. Below age 4, the absorptive capabilities of the pleura are such that inadequate absorption may lead to a progressive pleural effusion sufficient to impair ventilation. A fourth alternative is the gallbladder, a site chosen in children who have abdominal adhesions that preclude a VP shunt, recurrent bacteremia that precludes a VA shunt, and a small or restricted ventilatory capacity that precludes a ventriculopleural shunt. Ventriculogallbladder shunts have a higher complication rate (50%) than other shunts, and the complications may be serious.[26] If a shunt infection causes bacterial cholecystitis, the shunt must be removed surgically, closing the catheter entrance to the gallbladder.

trimester demonstrates marked fetal hydrocephalus, an MRI scan done near the time of delivery may aid in decision-making. Once the fetal head is engaged in the pelvis, motion is reduced so that adequate MRI scans can be obtained to define cerebral morphology (Fig. 6.19). If the MRI scan demonstrates a severe brain malformation (e.g., holoprosencephaly or hydranencephaly) always associated with profound retardation, the hydrocephalus can be treated by cephalocentesis, which results in fetal death in 90% of cases but allows delivery of the fetus without subjecting the mother to the risks of an extensive uterotomy.

Fetal hydrocephalus has been treated with in utero ventriculoamniotic shunts, but the results have been discouraging.[27] Fetal hydrocephalus is often accompanied by cerebral malformations, and the prognosis is not improved by treating the hydrocephalus. Currently, babies with hydrocephalus in utero who appear to have normal cerebral morphology are followed with serial ultrasound examinations. They are delivered by Caesearean section when fetal lung maturity is documented by the foam-stability index or the lecithin-sphingomyelin ratio (<2 suggests maturity), then treated with a CSF shunt.

TREATMENT OF HYDROCEPHALUS DIAGNOSED IN UTERO

In utero hydrocephalus can produce fetal head circumferences of 40 to 50 cm, causing cephalopelvic disproportion and inhibition of labor. If ultrasound in the last

TREATMENT OF POSTHEMORRHAGIC HYDROCEPHALUS

Premature babies weighing 500 to 1500 g often develop intraventricular hemorrhages that obstruct the CSF pathways. A treatment algorithm for this type of hydro-

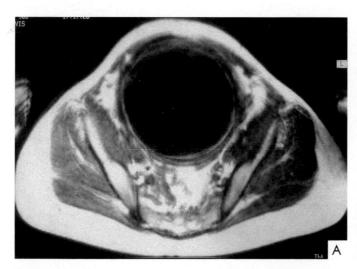
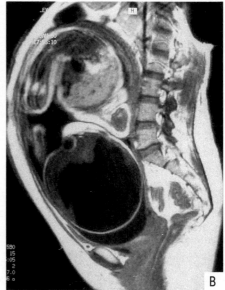

Figure 6.19 Fetal MR scan demonstrating holoprosencephaly (A) and severe hydrocephalus (B).

cephalus (Fig. 6.20) begins with serial lumbar punctures. These lumbar punctures need to remove an adequate volume of CSF, usually 7 to 15 mL daily, to normalize ICP as assessed by the anterior fontanelle and to reduce ventriculomegaly as assessed by ultrasound. External ventricular catheters can be inserted to remove bloody CSF; the infection rate of those catheters is high unless the catheter is tunnelled subcutaneously to exit over the neck or chest. The risk of infection of subcutaneous reservoirs is less than 5%, even if the reservoirs are aspirated daily.[28] VP shunts are not generally inserted until the CSF is cleared of debris and has a protein less than 200 mg%, and the infant weighs over 2 kg. Low-pressure shunts are usually inserted in these infants; medium pressure valves provide more resistance to CSF flow than the poorly myelinated brain, so the ventricles remain large, or even enlarge, in spite of a patent shunt.

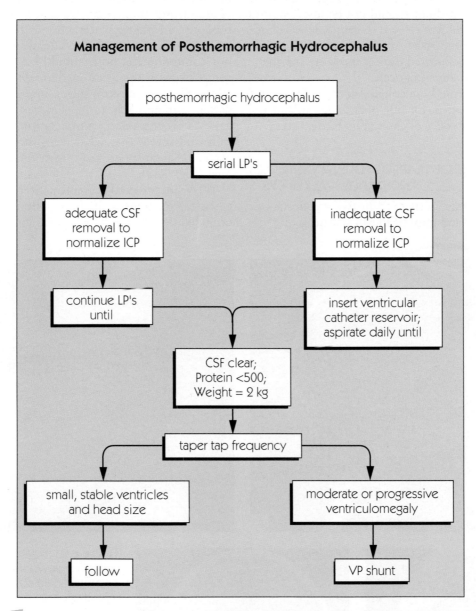

Figure 6.20 Algorithm for management of posthemorrhagic hydrocephalus.

TREATMENT OF HYDROCEPHALUS ASSOCIATED WITH MYELOMENINGOCELES AND ENCEPHALOCELES

Hydrocephalus develops in 90% of infants with myelomeningocele and is obvious at birth in approximately half of these infants. Treatment is usually a VP shunt. Third ventriculostomies have not reliably treated the hydrocephalus in these infants. Although the site of CSF obstruction in most infants with myelomeningoceles is at the craniovertebral junction,[18] their hydrocephalus has not been treated by craniovertebral decompressions. It has been taught that a shunt should not be inserted until the myelomeningocele was closed. Recently, however, reports indicate that the risks of shunt infection are no greater if the shunt is inserted during the same anesthetic used to close the myelomeningocele.[29,30]

Infants with occipital encephaloceles usually do not have hydrocephalus at birth, but it develops within the first month in 50% to 60% of cases (Fig. 6.21).

TREATMENT OF TRAPPED FOURTH VENTRICLES AND DANDY-WALKER CYSTS

Fourth ventricle shunts are needed in two circumstances: Dandy-Walker cysts and trapped fourth ventricles (TFVs).

Some Dandy-Walker cysts communicate with the lateral ventricles and some do not. After a contrast study is performed to determine if the two communicate, a shunt procedure is needed. If the lateral ventricles communicate with the cyst, a single shunt is usually adequate to drain both. Neurosurgeons insert the single shunt into either the lateral ventricles or the Dandy-Walker cyst.[17,31,32] The latter may have a somewhat higher likelihood of decompressing both the lateral ventricles and the cyst, but the complication rate of posterior shunts—in terms of shunt migration, CSF leakage around the shunt, and suboptimal catheter placement—is higher than with lateral ventricle shunts. If the lateral ventricle and cyst do not communicate, both should be shunted, the lateral ventricles with the usual medium-pressure valve and the cyst with a low-pressure valve, since substantial cyst evacuation is more likely to be achieved with a low-pressure valve. This treatment can decompress the cyst dramatically and reveal that what were thought to be atrophic cerebellar hemispheres are, in reality, badly compressed ones (Fig. 6.22).

TFVs occur predominantly after IVH but occasionally after meningitis, if the cerebral aqueduct has been occluded by subependymal gliosis and the basal foramina

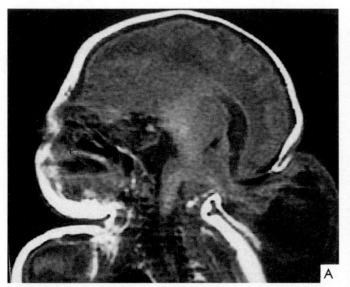
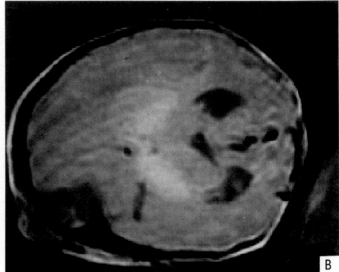
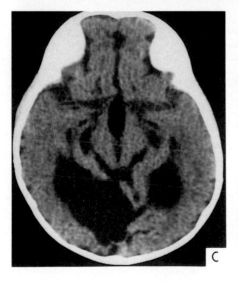
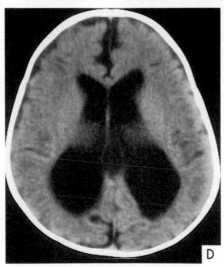

Figure 6.21 Sagittal (A) and axial (B) MR scans of a newborn with an occipital encephalocele. CT scans (C,D) 1 month later demonstrate hydrocephalus.

have been occluded by arachnoidal fibrosis. TFVs become evident after a lateral ventricular shunt has been inserted; the lateral and third ventricles decrease and the fourth ventricle enlarges. Symptoms include lethargy, increasing ataxia, nystagmus, diplopia, and dysarthria.[33,34] The treatment of TFVs can be surprisingly complicated. Catheters are inserted into the trapped fourth ventricle by a paramidline approach. The exact midline is avoided because of the midline occipital sinus, a structure that is often of substantial vascularity in an infant. Catheter length can be estimated from the CT scans.

The trajectory toward the fourth ventricle is estimated from the CT scan and from external landmarks, but there are no reliable external skull landmarks for the site of catheter insertion or for the trajectory. Intraoperative fluoroscopy is of little benefit since there are no reliable bony landmarks. Intraoperative ultrasound, if available, may demonstrate the fourth ventricle, but the heads of most current ultrasound probes are larger than 15 mm and require a considerably larger craniectomy than that desired for a shunt. After the catheter is inserted into the fourth ventricle, it can be connected directly to the shunt tubing from the lateral ventricle to the peritoneal shunt,

if there is a distal slit valve. If the valve is located proximally (in the coronal region) an additional valve must be inserted with the fourth ventricle catheter to approximate the pressure of the lateral ventricle valve.

TREATMENT OF HYDROCEPHALUS CAUSED BY ARACHNOID CYSTS

Most arachnoid cysts do not cause hydrocephalus and are treated by cystoperitoneal shunts, if they require treatment. Arachnoid cysts that cause hydrocephalus are treated either by cystoperitoneal shunts, in which case the hydrocephalus may resolve as the cyst is evacuated, or simultaneous cyst and lateral ventricle-peritoneal shunts. Shunts into arachnoid cysts often have low or ultra low pressure valves to promote cyst resolution.

TREATMENT OF HYDROCEPHALUS SECONDARY TO POSTERIOR FOSSA TUMORS

Children with hydrocephalus secondary to posterior fossa tumors rarely need precraniotomy shunts. Their hydrocephalus can be treated by an external ventricular

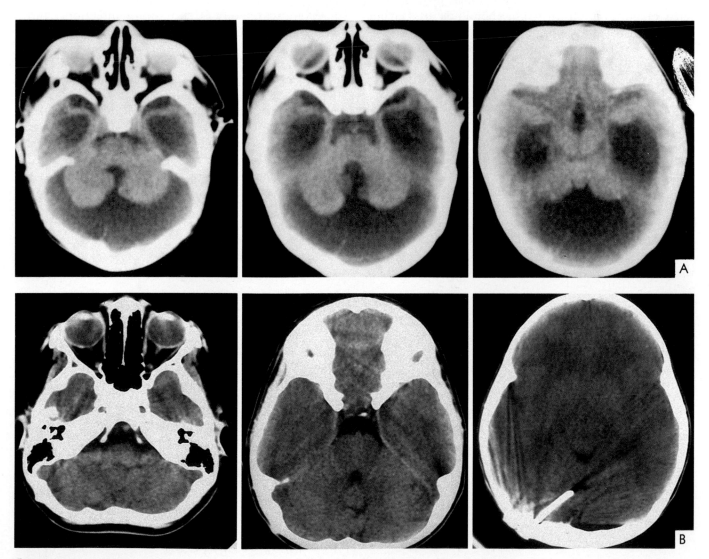

Figure 6.22 Axial CT scans demonstrating Dandy-Walker cyst before (**A**) and after (**B**) shunting.

drain (EVD) inserted after induction of anesthesia for craniotomy and tumor removal.[35] The EVD is left in place for several days after craniotomy, while edema resolves and CSF clears. Then the height of the drainage bag is progressively elevated to 25 to 30 cm above ventricular level and left for 24 hours. If children do not develop symptoms of increased ICP, the catheter can be withdrawn; if they develop symptoms or do not tolerate the elevated chamber, a shunt is required. Approximately 25% to 35% of children need shunts after removal of posterior fossa tumors.[36]

TREATMENT OF OTHER CONDITIONS

Children with hydranencephaly or holoprosencephaly present ethical dilemmas because their prognosis is dismal with or without a shunt. If these infants are not treated, however, their heads expand enormously, making care difficult and predisposing them to scalp ulceration (which is not a life-threatening problem). Shunts are often inserted in these children solely to normalize their head size. The shunts generally function well for long times; the proximal shunt catheters lie in large CSF compartments and are rarely outgrown or obstructed by choroid plexus. Percutaneous choroid plexus coagulation has been reported to decrease CSF production and prevent the need for a shunt in infants with hydranencephaly, but few patients thus treated have been reported.[37]

The treatment of hydrocephalus in achondroplastic children is debated. Treatment is needed if they are symptomatic from increased ICP, but this is unusual. Treatment is controversial if they have only progressive ventriculomegaly or macrocephaly but are asymptomatic and neurologically normal. Traditionally, these children's hydrocephalus has been treated with shunts, but recently they have been treated by decompression of the jugular foramen, which treats the cause of the hydrocephalus.[38]

Theoretically, lumboperitoneal shunts are appropriate for some children with communicating hydrocephalus, but they are infrequently used in childhood, except in those with pseudotumor cerebri. The lumbar catheters can be inserted intrathecally percutaneously via Touhy needles. It is considerably more difficult to assess lumboperitoneal shunt function than VP shunt function, and lumboperitoneal shunts may induce a Chiari malformation.

SHUNT COMPLICATIONS

Shunt complications are listed in Figure 6.23. There are two common shunt complications—infection and obstruction—and many uncommon ones. Approximately 5% to 10% of all shunt operations are complicated by infection in spite of the fact that neurosurgeons take numerous measures to decrease the risk of infection, including prescribing systemic and intrashunt antibiotics, covering exposed skin with an iodine-impregnated transparent drape, lining exposed incisions with Betadine-soaked sponges, and avoiding touching the shunt except with instruments. The risk of shunt infection is 2.6 times higher in children less than 6 months old.[39]

Shunt infections are almost always caused by colonization with skin bacteria at the time of shunt insertion. Staphylococci cause most shunt infections: *S epidermidis* causes approximately 60% of shunt infections, and *S aureus* causes approximately 30%; the remaining 10% are caused by coliform bacteria, propionibacteria, streptococci, or *Haemophilus influenzae* organisms. Approximately 75% of shunt infections become apparent within one month after shunt insertion. Symptoms of shunt infection include irritability and anorexia, and signs include fever (usually 37° to 38°C) and, in cases of *S aureus* infection, erythema along the shunt tract. The risk of shunt infection is similar for VA and VP shunts. Two common complications of infected VA shunts are subacute bacterial endocarditis and shunt nephritis, an immune-complex disorder that resembles acute glomerulonephritis.

Data about the value of prophylactic antibiotics are conflicting. In one randomized, prospective, double-blind trial, children treated with trimethoprim-sulfamethoxazole had a significant decrease in infection rate.[40] A

Figure 6.23 Shunt Complications

Common	Cranial	Uncommon		
		Subcutaneous	Peritoneal	Atrial
Infection	Subdural hygromas	Shunt migration	Peritonitis	Endocarditis
Obstruction	Subdural hematomas	Shunt disconnection	Pseudocysts	Nephritis
	Hemiparesis	Shunt fracture	Perforation	
	Hematoma		Hernias	

prospective randomized study using methicillin showed no significant reduction of infection, but the trial had a large beta error.[41] A recent review of the published literature on prophylactic antibiotics concluded that there was no definitive evidence supporting their use to prevent shunt infections.[42] Nevertheless, the use of prophylactic antibiotics is widespread. Most prophylactic regimens include antibiotics, such as vancomycin or methicillin, that kill staphylococci. Bayston believes that macrophages are able to remove bacteria on the exterior of shunts but those in the interior are not effectively treated with systemic antibiotics, only by intrashunt antibiotics.[43]

Treatment is by removal of the infected shunt, insertion of an external ventricular drain, and intravenous and intraventricular antibiotics. In the past, neurosurgeons have treated shunt infections by administering intravenous antibiotics for 2 weeks, with or without intraventricular antibiotics,[44,45] and not removing the shunt. Success rates range from 66% to 93%, but CSF infection persists longer than if the shunt had been removed, and therefore the sequelae of infection may be more serious. Shunt infections caused by *H influenzae*, however, can reliably be eradicated by intravenous antibiotics alone;[46] CSF usually becomes sterile within 48 hours. Intraventricular antibiotics, usually vancomycin 10 to 20 mg or methicillin 25 to 50 mg are given intrathecally through the EVD to clear staphylococcal infections faster, since the sequelae of ventriculitis are related to the duration of infection as well as to the infecting organism. *S epidermis* organisms are usually cleared from CSF within 3 days, if both intravenous and intraventricular antibiotics are given.

Criteria for the timing of shunt reinsertion vary, but usually require sterile CSF cultures for 3 consecutive days or longer, CSF white blood cell counts less than 50, and CSF protein less than 500 mg/dL at the maximum and ideally less than 200 mg/dL. CSF glucose remains low (<25 mg/dL) for weeks after CFS becomes sterile and does not need to normalize before a shunt is reinserted.

The second common shunt complication is obstruction. In the unusual case—a ventricular catheter is inadvertently inserted in a paraventricular location or the distal catheter is in the preperitoneal space—symptoms of obstruction are evident within 2 to 3 days after shunt insertion. More commonly, however, shunt obstruction occurs more than a year after insertion, usually because choroid plexus has occluded the ventricular catheter.

The symptoms of shunt malfunction—headache, drowsiness, and vomiting—are the same regardless of whether the obstruction is proximal or distal. In approximately 75% of cases of shunt malfunction, those symptoms last for a few hours, disappear, then recur with gradually increasing frequency and severity. In the remaining 25% of cases, headache persists and worsens, drowsiness and vomiting develop, and the symptoms remain until the shunt is revised. Children with suspected shunt malfunction should not be given narcotics because of the possibility of respiratory depression or arrest. "Pumping" the shunt valve, i.e., compressing it three or four times against the skull, provides some information about the patency of the proximal and distal ends of the shunt. Easy emptying suggests patency of the distal end and rapid refill suggests patency of the ventricular catheter. This information can be helpful, although even the experienced surgeon can find it misleading.

Children who present with symptoms of malfunction need x-rays of the head and abdomen to determine if the shunt has become disconnected or if growth has caused the peritoneal catheter to ascend out of the abdomen. CT scans should be obtained; if they demonstrate an interval increase in ventricular size, they confirm the clinical impression of shunt malfunction. However, the diagnosis of shunt malfunction is based on a combination of clinical and radiographic information. Shunt malfunction can be present even if the ventricles remain small, particularly in children who had large ventricles that disrupted the ependyma and received a shunt that functioned well for several years, causing them to develop small ventricles surrounded by periventricular gliosis, which inhibits ventricular dilatation. Symptoms indicative of shunt malfunction in the presence of small ventricles have been termed the "slit-ventricle" syndrome.[47] This disorder occurs in less than 5% of children with shunt malfunctions and can sometimes be diagnosed by CT during symptomatic episodes because the ventricles are larger. The syndrome is treated sequentially, first by excluding migraine,[48] then changing the valve to one of higher pressure. If that fails, an antisiphon device is often inserted into the shunt system just distal to the valve, and if that fails, subtemporal craniectomies are performed.

At times, neither the clinical picture nor the CT results are diagnostic of shunt malfunction. In these situations, shunt function can be evaluated by puncturing the shunt reservoir with a 25-gauge butterfly needle; free flow of CSF into the tubing behind the needle suggests patency of the ventricular catheter. Once the tubing is filled with CSF, it is connected to a manometer or pressure transducer, and the intracranial pressure is measured. Following that, radioactive indium can be injected into the reservoir while the valve is occluded. The needle is then removed and the shunt tract scanned for migration of isotope into the abdomen, a passage that should be evident within 30 minutes.

Shunt malfunction is treated by replacing either the malfunctioning component or the entire system. Barium-impregnated shunts in place for several years may become brittle and break easily; such shunts are usually replaced during shunt revisions, even if they are still patent. Serial shunt x-rays may demonstrate that the distal end of a VP shunt is becoming "short," i.e., migrating out of the abdomen, because of the child's growth. In these cases, some neurosurgeons electively lengthen the catheter, while others wait until symptoms develop, since some children outgrow the need for a shunt, especially children with posthemorrhagic hydrocephalus.

Other complications of VP shunts include subdural hygromas and hematomas, shunt migration, abdominal pseudocysts, ascites, hernias, and perforations. Subdural hygromas may develop after insertion of shunts into infants with very large ventricles. Effusions vary in size and need to be treated if they increase ICP or cause neurologic deficits. If they deform the cortex but cause no deficits, treatment is optional. Treatment consists of changing the shunt valve to a higher pressure or by inserting a catheter into the effusion and connecting it to the shunt system distal to the valve, or both.

Shunt migration out of the head and downward toward or into the abdomen occurs if the shunt is not fixed at the site where it exits the skull. Shunt migration, disconnection or fracture occurred in 25% of patients in one series.[49] The risk of migration and disconnection is probably lower if unishunts (without connectors in the tubing) are used, and if the catheters are inserted frontally but tunnelled directly posteriorly several centimeters before making the bend toward the abdomen, to lessen downward traction on the shunt when the neck rotates.

Abdominal pseudocysts may develop around the peritoneal end of VP shunts. Many pseudocysts are secondary to an indolent CSF infection with *S epidermidis* or propionibacteria, and most (62%) develop in children who have had a previous shunt infection.[50] The average age of children with pseudocysts was 4.5 years in one study.[51] Pseudocysts cause indolent symptoms of shunt malfunction, and they may cause abdominal pain and distention. They are diagnosed by abdominal ultrasound or CT. The cysts can be percutaneously aspirated; the fluid should be cultured for up to 10 days because of the indolent nature of some organisms, e.g., *Propionibacterium*, which cause pseudocysts. If infection is documented, the shunt is treated like any other infected shunt. If the pseudocyst fluid is sterile, the peritoneal catheter is placed in another site within the abdominal cavity. Ascites may indicate indolent peritonitis, inadequate absorptive capability, or CSF overproduction. Hernias develop within 3 months of shunt insertion in perhaps 15% of infants[49] and are treated as any other hernia. Perforations of the intestine, bladder, and even abdominal wall have occurred, but almost all have been caused by wire-reinforced peritoneal catheters that are used less frequently now. The risk of a postoperative hemiparesis after shunt insertion due to the ventricular catheter injuring the internal capsule is low—twice in over 2000 shunts in my experience. The risk of a major hemorrhage at the site of catheter insertion is approximately the same.

FOLLOW-UP

There is no fixed schedule for following patients with shunted hydrocephalus. I examine these children every 3 months during the first year, every 6 months in the second year, then yearly. A CT scan is needed for a postshunt baseline evaluation of ventricular size. Ventricles massively dilated at birth may take several years to decrease in size maximally (Fig. 6.24). Unless the ventricles

were initially extremely dilated, a CT at 1 year will usually provide the baseline information. Thereafter, scans are needed whenever children have symptoms that herald malfunction; they are obtained by some practitioners at 1- to 2-year intervals to detect occult shunt malfunctions, a relatively infrequent occurrence. Children with VA shunts need yearly chest x-rays to monitor location of the atrial catheter; when it rises to T-4, obstruction is likely. In my experience, approximately half the children with posthemorrhagic hydrocephalus and 15% of those with myelomeningoceles, but almost none of those with congenital aqueductal stenosis, appear to outgrow their need for shunts. Most children require two to five shunt revisions before they are 21 years old.[49] Approximately 70% of frontally inserted shunts function for 10 years without a revision.[24]

OUTCOME

The prognosis of infantile hydrocephalus depends more on brain morphology and on factors such as perinatal ischemia, IVH, or ventriculitis than on hydrocephalus per se. If the brain is structurally normal, even if it is badly compressed by hydrocephalus, the prognosis is reasonably good. If the parenchyma is disorganized, the outlook is guarded even if the hydrocephalus is treated promptly.

The 5-year survival rate of children with congenital hydrocephalus is 80% to 90%.[52] The value of cortical mantle thickness in predicting intellect is dubious. Normal intellect has been reported in 40% to 65% of treated children with all varieties of infantile hydrocephalus.[53,54] Approximately two thirds of treated children with overt neonatal hydrocephalus have normal or borderline intellect.[55] The prognosis of Dandy-Walker syndrome has historically been considered dismal, but recent reports indicate normal intellect in at least 75% of patients.[31,32] The mean IQ of children with shunted hydrocephalus associated with spina bifida was 95 in children who did not develop shunt infections and 73 in children who did develop shunt infections.[56] The outcome for children with posthemorrhagic hydrocephalus is abnormal in at least one third; the effects of hydrocephalus cannot be easily separated from those of perinatal ischemia. In 182 children with untreated hydrocephalus, 50% died and 50% developed "arrested hydrocephalus"; of the children with "arrested hydrocephalus," 75% had IQs >50 (educable) and 45% had IQs >85.[57]

Arrested hydrocephalus is a condition of nonprogressive hydrocephalus in which compensatory mechanisms have developed to the point that intracranial pressure is normal or only mildly increased without a functioning shunt; the ventricles often remain larger than normal. If the patient is asymptomatic and neurologically normal with mild ventriculomegaly, there is little evidence that shunt insertion or revision is beneficial. If the ventricles are moderate or large, the problem is more difficult: There is greater concern that retardation will develop if a shunt is not inserted but greater risk of subdural hygromas and hematomas if a shunt is inserted. I believe it is appropriate to treat these children. If the patient is asymptomatic but developmentally delayed, a shunt is probably indicated.[58] The decision to treat hydrocephalus with a shunt requires carefully weighing the symptoms, signs, scan findings, and prognosis. The surgical goal is to have each child develop to the maximum of its potential. Surgical benefits must be weighed against the attendant risks.

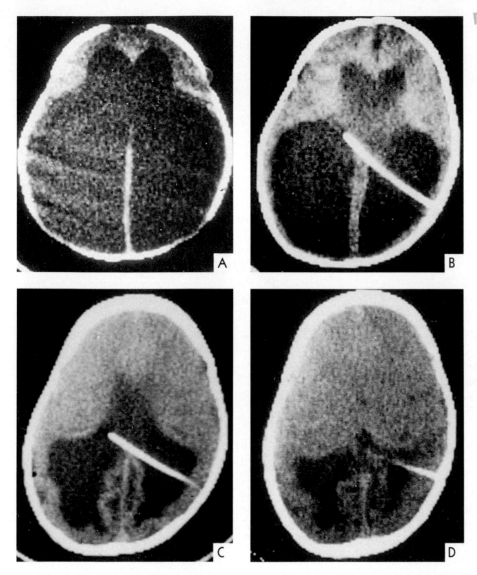

Figure 6.24 (A–D) Serial CT scans at approximately yearly intervals after a VP shunt was inserted for massive neonatal hydrocephalus.

REFERENCES

1. Cutler RWP, Page L, Galicich J, et al. Formation and absorption of cerebrospinal fluid in man. *Brain.* 1968;91:707–720.
2. Lorenzo AV, Page LK, Watters GV. Relationship between cerebrospinal fluid formation, absorption and pressure in human hydrocephalus. *Brain.* 1970; 93:679–692.
3. Milhorat TH, Hammock MK, Davis DA, et al. Choroid plexus papilloma. Proof of cerebrospinal fluid overproduction. *Childs Brain.* 1976;2:273–289.
4. Eisenberg HM, McComb JG, Lorenzo AV. Cerebrospinal fluid overproduction and hydrocephalus associated with choroid plexus papilloma. *J Neurosurg.* 1974;40:381–385.
5. Welch K, Strand R, Bresnan M, et al. Congenital hydrocephalus due to villous hypertrophy of the telencephalic choroid plexus. *J Neurosurg.* 1983; 59:172–175.
6. Chadduck WM, Glasier CM. Megachoroid as a cause of isolated ventricle syndrome. *Pediatr Neurol.* 1989;5:194–196.
7. Habballah MY, Hoffman HJ. The isolated lateral ventricle. *Surg Neurol.* 1987;27:220–222.
8. Hall WA, Lunsford LD. Changing concepts in the treatment of colloid cysts. *J Neurosurg.* 1987;66: 186–191.
9. Camacho A, Ahernathey CD, Kelley PJ, et al. Colloid cysts: experience with the management of 84 cases since the introduction of computed tomography. *Neurosurgery.* 1989;24:693–700.
10. Albright L. Treatment of bobble-head doll syndrome by transcallosal cystectomy. *Neurosurgery.* 1981; 8:593–595.
11. Wiese JA, Gentry LR, Menezes AH. Bobble-head doll syndrome: review of the pathophysiology and CSF dynamics. *Pediatr Neurol.* 1985;1:361–366.
12. Pierre-Kahn A, Capelle L, Brauner R, et al. Presentation and management of suprasellar arachnoid cysts. *J Neurosurg.* 1990;73:355–359.
13. Emery JL. Intracranial effects of longstanding decompression of the brain in children with hydrocephalus, and myelomeningocele. *Dev Med Child Neurol.* 1965;7:302–309.
14. Milhorat TH, Hammock MK, Chandra RS. The subarachnoid space in congenital obstructive hydrocephalus, II: microscopic findings. *J Neurosurg.* 1971;35:7–15.
15. Faivre J, Lemarec B, Betagne J, et al. X-linked hydrocephalus, with aqueductal stenosis, mental retardation, and adduction-flexion deformity of the thumbs. *Childs Brain.* 1976;2:226–233.
16. Spadaro A, Ambrosio D, Moracic A, et al. Nontumoral aqueductal stenosis in children affected by von Recklinghausen's disease. *Surg Neurol.* 1989; 26:487–495.
17. Asa A, Hoffman HJ, Hendrick EB, et al. Dandy-Walker syndrome: experience at the Hospital for Sick Children, Toronto. *Pediatr Neurosci.* 1989; 15:66–73.
18. Yamada H, Nakamura S, Tanaka Y, et al. Ventriculography and cisternography with water-soluble contrast media in infants with myelomeningocele. *Radiology.* 1982;143:75–83.
19. Shinnar S, Gammon K, Bergman EW, et al. Management of hydrocephalus in infancy: use of acetazolamide and furosemide to avoid cerebrospinal fluid shunts. *J Pediatr.* 1985;107:31–37.
20. Pudenz RH. The surgical treatment of hydrocephalus—a historical review. *Surg Neurol.* 1980; 15:15–26.
21. Kelly PJ. Stereotactic third ventriculostomy in patients with nontumoral adolescent/adult onset aqueductal stenosis and symptomatic hydrocephalus. *J Neurosurg.* 1991;75:865–873.
22. Jones RFC, Stening WA, Brydon M. Endoscopic third ventriculostomy. *Neurosurgery.* 1990; 26:86-92.
23. Hirsch JF. Percutaneous ventriculostomies in noncommunicating hydrocephalus. *Monogr Neural Sci.* 1982;8:170–178.
24. Albright AL, Haines SJ, Taylor FH. Function of parietal and frontal shunts in childhood hydrocephalus. *J Neurosurg.* 1988;69:883–886.
25. Bierbraure KS, Storrs BB, McLone DG, et al. A prospective randomized study of shunt function and infections as a function of shunt placement. *Pediatr Neurosci.* 1990–91;16:287–291.
26. West KW, Turner MK, Vane DW. Ventricular gallbladder shunts: an alternative procedure in hydrocephalus. *J Ped Surg.* 1987;22:609–612.
27. Report of the International Fetal Surgery Registry. Catheter shunts for fetal hydronephrosis and hydrocephalus. *N Engl J Med.* 1986;315:336–340.
28. McComb JG, Ramos AD, Platzker ACG, et al. Management of hydrocephalus secondary to intraventricular hemorrhage in the preterm infant with a subcutaneous ventricular catheter reservoir. *Neurosurgery.* 1983;13:295–300.
29. Bell WO, Arbit E, Fraser RAR. One-stage myelomeningocele closure and ventriculoperitoneal shunt placement. *Surg Neurol.* 1987;27:233–236.
30. Chadduck WM, Reding DL. Experience with simultaneous ventriculo-peritoneal shunt placement and myelomeningocele repair. *J Pediatr Surg.* 1988; 23:913–916.
31. Golden JA, Rorke LB, Bruce DA. Dandy-Walker syndrome and associated anomalies. *Pediatr Neurosci.* 1987;13:38–44.
32. Maria BL, Zinreich SJ, Carson BC, et al. Dandy-Walker syndrome revisited. *Pediatr Neurosci.* 1987; 13:45–51.

33. O'Hare AE, Brown JK, Minns RA. Specific enlargement of the fourth ventricle after ventriculoperitoneal shunt for post-hemorrhagic hydrocephalus. *Arch Dis Child.* 1987;62:1025–1029.

34. Scotti G, Musgrave MA, Fitz CR, et al. The isolated fourth ventricle in children: CT and clinical review of 16 cases. *Am J Roentgenol.* 1980;135:1233–1238.

35. Dias MS, Albright AL. The management of hydrocephalus complicating childhood posterior fossa tumors. *Pediatr Neurosci.* 1989; 15:283–290.

36. Albright AL, Wisoff J, Zeltzer P, et al. Current neurosurgical treatment of medulloblastomas in children. *Pediatr Neurosci.* 1989;15:276–282.

37. Albright AL. Percutaneous choroid plexus coagulation in hydranencephaly. *Childs Brain.* 1981;8:134–137.

38. Aryanpur J, Hurko O, Francomanu C, et al. Craniocervical decompression for cervicomedullary compression in pediatric patients with achondroplasia. *J Neurosurg.* 1990;73:375.

39. Renier D, Lacombe J, Pierre-Kahn A. Factors causing acute shunt infection. *J Neurosurg.* 1984;61:1072–1078.

40. Blomstedt GC. Results of trimethoprim-sulfa-methoxazole prophylaxis in ventriculostomy and shunting procedures. *J Neurosurg.* 1985;62:694–697.

41. Schmidt K, Gjerris F, Osgaard O, et al. Antibiotic prophylaxis in shunting: a prospective randomized trial in 152 hydrocephalic patients. *Neurosurgery.* 1985;17:1–5.

42. Quigley M, Reigel DH. Cerebrospinal fluid shunt infections. *Pediatr Neurosci.* 1989;15:11–20.

43. Bayston R. Treatment of shunt infections. In: Bayston R. *Hydrocephalus Shunt Infection.* London: Chapman and Hall; 1989;97–125.

44. Wald SL, McLaurin RL. Cerebrospinal fluid antibiotic levels during treatment of shunt infections. *J Neurosurg.* 1980;52:41–46.

45. Mates S, Glaser J, Shapiro K. Treatment of cerebrospinal fluid shunt infections with medical therapy alone. *Neurosurgery.* 1982;11:781–783.

46. Lerman SJ. Haemophilus influenzae infections of cerebrospinal fluid shunts. *J Neurosurg.* 1981;54:261–263.

47. Epstein F, Lapras C, Wisoff JH. "Slit-ventricle syndrome": etiology and treatment. *Pediatr Neurosci.* 1988;14:5–10.

48. Obana WG, Raskin NH, Cogen PH, et al. Antimigraine treatment for slit-ventricle syndrome. *Neurosurgery.* 1990;27:760–763.

49. McCullough DC. Hydrocephalus treatment. In: Wilkins RH, Rengachary SS, eds. *Neurosurgery.* New York, NY: McGraw-Hill Book Co; 1985;3:2140–2150.

50. Hahn YS, Engelhart H, McLone DG. Abdominal CSF pseudocyst: clinical features and surgical management. Pediatr. Neurosci. 1985–86;12:75–79.

51. Gaskill SJ, Marlin AE. Pseudocysts of the abdomen associated with ventriculoperitoneal shunts: a report of twelve cases and a review of the literature. *Pediatr Neurosci.* 1989;15:23–27.

52. Amacher AL, Wellington J. Infantile hydrocephalus: long-term results of surgical therapy. *Childs Brain.* 1984;11:217–229.

53. Dennis M, Fitz CR, Netley CT, et al. The intelligence of hydrocephalic children. *Arch Neurol.* 1981;38:607–615.

54. Raimondi AJ, Soare P. The intellectual development in shunted hydrocephalus. *Am J Dis Child.* 1974;127:664–671.

55. McCullough DC, Balzer-Martin LA. Current prognosis in overt neonatal hydrocephalus *J Neurosurg.* 1982;57: 378–383.

56. McLone DG, Czyzewski D, Raimondi AJ, et al. Central nervous system infections as a limitary factor in the intelligence of children with myelomeningocele. *Pediatrics.* 1982;70:338–342.

57. Laurence KM, Cortes S. Spontaneously arrested hydrocephalus. *Dev Med Child Neurol.* 1967; 13:4-13.

58. Torkelson RD, Gleibrock LG, Gustavson JL, et al. Neurological and neuropsychological effects of cerebral spinal fluid shunting in children with assumes arrested ("normal pressure") hydrocephalus. *J Neurol Neurosurg Psychiatry.* 1985;48:799–806.

Chapter 7

Hydrocephalus in Adults

Peter McL. Black, Mitsunori Matsumae

CLASSIFICATION AND ETIOLOGY

Hydrocephalus in adults can be classified as acute or chronic, compensated or uncompensated, normal-pressure or high-pressure, communicating or noncommunicating, and obstructive or nonobstructive. *Acute* and *chronic* refer to time course. In acute hydrocephalus there is a time course of days or weeks with symptoms of high intracranial pressure (see below). In chronic hydrocephalus the findings have been present for months or years. *Active, compensated,* or *arrested* refers to whether the hydrocephalus is still producing symptoms; *normal-pressure* or *high-pressure* refers to the CSF pressure; *communicating* or *noncommunicating* refers to whether the ventricles communicate with the subarachnoid space; and *obstructive* or *nonobstructive* refers to whether there is a block to CSF flow (Fig. 7.1).

The causes of hydrocephalus are shown in Figure 7.2. Communicating hydrocephalus can be caused by trauma, subarachnoid hemorrhage, or infection, or it may be idiopathic. Noncommunicating hydrocephalus may be caused by intraventricular hemorrhage, tumors of the ventricular system, aqueductal stenosis, posterior fossa tumors or hemorrhage, Paget's disease, or spinal cord tumors producing a high protein concentration in CSF.

With acute hydrocephalus the patient is ill, with drowsiness, headache, vomiting, and papilledema. In chronic hydrocephalus the patient has a chronic disorder characterized by walking difficulty, slowness of thought and action, memory loss, and urinary incontinence. The symptoms and signs of hydrocephalus are outlined in Figure 7.3.

DIAGNOSIS

The term *hydrocephalus* indicates that the ventricles are enlarged; thus, either CT or MRI must show ventricular enlargement for the diagnosis to be made (Fig.

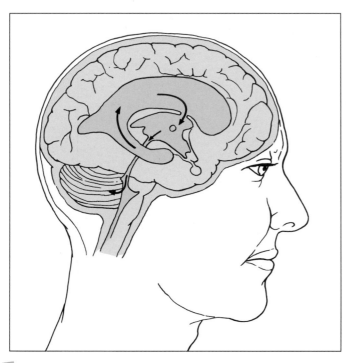

Figure 7.1 Normal cerebrospinal fluid pathway. The arrows indicate the direction of CSF flow. Noncommunicating hydrocephalus results from obstruction to CSF pathway within the ventricular system. Communicating hydrocephalus results from obstruction to the flow of CSF in the subarachnoid space.

Figure 7.2 Some Causes of Hydrocephalus

Noncommunicating
Tumors or cysts of the ventricular system
Aqueductal stenosis
Posterior fossa malformations, including tumors
Paget's disease

Communicating
Trauma
Subarachnoid hemorrhage
Infection
Idiopathic
Subdural hematoma
Extraaxial tumors

Figure 7.3 Symptoms and Signs of Hydrocephalus

Acute
Headache
Vomiting
Papilledema
Drowsiness
Ataxia

Chronic
Gait disorder
Memory loss

Urinary incontinence
Slowing of thought and action

7.4A,B). It is important for the neurosurgeon to know the patient's CSF pressure because patients with high pressure usually respond well to shunting while those with low pressure may not. Although a lumbar puncture may provide information about CSF pressure, it is not safe to perform in the presence of noncommunicating hydrocephalus because of the potential for downward herniation (Fig. 7.4C). Continuous monitoring of intracranial pressure may reveal elevations of pressure not noted on a single lumbar or ventricular puncture.

The work-up of a patient with suspected high-pressure hydrocephalus should include a CT scan and/or an MRI. MRI is more valuable as a single test because it may show ventricular volume and CSF flow through the foramen of Monro or aqueduct of Sylvius as well as the source of the hydrocephalus. A lumbar puncture may also be done if the hydrocephalus is known to be communicating.

The diagnosis of normal-pressure hydrocephalus is more complex. It is made best by history and physical examination. The history should include documentation of any loss of memory or urinary incontinence as well as any gait disorder. Occasionally there will be only gait difficulty, which, on examination, will be characterized by small steps and loss of balance—not the profoundly ataxic gait of cerebellar dysfunction. The memory disorder is for recent events and is usually mild. Patients who have striking dementia without much walking difficulty are usually poor candidates for shunting. There is also a general slowing of activity and affect as part of this process.

Overnight monitoring of CSF pressure and lumboventricular perfusion may be helpful in the work-up of suspected normal-pressure hydrocephalus. For example, one may place a ventricular catheter, monitor pressure overnight, and do lumboventricular perfusion the next morning.

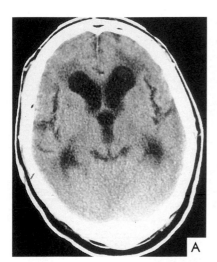
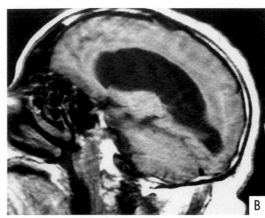

Figure 7.4 CT (A) and MRI (B) are used to diagnose normal-pressure hydrocephalus. A lumbar puncture (C) should not be performed in the presence of noncommunicating hydrocephalus, as illustrated here.

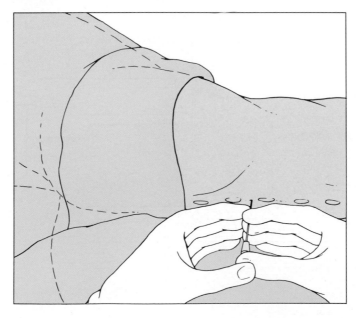

Adults generally tend to have less acute symptoms than children with hydrocephalus, but the diagnosis is otherwise made in the same way.

TREATMENT

There is no satisfactory medical treatment for hydrocephalus. The usual surgical treatment option is placement of a CSF shunt. Puncture of the floor of the third ventricle under direct vision through a ventriculoscope may be attempted if the hydrocephalus is noncommunicating. Figure 7.5 outlines some common shunt components. It is more important that the surgeon use a valve with which he or she is familiar than that it be of a particular type. The programmable pressure valve makes it possible to set the valve pressure at any desired level without shunt revision after the shunting system has been implanted. The common shunt components include the ventricular catheter, which may be curved or straight; the valve, which may be a slit valve or a ball valve; and a variety of other components, including in-line reservoirs, antisiphon devices, and on–off valves.

Ventriculoperitoneal shunting is by far the most commonly used method. For the ventricular catheter either a frontal or an occipital burr hole can be used (Fig. 7.6). If a frontal burr hole is used, the catheter is aimed at the medial canthus of the right eye and is inserted 10 cm behind the nasion and 2.5 cm to the right of the midline. In the sagittal plane it should be aimed 1 cm in front of the tragus. If an occipital burr hole is used, the catheter should be placed 7 cm above

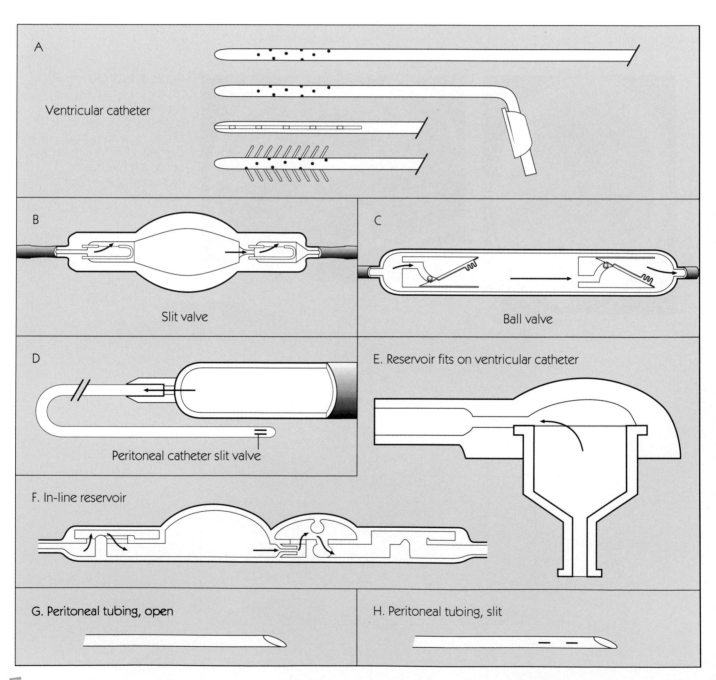

Figure 7.5 Some shunt components. Ventricular catheters (**A**), slit valve (**B**), ball valve (**C**), peritoneal catheter slit valve (**D**), reservoir that fits on ventricular catheter (**E**), in-line reservoir (**F**), peritoneal tubing (**G**), peritoneal tubing with slits (**H**).

Principles of Neurosurgery

the inion and 2.5 cm to the right of midline. The catheter should be aimed 1 cm above the nasion. Great care must be taken in marking out the landmarks for placement occipitally, as the catheter may end up in unusual places. The peritoneal catheter may be placed in the midline of the epigastrium, in which case finding the peritoneum beneath properitoneal fat may be a problem. Alternatively it may be placed in the right upper or right lower quadrant. In these cases a muscle-splitting incision should be used and the posterior fascia should be repaired after the peritoneum is opened.

Ventriculoatrial shunting (Fig. 7.7) uses the common facial vein as the insertion site for the catheter. The catheter is usually placed at the level of T-6 and should be confirmed by intraoperative x-ray. It should sit at the junction of the superior vena cava and the right atrium. The ventricular catheter placement is the same as for ventriculoperitoneal shunting.

Ventriculopleural shunting (Fig. 7.8) uses insertion of the catheter between the second and third ribs, usually in a midcostal line. Care must be taken not to create a pneumothorax, and the puncture through the pleura should be small.

Lumboperitoneal shunting (Fig. 7.9) can be done either with a trocar or by incision. There are a variety of shunt devices for this. Often the lumbar catheter can be placed percutaneously through a large Tuohy spinal needle, but the back may be incised at least to the spinous process to be certain that the catheter is placed in the midline. It is crucial to have the catheter in the midline so it does not go into a nerve root sheath, and it is usually placed at least 5 cm into the subarachnoid space, directed upward. The peritoneal catheter is best placed by direct incision rather than by a trocar, although some authors have advocated trocar placement. A muscle-splitting incision is usually made in the right or left lower quadrant. The incision must go into

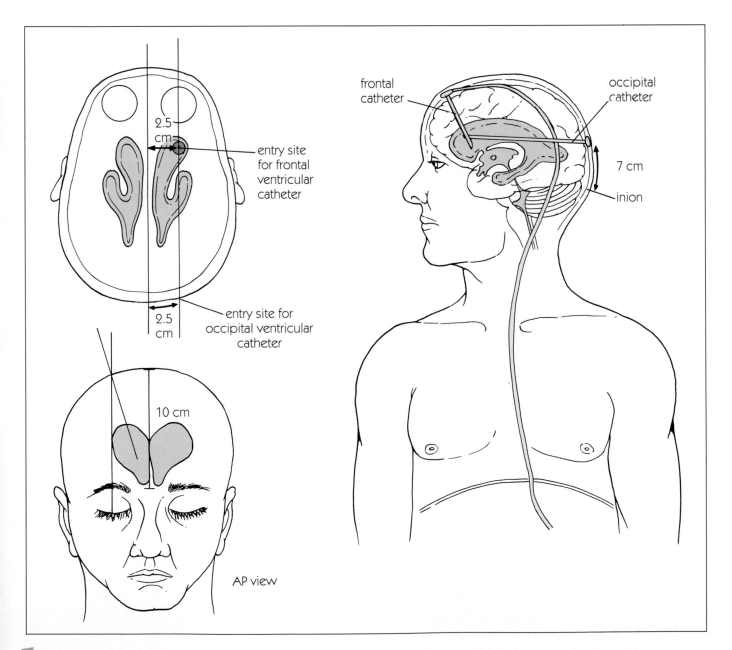

Figure 7.6 Ventriculoperitoneal shunt with a frontal placement. Alternatively, an occipital placement may be used.

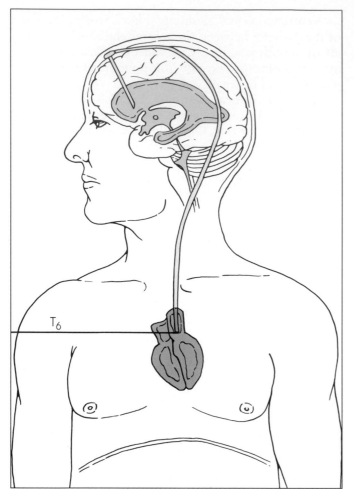

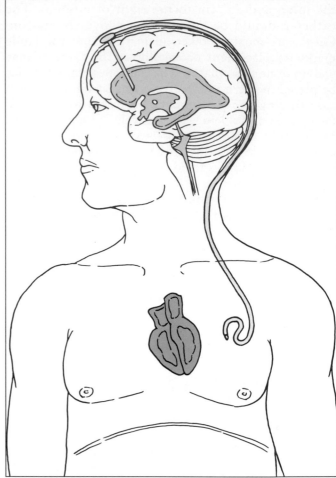

Figure 7.7 Ventriculoatrial shunt placement.

Figure 7.8 Ventriculopleural shunt placement.

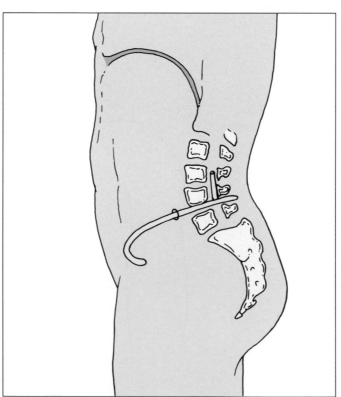

Figure 7.9 Lumboperitoneal shunt placement (for communicating hydrocephalus only).

the peritoneal cavity, so care must be taken that it is not retroperitoneal.

In the Torkildsen shunt a ventricular catheter is placed from the ventricle into the cisterna magna (Fig. 7.10). This is especially useful for obstructive hydrocephalus in aqueductal stenosis.

Treatment of hydrocephalus by shunting is essentially the same in adults and in children.

One of the goals to be achieved in treating hydrocephalus by shunting is to obtain the optimal CSF flow rate through the system, even though the flow rate must differ from time to time and CSF dynamics and the shunt flow rate are likely to be greatly influenced by changing posture. It is helpful, therefore, to provide a reliable way of measuring the shunt flow rate in vivo.

COMPLICATIONS

In all, the success rate of shunting is about 70% by clinical criteria, supplemented by CSF studies where necessary. The complication rate is about 20% if all subdural collections are included (Fig. 7.11).

OVERDRAINING

In shunt overdrainage the patient has a headache and may develop a subdural hematoma. Although the cause of these subdural hematomas is not definitely known, they may result from removing too much CSF with a shunt whose pressure is too low. This problem is more common in adults than children. In children slit ventricles result, in adults chronic or acute subdural collection.

INSUFFICIENT DRAINING

A second problem is failure of the ventricles to shrink with shunt placement. This also may be a result of mismatching valve pressure to ventricular pressure, although the reasons for persistently enlarged ventricles and subdural hematomas are not really understood. This problem may be greatly improved with a variable-pressure valve.

SHUNT MALFUNCTION

Failure of the ventricles to shrink may also herald shunt malfunction due to valve malfunction, plugging of the ventricular catheter with choroid plexus or other tissue, or, most commonly, peritoneal catheter dysfunction. In adults, especially those with normal-pressure hydrocephalus, this is often overlooked, and if symptoms do not regress, this possibility should be checked by shunt tapping or lumbar puncture to make certain the shunt is working. A telesensor can also indicate whether the shunt is working.

INFECTION

Shunt infections may occur, often with low-grade pathogens such as *Staphylococcus epidermidis* or diphtheroids. These are diagnosed by tapping the shunt. The treatment is removal of the shunt and later replacement.

OTHER COMPLICATIONS

Less common complications, such as viscus perforation or intracerebral hemorrhage, may occur as well.

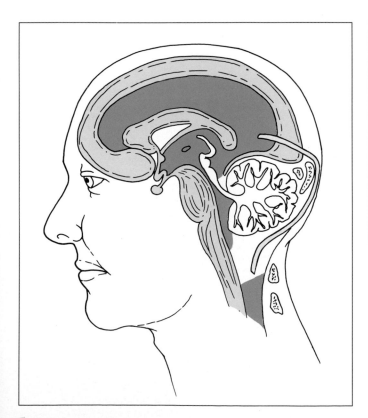

Figure 7.10 Torkildsen shunting.

Figure 7.11 Complications of Shunting

Subdural hematoma
Failure of ventricles to shrink
Infection
Shunt obstruction
Overdrainage and slit ventricle syndrome
Disconnection of shunt components
Perforation of hollow viscus by the peritoneal
  catheter

Chapter 8

Craniosynostosis

Mark E. Shaffrey, John A. Persing,
Christopher I. Shaffrey, John A. Jane

Our present understanding of the pathogenesis of craniosynostosis dates to 1791, when Sömmerring observed that bone growth in the skull occurred at suture lines.[1] He noted that when the sutures were fused prematurely, growth perpendicular to the suture's axis was reduced. These observations were confirmed by Otto in 1830[2] and later by Virchow in 1851.[3,4] Additionally, Virchow noted patterns of compensation in the skull to accommodate brain growth. He observed that growth in the skull was reduced in the plane perpendicular to the fused suture and increased in the plane parallel to it.[4] Virchow's observations became the principal guide to understanding craniosynostosis-related skull deformities for 100 years.

The importance of the prematurely fused calvarial suture in the development of cranial vault deformities was questioned by van der Klaauw in 1946[5] and later by Moss.[6,7] Moss based his criticisms on four basic findings: 1) Clinical observations showed occasional patency of a suspected premature suture despite a skull configuration that heralds the suture's stenosis; 2) characteristic cranial base abnormalities associated with an individual vault suture stenosis; 3) the experimental observation that removal of a normal cranial vault suture in the laboratory animal did not result in a significant change in overall skull shape; and 4) the cranial base develops and matures prior to the cranial vault.[8] Thus, Moss proposed that the cranial base was the locus of a primary abnormality that secondarily deformed the cranial vault.

However, despite these observations, the critical test to determine the role of premature closure of a cranial vault suture is to fuse the suture experimentally and then document alterations in cranial vault growth. Skull deformities have been documented following growth restriction of cranial vault sutures in animals.[9,10] With selective restriction of other individual cranial vault sutures, skull deformities have developed that closely mimic the clinical conditions of nonsyndromic craniosynostosis in humans.[11-13] Moreover, cranial base and facial deformities develop secondarily to cranial vault suture restrictions.[14] This suggests that cranial vault sutures probably play a major role in at least the development of the nonsyndromic craniosynostoses (i.e., metopic, coronal, sagittal, and lambdoid).

HYPOTHESIS

Regardless of the origin of the abnormalities that result in skull shape deformity, consistent patterns of deformity for individual vault suture stenosis do exist. However, it is clear that neither Virchow's nor Moss's clinical observations fully explain the range and pattern of abnormalities. Delashaw et al. undertook a retrospective analysis of patients with individual cranial vault suture stenosis to define fully the extent of abnormality in the cranial vault and to hypothesize the mechanism whereby these abnormalities may develop.[15] Through this analysis it has been found that all of the developed deformities in the skull may be explained by four basic tenets: 1) Cranial vault

bones directly adjacent to the prematurely fused suture act as a single (combined) bone plate with an overall reduced growth potential; 2) abnormal and asymmetric bone deposition occurs at vault sutures along the perimeter of a bone plate, with increased bone deposition occurring at the suture margin located further away from the plate; 3) nonperimeter sutures "in line" with a fused suture deposit bone symmetrically at their sutural edges; and 4) perimeter and abutting "in line" sutures nearest to the prematurely fused suture compensate with greater amounts of bone deposition than distant sutures. These observations help to delineate the full range of skull deformities so that the deformities may be more fully accounted for therapeutically.

PATIENT CLASSIFICATION

Individualization of surgical techniques has proven beneficial for the treatment of craniosynostosis. Emphasis has been placed on the location and degree of sutural involvement to determine the extent of cranial vault reshaping necessary for optimal results. However, in addition to the degree of sutural involvement, individualization also needs to be made according to the patient's age.[16] Two factors must be taken into account when considering patient age. First, under the age of 1 year, cranial vault bone is ordinarily easy to reshape using a number of techniques that will be described fully later. After 1 year, the calvarial bone becomes relatively brittle and a different set of approaches for reshaping bone must be undertaken.

The second consideration is that children under 3 years have a rapid rate of brain growth. Approximately 85% of total cranial vault and brain growth occurs by the age of 3 and bony remodeling must exclude fixation techniques that would impede brain growth.[17] Thus, the surgical treatment of craniosynostosis is generally divided into three treatment protocols according to age: 1) Children younger than 1 year, in whom significant brain growth remains and whose calvarial bone is malleable and amenable to large segment reshaping; 2) patients who are older than 3 years, in whom the reduced rate of brain growth allows more rigid fixation but whose brittle skull bone must be cut into smaller segments for adequate remodeling; and 3) children between 1 and 3 years, in whom the fixation techniques of the less than 1 year group must be employed but whose calvarial bone physical characteristics stipulate the remodeling methods used in the older than 3 years group.

METOPIC SYNOSTOSIS

Metopic synostosis is relatively uncommon and accounts for less than 10% of isolated suture, nonsyndromic craniosynostoses.[18,19] The metopic suture normally closes at approximately 2 years of age. However, when premature closure of the metopic suture occurs, the skull of the patient develops ridging of the stenotic metopic suture, flattening of the frontal bones, and flaring of the parietal bones, which results in a characteristic triangular shape. This triangular skull appearance, or trigonocephaly, is exaggerated by the lack of projection and flattening of the supraorbital rims laterally and narrowing of the temporal regions bilaterally. In addition, hypotelorism (reduction from the normal intercanthal distance) is a common facial characteristic of children with metopic synostosis.[20] The hypotelorism is often accompanied by elevation of both of the lateral canthi and the lateral portions of the eyebrows.

SURGICAL TECHNIQUES

Children Younger Than 1 Year

The term "early" metopic synostosis has been used to describe children aged less than 1 year. Surgical correction is performed with the patient in the supine position. A coronal incision is made bilaterally to the superior portion of each tragus. Dissection is carried out in the supraperiosteal plane, which is less vascular than the subperiosteal plane, to a level approximately 1 cm above the supraorbital ridges. An intact periosteum is advantageous because, by its adherence to the outer table of the skull, it permits better alignment of the bone fragments when the bone is being reshaped by fracture techniques. A horizontal periosteal incision is made above the orbital rims, and dissection continues in a subperiosteal fashion to expose the orbital rims superiorly, laterally, and inferiorly. When temporal narrowing and orbital rim hypoplasia are evident, the temporalis musculature adjacent to the lateral orbital rim is elevated subperiosteally and retracted posteriorly. Subperiosteal dissection is continued over the surface of the frontal process of the zygoma and the inferior orbital rim, ultimately exposing the lateral surface of the zygoma. A bifrontoparietal craniotomy is performed (Fig. 8.1A). Burr holes are placed in the pterional regions bilaterally and parasagittally. The frontal and anterior parietal bone is removed as a single bone graft. Following bilateral orbital roof osteotomies, an oblique osteotomy is made through the lateral orbital wall, below the level of the frontozygomatic suture (Fig. 8.1B). The portion of bone superior to the orbital wall osteotomy may be advanced over the inferior lip to project the lateral portion of the orbital rim anteriorly (Fig. 8.1B,C). The oblique cut serves to "lock" the advanced portion of the orbital rim in place.

The dura is plicated over the paramedian frontal lobes, which reduces the anterior prominence and encourages greater lateral convexity in the frontal region. "Barrel stave" osteotomies are made in the lateral sphenoid and squamous temporal regions bilaterally by performing parallel, vertically oriented osteotomies (Fig. 8.1D). The depth of the osteotomies is to the floor of the middle cranial fossa. The individual staves are then outfractured.

Reshaping the midline bony ridge in the glabellar region and on the bifrontoparietal bone graft is accomplished with a shaping burr on an air-driven power drill (Fig. 8.1E,F). The bifrontoparietal bone graft is remodeled by radial osteotomies (Fig. 8.1G). Controlled fractures using the mallet and Tessier rib-bender are employed adjunctively to attain the appropriate contour of the frontal bone (Fig. 8.1H). The bifrontal bone graft is secured with absorbable suture to the rostral supraorbital rims (Fig. 8.1I). This procedure creates a free-floating bone segment that permits anterior migration of the supraorbital rims as the brain enlarges. The temporalis muscle is rotated forward and attached to the lateral frontal bone and orbital rims.

Children Older Than 3 Years

In children older than 3 years, there is less concern about restrictive forces on brain growth; therefore more secure fixation may be elected. Likewise, the surgical techniques for reshaping bone are modified because the bone is less pliable. Thus, correction of metopic synostosis in the older than 3 years group relies on more direct reshaping and repositioning of formed bone segments and less on the "free-floating" bone concept.

Following supine positioning and a coronal incision, supraperiosteal dissection is carried out anteriorly to the level of the supraorbital rims. The temporalis muscle is elevated subperiosteally.

Deficiences in projection of the lateral frontal bone and supraorbital rims must be addressed; however, hypotelorism is rarely severe enough to require lateral orbital translocation. A bifrontal craniotomy is performed with burr hole placement as previously described (Fig. 8.2A). The bifrontoparietal bone graft is removed as a single bone segment, and the dura is plicated bifrontally adjacent to the midline. Barrel stave osteotomies are performed bilaterally in the squamous portion of the temporal bone and the lateral sphenoid wing (Fig. 8.2B). The individual staves are outfractured to achieve more lateral projection.

The supraorbital ridge recession in the older child is addressed by an orbital "C-shaped" osteotomy procedure.[21] After retracting the periorbita and frontal lobes, an orbital roof osteotomy is performed, extending from the junction of the medial and middle thirds of the orbital roof to the inferolateral portion of orbital rim (Fig. 8.2C). The osteotomy is made 5 to 10 mm posterior to the superior orbital rim. The orbital rim segments undergoing osteotomy are then "greenstick" fractured forward. Kerfs, or channels, are placed on the internal surface of the superior orbital rim, particularly laterally, to allow for bending of the orbital rim to a contour that is more convex anteriorly (see Fig. 8.2C). Bone grafts are placed between the inferolateral aspect of the orbit and the zygoma are secured in place using wire, bridging the osteotomy to the zygoma (see Fig. 8.2B). A lateral flange of sphenoid and temporal bone is left attached to the lateral orbital rim, which, when reshaped to a more convex form, augments the lateral projection of the temporal region (see Fig. 8.2C).

Remodeling of the frontoparietal region requires modification. The frontoparietal bone plate undergoes vertically oriented osteotomies in approximately 2 cm wide "slats" (Fig. 8.2D). Kerfs are placed on the inner table of the skull perpendicular to the plane of the osteotomy (see Fig. 8.2D). The slats are reshaped with the Tessier rib bender to achieve an appropriate contour and sutured together. These segments of bone are attached to the supraorbital rims using microfixation plates (Fig. 8.2E). Bone chips harvested from the parietal area are used to fill in the space posterior to the lateral orbital rim to prevent postoperative "hour-glass" deformity (see Fig. 8.2E). The temporalis muscle is translocated forward and attached to the superior lateral orbital rim (Fig. 8.2F).

Children 1 to 3 Years

In the child 1 to 3 years of age, the bony remodeling techniques are altered to allow reshaping of the more mature cranial vault. In this age group, bone tends to be more brittle and thus simple bending techniques are less effective. However, emphasis must still be placed on allowing free movement of bone to accommodate the growing brain.

The coronal incision, supraperiosteal dissection, bifrontal craniotomy, and dural plication are similar to the previous age groups. The midline prominence of the frontal bone in the region of the frontonasal suture is

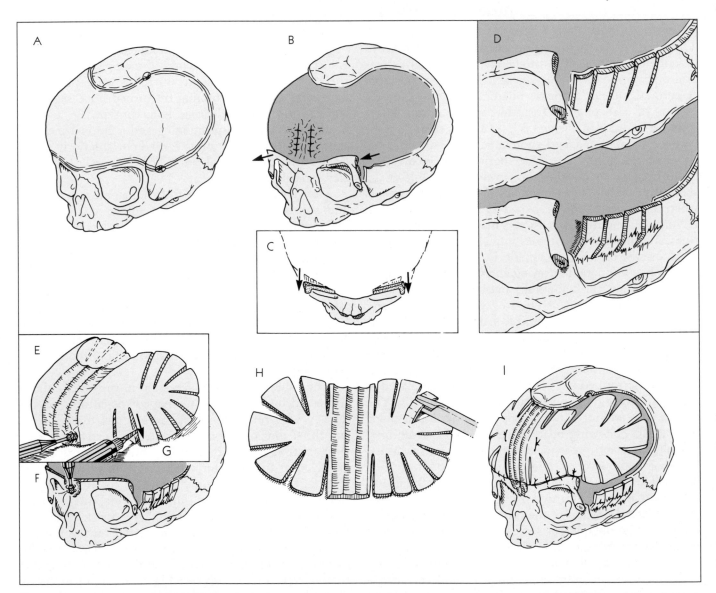

Figure 8.1 Metopic synostosis: children younger than 1 year. **(A)** A bifrontoparietal craniotomy is performed. **(B,C)** Orbital rim advancement technique used to address the orbital rim hypoplasia. **(D)** Barrel stave osteotomies are made in the lateral sphenoid and squamous temporal bone. The bony midline ridge is reduced on the bone graft **(E)** and in the glabellar region **(F)**. The bone graft undergoes radial osteotomies **(G)** and remodeling by controlled fractures **(H)**. **(I)** The remodeled bifrontoparietal bone is secured to the dura and the supraorbital rims. (Modified after Luce)

burred down (Fig. 8.3A). The bifrontoparietal bone graft undergoes vertically oriented osteotomies to create approximately 2 cm wide slats (Fig. 8.3B). Kerfs are placed on the inner table of the graft, oriented perpendicular to the plane of the osteotomy (Fig. 8.3C). The slats may then be remodeled to flatten the anterior parasagittal region and, conversely, to increase the convexity of the frontal bone laterally. The bone graft that has undergone osteotomy is pieced together using absorbable suture to the desired skull shape (Fig. 8.3D). Barrel stave osteotomies are performed in the squamous portion of the temporal bone and sphenoid wing bilaterally. The individual staves are outfractured using the Tessier rib-bender to increase lateral skull prominence.

Recession of the supraorbital rim is addressed with a modified C-shaped osteotomy similar to that described in children over 3 years (Fig. 8.3E,F). In modification of this technique the stacked bone grafts are attached to the inferolateral aspect of the advanced orbital rim but not posteriorly to the zygoma (Fig. 8.3G). This allows support of the advanced orbital rim but also allows the rim to free-float with subsequent brain growth.

The rostral portion of the bone flap is attached with wire to the remodeled orbital rim. However, the posterior frontal and anterior parietal bones are allowed to float free (Fig 8.3H). A gap of approximately 5 mm between the intact parietal bone and the remodeled bifrontoparietal bone graft is desirable, and removal of

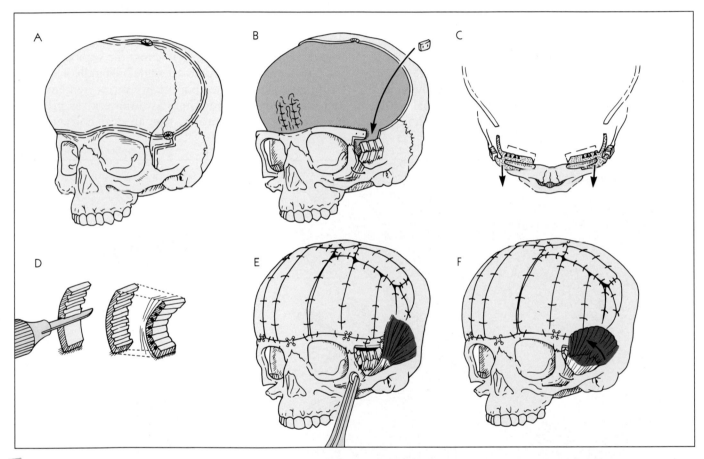

Figure 8.2 Metopic synostosis: children older than 3 years. (**A**) A bifrontoparietal craniotomy is performed with a lateral flange of sphenoid and temporal bone left attached to the lateral orbital rim. (**B,C**) Barrel stave osteotomies are made temporally and the orbital rim is advaced using a C-shaped osteotomy procedure. (**D**) The bifrontoparietal bone graft is remodeled by use of vertical osteotomies and kerfs. (**E**) Remodeled bony slats are sutured together and attached to the supraorbital rims using microfixation plates. (**F**) The temporalis muscle is attached to the supraorbital rim. (Modified after Luce)

parietal bone with rongeurs may be necessary. The temporalis muscle is advanced and secured to the lateral rim of the orbit and the frontal bone.

CORONAL SYNOSTOSIS

Synostosis of the coronal suture may involve all or a portion of the suture. Varying degrees of involvement of the coronal suture result in distinctly different skull shape abnormalities.

Clinically, the patient with unilateral coronal synostosis is characterized by ridging of the prematurely fused half of the coronal suture, flattening of the ipsilateral frontal (including supraorbital rim) and parietal bones, bulging of the ipsilateral squamous portion of the temporal bone, and bulging of the contralateral, frontal, and parietal bones. The orbits are asymmetric, with narrowing of the mediolateral dimension and widening of the vertical dimension ipsilateral to the fused suture as compared to the contralateral side. Radiographically, in addition to sutural sclerosis, the harlequin abnormality (relative elevation of the greater wing of the sphenoid bone

ipsilateral to the fused suture) is present. Basal CT scan demonstrates narrowing of the sphenopetrosal angle ipsilateral to the fused coronal suture and deviation of the anterior cranial base from the midline toward the side of the fused suture.

The patient with bilateral coronal synostosis has a characteristic clinical appearance that includes ridging of the coronal suture bilaterally, flattening of the caudal portion of the frontal bones and supraorbital ridges, and bulging of the cephalad portions of the frontal bones. The squamous portion of the temporal bone is excessively prominent and the vertex of the skull is more anteriorly situated and normal. The skull takes on the turribrachycephalic, or "tower-shaped" skull appearance. The diagnosis of bilateral coronal synostosis is made largely clinically but supported radiographically, showing sclerosis of the coronal suture associated with the bilateral harlequin deformity of the greater wings of the sphenoid bones. CT scan demonstrates bony fusion across the sutural margins and a narrowed sphenopetrosal angle bilaterally.

Because skull shape abnormality varies tremendously depending on whether there is unilateral or bilateral involvement of the suture, the surgical correction of

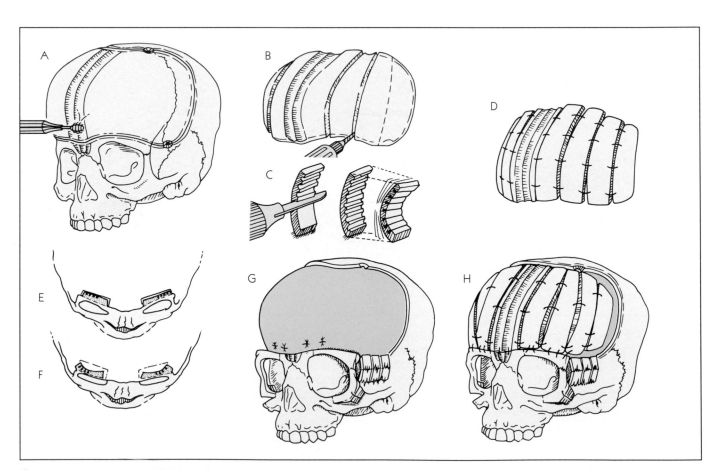

Figure 8.3 Metopic synostosis: children 1 to 3 years. **(A)** A similar bifrontoparietal craniotomy is made with reduction of the midline bony ridge. **(B–D)** The calvarial bone is remodeled with the "slat-and-kerf" technique for more mature bone. **(E,F)** The orbital rim is advanced with a C-shaped osteotomy.

(G) Stacked bone grafts support the advanced orbital rim but are attached only to the zygoma anteriorly. **(H)** The bifrontoparietal bone graft is secured anteriorly; rigid fixation is avoided in this age group. (Modified after Luce)

these abnormalities is individualized. The timing of surgery in patients with coronal synostosis is optimally within the first few weeks or months of life, so as to reduce potential deleterious effects of increased intracranial pressure on brain growth and take advantage of the ameliorative effect on skull shape by the remaining normal growth of the brain.[22] As in other forms of craniosynostosis treatment, a distinction is made between children under 1 year, 1 to 3 years, and over 3 years with respect to bone remodeling and fixation techniques.

SURGICAL TECHNIQUES

Unilateral Coronal Synostosis: Children Younger Than 1 Year

The patient is placed in the supine position on the operating table, and the face is prepped into the field in order to judge orbital and frontal symmetry intraoperatively. A coronal incision with supraperiosteal dissection is performed. Burr holes are placed bilaterally at the pterion and parasagittally (Fig. 8.4A). If the anterior fontanelle is patent, entry into the epidural space may be gained at the fontanelle's margin in the place of a separate burr

hole. A bifrontal craniotomy incorporating the coronal suture is performed (see Fig. 8.4A). In young patients, a bifrontal craniotomy yielding a solid single bone segment may not be possible due to patency of the metopic suture. This patency allows the two frontal bone segments to be independently mobile. However, if the periosteum is left intact, this helps to tether the bone segments and keep them in relative alignment.

Ipsilateral to the fused coronal suture, the greater wing of the sphenoid bone is thickened and displaced superiorly. This thickened sphenoid bone is rongeured away to the level of the lateral superior orbital fissure (Fig. 8.4B). This removes the lateral aspect of the abnormal basal portion of the "coronal ring" (i.e., the frontosphenoid suture) and may increase intraorbital volume. The orbit ipsilateral to the fused suture is shortened in the mediolateral dimension. The superior rim is augmented by interposition, and onlay bone grafts are placed following osteotomy in the roof and lateral orbital wall (Fig. 8.4C). Since the superior orbital rim is often displaced cephalad compared to the contralateral side, the rim is placed in a caudal position to equal the height of the opposite orbital rim. The orbital rim is advanced

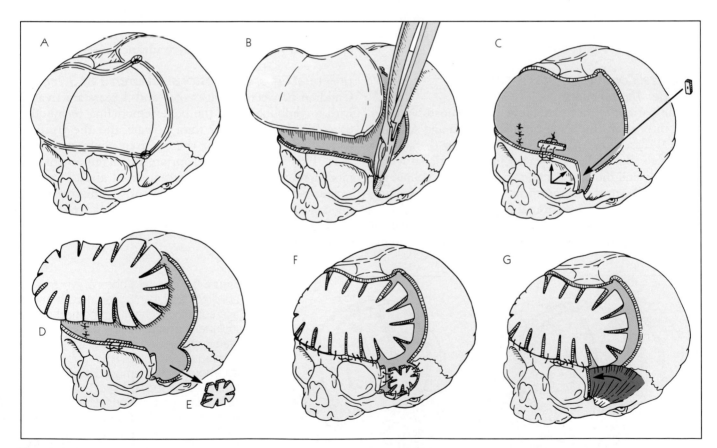

Figure 8.4 Unilateral coronal synostosis: children younger than 1 year. **(A,B)** A bifrontal craniotomy is performed and the thickened sphenoid wing is removed. **(C)** The "ipsilateral" orbital dimension discrepancy with the contralateral orbital rim is corrected using orbital roof and lateral wall osteotomies supported with superior orbital rim interposition and poste rior orbital rim onlay bone grafts. **(D)** The bifrontal bone graft is remodeled with radial osteotomies and controlled fractures. **(E,F)** The squamous portion of the temporal bone undergoes craniotomy and is remodeled and attached anteriorly, posteriorly, and inferiorly. **(G)** The temporalis muscle is attached anteriorly to the superior orbital rim. (Modified after Luce)

to a slightly overcorrected position but is not rigidly fixed to the cranial base or to the posterior body of the zygoma. Rather, bone grafts harvested from the parietal region are inserted posteriorly to the advanced orbital rim to support its advanced position (Fig. 8.4C).

The dura is plicated in the frontal region contralateral to the fused suture to yield frontal symmetry (see Fig. 8.4C). Radial osteotomies are placed into the center of the convex "contralateral" (to the fused suture) frontal bone and the flattened "ipsilateral" frontal and parietal bones (Fig. 8.4D). Each bone graft (or single bone graft if metopic suture is closed) is remodeled by controlled fractures using the Tessier rib-bender to achieve the desired form. The squamous portion of the temporal bone ipsilateral to the fused suture is removed by osteotomy and also cut radially to allow for recontouring (Fig. 8.4E). The temporal bone is attached by absorbable suture to the surrounding bone anteriorly, inferiorly, and posteriorly to deter recurrence of temporal bulging (Fig. 8.4F). The bifrontal bone plate is attached to the orbital rims superiorly and laterally but is not reattached posteriorly to the parietal bone (see Fig. 8.4F). A rim of parietal bone approximately 5 to 10 mm wide is excised to create, in effect, a "neo"-coronal suture. The temporalis muscle is reflected anteriorly to fill in the gap between the advanced orbital rim and the squamous portion of the temporal bone (Fig. 8.4G).

Unilateral Coronal Synostosis: Children Older Than 3 Years

In the patient with unilateral coronal synostosis, older than three years, the same coronal incision and supraperiosteal dissection is carried out to develop the anterior scalp flap. Burr holes are placed in the pterional region bilaterally and the parasagittal region medially behind the hairline. A frontal craniotomy is performed, leaving approximately 5 mm of frontal bone height cephalad to the apex of the orbital rim. The frontal dura contralateral to the fused suture is plicated in the area of excess frontal

prominence. A C-shaped osteotomy of the orbital rim ipsilateral to the fused suture is then performed as described earlier (Fig. 8.5A). The orbital rim is advanced to a slightly overcorrected position compared to the contralateral side. The hollow region, posterior to the advanced rim is filled in with bone chips harvested from parietal bone and either a split or a full segment cranial bone graft (Fig. 8.5B). The bulging in the squamous portion of the temporal bone is addressed by elevating this bone by craniotomy and radially cutting it (see Fig. 8.5A). Kerfs are oriented transverse to the radial osteotomies on the concave surface of the bone. The dura is plicated locally, and the bone is flattened by mallet and returned in place.

The frontal bone is cut into vertically oriented "slats" approximately 2 cm in width (see Fig. 8.5A). Periosteum that has been allowed to remain intact on the external surface aids in alignment of this more brittle bone when controlled fracture procedures are necessary. Kerfs are placed transversely to the long axes of the bony slats intracranially to allow more accurate remodeling of the bone in achievement of frontal symmetry (see Fig. 8.5A). The newly shaped frontal bone is then attached to the supraorbital rims and to the more posteriorly located temporal and parietal bones (see Fig. 8.5A). This more rigid fixation is acceptable since the child's brain and cranial vault growth is more advanced.

Unilateral Coronal Synostosis: Children 1 to 3 Years

Children between the ages of 1 and 3 years are treated with a combination of the bone remodeling techniques used for children older than 3 years and the fixation techniques described for the children younger than 1 year. This will allow appropriate management of the more mature calvarial bone encountered after 1 year of age (as described for metopic synostosis). The free-floating concept is employed and rigid fixation is avoided due to the rapid brain and skull growth that is ongoing during this age range.

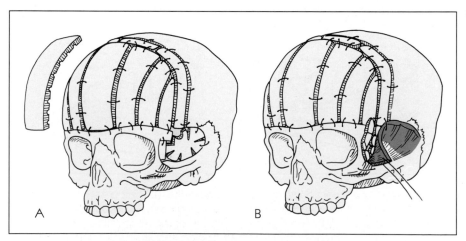

Figure 8.5 Unilateral coronal synostosis: children older than 3 years. Notable age-adjusted technique modifications include: the more mature bifrontal bone graft is remodeled with "slat-and-kerf" techniques, a minimal amount of lateral sphenoid wing is removed, the orbital rims are advanced using a C-shaped osteotomy, and fixation techniques are more rigid (**A**). Additional bone grafts are placed in the region of the pterion to prevent postoperative hollowing (**B**). (Modified after Luce)

Bilateral Coronal Synostosis: Children Younger Than 1 Year

In order to correct the full range of abnormalities associated with bilateral coronal synostosis, it will be necessary to place the patient in the modified prone position to address both the frontal and occipital abnormalities. Before placing the patient in this position, however, it is important to assess the stability of the cervical spine and determine whether craniovertebral junction anomalies exist preoperatively. Significant anomalies such as the Chiari malformation may preclude positioning in this manner. Positioning of the patient on the operating table is greatly aided by a vacuum-stiffened beanbag used adjunctively with the anterior segment of a Philadelphia collar (Philadelphia Collar, Westville, NJ).

A coronal incision is made extending to the pretragal regions bilaterally. A supraperiosteal dissection is performed to expose the frontoparietal and occipital regions bilaterally. A transversely oriented periosteal incision is placed 1 cm above the orbital rims, and then a subperiosteal dissection of the mediosuperior and lateral orbital rims is performed. The temporalis musculature is elevated out of the temporal fossa and the occipital musculature from the nuchal line in the occipital bone to the level of the superior rim of the foramen magnum caudally.

Burr holes are placed in the pterional region bilaterally and parasagittally in the anterior parietal bone just posterior to the coronal suture (Fig. 8.6A). Similarly, a biparietooccipital bone graft is outlined with multiple burr holes adjacent to the sagittal and transverse sinuses (see Fig. 8.6A). If the metopic or sagittal sutures are widely patent and preclude the elevation of the frontal or parietal occipital bones as a single piece, separate frontal or parietooccipital bone grafts should be elevated on each half of the skull. Once the bone is elevated both frontally and parietooccipitally, further dissection may be carried out below the level of the transverse sinus to allow the placement of barrel stave osteotomies in the occipital bone, 1 to 2 cm above the level of the foramen magnum medially and 2 to 4 cm laterally (see Fig. 8.6A). Outfracturing of the barrel staves enlarges the anteroposterior axis of the skull locally, which allows brain and dural displacement into this region as the height of the skull is reduced. The barrel stave osteotomies in the occipital bone in the

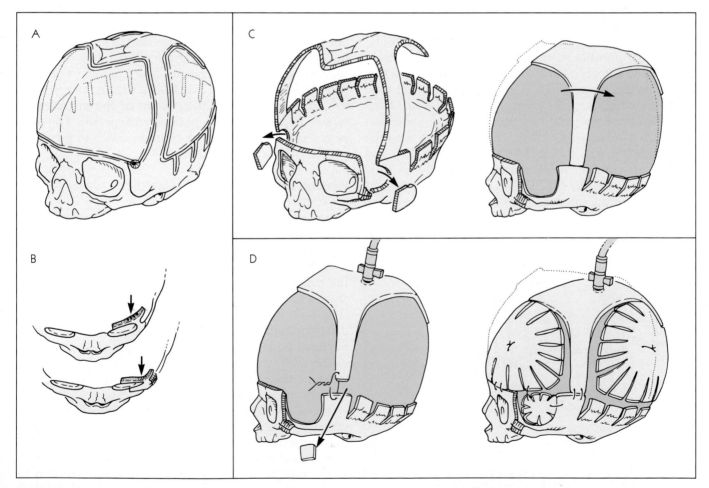

Figure 8.6 Bilateral coronal synostosis: children younger than 1 year. Bifrontal and biparietooccipital bone grafts are developed with a bony bridge left between the hemicrania; barrel stave osteotomies placed in the remaining occipital bone (A). (B) The orbital rims are advanced by C-shaped osteotomy. (C) The vertex of the skull is shifted posteriorly by severing the parietal bone struts and relocating them posteriorly. (D) Skull height is reduced by removing a segment of bone from the inferior portion of the parietal strut, cinching the basal and parietal bone segments together while intracranial pressure is monitored. (Modified after Luce)

median and paramedian regions are longer than those placed further laterally to achieve elongation of the anteroposterior axis of the skull without further widening of the parietoocciput. The individual staves are fractured outwardly at the base of the skull and then inwardly at their distal aspect so as not to create a pressure point on the overlying scalp.

In the lateral sphenoid region, the thickened and abnormally elevated superior portions of the sphenoid bone are removed by rongeur to the level of the lateral supraorbital fissure. With this bone removal, the basal extension of the coronal suture and the laterofrontal sphenoid suture is removed. C-shaped osteotomies are performed bilaterally to increase orbital rim projection (Fig. 8.6B). The advanced orbital rims are held forward by parietal bone grafts that are wedged in the osteotomy site in the body of the zygoma and secured to the rim anteriorly (see Fig. 8.6B). A craniotomy is performed to remove the abnormal convex squamous portion of the temporal bone (Fig. 8.6C). The bone is reshaped by a combination of radial osteotomies into the center of the convexity and controlled fractures of the bone segments with the Tessier rib bender. The dura is plicated bilaterally, and the temporal bone is returned to be secured to the surrounding skull base posteriorly and inferiorly (Fig. 8.6D).

Prior to reduction of the skull height, a fiber-optic intracranial pressure monitor is placed through a twist drill hole in the right paramedian parietal bone (see Fig. 8.6D). At this juncture, one is left with two parietal bone struts extending from the vertex of the skull to the basal portions of the temporal and parietal bones. These two bony struts are severed at their caudal interface with the skull base (see Fig. 8.6C). The vertex of the skull and bony struts are then slowly shifted posteriorly approximately 1 to 2 cm (see Fig. 8.6C). The shift is performed in order to reduce the bulging contour of the dura in the

superofrontal region and to replace posteriorly the elevated vertex point, which has become displaced anteriorly. The wire passed through drill holes in the struts and basal skull is slowly cinched down over 30 to 60 minutes and the intracranial pressure is continuously monitored under conditions of normocapnia and normotension (see Fig. 8.6D). We currently recommend that while the cranial vault is undergoing this reduction in height, cerebral perfusion pressure of approximately 60 mm Hg be maintained. During initial stages of height reduction, however, it is not unusual for intracranial pressures to be elevated greater than 20 mm Hg for short periods of time. If the surgeon does not observe a rapid reduction in intracranial pressure over a course of 1 to 2 minutes, then a smaller increment in reduction of cranial vault height is necessary over a longer period of time. Caution must be exercised during this maneuver to prevent brain injury.

While the incremental skull height reduction process is being achieved, the frontal and parietal bone segments can be remodeled to the desired contour. Radial osteotomies in the frontal and parietooccipital bones allow reshaping by a series of controlled fractures with the mallet and Tessier rib bender. After completion of the frontal bone reshaping, it is reattached to the orbital rims bilaterally (see Fig. 8.6D). The posterior aspect of the frontal bone is not secured and is allowed to free-float. The parietooccipital bone graft is attached to the surrounding dura after shortening the occipital bone to allow a gap of 5 to 10 mm between bone edges (see Fig. 8.6D). This is done in order to encourage further displacement of the neurocranial capsule posteriorly in the postoperative period. The temporalis muscle is advanced forward to attach to the lateral portion of the supraorbital rim.

Bilateral Coronal Synostosis: Children Older Than 3 Years

The patient with bilateral coronal synostosis who is older than 3 years is treated similarly in terms of positioning and craniotomy lines to those under 1 year.

Following bifrontal and biparietooccipital craniotomy, the orbital rims are advanced forward using the C-shaped orbital osteotomy technique described previously (Fig. 8.7). Barrel stave osteotomies are performed in the parietooccipital region, with the individual staves being fractured posteriorly to elongate the anteroposterior axis of the skull (see Fig. 8.7). The squamous portion of the temporal bone is removed by craniotomy. The cephalocaudally oriented parietal bone struts extending from the vertex of the skull are severed at the level of the caudal extent of the craniotomy. An intracranial pressure monitor is inserted in the right parietal bone. The parietal bone struts are displaced approximately 1 to 2 cm posteriorly, and the height of the skull is slowly reduced by cinching down on the wire loops in the basal, parietal, and squamous temporal bones. We have noted that it requires a longer time for elevated intracranial pressure reduction to occur in the older children when compared to similar incremental reduction in vault height in younger children.[22] Therefore, smaller increments of

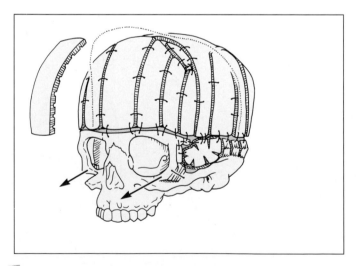

Figure 8.7 Bilateral coronal synostosis: children older than 3 years. Age-adjusted technique modifications include: bone graft remodeling by the "slat-and-kerf" method and more rigid fixation of the calvarial bone grafts and the advanced orbital rims. (Modified after Luce)

adjustment should be anticipated over a longer period of time. The cerebral perfusion pressure should be maintained at approximately 60 mm Hg under conditions of normocapnia and normotension.

The frontal and parietooccipital bone grafts are then cut into vertically oriented slats approximately 2 cm in width, leaving the periosteum attached to the external surface of the skull bone (see Fig. 8.7). Transversely oriented kerfs are placed through the inner table of the skull and controlled fractures are performed on the slats for reshaping. The individual bone segments are wired or sutured with long-acting absorbable suture to give the desired form (see Fig. 8.7). Due to its thinness, the temporal bone can ordinarily be molded by radial osteotomies and kerfing on the inner table without cutting the bone into slats (see Fig. 8.7). This allows easier fixation to the basal skull posteriorly and inferiorly. Bone chips from the parietal region are used to fill in the temporal hollow behind the advanced orbital rim and the temporalis muscle is transferred anteriorly and attached to the supralateral orbital rim. Patients who are over 3 years may have their bone fixed in a slightly overcorrected position to allow for further brain growth yet still provide the stability necessary for reconstruction of the skull.

Bilateral Coronal Synostosis: Children 1 to 3 Years
The child who is 1 to 3 years old with bilateral coronal synostosis is positioned in the modified prone position, and frontal and parietooccipital craniotomies are performed. The orbital rims are advanced using the C-shaped osteotomy procedure, but the rim is not fixed to the cranial base. The squamous portion of the temporal bone is remodeled and made planar, rather than convex, and secured to the posterior and inferior aspects of the osteotomy margin in the temporal region. The frontal and parietooccipital bone grafts are cut into slats, and controlled fractures are created at the abnormal curvature sites.

Fixation is different in these patients when compared to those who are older than 3 years because the frontal slats are secured only to the supraorbital rim anteriorly and laterally to each other but not posteriorly along the course of the coronal suture. After remodeling, the parietal bone is reattached with long-acting absorbable suture. The parietooccipital bone, however, is attached primarily to the underlying dura, leaving a gap of approximately 1 cm between the occipital barrel staves and the posterior margin of the parietooccipital bone graft.

SAGITTAL SYNOSTOSIS
Premature closure of the sagittal suture throughout its course typically results in a long, narrow skull. More focal deformities can result from only the anterior or posterior half of the sagittal suture fusing prematurely. In anterior sagittal synostosis, the anterior portion of the parietal bones is restricted in lateral growth, which results in a compensatory frontal bulge. Enhanced bony deposition of the occipital bone at the lambdoid suture creates the occipital prominence of posterior sagittal synostosis without an associated significant anterior cranial vault deformity.

Successful surgical correction of sagittal synostosis skull deformity includes consideration of two factors: the degree of skull shape abnormality and, as previously described, the patient's age. Whereas partial stenosis of the sagittal suture may result in frontal or occipital compensatory bulging, in addition to biparietal narrowing, complete sagittal suture stenosis characteristically results in frontal and occipital abnormalities. In this case, both regions of restrictive and compensatory vault abnormality (i.e., the whole cranial vault) need to be reshaped to achieve a normal cranial form.

SURGICAL TECHNIQUES
Children Younger Than 1 Year
In children less than 1 year of age, the patient is placed in a modified prone position on the operating room table, allowing simultaneous access to the frontal and occipital regions. A coronal incision is made and a supraperiosteal dissection is performed from the region of the glabella anteriorly to the region of the posterior lip of the foramen magnum posteriorly. Burr holes are placed bilaterally at the pterion and the paramedian position posterior to the coronal suture. A bifrontal craniotomy is performed and separate parietal craniotomies follow (Fig. 8.8A). A biparietooccipital craniotomy completes the exposure.

A major residual abnormality present in skull shape is flattening in the low temporal and parietal regions. To correct this, barrel stave osteotomies are placed in the lateral sphenoid bone, squamous portion of the temporal bone, and low parietal bone (see Fig. 8.8A). The bone is fractured outward to increase the flare in the basal skull (Fig. 8.8B). The occipital bone is remodeled by radial osteotomy to weaken the perimeter of the bone (see Fig. 8.8B). Using a mallet and Tessier rib bender, the bone is reshaped to reduce the acutely angled, conelike appearance and make it more blunted. This achieves two objectives: It restores normal contour and it increases the capacity of the occiput to allow subsequent shifting of the cranium posterolaterally.

The bifrontal bone graft is similarly remodeled, expanding the frontal bone laterally to increase the flare toward the temporal region (Fig. 8.8C). In order to allow posterior angulation of the protuberant frontal bone, a triangular wedge of frontal bone is removed laterally to allow this posterior inclination (see Fig. 8.8C). This is similar to a technique used by Marchac and Renier in dealing with more mature scaphalocephalic bone.[23]

Active shortening of the anterior-posterior dimension of the skull is performed next to achieve two goals: immediate improvement in skull shape and encouragement of secondary increase in convex lateral projection of the neurocranial capsule in the parietal region. Approximately 1 to 1.5 cm of bone is removed from the anterior portion of the parietal bone overlying the sagittal sinus.

Stripping of the sagittal sinus beneath the anterior surface of the parietal bone is performed in order to allow shifting of the sagittal sinus without kinking (see Fig. 8.8B).

The remaining parietal bone undergoes radial osteotomy and contouring to conform to the greater convexity in the parietal area. The parietal bone grafts are shortened to create "neosagittal" sutures to be developed adjacent to the true sagittal suture. Fixation of the parietal bone graft is to the dura alone, for the purpose of orientation and not for rigid fixation (see Fig. 8.8C). The goal is to allow this area to become a region of lesser resistance to lateral migration of bone with further brain development.

Children Older Than 3 Years
The patient is placed in the modified prone position. A coronal incision is made and the supraperiosteal dissection is carried to the level of the orbits anteriorly and to the lip of the foramen magnum posteriorly. Burr holes are placed in the pterional region bilaterally and posterior to the hairline frontally (Fig. 8.9A). A bifrontal craniotomy is performed. The parietal bone is removed as two separate bone plates. Subsequently, a parietooccipital craniotomy is performed. Lateral barrel stave osteotomies are placed in the temporoparietal region of the skull with outward fracturing of this basal skull bone (Fig. 8.9B).

The occipital bone ordinarily may be remodeled by placing radially oriented osteotomies into the large section of bone (see Fig. 8.9B). Kerfs are placed on the intracranial surface of the bone perpendicular to the long axis of the parietal bone strips. This facilitates the bending and reshaping of the parietooccipital area by selective weakening of the bone. After the occipital bone has been reshaped to a more rounded form, it is again secured with suture fixation (see Fig. 8.9B). The bifrontal bone is remodeled by removing triangular wedges of bone laterally to allow for posterior tilting of the protuberant frontal bone (Fig. 8.9C). The lateral portion of the

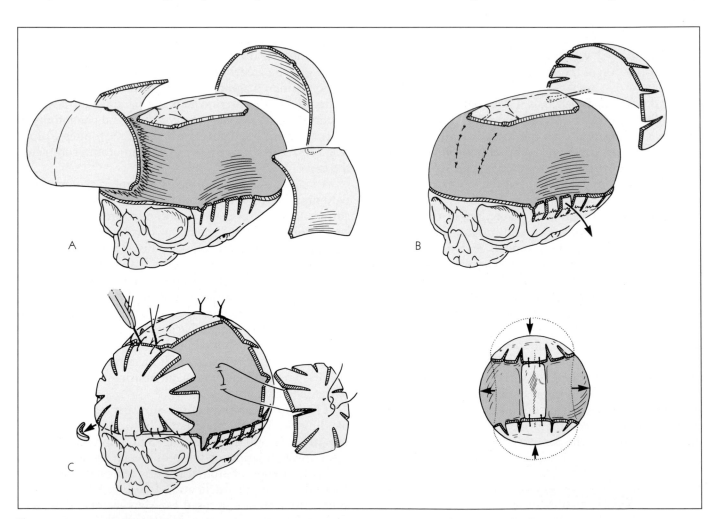

Figure 8.8 Sagittal synostosis: children younger than 1 year. (A) Bifrontal, separate parietal, and biparietooccipital craniotomies are performed and lateral barrel stave osteotomies are placed in the low temporal bone region. (B) The "barrel staves" are fractured outwardly; paramedian frontal dura is plicated; the midline parietal bone is separated from the sagittal sinus to avoid sinus kinking while reducing the anteroposterior dimension of the skull; and the biparietooccipital bone is remodeled using radial osteotomies and controlled fractures. (C) Reduction in the anteroposterior skull is achieved by removing a segment of midline frontal bone; triangular wedges of frontal bone are removed cephalad to the supraorbital margins to allow for posterior inclination of the forehead. (Modified after Luce)

frontal bone receives intracranial kerfs to allow more lateral bending without gross fracture. A sagittal segment of parietal bone is removed to allow active anteroposterior shortening of the cranial vault. The parietal bone is cut into slats approximately 2 cm in width. This aids in the precision of bone remodeling to achieve more accurately the desired skull shape. In addition, segments of parietal bone are added to the inferior portion of the slats to allow more of an increase in the lateral convexity (see Fig. 8.9C). This bone is obtained from the shortening of the anteroposterior dimensions of the skull and is used as a full-thickness graft. The bone is fixed in position with suture and wire with an over-correction allowing for remaining brain growth (Fig. 8.9D).

Children 1 to 3 Years
In the child 1 to 3 years of age, the bony remodeling techniques are changed to allow full reshaping of the more mature cranial vault. In this group, however, emphasis still must be placed on allowing free movement of bone to accommodate the growing brain.

The patient is placed in the modified prone position, a coronal incision is made, and supraperiosteal dissection of scalp flaps is performed to the glabella anteriorly and to the lip of the foramen magnum posteriorly. A submuscular dissection is performed temporally and occipi-

tally. Bifrontal, parietal, and occipital craniotomies are performed as described earlier for the child older than 3 years. Lateral barrel stave osteotomies are placed in the inferolateral, temporal, and parietal bones, as well as in the lateral portion of the sphenoid bone.

The occipital and frontal bones are remodeled (as in the patient older than 3 years) with lateral triangular wedges removed from the frontal bone with lateral bending performed before angulation of the frontal bone posteriorly to shorten the anteroposterior axis of the skull. The occipital bone is cut radially and kerfs are placed on the intracranial surface to allow a more controlled bending of the bone segments laterally. The bone grafts are secured only in the midline from the frontal to the occipital region. Lateral bending is performed in the individual posterior, frontal, and anterior and posterior parietal struts. The inferolateral portions of the parietal bones are removed to allow for further postoperative migration of the brain into the parietal region.

LAMBDOID SYNOSTOSIS
There are three basic components of lambdoid synostosis deformities: 1) the occipital abnormality, where flattening occurs unilaterally or bilaterally, depending on

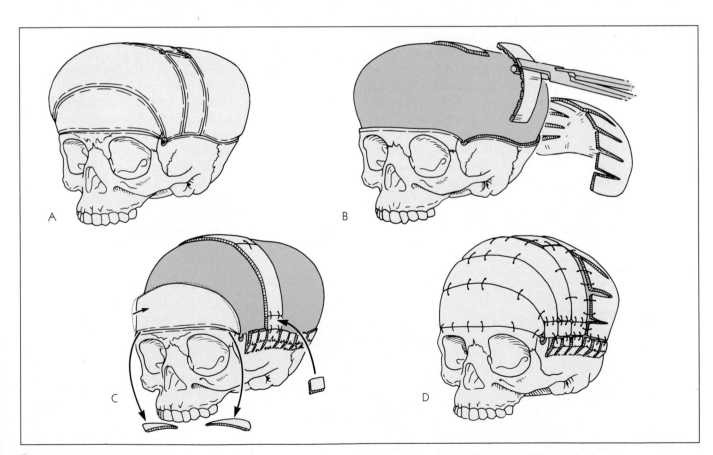

Figure 8.9 Sagittal synostosis: children older than 3 years. (A–D) Age-adjusted technique modifications include calvarial remodeling by the "slat-and-kerf" method, more rigid fixation techniques, and the addition of segments of parietal bone to increase the lateral convexity. (Modified after Luce)

whether the lambdoid suture is fused unilaterally or bilaterally, 2) asymmetric or symmetric frontal bulging, and/or 3) elevation of the absolute height of the skull. The treatment of lambdoid synostosis varies as to whether the condition is unilateral or bilateral, but the operative exposure and craniotomy lines are similar. As a result, the treatment of both unilateral and bilateral lambdoid synostosis will be addressed simultaneously.

Due to the tendency of severe lambdoid synostosis to present early and more mild deformity to go unrecognized or untreated, our experience with treatment of lambdoid synostosis after 1 year of age is very limited. However, a general description of the surgical correction follows, and one may apply the principles of age-adjusted treatment previously described to an older population.

SURGICAL TECHNIQUE

If the cranial vault abnormalities are confined to the parietooccipital area, the patient is placed in the prone position and a coronal incision is carried out to a level just above the pinna bilaterally. Dissection is performed in a supraperiosteal plane. The plane of dissection is extended subperiosteally at the origin of the occipital muscles and is carried down to the level of the lip of the foramen magnum posteriorly. This exposure allows full visualization of the occipital bone abnormality. For either asymmetric (unilateral) and symmetric (bilateral) deformity, burr holes are placed in the paramedian position in the posteroparietal bone and superior to the level of the transverse sinus (Fig. 8.10). A bilateral parietooccipital bone segment is elevated with the caudal extent reaching approximately 1 cm above the level of the transverse sinus. Barrel stave osteotomies are performed laterally in the flattened basal occipital bone to increase convex projection of the occipital bone locally (see Fig. 8.10). In patients with moderate unilateral lambdoid synostosis deformity, the barrel staves are placed primarily ipsilateral to the fused suture in the occipital bone. In more severe cases, bilateral barrel stave osteotomies are performed, infracturing the abnormally convex portion and outfracturing the flattened portion of occipital bone.

The biparietooccipital bone graft is cut radially and remodeled with the Tessier rib bender to achieve a normally rounded and symmetrical posterior skull (see Fig. 8.10). The dura is plicated in areas of excess projection prior to bone remodeling to assist in achieving bone symmetry. The bone graft is replaced and secured to the dura without attaching it to surrounding bone. A 5 to 10 mm gap is created at the posterior margin of the parietooccipital bone graft to simulate a "neolambdoid" suture.

If the parietooccipital abnormality is accompanied by a frontal abnormality, the patient is placed in the modified prone position so that both anterior and posterior skull abnormalities may be addressed simultaneously. A coronal incision is made and supraperiosteal dissection carried out to the level of the supraorbital rims anteriorly and the occipital musculature posteriorly. The parietooccipital bone is exposed by subperiosteal and submuscular dissection as described above.

To correct the frontal bone abnormality, a bifrontal craniotomy is performed. Characteristically, the frontal bone is mildly protuberant ipsilateral to the fused lambdoid suture. Burr holes are placed bilaterally at the pterion and one burr hole is placed parasagittally posterior to the coronal suture. The dura is plicated in the frontal and parietooccipital regions with abnormal convexity. The frontal and parietooccipital bone grafts are remodeled by radial osteotomies and controlled fracturing with the Tessier rib bender to develop normal symmetry. The frontal bone is secured to the orbital rims using long-acting absorbable suture. The parietooccipital bone is attached only to the dura to maintain the correct orientation of the bone graft. Allowing the parietooccipital bone to free-float offers less resistance to displacement and encourages further bone projections occipitally.

If frontal and parietooccipital abnormalities are accompanied by turricephaly (abnormally tall skull), the abnormal height may be reduced by a combination of techniques. The patient is placed in the modified prone position and frontal and parietooccipital craniotomies are performed as described above (Fig. 8.11). Barrel stave osteotomies are made in the occipital region and outfractured. In addition, the midparietal bone struts that

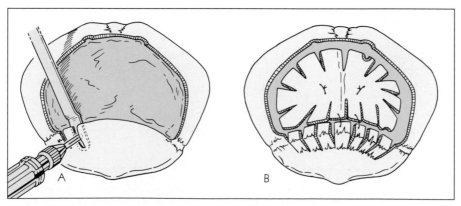

Figure 8.10 Lambdoid synostosis. (A,B) Barrel stave osteotomies are performed in the occipital bone to increase projection ipsilateral to the fused suture(s). A retractor is used to protect the transverse and sagittal sinuses during osteotomies. (A) The parietooccipital bone graft is remodelled following weakening radial osteotomies. (Modified after Luce)

remain attached to the vertex of the skull are severed basally as in correction of skull height abnormalities in coronal synostosis (see Fig. 8.11). An intracranial pressure monitor is placed in the parietal bone strut and the height of the skull is gradually reduced by cinching down on wire placed through the bone in the basal skull to achieve a normal configuration (see Fig. 8.11). There is no need for shifting of the vertex of the skull either anteriorly or posteriorly in lambdoid synostosis, as we have not observed displacement of the vertex to be a feature of this deformity. The degree of height reduction is usually less than 10 mm. Final contouring of the bifrontal or biparietooccipital bone grafts is made after skull height

reduction. The bone grafts are reshaped by radial osteotomies and controlled fractures using the Tessier rib bender. Fixation of bone grafts is secured anteriorly and free-floating posteriorly. A neolambdoid suture is created by leaving a gap of 5 to 10 mm between the posteroparietal and anteroooccipital bones.

As previously mentioned, our experience with treatment of lambdoid synostosis after 1 year of age is restricted. However, one may apply the principles of age-adjusted treatment previously described to this older population. Specifically, remodeling of more brittle bone would be done by use of the "slat-and-kerf" technique as opposed to the radial osteotomies and controlled fractures used in the younger age group. Fixation of remodeled bone to the cranial base should be restricted until the age of three.

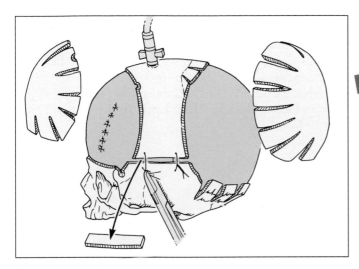

Figure 8.11 Lambdoid synostosis with significant turribrachycephaly. Following bifrontal and biparietooccipital craniotomies and creation of basal occipital barrel staves, the height of the skull is reduced by removing a segment of parietal bone and cinching it to basal skull.

CONCLUSION

The surgical treatment of craniosynostosis has evolved over many years. Since the earliest treatment attempts by removal of a stenotic suture by linear craniectomy, the sophistication of the surgical correction of craniosynostosis has increased tremendously. The recognition of significant compensatory changes distant to an isolated sutural stenosis has lead to a more holistic approach to surgical treatment. Optimal results in the treatment of skull deformities associated with craniosynostosis require accurate assessment of the full range of craniofacial defects and a treatment plan that addresses each observed abnormality. As well, we believe further technique modification should occur depending on the age of the child, which is directly related to brain development and the physical properties of bone.

REFERENCES

1. Sömmerring ST. *Vom Baue des menschlichen Körpers.* 2nd ed. Leipzig: Voss; 1839

2. Otto AW. *Lehrbuch der pathologischen des Menschen und der Thiere.* Berlin: Rücker; 1830.

3. Virchow R. Über den Cretinismus, namentlich in Franken. Und über pathologische Schädelformen. *Verh Phys Med Gesante Wurzburg.* 1851;2:230–271.

4. Persing JA, Jane JA, Shaffrey M. Virchow and the pathogenesis of craniosynostosis: a translation of his original work. *Plast Reconstr Surg.* 1989;83:728–742.

5. Klaauw CJ van der. Cerebral skull and facial skull. *Arch Neerl Zool.* 1946;7:16–37.

6. Moss ML. The pathogenesis of premature cranial synostosis in man. *Acta Anat (Basel).* 1959;37: 351–370.

7. Moss ML. Functional anatomy of cranial synostosis. *Childs Brain.* 1975;1:22–33.

8. Persing JA, Jane JA, Edgerton MT. Surgical treatment of craniosynostosis. In: Persing JA, Edgerton MT, Jane JA, eds. *Scientific Foundations and Surgical*

Treatment of Craniosynostosis. Baltimore, Md: Williams & Wilkins; 1989:117–238.

9. Christensen FK, Clark DB. The effect of restricted suture growth on brain growth in dogs. *Surg Forum.* 1970;21:439–440.

10. Laitinen L. Craniosynostosis. *Ann Paediatr Fenn.* 1956;2 (Suppl 6):1–130.

11. Persson KM, Roy WA, Persing JA, et al. Craniofacial growth following experimental craniosynostosis and craniectomy in rabbits. *J Neurosurg.* 1979;50: 187–197.

12. Babler WJ, Persing JA. Alterations in cranial suture growth associated with premature closure of the sagittal suture in rabbits. *Anat Rec.* 1985;211:14A.

13. Persing JA, Babler WJ, Jane JA, et al. Experimental unilateral coronal synostosis in rabbits. *Plast Reconstr Surg.* 1986;77:369–376.

14. Babler WJ, Persing JA. Experimental alteration of cranial suture growth: effects on the neurocranium, basicranium, and midface. In: Dixon AP, Sarnat

BG, eds. *Factors and Mechanisms Influencing Bone Growth.* New York, NY: Alan R Liss; 1982: 333–345.

15. Delashaw JB, Persing JA, Broaddus WC, et al. Cranial vault growth in craniosynostosis. *Neurosurgery.* 1989;70:159–165.

16. Persing JA, Shaffrey M, Angel M, et al. Age related technique modifications in the treatment of sagittal synostosis. In: Caronni EP, ed. *Craniofacial Surgery.* Bologna: Monduzzi Editore; 1991:237–242.

17. Boyd E. Organ weights from birth to maturity: man, North American. In: Altman PL, Dittmer DS, eds. *Growing Including Reproduction and Morphological Development.* Washington, DC: Federation of American Societies for Experimental Biology; 1962:346.

18. Albin RE, Hendee RW Jr, O'Donnell RS, et al. Trigonocephaly: refinements in reconstruction: experience with 33 patients. *Plast Reconstr Surg.* 1985;76:202.

19. Renier D. Intracranial pressure in craniosynostosis: pre- and postoperative recordings, correlation with functional results. In: Persing JA, Edgerton MT, Jane JA eds. *Scientific Foundations and Surgical Treatment of Craniosynostosis.* Baltimore, Md: Williams & Wilkins; 1989:263–269.

20. Shaffrey ME, Persing JA, Delashaw JB, et al. Surgical treatment of metopic synostosis. In: Persing JA, Jane JA, eds. *Neurosurgery Clinics of North America. Craniofacial Disorders.* Philadelphia, Pa: WB Saunders Co; 1991;2:621–627.

21. Persing JA, Jane JA, Park TS, et al. Floating C-shaped orbital osteotomy for orbital rim advancement in craniosynostosis: preliminary report. *J Neurosurg.* 1990;72:22–26.

22. Persing JA, Jane JA. Treatment of syndromic and nonsyndromic bilateral coronal synostosis in infancy and childhood. *Neurosurgery Clinics of North America. Craniofacial Disorders.* Philadelphia, Pa: WB Saunders Co; 1991;2:655–663.

23. Marchac D, Renier D. *Craniofacial Surgery for Craniosynostosis.* Boston, Mass: Little Brown & Co; 1982.

Chapter 9

Chiari Malformations and Syringohydromyelia

W. Jerry Oakes

Chiari malformations are a group of conditions originally described in the 1890s by H. Chiari, a German pathology professor. He outlined three degrees of hindbrain herniation, labeling them I, II, and III (Fig. 9.1), with I being the mildest degree of herniation and III the most severe.

A fourth type of malformation was originally included in this classification. This category, characterized by severe cerebellar hypoplasia or aplasia and a small posterior fossa (Figs. 9.2, 9.3), has been removed from the classification by most authors since no hindbrain herniation is involved. Patients with the Chiari IV malformation may appear amazingly well and have only mild to moderate neurologic deficits despite a striking radiographic appearance.

Type I and II lesions are the most common. Fortunately, Chiari III malformations rarely occur—infants with this lesion (Fig. 9.4) are severely disadvantaged neurologically. The lesion consists of a saclike structure emanating from the upper cervical/occipital area and contains components of brain stem and cerebellum. Surgical therapy to excise the sac, replace the neural tissue within the posterior fossa, and provide adequate dural and skin coverage is routinely offered to these patients. If progressive hydrocephalus supervenes, ventriculoperitoneal shunt insertion is advised.

Figure 9.1 Chiari Malformations

Type I
Caudal descent of the cerebellar tonsils into the cervical spine
Rarely seen below C-2
Not associated with myelomeningoceles
Hydrocephalus seen in <10% of patients

Type II
Caudal descent of the cerebellar vermis and lower brain stem into the cervical spine
Commonly seen below C-2
Multiple posterior fossa and cerebral anomalies associated with the hindbrain hernia, including "beaking" of the dorsal midbrain, enlargement of the massa intermedia, medullary "kinking," and hypoplasia of the tentorium
Hydrocephalus almost always present
Very commonly seen in conjunction with myelomeningoceles

Type III
Protrusion of a sac from the craniocervical junction that contains portions of the cerebellum and brain stem
Commonly associated with hydrocephalus

Type IV
Severe hypoplasia or aplasia of the cerebellum associated with a diminutive posterior fossa

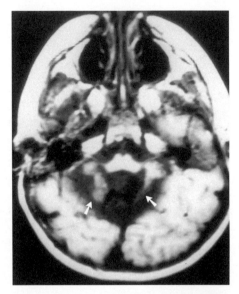

Figure 9.2 Axial MRI scan through the posterior fossa without contrast. The cerebellum is severely hypoplastic with only rudimentary development (arrows).

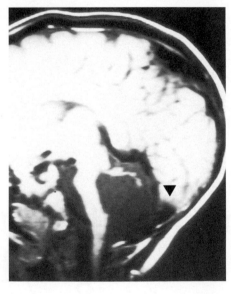

Figure 9.3 Sagittal MRI through the midline demonstrating minimal development of the cerebellum. Of note is the caudal displacement of the torcula (arrowhead). This child was evaluated for relatively mild coordination difficulty and is intellectually normal. The virtual absence of a cerebellum was truly surprising.

CHIARI I

Patients with more than 3 mm of caudal displacement of the cerebellar tonsils below the plane of the foramen magnum are generally considered to have a Chiari I malformation.[1] A pointed or "pegged" appearance of the tonsillar tips and crowding of the soft tissues at the foramen magnum is associated with the asymmetric descent of the cerebellar tonsils (Figs. 9.5–9.7). The brain stem is positioned normally in the majority of patients and syringohydromyelia is commonly seen. A new classification was recently proposed that emphasizes these findings.[2]

Many theories have been developed to explain this anomaly. Currently the most appealing emphasizes difficulty in rapidly equilibrating the CSF pressure wave seen following the Valsalva maneuver.[3] During this

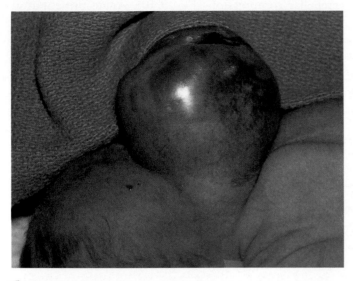

Figure 9.4 Neonate with a large cystic mass emanating from the craniocervical junction that contained both cerebellum and brain stem. This is a Chiari III malformation. On long-term follow-up this child was seen to have multiple severe neurologic deficits and developed hydrocephalus soon after closure of the lesion.

Figure 9.5 Radiographic Criteria for Chiari I Malformation

Caudal descent of the cerebellar tonsils >3 mm below the plane of the foramen magnum

"Pegged" or pointed appearance of the tonsillar tips

Crowding of the subarachnoid space in the area of the craniocervical junction

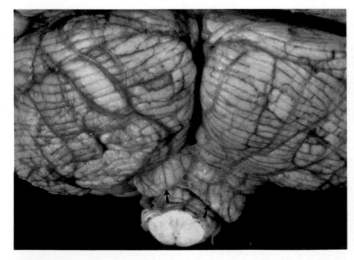

Figure 9.6 Posterior view of a specimen demonstrating asymmetric descent of the cerebellar tonsils (Chiari I malformation). The tonsils can be identified by their vertically oriented folia (arrows). This adult presented with downbeat nystagmus and difficulty with ambulation. There was no evidence of syringohydromyelia. She died abruptly of an unrelated cause prior to intervention for this lesion.

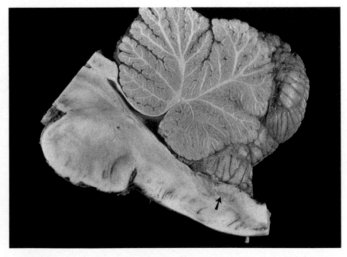

Figure 9.7 Sagittal view of the patient in Figure 9.6. Histologically confirmed necrosis of the dorsal medulla (arrow) due to the soft-tissue impaction existed beneath the area of tonsillar herniation.

delay in achieving equilibrium there is a vector of force out of the intracranial cavity (Fig. 9.8). The prolonged intracranial hypertension relative to the intraspinal compartment may last several seconds or minutes. With time this force results in the caudal migration of the soft tissues at the foramen magnum (cerebellar tonsils). Conditions that impede the physiologic flow of CSF at the foramen of Magendie enhance the formation of this malformation. This could include veils or septations in this region (Fig. 9.9) as well as adhesions. Alternatively, conditions that artificially lower the intraspinal pressure relative to the intracranial pressure (lumboperitoneal shunts) have been seen to "cause" the Chiari I malformation with the subsequent development of syringohydromyelia.[4]

The clinical presentation of patients with Chiari I malformations is one of the most protean in medicine. Their symptoms can be thought of as those attributable to dysfunction of the spinal cord through the syringohydromyelia and those due to primary brain stem and cerebellar compression (Fig. 9.10). Acute presentation with catastrophic neurologic compromise is unusual but

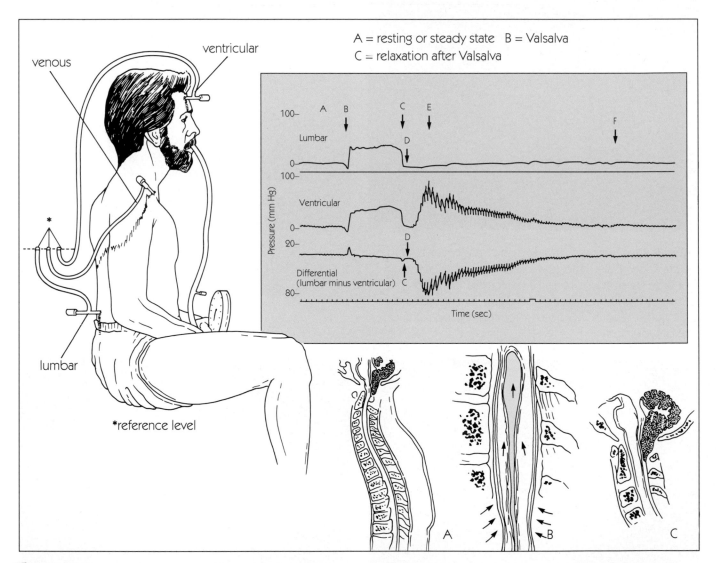

Figure 9.8 When ventricular and lumbar subarachnoid pressure are simultaneously monitored in a patient with a Chiari I malformation the pressures are the same in the resting state when calibrated against a reference (**A**). With Valsalva there is an abrupt rise of lumbar pressure (**B**) exceeding that seen in the ventricular system. With relaxation (**C**) the lumbar space has its pressure rapidly fall and return to the baseline. The ventricular pressure, on the other hand, cannot equilibrate, and sustained intracranial hypertension relative to the intraspinal compartment is maintained for several seconds to a few minutes. This vector of force is the pathophysiologic mechanism for the development of progressive displacement of the cerebellar tonsils into the cervical spine and the development of syringohydromyelia (after B. Williams).

does occur.[5] The headache associated with the Chiari malformation deserves special comment. This pain is nonradicular in its description but is frequently associated with a dysesthetic component in the C-2 dermatome. The neck pain/headache is frequently brought on by exertion or by coughing or sneezing.[6] This Valsalva-induced component is striking by history and should quickly lead the clinician to evaluate the patient for the presence of a Chiari malformation.

The diagnosis can easily be confirmed with MRI. This allows direct sagittal as well as axial imaging without invasive contrast material. In addition to assessing the anatomy of the craniocervical junction, the presence and extent of a syringohydromyelia can easily be determined (Fig. 9.11). Evidence of dynamic ventral compression can also be obtained with this modality. Routine CT without subarachnoid contrast is an inadequate technique for assessing the presence of a Chiari malformation or syringohydromyelia. Bony anatomy may not be easily appreciated by MRI, and dynamic cervical radiographs with or without tomography may be useful in the initial evaluation and assessment. Additional physiologic testing is not generally useful and should not replace MRI as a screening tool.

The therapeutic options available include further clinical observation and surgical intervention (Fig. 9.12). At times spontaneous resolution of large syrinx cavities has been reported.[7] However, this is unusual. If

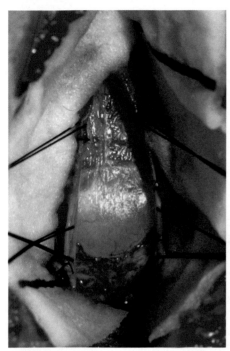

Figure 9.9 Intraoperative view of the craniocervical junction of a Chiari II patient with the bony removal complete and the dura tented laterally (sutures). A veil is apparent over the area of the foramen of Magendie. The horizontal folia of the cerebellar vermis (arrow) are apparent at the superior end of the opening while the displaced medulla is present below. In this particular case there is unimpressive herniation of the cerebellar vermis, although a huge syrinx was present below this point. This veil acted as an obstruction to the dissipation of the water hammer CSF pulse. In this pathologic condition the CSF pressure wave within the fourth ventricle was redirected within the cord rather than into the subarachnoid space.

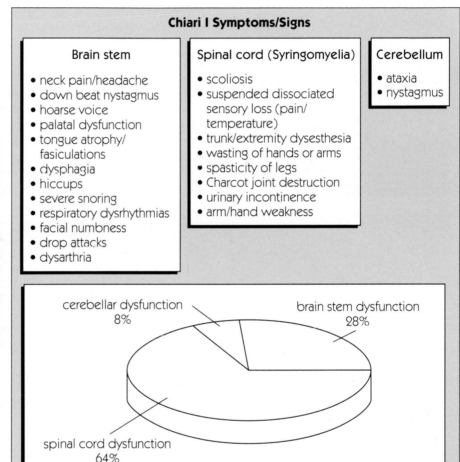

Figure 9.10 Symptoms and signs of patients with Chiari I malformations.

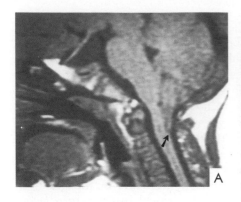

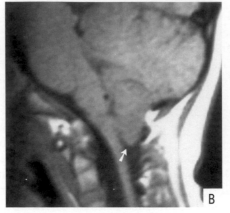

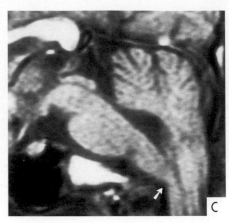

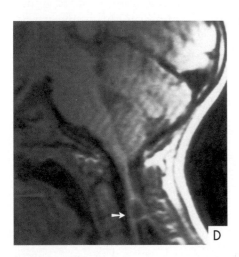

Figure 9.11 (A) Midsagittal MRI of a patient who meets all criteria for a Chiari I malformation, including caudal descent of the tonsils (arrow). The patient is asymptomatic and has no syrinx. This patient was followed expectantly for more than 4 years but did not develop any problem attributable to the lesion. **(B)** Midsagittal MRI of a 5-year-old with cough-induced neck and head pain due to caudal displacement of the cerebellar tonsils (arrow). His physical examination was normal. Following the opening and stenting of the foramen of Magendie the headaches completely disappeared. **(C)** Midsagittal MRI of a patient with significant caudal displacement of the cerebellar tonsils as well as significant ventral compression of the medulla (arrow). This patient should undergo decompression of the bone and soft tissues compromising the ventral brain stem through a transoral procedure rather than directing attention to the Chiari malformation. **(D)** Midsagittal MRI of a 5-year-old male presenting with very dysesthetic arms, spasticity, and marked difficulty with his gait. The Chiari I malformation is apparent, but a huge syrinx beginning just below C-2 is also obvious (arrow).

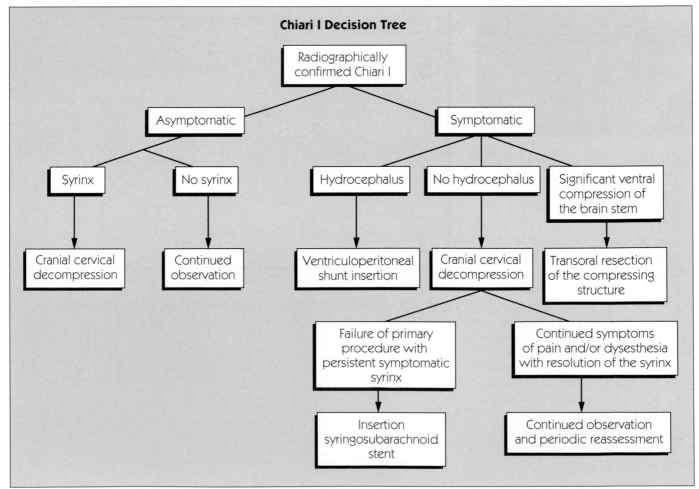

Chiari I Decision Tree

```
                    Radiographically
                    confirmed Chiari I
                    /                \
           Asymptomatic            Symptomatic
            /        \            /      |        \
      Syrinx      No syrinx   Hydrocephalus  No hydrocephalus  Significant ventral
        |            |            |              |             compression of
                                                               the brain stem
   Cranial cervical  Continued  Ventriculoperitoneal  Cranial cervical  Transoral resection
   decompression     observation  shunt insertion     decompression     of the compressing
                                                       /         \           structure
                                        Failure of primary    Continued symptoms
                                        procedure with        of pain and/or dysesthesia
                                        persistent symptomatic with resolution of the syrinx
                                        syrinx                     |
                                          |                  Continued observation
                                     Insertion              and periodic reassessment
                                     syringosubarachnoid
                                     stent
```

Figure 9.12 Therapeutic options for treating Chiari I malformations.

Principles of Neurosurgery

the patient is asymptomatic and no syrinx is present, continued observation is appropriate. A significant number of patients in this category are being followed since the advent of MRI. Their natural history is unknown, but surgical intervention without symptoms or the presence of a syrinx seems unjustified at this time. Progressive or functionally significant symptoms demand operative intervention. Because of MRI, a group of patients without obvious symptoms but with large "asymptomatic" syringohydromyelia have been discovered during the investigation of unrelated problems. It is my practice in this situation to discuss intervention with the patient and family in terms of risk versus benefit and to favor intervention in an attempt to prevent the likely neurologic deterioration associated with a syrinx. In less than 10% of patients, hydrocephalus is associated with the Chiari I malformation, in which case a ventriculoperitoneal shunt should be the initial form of therapy. Similarly, if there is significant ventral compression on the brain stem, relief of compression should be the initial form of therapy. Posterior fossa craniectomy and cervical laminectomy in the face of ventral compression frequently intensifies the rate of neurologic deterioration.

SURGICAL TECHNIQUE

Once operative intervention has been decided upon, the patient is positioned prone with the neck flexed (Fig. 9.13). A limited suboccipital craniectomy and C-1 laminectomy are performed.[8] C-2, with its important muscular attachments, can usually be left intact. The dura is opened widely and the tonsils separated (Fig. 9.14). To maintain free egress from the foramen of Magendie a stent or conduit of plastic tubing and/or sheeting can be fashioned. It is passed through the foramen of Magendie and sewn to the pia of the tonsil. This maximizes the likelihood of continued patency of the outlet foramen of the fourth ventricle. In general I have not found the placement of a fat or muscle plug into the obex to be useful. With the outflow from the fourth ventricle to the subarachnoid space re-established, the dura is grafted and the wound closed. Simultaneous syringostomy should be avoided during

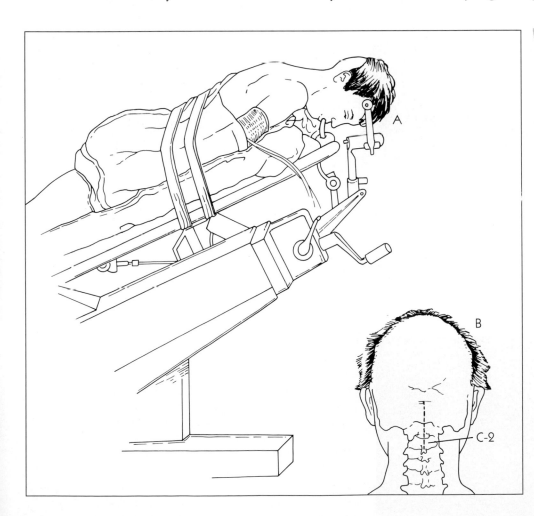

Figure 9.13 Operative position for Chiari decompression. **(A)** The operative field is maintained horizontally with the head flexed and held in a pin fixation device. **(B)** Preparation is made for a midline linear incision 2 cm below the external occipital protuberance and extending to the spinous process of C-2.

the initial procedure; it commonly results in a dysesthetic area in the upper cervical dermatomes where the cord has been disrupted, and it is not necessary in the majority of patients since the syrinx cavity is likely to resolve spontaneously by allowing adequate egress of fluid through the foramen of Magendie.

RESULTS

Postoperative MRI has demonstrated relatively rapid resolution of the syringohydromyelia cavity in the majority of patients.[9] If craniocervical decompression fails to resolve an extensive syrinx cavity completely, and motor symptoms persist or sensory symptoms worsen, and the level of dysfunction is appropriate to the anatomic position of the retained cavity, consideration can be given to drainage of the syrinx. If the subarachnoid space is pristine, a syringosubarachnoid stent can be placed at the caudal end of the cavity. If the subarachnoid space is compartmentalized, a syringopleural or syringoperitoneal shunt should be considered.

The results of craniocervical decompression are encouraging in long-term follow-up.[10] The likelihood of resolution of the syrinx is high. Advanced symptoms of medullary dysfunction, muscle wasting, and dysesthesia in the extremities or trunk are unlikely to resolve but should not progress. Mild to moderate scoliosis, spasticity, and Valsalva-induced pain are likely to improve.

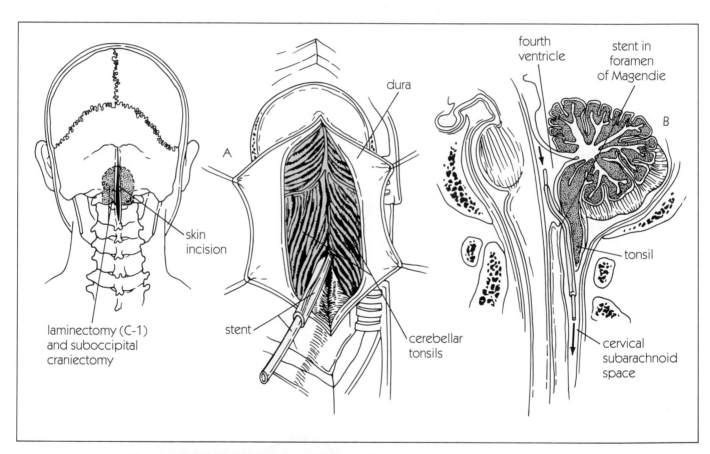

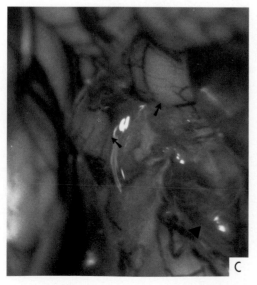

Figure 9.14 (A) Intraoperative view following the suboccipital craniectomy and C-1 laminectomy. The dura has been opened and the caudally descended cerebellar tonsils are in view. They are separated, and a stent composed of plastic tubing surrounded by sheeting is inserted through the foramen of Magendie. (B) Sagittal view following placement of the stent. Free egress of fluid from the fourth ventricle to the cervical subarachnoid space is possible once the stent is in place. (C) Intraoperative view of the craniocervical junction with the dura open. Arachnoidal scarring at the foramen of Magendie (upper arrows) is seen, which effectively occluded this outlet. The right posterior inferior cerebellar artery is seen (arrowhead). (Same patient as in Figure 9.11D.)

CHIARI II

The caudal displacement of the cerebellar vermis and lower brain stem is seen almost exclusively in conjuction with myelomeningoceles. In addition to the changes of the craniocervical junction, other dysmorphic areas of the brain and spinal cord are abundant (Fig. 9.15). Changes caused by the Chiari II malformation vary according to the individual.

The pathophysiology of the malformation has been postulated to be similar to the Chiari I malformation, that is, difficulty equilibrating the dynamic CSF pulse pressure induced by Valsalva.[11] In this case the intraspinal pressure is lowered in utero by CSF leakage at the myelomeningocele site. The rudimentary cerebellar vermis is caudally displaced along with the developing brain stem. At the embryologic time of this displacement the cerebellar tonsils have not yet developed.

Some aspects of the posterior fossa seem almost to have arrested development, with the choroid plexus retaining its embryonic extraventricular position. Knowing this fact will prove useful in the discussion of surgical technique. Recently, efforts have been made to assimilate the anatomic and embryologic descriptions into a "unified theory" of development,[12] which attributes associated CNS anomalies to the lack of distention of the ventricular system by leakage of CSF at the myelomeningocele site. This appealing theory is gaining support.

Symptoms produced by the Chiari II malformation are best considered according to the area demonstrating disturbed function[13] (spinal cord, cerebellum, or brain stem) (Fig. 9.16). Although spinal cord dysfunction with development of spasticity of the upper extremities may be present at birth, it characteristically develops later in life. When present in infancy the increased tone of the

Figure 9.15 Chiari II Neuropathologic Changes

"Beaking" of the dorsal midbrain through fusion of the superior and inferior colliculi
"Kinking" of the medulla
Enlargement of the massa intermedia
Hypoplasia of the tentorium and falx cerebri
Polygyria
Inversion of the cerebellum
Scalloping of the petrous ridges
Lückenschädel of the skull
Hydrocephalus

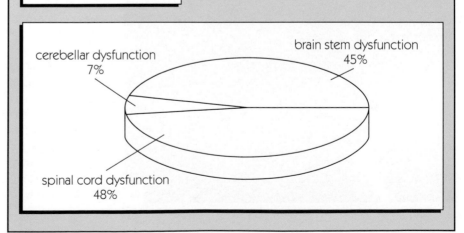

Brain Stem

- dysphagia, poor suck response
- nasal vocalization, palatal weakness
- aspiration pneumonia
- gastroesophageal reflux
- tongue fasiculations/atrophy
- opisthotonos
- central apnea, especially during sleep
- poor or weak cry
- severe prolonged breath-holding spells
- inspiratory wheezing
- nerve VI palsy
- facial weakness
- lack of response to inspired CO_2
- tracheal anesthesia
- depressed or absent gag response
- prolonged hiccups

Spinal Cord

- upper extremity spasticity
- persistent cortical thumbs
- suspended dissociated sensory loss (pain/temperature)
- upper extremity weakness and hand muscle wasting
- scoliosis

Cerebellum

- appendicular/truncal ataxia
- nystagmus

cerebellar dysfunction 7%

brain stem dysfunction 45%

spinal cord dysfunction 48%

Figure 9.16 Symptoms and signs of patients with Chiari II malformations.

arms can be appreciated along with persistent cortical thumbs. Cerebellar dysfunction may be more elusive to detect during clinical examination since it primarily involves truncal ataxia and many of the patients are already confined to wheelchairs. Nystagmus is commonly present and may be quite severe; it may be the only obvious clinical herald of a cerebellar disturbance.

The primary cause of death in the treated myelodysplastic population today is lower brain stem dysfunction, which causes central respiratory depression[14] and/or aspiration. Some debate has occurred as to whether this is a primary hypoplasia of the medullary neurons[15] or is caused by compression and/or secondary ischemia. If the dysfunction is secondary, appropriate surgical therapy directed at the primary abnormality might prove successful. If the problem is primarily cellular hypoplasia, obviously no therapy will prove useful. Since many patients who eventually develop life-threatening difficulties have weeks or months of adequate medullary function prior to deterioration, primary hypoplasia must be a minor factor in most symptomatic patients.

Scoliosis that accompanies the myelomeningocele patient is usually multifactorial in its causation. The presence of syringohydromyelia may be a contributing factor.[16] It may be difficult to determine the degree of responsibility that each factor plays in the development of the scoliosis.

MRI has revolutionized the evaluation of the patient with Chiari II malformation. No other imaging technique gives the anatomic detail of MRI (Fig. 9.17).[17]

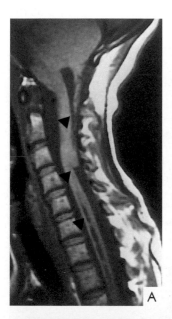
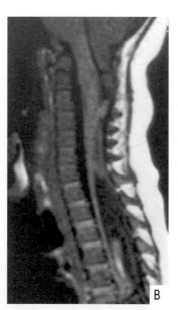
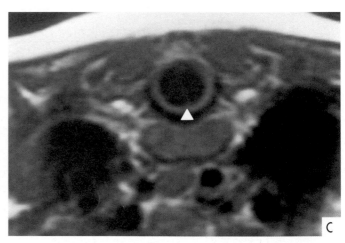
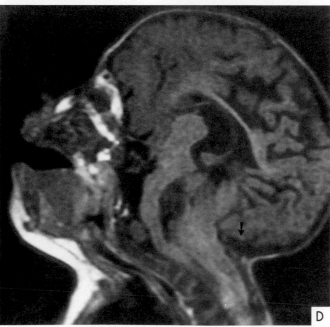

Figure 9.17 (A) Midsagittal MRI of the craniocervical junction in a patient with a Chiari II malformation. The brain stem and cerebellar vermis are caudally displaced. The choroid plexus (upper arrowhead) and medullary kink (middle arrowhead) are apparent. A moderate-sized syrinx (lower arrowhead) is also seen. (B) Midsagittal MRI of a patient with a Chiari II malformation. Again the medullary kink and caudally displaced vermis are apparent. The syrinx, however, is massively dilated in the lower cervical and upper thoracic region. Interestingly, this patient's neurologic function was not seriously compromised with regard to hand function despite this massively dilated syrinx. (C) Axial MRI of the patient in B, showing thin rim of cord tissue (arrowhead) surrounding a massively dilated syrinx. With time, serious compromise of motor and sensory function of the arms developed. (D) Severe Chiari II malformation with much of the brain stem and cerebellum displaced into the cervical spine. The torcula is positioned at the foramen magnum. The upper cervical spine is deviated markedly anteriorly, compromising the trachea and esophagus. The spine is widely bifid posteriorly. This lesion is beyond our ability to influence.

Principles of Neurosurgery

Flexion-extension cervical spine radiographs complement the MRI nicely. Although physiologic testing of various medullary functions has proven interesting from an investigational standpoint, none have consistently proven to be useful clinically.

Since virtually all patients with a myelomeningocele have some element of hindbrain herniation, surgery should be done on the basis of clinical criteria, not radiographic criteria (Fig. 9.18). In general, progressive or life-threatening difficulties warrant intervention. Quick recourse to operative intervention in symptomatic infants is the most likely way to alter the natural history of this condition. As neurosurgeons have become aware of the safety of the procedure, increasingly liberal criteria have been developed. With more sensitive criteria for decompression, between 20% and 30% of myelomeningocele patients are offered surgery by age ten. It should be emphasized that good function of the existing shunt system is a necessary prerequisite for considering surgical decompression of the posterior fossa (Fig. 9.19).

Figure 9.18 Indications for Surgical Decompression in Chiari II Patients

Functionally significant or progressive spasticity of the upper extremities
Functionally significant or progressive truncal and/or appendicular ataxia
Inspiratory stridor at rest or progressive by history
Recurrent aspiration pneumonia due to palatal dysfunction or gastroesophageal reflux
Central apnea with or without cyanosis, especially during sleep
Significant opisthotonos

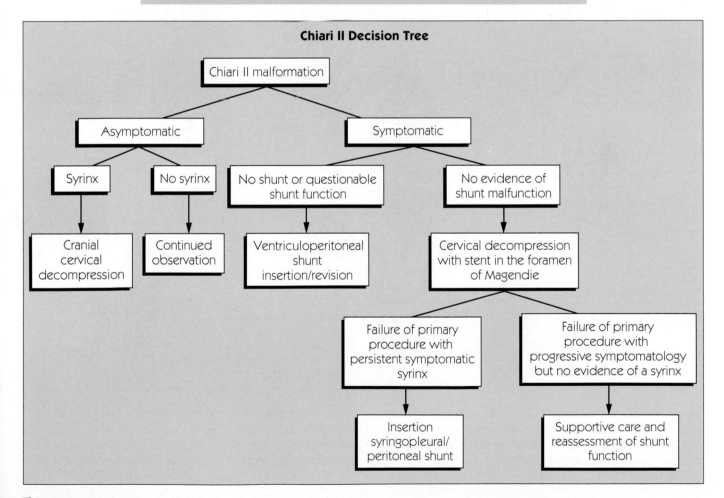

Figure 9.19 Therapeutic options for treating patients with Chiari II malformations.

SURGICAL TECHNIQUE

When surgery is elected, patients are positioned prone with the neck flexed. There is rarely need for suboccipital craniectomy, but the laminectomy portion of the procedure must include the entire area of the displaced vermis (Fig. 9.20). This frequently means the laminectomy must be extended to include at least C-4 or below. With a small posterior fossa the dural sinuses may also be significantly displaced toward the foramen magnum. This fact is important in planning the bony exposure and dural opening. The dura is opened widely, with grafting anticipated at the time of closure. The goal of the intradural exploration is to open and stent the foramen of Magendie. Finding the fourth ventricle in these patients can prove technically challenging (Fig. 9.21). If the choroid plexus can be located it will lead the operator into the ventricle. At times this structure may be difficult to visualize through the dense arachnoidal scarring. Intraoperative ultrasound guidance has proven useful.[18] The unwary may mistake the medullary kink for the cerebellar vermis and attempt to dissect through the medulla. The likelihood of this can be minimized by carefully analyzing the anatomic detail on the MRI, liberal use of intraoperative ultrasound, and strict microdissection through anatomic planes under high magnification. Once located, a stent is placed from the avascular floor of the fourth ventricle to the subarachnoid space. This stent is composed of plastic tubing and sheeting and is fashioned to maintain the integrity of the foramen of Magendie. Care is taken to position the distal end of the stent in the subarachnoid—not the subdural—space.

RESULTS

Outcome following surgery is largely dependent on the degree of disability prior to intervention. Patients with upper extremity spasticity and nystagmus can expect no further deterioration and are likely to improve functionally. Young infants unable to maintain adequate spontaneous ventilation associated with aspiration and dysphasia may not have their natural history affected by surgical intervention.

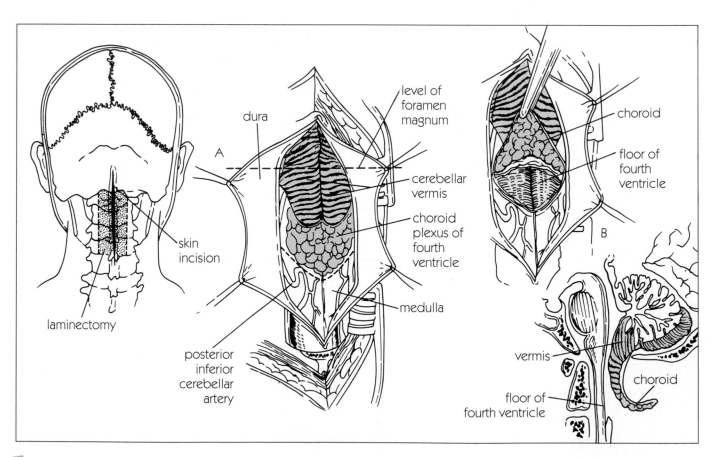

Figure 9.20 (A) Intraoperative view following upper cervical laminectomy in a patient with Chiari II malformation. The granular yellow-orange choroid plexus may be visualized through the arachnoid. The horizontal folia of the cerebellar vermis are apparent and the caudally displaced medulla and posterior inferior cerebellar artery immediately below the choroid plexus can also be seen. (B) With dissection of the thickened arachnoid in the area of the choroid plexus the avascular floor of the fourth ventricle can be visualized. Again, a stent is placed through this opening to maintain its integrity.

SYRINGOHYDROMYELIA

The accumulation of fluid within the spinal cord is not thought to be the primary manifestation of any disease process. Syringohydromyelia is a secondary process with many causes. The mechanism by which the fluid accumulates varies significantly from one disease process to another. One useful classification divides instances into communicating and noncommunicating causes. Those with CSF-like fluid in the cavity are "communicating" and could be associated with a Chiari malformation or occult spinal dysraphism, for example.

Highly proteinaceous fluid is found secondary to neoplasms, vascular anomalies, arachnoiditis, and trauma. These lesions are thought to be "noncommunicating." This difference in the character of the cyst fluid can sometimes be useful in helping to ascertain the cause of an "idiopathic" syrinx.

When symptoms come from a syrinx they are relatively stereotyped, with loss of pain and temperature appreciation usually occurring in the arm or chest, absent or diminished deep tendon reflexes, and spasticity of the lower extremities. These symptoms are gener-

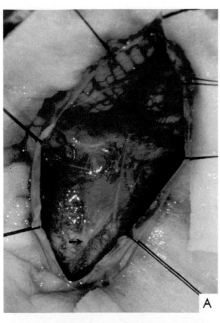
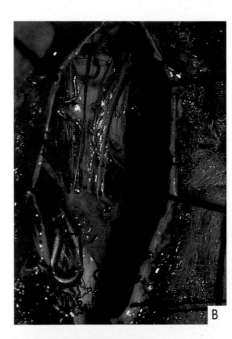
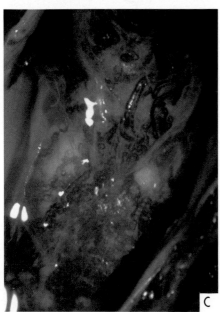
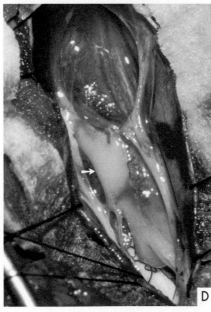

Figure 9.21 (A) Intraoperative view of a Chiari II malformation with the dura open. The cerebellar vermis is displaced minimally; however, the brain stem with its fourth ventricle is displaced well below the foramen magnum. The triangular appearance of the lower brain stem is apparent with a veil over its opening (arrows). (B) Intraoperative view of a Chiari II malformation with the horizontal folia of the cerebellar vermis (upper arrow) and yellow-orange appearance of the choroid plexus (lower arrow) apparent. The redundant left posterior inferior cerebellar artery can also easily be seen lying on the dorsal aspect of the medulla. (C) Intraoperative intradural view of a Chiari II malformation with significant thickening of the arachnoid and neovascularity over the dorsal vermis and brain stem. In this patient the plane of dissection to allow opening of the foramen of Magendie is much less obvious. (D) Severe caudal displacement of the vermis and brain stem to the level of T-4. The waxy avascular yellow appearance of the cerebellar vermis (arrows) is apparent. These tissues have been displaced to such a severe degree that they have become ischemic and gliotic.

ally of gradual onset. Variations on this theme include the development of scoliosis, dysesthesia, and wasting of the intrinsic muscles of the hand. The symptoms from the syrinx itself can generally be differentiated from symptoms caused by the underlying condition. As the cavity expands in the central portion of the cord, the early loss of pain and temperature sensitivity is secondary to disruption or compromise of the crossing spinothalamic tract fibers (Fig. 9.22).

At times patients with syringohydromyelia develop acute loss of neurologic function with a bout of cough-ing or straining. The reason for this change can be understood when one realizes the degree of compress-ibility of a cord expanded with fluid (Fig. 9.23). When the Valsalva maneuver causes the epidural venous com-plex to expand, the cavity may be forced to dissect through white matter within the cord.

Also worthy of mention is the method of distention that the fluid uses to leave the expanded central canal (hydromyelia), which is lined by ependyma, and dissect into the surrounding cord substance (syringomyelia), which is not lined by ependyma (Fig. 9.24). To some

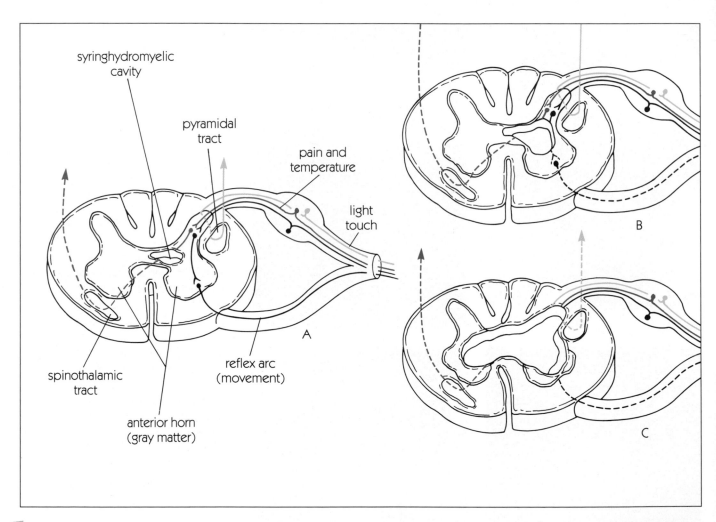

Figure 9.22 (A) Axial section through the spinal cord with progressive enlargement of a syringohydromyelic cavity. (B) The crossing fibers of the spinothalamic tract are first to be affected by this cystic expansion. (C) Next affected are the anterior horn cells, resulting in wasting, fasciculations, and atrophy characteristically in the hands.

Principles of Neurosurgery

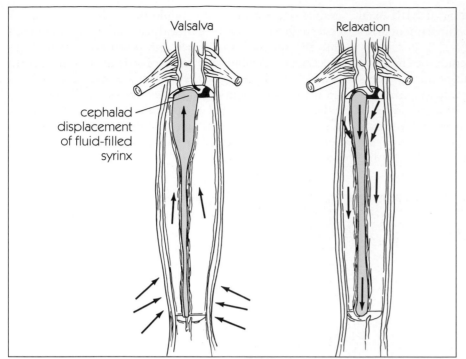

Valsalva

Relaxation

cephalad
displacement
of fluid-filled
syrinx

Figure 9.23 Increased intraabdominal pressure caused by the Valsalva maneuver forces blood into the epidural venous complex. When the epidural veins are forcefully expanded against the enlarged cystic cord they may force the cyst to be displaced (usually cephalad). This sudden displacement with forceful coughing or sneezing may actually be associated with a significant worsening of the patient's neurologic condition.

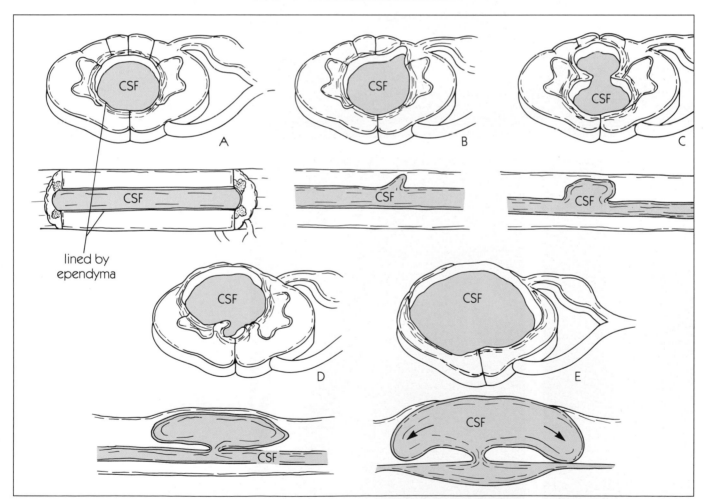

lined by
ependyma

Figure 9.24 (A–E) Stages in the progressive expansion of an ependyma-lined hydromyelia to a larger cavity compressing the central canal. This large cavity has no ependymal lining and so could be termed a syrinx.

degree this can be confirmed by looking at MRI axial views of a syrinx demonstrating the compartmentalization within the cavity (Fig. 9.25).

MRI reigns as the diagnostic procedure of choice in this condition also (Fig. 9.26). It enables one to assess the extent of the cyst, and sometimes comparing the signal characteristics of the CSF and the syrinx fluid helps identify the etiology. If a neoplasm is suspected, contrast enhancement may prove useful. If the cause cannot be determined by the history or a routine radiographic

evaluation, consideration should be given to doing a CT cisternogram. This test introduces radiopaque contrast into the subarachnoid space and positions it at the craniocervical junction. Free reflux of contrast into the fourth ventricle indicates that the outlets are open and there is no reason for craniocervical decompression. If no alternative explanation for a surgically significant syrinx is seen and there is no reflux of contrast into the fourth ventricle, exploration of the craniocervical junction should be considered.

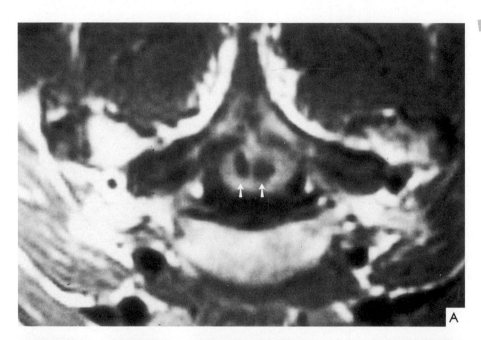

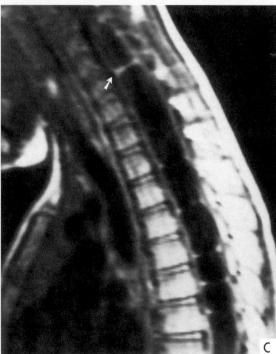

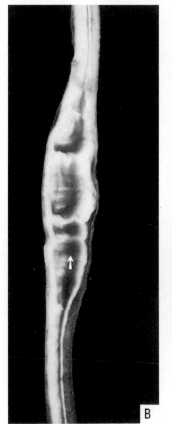

Figure 9.25 (A) Axial MRI of a Chiari I patient demonstrates two areas of dissection within the cord (arrows). (B) Pathologic specimen demonstrating the haustra within a syrinx cavity. (C) Midsagittal MRI of a markedly expanded syrinx, again demonstrating radiographically the septations or haustra between the compartments within the syrinx. These cavities may or may not communicate with each other.

If symptoms are functionally significant or progressive, intervention should be considered, with the recommended procedure varying widely depending on the underlying condition (Fig. 9.27).[19,20]

Outcome is again dependent on the degree of disability prior to intervention and the cause of the syrinx. Follow-up MRI can readily evaluate the recurrence of fluid. Some syrinxes are multicompartmental and may require drainage at multiple sites. This too can readily be appreciated in follow-up.

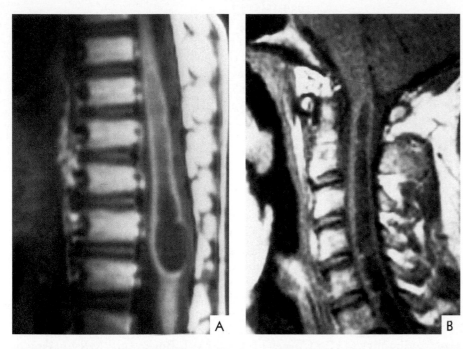

A B

Figure 9.26 (A) Midsagittal MRI of a patient with occult spinal dysraphism including a tethered spinal cord and diastematomyelia without a fibrous septum. In the upper lumbar region a terminal syrinx can easily be appreciated. This patient was "asymptomatic" at this time. Following drainage of the syrinx, however, significant improvement in the patient's spontaneous gait and urinary stream was noted. (B) Patient who developed a traumatic thoracic fracture and posttraumatic syringomyelia that extends to the craniocervical junction. In this patient progressive weakness of the arms and hands was the primary clinical manifestation.

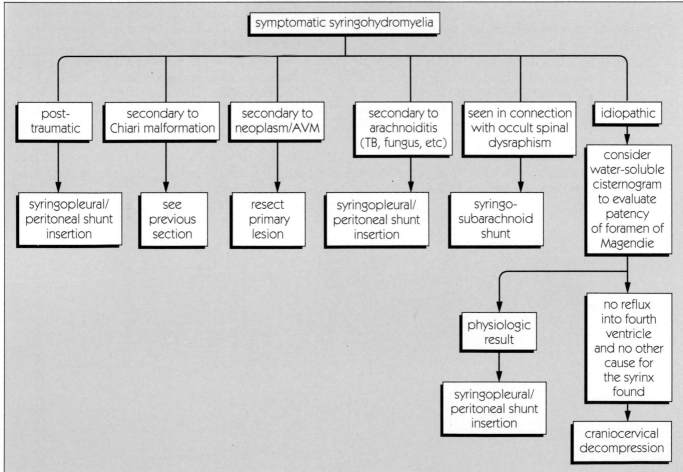

Figure 9.27 Therapeutic options for patients with symptomatic syringohydromyelia.

REFERENCES

1. Aboulezz AO, Sartor K, Geyer CA, Gado MH. Position of cerebellar tonsils in the normal population and in patients with Chiari I malformation: a quantitative approach with MR imaging. *J Comput Assist Tomogr.* 1985;9:1033–1036.

2. Pillay PK, Awad IA, Little JR, Hahn JF. Symptomatic Chiari malformation in adults: a new classification based on magnetic resonance imaging with clinical and prognostic significance. *Neurosurgery.* 1991;28:639–645.

3. Williams B. Simultaneous cerebral and spinal fluid pressure recordings, II: cerebrospinal dissociation with lesions at the foramen magnum. *Acta Neurochir.* 1981;59:123–142.

4. Welch K, Shillito J, Strand R, Fischer EG, Winston KR. Chiari I malformation—an acquired disorder? *J Neurosurg.* 1981;55:604–609.

5. Zager EL, Ojemann RG, Poletti CE. Acute presentations of syringomyelia. *J Neurosurg.* 1990;72:133–138.

6. Nightingale S, Williams B. Hindbrain hernia headache. *Lancet.* 1987;1:731–734.

7. Jack CR, Komen E, Onofrio BM. Spontaneous decompression of syringomyelia: magnetic resonance imaging findings. *J Neurosurg.* 1991;74:283–286.

8. Oakes WJ. Chiari malformations and syringohydromyelia in children. In: Rengachary SS, ed. *Neurosurgical Operative Atlas.* Chicago, Ill: AANS; 1991;1:59–65.

9. Batzdorf U. Chiari I malformation with syringomyelia: evaluation of surgical therapy by magnetic resonance imaging. *J Neurosurg.* 1988;68:726–730.

10. Dyste GN, Menezes AH, VanGilder JC. Symptomatic Chiari malformations: an analysis of presentation, management, and long-term outcome. *J Neurosurg.* 1989;71:159–168.

11. Williams B. Cerebrospinal fluid pressure-gradients in spina bifida cystica, with special reference to the Arnold-Chiari malformation and aqueductal stenosis. *Dev Med Child Neurol Supp.* 1975;17:138–150.

12. McLone DG, Knepper PA. The cause of Chiari II malformation: a unified theory. *Pediatr Neurosci.* 1989;15:1–12.

13. Oakes WJ, Worley G, Spock A, Whiting K. Intervention in twenty-nine patients with symptomatic Type II Chiari malformations: clinical presentation and outcome. *Concepts Pediatr Neurosurg.* 1988;8:76–85.

14. Davidson Ward SL, Nickerson BG, vanderHal A, Rodriguez AM, Jacobs RA, Keens TG. Absent hypoxic and hypercapneic arousal responses in children with myelomeningocele and apnea. *Pediatrics.* 1986;78:44–50.

15. Gilbert JN, Jones KL, Rorke LB, Chernoff GF, James HE. Central nervous system anomalies associated with meningomyelocele, hydrocephalus, and the Arnold-Chiari malformation: reappraisal of theories regarding the pathogenesis of posterior neural tube closure defects. *Neurosurgery.* 1986;18:559–564.

16. Hall PV, Lindseth RE, Campbell RL, Kalsbeck JE. Myelodysplasia and developmental scoliosis: a manifestation of syringomyelia. *Spine.* 1976;1:48–56.

17. Curnes JT, Oakes WJ, Boyko OB. MR imaging of hindbrain deformity in Chiari II patients with and without symptoms of brainstem compression. *AJNR.* 1989;10:293–302.

18. Venes JL, Black KL, Latack JT. Preoperative evaluation and surgical management of the Arnold-Chiari II malformation. *J Neurosurg.* 1986;64:363–370.

19. Caplan LR, Norohna AB, Amico LL. Syringomyelia and arachnoiditis. *J Neurol Neurosurg Psychiatry.* 1990;53:106–113.

20. Davis CHG, Symon L. Mechanisms and treatment in post-traumatic syringomyelia. *Br J Neurosurg.* 1989;3:669–674.

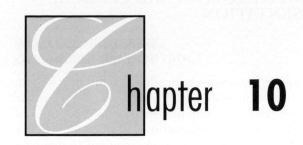

Chapter 10

Cerebrovascular
Occlusive Disease

Issam A. Awad

PATHOPHYSIOLOGY AND CLINICAL PRESENTATION

CEREBRAL BLOOD FLOW AND ISCHEMIC THRESHOLDS

Brain mass represents approximately 2% of body weight, but its circulation is endowed with 20% of the cardiac output and its energy requirements account for 20% of total body oxygen consumption (Fig. 10.1).[1] These tremendous metabolic demands are required to maintain the high degree of order required for control of body functions and behavior. Among the brain's metabolic requirements are: 1) the synthesis and transport of substrates and macromolecules, including neurotransmitters; 2) the maintenance of strict osmotic compartmentalization and integrity of cellular and support structures; and 3) the orderly execution of biochemical reactions involving various biomolecules. A substantial amount of energy

in the brain is also required for heat production. Such heat is by no means "wasted," since its release is necessary for the unidirectional flow of various biochemical reactions (away from equilibrium) and the maintenance of an optimal temperature for enzymatic function.

To function metabolically, the brain needs a steady flow of oxygen and substrate delivered by the cerebral circulation.[1] *Ischemia* is the condition where cerebral blood flow is not sufficient to maintain cerebral metabolic functions. Ischemia may be complete (absent cerebral blood flow) or incomplete (insufficient cerebral blood flow), global (affecting the whole brain) or focal (affecting a region of the brain). Regional cerebral blood flow (rCBF) is usually expressed in milliliters per 100 grams of brain tissue per minute (mL/100 g/min). Normal rCBF is typically in the range of 50 to 60 mL/100 g/min, is greater in gray than in white matter, and may be higher during functional activation of individual brain regions.

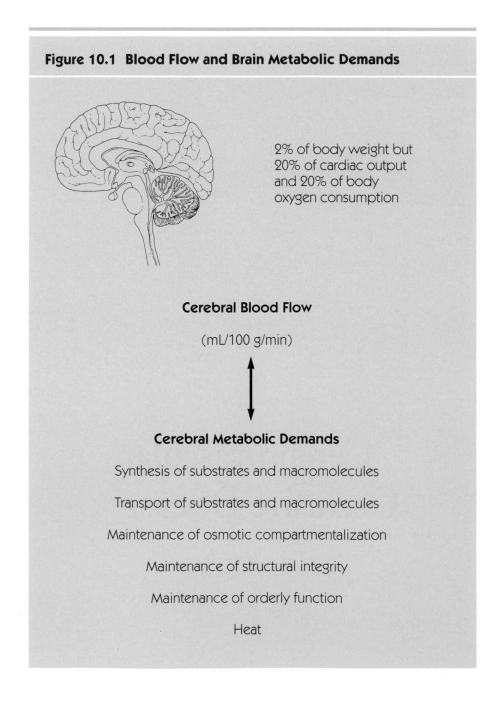

Figure 10.1 Blood Flow and Brain Metabolic Demands

2% of body weight but 20% of cardiac output and 20% of body oxygen consumption

Cerebral Blood Flow

(mL/100 g/min)

↕

Cerebral Metabolic Demands

Synthesis of substrates and macromolecules

Transport of substrates and macromolecules

Maintenance of osmotic compartmentalization

Maintenance of structural integrity

Maintenance of orderly function

Heat

Specific *ischemic thresholds* have been identified in humans and experimental animals (Fig. 10.2).[2] Intact cellular structure and function are well maintained whenever the rCBF exceeds 20 to 25 mL/100 g/min. Below this threshold, there is impaired cellular function characterized by slowing and decreased amplitude of the electroencephalogram, disruption of evoked cortical responses, and degraded clinical function related to the particular region of the brain. Intact cellular structure appears to be maintained unless the rCBF drops below 5 to 10 mL/100g/min. This threshold for tissue infarction depends not only on the the rCBF level but also on the duration of ischemia (see Fig. 10.2). Higher ranges of rCBF may still result in tissue infarction, if they persist for long periods of time.[2]

This concept of ischemic thresholds accounts for the transient cerebral dysfunction without residual tissue infarction that is sometimes observed clinically. Also, it indicates that a region of the brain can be functionally impaired indefinitely without adequate rCBF but still remain structurally intact as long as it receives enough blood flow for cellular maintenance ("idling neurons").

Global brain ischemia is encountered with hemodynamic failure or cardiac arrest. Focal brain ischemia may result from a variety of mechanisms (Fig. 10.3). Cardiogenic emboli may arise from dysfunctional valves or mural thrombi and lodge in cerebral arteries, resulting in focal ischemia. Artery-to-artery embolism may result from atherosclerotic disease in large cerebral arteries, with platelet, calcific, or thrombotic emboli lodging in smaller arteries downstream. Embolic arterial occlusions typically result in infarction in the territory of the occluded artery. However, collateral circulation (see below) or fragmentation of the embolus (with reperfusion) can limit the size of such infarctions.

Occlusion of large cerebral arteries may cause thromboembolism to propagate in more distal vessels. Also, large vessel occlusions can cause hemodynamic insufficiency in the watershed zones of the territory supplied by the occluded artery. Lastly, occlusion of small penetrating arteries can result in small infarctions within the territory of such deep penetrating vessels. These are known as lacunar infarctions.

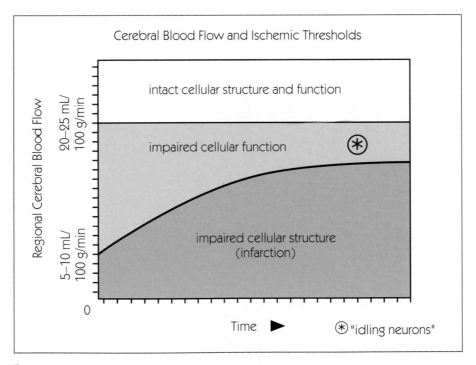

Figure 10.2 Cerebral blood flow and ischemic thresholds. Several lines of evidence from humans, primates, and higher mammals demonstrate clear thresholds for impaired cellular function and tissue infarction. Such thresholds depend on the level of regional cerebral blood flow and also the duration of ischemia. Longer periods of hypoperfusion increase the likelihood of tissue infarction. This concept explains clinical observations of transient ischemia, and also the possibility of preserved but dysfunctional tissue in moderate ischemia ("idling neurons"). (Figure modified from Jones TH, et al., 1981)

The occlusion of a given cerebral artery does not always result in a predictable infarction. Collateral pathways (Fig. 10.4) may redistribute blood flow sufficiently to prevent infarction in particular regions of the brain.[3] The competence of the collateral pathways depends on individual vascular anatomy (collateral pathways may be atretic or particularly prominent in certain individuals) and on the chronicity of ischemia (certain collateral pathways may become more prominent with longer durations of chronic ischemia).

Major collateral pathways include the epicerebral leptomeningeal circulation (consisting of the network of small arteries in the subarachnoid space surrounding the brain), the anterior circle of Willis (anterior cerebral and communicating arteries), the posterior circle of Willis (posterior communicating artery), and the ophthalmic artery (allowing communication between the external and internal carotid circulations). Less prominent collateral pathways may be operative in pathologic situations of chronic ischemia. These include transdural transcerebral (across the dura mater), cervical muscular collaterals, and a proliferation of deep cerebral arteries (often resembling a puff of smoke on angiography, hence the Japanese term "moyamoya collaterals").

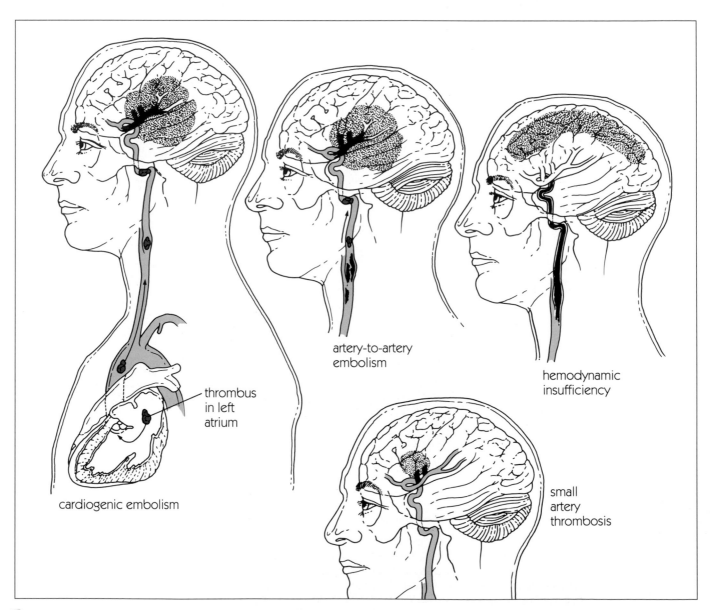

Figure 10.3 Mechanisms of focal ischemia. *Cardiogenic embolism* results from a variety of cardiac pathologies, including valvular disease, mural thrombus, and atrial myxoma, and can lead to occlusion of cerebral arteries with resulting territorial infarctions. Artery-to-artery embolism involves platelet aggregates, thrombi, or fragments of atheroma originating in atherosclerotic large arteries and leads to occlusion of smaller cerebral arteries downstream with territorial infarctions. Hemodynamic insufficiency results from occluded large vessels and impaired collateral pathways, causing "watershed" infarctions. *Small artery thrombosis* is caused by occlusion of sclerotic small cerebral vessels with lacunar infarctions involving the respective territories of these deep arteries.

A wide spectrum of clinical manifestations and vascular and parenchymal pathologic changes are associated with brain ischemia (Fig. 10.5).

Clinical Spectrum

Occlusive cerebrovascular disease may be totally asymptomatic or it may be accompanied by subtle clinical signs such as a cervical bruit (on ausculation). A cervical bruit is an index of systemic vasculopathy, including coronary and carotid occlusive disease, and is not a reliable herald of severe or clinically relevant carotid occlusive disease.

Transient (less than 24 hours) or reversible (less than 3 days) clinical symptoms of ischemia may include a temporary focal neurologic dysfunction in which there is complete clinical recovery between or following the spell(s). Transient ischemic attacks (TIAs) or reversible ischemic neurologic deficits (RINDs) affecting the carotid circulation include temporary focal paresis, dysphasia, focal sensory disturbance, or amaurosis fugax (transient monocular blindness). TIAs or RINDs affecting the vertebrobasilar circulation include crossed motor or sensory symptoms (affecting one side of the face and the contralateral half of the body), drop attacks (sudden falls), tinnitus, vertigo, diplopia, dysarthria, dysphagia, or homonomous visual field disturbances. Such reversible symptoms may result from temporary cerebrovascular circulatory compromise (embolus with rapid fragmentation or transient hemodynamic insufficiency) or minute cerebral infarctions (with rapid recovery of clinical symptoms).

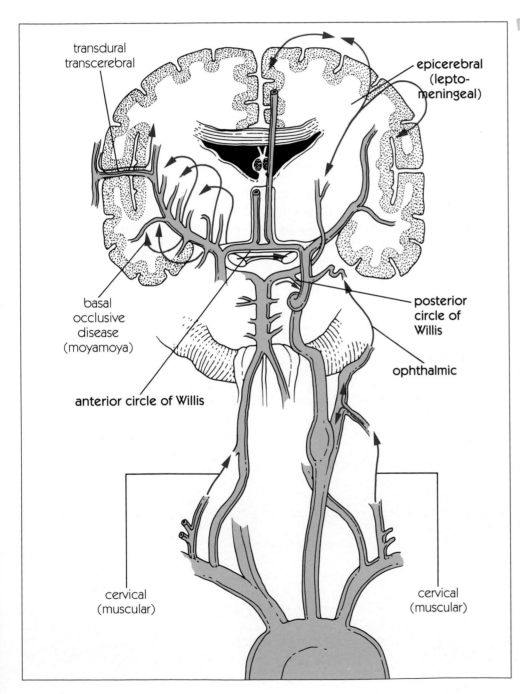

transdural
transcerebral

epicerebral
(lepto-
meningeal)

basal
occlusive
disease
(moyamoya)

posterior
circle of
Willis

ophthalmic

anterior circle of Willis

cervical
(muscular)

cervical
(muscular)

Figure 10.4 The collateral pathways. Collateral pathways allow redistribution of blood flow in the presence of arterial insufficiency, which prevents infarction in particular regions of the brain. Major collateral pathways include the epicerebral (leptomeningeal) collaterals (providing communication between various vascular territories), the anterior circle of Willis (providing communication between cerebral hemispheres), the posterior circle of Willis (providing communication between the vertebrobasilar and carotid circulations), and the ophthalmic collaterals (providing communication between the external carotid and internal carotid circulations). Less prominent collateral pathways may be operative in pathologic situations of chronic ischemia and include transdural transcerebral collaterals from arteries of the dura mater, and basal occlusive collaterals (proliferation of arterial channels in the region of the perforating arteries).

Ischemic stroke results in a permanent focal functional neurologic deficit referable to the region of brain infarction. An ischemic infarct may be totally asymptomatic if it affects noneloquent regions of the brain. Subtle or reversible symptoms may occur with smaller infarctions. Minor stroke results in persistent residual symptoms that are not severely disabling (incomplete paresis, partial dysphasia, etc.). Major stroke typically results in profound multimodal neurologic deficits, such as hemiplegia, hemisensory deficit, hemineglect, and hemianopsia.

A possible cumulative effect of multiple infarctions is mental deterioration and cognitive decline. In general, the larger the area of parenchymal infarction the more prominent the clinical symptoms. However, the location of the infarction and other factors, including age and general medical condition, also play a role in the functional sequelae of stroke. Therefore, the clinical spectrum of symptomatic brain ischemia does not necessarily correspond to proportional parenchymal brain damage.

Vascular Pathologic Spectrum

As with brain infarction, a spectrum of vascular pathologies can cause brain ischemia.[3]

Cardiac disease can cause brain ischemia through a variety of mechanisms. Cardioembolic stroke may result from atrial fibrillation, atrial or ventricular mural thrombus, mural myxoma, and infected or noninfected valvular vegetations. Cardiac dysrhythmia or aortic stenosis may result in global cerebral ischemia or in the accentuation of focal cerebrovascular occlusive disease. There is also a noncausal association between coronary artery disease and cerebrovascular occlusive disease as both pathologic processes share many risk factors (see below).[4]

Large-vessel atherosclerotic disease preferentially affects the carotid bifurcation in the neck, but it may involve the intrapetrous and intracavernous carotid arteries or more distal cerebral arteries less frequently. Large-vessel atherosclerosis may be responsible for artery-to-artery embolism of calcific fragments, thrombi, or platelet aggregates originating at the atherosclerotic plaque. In addition, large-vessel atherosclerosis may result in thrombotic arterial occlusion with subsequent hemodynamic compromise (depending on collateral circulation), thrombotic propagation (beyond collateral pathways), or tail embolism from the fresh occluding thrombus.

Small-vessel arteriosclerosis may affect perforating branches of the cerebral arteries at the base of the brain. Pathology in these vessels typically consists of lipohyalinosis, which is strongly associated with long-standing arterial hypertension.

Other arteriopathies that may affect the cerebral circulation include congenital, inflammatory, and idiopathic arteriopathies. A peculiar form of basal idiopathic occlusive vasculopathy affects arteries at the circle of Willis and their branches, with secondary proliferation of collateral vessels at the base of the brain, simulating a puff of smoke on angiography and hence the term "moya-moya" disease from the Japanese language.

Parenchymal Pathologic Spectrum[5]

As mentioned previously, occlusive cerebrovascular disease may be present without parenchymal damage or clinical symptoms. In other situations, it may result in complete arterial territorial infarction (typically a wedge-shaped infarction outlining the territory of a major cerebral artery). Such arterial territorial infarction is usually

---

Figure 10.5 Clinical and Pathologic Spectrum of Brain Ischemia

Clinical Spectrum	Vascular Pathologic Spectrum	Parenchymal Pathologic Spectrum
Asymptomatic	Cardiopathies	Vascular disease without parenchymal damage
Transient ischemia	Large vessel atherostenosis	Arterial territorial infarction (complete or incomplete)
Reversible ischemia	Large vessel occlusion (atheromatous, thrombotic, or embolic)	Watershed infarction (cortical or periventricular)
Minor stroke		
Major stroke	Small vessel arteriosclerosis	Lacunar infarction
Multiinfarct state	Other arteriopathies	Subcortical arteriosclerotic encephalomalacia
		Cortical atrophy
		Binswanger's disease

thromboembolic in etiology and implies occlusion of the major vessel and impairment of the collaterals to that territory. An incomplete arterial territorial infarction may be present, depending on the pattern and competence of collateral pathways.

Watershed infarctions affect the most distal territory of vascular supply. Watershed territories include the border zone of supply of the anterior, middle, and/or posterior cerebral arteries (usually high over the cerebral convexity). Another watershed territory may exist in periventricular regions between the penetrating branches of cortical vessels and perforating arteries that arise at the base of the brain.

Lacunar infarction refers to a small cavitation necrosis in the brain, corresponding to the territory of a deep parenchymal vessel. They have been shown to occur with occlusion of lipohyalinotic perforating arteries. Lacunar-like ischemic cavitations also occur in the watershed territories (hemodynamic) or as a result of embolism.[5]

Other parenchymal changes secondary to ischemia include cortical atrophy, subcortical arteriosclerotic encephalomalacia (leukoaraiosis), and the multiinfarct state, including Binswanger's disease.

Natural History

The natural history of many cerebrovascular disease entities has been elucidated with the advent of reliable diagnostic techniques (see below). It has been convincingly demonstrated that transient, reversible, or other ischemic insults predispose the patient to further brain ischemia, including massive devastating stroke.[6] The precise pathophysiology of the ischemic event greatly influences the prognosis.[7] Of patients with TIA, 20% to 30% will sustain a major ischemic stroke in the same territory in the subsequent 3 to 5 years. Patients with severe preocclusive carotid stenosis and TIA appear to be at much higher risk of subsequent stroke (up to 30% per year), while patients with completed carotid occlusion and a flurry of TIAs (around the time of occlusion) are very unlikely to sustain delayed ischemic infarction in the same territory.

Carotid stenoses are not static lesions.[7,8] Once a diagnosis of carotid stenosis has been established, it is likely that the lesions will progress in more than 50% of cases over the subsequent 1 to 5 years. This progression may be accelerated by uncontrolled vascular risk factors (see below).

The most risky phase following symptomatic brain ischemia is immediately after the ischemic spell. Up to one third of patients with ischemic symptoms may suffer further neurologic deterioration during the same hospitalization.[6] Again, the pathophysiologic mechanism of ischemia will largely determine the likelihood of further symptoms. Several lines of evidence indicate that the most critical periods in the natural history of an arterial stenosis are immediately preceding and immediately following arterial occlusion.[5,7-10] Therefore, the most serious lesions are those that are preocclusive or have recently

occluded. This is mostly related to the ominous prognosis of propagating thrombosis and thromboembolism.

Thirty percent to 60% of major (disabling) strokes are preceded by a temporary or minor ischemic insult.[6] It is therefore cardinal to identify the pathophysiologic mechanism of ischemia even when there are only minor symptoms, since many patients have much to lose from subsequent infarction in the same territory. Also, minor symptoms are often misinterpreted by patients and misdiagnosed by physicians, and transient symptoms can be missed if they occur during sleep.[6] Asymptomatic disease cannot be ignored because ominous occlusive cerebrovascular disease can well occur in the absence of any overt clinical symptoms.[6,11] In fact, a substantial fraction of disabling infarctions are not preceded by symptoms.

DIAGNOSTIC STUDIES

DOPPLER ULTRASONOGRAPHY

Noninvasive examination of the cerebral circulation has been made possible by ultrasound applications of the Doppler principle[12] (i.e., the frequency shift of echoed signals in relation to signals emitted by the instrument, thereby revealing the velocity of moving blood in the insonated artery). It is known that blood velocity increases substantially at and just beyond a stenotic lesion. In addition, B-mode ultrasonography allows visualization of arterial walls based on relative density to ultrasound beams.

Duplex sonography allows real-time imaging of extracranial carotid arteries using B-mode scanning of the vessel wall with simultaneous Doppler information about intravascular blood velocity. The resulting reconstruction provides an accurate representation of arterial stenosis and its resulting hemodynamic impact. Duplex ultrasonography of extracranial carotid arteries is highly sensitive to stenotic changes in the carotid arteries. However, ulcerative lesions may be missed unless heavily calcified or associated with local hemodynamic changes. Also, an artery can be assumed to be obstructed when the external and internal arteries are superimposed in one plane or when there is severe preocclusive stenosis and sluggish antegrade flow.[12]

Transcranial Doppler ultrasonography uses a low frequency probe for improved tissue penetration (2 MHz as opposed to 7 to 10 MHz for Doppler study of extracranial vessels). The majority of the skull is opaque to ultrasound signals except for the thin squamosal portion of the temporal bone (temporal window), the orbits (orbital window), and the foramen magnum. These three windows allow insonation of vessels leading to and arising from the circle of Willis. Directional flow in these vessels can be accurately evaluated using transcranial Doppler, thereby providing a noninvasive index of collateral pathways. Also, flow velocities in the intracranial vessels may indicate hyperdynamic flow states or focal stenoses. Lastly, transcranial Doppler has been used to detect embolism in the intracranial cerebral circulation.

Both extracranial and transcranial Doppler studies are strongly technician-dependent. They need to be interpreted in conjunction with other diagnostic studies to avoid errors. Ultrasound evaluation of the cervical carotid arteries is an excellent way to rule out large-vessel carotid occlusive disease in the presence of symptomatic brain ischemia. However, this method cannot reliably assess the precise severity and extent of stenosis and there will be significant errors in evaluating severe preocclusive stenosis.

Injecting radiographic contrast material into cerebral arteries provides an excellent view of large and small cerebral arteries and facilitates a survey of flow dynamics and collateral pathways into various vascular territories (Figs. 10.6, 10.7). These studies reliably show stenotic lesions in vessels larger than 1 to 2 mm and also can reveal embolic sources, including luminal thrombi and ulcerations. A complete survey of the cerebral circulation allows evaluation of collateral pathways, including their patency and contribution to the particular pathophysiologic situation, and determines the presence of occlusive disease, which

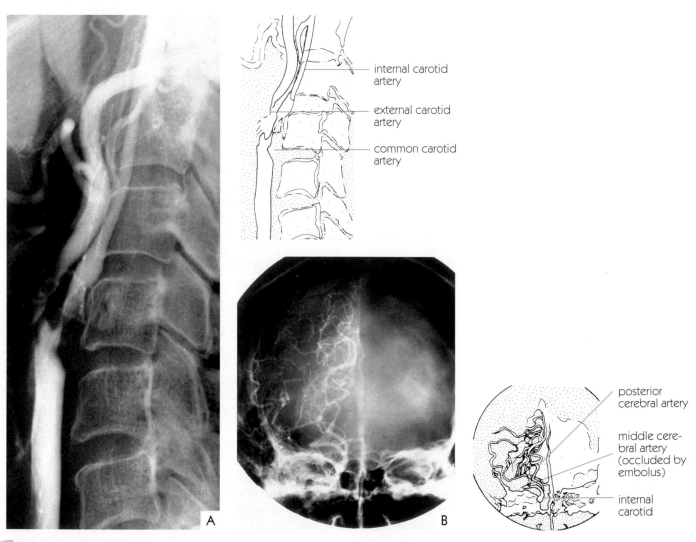

Figure 10.6 Cerebral angiography. (A) Right common carotid arteriogram showing severe right internal carotid artery stenosis from atheroma at the carotid bifurcation. (B) Anteroposterior intracranial view of the same injection, revealing occlusion of the middle cerebral artery from embolism presumably originating from the atheroma upstream. The posterior cerebral artery fills from this same injection, indicating patency of the posterior circle of Willis.

might affect the collateral pathways. Many centers currently perform arterial digital subtraction angiography, which provides excellent visualization of arterial anatomy using small catheters and low contrast volume, resulting in lower procedure-related morbidity than conventional angiographic techniques. Transfemoral retrograde arterial catheterization has all but eliminated complications related to direct puncture of cerebral arteries. Finally, newer flow-directed catheters allow superselective arteriography as well as selective injection of therapeutic agents into small arterial branches.

A typical angiographic study in a case of brain ischemia would include selective injection of both carotid circulations (with extracranial and intracranial views in at least two planes) as well as visualization of the aortic arch, the origin of the great vessels, and preferably a view of the posterior circulation (essential if posterior circulation ischemia is suspected). In the presence of an arterial lesion, a careful evaluation of the cerebral angiogram should estimate dynamic flow rate and patterns of collateral circulation and rule out pseudoocclusion (the false angiographic appearance of an occlusion due to exceedingly low flow rates). Pseudoocclusion is demonstrated by obtaining late views of the apparently occluded artery to show the faint appearance of sluggish antegrade flow. In the setting of arterial branch occlusions, upstream vessels should be closely examined for potential emboligenic sources (e.g., atherosclerotic ulcers).

COMPUTED TOMOGRAPHY

The advent of CT scanning of the brain has revolutionized the diagnosis of brain ischemia.[13] A patient with acute ischemic insult will usually have a negative CT scan, thereby ruling out other structural pathology, including hemorrhage, as a cause of the symptoms. Within hours of the ischemic spell (longer for small regions of ischemia), the CT shows decreased density in the infarcted parenchyma. This becomes more evident and well demarcated by 24 to 48 hours. Upon intravenous contrast administration, there may be enhancement of the infarcted tissue, indicating breakdown of the blood-

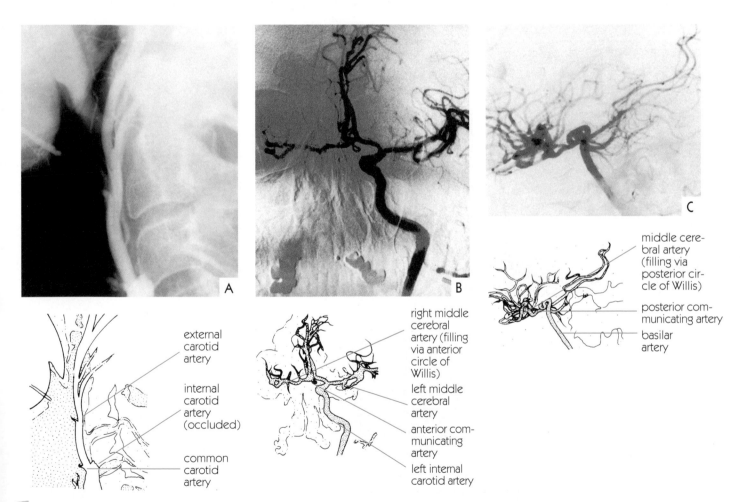

Figure 10.7 Cerebral angiography. (A) Right common carotid arteriogram injection revealing occlusion of the internal carotid artery just distal to its origin. (B) Anteroposterior intracranial (subtracted) view of the contralateral internal carotid artery injection showing filling of both cerebral hemispheres via a patent anterior circle of Willis. (C) Injection of the vertebrobasilar system (lateral view) in same case reveals filling of the right middle cerebral artery distribution via the posterior communicating artery, indicating patency of the posterior circle of Willis. This patient tolerated internal carotid artery occlusion without infarction and in view of excellent collateral filling is at low risk of subsequent brain ischemia in the same territory.

brain barrier. This is noticeable several days after the onset of ischemia and remains prominent for several weeks. Chronic cerebral infarctions do not reveal contrast enhancement and essentially consist of cavitated lesions filled with CSF.

The location of cerebral infarction can often be correlated with clinical symptoms.[13,14] Also, the CT may reveal evidence of prior remote ischemic insults. The appearance of cerebral infarction on CT scan can suggest a probable pathophysiologic mechanism (Fig. 10.8).[14] Small lacunar cavitations are usually due to small vessel occlusive disease, and rarely to hemodynamic ischemia or embolism. Large wedge-shaped infarctions suggest thromboembolism and territorial arterial infarction. Ill-defined infarctions at the border of arterial territories (high convexity or periventricular regions) could suggest hemodynamic ischemia.[14]

Other changes on the CT scan may indicate chronic cerebrovascular disease. Focal sulcal atrophy may indicate chronic hemodynamic insufficiency. Also, radiolucencies in the periventricular regions have been associated with cerebrovascular disease risk factors and subtle dementia.

These have been referred to as "leukoaraiosis" and can represent an index of brain parenchymal changes caused by chronic cerebrovascular disease.[15]

MAGNETIC RESONANCE IMAGING

All ischemic lesions visible on CT scan are more sensitively visualized by MRI. In addition, MRI can reveal evidence of parenchymal infarction several hours before CT scan.[16] In patients with cerebrovascular disease many lesions that cannot be seen on the CT scan are evident on MRI. Some of these MRI lesions represent subtle infarctions missed by the CT scan; however, the majority correlate with the appearance of leukoaraiosis on the CT scan (Fig. 10.9)[16,17] as well as various risk factors of cerebrovascular disease (including age). The lesions may indicate parenchymal brain changes caused by chronic cerebrovascular disease.[17]

More recently, flow imaging using MRI has enabled the cervical and intracranial vessels to be seen with a sensitivity, specificity, and spatial resolution exceeding that of ultrasound studies. This technique, magnetic res-

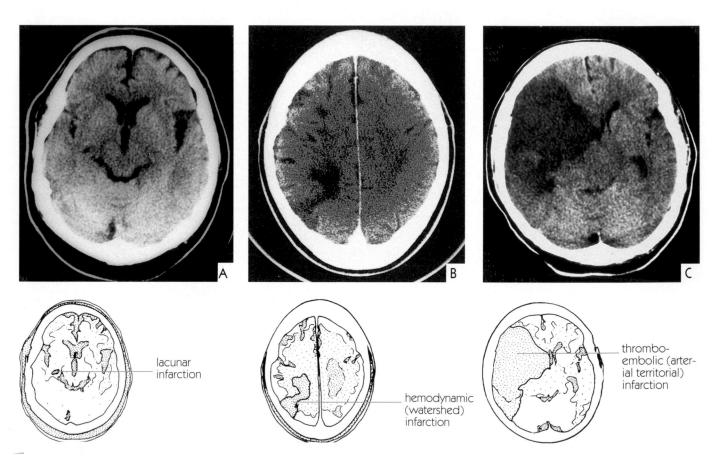

Figure 10.8 CT scan of cerebral infarction. (A) Lacunar infarction in the posterior limb of the internal capsule, presumed secondary to small vessel disease; larger lacunar infarctions may also result from cerebral embolism. (B) Watershed infarction, presumably hemodynamic, in the territory bordering the middle cerebral and posterior cerebral arterial circulations.

(C) Complete middle cerebral artery territorial infarction, presumed to be thromboembolic. Other embolic infarctions may result in partial arterial territorial parenchymal damage, depending on the size of the occluded branch, subsequent fragmentation of the embolus, and collateral pathways.

onance angiography, is in its infancy but may soon be perfected, replacing conventional angiography in certain situations. MRI's more modern diffusion, perfusion, and spectroscopic imaging can reveal ischemic changes minutes after the onset of symptoms. These techniques are not yet widely available to the clinician.

CEREBRAL BLOOD FLOW AND METABOLISM

The above diagnostic methods do not provide a direct measure of rCBF or metabolism. Direct measurements can be useful in individual clinical situations when there is a difficult differential diagnosis or when therapeutic choices depend on or are titrated against cerebral blood flow and metabolic rates. It must be emphasized that this is rarely the case in routine clinical practice.[18]

The rCBF can be measured using the washout technique of inhaled or intravenously administered substances. This is the basis for various xenon rCBF measurements, including the CT technique that provides a quantified measure of rCBF with a tomographic spatial resolution of several millimeters.[19] The dynamic accumulation and/or washout of photon-emitting substances administered intravenously are the basis for single photon emission computed tomography (SPECT) (Fig. 10.10). The regional cerebral metabolic rate of glucose and oxygen can be quantified tomographically using positron emission tomography (PET). These sophisticated and highly expensive instruments are available at few institutions and currently have limited clinical application. However, such instruments are powerful research tools that have significantly advanced our knowledge of pathophysiologic phenomena in brain ischemia.

PREVENTION AND MEDICAL MANAGEMENT

RISK FACTOR MODIFICATION

Several factors associated with a statistically increased risk of symptomatic brain ischemia[4] are age, essential hypertension, heart disease, and a prior history of symptomatic brain ischemia. Other risk factors for stroke

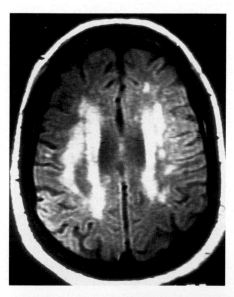
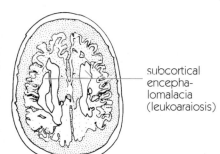

subcortical encepha-lomalacia (leukoaraiosis)

Figure 10.9 MRI in brain ischemia. This modality is highly sensitive to parenchymal changes of ischemia. In this case, there are multiple focal confluent regions of increased signal in the centrum semiovale and periventricular regions. These changes, typical of subcortical encephalomalacia (leukoaraiosis), correlate with age and cerebrovascular risk factors. These changes may be an index of parenchymal brain changes with chronic cerebrovascular disease.

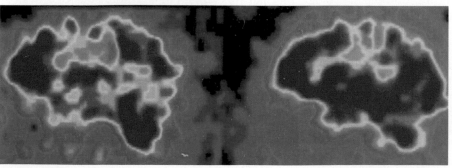

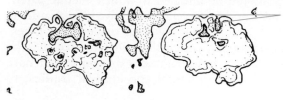

areas of hypoperfusion in the watershed zone

Figure 10.10 Single photon emission computed tomographic (SPECT) cerebral blood flow scan in a patient with carotid occlusion and frequent spells of hemiparesis but no evidence of infarction on CT or MRI scan. The parasagittal cuts demonstrate focal hypoperfusion in the watershed border zone between the territories of the anterior cerebral and middle cerebral arteries.

include diabetes, smoking, hyperlipemia, peripheral atherosclerotic occlusive disease, and the use of certain birth control pills. Controversy exists as to whether each of these factors independently increases the risk of stroke; clearly, many of these risks are interrelated.

Modification of risk factors (e.g., controlling arterial hypertension and discontinuing smoking) has been shown to alter the risk of subsequent stroke.[20] Risk factor modification may slow the progression of atherogenesis and alter hematologic and rheologic factors, lessening the risk of further ischemic insults. Risk factor modification alone will not reverse severe arterial stenosis and cannot per se eliminate all risk of subsequent stroke. However, it can be part of a comprehensive strategy of stroke prevention used in conjunction with other medical and surgical therapeutic options.

MEDICAL THERAPY FOR STROKE PREVENTION

Antiplatelet therapy (usually aspirin 325 to 975 mg daily) has been shown to decrease the risk of ischemic stroke in several clinical settings,[21] an effect that seems more pronounced in males. But the risk of stroke is not altogether eliminated. In fact, given the pathophysiologic heterogeneity of stroke discussed previously, aspirin alone would not be expected to eradicate the risk of ischemic brain damage. Antiplatelet therapy can prevent the formation of mural fibrin-platelet clumps, which may play a role in retinal and cerebral emboli. Antiplatelet therapy also can inhibit the process of mural thrombosis in the heart and large vessels and improve blood flow characteristics in the cerebral microcirculation. More recently, aspirin has been shown to reduce (but not eliminate) the risk of cerebral embolism from atrial fibrillation.[22]

Anticoagulation therapy with heparin or warfarin inhibits the process of thrombosis and may prevent propagating thromboembolism when there is acute large vessel occlusion and stroke-in-evolution.[21,23] Several clinical trials in progress address specific issues in various ischemic situations. A recently completed multiinstitutional trial has demonstrated the effectiveness of warfarin therapy in the prevention of cerebral embolism from atrial fibrillation.[22] The beneficial effect of anticoagulation in this setting was far greater than the protection provided by antiplatelet therapy; however, the risks of anticoagulation therapy (especially prolonged anticoagulation) should be weighed against any proven or suspected benefits.[24] Risks of systemic or cerebral hemorrhage are in the range of 1% to 5% per year depending on the anticoagulation regimen and patient population. Anticoagulation is contraindicated when there is extensive brain infarction (high risk of hemorrhagic sequelae) or evidence of central nervous system or systemic bleeding. Chronic anticoagulation is contraindicated in unreliable or noncompliant patients and in those who are subject to frequent falls or trauma. Little consensus exists about the optimal regimen of anticoagulation for brain ischemia. There is no evidence that vigorous anticoagulation (beyond 1.5 to 2 times control values on clotting tests) provides any additional protection, yet it subjects the patient to increased hemorrhagic risk compared to lesser degrees of anticoagulation.

In summary, antiplatelet therapy is indicated in the presence of asymptomatic cerebrovascular disease and following TIA, RIND, or previous stroke. Antiplatelet therapy is not a substitute for other therapeutic intervention for cardiac disease or preocclusive large vessel stenosis. Anticoagulation therapy may be useful in the setting of cardioembolism, preocclusive large vessel stenosis (as a temporary measure or in patients who are not candidates for surgery), and in certain cases of stroke-in-evolution if there is suspicion of propagating thrombosis and thromboembolism. This therapy may also be indicated if hypercoagulability predisposes the patient to cerebral ischemia.

MANAGEMENT OF ACUTE BRAIN ISCHEMIA

General medical measures are indicated in the management of each case of acute brain ischemia (Fig. 10.11). Whenever necessary, airway support must be established. There should be careful attention to hemodynamic and rheologic optimization, electrolyte balance, and nutritional maintenance. Deep vein thromboembolic and gastrointestinal bleeding prophylaxis and respiratory and physical therapy are indicated in all cases of major stroke and should be initiated as soon as possible.[25]

Regardless of the extent of clinical symptoms, diagnostic studies should be undertaken following immediate medical stabilization. Most clinicians agree that a TIA or RIND should be treated as a medical emergency until the possibility of serious impending progression has been eliminated. Initial diagnostic studies should include parenchymal neuroimaging (CT or MRI) and vascular evaluation. Duplex ultrasonography with or without transcranial Doppler examination or magnetic resonance angiography (where available) can be used as a screening measure. Cerebral angiography is performed whenever large-vessel disease has not been reliably ruled out by noninvasive studies or when the diagnosis or pathophysiologic mechanisms remain in question. A cardiac evaluation is performed in every case and should at least include an electrocardiogram and an echocardiogram. Patients with strongly suspected cardioembolism should probably be studied by transesophageal echocardiography because of its higher sensitivity. Patients considered for major surgical procedures should undergo a cardiology clearance, including a thorough evaluation of cardiac risks and possible coronary angiography.

Stroke is a powerful risk factor of subsequent myocardial infarction and cardiac death.

Therapy should be initiated to limit ischemic parenchymal damage and to prevent progressive ischemia. In all cases in which a significant region of tissue injury is suspected, consideration should be given to treating the patient with one or more regimens or agents that have been shown, in experimental and clinical studies, to reduce parenchymal damage from brain ischemia[26] (i.e., mannitol, dextran, hypertensive hypervolemic therapy, avoidance of hemoconcentration and, possibly, anticonvulsants and calcium channel blockers).

Therapy to prevent recurrent ischemia should be initiated according to suspected or demonstrated pathophysiologic mechanisms. The type of therapy depends on the nature and extent of vascular and parenchymal pathology. Such therapy may include antiplatelet drugs, anticoagulants, surgical intervention, and, possibly, endovascular therapy. Risk factor modification and long-term rehabilitation should be instituted in every case.[25]

SURGERY FOR EXTRACRANIAL CAROTID DISEASE

INDICATIONS

Convergent evidence from clinical registries, natural history studies, and at least two recent multiinstitutional prospective randomized trials have demonstrated the effectiveness of carotid endarterectomy for stroke prevention in severe (greater than 70%) cervical internal carotid artery stenosis and previous ipsilateral cerebral or retinal ischemic symptoms. Carotid artery surgery in this setting has been shown to decrease significantly the risk of subsequent stroke compared to the best medical therapy alone.[27]

Other possible indications for carotid endarterectomy include less severe stenosis in the presence of deep shaggy ulceration and definite attributable symptoms and preocclusive asymptomatic stenosis (Fig. 10.12).[28] Possible contraindications to carotid endarterectomy include serious medical risk (consider regional anesthesia) and recent large parenchymal infarction (high risk of perfusion breakthrough and brain hemorrhage). Recent limited parenchymal infarction is not a contraindication to carotid endarterectomy.

Carotid artery surgery has also been used when the patient has acute carotid occlusion and minor stroke (thrombectomy and endarterectomy). External carotid endarterectomy is indicated for ipsilateral retinal or cerebral symptoms in the setting of chronic carotid occlusion and impaired external carotid collaterals (or ulcerated carotid bifurcation stump and proximal external carotid

Figure 10.11 Management of Acute Brain Ischemia

General Medical Measures	Diagnostic Studies	Therapy to Limit Parenchymal Damage	Therapy to Prevent Recurrent Ischemia
Airway support	Parenchymal neuroimaging (CT or MRI)	Mannitol	Antiplatelet therapy
Nutritional support		Anticonvulsants (?)	Anticoagulant therapy
Electrolyte balance	Vascular evaluation (ultrasound, angiography)	Calcium channel blockers (?)	Surgery
Hemodynamic optimization			Endovascular therapy (?)
Hemostatic optimization	Cardiac evaluation	Dextran (or related agents) (?)	Risk factor modification
Rheologic optimization	Hemostatic optimization	Hypertensive therapy (?)	
Deep vein thromboembolic prophylaxis		Hypervolemic therapy (?)	
Gastrointestinal bleeding prophylaxis		Hemodilution (?)	
Respiratory therapy		Thrombolysis (?)	
Physical therapy			

artery emboligenic sources).[28] These indications have not been thoroughly examined in scientific studies.

CAROTID ENDARTERECTOMY

The technique of carotid endarterectomy is illustrated in Figure 10.13. A cervical incision is made along the anterior border of the sternocleidomastoid muscle. Dissection then proceeds through the platysma layer and medial to the sternocleidomastoid muscle along its length (with interruption of the common facial and other bridging veins). The carotid sheath is entered medial to the internal jugular vein, exposing the distal common carotid artery and the proximal several centimeters of internal and external carotid arteries. The carotid body may be anesthetized to blunt hemodynamic instability during the remainder of the operation. Systemic anticoagulation is administered (typically 100 IU heparin per kilogram of body weight) followed by temporary cross-clamping of the carotid bifurcation. An arteriotomy is performed at the distal common carotid artery and along the proximal internal carotid artery to a

---

Figure 10.12 Carotid Endarterectomy Indications

Proven Indication	Other Possible Indications	Possible Contraindications
Severe (>70%) internal carotid artery cross-sectional stenosis* and previous ipsilateral cerebral or retinal ischemic symptoms	Less severe stenosis in presence of deep shaggy ulceration and definite attributable symptoms Preocclusive asymptomatic stenosis	Serious medical risk (consider regional anesthesia) Recent large parenchymal infarction

*Measured as angiographic vessel diameter at narrowest point, divided by normal distal vessel diameter beyond the atheromatous plaque

---

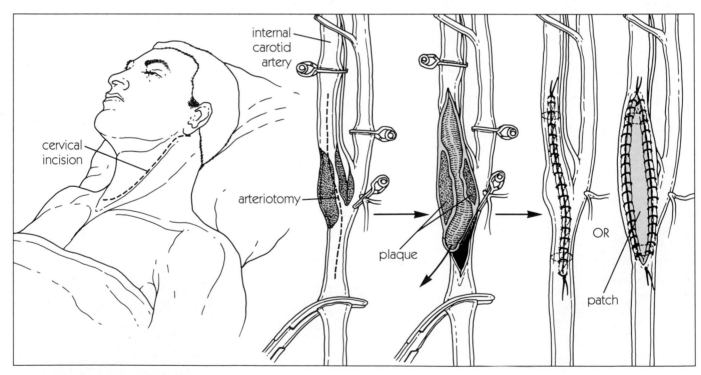

Figure 10.13 Technique of carotid endarterectomy. An oblique cervical incision allows dissection of the carotid bifurcation. Following heparinization, the arteries of the bifurcation are cross-clamped and an arteriotomy is performed. The plaque is dissected precisely in the subintimal plane, with a subsequent closure (primary or via patch reconstruc-tion) of the arteriotomy. Other adjuvant technical aspects of the operation include intraoperative monitoring during cross-clamping, microsurgical technique allowing optimal lighting and magnification, patch angioplasty, shunting, and verification of patency.

point just beyond the stenotic plaque. Endarterectomy is then performed in the subintimal plane, separating the plaque from the underlying arterial media. This portion of the operation is performed with technical precision so that all potential intimal flaps and sources of emboli are removed. The distal intima along the internal carotid artery is tacked down with carefully placed 7-0 vascular sutures unless it is absolutely adherent to the underlying vessel wall. The arteriotomy is closed with a continuous 5-0 or 6-0 vascular suture. A vein or synthetic patch may be incorporated in the arteriotomy closure to widen the vessel lumen.

The success of carotid endarterectomy clearly depends on the technical precision of the operation and meticulous prevention of cerebral complications during the procedure. Anesthetic technique should maximize cerebral and cardiac protection, and intraoperative hypotension must be avoided, especially during carotid cross-clamping. Intraoperative monitoring using electroencephalography, evoked potential monitoring, transcranial Doppler, cerebral blood flow, or other modalities enhances operative safety. Electroencephalography is widely used, and has been shown to be a reliable predictor of intraoperative brain ischemia.[28]

Technical adjuncts to this operation include meticulous hemostatic dissection and optimal illumination and magnification. The operating microscope enables neurosurgeons to pay meticulous attention to intimal flaps and arteriotomy closure. Luminal shunting may prevent hemodynamic cerebral insufficiency during carotid cross-clamping; however, it hinders visualization and technical perfection of the endarterectomy itself and may increase the chance of intraoperative cerebral embolism. Selective shunting, indicated by electroencephalographic changes during carotid cross-clamping, allows selection of patients whose circulation requires a shunt (and enables an easier and technically superior operation), while sparing a shunt in the majority of patients.[28]

Patching during arteriotomy closure increases luminal diameter. It may decrease the likelihood of postoperative carotid occlusion[29] and carotid restenosis. Patching may increase the likelihood of suture line disruption and lengthen the duration of cross-clamping. Many surgeons use patch angioplasty in endarterectomies, except with large vessels and very focal stenoses.[29]

Many surgeons advocate intraoperative verification of arterial patency, which can be done using ultrasonography or intraoperative angiography. Reversal of anticoagulation is optional, and there are many theoretical arguments against it (the endarterectomized vessel is most thrombogenic in the first 90 minutes following carotid endarterectomy). However, this consideration must be balanced against the risk of bleeding from the arteriotomy and other sites. The majority of surgeons drain the wound but this too must be viewed in light of the overall hemostatic aspects of the dissection.

Outstanding results have been reported with carotid endarterectomy whether or not one or more of the above technical adjuncts is used. The routine or selective use of most of the aforementioned modalities continues to be debated. However, the common denominator of operative success is careful anesthetic management and compulsive attention to the technical details of vascular repair.

SURGICAL RESULTS

A combination of judicious patient selection and superior surgical technique should insure an operative mortality rate of less than 2% and stroke rate of less than 4%. This outcome has been consistently accomplished by experienced and well-trained surgeons in symptomatic and asymptomatic patients (morbidity rates are slightly higher in symptomatic cases). A preoperative grading of medical, angiographic, and neurologic risks may help one predict the surgical outcome. It is unlikely that the operation will provide a significant overall benefit unless the surgical team can achieve this standard of surgical performance. Carotid artery surgery should be used judiciously in conjunction with other medical treatment modalities and risk factor modification programs for optimal stroke prevention.

Carotid artery surgery helps prevent subsequent brain ischemia secondary to hemodynamic insufficiency, arterial embolism, or propagating thrombosis from the diseased artery. The surgery does not necessarily protect against other mechanisms of brain ischemia, and it does not eliminate the risk of subsequent stroke altogether.

The benefits of carotid artery surgery appear to be durable. Recurrent stenosis (50% narrowing) occurs at a rate of 5% to 10% per year following operation but is not always symptomatic.[30] Symptomatic brain ischemia attributable to a previously operated artery is rare and may be amenable to successful reoperation. The use of patch angioplasty, risk factor modification, and medical therapy may decrease the likelihood of symptomatic restenosis.[29,30]

NONATHEROSCLEROTIC CAROTID OCCLUSIVE DISEASE

Carotid occlusive disease can be documented in the absence of atherosclerotic risk factors. Fibromuscular dysplasia is a vasculopathy affecting multiple large and medium sized arteries, including renal and carotid arteries.[31] When affecting the cervical carotid circulation, it may result in a bead-like, string-like, or pseudoaneurysmal appearance of the carotid artery. This may predispose the patient to carotid dissection or hemodynamic insufficiency.

Carotid dissection results from disruption of the intimal vascular plane, with blood flow partially directed in the subintimal, intramedial, or subadventitial plane.[32] Carotid dissection may occur spontaneously or following blunt trauma, and it has also been associated with fibromuscular dysplasia. The most frequent location of vessel disruption is at the level of the second vertebral body, usually well beyond the carotid bifurcation and just proximal to the carotid canal of the skull. It has been postulated that this location predisposes the artery to tethering against the bony lateral mass of the axis.

Carotid dissection can result in occlusion, near-occlusion, and/or intraluminal or subintimal thrombosis. In fact, the angiographic appearance of a tapered occlusion or stenosis of the internal carotid artery beyond a normal (nonatheromatous) bifurcation is nearly pathognomonic of dissection. Pseudoaneurysmal outpouching may occur at the level of dissection.

Carotid dissection should be treated medically since surgical correction of the intimal flap is typically too risky (the dissection usually extends into the bony carotid canal). Anticoagulation therapy appears to provide excellent protection against thromboembolic complications and may enhance vascular healing.[32] If anticoagulation therapy is used, a large number of carotid dissections will heal, so angiographically the vessel returns to normal or near-normal appearance. A small number will undergo complete carotid occlusion, while the remainder will continue to show varying degrees of stenosis, irregularity, and aneurysmal appearance. Upon vascular healing and resolution of the severe stenotic appearance of a dissection, anticoagulation therapy may be converted to antiplatelet therapy, which is usually continued indefinitely.

VERTEBRAL ARTERY OCCLUSIVE DISEASE

Infarctions of the vertebrobasilar territory carry a grave prognosis, with acute mortality ranging between 20% and 30%. Nearly half of the patients suffer previous TIAs or minor strokes in the same distribution, while subsequent stroke occurs within 5 years in 26% to 35% of patients with vertebrobasilar TIA. This rate is comparable to that following TIAs in the carotid territory.[28]

Isolated stenosis at the origin of a single vertebral artery is usually well tolerated, and many patients remain asymptomatic despite absence or occlusion of one vertebral artery. However, extracranial vertebral artery disease is not always benign. At autopsy more than half of posterior circulation infarctions are associated with extracranial occlusion or stenosis of a single vertebral artery. Less commonly, vertebrobasilar ischemia results from traumatic or spontaneous dissection of a vertebral artery, tethering by a fibrous cervical band, or extensive compression by an osteophyte. Occasionally, obstruction of the subclavian artery proximal to the origin of the vertebral artery will reverse flow in the vertebral artery and produce a steal of blood from the vertebral artery to the ipsilateral brachial artery. This subclavian steal is often asymptomatic and has rarely been convincingly associated with serious neurologic morbidity. While embolism occurs in certain patients, hemodynamic mechanisms are thought to be the major etiologic factors in vertebrobasilar ischemia. Propagating thrombosis from fresh occlusion of an artery also plays a role in cases with serious infarction.

No medical or surgical therapy has been demonstrated to be effective in preventing vertebrobasilar ischemia. Due to the wide variety of possible mechanisms, it is not likely that a single modality will be beneficial in all cases. Rational therapeutic approach to the individual patient requires accurate delineation of pathophysiologic mechanisms. Antiplatelet therapy is likely to be effective when there are mild atherosclerotic plaques in the vertebrobasilar circulation with or without symptoms. Antiplatelet therapy is not likely to improve the hemodynamic consequences of severe stenosis or vascular occlusion. Antiplatelet therapy does not protect against vascular occlusion or propagating thrombosis. Anticoagulant therapy is indicated when there is severe hemodynamically significant stenosis or fresh luminal thrombosis and propagating thromboembolism.

Surgical intervention should be considered in situations of accessible focal stenoses of the vertebral artery, especially when contralateral vertebral artery occlusion is present.[28] The goals of surgical intervention in extracranial vertebral artery disease are to reverse hemodynamic compromise and eliminate embolic sources. Indications for surgery include persistent clinical symptoms of vertebrobasilar ischemia and angiographic evidence of hemodynamic compromise. Lesions without hemodynamic compromise are considered for surgery only after the failure of antiplatelet or anticoagulant therapy. Surgical options include vertebral artery transposition, vertebral endarterectomy, and other more specialized procedures.

Vertebral artery transposition is indicated in focal vertebral artery origin stenosis or in the rare situations of subclavian steal with demonstrated symptoms of vertebrobasilar ischemia. The goal of the operation is to transpose the vertebral artery (distal to stenotic segment) onto the common carotid artery in an end-to-side fashion. This results in vertebral artery flow arising from the common carotid artery, thereby bypassing the stenotic lesion (Fig. 10.14). The operation is performed via a transverse incision 2 cm above the clavicle, and extending approximately 6 to 8 cm behind the anterior border of the sternocleidomastoid muscle. The sternocleidomastoid muscle is divided transversely and the carotid sheath is entered by retraction of the jugular vein. The common carotid artery is isolated and followed proximally in order to locate the subclavian artery. Then the vertebral artery is identified (usually 1 to 2 cm proximal to the origin of the thyrocervical trunk) and dissected from its origin at the subclavian artery to its point of entrance into the bony foramen transversarium. After full heparinization (see carotid endarterectomy), the origin of the vertebral artery is double clipped and the artery is transected just distal to the stenotic lesion. After microvascular preparation and tapering of the vessel end, it is transposed in an end-to-side fashion onto the nearby common carotid artery. The latter is cross-clamped for the duration of anastomosis, with monitoring undertaken as in carotid endarterectomy. End-to-side anastomosis is performed using 7-0 suture under microsurgical magnification.

In various series the reported outcome of this procedure, including prevention of further symptomatic ischemia, is comparable to that of carotid endarterectomy.[28]

Other extracranial vertebral artery procedures include endarterectomy of a focal arterial segment, untethering of stenosing fibrous bands, or resection of compressing osteophytes. These procedures are performed via a direct approach, insuring adequate surgical exposure for proximal and distal control on the vertebral artery.

INTRACRANIAL OCCLUSIVE DISEASE

Atherosclerotic occlusive disease may affect vessels that are inaccessible to direct extracranial endarterectomy. Such intracranial stenoses have a serious prognosis and are associated with a significant risk of subsequent stroke and myocardial infarction.[33] Extracranial-to-intracranial (EC-IC) bypass surgery in the setting of symptomatic stenoses has not been effective. In fact, there is a significant likelihood of a bypass converting a stenotic lesion into a symptomatic occlusion with disastrous consequences.[34] Intracranial arterial stenoses are best treated medically. Rare surgical options include extracranial endarterectomy of upstream tandem stenoses and EC-

IC bypass after all medical therapy has failed and convincing hemodynamic compromise has been demonstrated (see below).

Occlusion of major cerebral arteries is associated with a significant risk of stroke at the time of vessel occlusion. Delayed ischemia is uncommon but may occur via a wide variety of mechanisms. These include thromboembolism via collateral pathways or progressive hemodynamic compromise because of impaired collaterals. Also, small vessel disease may occur incidentally in the same territory as an occluded artery.[35]

Bypass surgery was designed to provide collateral blood flow to the territory of occluded or severely stenosed cerebral arteries. A large international cooperative study, however, failed to reveal any benefit of EC-IC bypass surgery in the setting of symptomatic arterial occlusions and inaccessible stenoses.[36] However, the study was not designed to assess, with statistical reliability, benefit or lack of benefit from the procedure in specific subgroups of patients. Two particular subgroups were not addressed: 1) Patients for whom the best available medical therapy failed. Over 50% of the patients admitted to the study did not have a trial on medical therapy and may have been less likely to benefit from additional revascularization than patients who had further brain ischemia despite antiplatelet therapy or anticoagulation. 2) Patients

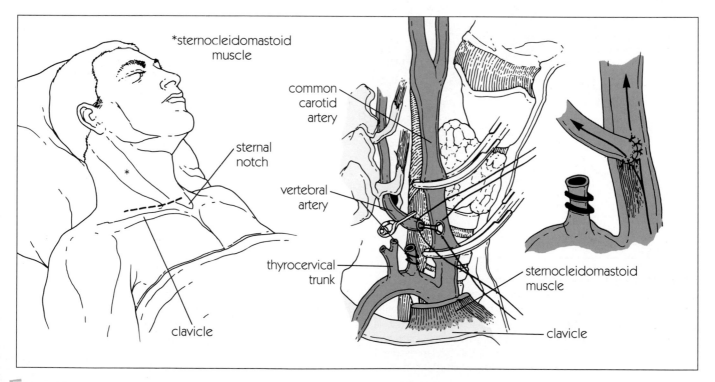

Figure 10.14 Technique of vertebral artery transposition for severe origin stenosis of the vertebral artery and hemodynamic insufficiency in the vertebrobasilar circulation. A transverse lateral cervical incision allows exposure of the vertebral artery and common carotid artery. The vertebral artery is transected just distal to the stenosis and transposed in an end-to-side fashion to the common carotid artery. This operation is also performed in rare cases of clearly symptomatic subclavian steal.

with clearly documented hemodynamic compromise. Over one third of the patients in the study had internal carotid artery occlusion without subsequent symptoms, while many others had hemodynamically insignificant lesions. Including all patients with brain ischemia without regard to the pathophysiologic mechanisms in each subgroup (i.e., including a large number of patients who by current understanding of the disease would not be candidates for the procedure) may have diluted the study. A limited number of patients who have clear hemodynamic compromise and/or for whom medical therapy has failed may benefit from the procedure, although the study was not designed to uncover benefit in these patients.[28,37]

There is a consensus among many cerebrovascular surgeons that a small group of patients with arterial occlusions, impaired collaterals, and demonstrated progressive ischemia despite anticoagulant therapy may benefit from revascularization surgery. Two strict criteria must be met to justify a bypass procedure in the era following the EC-IC bypass study: demonstrated hemodynamic compromise (impaired collaterals and preferably a confirmatory study demonstrating rCBF compromise) and failed maximal medical therapy.[28,37]

Several techniques provide a bypass graft between the extracranial and intracranial circulations,[28,37] including direct anastomoses of the superficial temporal artery to cortical branches of the middle cerebral artery. Also, long segments of high-flow grafts can be established between the cervical carotid arteries and more proximal segments of the middle cerebral artery. The preferred procedure currently performed at our institution interposes a reversed short segment of saphenous vein between the superficial temporal artery at the level of the zygoma (in an end-to-side fashion) to an M2 segment of the middle cerebral artery within the sylvian fissure (also in an end-to-side fashion) (Fig. 10.15). This allows the creation of a high-flow conduit with high short-term and long-term patency rates and low operative morbidity.[28,37]

Other clinical situations in which an EC-IC bypass procedure might be considered include giant cerebral aneurysms not amenable to direct clipping and vascular reconstruction (where the parent vessel must be sacrificed),

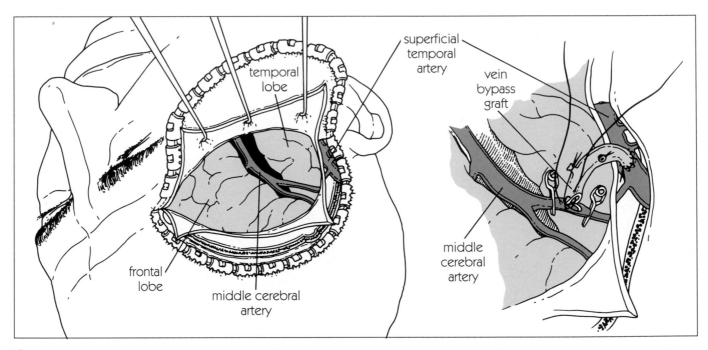

Figure 10.15 Superficial temporal artery-to-middle cerebral artery bypass technique. This is one of many possible technical methods of providing a bypass between the extracranial and intracranial circulations. The superficial temporal artery is exposed at the level of the zygomatic arch. A small pterional craniotomy is performed with splitting of the sylvian fissure, and exposure of the middle cerebral artery bifurcation. An interpositional vein bypass graft is then performed in an end-to-side fashion to both arteries. Other technical approaches for bypass include direct artery-to-artery end-to-side anastomosis, the use of more peripheral middle cerebral artery branches, and modifications of the technique for posterior circulation bypass.

extensive brain tumors invading cerebral arteries, and progressive occlusive vasculopathies (including "moyamoya" disease). Bypass surgery in these cases is individualized according to the angiographic collateral pattern, rCBF measurements, and tolerance of temporary occlusion tests (which may be performed using intravascular balloons with the patient awake and anticoagulated).[38]

An EC-IC bypass procedure is rarely considered for progressively symptomatic intracranial vertebrobasilar occlusive disease that occurs despite anticoagulant therapy. In such instances, anastomosis of the occipital or superficial temporal artery may be performed (directly or via an interpositional vein graft) to the posterior inferior cerebellar artery, anterior inferior cerebellar artery, superior cerebellar artery, or posterior cerebral artery, depending on the site of arterial stenosis and collateral pathways.[28]

CONCLUSION

Brain ischemia is the result of complex interactions between the brain parenchyma, vascular occlusive disease, and cerebral blood flow. Multiple pathophysiologic mechanisms are frequently operating, and interact closely to determine eventual clinical prognosis. Therapeutic modalities include a variety of medical treatments and selected surgical procedures, which should be judiciously combined and/or individualized in each case, and which must be guided, whenever possible, by a rational analysis of pathophysiologic mechanisms and natural history. It is not likely that any single treatment will benefit all patients with brain ischemia. Further studies are likely to clarify the role of individual treatment modalities in light of such pathophysiologic heterogeneity.

REFERENCES

1. Siesjo BK. *Brain Energy Metabolism*. New York, NY:John Wiley & Sons; 1978:1–149.
2. Jones TH, Morawetz RB, Crowell RM, et al. Thresholds of focal cerebral ischemia in awake monkeys. *J Neurosurg*. 1981;54:773–782.
3. Raichle MF. The pathophysiology of brain ischemia and infarction. *Clin Neurosurg*. 1982; 29:379–389.
4. Wolf PA, D'Agostino RB, Belanger AJ, et al. Probability of stroke: a risk profile from the Framingham Study. *Stroke*. 1991;22:312–318.
5. Ringelstein EB, Zeumer H, Angelou D. The pathogenesis of strokes from internal carotid artery occlusion: diagnostic and therapeutical implications. *Stroke*. 1983;14:867-875.
6. Toole JF. Transient ischemic attacks. In: Toole JF, ed. *Cerebrovascular Disorders*. New York, NY: Raven Press; 1984:101–116.
7. Bogousslavsky J, Despland PA, Regli F. Prognosis of high-risk patients with nonoperated symptomatic extracranial carotid tight stenosis. *Stroke*. 1988;19:108–111.
8. Javid H, Ostermiller WE, Hengesh JW, et al. Natural history of carotid bifurcation atheroma. *Surgery*. 1970;67:80–89.
9. Pessin MS, Hinton RC, Davis KR, et al. Mechanisms of acute stroke. *Ann Neurol*. 1979;6:245-251.
10. Norrving B, Nilsson B. Carotid artery occlusion: acute symptoms and long-term prognosis. *Neurol Res*. 1981;3:229–236.
11. Bogousslavsky J, Despland PA, Regli F. Asymptomatic tight stenosis of the internal carotid artery: long-term prognosis. *Neurology*. 1986;36:861–863.
12. Smith R, Brown R, Martin J, et al. Noninvasive carotid artery testing: an expanding science. In: Wood JH, ed. *Carotid Artery Surgery in Stroke*. Philadelphia, Pa: Hanley and Belfus; 1989:27–42.
13. Savoiardo M. CT scanning. In: Barnett HJM, Stein BM, Mohr JP, Yatsu FM, eds. *Stroke: Pathophysiology, Diagnosis and Management*. New York, NY: Churchill Livingstone; 1986:189–219.
14. Wozard R. Watershed infarctions and computed tomography: a topographical study in cases with stenosis or occlusion of the carotid artery. *Neuroradiol*. 1980;19:245–248.
15. Hachinski VC, Potter P, Merskey H. Leuko-araiosis. *Arch Neurol*. 1987;44:21–23.
16. Awad IA, Modic M, Little JR, et al. Focal parenchymal lesions in transient ischemic attacks; correlation of CT and MRI. *Stroke*. 1986;17:399–403.
17. Awad IA, Spetzler RF, Hodak JA, et al. Incidental subcortical lesions identified on MRI in the elderly, I: correlation with age and cerebrovascular risk factors. *Stroke*. 1986;17:1084–1089.
18. Yanagihara T, Wahner HW. Cerebral blood flow measurement in cerebrovascular occlusive disease. *Stroke*. 1984;15:816–822.
19. Yonas H, Goode WF, Gur D, et al. Mapping central blood flow by xenon-enhanced computed tomography: clinical experience. *Radiology*. 1984; 152:435–442.
20. Hypertension Detection and Follow-up Program Cooperative Group. Five-year findings of the Hypertension Detection and Follow-up Program, III: reduction in stroke incidents among persons with high blood pressure. *JAMA*. 1982;247:633–638.
21. Dykan ML. Anticoagulant and platelet antiaggregating therapy in stroke and threatened stroke. *Neurol Clin*. 1983;1:223–242.
22. Kelly RE. Stroke prevention in Atrial Fibrillation Study preliminary results. Presented at 16th International Joint Conference on Stroke and Cerebral Circulation; February 21, 1991; San Francisco, Calif.
23. Putnam SF, Adams HB, Usefulness of heparin in initial management of patients with recent transient ischemic attacks. *Arch Neurol*. 1985;42:960–962.
24. Levine M, Hirsch J. Hemorrhagic complications of

long-term anticoagulant therapy for ischemic cerebral vascular disease. *Stroke*. 1986;17:111–116.

25. Hachinski V, Norris JW. *The Acute Stroke*. Philadelphia, Pa: FA Davis; 1985. Contemporary Neurology Series 27.

26. Siesjo BK, Wieloch T. Cerebral metabolism in ischemia: neurochemical basis for therapy. *Br J Anaesth*. 1985;57:47–62.

27. NASCET Investigators. Clinical Alert. Benefit of carotid endarterectomy for patients with high grade stenosis of the internal carotid artery. National Institute of Neurological Disorders and Stroke; February 25, 1991.

28. Spetzler RF, Nehls DG, Awad IA. Ischemia and infarction: surgical treatment. In: Toole JF, ed. *Handbook of Clinical Neurology: Vascular Diseases, Part I*. New York, NY: Elsevier Science; 1989: 441–458.

29. Awad IA, Little JR. Patch angioplasty in carotid endarterectomy: advantages, concerns and controversies. *Stroke*. 1989;20:417–422.

30. Clagett GP, Rich NM, McDonald PT, et al. Etiologic factors for recurrent carotid artery stenosis. *Surgery*. 1983;93:913–918.

31. Olivi A, Tew JM, Van Loveran HR. Fibromuscular dysplasia. In: Wood JH, ed. *Carotid Artery Surgery in Stroke*. Philadelphia, Pa: Hanley and Belfus; 1989:

193–200. Neurosurgery: State of the Art Reviews.

32. Hart RG, Easton JD. Dissections and trauma of cervico-cerebral arteries. In: Barnett HJM, Stein BM, Mohr JP, Yatsu FM, eds. *Stroke: Pathophysiology, Diagnosis, and Management*. New York, NY: Churchill Livingstone; 1986:775–788.

33. Marzewski DJ, Furlan AJ, St Louis P, et al. Intracranial internal carotid artery stenosis: long-term prognosis. *Stroke*. 1982;13:821–824.

34. Awad IA, Furlan AJ, Little JR. Changes in intracranial stenotic lesions after extracranial-intracranial bypass surgery. *J Neurosurg*. 1984;60:771–776.

35. Furlan AJ, Whisnant JP, Baker HL. Long-term prognosis after carotid artery occlusion. *Neurology*. 1980;30:986–988.

36. EC-IC Bypass Study Group. Failure of extracranial-intracranial arterial bypass to reduce the risk of ischemic stroke, results of an international randomized trial. *N Engl J Med*. 1985;313:1191–1200.

37. Awad IA, Spetzler RF. Extracranial-intracranial (EC-IC) bypass surgery: a critical analysis in light of the International Cooperative Study. *Neurosurgery*. 1986;19:655–664.

38. Little JR, Rosenfeld J, Awad IA. Internal carotid artery occlusion for cavernous segment aneurysm. *Neurosurgery*. 1989;25:398–404.

Principles of Neurosurgery

Intracranial Aneurysm

H. Hunt Batjer

Intracranial aneurysmal disease encompasses a surprisingly broad spectrum of hemorrhagic and ischemic cerebrovascular entities. Clinical syndromes range from a completely silent and asymptomatic state to sudden death. This chapter provides an overview of the disease and discusses how to manage patients suffering from the various symptoms produced by aneurysms as well as some of the technical aspects of surgical treatment. While a number of types of aneurysm are known to occur on the intracranial vessels (including those that are atherosclerotic, tumor-related, infectious, and traumatic), the major thrust of this discussion is the most common type, the saccular or berry aneurysm.

EPIDEMIOLOGY

The actual incidence of aneurysms in the general population is difficult to estimate as autopsy series vary depending on the age of the individuals studied. It is clear, however, that the frequency with which aneurysms are detected increases with age.[1] The risk of developing aneurysms may differ among racial groups. Based on extrapolation from an autopsy series reported by McCormick, it is likely that 10 to 15 million Americans harbor aneurysms,[1] an incidence of more than 5% of the adult population. Kassell and Drake's 1982 study estimated that in North America approximately 28,000 people a year suffer subarachnoid hemorrhage (SAH) from a ruptured aneurysm.[2] Sadly, fewer than 40% of patients so stricken return to functional life despite modern treatment.[2] To add to this catastrophic loss to society, the age of SAH patients (the mean age is approximately 50 years[2]) is considerably less than that of patients disabled from occlusive cerebrovascular disease. In addition to the large number of patients who suffer from a ruptured aneurysm, neurosurgeons frequently see patients who have developed neurologic deficits from intracranial mass effect due to enlarging aneurysms or who present with focal cerebral ischemic symptoms due to embolization from the lumen of large or giant aneurysms.

PATHOLOGY

The histology of cerebral arteries, particularly at points of bifurcation (either vestigial or persistent), is germane to the various theories of aneurysmal development. An outer layer of fibrous adventitia overlies the muscular media, which contributes most of the strength in main-

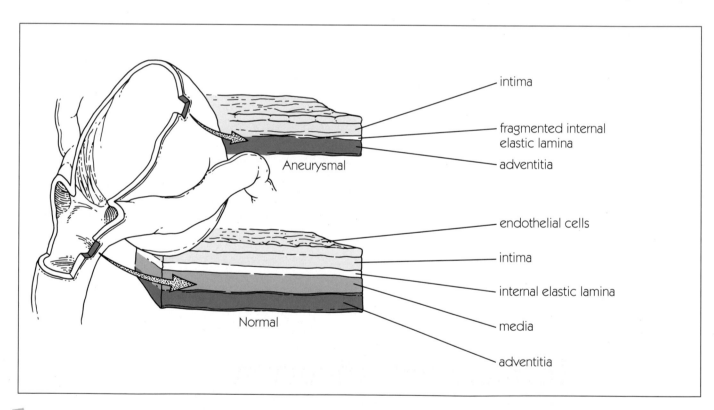

Figure 11.1 Histologic layers of cerebral arteries. Note the absence of media in the aneurysmal wall and the fragmented internal elastic lamina. The wall may be quite sclerotic in some areas and extremely thin in others.

taining vessel integrity. Deep to the media lies the intima, whose lumenal surface is lined by a layer of endothelial cells. The internal elastic lamina separates the intima from the media, but the external elastic lamina present in extracranial vessels is absent in arteries (Fig. 11.1).[3] Sekhar and Heros summarized available histological data and noted that a number of congenital factors have been implicated in the pathogenesis of these lesions: medial defects, elastic defects, sites of origin of small vessels, and failure of branch involution. They suggest that acquired factors may also play a role, including degenerative changes, thinning of the media, inflammation, atherosclerosis, hypertension, and hemodynamic stress.[3]

It is likely that aneurysms arise from a complex multifactorial set of circumstances involving a congenital anatomic predisposition enhanced by local or systemic environmental factors that further weaken the arterial wall and lead to aneurysmal dilation. The overwhelming majority of such lesions are found at the branching points of large subarachnoid conducting arteries, indicating that the point of bifurcation is an extremely vulnerable site. Evidence strongly supports the role played by hemodynamic stress in creating new aneurysms. *De novo* aneurysms commonly develop in the anterior communicating artery region several years following occlusion of one carotid artery, a phenomenon described by Somach and Shenkin.[4] Also seen are acute distension and fatal rupture of a distal basilar aneurysm after carotid ligation for giant cavernous aneurysms, an event precipitated by recruitment of retrograde flow through the posterior communicating artery.[5] In addition, regrowth of an imperfectly clipped aneurysm as a result of induced hypertension postoperatively has been noted.[6] A final point of supporting evidence can be found in patients harboring high flow arteriovenous malformations: A higher than expected incidence of aneurysms, especially on feeding arteries, has been noted in this population, and often the aneurysms are in atypical distal sites close to the malformation (Fig. 11.2).[7]

As an aneurysm enlarges, its complexity often increases in relation to its wall and to the efferent circulation. The wall of a large (12 to 25 mm) or giant (>25 mm in diameter) aneurysm usually has regions of extremely tough hyalinized tissue as well as regions of extremely attenuated transparent tissue, a phenomenon that can complicate obliteration. Furthermore, efferent vessels are further displaced from the parent arterial trunk, often appearing to arise from the aneurysm itself

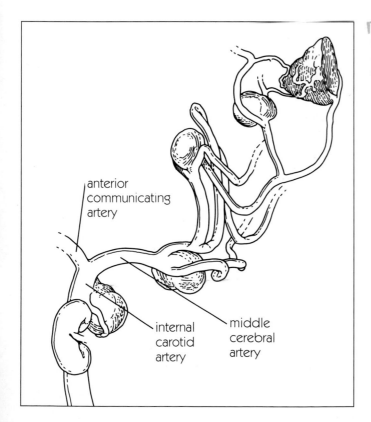

Figure 11.2 When high-flow situations complicate cerebral hemodynamics, such as an intracranial arteriovenous malformation, aneurysms are found with a relatively high frequency on feeding arteries and often in atypical distal sites.

(Fig. 11.3). Dissection usually permits accurate reconstruction, although occasionally a large efferent branch actually arises from the fundus of the aneurysm itself.

Intracranial aneurysms have been associated with intracranial vascular malformations as well as other systemic conditions, such as coarctation of the aorta, polycystic kidney disease, extracranial fibromuscular dysphasia, Marfan's syndrome, tuberous sclerosis, and Ehlers-Danlos syndrome.[8]

NEUROLOGY

SYMPTOMS

Few physicians would fail to diagnose accurately a 50-year-old housewife who collapsed at home with the sudden onset of the worst headache of her life, subsequently vomited, briefly lost consciousness, and was noted to have subhyaloid ocular hemorrhages and a rigid neck. Unfortunately, for many patients this catastrophic episode of SAH sets in motion a cascade of neurologic events that ultimately prove fatal, even if rebleeding does not occur. For this reason, it is of paramount importance to identify premonitory symptoms that herald either sudden enlargement of an aneurysm or a minor leak. In most surgeons' experience, between 25% and 50% of patients give a history of a warning leak a few days or weeks prior to a major SAH.[8] While the symptoms of a warning leak can be distressingly mild, the sudden onset of headache (even if short-lived) or minor focal neurologic deficit should heighten the physician's suspicions. Diagnosis is usually difficult; consequently, a number of patients, sent home from the physician's office or emergency room and instructed to take analgesics, ultimately suffer catastrophic rebleeding episodes several days later.

A number of patients experience sentinel symptoms more consistent with acute distention or enlargement of

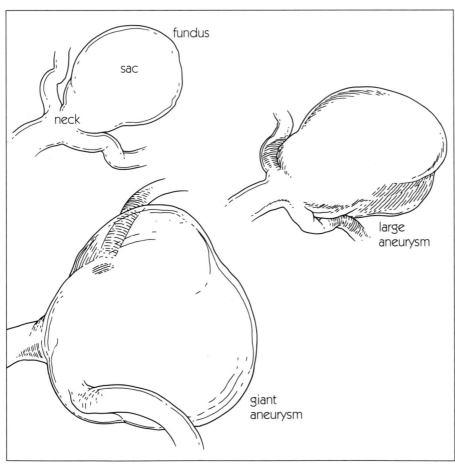

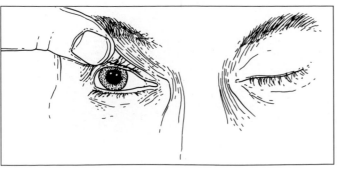

Figure 11.3 This figure depicts the potential evolution of a small aneurysm into a large and finally giant aneurysm. With each stage of enlargement, the efferent branches migrate farther out onto the sac itself.

Figure 11.4 A patient with a third cranial nerve palsy will exhibit some or all of the following signs: ptosis, pupillary dilation, and inability to elevate, depress or medially deviate (adduct) the eye. These findings (particularly pupillary dilation) strongly suggest focal mass effect.

the aneurysm. While the exact type of focal sign that develops depends on the aneurysmal site, the patient most commonly notes eye, facial, or head pain, visual loss, or double vision. The onset of a third cranial nerve palsy (Fig. 11.4), particularly with a fixed dilated pupil, mandates diagnostic studies to rule out a posterior carotid wall aneurysm or a distal basilar aneurysm (Fig. 11.5). Thus, the minimum diagnostic workup of a new third cranial nerve palsy includes CT scan to rule out minor or frank SAH and an ipsilateral carotid and single vertebral arteriogram. Oculomotor palsy with pupillary sparing may be seen without a focal mass in patients with diabetes and hypertensive cerebrovascular disease.

The diagnostic workup of a patient presenting with classic SAH includes a CT scan without enhancement, which in the first few days after SAH detects blood in the subarachnoid, subdural, or interventricular spaces or within the brain parenchyma in over 95% of cases (Fig. 11.6).[9,10] If the CT is negative and the history is extremely suggestive, the physician can elect to proceed with lumbar puncture to look for evidence of red blood cells or xanthochromia. Despite a negative CT scan, I often proceed with 4-vessel cerebral angiography, if the history is substantially suggestive. It is possible that a small leakage of

blood could be loculated around the aneurysmal fundus and not disseminate into the CSF. When a patient is first evaluated several days after a suggestive headache, the CT is often negative because the blood is isodense with brain tissue. Four-vessel angiography is indicated in these cases—with or without supportive CSF findings.

The initial neurological examination is critical for determining the patient's fitness for early surgical intervention (see below) and for acquiring prognostic data. A variety of grading scales are used; we continue to use the original Hunt-Hess scale with minor modifications (Fig. 11.7).[11] As seen in the original report by Hunt and Hess, morbidity and mortality clearly increase with each ascending category.[11]

As previously mentioned, aneurysms may slowly enlarge over time and become extremely large. The clinical signs and symptoms may mimic other conditions that result in local brain distortion or generalized elevations of intracranial pressure. A CT scan with and without enhancement detects the presence and location of such lesions and calcification in the wall. While the distribution of contrast material within the lesions may suggest intraluminal thrombosis, in our experience MRI is considerably more helpful in this regard. These imaging

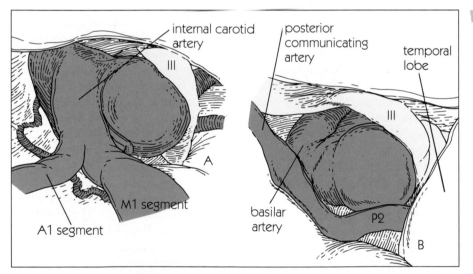

Figure 11.5 The presence of a third cranial nerve palsy (especially with pupillary involvement) may be due to an ipsilateral posterior carotid wall aneurysm (**A**) or a distal basilar artery aneurysm (**B**).

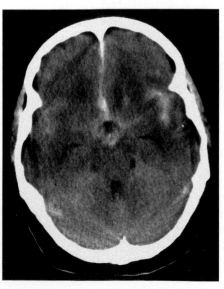

Figure 11.6 CT scan performed shortly after SAH reveals diffuse blood in the subarachnoid cisterns.

Figure 11.7 Subarachnoid Hemorrhage Grading Scale

I	Alert, oriented, asymptomatic
II	Alert, oriented, headache, stiff neck
III	Lethargy or confusion, may have minor neurologic deficit (hemiparesis)
IV	Stupor or dense focal deficit (hemiplegia)
V	Comatose

Modified from Hunt WE, Hess RM, 1968

studies should be followed by formal four-vessel diagnostic angiography to identify the afferent and efferent vessels involved and determine the presence of other aneurysms, because 15% of aneurysm patients harbor multiple lesions.

Patients with large aneurysms may develop a stuttering or progressive neurologic course due to embolization from within the lumen. CT, MRI, and angiography, as mentioned above, are important for locating and quantifying intraluminal debris as well as determining if significant infarction or brain edema is present, because these factors affect the timing of surgery.

ACUTE SUBARACHNOID HEMORRHAGE

Natural History

In order to formulate rational treatment strategies for SAH, it is necessary to understand its natural history and common sequelae. For those surviving their initial hemorrhage, the peak risk of rebleeding occurs during the first 48 hours.[9,12,13] On the first day of SAH, there is a 4.1% risk of rebleeding, which decreases steadily until the third day when there is a 1.5% per day risk of rebleeding.[12] By day 14, a cumulative rebleeding incidence of 19% was noted in the Cooperative Aneurysm Study.[12] Six months following SAH, 50% of patients have rebled and the long-term risk stabilizes at 3% per year.[13]

Complications

Symptomatic cerebral ischemia secondary to cerebral vasospasm peaks in onset between 7 and 10 days post-SAH.[14–16] The risk of symptomatic vasospasm can be accurately predicted by the admission CT scan. Those with a thick clot within the subarachnoid cisterns have a much higher risk than those with thin layering.[17] Using modern and current medical and surgical technology to treat SAH, vasospasm is the leading cause of death and disability, accounting for 14% of poor outcomes while rebleeding accounts for only 7%.[9,16]

Hydrocephalus, either communicating or noncommunicating, develops frequently in the first few days after SAH and partly explains the "tight, swollen brain" frequently encountered when surgery is performed on acute conditions. In most patients this condition resolves with time and requires no specific therapy. In about 10% of patients permanent CSF diversion is necessary.

Medical Complications

A multitude of medical complications may develop during the patient's acute illness. While it is beyond the scope of this chapter to deal thoroughly with each of these entities, brief mention will be made of the most common.

Pulmonary complications are not infrequent in SAH patients, particularly elderly individuals with pre-existing chronic obstructive lung disease. These patients, particularly those in poor neurologic grade, are often difficult to wean from ventilators postoperatively because of their abnormal pulmonary physiology and decreased level of consciousness. Pulmonary edema is occasionally evident on admission to the hospital. In my experience this phenomenon occurs more frequently in the severely neurolog-

ically injured (grades III, IV, V) patient. It is not known whether this condition represents "neurogenic" pulmonary edema or is secondary to acute cardiac dysfunction. Due to the frequent transient loss of consciousness associated with SAH, a moderate number of patients have aspiration pneumonitis shortly after admission. Occasionally this complication progresses to full blown adult respiratory distress syndrome with pulmonary failure.

Cardiac physiology is tightly linked to neurophysiology and most acute neurologic conditions are followed by various ECG changes. The outpouring of catecholamines during SAH probably induces some subendocardial damage on occasion. Rarely, acute myocardial infarction and even cardiogenic shock accompany SAH, gravely complicating management. Most neurosurgeons consult a cardiologist to assist in the perioperative care of the patient when significant ECG changes are noted.

Electrolyte disturbances are quite common after SAH, especially inappropriate secretion of antidiuretic hormone (SIADH) with hyponatremia. Doczi noted a 10% incidence in anterior communicating aneurysm patients and only a 3% incidence in patients who bled from other sites.[18] Hyponatremia can develop several days after hemorrhage and can depress the levels of consciousness and lower the seizure threshold. Since fluid restriction is the cornerstone of therapy for this disorder, care should be taken with patients inclined to develop delayed cerebral ischemia.[8] Diabetes insipidus with progressive hypernatremia is frequently seen in comatose patients with lethal hemorrhages and massively elevated ICP. Much less frequently, this disorder can be seen in patients who have suprasellar giant aneurysms, are in good neurologic condition, but have hypothalamic injury from the SAH or surgical injury to perforating vessels or eloquent tissue.

Infectious systemic complications are common because of the high incidence of patients who are on controlled ventilators and have catheters placed in their veins, arteries, and urinary bladder. Postoperative meningitis is uncommon but its presence signals the possibility of CSF leak into the frontal or ethmoid sinuses. Isolated organisms commonly inhabit the paranasal sinuses.

After SAH, venous thrombosis occurs in about 2% of patients and has been implicated in pulmonary embolism in 1%.[19] Our method of prevention includes hose and pneumatic compression devices for all patients in the intensive care unit with early postoperative ambulation when possible. Figure 11.8 summarizes the major medical and neurologic complications that may accompany SAH.

TREATMENT

This section will provide a conceptual framework from which management strategies can be developed for the individual patient. It should be emphasized that no two patients are truly similar or have identical systemic physiology. Therefore, despite the plethora of diagnostic information, the most effective way to time surgery is by acquiring a critical subjective "feel" for the patient's neurologic and systemic status. For the purposes of discussion, "good grade" will refer to Hunt-Hess grades I and II and grade III patients who are confused but have a normal level of consciousness.

Since the peak incidence of rebleeding occurs within the first 48 hours posthemorrhage, the most effective strategy to minimize this risk is to secure the ruptured aneurysm surgically as soon as possible. Unfortunately, most patients referred to neurosurgical centers arrive one or more days after the original SAH, thus surgery within the first 48 hours is not possible. Secondly, it is not in the patient's best interest to undergo aneurysm surgery at night, when the surgeon is tired and the operating room staff (including the anesthesiology staff and scrub and circulating nurses) may be suboptimal. The heightened risk to the patient under these circumstances far outweighs the risk of rebleeding while waiting for the first elective surgical day, when the proper team is assembled. Thirdly, not all aneurysms are alike; some require extensive retraction and dissection, which may not be tolerated well by the freshly injured brain. It is likely that patients in poor neurologic condition are often worsened by a hasty operation and would be better served by allowing the brain a few days to recover. However, the neurosurgeon should secure ruptured aneurysms prior to the onset of delayed ischemia from vasospasm because the most effective forms of therapy for vasospasm involve hypervolemia and hypertension, highly dangerous maneuvers when unsecured aneurysms are present. Therefore, in general we attempt to achieve obliteration of the offending aneurysm prior to days 5 to 7, especially if the CT suggested a high likelihood of vasospasm. The entire issue of surgical timing, however, remains highly controversial.[2,9,12,20–22]

Antifibrinolytic therapy (epsilon aminocaproic acid) became available more than 20 years ago. It provided great hope that patients with ruptured aneurysms could be prevented from rebleeding or that rebleeding could be delayed, allowing time for surgical intervention. The Cooperative Aneurysm Study found that the rebleeding rate at 14 days was 11.7% if antifibrinolytics were used and 19.4% if no antifibrinolytics were used. However,

cerebral ischemia from vasospasm was more frequent if antifibrinolytics were used (32.4%) than if no antifibrinolytics were used (22.7%). Thus, the mortality rate of the two groups over the first month was identical.[23] We tend to use antifibrinolytic therapy in the poor grade patient who clearly will not be an operative candidate for some time, despite the knowledge that we are increasing his risk of symptomatic vasospasm.

Symptomatic vasospasm is the leading cause of disability and death following SAH and, to date, eludes definitive treatment. While most known vasoactive compounds have been tried in this condition, very few modalities have lasting value. Kosnik and Hunt observed a striking response in patients with induced hypertension.[24] The use of pressors remains a mainstay of therapy. The efficacy and safety of pressors seems to be markedly enhanced by volume expansion, and the combination of hypervolemia and hypertension remains the most effective medical means of reversing these neurologic deficits.[25] One large series reported clinical response in 70% of patients treated in this way.[26] Complications have resulted, however, including systemic cardiopulmonary decompensation, conversion of ischemic infarction to hemorrhagic infarction, hematomas, progressing brain edema, and new aneurysms.[26–29] Calcium channel blockers have been widely studied and used clinically during the 1980s, but convincing evidence of their efficacy has not been clearly shown in my opinion. Angiographic arterial narrowing is not prevented or reversed by these agents. Recently interventional radiologists have developed technology that has significant value for medical failures in our unit[30]; their technique, transluminal angioplasty, has the potential to reverse arterial narrowing in the major cerebral conducting vessels.

Our current strategy for managing delayed ischemic complications involves mild to moderate volume expansion with crystalloid and colloid solutions followed by early craniotomy to secure the ruptured aneurysm. We attempt to maintain this status through the period of maximal risk of vasospasm (days 5 to 10). Concurrently, we attempt to maximize blood rheologic properties to improve tissue perfusion by maintaining mild hemodilu-

Figure 11.8 Summary of Major Medical and Neurologic Complications of Subarachnoid Hemorrhage

Venous thromboembolism	Pulmonary failure
Infection	Hydrocephalus
Diabetes insipidis	Vasospasm
SIADH	Rebleed
Cardiac injury	Direct brain injury

tion (hematocrit 30 to 34). Should a focal neurologic deficit develop we immediately add a vasopressor (dopamine) and raise the systolic blood pressure up to the 200 mm Hg range or until the deficit reverses. If this medical therapy fails to improve the patient's condition and the CT scan does not show obvious infarction, we proceed immediately with angiography with plans for angioplasty. To date, this protocol has been fairly effective, although some patients have a virulent course that is often fatal, regardless of therapy (Fig. 11.9).

The ability temporarily to occlude cerebral arteries safely and reliably is of considerable value for two reasons. First, the frequent use of temporary clips to soften or "defuse" an aneurysm during final dissection and clipping has decreased the risk of premature intraoperative rupture. The occurrence of significant premature bleeding converts an orderly, precise microsurgical procedure into a stressful situation that often adversely affects the patient.[31] Second, many large and giant aneurysms, particularly those with calcific walls and mural thrombus, must be temporarily excluded from the cerebral circulation to allow definitive arterial reconstruction (Fig. 11.10). Regrettably, this temporary interruption is prolonged in some cases, thus exceeding the ischemic threshold and leading to infarction.

Barbiturates are effective in protecting the brain from ischemic and hypoxic insults both experimentally and clinically.[32–34] This protective effect is likely caused by a substantially depressed cerebral metabolic rate, evidenced by the lack of EEG activity. Unfortunately, some elderly patients—especially those with significant heart disease—may become significantly hypotensive at the dosage required for cerebral metabolic depression. This toxic effect substantially diminishes potential available collateral circulation during occlusion of a major cerebral vessel. Also, the prolonged anesthetic effect of high doses of a barbiturate can obscure important neurologic changes in the immediate postoperative period. For these reasons, we have used etomidate to accomplish the same degree of metabolic suppression without cardiotoxicity.[35] Before placing temporary arterial clips, our anesthesiologists insure normotension, accomplish EEG burst suppression with etomidate, and maintain EEG suppression throughout the duration of temporary arterial occlusion.

SURGICAL MANAGEMENT OF SPECIFIC ANEURYSMS

The following discussion, an overview of some general problems caused by aneurysms in various locations, illustrates the anatomic complexities and unique features found by the neurosurgeon treating these various lesions. It is important to understand that generalities regarding the care of SAH patients are difficult to apply to the individual case. The treatment of aneurysmal disease has been aided by development of the surgical microscope; its ability to magnify and brilliantly illuminate very narrow exposures has had an incredible impact on neurosurgery in general and aneurysmal disease in particular. Tiny vessels that serve as end arteries for eloquent brain regions, including the brain stem and diencephalon, are simply not visible to the naked eye, but can now be safely and elegantly spared during the clipping of difficult aneurysms.

THE PTERIONAL "FRONTOTEMPORAL" CRANIOTOMY

The pterional craniotomy is an extremely versatile procedure that has become fundamental to managing a variety of neoplastic, congenital, and vascular processes. Neurosurgeons must become intimately familiar with the advantages of this approach and its many modifications and develop an appreciation for the neurovascular anatomy viewed from this unusual perspective. In this exposure the anatomy is viewed in an oblique and inverted orientation. Fortunately, experience quickly renders the microanatomy viewed from this perspective familiar, predictable, and natural.

A key element of this operative approach is patient position. Careful attention to this basic first step facilitates exposure and allows complex procedures to be done through small bony windows, a limited dural opening, and with a minimum of cerebral cortex exposed. The Mayfield-Keys three-point skull fixation device should be employed in virtually all aneurysm procedures as it provides almost absolute head stability in the event of sudden patient movement or coughing during inadvertent emergence from anesthesia (Fig. 11.11). In general, it is most convenient to apply the three-point fixation with two pins anteriorly contralateral to the planned

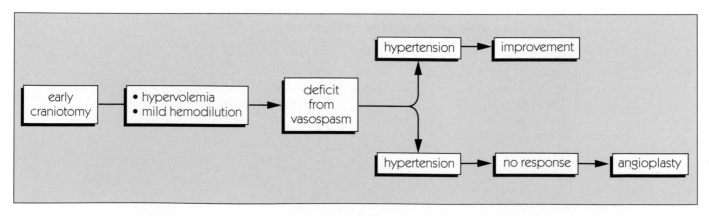

Figure 11.9 Prophylactic and therapeutic strategy for vasospasm at the University of Texas Southwestern Medical Center.

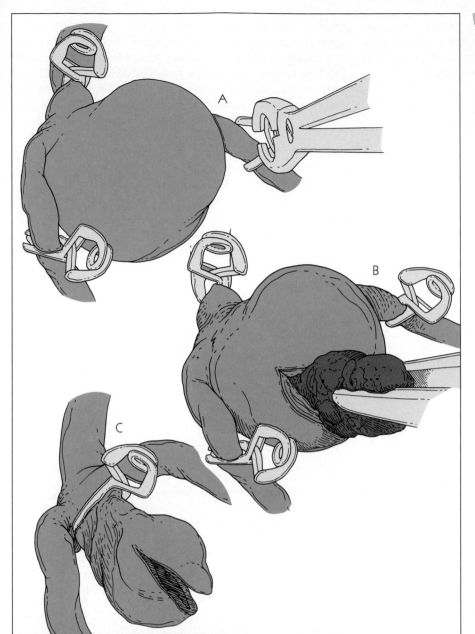

Figure 11.10 (A–C) Temporary arterial occlusion is often necessary in repairing complex large or giant aneurysms. Not infrequently, the aneurysm must be widely opened to allow evacuation of debris and thrombus before definitive clip reconstruction can be performed.

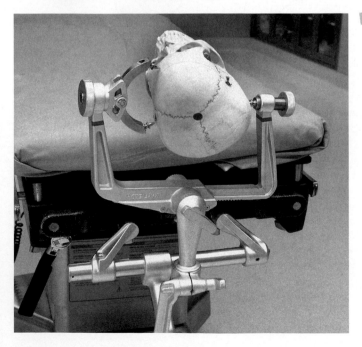

Figure 11.11 The Mayfield-Keys three point skull fixation device provides optimal head stability so that inadvertent patient movement will not result in catastrophic injury to neural or vascular structures.

exposure and one pin posterior to the planned surgical incision just above the mastoid region. After inserting the pins, the surgeon performs three distinct maneuvers to position the head optimally for the procedure.[36]

Rotation

The head is rotated toward the contralateral or nonoperated side to an angle determined by the target anatomic site. In general, when treating internal carotid or distal basilar artery aneurysms, minimal head rotation (20°) is employed because with further rotation the temporal lobe gravitationally migrates posteriorly and thus encroaches upon the operative field. Aneurysms of the middle cerebral artery bifurcation require somewhat more rotation (45°) to expose the sylvian fissure maximally for a convenient transsylvian dissection. For aneurysms of the anterior communicating artery, even more rotation is necessary (45° to 60°) in order to simplify the exposure of the medial gyrus rectus and interhemispheric fissure. In this dissection, temporal lobe encroachment does not limit exposure of the anterior communicating region due to its anterior location in the skull (Fig. 11.12A).

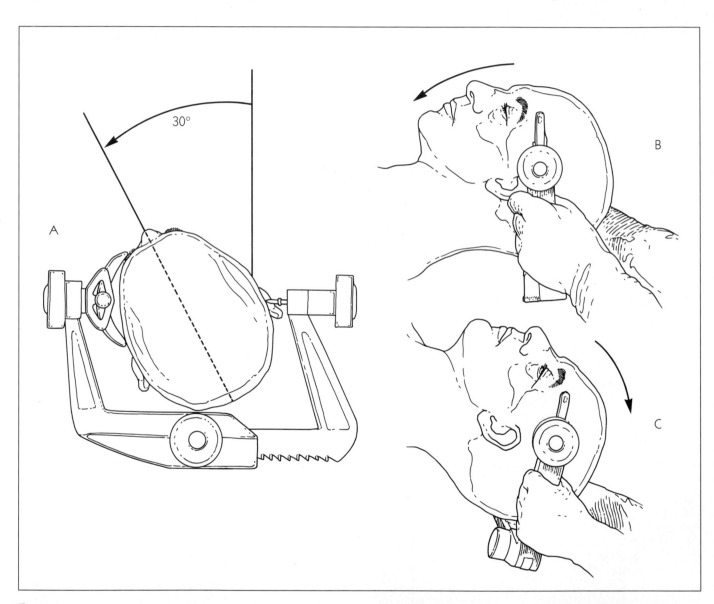

Figure 11.12 Patient positioning for pterional craniotomy. (A) Rotation. The head is elevated slightly relative to the thorax and rotated contralaterally by an extent dictated by the specific operative target (less rotation for carotid and basilar bifurcation aneurysms and more rotation for aneurysm of the middle cerebral artery or anterior communicating region). (B) Flexion. The neck should then be gently flexed, bringing the chin toward the contralateral clavicle. This subtle maneuver orients the floor of the anterior cranial fossa perpendicularly with the long axis of the patient's body, maximizing the surgeon's access to the anatomic target without encroachment on the patient's ipsilateral shoulder. (C) Extension (tilt). While maintaining the previous elements of rotation and flexion, the vertex is tilted inferiorly so that the maxillary eminence rises superior to the brow. The degree of extension will vary somewhat with the target aneurysm (less for paraclinoidal aneurysms and more with distal basilar aneurysms).

Flexion

This subtle maneuver is designed to maintain a perpendicular relationship between the floor of the anterior cranial fossa and the long axis of the patient's body. The maneuver is accomplished by achieving the degree of desired rotation, then flexing the neck gently, bringing the chin toward the contralateral clavicle. Be careful to avoid compromising cervical venous return. Successful accomplishment of this maneuver allows the seated surgeon comfortable access to the target region without awkwardly encroaching on the patient's ipsilateral shoulder (Fig. 11.12B).

Extension "Tilt"

When this critical manipulation is successful, the frontal lobe gravitationally falls away from the floor of the anterior cranial fossa. To minimize necessary retraction and optimally display the vascular structures at the skull base, the vertex of the skull is tilted inferiorly so the maxillary eminence rises superior to the brow (Fig. 11.12C). After this final maneuver, the Mayfield device is secured to the operating table. With experience, the surgeon can literally see the vascular anatomy with its associated target aneurysm as the head is manipulated externally. Once the surgeon has this level of experience, measuring degrees of rotation and extension is unnecessary, and he or she simply positions the head for optimal exposure of the lesion.

The surgical incision is begun about 1 cm anterior to the tragus at the level of the zygoma and extends superiorly immediately behind the hairline and gently curves anteriorly to the midline (Fig. 11.13). Every attempt is made to keep the incision behind the hairline for cosmesis, although this can be difficult in a balding man. Numerous options are available for reflecting the scalp flap, including an interfascial dissection described by Yasargil. Perhaps the most widely used is an incision through the galea, temporalis fascia, and muscle to the bone, reflecting the scalp flap in a single layer (Fig. 11.14). It is important to preserve the frontalis branch of the facial nerve and mobilization of the temporalis muscle anteriorly and inferiorly enough for the anatomic key to be well exposed. Certain surgical targets require aggressive exposure of the temporal squama. While the craniotomy flap varies somewhat depending on the surgical target, in general a power craniotome is used to

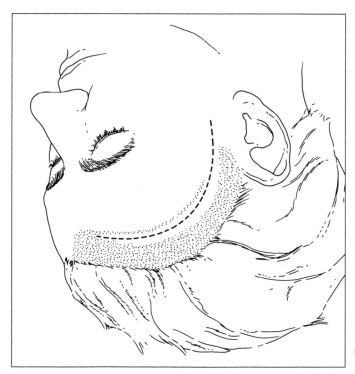

Figure 11.13 The skin incision for the pterional craniotomy extends from the zygoma to the midline, curving gently just posterior to the hairline.

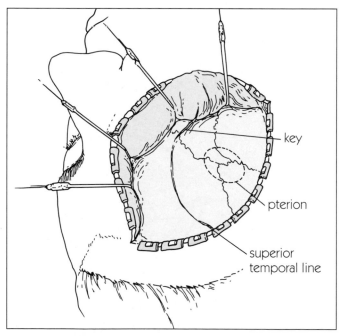

Figure 11.14 A commonly employed means of opening the scalp involves incision of the skin, galea, temporalis fascia, and muscle with reflexion of the resultant flap in a single layer.

fashion a frontal temporal craniotomy by connecting three burr holes (Fig. 11.15). Placing the posterior burr hole immediately inferior to the superior temporal line allows a cosmetic closure of the temporalis muscle over this bony defect. After the bone flap is removed, the anterior temporal bone is extracted with rongeurs as is the lateral third of the sphenoid ridge (Fig. 11.16). Often it is necessary to remove the deepest portion of the

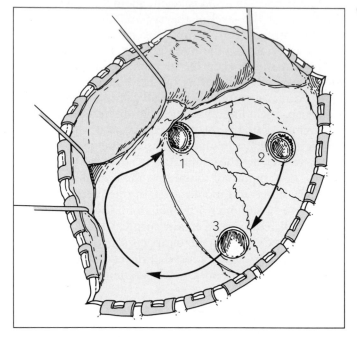

Figure 11.15 The pterional craniotomy is performed with power instruments so that three burr holes are placed, one at the anatomic key, one inferiorly on the temporal squama, and one posteriorly just inferior to the superior temporal line. The bone is cut as shown, exposing the frontal and temporal dura and the sphenoid ridge.

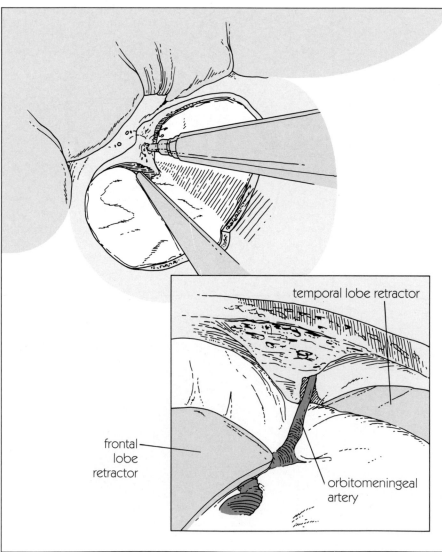

Figure 11.16 After removal of the bone flap, the sphenoid ridge is resected to the level of the orbitomeningeal artery. The inner table of the frontal bone can also be resected. This maneuver is particularly useful in exposing the anterior communicating region.

temporal lobe retractor

frontal lobe retractor

orbitomeningeal artery

sphenoid ridge with a power drill. The drill is also used to resect the inner table of the frontal bone medially; the resultant bony removal enables excellent access to the parasellar region with a minimum of frontal retraction. The dura mater is opened in a semilunar fashion and reflected over the sphenoid ridge to maximize cortical exposure (Fig. 11.17).

After satisfactory exposure of the parasylvian region, the surgical microscope is brought into the field and the remainder of the procedure is accomplished with magni-fied vision. The initial brain retraction involves the progressive elevation of the posterior frontal cortex immediately anterior to the sylvian fissure from the sphenoid ridge (Fig. 11.18). Keeping the sphenoid ridge as a directional indicator will insure safe arrival at the carotid cistern. Once this cistern is reached, the optic nerve can be viewed medially through the arachnoid even after a brisk SAH (Fig. 11.19).

At this point, either a microknife or microscissors is used to open sharply this dense arachnoid extending

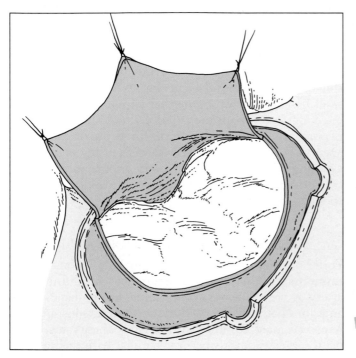

Figure 11.17 The dura is opened in a semilunar fashion and reflected with stay sutures.

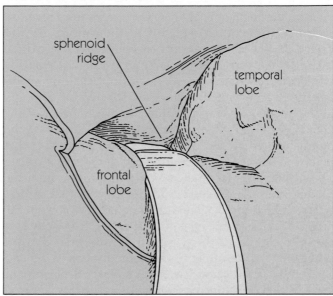

Figure 11.18 As the retractor is deepened medially, the posterior frontal cortex is elevated. Gently following the course of the sphenoid ridge helps keep the direction of retraction correct.

Figure 11.19 Safe arrival at the carotid cistern is heralded by visualizing the optic nerve through the arachnoid medially. The retractor is stabilized just lateral to the nerve so the arachnoid of the carotid cistern and medial sylvian fissure is placed on gentle stretch.

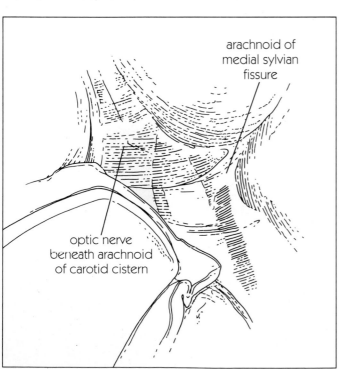

from the prechiasmatic region across the carotid cistern and laterally to dissect fully the medial aspect of the sylvian fissure (Fig. 11.20). Once this arachnoid is fully dissected, the entire subarachnoid course of the carotid artery will be seen, including its bifurcation into the middle and anterior cerebral arteries. From this point, the principles of further dissection are governed by the specific aneurysmal site.

ANEURYSMS OF THE PROXIMAL CAROTID (PARACLINOIDAL) ARTERY

This interesting family of aneurysms arises from the most proximal intracranial segment of the internal carotid artery. It is not uncommon to see bilateral proximal carotid aneurysms, particularly in women. These aneurysms are often termed carotidophthalmic artery aneurysms, implying a distinct relationship to the origin of the ophthalmic branch. More commonly, however, the aneurysms arise some distance from the origin of the ophthalmic artery and occasionally have projections that make the ophthalmic artery unlikely as the site of origin. Dr. Arthur Day has studied aneurysms arising from the medial and inferomedial wall of the proximal carotid artery and has nicely related their pathophysiology to the origin of the superior hypophyseal artery. It is likely that the presence of a third group of proximal carotid aneurysms is due simply to the hemodynamic stress of a sharp bend in the carotid artery as it leaves the cavernous sinus, which over time can weaken the vessel wall tissue. Regardless of their configuration, these aneurysms present several unique technical problems to the neurosurgeon. Their extremely proximal intracranial location makes the essential vascular principle of proximal control difficult if not impossible to achieve intracranially. Secondly, when these aneurysms reach significant size, they routinely attenuate the optic nerve traumatically and often cause associated visual neurologic deficit. This fac-

tor frequently mandates that the surgeon not only exclude the aneurysm from circulation but deflate it to decompress the optic nerve. This is difficult, particularly in large and giant aneurysms whose walls may be calcific. The multiple clips that aneurysms of this type require often distort or compress the optic nerve. A third unique feature of this particular aneurysm is its relationship to the bony floor of the skull. The anterior clinoid process often hoods the origin of the ophthalmic artery and it frequently obscures the proximal neck of these aneurysms. While it is occasionally possible to secure safe exposure of the proximal neck by simply incising the dura overlying the optic canal and its underlying falciform ligament, more commonly some degree of bony resection is needed to insure that the lumen of the carotid artery is not jeopardized.[36,37] Figure 11.21 illustrates the unique relationship of proximal carotid aneurysms to the optic nerve and skull base as well as a potential clipping solution after resecting a portion of the anterior clinoid process. In the majority of large and giant ruptured proximal carotid aneurysms, the patient is served well, in my opinion, by exposing the cervical internal artery prior to initiating the craniotomy. This guarantees early proximal control should difficulties arise.

ANEURYSMS OF THE POSTERIOR CAROTID WALL

Posterior carotid wall aneurysms include lesions arising immediately distal to the posterior communicating artery as well as those arising immediately distal to the anterior choroidal artery. Because these lesions are perhaps the most common intracranial aneurysms, most neurosurgeons quickly become familiar with the involved microanatomy and treat these lesions successfully in the majority of cases. Enlarging aneurysms at this site can become symptomatic prior to frank SAH by compression of the tentorial incisura, which produces pain, and of the third cranial nerve (see Fig. 11.5). In my experi-

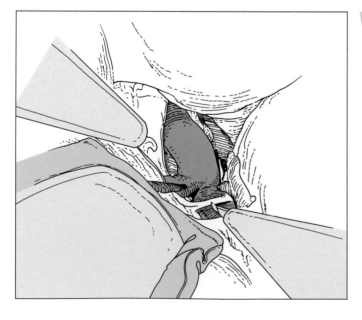

Figure 11.20 Sharp microinstruments are used to fully dissect the parasellar cisterns from the prechiasmatic cistern across the carotid cistern into the medial aspect of the sylvian fissure.

ence, early warning signs of some type are more frequently seen with aneurysms of the posterior carotid wall than with any other intracranial aneurysm. The relative simplicity of the anatomy of these aneurysms as well as the frequency with which they are exposed and treated should not induce a sense of complacency in the operating surgeon. The intimate association between the distal neck of the common carotid-posterior communicating artery aneurysm to the anterior choroidal artery together with the fragility of the anterior chor-

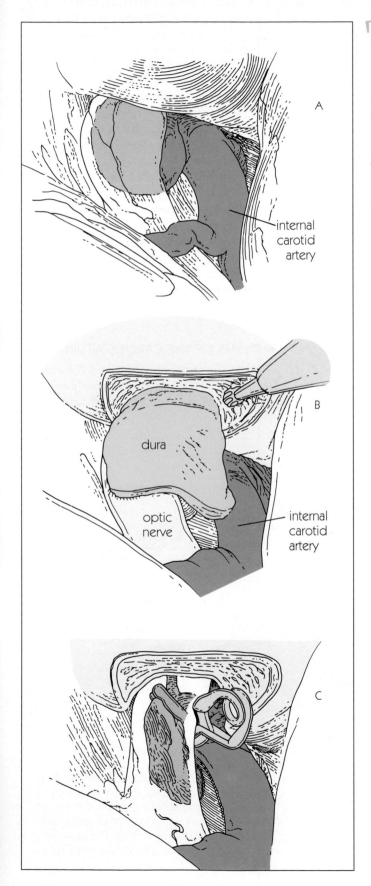

Figure 11.21 Proximal carotid (paraclinoidal) aneurysm.
(A) These aneurysms often distort and attenuate the optic nerve and may have their proximal neck obscured by the dura covering the lateral aspect of the optic canal or by the bony anterior clinoidal process. Without securing proximal control in the neck, it is obvious that true control of this aneurysm may be achieved intracranially only at some peril.
(B) In order to resect the anterior clinoid process, a dural flap is fashioned and reflected over the fundus of the aneurysm. A high-speed drill is then used to remove as much bone as is necessary to expose the proximal neck of the aneurysm.
(C) The specific clip placement chosen must not jeopardize the optic nerve or the patency of the internal carotid artery.

oidal artery places it very much "in harm's way" (Fig. 11.22). The anterior choroidal artery supplies the posterior limb of the internal capsule, the lentiform nucleus, the optic tract, the amygdala, and the choroid plexus of the temporal horn. Injuring it by aggressive dissection techniques or placing a small piece of cotton in the distal neck of the aneurysm to control minor intraoperative bleeding can result in profound and devastating neurologic deficit. It should be stressed that the distal course of the anterior choroidal as it travels posteriorly must be carefully freed from the aneurysmal fundus so the distal clip blade does not compromise this vital structure. The posterior communicating artery usually arises just proximal to the origin of a carotid posterior communicating artery aneurysm and every attempt should be made to preserve this vessel. Important anterior thalamoperforating branches ramify from the posterior communicating artery. Occasionally patients have persistent fetal circulation in which the posterior cerebral artery originates from the carotid, and the P1 segment is nonexistent. This phenomenon can be discerned from the preoperative arteriogram and, when approaching the posterior carotid wall aneurysm, the neurosurgeon should know whether or not the posterior cerebral artery is fetal. It is often acceptable to include the posterior communicating artery in the clip, assuming the anterior thalamoperforates will be irrigated retrograde from the P1 segment off the basilar artery. Nevertheless, when possible, all components of the circle of Willis should be preserved, particularly in the SAH patient who may subsequently develop vasospasm and increase reliance on available natural collateral pathways. The most common clip arrangement for a posterior communicating artery aneurysm is perpendicular to the carotid artery (Fig. 11.23A). In relatively small aneurysms, the resultant degree of shortening of the carotid artery is trivial and thus acceptable. In larger broad-based aneurysms, clipping perpendicular to the carotid artery can substantially foreshorten and even wrinkle the carotid and imposed shear forces on the fragile neck of the aneurysm during closure of the clip. The aperture clip originally developed by Drake[38,39] allows clip placement so the blades close parallel to the carotid artery, minimizing the shear forces (Fig. 11.23B). Regardless of the clip chosen, it is critical to inspect the course of the anterior choroidal and posterior communicating arteries to insure that these vessels have not been compromised.

For patients presenting with acute or chronic third nerve palsies, it has been our policy to evacuate the aneurysmal contents but not develop the dissection plane between the aneurysmal fundus and the third cranial nerve, to avoid further damage to this already diseased and fragile structure. Many neurosurgeons believe that eliminating the direct pulsations from the arterial tree does as much as any other maneuver to allow recovery of the nerve's function.

ANEURYSMS OF THE CAROTID BIFURCATION

Despite the fact that the intracranial carotid bifurcation is major and frequently tortuous, it is a relatively rare site for aneurysmal development. Aneurysms of this region

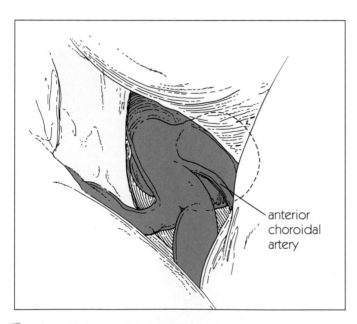

Figure 11.22 Posterior carotid wall aneurysm. Despite their frequency and relative simplicity, especially the ease of achieving early proximal control intracranially, the neurosurgeon should not be nonchalant or complacent. The anterior choroidal artery is in intimate relationship with the distal neck and simple retraction and mild compression can have devastating consequences.

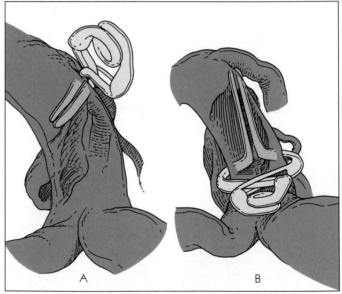

Figure 11.23 Alternatives for clipping posterior carotid wall aneurysms. **(A)** For small aneurysms, a direct clip placement perpendicular to the carotid artery is often the best alternative. **(B)** For larger aneurysms in this location, the degree of "gathering" of tissue by a perpendicular clip placement can jeopardize the carotid artery as well as apply serious shear stresses to the aneurysm neck during closure. The aperture clip allows blade closure parallel to the carotid artery minimizing these deleterious events.

Principles of Neurosurgery

typically project superiorly and occasionally superoposteriorly. An occasional patient presents with a primarily intracerebral hemorrhage and a hematoma anterior and inferior to a classic putaminal hypertensive hemorrhage. These hematomas may be associated with a paucity of true subarachnoid blood. This CT picture in a nonhypertensive patient should immediately alert the clinician to the presence of an ominous vascular condition.

The operative exposure and definitive clipping of aneurysms at this site requires considerable dissection of the carotid cistern and the sphenoidal portion of the sylvian fissure. The proximity of the distal anterior choroidal artery and the infinite variability of the subarachnoid course of the medial lenticulostriate branches from the middle cerebral and anterior cerebral arteries explains the often intimate association of these vessels with the aneurysmal neck (Fig. 11.24). When the surgeon uses a clip with long blades, particularly in large and broad-based aneurysms of the carotid bifurcation, he or she must be able to see these penetrating vessels in the depths of the exposure.

There are two key aspects to surgical dissection: proximal control of the internal carotid artery in the carotid cistern must be achieved, and the sphenoidal portion of the sylvian fissure must be opened widely. As the dissection is carried more distally along the internal carotid, simultaneous extension of the sylvian dissection along the M1 segment from distal to proximal assures an atraumatic arrival at the carotid bifurcation and control of the afferent and efferent circulation. It is essential that the surgeon enter the operating room knowing whether the anterior communicating artery is patent. Sacrifice of the ipsilateral A1 segment is a valuable ther-

apeutic option in difficult large and giant aneurysms as well as a life-saving maneuver in the event of an untimely intraoperative rupture. Knowing that the anterior communicating artery is patent enables definitive clipping, which incorporates the A1 segment if premature rupture develops (Fig. 11.25).[36] A small clip can then be added to the A1 segment to insure against retrograde irrigation of the aneurysm. It should be emphasized that medial sylvian dissection is critical to minimize the degree of frontal lobe retraction required for the exposure of this particular aneurysm.

ANEURYSMS OF THE MIDDLE CEREBRAL ARTERY BIFURCATION

Aneurysms of the middle cerebral artery bifurcation are quite common and hemorrhage from these lesions can produce several unique features. As aneurysms become relatively large at this site, they can erode through the lateral aspect of the sphenoidal portion of the sylvian fissure, occasionally causing hemorrhage directly into the subdural space. Acute subdural hematoma with relatively less blood directed into the subarachnoid space occurs in 5% to 10% of these patients. Knowledge of this phenomenon should alert the neurosurgeon evaluating a patient who had an unwitnessed motor vehicle accident and was found to have an acute subdural hematoma. It is possible that the hemorrhage caused a loss of consciousness, which precipitated the car accident. Additionally, the anatomy of the middle cerebral artery bifurcation just medial to the limen of insula allows aneurysmal growth to occur in the substance of the temporal lobe or invaginate the pia

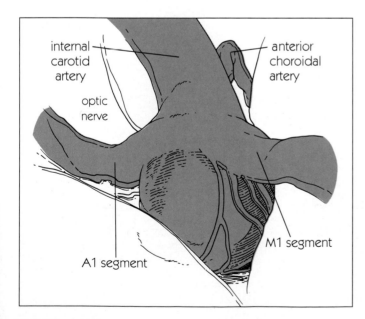

Figure 11.24 Aneurysms of the internal carotid artery bifurcation are frequently in intimate association with the distal course of the anterior choroidal artery as well as the medial lenticulostriate arteries arising from the middle and anterior cerebral arteries.

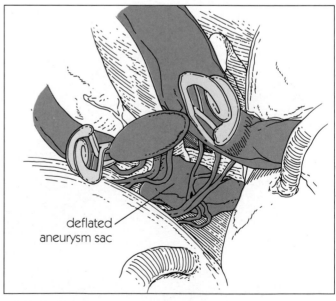

Figure 11.25 Carotid bifurcation aneurysm. If the anterior communicating artery is known to be patent, a valuable option for ceasing untimely intraoperative rupture is to incorporate the ipsilateral A1 segment into the definitive clipping, thus relying on the contralateral carotid to irrigate the anterior cerebral artery territory bilaterally.

arachnoid of the medial temporal lobe (Fig. 11.26). When rupture occurs at the distal aspect of the fundus, a hematoma frequently develops primarily within the temporal lobe. This complication can be an acute life-threatening emergency simply because of mass effect from the hematoma. If a patient is found to have striking mass effect from a temporal hematoma after becoming immediately comatose or deteriorating upon arrival in the emergency room, he or she should not be evaluated as a standard SAH patient by the Hunt-Hess criteria. The surgeon should consider the patient to have a life-threatening mass and perform immediate surgical therapy to remove the hematoma and definitively clip the aneurysm. If possible, a diagnostic angiography should be obtained before exploring these lesions, although this can be deferred in the rapidly deteriorating patient.

Significant controversy exists in the neurosurgical community regarding the most appropriate means to dissect these aneurysms. Many surgeons prefer to isolate proximal control at the carotid cistern and dissect from proximal to distal through the sylvian fissure until the bifurcation is reached. This type of maneuver requires a tremendous amount of frontal lobe retraction but has the theoretical advantage of enabling early proximal control. Other surgeons advocate an approach through the temporal lobe itself; this type of superior temporal gyrus approach is especially useful in patients with a temporal lobe hematoma. Nevertheless, it does require re-entry into the subarachnoid space as the region of the limen of insula is

approached. In my opinion, the preferred approach to most lesions of the middle cerebral bifurcation (with the exception of those associated with large hematomas) lies in a direct transsylvian approach. The dissection is initiated through the lateral aspect of the sylvian fissure 2 to 3 cm from the sphenoid ridge (Fig. 11.27). Dissection via this route allows the surgeon to stay within the subarachnoid space from the outset, minimizes the degree of brain tissue retraction necessary and, with experience, allows proximal control to be achieved safely. As the dissection deepens within the sylvian fissure, the small middle cerebral branches are dissected down to the M2 segments and, using knowledge of the aneurysmal anatomy and how it projects, a safe dissection plane (usually posterosuperiorly) is followed, until the M1 segment is clearly visualized, at which point proximal control is assured. On initial exposure, aneurysms at this site frequently appear to have substantially widened the true bifurcation region, with the M2 segments appearing to emerge from the aneurysmal fundus itself. These vessels should be dissected from the aneurysmal neck to the point at which definitive clip reconstruction can be accomplished.

ANEURYSMS OF THE ANTERIOR COMMUNICATING ARTERY

Aneurysms in the region of the anterior communicating artery are perhaps the most common cause of SAH and represent approximately 30% of all cases of SAH in the

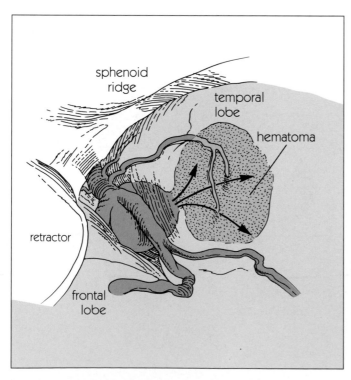

Figure 11.26 Aneurysms arising from the middle cerebral artery bifurcation often project into the medial aspect of the temporal lobe. Upon rupture, a hematoma may develop primarily within the temporal lobe itself and only minimally involve the subarachnoid space.

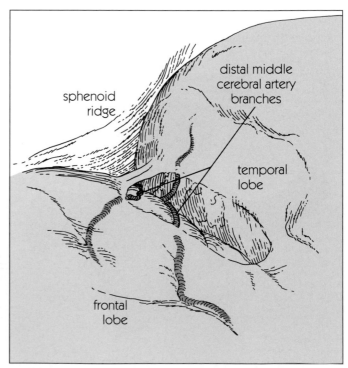

Figure 11.27 The transsylvian approach to middle cerebral artery bifurcation aneurysms minimizes brain retraction but defers achievement of proximal control until somewhat late in the dissection.

Principles of Neurosurgery

early Cooperative Aneurysm Study.[40] The anterior communicating artery as well as the A1 segments of the anterior cerebral artery are some of the most variable components of the circle of Willis and frequent anomalies (i.e., irregularities in size, the tendency of one A1 segment to be dominant over the contralateral one, and fenestration, duplication, or triplication of the anterior communicating artery itself) are the rule rather than the exception. Each of these circumstances produces a hemodynamic predisposition to the development of aneurysms. In fact, most anterior communicating aneurysms arise from the junction of the dominant A1 segment with the anterior communicating artery. Hemorrhage from this region is only very rarely preceded by local signs of mass effect as aneurysms must be extremely large before neurologic symptoms manifest. Once hemorrhage occurs, the unique anatomic relationships predispose the individual to diffuse SAH, focal interhemispheric SAH, intraventricular hemorrhage (by rupture of the aneurysm up through the lamina terminalis into the anterior third ventricle), and intracerebral hemorrhage (typically a flame-shaped frontal lobe hematoma). When two or more of these patterns occur together, the study is virtually diagnostic of hemorrhage from an anterior communicating artery aneurysm.

Several points about the operative treatment of these patients deserve mention. In general the bony craniotomy should be carried somewhat more medially and inferiorly than the craniotomy designed for other lesions. This is because the anterior communicating complex is located slightly anterior to the carotid cistern. By enlarging the craniotomy to the midpupillary line and carrying the bony incision down to the brow (with every attempt made to avoid the frontal sinus), the surgeon has maximal flexibility in terms of instrument usage and will not be impeded by contacting bone. The microsurgical procedure is focused less on the medial sylvian fissure than on opening the carotid cistern, at which point a decision must be made either to isolate the A1 segment at the carotid bifurcation or to create a more medial exposure of this vessel. Considerable difference of opinion exists but, generally, mobilization of gyrus rectus from the optic nerve is thought to allow safe proximal dissection of the A1 segment without the additional brain retraction necessary to expose the carotid bifurcation (Fig. 11.28). The A1 is then followed to the point at which it angles superiorly and heads into the interhemispheric fissure. Attention is then directed not to the anterior communicating artery, but to the contralateral A1 segment, which often enters the interhemispheric fissure at a mirror image site from the ipsilateral vessel (Fig. 11.29). Once definitive proximal control has been obtained, the retractor is withdrawn by about 1 to 1.5 cm, allowing a small amount of gyrus rectus to herniate over the retractor blade, which immediately obscures the anterior communicating region.

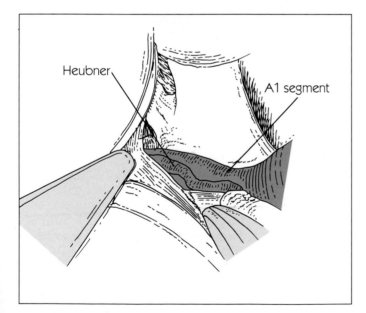

Figure 11.28 In approaching anterior communicating artery aneurysms, the additional brain retraction needed to isolate the origin of the A1 anterior cerebral segment at the carotid bifurcation can be avoided by dissecting the gyrus rectus from the optic nerve and tract. Deepening this plane will expose the A1 proximal to the anterior communicating artery.

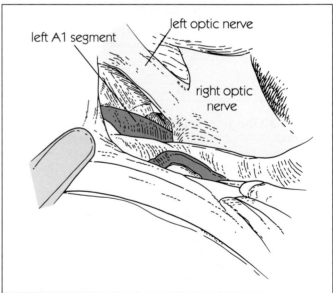

Figure 11.29 Isolation of the contralateral A1 segment completes acquisition of proximal control.

This tissue is aggressively resected with cautery and suction (Fig. 11.30). The overlying veil of pia arachnoid is then opened sharply, allowing full definition of the ipsilateral A2 segment. Subsequent dissection is defined by the orientation of the aneurysm but must focus on the identification of the A2 segment on the contralateral side. Once this vessel is seen, definitive dissection of the anterior communicating artery and neck of the aneurysm is possible. Great care must be taken to avoid occluding perforating arteries that emanate from the posterior aspect of the anterior communicating artery in the clip (Fig. 11.31). This technical error can produce serious psychological and hypothalamic sequelae.

Injury to these penetrating arteries as well as inadvertent injury to the aneurysm and the major parent vasculature can be avoided by a very thorough dissection in each case. All aspects of the complex, including both A1 and A2 segments and both sides of the anterior communicating artery, should always be seen and understood prior to definitive neck dissection and clipping.

ANEURYSMS OF THE VERTEBRAL ARTERY- POSTERIOR INFERIOR CEREBELLAR ARTERY

Aneurysms of the proximal intracranial vertebral artery typically occur immediately distal to the origin of the posterior inferior cerebellar artery (PICA). This variety of posterior circulation aneurysm is second only to the distal basilar artery in frequency of occurrence. CT scanning following SAH often localizes the hemorrhage to the appropriate lateral aspect of the brain stem and sometimes a small portion of the hemorrhage will extend into

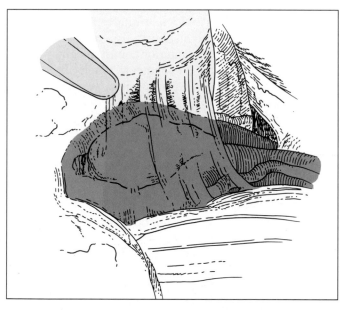

Figure 11.30 The gyrus rectus tissue immediately overlying the anterior communicating complex is aggressively resected leaving a layer of pia arachnoid obscuring the distal anterior cerebral branches (A1) and the aneurysm.

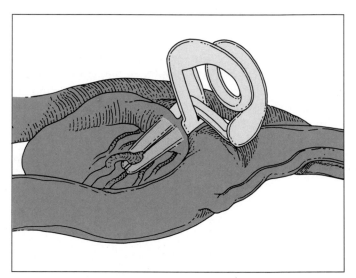

Figure 11.31 Multiple penetrating vessels arise from the posterior aspect of the anterior communicating artery. This schematic illustration shows that the use of excessive clip length and poor visibility behind the aneurysm can cause injury to these important vessels.

Figure 11.32 For exposure of vertebral-PICA aneurysms the patient is positioned laterally on the operating table with the vertex tilted slightly toward the floor with approximately 10° of rotation of the chin to the floor.

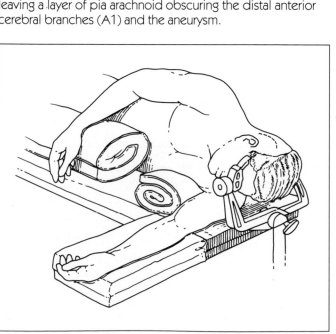

the fourth ventricle (through the foramen of Luschka). Surgery of aneurysms in this region is complicated by the intimate relationship of the aneurysm to the brainstem and to the critical lower cranial nerves (cranial nerves IX, X, XI).

To expose this region, the patient can be positioned in the lateral position with a small roll or gel pad under the dependent axilla. The vertex is tipped slightly inferiorly and the chin is rotated approximately 10° toward the floor (Fig. 11.32). This so-called park bench position allows the seated surgeon comfortable access to the subarachnoid space lateral to the medulla. A craniotomy or craniectomy is performed that includes the foramen magnum and generously exposes the ipsilateral cerebellar hemisphere. The subarachnoid dissection begins in the cisterna magna, progressively elevating the cerebellar tonsil to allow identification of the vertebral artery proximal to the PICA origin. The fibers of the 10th cranial nerve are gently dissected and they usually separate, allowing adequate room for exposure between these fibers (Fig. 11.33). Great care is used in dissection as undue trauma to these delicate fibers can result in vocal cord paralysis, a potential cause of dangerous postoperative aspiration. Fortunately, the vertebral artery typically travels almost due medially after the PICA origin, making it relatively protected, even from a blind clip application. When necessary, small groups of fibers of the 12th cranial nerve may be either sectioned or included in a difficult clip placement, a maneuver safer than the aggressive dissection necessary to completely free them; its use is associated with either no neurologic deficit or a trivial one.

ANEURYSMS OF THE VERTEBRAL CONFLUENS AND LOWER BASILAR TRUNK

This group of extremely difficult aneurysms taxes the ingenuity of the most experienced vascular neurosurgeons due to the depth of exposure, the requirement for optimal exposure ventral to the brain stem, and the frequent need for innovative skull base exposures. The vertebral confluens is a unique arterial site, in which two large vessels join to form a larger vessel. Taking the direction of normal flow into account, the previous discussion of pathophysiology of aneurysms suggests that aneurysmal dilation would not occur at this site. Unfortunately, the anatomy of distal vertebral arteries and the lower basilar trunk only rarely occurs in the textbook configuration. Tremendous asymmetry between the sizes and lengths of the vertebral arteries can occur and the confluens itself can be extremely tortuous and, on occasion, located well into the cerebellar pontine angle. In addition, fenestrations of the lower basilar trunk are not uncommon in patients who develop aneurysms in these sites. Obviously, the anatomic anomalies that seem to predispose aneurysmal development also gravely complicate dissection in a very deep wound, which is often packed with fresh subarachnoid blood. In general, lesions in this area are exposed through a lateral patient position and the early portion of the dissection is simply a continuation of what was previously described for vertebral-PICA aneurysms. Dissection is usually carried out between the fibers of the ninth cranial nerve below and the seventh and eighth cranial nerves above (Fig. 11.34). Aneurysms of the lower basilar trunk are usually associated with the origin of the anterior

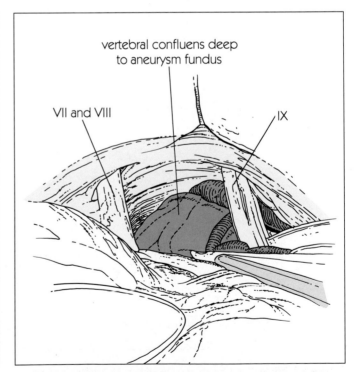

Figure 11.33 The typical vertebral-PICA aneurysm is dissected between the fibers of the lower cranial nerves, which exit at the jugular foramen.

Figure 11.34 The region of the vertebral confluens is typically defined between the seventh and eighth cranial nerves superiorly and the ninth nerve inferiorly. The depth of exposure, relationship to the brain stem, and frequency of arterial anomalies make this a very difficult exposure.

inferior cerebellar artery (ICA) and the sixth cranial nerve. Their exposure is beyond the scope of this text but typically involves a skull base approach, either by sectioning the tentorium from a subtemporal approach or by an exposure anterior to or through the sigmoid sinus. These are involved multidisciplinary procedures that should be done at a center that has an involved and committed skull base and neurovascular program.

ANEURYSMS OF THE DISTAL BASILAR ARTERY

Aneurysms arising from the basilar apex or immediately distal to the origin of the superior cerebellar arteries comprise the most common form of posterior circulation aneurysm. Definitive surgical treatment became possible significantly later than it did for other types of aneurysmal disease, and it reflects the outstanding contributions made by Drs. Charles Drake and Gazi Yasargil.[38,39,41,42] Access to the distal basilar artery in the interpeduncular cistern, which requires deep exposure from any approach, is complicated by the myriad of vital perforating arteries arising from the posterior aspect of the distal basilar artery and both P1 segments (Fig. 11.35).[43] Failure to design specific operative strategies to insure preservation of these vessels invariably results in clip occlusion and an almost certain likelihood of the patient suffering mesencephalic or diencephalic infarction (Fig. 11.36). Three specific operative approaches have been designed to expose and treat aneurysms of the distal basilar artery, each with advantages, disadvantages, and limitations.

Pterional (Transsylvian) Approach

The pterional approach, particularly with wide sylvian fissure dissection, is extremely versatile and used for many aneurysms of the distal basilar complex. Wide dissection of the parasellar cisterns enables access to the interpeduncular cistern by one or multiple routes (Fig. 11.37). The dissection plane and the approach can be developed lateral to the internal carotid artery wherein the posterior communicating artery is followed to the junction of the P1 and P2 segments of the posterior cerebral artery. The P1 is then followed proximally to isolate proximal control on the distal basilar artery. Similarly, a dissection plane can be developed medial to the carotid artery that separates the small perforating arteries to the hypothalamic region and optic tract, opening the membrane of Liliequist, therefore directly exposing the basilar trunk in the interpeduncular cistern. In particularly high basilar bifurcation aneurysms, it may be necessary to gain additional superior exposure by developing the plane immediately above the carotid bifurcation. This can be done by carefully dividing the arachnoidal fibers that bind together the small lenticulostriate vessels and, with patience, adequate separation of this tissue can be developed, allowing elevation of the optic tract with workable space within the interpeduncular cistern. In fact, regardless of the procedure, defining each of these planes minimizes obscuration of vital anatomy by instruments placed in the exposure. Figure 11.38 illustrates a technique whereby a right-handed surgeon can approach the bifurcation region by using the microscope's line of sight medial to the carotid artery and passing the clip applier lateral to the carotid artery, minimizing obscuration of this narrow space. This transsylvian exposure can be used to treat a wide variety of aneurysms in this location, because it allows the surgeon a good view of the anatomy. It also enables exquisite access to the proximal basilar trunk and both P1 segments for definitive tempo-

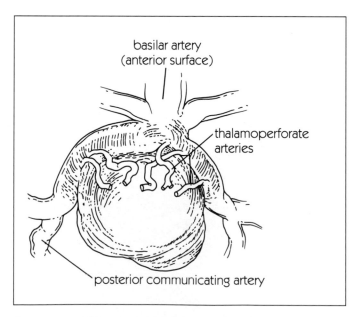

Figure 11.35 Aneurysms of the distal basilar artery must be treated with a precise awareness of the constant presence and infinite variability of the posterior thalamoperforating arteries supplying the mesencephalon and diencephalon.

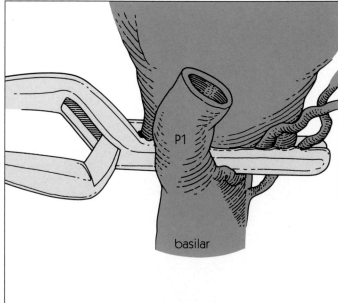

Figure 11.36 Clip applied to a basilar bifurcation aneurysm with inadvertent occlusion of thalamoperforating vessels. This error is almost always devastating to the patient.

Principles of Neurosurgery

rary occlusion with aneurysmal decompression, if necessary, to control intraoperative bleeding or facilitate the dissection of difficult large and giant lesions.

Half and Half Approach

Drake has described this modification of the pterional exposure to improve access to the posterior reaches of the interpeduncular cistern through a slightly more lateral viewpoint.[39] This approach involves rotating the head a bit more than in a direct transsylvian exposure

and mobilizing the temporal lobe with superior and slightly lateral displacement of the uncus (Fig. 11.39). In addition to the improved posterior exposure, this approach offers an improved view of the entire interpeduncular fossa. In many circumstances, it is a very desirable approach to plan from the outset of the procedure.

Subtemporal Approach

The lateral view of the interpeduncular cistern, which was highly developed by Drake,[39] offers perhaps the

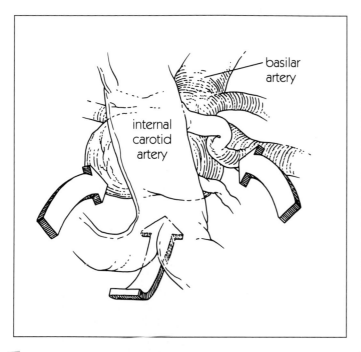

Figure 11.37 The pterional exposure of the distal basilar artery may be accomplished by an approach lateral to the internal carotid, medial to the internal carotid, or superior to the carotid bifurcation.

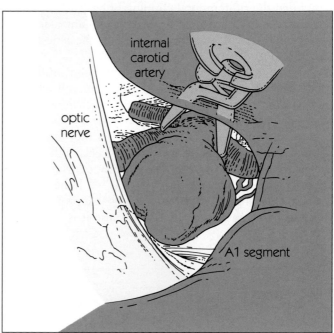

Figure 11.38 The surgeon can take advantage of the versatility of the pterional exposure by directing the microscope and thus the line of sight medial to the carotid artery and inserting the clip lateral and posterior to the carotid so the bulk of the clip and applier do not obscure the view.

Figure 11.39 The half and half approach to basilar bifurcation improves access to the posteriorly located thalamoperforating arteries and improves illumination. The uncus is mobilized out of the tentorial incisura with a second retractor.

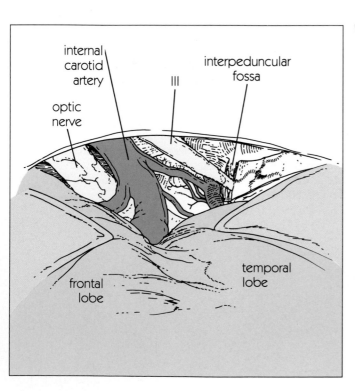

ideal view of the vital perforators posterior to the aneurysmal fundus (Fig. 11.40). For the typical superior projecting aneurysm, this viewpoint maximizes one's ability to salvage the perforating arteries, although the contralateral posterior cerebral artery is more difficult to see and quite difficult, if not impossible, to occlude temporarily. For a standard subtemporal clipping, however, the space anterior to the aneurysmal neck can usually be retracted gently so that the contralateral P1 segment with its initial anterior course can be definitively seen. Drake's innovation of the aperture or fenestrated clip has greatly simplified the subtemporal clipping of basilar bifurcation aneurysms such that the P1 segment and any associated perforating arteries may be included in the fenestration (Fig. 11.41).

Great familiarity with these approaches and their modifications is a prerequisite to successful and relatively safe treatment of patients with these treacherous lesions. A management strategy evolved over several years that has proven valuable at our institution favors the transsylvian approach for most aneurysms of the basilar bifurcation, except for those that project posteriorly or whose necks arise inferior to the midsellar depth.[36,44] It has proven extremely hazardous to treat aneurysms that project posteriorly from an anterior approach because it is impossible to see perforating arteries behind the basilar trunk. A subtemporal approach is preferred because the penetrating vessels and associated posterior projecting aneurysm can be seen well.[29] For low-lying basilar bifurcation aneurysms that arise inferior to the midsellar depth, the posterior clinoid and clivus often obscure adequate proximal exposure, thus the subtemporal approach with opening of tentorial incisura is a successful alternative.

CONCLUSION

Intracranial aneurysms can be catastrophic. The events set in motion by the rupture of an intracranial aneurysm often preclude a successful neurologic outcome despite the best medical and surgical management. Microsurgical technology, along with the variety of temporary and permanent aneurysm clips, has revolutionized therapy for these lesions. Intimate familiarity with the unique aspects of the microsurgical anatomy at each aneurysm site together with the development of skilled microsurgical technique is the cornerstone in surgical treatment of intracranial aneurysms. There is little evidence that less than definitive and precise clipping of intracranial aneurysms provides significant long-term protection to the patient.[29,45–49]

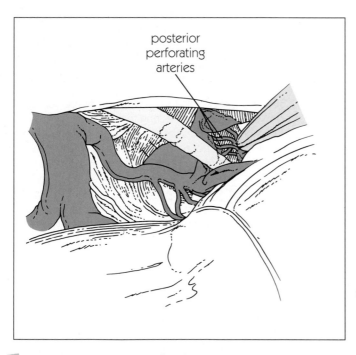

Figure 11.40 The subtemporal approach maximizes the surgical view of the thalamoperforating arteries while rendering the access to the contralateral posterior cerebral artery more difficult.

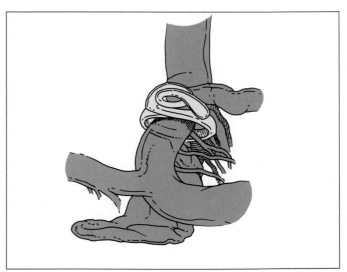

Figure 11.41 Aperture or fenestrated clips for subtemporal clipping of basilar bifurcation aneurysms have proven to be immensely valuable. The ipsilateral P1 segment with associated perforating arteries may be safely included in the fenestration.

REFERENCES

1. McCormick WF, Acosta-Rua GJ. The size of intracranial saccular aneurysms: an autopsy study. *J Neurosurg.* 1970;33:422–427.
2. Kassell NF, Drake CG. Timing of aneurysm surgery. *Neurosurgery.* 1982;10:514–519.
3. Sekhar LN, Heros RC. Origin, growth, and rupture of saccular aneurysms: a review. *Neurosurgery.* 1981; 8:248–260.
4. Somach FM, Shenkin HA. Angiographic end-results of carotid ligation in the treatment of carotid aneurysm. *J Neurosurg.* 1966;24:966–974.
5. Batjer HH, Mickey BE, Samson D. Enlargement and rupture of distal basilar aneurysm following iatrogenic carotid occlusion. *Neurosurgery.* 1987; 20:624–628.
6. Adamson T, Batjer HH. Aneurysm recurrence associated with induced hypertension and hypervolemia. *Surg Neurol.* 1988;29:57–61.
7. Batjer HH, Suss RA, Samson DS. Intracranial arteriovenous malformations associated with aneurysms. *Neurosurgery.* 1986;18:29–35.
8. Weir B. *Aneurysms Affecting the Nervous System.* Baltimore, Md: Williams & Wilkins; 1987:54–133.
9. Kassell NF, Torner JC. The International Cooperative Study on timing of aneurysm surgery: an update. *Stroke.* 1984;15:566–570.
10. Adams HP, Kassell NF, Torner JC. Usefulness of computed tomography in predicting outcome after aneurysmal subarachnoid hemorrhage: a preliminary report of the Cooperative Aneurysm Study. *Neurology.* 1985;35:1263–1267.
11. Hunt WE, Hess RM. Surgical risk as related to time of intervention in the repair of intracranial aneurysms. *J Neurosurg.* 1968;28:14–19.
12. Kassell NF, Torner JC. Aneurysmal rebleeding: a preliminary report from the Cooperative Aneurysm Study. *Neurosurgery.* 1983;13:479–481.
13. Jane JA, Kassell NF, Torner JC, et al. The natural history of aneurysms and arteriovenous malformations. *J Neurosurg.* 1985;62:321–323.
14. Weir B, Grace M, Hansen J, et al. Time course of vasospasm in man. *J Neurosurg.* 1978;48:173–178.
15. Kwak R, Niizuma H, Takatsugu D, et al. Angiographic study of cerebral vasospasm following rupture of intracranial aneurysms, I: time of the appearance. *Surg Neurol.* 1979;11:257–262.
16. Kassell NF, Sasaki T, Colohan ART, et al. Cerebral vasospasm following subarachnoid hemorrhage. *Stroke.* 1985;16:562–572.
17. Fisher CM, Kistler JP, Davis JM. Relation of cerebral vasospasm to subarachnoid hemorrhage visualized by computerized tomographic scanning. *Neurosurgery.* 1980;6:1–9.
18. Doczi T, Bende J, Huzka E, et al. Syndrome of inappropriate secretion of antidiuretic hormone after subarachnoid hemorrhage. *Neurosurgery.* 1981; 9:394–397.
19. Kassell NF, Boarini DJ. Perioperative care of the aneurysm patient. *Contemp Neurosurg.* 1984;6:1–6.
20. Ljunggren B, Brandt L, Kagstrom E, et al. Results of early operations for ruptured aneurysms. *J Neurosurg.* 1981;54:473–479.
21. Ljunggren B, Saveland H, Brandt L, et al. Early operation and overall outcome in aneurysmal subarachnoid hemorrhage. *J Neurosurg.* 1985;62: 547–551.
22. Winn HR, Newell DW, Mayberg MR, et al. Early surgical management of poor-grade patients with intracranial aneurysms. *Clin Neurosurg.* 1990; 36:289–298.
23. Kassell NF, Torner JC, Adams HP. Antifibrinolytic therapy in the acute period following aneurysmal subarachnoid hemorrhage: preliminary observations from the Cooperative Aneurysm Study. *J Neurosurg.* 1984;61:225–230.
24. Kosnik EJ, Hunt WE. Postoperative hypertension in the management of patients with intracranial aneurysms. *J Neurosurg.* 1976;45:148–154.
25. Finn SS, Stephenson SA, Miller CA, et al. Observations on the perioperative management of aneurysmal subarachnoid hemorrhage. *J Neurosurg.* 1986;65:48–62.
26. Kassell NF, Peerless SJ, Durward QJ, et al. Treatment of ischemic deficits from vasospasm with intravascular volume expansion and induced arterial hypertension. *Neurosurgery.* 1982;11:337–343.
27. Gentleman D, Johnston R. Postoperative extradural hematoma associated with induced hypertension. *Neurosurgery.* 1985;17:105–106.
28. Terada T, Komai N, Hayashi S, et al. Hemorrhagic infarction after vasospasm due to ruptured cerebral aneurysm. *Neurosurgery.* 1986;18:415–418.
29. Batjer HH, Samson DS. Causes of morbidity and mortality from surgery of aneurysms of the distal basilar artery. *Neurosurgery.* 1989;25:904–916.
30. Higashida RT, Hieshima GB, Tsai FY, et al. Transluminal angioplasty of the vertebral and basilar artery. *AJNR.* 1987;8:745–749.

31. Batjer HH, Samson DS. Intraoperative aneurysmal rupture: incidence, outcome, and suggestions for surgical management. *Neurosurgery*. 1986;18: 701–707.

32. Michenfelder JD, Theye RA. Cerebral protection by thiopental during hypoxia. *Anesthesiology*. 1973; 39:510–517.

33. Michenfelder JD, Milde JH. Influence of anesthetics on metabolic, functional and pathological responses to regional cerebral ischemia. *Stroke*. 1975; 6: 405–410.

34. Michenfelder JD, Milde JH, Sundt TM Jr. Cerebral protection by barbiturate anesthesia. *Arch Neurol*. 1976;33:345–350.

35. Batjer HH, Frankfurt AI, Purdy PD, et al. Use of etomidate, temporary arterial occlusion, and intraoperative angiography in large and giant cerebral aneurysm surgery. *J Neurosurg*. 1988;68:234–240.

36. Samson DS, Batjer HH. *Intracranial Aneurysm Surgery: Techniques*. Mount Kisco, NY: Futura Publishing Co; 1990.

37. Heros RC, Nelson PB, Ojemann RG, et al. Large and giant paraclinoid aneurysms: surgical techniques, complications, and results. *Neurosurgery*. 1983;12:153–163.

38. Drake CG. Giant intracranial aneurysms: experience with surgical treatment in 174 patients. *Clin Neurosurg*. 1979;26:12–95.

39. Drake CG. The treatment of aneurysms of the posterior circulation. *Clin Neurosurg*. 1979;26:96–144.

40. Locksley HB. Report on the Cooperative Study of Intracranial Aneurysm and Subarachnoid Hemorrhage, section V, part 1: natural history of subarachnoid hemorrhage, intracranial aneurysms and arteriovenous malformations: based on 6368 cases in the cooperative study. *J Neurosurg*. 1966;25:219–239.

41. Yasargil MG. Operative anatomy. In: Yasargil MG. *Microneurosurgery*. Stuttgart: Georg Thieme Verlag; 1984;1:5–168.

42. Yasargil MG. Pathological considerations. In: Yasargil MG. *Microneurosurgery*. Stuttgart: Georg Thieme Verlag; 1984;1:279–349.

43. Grand W, Hopkins LN. The microsurgical anatomy of the basilar artery bifurcation. *Neurosurgery*. 1977; 1:128–131.

44. Samson DS, Hodosh RM, Clark WK. Microsurgical evaluation of the pterional approach to aneurysms of the distal basilar circulation. *Neurosurgery*. 1978;3: 135–141.

45. Drake CG, Vanderlinden RG. The late consquences of incomplete surgical treatment of cerebral aneurysms. *J Neurosurg*. 1967;27:226–238.

46. Drake CG, Friedman AH, Peerless SJ. Failed aneurysm surgery: reoperation in 115 cases. *J Neurosurg*. 1984;61:848–856.

47. Feuerberg I, Lindquist C, Lindqvist M, et al. Natural history of postoperative aneurysm rests. *J Neurosurg*. 1987;66:30–34.

48. Todd NV, Tocher JL, Jones PA, et al. Outcome following aneurysm wrapping: a 10-year follow-up review of clipped and wrapped aneurysms. *J Neurosurg*. 1989;70:841–846.

49. Lin T, Fox AJ, Drake CG. Regrowth of aneurysm sacs from residual neck following aneurysm clipping. *J Neurosurg*. 1989;70:556–560.

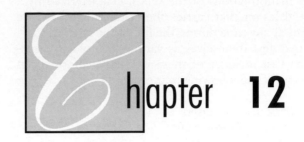

Chapter **12**

Vascular Malformations Affecting the Nervous System

Robert A. Solomon

Vascular malformations of the CNS, characterized by a congenital lesion that carries the potential to produce symptoms at any time during the life of the affected individual, manifest themselves as various neurologic disorders. The vast majority of these vascular malformations fall into one of the following four groups:

1. Capillary telangiectasias
2. Cavernous malformations
3. Venous malformations
4. Arteriovenous malformations (AVMs)

A considerable amount of information indicates that the boundaries between the lesion types are not well defined, and transitional forms of vascular anomalies may exist between the subgroups.

This chapter focuses on lesions that are viewed as developmental malformations rather than neoplastic lesions. Many volumes have been written on this type of vascular malformation; this chapter is designed to give an overview of the salient clinical aspects. The pathology, clinical behavior, and therapeutic options for vascular malformations of the nervous system will be explored.

PATHOLOGY AND CLASSIFICATION

Morphologically, vascular malformations resemble the early anastomotic plexuses formed during embryogenesis of the vascular system of the CNS.[1] Nevertheless, it is very difficult to correlate vascular malformations with specific adverse events during the vasculogenesis of the nervous system. Making it more difficult to relate their appearance when they become symptomatic to events in the embryonic stage is the fact that these lesions are dynamic, that is, characterized by constant change in size and configuration.

Although AVMs are the most common vascular anomalies seen clinically, autopsy studies reveal that venous malformations and telangiectasias are far more prevalent.[2] The clinician rarely encounters these latter lesions because they do not have the same propensity for hemorrhage as AVMs.

CAPILLARY TELANGIECTASIAS

Capillary telangiectasias are very small vascular malformations most commonly seen in the pons (Fig. 12.1). This type of malformation is composed solely of small capillary-type blood vessels, and the entire malformation usually measures no more than 1 cm in diameter. The histology of the vessel walls that compose the malformation is identical to that of normal capillaries, and normal neural parenchyma are found between the capillaries. Although capillary telangiectasias can be multiple, these lesions rarely show pathologic alterations such as hemorrhage or thrombosis. The diagnosis is made during an autopsy, usually as an incidental finding. Telangiectasias can rarely be seen on CT and MRI. These lesions are not visualized by angiography. Capillary telangiectasias are clinically interesting only because these lesions may represent an earlier stage of cavernous malformations.[3]

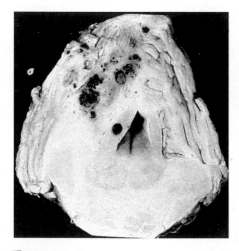

Figure 12.1 Gross autopsy specimen with cross-sectional view of pons, demonstrating capillary telangiectasia.

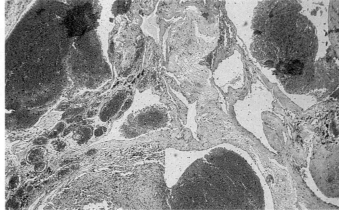

Figure 12.2 Hematoxylin and eosin (H&E) stained micrograph of surgically removed cavernous malformation. Note large cystic vascular spaces.

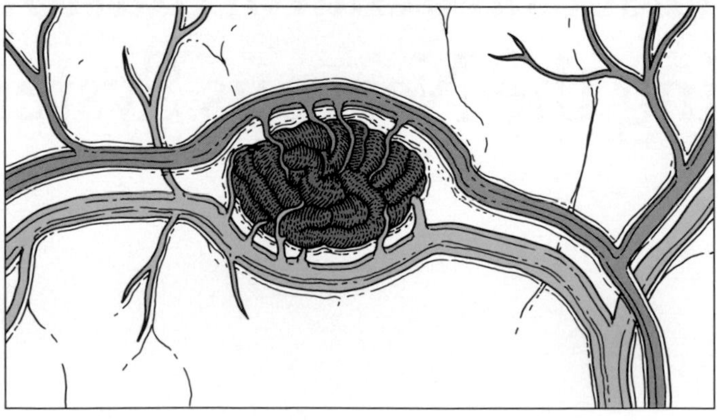

Figure 12.3 The vascular structures of a cavernous malformation.

CAVERNOUS MALFORMATIONS

Cavernous malformations are often much larger than capillary telangiectasias. These lesions are composed of cystic vascular spaces lined by a single layer of endothelial cells. These sinusoidal vessels form a compact mass with no intervening neural parenchyma between the vascular structures (Fig. 12.2). No recognizable arteries or veins can be found within the interstices of the malformations, and therefore the vessels resemble those in capillary telangiectasias (Fig. 12.3). Unlike the telangiectasias, however, cavernous malformations have a propensity to cause hemorrhage. Although hemorrhage is rarely massive, cavernous malformations invariably show areas of recent and old hemorrhage with hemosiderin deposition, gliosis, and focal areas of calcification. Ossification may even be seen in the larger cavernous malformations.

These lesions are generally not well visualized on conventional angiography because there is an absence of direct arterial input. However, their appearance on MRI is very characteristic, allowing reasonable accuracy in preoperative diagnosis (Fig. 12.4). Their contents are variegated, owing to varying amounts of hemosiderin, clotted and nonclotted blood, and calcium. They usually have low-signal rims interspersed with high-signal crescents. These lesions are found in all parts of the central nervous system and are often multiple. Sometimes they are associated with other vascular malformations such as venous malformations or capillary telangiectasias.

VENOUS MALFORMATIONS

In McCormick's autopsy series, venous malformations were found to be the most common type of vascular malformation.[2] These lesions are composed of anomalous veins separated by normal neural parenchyma. The malformations may be composed of a single, greatly dilated, tortuous vein or a number of smaller veins coalescing at a single point. Often a single draining vein forms the most conspicuous aspect of the malformation. There is never direct arterial input (Fig. 12.5).

Clinically, these lesions are considered benign without risk of major hemorrhage or neurologic problems. Rare cases of hemorrhage have been reported, but usually in cases of coexisting cavernous malformations. Au-

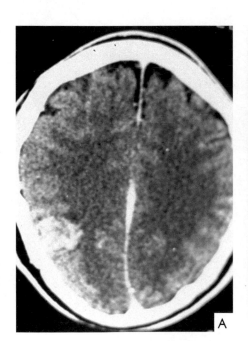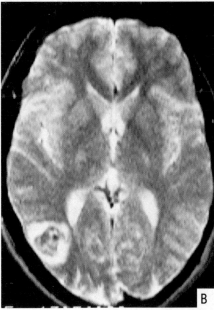

Figure 12.4 (A) Contrast enhanced CT scan of patient with right parietal cavernous malformation. (B) MRI of the same patient, demonstrating the characteristic appearance of a cavernous malformation.

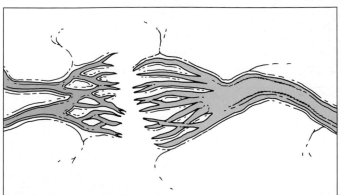

Figure 12.5 Anatomy of a venous malformation.

topsy studies generally fail to reveal evidence of old hemorrhage, even microscopic hemorrhage. These lesions have a characteristic appearance in the venous phase of an angiogram, described as a *caput medusae* (Fig. 12.6). Venous malformations can also be appreciated as linear signals in abnormal locations during contrast-enhanced CT scans or conventional MRI scans (Fig. 12.7).

ARTERIOVENOUS MALFORMATIONS

AVMs are complex lesions whose primary feature is direct shunting of arterial blood to the venous system. The lesions are composed of abnormally developed arteries and veins with no capillary component. Most of the vascular channels within an AVM are venous in morphology, but there are usually examples of transitional vessels (Fig. 12.8). The vascular channels are tightly compacted, usually with no intervening neural parenchyma (Fig. 12.9). However, this is by no means a universal finding, and some AVMs are diffuse in nature with significant areas of functional neural tissue intertwined among vascular structures. The compactness of the component vessels, therefore, varies considerably from specimen to specimen.

These lesions are well known for their propensity to hemorrhage. Even in patients without any clinical history of ictal events, pathologic examination of removed AVMs often reveals areas of hemosiderin deposition and abnormal gliotic parenchyma, indicative of numerous microhemorrhages. Thrombosis and reparative fibrosis, also important features of AVMs, may cause consider-

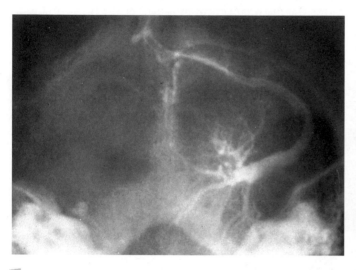

Figure 12.6 Typical angiographic appearance of a venous malformation described as a *caput medusae.*

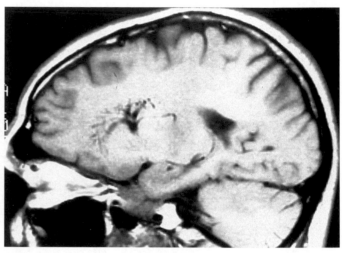

Figure 12.7 MRI of patient with a deep frontal venous malformation.

Figure 12.8 AVM showing various arterial feeders and primary draining vein.

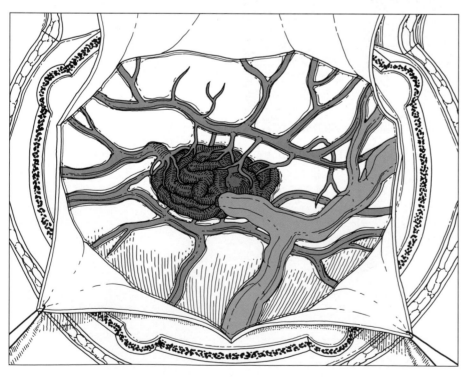

Principles of Neurosurgery

able scar tissue in and around the lesion. They have the potential for extensive calcification.

Since AVMs are true artery-to-vein fistulae, they have a characteristic MRI (Fig. 12.10) and angiographic (Fig. 12.11) appearance. In fact, if a fistulous connection cannot be seen angiographically, the diagnosis cannot be made. AVMs receive direct arterial supply, usually from multiple feeding arteries, and the venous drainage is subserved by veins that vary considerably in terms of number, size, and configuration. Venous aneurysms are not uncommon, and arterial aneurysms are seen in as many as 15% of cases, usually on the feeding arteries.

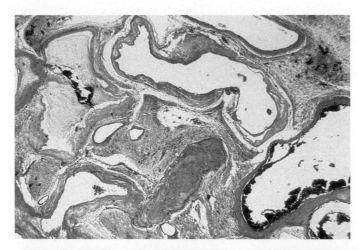

Figure 12.9 H&E stained micrograph of surgically removed AVM. Note the transitional morphology of vessels.

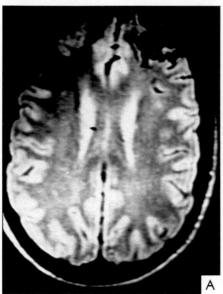

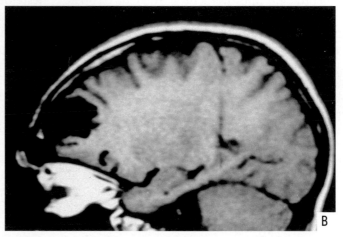

Figure 12.10 Typical MRI appearance of left frontal AVM showing axial (**A**) and parasagittal (**B**) views. Signal void is evidence of high flow through the malformation.

Figure 12.11 Angiographic appearance of AVM (same case as Figure 12.10). Lateral (**A**) and AP (**B**) views indicate direct AV shunting.

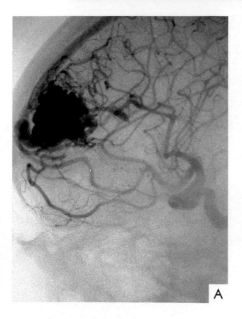

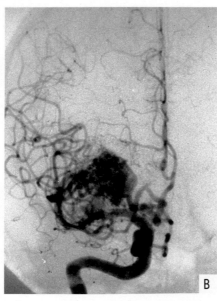

CLINICAL PRESENTATION AND NATURAL HISTORY

INTRACEREBRAL HEMORRHAGE

Intracranial hemorrhage is by far the most frequent presenting symptom for patients with intracranial vascular malformations. Depending on the series, between 50% and 75% of patients have a hemorrhage as the initial symptom related to an intracranial AVM. Because most of the malformations lie within the cerebral parenchyma, hemorrhages from these lesions are most often of the intracerebral type (Fig. 12.12). Ventricular and subarachnoid hemorrhages frequently accompany rupture of AVMs. These hemorrhages usually come from the venous channels that carry blood with arterial pressure and are rarely of the catastrophic nature seen with ruptured intracranial aneurysms. The great majority of patients with AVMs who suffer a hemorrhage survive. Vasospasm and rebleeding, deadly and frequent complications of aneurysmal rupture, are almost never a problem in patients with ruptured AVMs.[4] In fact, 90% of patients will survive an initial hemorrhage from an AVM and show neurologic improvement as the clot resolves. Recurrent hemorrhages are usually separated by years and sometimes decades.[5-7]

Nonetheless, natural history studies indicate the treacherous nature of AVMs. In several studies the yearly incidence of death and disability diagnosed by AVMs left untreated approached 4%.[6,8-11] The best natural history study, performed by Ondra et al.[6] prospectively followed 166 unoperated patients with symptomatic AVMs over a mean period of 23.7 years: 23% of the patients died from the effects of hemorrhage caused by the malformations, and the rate of major rebleeding was 4% per year.

SEIZURES

Seizures are the second most common symptom that herald the presence of an intracranial vascular anomaly. Approximately 25% to 50% of all patients with AVMs present with focal or generalized seizures without obvious hemorrhage. Malformations located in the posterior fossa are not associated with seizures. However, when the lesions are located in the temporal, frontal, and parietal areas, seizures are a common presenting symptom.

For the most part, epilepsy related to intracranial vascular anomalies can be controlled with effective medical management. The presence of a seizure disorder alone is not sufficient to warrant radical surgical treatment of an AVM or cavernous malformation. Although in many instances seizure disorders will improve following surgical resection, often the severity of the seizure is not changed by the operation. The selection of patients for surgical treatment should be based on the risk of future hemorrhage, an issue that will be discussed subsequently.

HEADACHES

Headaches are a frequent problem in patients with AVMs but are rarely encountered in other vascular anomalies without evidence of hemorrhage. A headache disorder similar to classical migraine headaches has been described for brain AVMs. Headaches associated with AVMs are usually unilateral and do not shift from side to side in true migrainous fashion. However auras, visual symptomatology, and severe debilitating intermittent headaches have been described in patients with AVMs. Migraine-like headache disorder is most commonly seen in patients who harbor AVMs of the occipital lobes, which can usually be cured by resection of the AVM.

More generalized headaches, often related to elevated venous pressures and stretching of venous sinuses and dura, have been reported. These types of headaches are less dramatic than those seen with the occipital lobe AVMs and are rarely of a debilitating nature.

STEAL SYNDROME

The final symptom often associated with AVMs of the brain is related to arterial steal phenomenon. Although

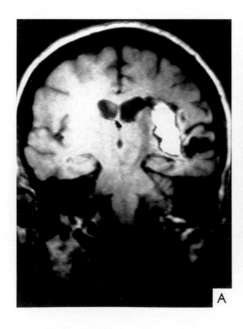

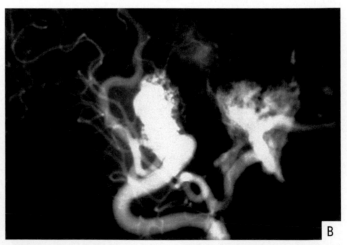

Figure 12.12 (A) Coronal MRI demonstrating intracerebral hemorrhage in a patient with AVM of the dominant motor area. (B) Lateral carotid angiogram of the same patient.

the clinical expression of this syndrome is rarely seen, a subgroup of patients develops progressive neurologic deficits without hemorrhage over many years in conjunction with a high-flow AVM.[13,14] Although a definitive explanation for this problem is lacking, most likely the deficit is related to the cumulative effect of steal from the normal perfusion of the surrounding brain by the AVM. Xenon flow studies have indeed confirmed hypoperfusion in normal brain regions surrounding high-flow AVMs. This chronic ischemia, which has been attributed to the severe postoperative problem of normal perfusion pressure breakthrough,[14,15] will be discussed subsequently.

THERAPEUTIC OPTIONS

Considering the therapeutic options available for treatment for intracranial vascular malformations, the neurosurgeon must constantly balance the risk of an untreated malformation against the risk of the various treatments available. Therapeutic alternatives include the following, either alone or in combination: 1) operative resection or obliteration, 2) endovascular embolization, and 3) radiosurgery.

Venous malformations and capillary telangiectasias do not require therapeutic intervention because of the relatively benign nature of these lesions. Cavernous malformations are best left untreated when they are found incidentally; however, if they present with a hemorrhage, they should be surgically removed (Fig. 12.13). Symptomatic cavernous malformations of the spinal cord and supratentorial compartment can often be excised and cured by surgery.[1,3,16] Cavernous malformations of the cerebellum are also readily excisable when hemorrhage has been the presenting symptom. The real problem lies with cavernous malformations of the brain stem. Although some heroic attempts to remove malformations in this location have been successful, removal of cavernous malformations of the brain stem is often extremely difficult. The wisdom of a surgical approach to this group of lesions remains highly controversial.[4]

The most important clinical decision making with regard to vascular malformations is related to the AVMs.

Although these lesions can produce the most devastating symptoms when left untreated, treatment also carries a very high risk to the patient.

SURGICAL EXCISION

Surgical removal of an AVM is the most definitive treatment. This form of therapy offers the patient the chance for an immediate cure and avoidance of possible side effects from the damages of radiation. Nevertheless, surgery carries significant risk of morbidity and mortality, and patients should be carefully selected for this form of treatment.[17,18]

The presenting symptoms of an AVM are probably the least important factor in deciding whether or not a patient should be subjected to an intracranial operation. Natural history studies show that even patients who present with headaches or seizures are still at significant risk for severe hemorrhagic complications from the malformations.[6] As well, patients who present with hemorrhage often can go years or decades without recurrent bleeding.

Age is is the most critical factor in deciding the patient's suitability for operative resection. Generally, the risk of operation cannot be justified in asymptomatic patients older than 55 years. At age 55 the risks of surgery are about equal to the risk of allowing the lesions to develop naturally over the projected lifetime of the individual.

A factor equally important to age is location of the lesion. If the malformation is located in an inaccessible area, such as the diencephalon or brain stem, the risk of neurologic damage becomes high. Such lesions should be operated on only by an experienced surgical team because of the difficulties in exposing and removing such malformations.[19-24] These AVMs should be treated surgically only in young individuals who have a hemorrhagic presentation. Lesions located in the medial hemisphere also have a higher degree of operative difficulty than those located in other supratentorial locations.[25-27] In contrast, malformations that are small, polar in location, and readily accessible can be treated surgically, even in older individuals.

The third important issue in deciding on the operability of an AVM regards the size and configuration of

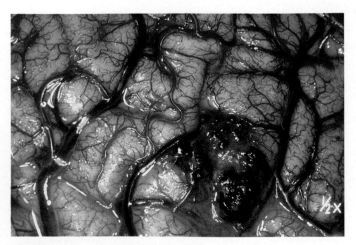

Figure 12.13 Operative appearance of a parietal lobe cavernous malformation. A distinct separation between the lesion and normal brain can be appreciated.

the lesion. Malformations that encompass multiple lobes of the brain can be removed only with great difficulty and the risk of postoperative neurologic complications is high. In older individuals, these lesions are best left untreated. In younger individuals, however, special techniques are required, including multiple operations and preoperative embolization therapy. Grading systems have been proposed in order to analyze the surgical risk of an AVM, taking into account the size of the malformation, the location in critical areas of the brain, and the number and complexity of feeding arteries and draining veins.[28,29] Lesions of a higher grade, indicating higher complexity, are associated with a higher incidence of surgical complications. This type of analysis reflects the need to consider multiple factors when deciding on the suitability of a patient for surgical resection of an AVM.

Operative Technique

The patient is prepared for surgery by achieving adequate anticonvulsant drug levels prior to surgery. Following surgical resection patients are often at a higher risk for seizures, possibly caused by changes in venous blood flow patterns. Therefore, it is essential that patients be loaded preoperatively and adequate anticonvulsant drug levels be maintained in the immediate postoperative period.

Maximum brain relaxation is absolutely essential for AVM surgery. Relaxation is achieved by a combination of proper patient position, with the head as high above the heart as possible, spinal drainage, hyperventilation, and mannitol. In most instances, the patient should be positioned so the surface of the malformation is not only high above the heart but also parallel to the floor, allowing a perpendicular approach. This position may be impractical in posterior fossa malformations or those located in the inner hemispheric surfaces. In these latter instances, the neurosurgeon must make adjustments for a tangential approach during operative resection.[24,27,30]

The craniotomy is made as large as possible, leaving generous space around the margins of the malformations. This is essential because it is necessary to identify all of the surface landmarks, including arteries and veins, to exactly locate the nidus of the malformation.

When opening the dura, the surgeon must take care that any large draining veins that adhere to or pass directly into the dura are not violated. A wide dural opening is essential when working over the convexity, and this applies to lesions in the posterior fossa as well as those that are interhemispheric. With interhemispheric lesions the dura must be reflected towards the sagittal sinus, and often the bridging veins between the brain and the sagittal sinus must be dissected or even divided in order to allow retraction of the hemisphere and exposure of the region around the falx.

The arterialized distended veins of an AVM are the best surface landmarks and can be correlated with the angiogram to pinpoint the location of arteries that often

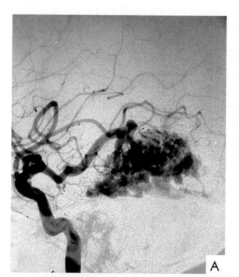 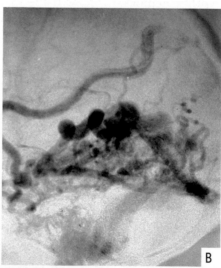

Figure 12.14 Lateral carotid angiogram in a patient with a high-flow posterior temporal AVM. **(A)** Early arterial phase showing large PCA feeder. **(B)** Late venous phase showing extensive venous involvement.

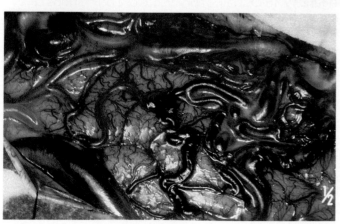

Figure 12.15 Operative photo of the patient in Figure 12.14 showing appearance of AVM on the surface prior to resection. The tentorial surface of the temporal lobe is at the top.

lie deeper (Figs. 12.14, 12.15). The bulk of the malformation may flare out under otherwise normal-appearing cortex so that only the tip of the lesion is seen. After exposure of the malformation's surface and a thorough review of the angiogram, a circumscribing incision is made, avoiding normal cortex. Care should be taken at this point not to disturb major draining veins. Smaller vessels may be interrupted but even with a major deep draining vein, the primary cortical vein should be left intact until much later in the operation (Fig. 12.16). Nutrient arteries are usually found deep in the sulcus. They are cauterized, clipped, and divided, working circumferentially around the margins of the malformations. Thus, the entire cortical margin and subcortical surface of the malformation are circumscribed, avoiding the major veins while securing the arterial supply (Fig. 12.17).

In general, the bipolar cautery is used to secure arterial feeders. Some larger vessels will need to be clipped, and

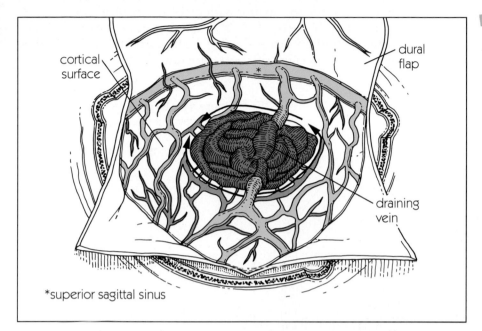

Figure 12.16 Circumscribing incision that interrupts arterial feeders while preserving the draining vein.

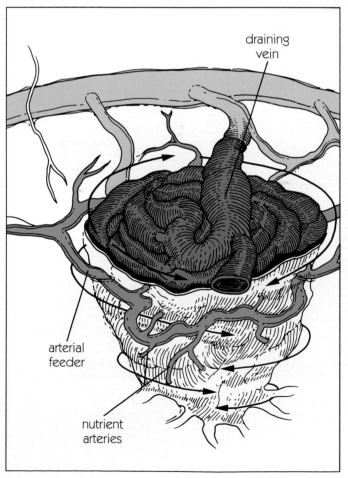

Figure 12.17 Circumferential dissection around the deep margins of an AVM.

smaller arteries can be cauterized and sectioned primarily. As deeper portions of the malformations are uncovered, the neurosurgeon encounters a gliotic area that surrounds the malformation and separates it from normal white matter. This often affords an excellent plane of dissection that is aided by previous hemorrhages. However, deep areas of the malformation are sometimes supplied by numerous tiny penetrating vessels transversing white matter, which can be extremely difficult to cauterize and divide. It is often the deep portions of the malformation that are most difficult for the neurosurgeon and most frustrating to deal with. Decreasing systemic blood pressure greatly facilitates the cauterization of the small white matter vessels supplying the deep surface of the malformation.

The surgeon should never cut across an AVM because of the risk of bleeding. Malformations are generally removed as a single piece with division of all arterial inputs followed by division of the venous connections (Fig. 12.18).

Special approaches and surgical techniques are required for a number of malformations located in complex areas of the nervous system. The special techniques for these malformations are beyond the scope of this brief overview, but special references should be addressed when considering malformations of the medial aspect of the hemispheres,[26,27,30–33] deep diencephalic or basal ganglion lesions,[22,24,34–37] malformations that follow the incisura of the tentorium,[26] and posterior fossa

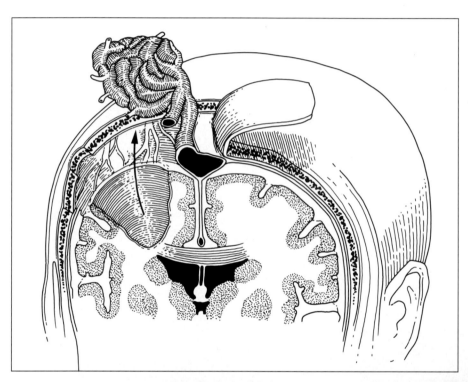

Figure 12.18 Final ligation and division of the major draining vein of a removed AVM. The coronal view shows the vein emptying into the superior sagittal sinus.

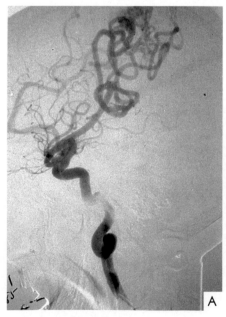

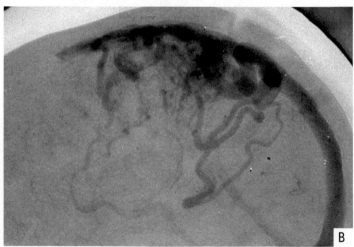

Figure 12.19 Lateral carotid angiogram of a patient with a high-flow AVM of right parietal lobe. (**A**) Early arterial phase. (**B**) Venous phase showing high degree of shunting.

malformations including lesions of the brain stem and cerebellum.[19,21–23,38]

Postoperative Management

Following total removal of an AVM, the two most feared complications are delayed hemorrhage and seizures. Significant postoperative hemorrhages are most likely to occur within the first 12 to 24 hours after the operative procedure. In most instances, clinically significant hemorrhages are the result of residual malformation left during the operative procedure. In these cases, the patient will deteriorate rapidly and must undergo emergency removal of the blood clot. Hemostasis must be obtained, and then a search for residual malformation must be undertaken using the operating microscope. The final piece of AVM must then be removed. Other causes for postoperative hemorrhage include insufficient occlusion of the major arterial inputs and the normal perfusion pressure breakthrough phenomenon.[15] Normal perfusion pressure breakthrough is usually manifested by small parenchymal hemorrhages and diffuse swelling of the brain or hemisphere surrounding the operative resection. Re-elevation is almost never required in this latter circumstance. Nonetheless, brain damage from swelling and herniation can, at times, be quite severe. It is important to control these complications with dehydration of the brain and lowering of systemic blood pressure (Figs. 12.19, 12.20).

Seizures may occur postoperatively even though adequate levels of anticonvulsants have been maintained before, during, and after the operation. The brain becomes extremely sensitive after surgery, especially if the patient has been subject to seizures previously. It is wise to provide high levels of anticonvulsant coverage, usually with more than one drug, during the operation. If seizures should occur postoperatively, control must be gained as rapidly as possible by using standard multiple drug therapy.

Following surgery, 24 hours of ICU monitoring is sufficient in uncomplicated cases. Patients can then be rapidly tapered off of dexamethasone, and they can begin ambulating. Seizure prophylaxis is generally advisable for approximately 3 months following uncomplicated surgery, but longer periods may be required in patients with a previous history of seizures or in patients who developed postoperative seizures. A postoperative angiogram is mandatory in all patients with resected AVMs. Documentation of complete removal is essential since small residual pieces of malformation can subsequently enlarge, making hemorrhage likely.

ENDOVASCULAR EMBOLIZATION

Embolization treatment can only rarely be expected to annihilate an AVM. There is also no indication that a partially treated AVM has a more benign natural history than an AVM left undisturbed. In fact, considerable evidence indicates that a partially treated AVM may be more dangerous than an AVM left untreated. Therefore, embolization should never be the primary or sole treat-

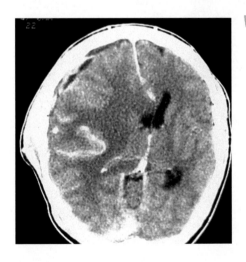

Figure 12.20 Postoperative CT scan of the patient in Figure 12.13 showing massive swelling of normal brain around operative site secondary to normal perfusion pressure breakthrough phenomenon.

ment of a vascular malformation.[39] Embolization treatment is generally used as an adjunct to surgical excision.[31,40–44]

Embolization can successfully remove deep feeders to the malformation, greatly facilitating a subsequent operative resection (Fig. 12.21). Moreover, by gradually occluding the flow through the malformation, the complication of normal perfusion pressure breakthrough, which is often seen following the abrupt removal of large AVMs, can be avoided. This factor is the most compelling reason to perform preoperative embolization treatment for large AVMs. Finally, embolization treatment can induce partial thrombosis of the malformation and further facilitate operative resection. In some instances, embolization treatment can reduce a large malformation down to a small size that may be amenable to radiosurgery. The value of this approach has yet to be proven since it has been well established that large thrombosed sections of an AVM can recanalize and re-establish AV shunting when complete excision has not been accomplished.

RADIOSURGERY

Radiosurgery is an exciting new approach to the treatment of AVMs of the brain.[45–47] Stereotactically focused, high-energy radiation is delivered to a well-defined volume containing the nidus of the malformation. This dose of radiation induces gradual sclerosis of the blood vessels, which causes obliteration of the malformation. Obliteration of an AVM seems to take 1 to 2 years fol-

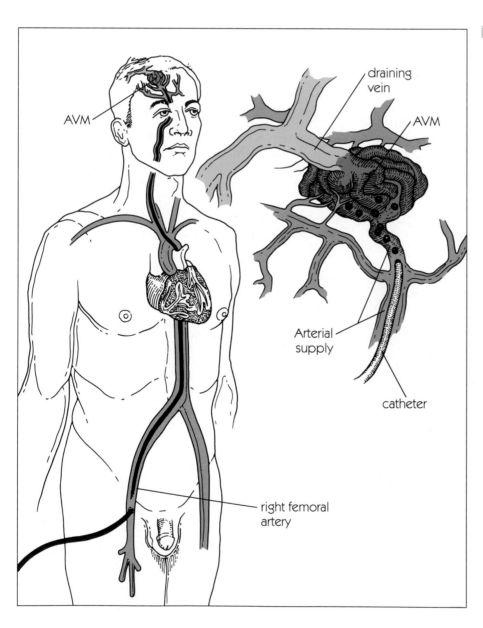

draining vein

AVM

AVM

Arterial supply

catheter

right femoral artery

Figure 12.21 Embolization procedure. The catheter is inserted in the right femoral artery and fluoroscopically directed into the feeding artery of the AVM. The close up shows delivery of embolic materials (wire coils, pellets, particulate slurries, or glue) to interstices of the malformation.

lowing the delivery of the therapeutic dose. Radiosurgery has been shown to be highly effective for treating small malformations, whereas malformations greater than 2 cm have a decreased response.[47]

With proper dosimetry the immediate side effects of radiosurgery have been moderate and limited to mild episodes of radiation necrosis.[46] However, the long-term side effects are unknown at this time, and it is conceivable that neoplastic changes may be induced in some patients who have had radiosurgery. The down side of radiosurgery has to do with the relatively long time between delivery of the radiation and obliteration of the malformation. During this time the patient continues to be at risk for hemorrhage, and therefore lesions that are amenable to surgical treatment should probably not be subjected to radiosurgery. However, radiosurgery should be a primary mode of treatment for patients with small lesions for whom surgical intervention is too risky (e.g., they are too old or the AVM is in a critical location).

Radiosurgery was first performed with a device called the *gamma-knife*.[47] However, because this instrument is expensive and depends on high-energy cobalt sources it is available at only a very few centers. Proton beams and linear accelerators have been effectively used for radiosurgery since these high-energy radiation sources are more readily available and can be easily interfaced with standard CT and angiography-directed stereotactic equipment.[45,46,48] All three types of radiation sources seem to be equally efficacious (Fig. 12.22).

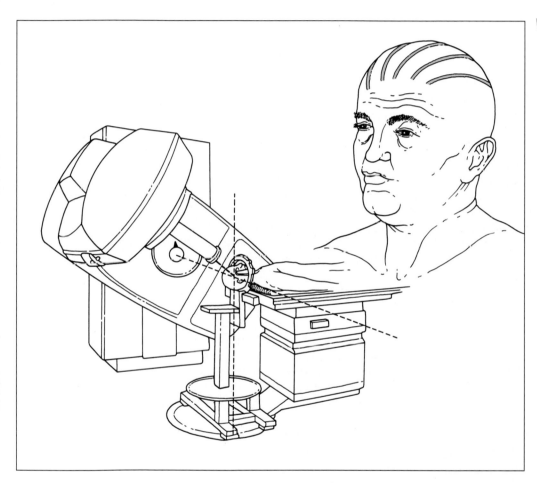

Figure 12.22 Radiosurgery set-up for a patient with a small inoperable AVM. Linear accelerator is poised to deliver stereotactically focused gamma irradiation. (Adapted with permission from Winston KR, 1988)

REFERENCES

1. Yasargil MG. AVM of the brain: history, embryology, pathological considerations, hemodynamics. In: Yasargil MG, ed. *Microneurosurgery.* New York, NY: Thieme Medical Publishers; 1987:48 IIIA.
2. McCormick WF. Pathology of vascular malformations of the brain. In: Wilson CB, Stein BM, eds. *Intracranial Arteriovenous Malformations.* Baltimore, Md: Williams & Wilkins; 1984:44–63.
3. Rigamonti D, Johnson PÇ, Spetzler RF, Hadley MN, Drayer BP. Cavernous malformations and capillary telangiectasias: a spectrum within a single pathological entity. *Neurosurgery.* 1991;28:60–64.
4. Ondra SL, Doty JR, Mahla ME, George ED. Surgical excision of a cavernous hemangioma of the rostral brain stem: case report. *Neurosurgery.* 1988; 23:490–493.
5. Jane J, Kassell N, Torner J, Winn HR. The natural history of aneurysms and arteriovenous malformations. *J Neurosurg.* 1985;62:321–323.
6. Ondra SL, Troupp H, George ED, Schwab K. The natural history of symptomatic arteriovenous malformations of the brain: a 24 year follow-up assessment. *J Neurosurg.* 1990;73:387–391.
7. Perret G, Nishioka H. Report on the cooperative study of intracranial aneurysms and subarachnoid hemorrhage, VI: arteriovenous malformations: an analysis of 545 cases of cranio-cerebral arteriovenous malformations and fistulae reported to the cooperative study. *J Neurosurg.* 1966;25:467–490.
8. Fults D, Kelly DL. Natural history of arteriovenous malformations of the brain: a clinical study. *Neurosurgery.* 1984;15:658–662.
9. Graf CJ, Perret G, Toner JC. Bleeding from cerebral arteriovenous malformations as part of their natural history. *J Neurosurg.* 1983;58:331–337.
10. Michelsen JW. Natural history and pathophysiology of arteriovenous malformations. *Clin Neurosurg.* 1979;26:307–313.
11. Wilkins RH. Natural history of intracranial vascular malformation: a review. *Neurosurgery.* 1985;16: 421–430.
12. Martin NA, Wilson CB. Medial occipital arteriovenous malformations, surgical treatment. *J Neurosurg.* 1982;56:798–802.
13. Costantino A, Vinters HV. A pathologic correlate of the "steal" phenomenon in a patient with cerebral arteriovenous malformation. *Stroke.* 1986;17: 103–110.
14. Solomon RA, Michelsen JW. Defective cerebrovascular autoregulation in regions proximal to arteriovenous malformations of the brain: a case report and topic review. *Neurosurgery.* 1984;14:78–82.
15. Spetzler RF, Wilson CB, Weinstein P, Mehdorn M, Townsend J, Telles D. Normal perfusion pressure breakthrough theory. *Clin Neurosurg.* 1978;25: 651–672.
16. Yasargil MG. AVM of the brain, clinical considerations, general and special operative techniques, surgical results, non-operated cases, cavernous and venous angiomas, neuroanesthesia. In: Yasargil MG, ed. *Microneurosurgery.* New York, NY: Thieme Medical Publishers; 1987:49 IIIB.
17. Drake CG. Cerebral Arteriovenous malformations: considerations for and experience with surgical treatment in 166 cases. *Clin Neurosurg.* 1979;26:145–208.
18. Stein BM, Solomon RA. Arteriovenous malformations of the brain. In: Youmans JR, ed. *Neurological Surgery,* 3rd ed. Philadelphia, Pa: WB Saunders & Co; 1990:1831–1863.
19. Batjer H, Samson D. Arteriovenous malformations of the posterior fossa: clinical presentations, diagnostic evaluation, and surgical treatment. *J Neurosurg.* 1986;64:849–856.
20. Chou SN, Erickson DL, Ortiz-Suarez HJ. Surgical treatment of vascular lesions in the brain stem. *J Neurosurg.* 1975;42:23–31.
21. Drake CG. Surgical removal of arteriovenous malformations from the brain stem and cerebellopontine angle. *J Neurosurg.* 1975;43:661–670.
22. Juhasz J. Surgical treatment of arteriovenous angiomas localized in the corpus callosum, basal ganglia and near the brain stem. *Acta Neurochir (Wein).* 1978; 40:83–101.
23. Solomon RA, Stein BM. Management of arteriovenous malformations of the brain stem. *J Neurosurg.* 1986;64:857–864.
24. Solomon RA, Stein BM. Interhemispheric approach for the surgical removal of thalamocaudate arteriovenous malformations. *J Neurosurg.* 1987;66:345–351.
25. Heros RC. Arteriovenous malformations of the me-

dial temporal lobe: surgical approach and neuroradiological characterizations. *J Neurosurg.* 1982;56: 44–52.

26. Solomon RA, Stein BM. Surgical management of arteriovenous malformations that follow the tentorial ring. *Neurosurgery.* 1986;18:708–715.

27. Stein BM. Arteriovenous malformations of the medial cerebral hemisphere and the limbic system. *J Neurosurg.* 1984;60:23–31.

28. Luessenhop AJ, Gennarelli TA. Anatomical grading of supratentorial arteriovenous malformations for determining operability. *J Neurosurg.* 1975;1:30–35.

29. Spetzler RF, Martin NA. A proposed grading system for arteriovenous malformations. *J Neurosurg.* 1986;65:476–483.

30. Almeida GM, Shibata MK, Nakagawa EJ. Contralateral parafalcine approach for parasagittal and callosal arteriovenous malformations. *Neurosurgery.* 1984;14:744–746.

31. Hilal SK. Endovascular treatment of arteriovenous malformations of the central nervous system. In: Wilson CB, Stein BM, eds. *Intracranial Arteriovenous Malformations.* Baltimore, Md: Williams & Wilkins; 1984:259–273.

32. Yasargil MG, Jain KK, Antic J, Laciga R. Arteriovenous malformations of the splenium of the corpus callosum: microsurgical treatment. *Surg Neurol.* 1976;5:5–14.

33. Yasargil MG, Jain KK, Antic J, Laciga R, Kletter G. Arteriovenous malformations of the anterior and middle portion of the corpus callosum: microsurgical treatment. *Surg Neurol.* 1976;5:67–80.

34. Kunc Z. Deep seated arteriovenous malformations: a critical review. In: Carrea R, ed. *Neurological Surgery with Emphasis on Non-invasive Methods of Diagnosis and Treatment.* Amsterdam: Excerpta Medica; 1978:188–193.

35. U HS. Microsurgical excision of paraventricular arteriovenous malformations. *Neurosurgery.* 1985;16: 293–303.

36. Viale GL, Turtas S, Pau A. Surgical removal of striate arteriovenous malformations. *Surg Neurol.* 1980; 14:321–324.

37. Wilson CB, Martin NA: Deep supratentorial arteriovenous malformations. In: Wilson CB, Stein BM, eds. *Intracranial Arteriovenous Malformations.* Baltimore, Md: Williams & Wilkins; 1984:184–208.

38. Viale GL, Pau A, Viale ES. Surgical treatment of arteriovenous malformations of the posterior fossa. *Surg Neurol.* 1979;12:379–384.

39. Luessenhop AJ, Presper JH. Surgical embolization of cerebral arteriovenous malformations through internal carotid and vertebral arteries: long-term results. *J Neurosurg.* 1975;42:443–451.

40. Debrun GM, Vinuela F, Fox A, Drake CG. Embolization of cerebral arteriovenous malformations with bucrylate: experience in 46 cases. *J Neurosurg.* 1982;56:615–627.

41. Klara P, George E, McDonnell D, Pevsner P. Morphological studies of human arteriovenous malformations: effects of isobutyl 12-cyanoacrylate embolization. *J Neurosurg.* 1985;63:421–425.

42. Luessenhop AJ, Rosa L. Cerebral arteriovenous malformations: indications for and results of surgery, and the role of intravascular techniques. *J Neurosurg.* 1984;60:14–22.

43. Stein BM, Wolpert SM. Arteriovenous malformations of the brain, I: current concepts and treatment. *Arch Neurol.* 1980;37:1–5.

44. Stein BM, Wolpert SM. Arteriovenous malformations of the brain, II: current concepts and treatment. *Arch Neurol.* 1980;37:69–75.

45. Kjellberg RN, Hanamura T, Davis KR, Lyons SL, Adams RD. Bragg-peak proton beam therapy for arteriovenous malformations of the brain. *N Engl J Med.* 1983;309:269–274.

46. Steinberg GK, Fabrikant JI, Marks MP, et al. Stereotactic heavy charged-particle Bragg-peak radiation for intracranial arteriovenous malformations. *N Engl J Med.* 1990;323:96–101.

47. Steiner L. Treatment of arteriovenous malformations by radiosurgery. In: Wilson CB, Stein BM, eds. *Intracranial Arteriovenous Malformations.* Baltimore, Md: Williams & Wilkins; 1984:295–313.

48. Winston KR, Lutz W. Linear accelerator as a neurosurgical tool for stereotactic radiosurgery. *Neurosurgery.* 1988;22:454–464.

Chapter 13

Spontaneous Intracerebral Hemorrhage

Neil A. Martin, Martin C. Holland

Spontaneous intracerebral hemorrhage (ICH) is defined as bleeding into brain parenchyma without accompanying trauma. The impact of ICH on the general population can be fully grasped when viewed within the broader category of stroke, currently the leading cause of neurologic deficit in the world and the third leading cause of death in the United States (behind cancer and heart disease), accounting for 15% of all U.S. deaths annually.[1] Significantly, ICH accounts for 10% to 17% of all strokes.[2-5] Moreover, the mortality for ICH is considerably higher than that for nonhemorrhagic or ischemic stroke (cerebral infarct) as seen in a study by the Machlachlan Acute Stroke Unit in Toronto. Of 1073 patients admitted with completed stroke, mortality at 30 days from supratentorial and infratentorial infarct was 15% and 18% respectively, compared to that for ICH which was 58% and 31% respectively.[6] Indeed, some studies quote a mortality figure as high as 90%.[7]

The incidence of stroke remains underreported due to the inherent shortcomings of epidemiologic, pathologic, and clinical studies. Even so, it is estimated that 500,000 people suffer a stroke each year, 150,000 of whom will die.[1] Moreover, with 2,000,000 stroke survivors requiring chronic care, the cost in terms of medical expense amounts to over 7 billion dollars annually[8] not to mention the cost in terms of physical and emotional suffering. It should be mentioned, however, that the incidence of both stroke and ICH has declined at an annual rate of 1% per year since 1915, with an acceleration in the decline to over 5% per year since 1975, reflecting an improvement in both the prevention and treatment of stroke.[7]

pressure, often leading to herniation syndromes. A *subdural hematoma* may result when cerebral bridging veins tear or when a subarachnoid or intraparenchymal bleed extends into the subdural space through a tear in the arachnoid. A *subarachnoid hemorrhage* involves the accumulation of blood between the arachnoid and the pia mater; it is often the result of an aneurysmal rupture, although arteriovenous malformations (AVMs) or trauma figure often in this entity. An *intraventricular hemorrhage* may be arterial or venous, it may be isolated or extend from an intraparenchymal bleed, it often leads to obstructive hydrocephalus, and it usually has a poor prognosis. *Intraparenchymal hemorrhages* can occur at any site within the CNS, though some areas are more susceptible than others. Eighty percent occur within the cerebral hemispheres while the remaining 20% are infratentorial. Of note, hypertensive bleeds occur in the deep gray matter (65%), pons (11%), and cerebellum (8%), whereas bleeds associated with other disorders are likely to be located in the subcortical white matter (45%), deep gray matter (36%), pons (10%), and cerebellum (3%).[2,9-11] Similarly, bleeds at any one particular location tend to be associated with certain conditions more than others (Fig. 13.2). For example, *lobar bleeds*—found in the subcortical white matter—are often associated with tumors, vascular malformations, and cerebral amyloid angiopathy; *basal ganglia* bleeds, which may extend to include the internal capsule and thalamus, are often associated with hypertension as are *brain stem* bleeds, though these are usually much more serious. Finally, *cerebellar* bleeds tend to accompany tumors, vascular malformations, blood dyscrasias, and hypertension.[2,12]

PATHOPHYSIOLOGY

Spontaneous ICH results from an intracerebral arterial or, less frequently, venous rupture, which leads to the formation of an intraparenchymal hematoma. The hematoma expands following the path of least resistance, usually along white matter tracts, and occasionally dissects its way into the ventricular system. In time, the bleeding slows and eventually stops as increasing tissue pressure leads to tamponade of the rupture site. Neurologic deficit results from both direct tissue destruction and indirect compression of neural structures, usually in proportion to both the volume of the hematoma and its rate of expansion. A slowly expanding lesion, for example, tends to dissect along white matter tracts, leaving functional units intact, whereas a rapidly expanding lesion tears through tissue planes and severs axons, permanently disrupting neural function.

Intracranial hemorrhages may be classified according to their location (Fig. 13.1). An *epidural hematoma* is usually the result of a meningeal artery tear in which blood accumulates between bone and dura mater. Because of its arterial origin, the hematoma grows under considerable

ETIOLOGY

By far the most important risk factor associated with ICH is hypertension, with 40% to 60% of all ICH patients found to have this disorder. Aneurysms (20%), vascular malformations (5% to 7%), coagulopathies (5% to 7%), and tumors (1% to 11%) as well as hemorrhagic infarcts, cerebral amyloid angiopathy, and drug reactions account for the remaining major etiologies of ICH (Fig. 13.3).[2,11]

HYPERTENSION

As previously noted, it has been established that patients who have chronic hypertension are predisposed to ICH. Compared to hemorrhages from other causes, this type of bleed is more frequently associated with a fatal outcome, reflecting both its high incidence and its tendency to occur in critical locations. To review, the most common location for hypertensive bleeds is the basal ganglia, followed by the pons and cerebellum, regions that are variously supplied by the lenticulostriate branches off the middle cerebral artery or the paramedian branches off the basilar artery. Much research has been done on the mechanism

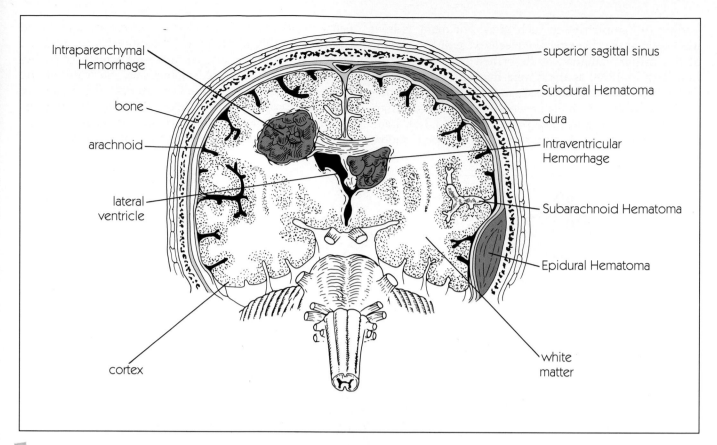

Figure 13.1 Types of intracerebral hemorrhage.

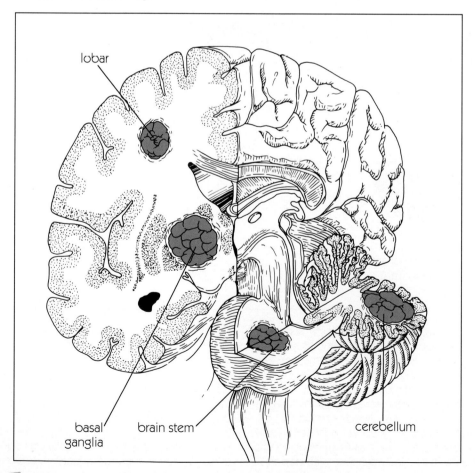

Figure 13.2 Locations of intraparenchymal hemorrhage.

leading to hemorrhage in such cases. For many years it was assumed that hypertensive bleeds were due to rupture of the miliary aneurysms described by Charcot and Bouchard in 1868, as these were frequently seen on the perforating arteries of the basal ganglia and pons of hypertensive patients, which, as previously noted, are common sites of hemorrhage in these patients (Fig. 13.3A). Later investigations, however, have shown these to be pseudoa-

neurysms, that is, small collections of extravasated blood covered by a thin fibrin layer,[13,14] presumably the result of an aborted or limited arterial rupture. Microscopic studies have since demonstrated changes in the walls of the lenticulostriates and paramedian arteries of hypertensive patients (alternately called "lipohyalinosis," "fibrinohyalinosis," or "angionecrosis"), which are characterized by the deposition of fat cells as well as a fibrinlike material within

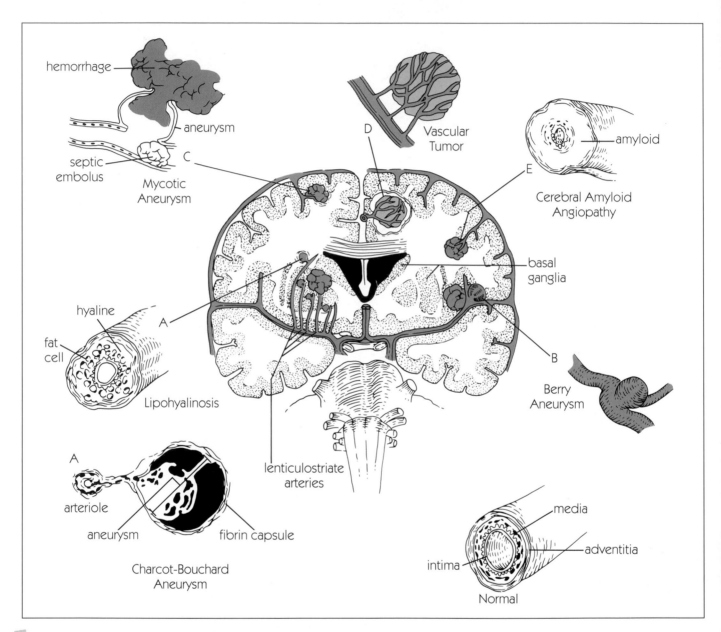

Figure 13.3 The major causes of ICH, the principal locations at which they present, and detailed morphologic or histologic features associated with the process. A normal vessel has an intima composed of a single layer of epithelial cells surrounded by a layer of smooth muscle and elastic tissue, both of which are enveloped by the adventitia, a thick layer of collagenous connective tissue. **(A)** Bleeds caused by hypertension occur in the basal ganglia and brain stem. Typical histologic changes are the formation of Charcot-Bouchard or miliary aneurysms as well as "lipohyalinosis" with deposition of hyaline and fat cells within the arterial wall. **(B)** Berry aneurysms form at the bi- or trifurcations of arteries and usu-

ally lead to subarachnoid hemorrhage, although they may rupture into the brain parenchyma. **(C)** When a septic embolus lodges in and infects a cortical arteriole, its wall weakens and a mycotic aneurysm forms, which may bleed, usually into the subcortical white matter. **(D)** Hemorrhage tends to occur at the periphery of tumors such as glioblastomas, melanomas, and bronchogenic carcinomas. **(E)** Cerebral amyloid angiopathy is characterized by weakening of the vessel due to deposition of amyloid within the media and adventitia and should be suspected in the elderly patient, especially when hypertension is not present.

the media of the affected vessels (see Fig. 13.3A). Furthermore, these changes are often seen closer to the bleeding site than are miliary aneurysms and are now considered the primary lesion leading to arterial wall weakness and subsequent rupture.[11,14] That these vessels are affected more than others may reflect the fact that they are small arterial twigs branching directly off major arteries (e.g., middle cerebral or basilar). As such, they are subjected to much higher pressures than the similar-sized cortical vessels that lie at the end of a multiple series of arterial splits, each of which lowers intraluminal pressure, thus affording these smaller vessels some measure of protection against the effects of systemic hypertension.

A great deal of controversy remains regarding the role of miliary aneurysms in hypertensive bleeds. Regardless, hypertension remains the major risk factor in the development of fatal or disabling ICH.

NONHYPERTENSIVE INTRACEREBRAL HEMORRHAGE

There are a number of conditions that are statistically less important than hypertension but are nonetheless the etiology of a significant number of spontaneous ICHs: aneurysms (20%), vascular malformations (5% to 7%), coagulopathics (5% to 7%), and tumors (1% to 11%) are the most common, with cerebral amyloid angiopathy, hemorrhagic infarcts, and drug-induced hemorrhages, among others, making up a small percentage of cases.[2,11]

Aneurysms

Aneurysms are saccular or fusiform arterial deformities, the result of dissection and protrusion of the intima through a structural defect in an artery's muscular layer, whose underlying cause may be embolic, neoplastic, traumatic, or atherosclerotic. Most aneurysms, however, are the so-called berry aneurysms whose etiology is likely a combination of congenital, hereditary, and acquired factors.

Berry Aneurysms

Berry aneurysms (Fig. 13.3B) are typically found at the bi- or trifurcations of major cerebral arteries—usually those forming the circle of Willis—and may be associated with inherited disorders such as Ehlers-Danlos syndrome or other diseases that weaken the media of cerebral arteries. Similarly, a tumor, vascular malformation, or any other process that alters cerebral hemodynamics by increasing arterial blood flow or raising intraluminal hydrostatic pressure may eventually lead to the formation of an aneurysm. There is a general disagreement over the exact process of aneurysm formation, however. One school of thought proposes that a congenital defect in the muscular layer leads to aneurysmal dilatation of arteries. A second claims that the primary lesion is the damage that normally occurs over time to the lamina elastica interna, with some people being more affected than oth-

ers. A third, holding a somewhat middle ground, states that both congenital and acquired processes are needed for an aneurysm to form. Especially susceptible to degenerative changes are the arterial branch points, where the normal near-laminar flow of blood gives way to high turbulence, creating higher-than-normal pressure points against the arterial wall. In time, the aneurysm may enlarge and rupture, spilling blood into the subarachnoid space, often with accompanying ICH. In particularly violent ruptures, the hematoma may either dissect its way into the ventricular system or rip the arachnoid forming a subdural hematoma.

Since berry aneurysms tend to occur in the large arteries at the base of the brain and posterior fossa, the neural structures at greatest risk for damage are the diencephalon and brain stem; when these structures are injured, the outcome may be fatal. The prevalence of ICH after berry aneurysm rupture has not been well established, though 5% to 25% of operative reports and 50% to 100% of autopsy reports indicate the presence if ICH after aneurysmal rupture.[15] This is significant to the neurosurgeon because the presence as well as location of the hematoma may alter the need, timing, and approach of surgery.

Mycotic Aneurysms

Mycotic aneurysms usually form in the smaller cortical arteries when septic emboli lodge in the vessel, extend their infection (usually bacterial, not fungal, despite the name) through the arterial wall, and damage the media; this sets the stage for subsequent aneurysmal dilatation and rupture (Fig. 13.3C). This is usually seen in the setting of subacute bacterial endocarditis, where up to 17% of patients develop cerebral emboli.[16] On occasion, the aneurysm thrombosis, and if the infection has been adequately treated, no further intervention is needed. If the aneurysm continues to enlarge, however, it should be surgically clipped and resected to prevent rupture and continued infection.

Neoplastic Aneurysms

Arterial invasion by a tumor rarely leads to muscular weakness and subsequent aneurysmal formation. On the rare occasion that one does form, it may require clipping with or without concomitant tumor removal.

Atherosclerotic Aneurysms

These usually occur in the setting of severe atherosclerosis with accompanying hypertension. The vertebrobasilar system is usually involved and rupture is extremely rare.

Vascular Malformations

There are four basic types of vascular malformations. The most common and most significant clinically is the arteriovenous malformation (AVM), a congenital vascular anomaly consisting of a tangle of vessels fed by one or more arteries and draining directly into the venous circulation without the benefit of intervening capillaries to decrease venous blood flow and pressure (Fig. 13.4A). Much less important are the cavernous and venous angiomas (Fig. 13.4B), which consist of large anomalous venous channels within the deep white matter. Cavernous angiomas differ from venous angiomas in that the latter contain normal brain tissue within their confines whereas the former have none. Also less important are the capillary telangiectasias (Fig. 13.4C), small, capillary-like vessels mostly found in the brain stem and cerebellum. These last three entities are of dubious clinical significance, though the telangiectasias, because of their location, may cause severe neurologic deficits if they hemorrhage.

AVMs, on the other hand, are notorious for bleeding; over one half of them present as a hemorrhage. ICH accounts for 60% of cases, subarachnoid hemorrhage for 30%, and intraventricular hemorrhage for less than 10%.[17] These bleeds are arteriovenous; as such they are less violent than aneurysmal ruptures and the accompanying neurologic deficits, usually focal, are more slowly progressive. Hemorrhage tends to occur during the second to fourth decade of life compared to hypertensive or aneurysmal bleeds, which occur in an older population.

Interventional radiographic embolization of these lesions has made their surgical removal considerably safer

and occasionally unnecessary, thus paving the way for better and safer treatment of these vascular abnormalities.

Coagulopathies

Approximately 5% to 7% of ICH cases are caused by an underlying coagulopathy.[2] Systemic disorders such as leukemia, thrombocytopenia, and liver and renal failure as well as anticoagulation therapy with warfarin, aspirin, or dipyridamole account for the majority of cases. Of significance is the fact that ICH is the primary complication of anticoagulation therapy, with approximately 2% of all such patients developing bleeds.[18] These types of hemorrhage tend to occur in cortical and subcortical regions, especially in the cerebellum, and usually follow a protracted course. In most cases, the underlying coagulopathy must be corrected prior to surgical evacuation of the hematoma unless the patient's life is in immediate danger. Most of these bleeds, however, can be followed with serial tomographic studies and tend to resolve once the underlying coagulopathy is corrected.

Tumors

Massive hemorrhage into a tumor is a rare event; in most studies about 1% of tumors develop bleeds.[18] These occur mostly in malignant neoplasms, either primary, such as

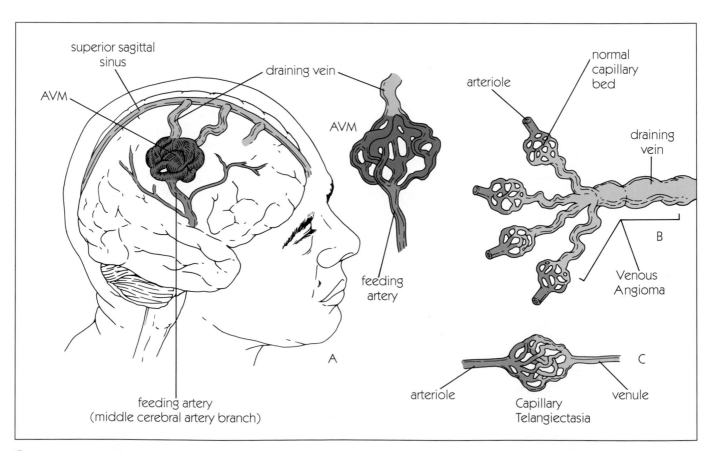

Figure 13.4 Vascular malformations. (A) The AVM is depicted here in a typical location within the brain. It is fed by a branch from the middle cerebral artery and its major draining vein is emptying into the superior sagittal sinus. In the simplified version of the AVM note that the arterial system drains directly into the venous system without an intervening capillary bed, which would normally reduce the pressure on the venous side. (B) In the venous malformation, a series of normal capillary beds drain into several abnormally dilated venous channels, all of which meet at a common draining vein, forming the typical caput medusae of the venous angioma. (C) Capillary telangiectasias consist of a series of dilated capillaries that lack normal elastic tissue, thus making them more susceptible to hemorrhage.

glioblastoma multiforme, or metastatic, especially bronchogenic carcinoma and malignant melanoma (see Fig. 13.3D). Reports of bleeds into oligodendrogliomas, choroid plexus papillomas, choriocarcinomas, and even benign meningiomas are found in the literature though these are indeed rare.

Cerebral Amyloid Angiopathy

Cerebral amyloid angiopathy (CAA) is a rare cause of ICH. It must, however, be suspected in the elderly patient with no history of hypertension. CAA is characterized by the deposition of amyloid in the media and adventitia of medium-sized hemispheric arteries (see Fig. 13.3E).

It is estimated that during the seventh decade of life 10% of the population develops CAA, and by age 90 the incidence increases to 60%. Of note, this entity may account for as much as 30% of senile dementia, and it may be one of the major etiologic factors of spontaneous ICH in the elderly.[18]

The typical clinical picture is one of multiple, recurrent subcortical lobar bleeds. These can be asymptomatic or massive, leading to acute neurologic deterioration and death. The diagnosis is one of exclusion and may be confirmed on biopsy or necropsy when other more common etiologies have been excluded.

Hemorrhagic Infarcts

Hemorrhagic infarcts occur when an area of infarction—the result of a recent thromboembolic event—is reperfused with blood that then leaks into brain tissue through broken down, necrotic vessel walls. Patients on anticoagulation therapy can have particularly severe courses, as is occasionally seen in the patient who, while taking warfarin after artificial valve replacement, develops valvular infectious or thrombotic vegetations and subsequent cardioembolic events. Managing these patients is particularly difficult. In order to prevent further bleeding one must correct the patient's coagulopathy. This, however, increases the patient's risk of developing further embolic events. These hemorrhages tend to be multicentric, are usually found in the subcortical white matter, and often extend into the cortex or, occasionally, subarachnoid space. They are often treated conservatively and may be followed closely with serial CT scans of the head.

Drugs

Both legal and illegal drugs can cause spontaneous ICH. The agents most likely to cause bleeds are the amphetamines, although others (e.g., cocaine, pseudoephedrine, and heroin) have also been associated with ICH. Two basic mechanisms for this exist: 1) a pharmacologically-induced rise in blood pressure leads to arterial rupture similar to that seen in the hypertensive patient and 2) an intravenous injection of a nonsterile substance leads to a condition known as necrotizing angiitis, which is characterized by chronic damage to the smaller cortical vessels, causing arterial wall degeneration and bleeding if the intraluminal pressure exceeds arterial wall strength. The hemorrhages tend to be subcortical in location and are

usually preceded by a hypertensive crisis that occasionally occurs without a known precipitating factor.

ICH has also been associated with chronic alcoholism and is often seen as petechial hemorrhage of the mamillary bodies. This, however, is thought to be more due to cirrhosis of the liver and the accompanying coagulopathy of liver disease than to a primary effect on the cerebral vasculature.

SIGNS AND SYMPTOMS

ICH has a wide range of presentations, ranging from asymptomatic or TIA-like to coma or death, each determined by the size and location of the hemorrhage. Early diagnosis of ICH can be extremely difficult without the help of modern radiographic studies such as CT or MRI, since the majority of patients present like cerebral infarct patients—hemiplegia is found in up to 95% of cases, stupor or drowsiness in 45% to 50% of cases, and coma in approximately 30% of cases. Other findings, which depend primarily on the location of the bleed, include headache, nausea, vomiting, seizures, cranial nerve deficits, ataxia, and aphasia. Overall, about one third of patients present with maximal deficits at onset while the remaining two thirds have a gradual presentation of symptoms and smooth progression of deficits over minutes or hours. It is diagnostically useful to know that there is never a regression of symptoms in the acute phase of ICH; thus a bleed can be effectively ruled out as a cause of stroke if symptom regression occurs. Other signs of ICH that help distinguish it from cerebral infarct are bilaterality of symptoms, persistent headache with nuchal rigidity, and neural deficits that localize over the distribution of two or more major arteries. Autonomic changes with vomiting and a rapid deterioration in neurologic status may suggest extension of the hemorrhage into the ventricular system.

In the days and weeks following the bleed, the patient's clinical course largely depends on several factors, the most important of which is the amount and location of permanent tissue loss occurring during the initial event. Other important prognostic factors include the patient's age, severity of neurologic deficits on the initial examination, the presence or absence of intraventricular hemorrhage, and/or obstructive hydrocephalus as well as the ensuing amount of cerebral edema, its subsequent impact on intracranial pressure, and its potential for causing a herniation syndrome. Systemic disorders such as hypertension and diabetes mellitus as well as individual organ dysfunction (i.e., cardiac, pulmonary, or renal) have an indirect yet significant impact on survival during the subacute period (2 to 4 weeks postictus), whereas CNS complications such as hydrocephalus and edema tend to influence the early clinical course.[10]

As mentioned above, the location of the bleed largely determines the observed neurologic deficits (Fig. 13.5). Basal ganglia and thalamic bleeds, for example, present as massive hemiplegia, with thalamic bleeds occasionally including a hemisensory loss. Cortical hemorrhages are often accompanied by seizures as well as *focal neurologic deficits* (see Fig. 13.5A) as local tissue damage secondary to the hemorrhage disrupts fiber tracts and causes symptoms referable to the area involved. Thus a patient presenting with a small hemorrhage in the posterior limb of the right internal capsule would likely exhibit contralateral (left) hemiplegia and possibly hemianesthesia if the thalamus were involved as well. Posterior fossa lesions are often accompanied by nausea, vomiting, decreased mentation, and hydrocephalus as well as cranial nerve deficits, plegia, paresis, autonomic abnormalities, and anesthesia from brain stem bleeds or ataxia, nystagmus, and dysmetria from cerebellar involvement. The extension of hemorrhage into the ventricular system is particularly important as it is associated with a high mortality (65% to 75% of all fatal hypertensive bleeds), autonomic abnormalities, neurologic deficits whose severity is out of proportion to the size of the bleed, as well as a decreased level of consciousness and the development of obstructive hydrocephalus.[18] *Hydrocephalus* is often associated with posterior fossa lesions or intraventricular hemorrhages which block ventricular outflow channels (see Fig. 13.5B). *Herniation* is usually the result of a signifi-

cant increase in intracranial pressure either from a hematoma swelling or hydrocephalus. Figure 13.5C shows transtentorial uncal herniation as a result of a massive right hemispheric bleed. This situation is a neurosurgical emergency and requires immediate intervention directed at relieving the increased pressure—evacuating the hematoma in this case.

RADIOGRAPHIC STUDIES

Prior to about 1975, before widespread use of CT, identifying the site of acute ICH greatly depended on the physician's skill in interpreting clinical signs and symptoms as well as reading angiograms. Today, in all but selected cases, CT is almost exclusively used in the acute setting. It allows quick and accurate assessment of anatomy and shows the presence of parenchymal shift, hydrocephalus, and hemorrhage, and in most cases suggests the underlying etiology.

Acute hemorrhage on CT appears brighter than normal brain tissue (Fig. 13.6A), and it changes over time to become isointense and within a period of weeks to months it becomes hypointense. Hemorrhage on MRI

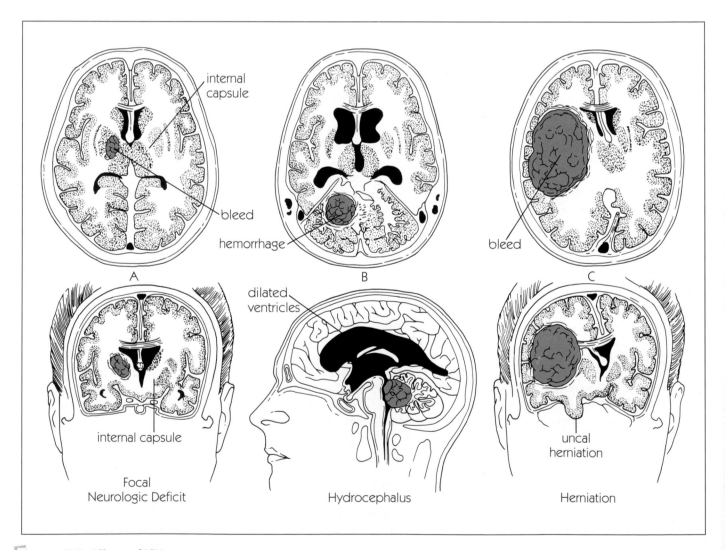

Figure 13.5 Effects of ICH.

(Fig. 13.6B) undergoes more complex changes depending on the image sequence (e.g., T1, T2, or proton density), the proportion of oxyhemoglobin, deoxyhemoglobin, and methemoglobin within the clot, and its distribution (i.e., intra- or extracellular). MRI has little advantage over CT in the acute setting and should be used only if CT is not available, although it may help narrow the differential diagnosis. Intravenous contrast agents are of limited value unless a tumor is suspected (though, on occasion, a vascular malformation may be detected). They are therefore usually not indicated in the acute setting of ICH.

Angiography is rarely used, especially in the rapidly deteriorating patient. It is usually reserved for cases in which a vascular malformation or aneurysm is suspected and must be visualized prior to surgery (Fig. 13.6C). Of note, when working up AVMs or aneurysms, there is a 10% incidence of false-negative angiograms on initial study, and a repeat angiogram is indicated 3 weeks later in order to rule out an AVM or aneurysm. Occasionally, the repeat angiogram is also negative and no source of bleed is ever found. This is sometimes due to obliteration of the AVM or thrombosis of the aneurysm during the initial bleed. As a result they become angiographically occult.

To summarize, CT remains the standard method of diagnosis in all cases of acute ICH. MRI and angiography are used only as secondary studies or in case CT is not available.

TREATMENT

ICH can be treated either medically or surgically. For the most part, surgery is performed only if the patient can no longer be managed medically.

Medical therapy is aimed at correcting any underlying systemic disorders, such as hypertension or a coagulopathy, and controlling high intracranial pressure using mannitol, hyperventilation, steroids, and barbiturates as indicated, and elevating the head of the patient's bed to insure optimal cerebral venous drainage. Frequent neurologic exams as well as serial CT scans are indicated, especially early in the clinical course, in order to modify the therapeutic plan appropriately and anticipate further deterioration by following neurologic and radiographic trends.

Surgical intervention is resorted to if the patient is deteriorating rapidly and immediate evacuation of the hematoma is needed to either reduce intracranial pressure or relieve local compression of neural structures (Fig. 13.7A). Ventriculostomy catheters are often used in the management of ICH both as a monitor of intracranial pressure and as a therapeutic modality since they can be used to drain fluid from the ventricular system (Fig. 13.7B). This is because patients with brain injury, intraventricular hemorrhage, or posterior fossa bleeds often develop hydrocephalus and an elevated intracranial pressure. Underlying lesions such as tumors, AVMs, and aneurysms may also be managed surgically. Surgery, however, is not done until the patient has been stabilized and adequate secondary studies have been obtained. Occasionally, ICH resolves spontaneously, leaving a cleft within the brain, and no further therapy is needed (Fig. 13.8).

The prognosis of ICH depends on several factors. Location and size of hemorrhage are of primary importance. They are closely followed by the patient's age, development and severity of posthemorrhagic complications such as cerebral edema, hydrocephalus, and herniation syndromes, as well as systemic disorders, including pulmonary emboli, myocardial infarcts, and pneumonia.

In general, brain stem and diencephalic bleeds herald a poor prognosis, especially if intraventricular hemorrhage is present, and every effort should be made to treat these patients aggressively early in their clinical course, if any chance for recovery exists.

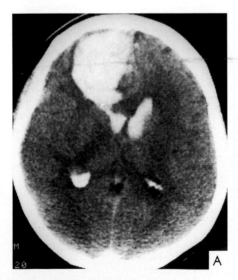 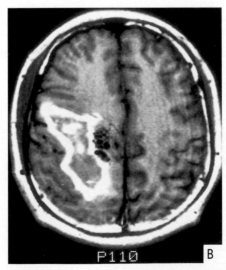 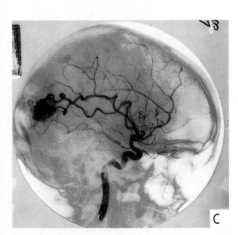

Figure 13.6 CT, MRI, and angiography are the three most important modalities used in managing spontaneous ICH. **(A)** CT scan showing an axial cut through the hemispheres with the hemorrhage appearing as a brightly lit area within the right frontal lobe with extension into the ventricular system. **(B)** T1-weighted axial MR image, showing a hemorrhage in the right frontoparietal region from an AVM. The effect of peripheral enhancement is due to differences in oxyhemoglobin, deoxyhemoglobin, and methemoglobin in the center and periphery of the clot as it resorbs. **(C)** Carotid angiogram in the lateral projection shows an AVM of the parietooccipital region with the feeding arteries and draining vein clearly seen.

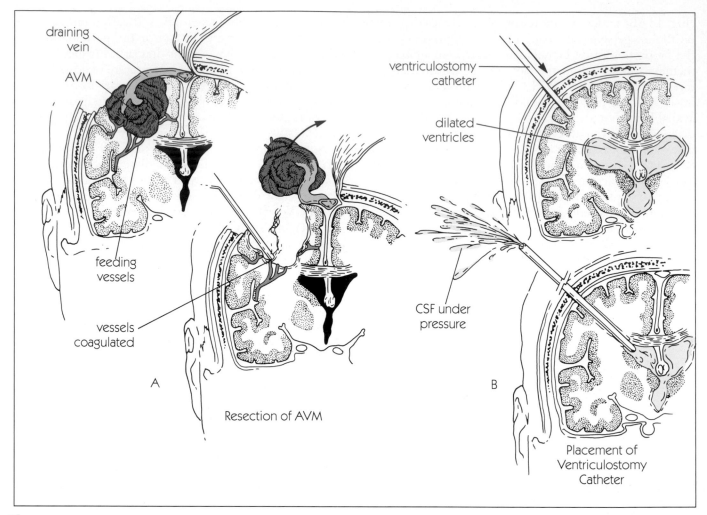

Figure 13.7 (A) Surgical evacuation of a hematoma. Once the underlying pathology and location of the clot have been determined, the patient is taken to the operating room. The head is shaved and positioned appropriately. The scalp incision should allow for maximal exposure with minimal dissection while keeping eloquent areas intact. Once the brain is exposed, a cortical incision is made using bipolar coagulation on the pial vessels overlying the clot. The hematoma is evacuated through the cortical incision using bipolar coagulation and suction. Brain retractors keep the cortical incision exposed. (B) Ventriculostomy catheters are used to monitor intracranial pressure and to drain fluid from the ventricular system.

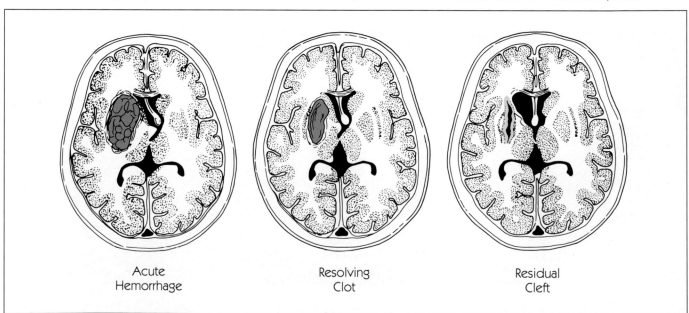

Figure 13.8 Spontaneous resolution of an ICH. The natural history of an ICH is characterized by liquefaction of both the clot and necrotic brain tissue with ensuing reabsorption of both.

Principles of Neurosurgery

REFERENCES

1. Kuller LH. Incidence, rates of stroke in the 80s. *Stroke.* 1989;20:841–843.
2. Cahill DW, Ducker TB. Spontaneous intracerebral hemorrhage. In: Weiss MH, et al, eds. *Clinical Neurosurgery: Proceedings of the CNS, Los Angeles, 1981.* Baltimore: Williams & Wilkins; 1982;29:722–779.
3. Kurtzke JF. *Epidemiology of Cerebrovascular Disease.* Berlin: Springer-Verlag; 1969.
4. Mohr JP, Caplan LR, Melski JW, et al. The Harvard Cooperative Stroke Registry: a prospective registry. *Neurology.* 1978;28:754.
5. Toole JF, Patel AN. *Cerebrovascular Disorders.* 2nd ed. New York, NY: McGraw-Hill; 1967.
6. Chambers BR, et al. Prognostic profiles in acute stroke. In: Hachinski V, Norris JW, eds. *The Acute Stroke.* Philadelphia, Pa: FA Davis Company; 1985:245–258. Contemporary Neurology Series 27.
7. Wolf PA, Kannel WB, et al. Epidemiology of stroke in North America. In: Barnett HJM, Mohr JP, Stein BM, Yatsu FM, eds. *Stroke: Pathophysiology, Diagnosis, and Management.* New York, NY: Churchill Livingstone; 1986:19–29.
8. Weinfeld FD, ed. The national survey of stroke. *Stroke.* 1981;12(suppl):I-71.
9. Freytag E. Fatal hypertensive intracerebral hematomas: a survey of the pathological anatomy of 393 cases. *J Neurol Neurosurg Psychiatry.* 1968;31:616.
10. Hachinski V, Norris JW. *The Acute Stroke.* Philadelphia, Pa: FA Davis Company; 1985. Contemporary Neurology Series 27.
11. Kase CS, Mohr JP. General features of intracerebral hemorrhage. In: Barnett HJM, Stein BM, Mohr JP, Yatsu FM, eds. *Stroke: Pathophysiology, Diagnosis, and Management.* New York, NY: Churchill Livingstone; 1986:497–523.
12. Kase CS, Robinson RK, et al. Anticoagulant-related intracerebral hemorrhage. *Neurology.* 1985;35:943.
13. Fisher CM. Cerebral miliary aneurysms in hypertension. *Am J Pathol.* 1972;66:313.
14. Okizaki H. *Fundamentals of Neuropathology: Morphologic Basis of Neurologic Disorders.* 2nd ed. New York, NY: Igaku-Shoin; 1989.
15. Fox JL. *Intracranial Aneurysms.* New York, NY: Springer-Verlag; 1983.
16. Mohr JP, Kistler JP, et al. Intracranial aneurysms. In: Barnett HJM, Mohr JP, Stein BM, Yatsu FM, eds. *Stroke: Pathophysiology, Diagnosis, and Management.* New York, NY: Churchill Livingstone; 1986:643–677.
17. Mohr JP, Tatemichi TK, et al. Vascular malformations of the brain. In: Barnett HJM, Mohr JP, Stein BM, Yatsu FM, eds. *Stroke: Pathophysiology, Diagnosis, and Management.* New York, NY: Churchill Livingstone; 1986:679–705.
18. Castel JP, Kissel P. Spontaneous intracerebral and infratentorial hemorrhage. In: Youmans J, ed. *Neurological Surgery.* 3rd ed. Philadelphia, Pa: WB Saunders Co; 1990:1890–1917.

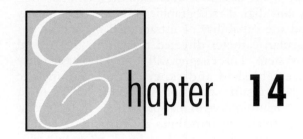

Interventional Neuroradiology (Endovascular Therapy)

Michael Brothers

Advances in the design of microcatheters, embolization devices, and digital radiographic software have greatly extended the capability of intracranial navigation for transvascular, catheter-directed therapy in the central nervous system. This chapter will review the basic techniques, established and experimental therapeutic approaches, results, and complications of the most important neurointerventional procedures in use today. Four basic treatment modalities are currently available: 1) *Embolization,* which, strictly defined, refers to occlusive material injected into the flowing blood stream, where it lodges to produce vascular occlusion. The advantages and disadvantages of the various embolic materials presently employed in embolization therapy must be considered when selecting the one best suited for a given application (Fig. 14.1). 2) *Detachable balloon therapy,* which can be considered a form of embolization, although detachable balloons usually are employed to occlude larger vascular lumina or cavities by carefully positioning the balloon in an ideal site. It is not usually intended to dislodge or move distally with flow after detachment. Using detachable balloons to occlude arteriovenous fistulae and major cerebral arteries is usually the method of choice. 3) *Angioplasty,* the therapeutic dilatation of arterial stenoses, although still experimental in neurovascular management techniques, shows considerable promise. This technique has been used for intra- and extracranial atheromatous stenosis as well as the management of medically intractable cerebral vasospasm following subarachnoid hemorrhage. 4) *Superselective intracranial infusion therapies*—rapid, safe catheterization of virtually any cerebral arterial territory—are now readily achieved and permit superselective perfusion of malignant brain tumor with chemotherapeutic agents. Limited experience with intracranial thrombolysis of acute cerebral thromboemboli has also shown promise.

Most procedures are carried out while the patient is awake, to allow moment-to-moment clinical neurologic assessment and early detection of complications. Mild neuroleptic anesthesia and local anesthesia are employed. Most are performed under systemic heparinization[1] to reduce thromboembolic complications. The vast majority of procedures can be accomplished with transfemoral access through routine guiding catheters, but occasionally, due to severe aortic arch tortuousity, it is necessary or desirable to access the intracranial circulation via direct carotid puncture. Both digital subtraction fluoroscopy and roadmapping fluoroscopy capabilities are

---

Figure 14.1 Various Emboli in Neurointerventional Procedures*

Particles
   1. Polyvinyl alcohol (PVA)
   2. Collagen–Avetene
   3. Gelfoam powder

Other mechanical occlusive materials
   1. Silk suture segments (e.g., 4-0 silk in 1.5 cm lengths)
   2. Occlusive "mini coils" (typically 0.018 in caliber)
      a. Platinum; steel
      b. Fiber-coated; noncoated
      c. Various shapes and sizes
   3. Detachable balloons
      a. Latex[†]
      b. Silicone[†]

Liquid agents
   1. Occlusive
      a. IBCA[†] (no longer available)
      b. NBCA[†]
      c. Liquid silicone[†]
   2. Sclerosing ethanol

*Includes only those in routine use in North America. Choice of agent is critical to safety and
   success; strategy is beyond the scope of this chapter.
[†]Not approved by United States Food and Drug Administration.

highly advantageous. Postprocedure monitoring of the patient is often best achieved in a neurological intensive care nursing unit.

Neurointerventional therapeutic strategies encompass:

1. Devascularization of hyperemic lesions (e.g., arteriovenous malformations [AVM] and vascular tumors)
2. Correction of anatomical (nonhyperemic) vascular lesions (e.g., cerebral aneurysm and arterial stenosis)
3. Inducement of biologic alteration (e.g., tumor chemotherapy infusion and intracranial thrombolysis)

Few large series have been published describing success rates and complication rates for neurointerventional procedures. In part, this is related to the rapid changes in techniques, precluding accumulation of a large patient population treated with a single approach. As such, many techniques described herein are viewed as partly experimental (e.g., intrasaccular balloon therapy of aneurysm and vasospasm angioplasty).

ARTERIOVENOUS MALFORMATION OF THE BRAIN

A variety of techniques are employed in brain AVM embolization[2-4]; choice of technique is predicated on the therapeutic goal (Fig. 14.2). AVMs are not commonly cured by embolization alone,[4-7] unless the lesions are small and have only a few feeders. Embolization's more common role is as a preoperative maneuver or adjunctive therapy in inoperable AVMs.

Large AVMs can be reduced by preoperative embolization so they are more amenable to surgical removal. Some authors[8,9] cite the importance of staged multisession reduction of the bulk of the AVM by embolization in order to reduce the risk of intraoperative "normal perfusion-pressure breakthrough" phenomenon. Preoperatively, the embolic material need not be permanently occlusive so there is a larger choice. Particulate embolization (usually using polyvinyl alcohol) is frequently employed[3,7,10] as it is more easily handled than liquid adhesives. Particle sizes can be chosen between 150 μm and 1000 μm or larger for use. Some workers also employ microfibrillar collagen particles. Both types can be injected (once mixed as a slurry in contrast material) through the intracranially positioned microcatheter. Recently, short segments of silk suture material, injected through the microcatheter, have been successful.[10,11] Liquid adhesive such as N-butyl cyanoacrylate (NBCA) is another preoperative option.[4,7]

When the AVM would not be rendered operable by embolization, palliation of progressive neurologic deficit can sometimes be achieved by partial therapy,[12] likely by

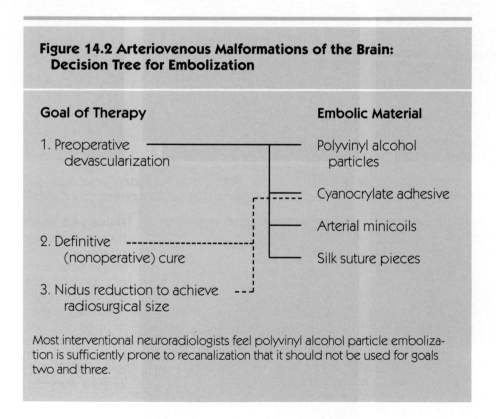

Figure 14.2 Arteriovenous Malformations of the Brain: Decision Tree for Embolization

Goal of Therapy

1. Preoperative devascularization

2. Definitive (nonoperative) cure

3. Nidus reduction to achieve radiosurgical size

Embolic Material

Polyvinyl alcohol particles

Cyanocrylate adhesive

Arterial minicoils

Silk suture pieces

Most interventional neuroradiologists feel polyvinyl alcohol particle embolization is sufficiently prone to recanalization that it should not be used for goals two and three.

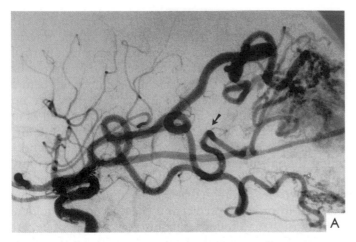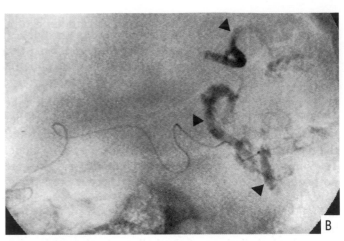

Figure 14.7 A parietooccipital brain AVM treated by glue embolization using the Magic catheter. **(A)** Lateral view, carotid arteriogram, before therapy. The Magic catheter is positioned in an MCA feeder (arrow) in preparation for glue embolization. **(B)** Spot film, lateral view. Multiple injections of glue into anterior and posterior cerebral feeders have been performed (arrowheads).

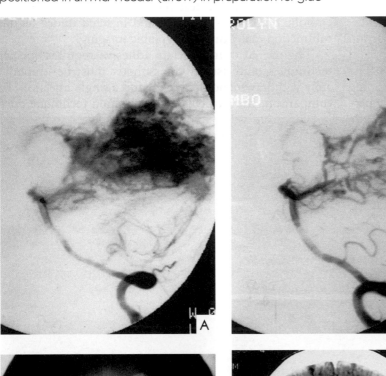

Figure 14.8 Preoperative glue embolization of an occipital brain AVM. **(A)** Lateral view, vertebral arteriogram, before treatment. A large AVM is visible. **(B)** After two sessions of embolization in which three injections of adhesive were made, marked reduction of AVM filling is evident. **(C)** Frontal skull film. The opacified glue emboli are apparent. **(D)** CT scan localizing the glue emboli within the AVM nidus. Residual AVM and draining veins are seen posteriorly (arrowheads).

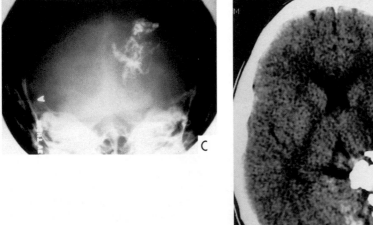

Principles of Neurosurgery

types of agents it is critical to avoid reflux of embolic material proximally once the flow in the pedicle has slowed or stopped. Additional risks are posed by the use of adhesive, wherein the polymerization time must be short enough to prevent passage of liquid glue into the venous side.[14,15] Rarely, a microcatheter becomes glued in place during the injection; the routine rapid withdrawal of the microcatheter at the termination of the glue injection usually results in catheter breakage. Retained ("glued-in") segments of broken microcatheters have not yet been found to produce neurologic complications.[16]

Regardless of the clinical setting or indication, ideally the goal is to deposit embolic material within the AVM nidus rather than the arterial feeder (Figs. 14.8, 14.9). Feeder occlusion alone leads to the development of collateral arterial supply, which may increase difficulty for the surgeon and the interventionist. In comparison, even partial filling of the nidus with embolic material may incite progressive thrombosis of the nidus.[15,17] When occlusion of arterial pedicles is performed immediately preoperatively, however, the surgeon may benefit from such "endovascular clipping" through reduced AVM pressure and bleeding. It may reduce the risk of "normal perfusion pressure breakthrough" bleeding at AVM surgery as well.[8]

When considering a patient for brain AVM embolization therapy, careful assessment of detailed cerebral angiography is required. Most brain AVMs are amenable to some form of embolotherapy. The complication rate for embolization has been variously reported to include mortality rates of 1% to 5%, permanent neurologic morbidity of 2% to 10%, and temporary deficits of 10%.[3,4,18–20] Careful consideration of the potential benefits and risks determines whether preoperative embolization of the operable lesion is warranted.

More common forms of complication[20] include stroke, rupture of the AVM nidus with intracerebral hemorrhage and, rarely, arterial rupture caused by a calibrated-leak balloon, or perforation[21] by a push-type guidewire/catheter combination system.

ARTERIOVENOUS MALFORMATION OF THE SPINAL CORD

These are difficult lesions to remove surgically or to approach neurointerventionally.[22] Most are fed in part or in whole by the anterior spinal artery (ASA). Management strategies include, as with brain AVM embolization: 1) palliative reduction of AVM size to reduce progressive neurologic deficit, 2) attempt at curative obliteration, and 3) preoperative partial embolization to reduce surgical morbidity. Embolization of non-ASA feeding pedicles (posterior spinal artery, meningeal branches) can be achieved with little morbidity but will in most instances have only a minor impact in reducing the AVM. Embolization in the ASA territory is much

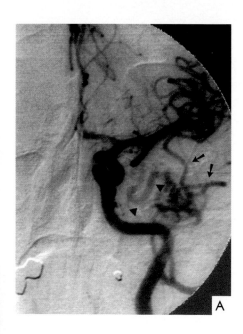
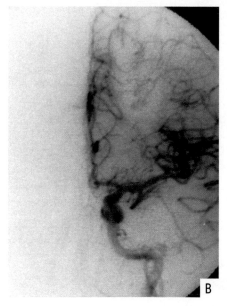

Figure 14.9 A small anterior temporal AVM with a single MCA feeder was completely obliterated with embolization using polyvinyl alcohol particles. (A) Pretreatment frontal view, left common carotid angiogram. Feeder noted by arrows; draining vein by arrowheads. (B) Immediately after embolization, no AVM filling is noted. Follow-up angiogram at 3 months also revealed no AVM.

riskier, as this critical vessel must remain patent to sustain spinal cord blood supply (Fig. 14.10). Two embolization strategies have been employed in the ASA territory: 1) Calibrated-size particle injection,[22-25] a technique that relies on high-quality spinal arteriography to measure the hypertrophied AVM feeding branches accurately. Polyvinyl alcohol particles of a predetermined size are chosen to enter the enlarged AVM perforators but not the smaller normal portion of the anterior spinal artery. Particles are injected, usually into the intercostal

artery (or radiculomedullary parent vessel, e.g., artery of Adamkiewicz). Such embolization is not curative, but has been successful in reducing progressive deficit,[26,29] and it can aid in subsequent surgical removal. 2) Liquid adhesive injection into the AVM perforating vessels superselectively,[23] a recent innovation that relies on safe navigation of the anterior spinal artery by a microcatheter to lodge a very small catheter tip superselectively in the perforating branches off the ASA that supply the AVM. Obviously, any reflux of embolic material

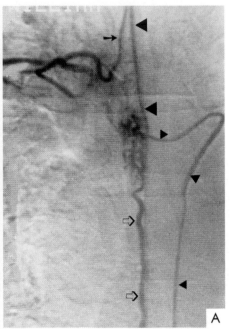

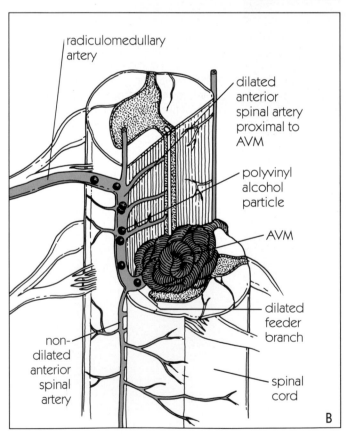

Figure 14.10 (A) Intramedullary spinal cord AVM. Early (left) and slightly later (right) frontal angiographic images obtained by arteriographic injection in right T-7 intercostal artery; note catheter (small arrowheads), artery of Adamkiewicz (arrow), anterior spinal artery (larger arrowheads), and draining vein (open arrows); curved arrow marks transient reflux of contrast material from intercostal orifice into aorta. The tiny perforating branches from ASA to nidus are visible. (B) Schematic illustration of particle embolization strategy for intramedullary AVM. ASA = anterior spinal artery. Particle size is chosen to be larger than the "normal" ASA diameter (undilated portion) but small enough to enter the dilated feeding branch to the AVM.

could occlude the anterior spinal artery and lead to cord injury.[26] The success and complication rates of these procedures are not yet well documented.[22]

ARTERIOVENOUS FISTULA OF THE SPINAL DURA

These lesions usually present in the thoracolumbar region angiographically, producing progressive myelopathy via spinal cord venous congestion. Typically, the lesion resides in the intervertebral foramen, which is fed by a dural branch of a single intercostal artery.[27] Particulate embolization in the arterial pedicle can obliterate the lesion, but it almost invariably recurs.[28] The most effective strategy is to occlude the fistula site itself or the venous outflow (Fig. 14.11). While this can be accomplished with direct neurosurgery, some success in permanent obliteration has been achieved using liquid adhesive embolization.[23,25] To be curative, the glue must reach the proximal venous side of the lesion and completely occlude the fistula or its vein.[23] Because the exact site at which the glue will polymerize when injected into a flowing system is uncertain, individual results are not entirely predictable. Occlusion of only the arterial side allows recurrence of the fistula when collaterals are recruited. If the glue passes too far distally, it can produce injury due to venous infarction in the spinal cord. Finally, even perfect deposition of glue in the first cen-timeter or two of the venous side of the fistula will fail to provide a cure, if the glue does not completely occupy the vascular lumen (allowing blood flow around the glue plug itself). At present, glue embolization of spinal dural AVF is a reasonable first maneuver in the management of the condition; if it fails, surgery is a more definitive option. The risk of embolization in this disorder appears low when care is taken to identify and avoid the artery of Adamkiewicz. If this important artery arises from the same intercostal artery that gives rise to the AVF, embolization is contraindicated.

CEREBRAL ANEURYSM

Three strategies (Fig. 14.12) have been employed in nonoperative obliteration of aneurysm: occlusion of the parent cerebral vessel and intrasaccular occlusion of the aneurysm by detachable balloons or thrombogenic coils.

OCCLUSION OF THE PARENT CEREBRAL VESSEL

This was the earliest approach devised and, while its applicability is limited, it is the safest. Occlusion of the internal carotid (ICA) or vertebral artery (VA) is highly effective for some types of aneurysm arising from them.[30,31] Permanent occlusion is carried out only if the patient can tolerate a temporary occlusion test. The test is usually carried out when the patient is awake, inflating

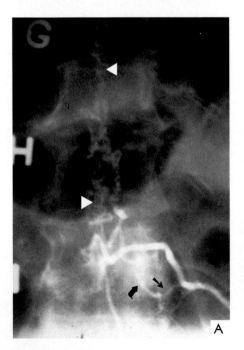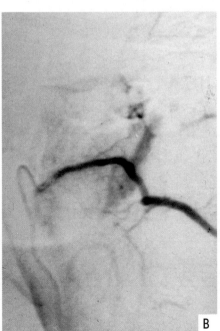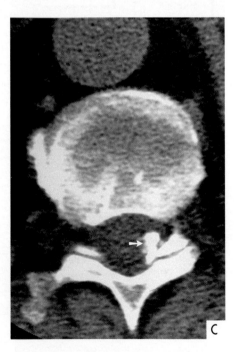

Figure 14.11 Spinal dural arteriovenous fistula. **(A)** Unsubtracted angiogram, frontal view, left T-11 intercostal injection, before treatment. Note feeder branching under vertebral pedicle (arrow); the single vein draining the fistula (curved arrow) connects to a network of engorged spinal cord veins (arrowheads). **(B)** The same patient immediately after embolization, using glue injected superselectively into the feeding branch. The intercostal is preserved, but the AVF no longer fills. **(C)** CT at the T-11 vertebral level shows that the radiopaque glue achieved an ideal, intradural position (arrow) in the vein segment draining the nidus.

a nondetachable balloon in a position approximating that intended for permanent occlusion (i.e., close to the aneurysm) so it produces flow arrest in the parent vessel.[30,31] Test occlusion is carried out with systemic heparinization and frequent clinical neurologic evaluations. Many workers also include ancillary assessments of cerebral perfusion, such as stable xenon CT,[32] during the test occlusion. Experience has shown that if a patient tolerates 15 minutes of complete internal carotid occlusion without neurologic deficit, subsequent permanent occlusion of the vessel will be uncomplicated in 80% to 90% of cases.[30,33] Aneurysms most amenable to parent vessel occlusion will be those of the internal carotid artery below its bifurcation, particularly those arising proximal to significant collateral vessels that might maintain aneurysm patency after ICA occlusion. Thus, best results are obtained for intracavernous carotid aneurysm and, similarly, vertebral aneurysm below the vertebral-basilar junction.[30] While surgical ligation of these arteries has been used effectively for years,[34,35] it is likely that the detachable balloon occlusion method has lower risk.

Aneurysms distal to a significant collateral entry point can sometimes be managed by parent vessel occlu-sion, but the success rate is lower. For example, by reducing the jet effect, which maintains aneurysm patency, internal carotid occlusion for a carotid termination aneurysm results in progressive thrombosis of its lumen, but the extent of obliteration is less predictable.[30] Occlusion balloons are not usually placed within cerebral vessels other than the internal carotid or vertebral artery (e.g., MCA, PCA, ACA) because the length of the inflated balloon might occlude the origin of significant perforator arteries,[36] which cannot be sacrificed. Also, the collateral blood supply with this type of occlusion is less often adequate to maintain brain viability.

The detachable balloons are carefully prepared prior to placement (Fig. 14.13). Those with a built in valve can be inflated and detached in vitro to test their integrity. The detachment force required depends on both the type of balloon and the diameter of the microcatheter tip on which the balloon is to be mounted. Using the type with a built-in valve allows the detachment strength to be tested as well. The balloon catheter system, once assembled, must be purged of air and flushed with contrast material, then loaded into the guiding catheter and advanced coaxially to achieve the desired position in the parent vessel. Usually the balloons

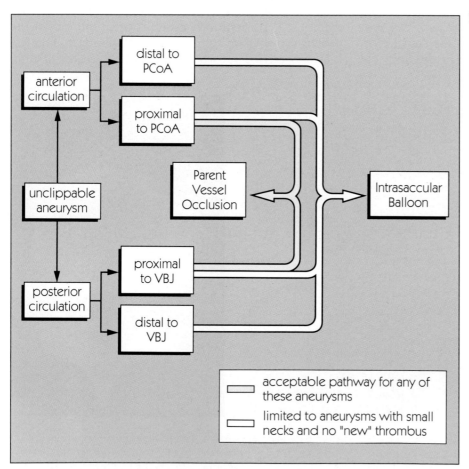

Figure 14.12 Decision tree for management of cerebral aneurysm by endovascular therapy. VBJ = vertebrobasilar junction; PCoA = posterior communicating artery. While unclippable aneurysms distal to PCoA (anterior circulation) or to VBJ (posterior circulation) can occasionally be effectively managed by parent vessel occlusion, more often other strategies, such as Drake tourniquet application, are appropriate. Aneurysms at the VBJ (involving both vertebral arteries) usually require vertebral artery occlusions bilaterally, if parent vessel occlusion is the treatment of choice.

are inflated with contrast material only; all types eventually deflate, but usually long after the desired thrombosis of the parent vessel (and aneurysm) has occurred. The deflated balloons then remain lodged permanently in the thrombus. Most workers now employ balloon/catheter assemblies that use a "pull-only" detachment mechanism, wherein the friction of the inflated balloon on the vessel wall keeps the balloon in position while the microcatheter is withdrawn from its neck by simple traction.* Many patients experience some headache or pain due to the pressure of the inflated balloon on the arterial wall, but this is temporary and easily managed with analgesics.

Only aneurysms that are unclippable or patients in whom operative risk is prohibitive are candidates for

*An alternative detachment technique employs a coaxial 4 Fr catheter slipped over a 2 Fr delivery microcatheter, on which the balloon has been loaded. The 4 Fr catheter can then be used to push the balloon off the 2 Fr catheter.

parent vessel occlusion (Fig. 14.14) (e.g., giant carotid or vertebral aneurysms). The progressive thrombosis of the aneurysm subsequent to parent vessel occlusion often induces headache, and some swelling of the aneurysm may occur occasionally, which may through local pressure phenomena induce cranial neuropathy.[30]

INTRASACCULAR BALLOON OCCLUSION OF ANEURYSM

This experimental intrasaccular therapy can be done on a much wider variety of aneurysms than parent vessel occlusion, but the risk is significantly greater and the long-term efficacy has not been documented. The goal

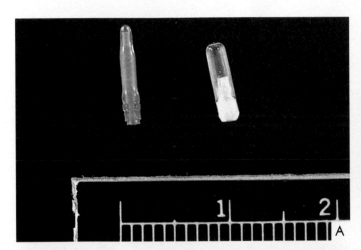

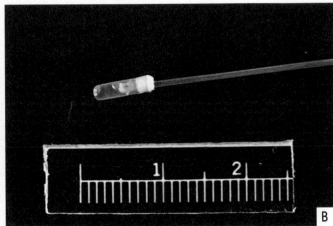

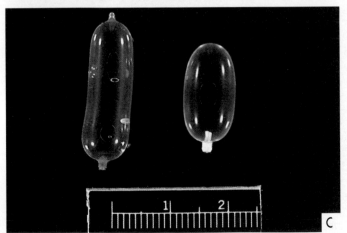

Figure 14.13 Two detachable balloon systems. A variety of balloon sizes and shapes is available. **(A)** Uninflated balloons. Ingenor "gold valve" (left) and ITC DSB1.8 (right). **(B)** Balloon assembled on a delivery microcatheter. **(C)** Detached balloons. Ingenor "gold valve" #16 (left) and ITC DSB1.8 (right).

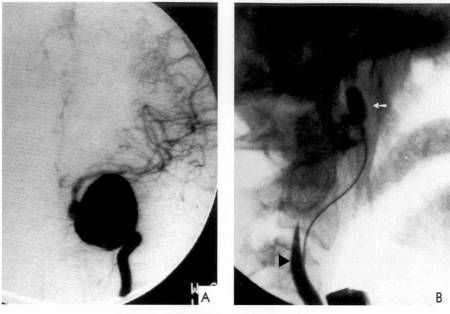

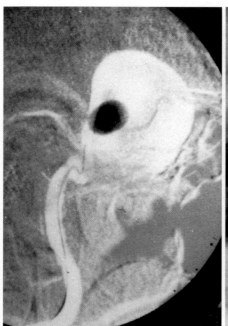

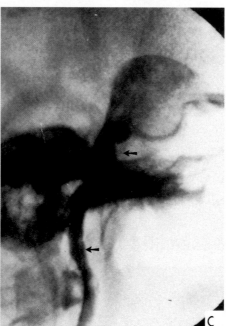

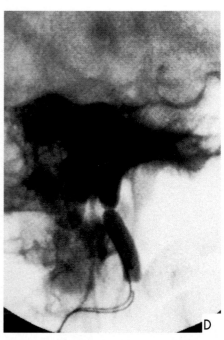

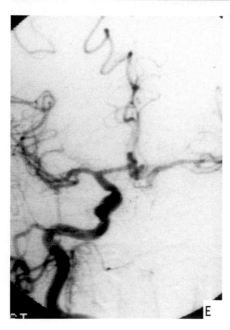

Figure 14.14 Carotid occlusion for giant intracranial aneurysm. **(A)** Frontal view, left internal carotid angiogram, reveals giant aneurysm of cavernous segment. **(B)** Temporary occlusion test of internal carotid artery, lateral spot film. A nondetachable balloon has been inflated in the high cervical carotid artery (arrow) to produce complete occlusion of flow. Note the stagnant column of contrast in the more proximal carotid artery (arrowhead). **(C)** Intrasaccular test occlusion of the aneurysm is attempted. The nondetachable balloon is guided into the aneurysm lumen using lateral roadmapping fluoroscopy and partly inflated (left). It is then snugged down into the aneurysm neck by gentle traction (right), but contrast injection into the proximal carotid artery reveals that the balloon has occluded the internal carotid; note the stagnant contrast column proximally (arrows). The aneurysm clearly has no "neck" to retain the balloon, but is instead a fusiform aneurysm requiring parent vessel occlusion. **(D)** Two detachable balloons, on their respective delivery microcatheters, have been advanced in tandem into the internal carotid just proximal to the aneurysm and inflated. They were then detached in situ by traction. **(E)** Postdetachment, contralateral right carotid arteriogram, frontal projection. Good crossfilling of the left hemisphere vessels via the anterior communicating artery is seen. The aneurysm does not fill.

is to exclude the aneurysm lumen from the parent vessel lumen by inflating a detachable balloon within the aneurysm itself (Fig. 14.15).[33,36,37] In order to retain the balloon within the aneurysm after detachment, the aneurysm must have a neck smaller than the inflated balloon diameter. Because the balloon must remain permanently inflated to effect a cure, the inflation material must be a polymerizing liquid plastic rather than contrast material. Both liquid silicone and HEMA (hydroxyethylmethacrylate) have been used to produce solidification of balloon contents; each has its problems. Critical to the technique's success is the close fit of the balloon to the aneurysm lumen or neck. This cannot be achieved without excellent fluoroscopic roadmapping technique and skill on the part of the operator. Slight overinflation of the balloon may result in aneurysm rupture, either early or delayed, which is often fatal.[36-38] Underinflation of the balloon allows blood to flow around it, which can displace the balloon and enlarge the aneurysm. In large aneurysms, where a single balloon cannot fill the lumen, multiple balloons have been placed, sometimes successfully producing lumen thrombosis, but some patients show residual lumen, shifting of the balloons, and even aneurysm growth.[33-39]

Besides the risk of aneurysm rupture, a frequent complication is thromboembolic stroke.[33,36-39] Many of the larger aneurysms treated by intrasaccular balloon placement contain preformed thrombus. Sometimes it is not

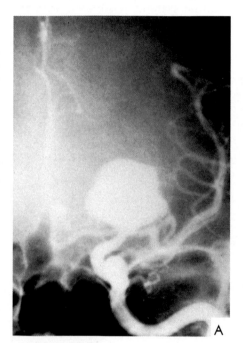

A

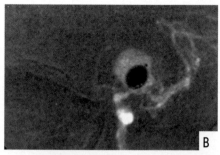

B

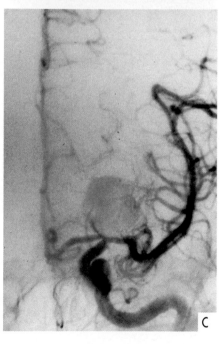

C

Figure 14.15 Intrasaccular balloon occlusion of giant aneurysm. **(A)** Frontal view, left carotid angiogram, shows giant left carotid "fork" aneurysm. **(B)** Roadmap image of detachable balloon partially inflated with contrast inside aneurysm. **(C)** The detachable balloon, when fully inflated, occludes the aneurysm lumen, isolating it from arterial flow. The contents of the balloon have been exchanged for a polymerizing liquid plastic (hydroxyethyl-methacrylate) and the balloon detached. Postdetachment subtraction arteriography reveals near-complete aneurysm occlusion (6 hours later, the patient suffered MCA thrombotic occlusion).

possible to determine whether thrombus is present or not, or whether it is loose or adherent. The balloon's impact on the thrombus during inflation and positioning frequently results in distal thromboembolism and stroke. Other causes of stroke in this procedure include premature detachment of balloons which can embolize distally, and distal embolization of partially solidified polymerizing liquids, which may leak from defective balloons or balloons that rupture during or after positioning.

To date, published results employing the intrasaccular technique have encountered a 37% to 50% combined morbidity/mortality rate, while complete occlusion of the aneurysm lumen, at least in the short term (1 to 2 year follow up), is achieved in about two thirds of cases.[33,36]

Intrasaccular balloon therapy of cerebral aneurysm is probably the riskiest neurointerventional procedure today. It is likely that safer techniques will replace this procedure in the future. A new, recently described, approach is packing the aneurysm lumen transvascularly with fine caliber occlusive metallic coils or wire (Fig. 14.16).[40,41] The long-term results and the complication rate are as yet undetermined, but incomplete occlusion is common.

ARTERIOVENOUS FISTULA OF MAJOR CEREBRAL ARTERIES

CAROTID CAVERNOUS FISTULA (CCF)

These high-flow lesions are typically posttraumatic and most commonly signify a rent in the intracavernous course of the internal carotid artery with direct communication established to the cavernous sinus. Symptoms depend in part upon the type of venous drainage—anteriorly into the ophthalmic system; posteriorly into the petrosal sinuses; or superiorly, refluxing into cortical veins.[42-44] Frequently, patients present with proptosis, bruit, chemosis, and cranial nerve palsies related to cav-

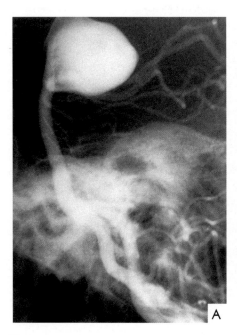
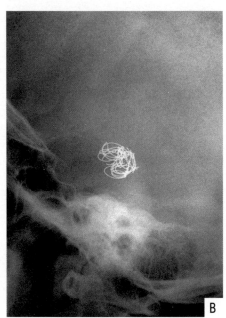
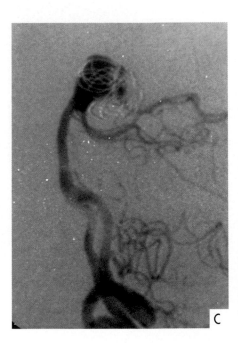

Figure 14.16 Embolization of unclippable aneurysm by occlusive minicoils. **(A)** Pretreatment lateral view, vertebral arteriogram, reveals giant basilar tip aneurysm. **(B)** After two treatment sessions, 17 lengths of C-shaped, fiber-coated platinum "coil," 3 cm each, have been deposited in the aneurysm lumen, using a Tracker catheter. **(C)** Lateral vertebral arteriogram immediately after the second embolization session shows marked reduction of blood flow into the aneurysm lumen. Further thrombosis is expected. Additional coils will likely be placed to reduce the aneurysm further.

ernous sinus syndrome. Indications for urgent treatment include rapidly deteriorating visual dysfunction, hemorrhage, intracranial hypertension, and transient ischemic attacks.[44,45] Direct neurosurgery[46] has now been almost entirely superseded by the intravascular approach. Endovascular occlusion has a greater than 90% success rate using detachable balloons,[43,44,47] usually placed transarterially, although occasionally a transvenous route is required.[45,48]

A detachable balloon, positioned on the microcatheter, is advanced coaxially through an internal carotid artery guiding catheter. Partial inflation of the balloon causes it to be sucked through the fistula connection into the cavernous sinus (Fig. 14.17). Further inflation and positioning on the cavernous side of the fistula will, in most cases, allow occlusion of the fistula while preserving the internal carotid patency. Sometimes two or more balloons are required to obliterate the fistula completely. Patients frequently experience some pain during inflation of the balloon in the cavernous sinus and occasionally cranial nerve palsies (ophthalmoplegia) are precipitated or worsened. Because the balloons are normally inflated

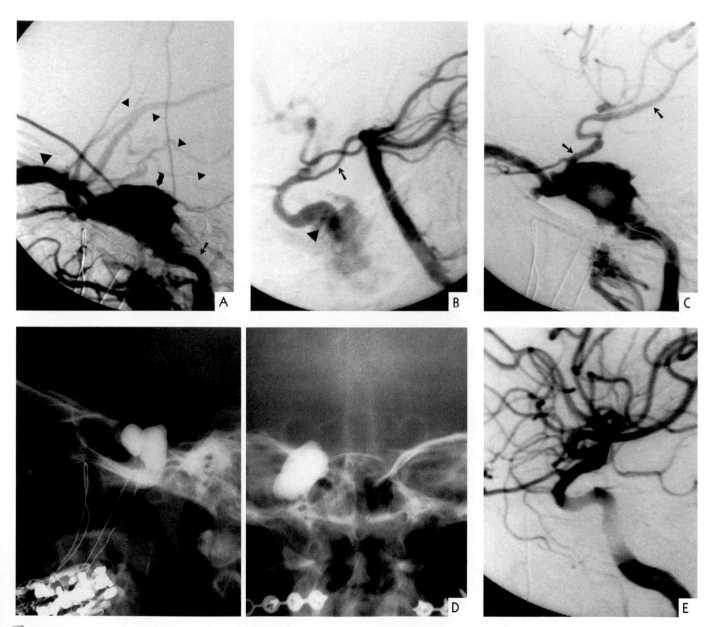

Figure 14.17 Carotid-cavernous fistula embolization. (A) Lateral view, carotid angiogram. Immediate massive shunting from carotid artery (arrow) to cavernous sinus (curved arrow) and ophthalmic vein (large arrowhead) with no visible opacification of cerebral arteries. The site of the carotid tear is obscured by the rapid shunting. Note reflux of flow into cortical veins (small arrowheads). (B) The site of the fistula is better revealed on vertebral arteriography when retrograde flow in the posterior communicating artery (arrow) fills the carotid artery above and down to the level of the fistula (arrowhead). (C) Partial inflation of a detachable balloon has caused it to be carried into the cavernous sinus. Further inflation there has reduced the shunt through the fistula, so that cerebral arteries are now opacified (arrows). Shunting to the veins is reduced. (D) Two large balloons were required to occlude the fistula fully. Skull films post-therapy: lateral view (left) and frontal view (right) showing balloons in cavernous sinus. (E) Postembolization carotid subtraction angiography. No shunting remains, the fistula is closed, and the carotid is patent.

only with contrast material, they ultimately deflate and in many cases the cranial nerve palsy resolves; they need to stay inflated only long enough for thrombosis of the fistula/sinus to occur (usually several days).

When this simple transarterial approach fails, a transvenous approach—in order to occlude the venous side of the fistula in the cavernous sinus—can be successful (Fig. 14.18).[45,48] Occasionally, it is necessary to occlude the internal carotid artery by trapping the fistula hole[41,46] with a pair of balloons. The patient, of course, must have tolerated temporary internal carotid occlusion.

A success rate of 85% to 97% has been described[42,43,47] for obliteration of CCF by endovascular means. Recurrence (1% to 3.9%) usually responds to a second balloon treatment.[43] A complication rate of 1% to 3% has been reported[42,43,47,50] and is typically attributed to the migration of balloons or thromboembolism resulting in stroke. In over three quarters of patients, carotid patency can be preserved[43,50] using an arterial-side approach. It is likely that most carotid occlusions for CCF can be avoided by the transvenous access route, when indicated.[45] Delayed ill effects of balloon therapy for CCF include pseudoaneurysm formation and persistent ophthalmoplegias.[51]

VERTEBRAL ARTERY FISTULA

These extracranial lesions can be congenital or posttraumatic in origin. Symptoms may be attributable to steal (vertebral basilar insufficiency or spinal cord ischemia) or venous congestion (cord ischemia or nerve root compression). Bruit with tinnitus is the most common presentation. While the natural history of untreated lesions has not been well documented, spontaneous thrombosis is unusual.[52,53] As with CCF, surgical treatment can be difficult,[54] while the intravascular approach with its low morbidity is highly successful.

Technique and strategy are analogous to those used in the treatment of CCF: Transarterial occlusion of the fis-

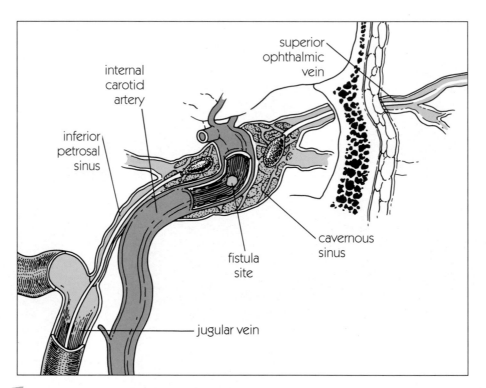

Figure 14.18 Strategies in transvenous access to CCF. Balloons (red) can be positioned in the cavernous sinus via 1) transfemoral access to the inferior petrosal sinus via the jugular vein or 2) surgical exposure of the dilated superior ophthalmic vein, allowing its direct retrograde catheterization.

tula site to preserve vertebral flow is attempted first (Fig. 14.19). The balloon is positioned on the venous side or across the arteriovenous connection. Occasionally, sacrifice of the parent vessel by trapping it between balloons or laying the balloon across the fistula opening is necessary.

Balloons are placed in a mobile portion of the anatomy for this disorder, therefore after treatment limitation of neck motion is usually recommended: bed rest for the first few days, followed by limited physical activity for several weeks (or until balloon deflation has been

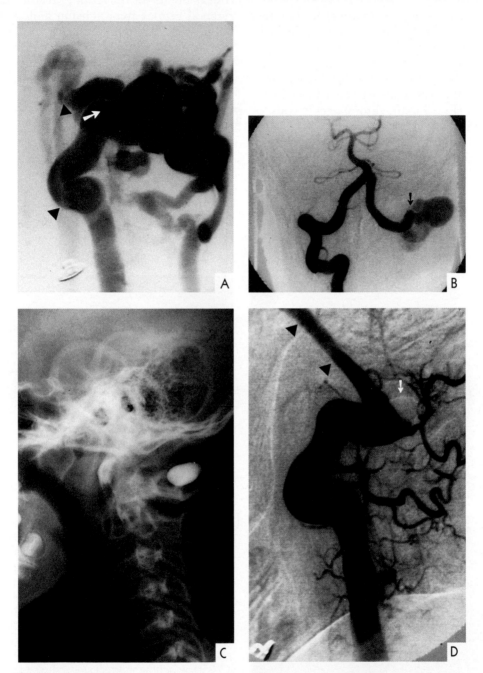

Figure 14.19 Congenital vertebral arteriovenous fistula at C-1 cervical level in a 10-year-old boy presenting with severe tinnitus. (**A**) Lateral view, ipsilateral left vertebral arteriogram. Immediate massive filling of variceal veins obscures the site of arterial leak (arrow) from the vertebral artery (arrowheads). No antegrade flow reaches intracranially. (**B**) Frontal view, contralateral right vertebral arteriogram, better defines the site of fistula (arrow) as blood flow has reversed down the left vertebral artery. (**C**) Lateral neck film after detachment of the silicone balloon (contrast filled) on venous side of fistula. Balloon was delivered transarterially up the left vertebral artery and passed through the fistula. (**D**) Lateral view, left vertebral arteriogram, after balloon detachment. The fistula is completely closed, and the patency of the vertebral artery is preserved. "Subtracted" shadow of balloon is visible (arrow). Note good filling of basilar artery (arrowheads).

documented). Successful obliteration is achieved in 95% to 100% of patients with virtually no serious complications.[52,53,55]

CEREBRAL ARTERIOVENOUS FISTULA

These fistulae may have single or multiple feeders that enter a large varix. In older children and adults, the "solitary" (single feeder) cerebral AVF is more frequent.[56,57] Presentation may result from the mass effect of the varix, hemorrhage, or seizure, or the patient may be asymptomatic. Occlusion of the fistula site can be achieved with detachable balloons (Fig. 14.20), thrombogenic coils, or liquid adhesive with excellent results.

In the neonatal "vein of Galen aneurysm" type (Fig. 14.21), however, the transarterial route is sometimes insufficient. Considerable success has been achieved with a transvenous route:[58] A length of thrombogenic metallic coil can be placed via the transtorcular or percutaneous transvenous route into the Galenic varix to incite thrombosis. Subtotal occlusion usually results, and therapy is directed at reversing high output cardiac failure. Subsequent treatments to occlude feeding pedicles are often required, either by transarterial embolization or direct surgical ligation. The long-term prognosis may be guarded, even when early intervention results in good control or cure of the lesion, because chronic intrauterine cerebral venous hypertension and/or arterial steal may induce significant brain injury and atrophy. Complications of interventional therapy are frequent,[58] but less so than for surgery alone and with better results.

DURAL ARTERIOVENOUS MALFORMATIONS (AND FISTULAE)

While brain AVMs have an associated dural component in 15% of cases, purely dural AVMs are a distinct entity.[59] These are normally acquired lesions, usually presenting in the adult, and most frequently associated with a major venous dural sinus. Symptoms are related to one or more of the following mechanisms: 1) high flow, caus-

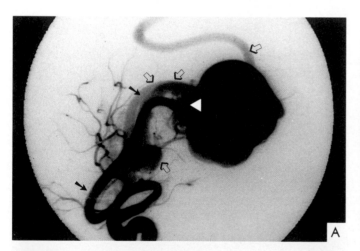

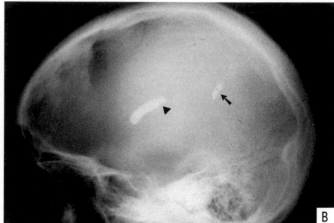

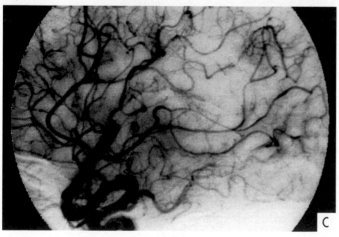

Figure 14.20 "Solitary" cerebral arteriovenous fistula in an adult presenting with grand mal seizures. **(A)** Lateral internal carotid arteriogram shows hypertrophied single middle cerebral branch feeder (arrows), filling a huge varix at site of fistula (arrowhead), and surface veins draining away from the varix (open arrows). **(B)** Transarterial embolization was initially unsuccessful using platinum minicoils, which were deposited in distal part of feeder but were carried off into the varix by flow (arrow). A balloon was successfully positioned in the feeder, across the fistula site (arrowhead), and detached. **(C)** Postdetachment arteriogram shows proximally preservation of MCA feeder, but occlusion of the fistula. No neurologic deficit resulted.

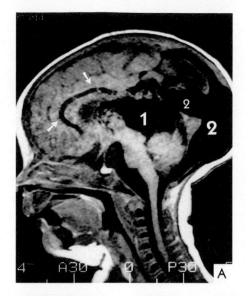

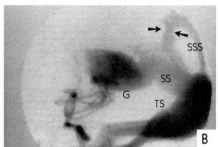

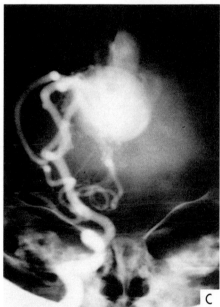

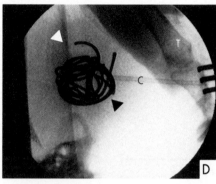

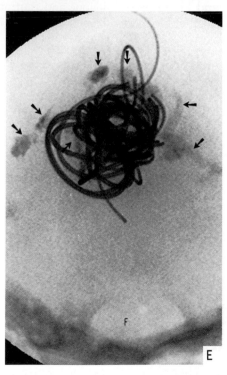

Figure 14.21 Two weeks after birth, congestive heart failure and cranial bruit led to diagnosis of "vein of Galen aneurysm." (**A**) Sagittal T1-weighted MR scan, showing huge vein of Galen (1) and draining dural sinuses (2), as well as hypertrophied feeding anterior cerebral arteries (arrow). (**B**) Lateral view, vertebral arteriogram, reveals massively dilated dural venous sinuses and feeding arteries arising from both posterior cerebrals, and superior cerebellars. Note anomalous accessory "falcine" sinus (arrows) draining to the superior sagittal sinus (SSS). G = vein of Galen; SS = straight sinus. (**C**) Frontal view, right carotid angiogram. Anterior and posterior choroidal feeders were found bilaterally. (**D**) Lateral spot film, intraoperative. Transtorcular puncture; the straight sinus was used to position a catheter in the vein of Galen, and large, fibercoated Gianturco thrombogenic coils (arrowhead) were deposited there to induce venous thrombosis. Arrow indicates skin retractor; C = catheter; T = surgeon's thumb. (**E**) Frontal skull film, after two sessions of transtorcular coil embolization, and three sessions of transarterial glue embolization of feeding arteries. Note seven glue casts (arrows) in bilateral anterior cerebral, bilateral posterior choroidal arteries. Marked clinical improvement resulted, and at 6 months, the infant is home with no need for other medications. Additional therapy is planned. F = foramen magnum.

ing bruit (Fig. 14.22); 2) venous hypertension, which may result in intracranial hemorrhage (Fig. 14.23); 3) neural compression by enlarged vascular structures. Because a rather extensive collateral network can supply the lesions, a transarterial approach frequently does not result in complete obliteration. Partial treatment can result in alleviation of symptoms and occasionally spontaneous thrombosis of the remaining lesion occurs. A more complete "anatomic" cure can sometimes be obtained by transvenous occlusion of the involved sinus using coils or adhesive (Fig. 14.24); the risks may be significantly higher with such an approach,[60] especially if normal cerebral veins drain into the section of sinus for planned occlusion. The method of therapy chosen will be dictated by the patient's symptoms and angiographic findings. When the dural AVM's venous drainage refluxes into the cortical veins, the patient is at increased risk for intracranial hemorrhage,[61,62] and an aggressive approach to effect an anatomic cure is mandated. However, when no cortical venous drainage is present and the patient suffers only from bruit, sometimes the risk of dural venous sinus occlusion cannot be justified, and treatment is usually limited to arterial side embolization. When indicated, surgical resection of the involved sinus is an alternative.[63,64]

CEREBRAL ARTERIAL VASOSPASM

While management of blood rheology and blood pressure and the administration of calcium channel blockers can reduce the incidence and severity of postsubarachnoid hemorrhage vasospasm,[65] there are still patients for whom medical prophylaxis and therapy do not work (Fig. 14.25). Progressive obtundation and neurologic deficit attributable to ischemia in the setting of chronic vasospasm has been successfully treated by percutaneous angioplasty. The technique is at present experimental (Figs. 14.26, 14.27), but in the few small series published to date, a number of patients have shown early clinical improvement.[66–68] Recurrence (without a repeated SAH) has not been reported. Selection criteria and contraindications, as well as the complication and success rates, have yet to be firmly established. Likely, there is a 10% to 15% incidence of major complications, including rupture of a cerebral artery, which is routinely fatal, and conversion of a fresh bland cerebral infarction into a hemorrhagic one.

ATHEROMATOUS ARTERIAL STENOSIS

There is a growing body of evidence that angioplasty of the extracranial internal carotid and vertebral arteries can alleviate atheromatous stenosis and possibly reduce ischemic symptoms, and it has a low morbidity rate.[69–72] However, no controlled, prospective, or randomized trial of this form of therapy has yet been published. Many workers express reservations that atheromatous and thrombus debris might be released by the splitting of plaque and caution that some form of cerebral protection be employed. At present, these precautions include expos-

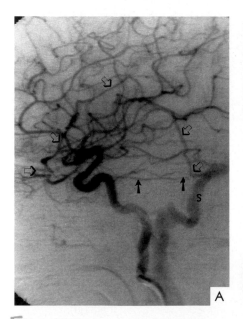
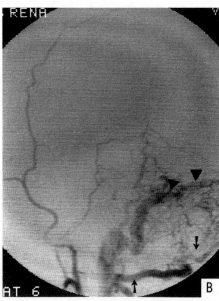
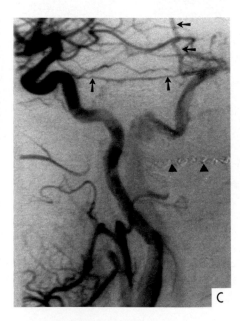

Figure 14.22 Dural AVM of the sigmoid sinus, causing tinnitus. (A) Internal carotid angiogram, showing dural supply from cavernous carotid branches (arrows) as well as anomalous origin of middle meningeal artery from the ophthalmic (open arrows). These ICA sources cannot be safely obliterated by embolization in this patient. S = sigmoid sinus. (B) Lateral view, external carotid angiogram. Marked hypertrophy of occipital artery, the dominant feeder, is noted (arrows), with early filling of the sigmoid sinus (arrowheads). (C) After embolization of the feeding occipital and posterior auricular arteries with glue, particles, and coils, the tinnitus resolved. This lateral view, common carotid arteriogram, shows residual supply to AVM from cavernous ICA, and anomalous middle meningeal arteries (arrows). Note coils in occipital artery (arrowheads).

ing the vessel during surgery so it can be temporarily occluded and flushed, or using tandem balloon catheter systems to occlude temporarily beyond the site of angioplasty so debris can be flushed out of the proximal arterial segment.[71,72] Other related experimental techniques include angioplasty of intracranial atheromatous stenoses[73-75] (with significantly greater risk anticipated).

ACUTE CEREBRAL THROMBOEMBOLISM

Emergency thrombolysis holds promise as a therapy for the acute stroke patient. Preliminary work has shown that a high rate of success can be achieved in reopening acutely occluded cerebral vessels[76,77]; however, improved clinical outcome has yet to be firmly documented. No prospective, controlled, randomized trials have been published. There are impressive, albeit few, anecdotal reports of major improvement in clinical status, particularly in the setting of basilar artery thrombosis. The logistic obstacles to delivery of thrombolytic therapy quickly enough following onset of stroke limit the salvage rate. Whether superselective intracranial intraarterial infusion of thrombolytic agents (tissue plasminogen activator, urokinase, streptokinase) will be more efficacious than intravenous administration has yet to be determined. The most significant risk to date appears to

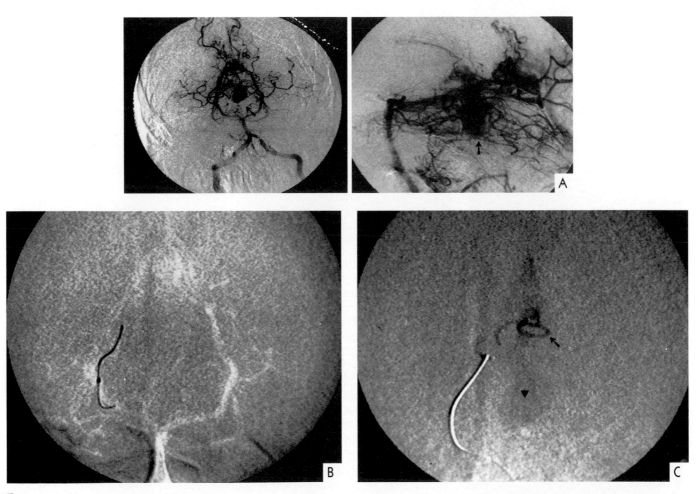

Figure 14.23 A middle-aged male presenting with repeated intraventricular hemorrhages was found to have a dural AVM of tentorial apex. (**A**) Left vertebral angiogram: venous varix (arrow) fills with A-V shunting in the early arterial phase and projects into the fourth ventricle. Extensive dural supply from bilateral middle meningeal and meningohypophyseal arteries was found. (**B**) Frontal roadmap image of posterior circulation, with Tracker catheter and guidewire positioned in a large dural feeder—the dural branch of the posterior cerebral artery (Davidoff-Schechter). No pial arteries supplied the lesion. (**C**) Superselective angiogram, same catheter position as in **B**. The tortuous feeder (arrow) empties into the veins that fill the varix (arrowhead). Glue embolization of this dural supply was next performed.

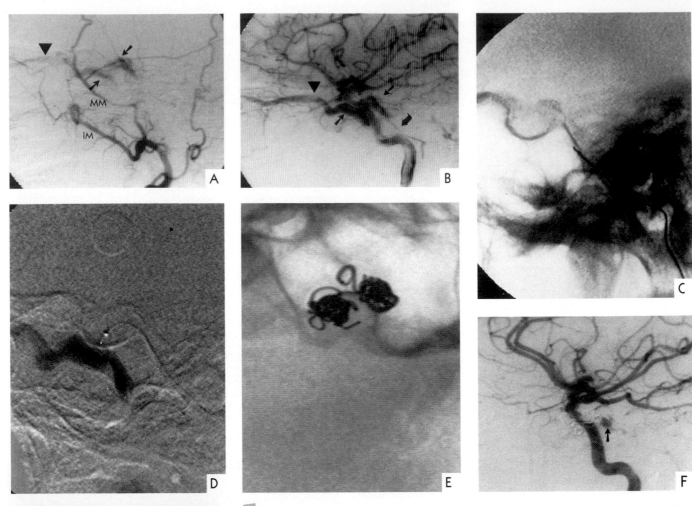

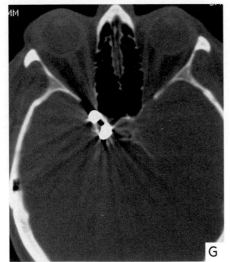

Figure 14.24 Dural AVM of cavernous sinus presenting with chemosis and orbital pain with ophthalmoplegia. A "slow-flow" type lesion is demonstrated. **(A)** Lateral view, external carotid angiogram. Early filling of the cavernous sinus (arrows) and superior ophthalmic vein (arrowhead) is seen. Supply is from middle meningeal (MM) and distal internal maxillary (IM) arteries. **(B)** Internal carotid angiogram, lateral view. Again, early filling of cavernous sinus (arrows) and ophthalmic vein (arrowhead) is seen, from cavernous carotid dural branches (obscured by sinus). The inferior petrosal sinus (curved arrow) drains towards the jugular bulb. **(C)** After particle embolization of external carotid supply, transvenous embolization was performed, accessing the cavernous sinus via a transfemoral approach to the inferior petrosal sinus (IPS). A lateral spot film shows Tracker catheter positioned in the IPS. **(D)** Contrast material injected directly into cavernous sinus via same catheter as in **C** to confirm position prior to embolization with platinum minicoils. **(E)** Nine minicoils have been packed into anterior and posterior cavernous sinus. **(F)** Postembolization internal carotid angiogram: slight filling of the cavernous sinus persists (arrow), but shunting is markedly reduced. **(G)** CT scan shows position of intracavernous coil emboli.

Principles of Neurosurgery

be conversion of bland stroke into an intracerebral hemorrhage; certain patterns of vascular occlusion appear to be at increased risk for this.[77]

PREOPERATIVE DEVASCULARIZATION OF INTRACRANIAL TUMORS

When reduced intraoperative blood loss is the goal, intra- and extraaxial neoplasms can be devascularized by embolization prior to their surgical removal, if they are hypervascular (that is, showing an angiographic "blush"). Typically, such embolization can be carried out at the same session as the diagnostic arteriogram.

The tumors most commonly considered for this therapy include meningiomas,[78] particularly those of the skull base, where surgical access to the dural arterial supply is more difficult to achieve, and hemangioblastomas.[79]

Embolization of meningiomas and other dural-based lesions involves injection of particulate or liquid agents

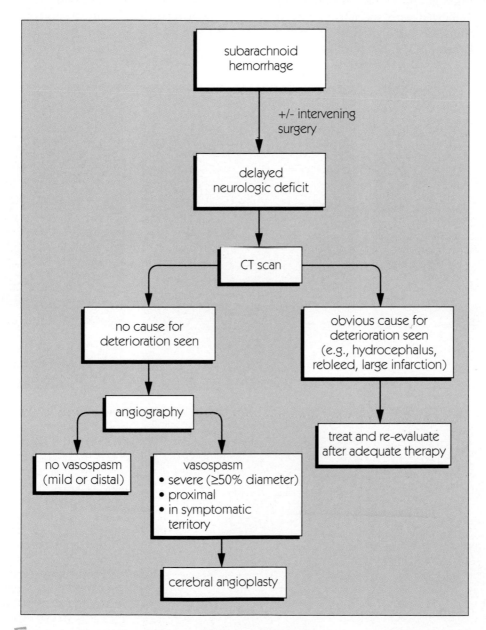

Figure 14.25 Decision tree for vasospasm angioplasty.

in the external carotid (ECA) and/or ICA branches (Figs. 14.28, 14.29). ECA territory embolization technique requires vigilance to prevent entry of occlusive materials into "dangerous anastomoses" with the cerebral or ocular circulations.[78] Also, careful consideration must be given to the cranial nerve blood supply and the vascular integrity of the skin and mucous membranes. Familiarity with the range of available embolic agents allows safe treatment planning and prevents complications.

Embolization of dural branches of the ICA (meningohypophyseal trunk, inferolateral trunk, and ophthalmic artery) can be safely achieved with special superselective catheterization techniques,[80] but it is difficult and has inherently greater risk (see Fig. 14.29). Such an approach is occasionally mandated when the surgeon feels preoperative devascularization is especially important.

Intraaxial tumor embolization has hazards similar to those in brain AVM embolotherapy. If an arterial feeding pedicle leading solely to the tumor can be superselectively catheterized, without risk to branches to normal brain, embolization can be safely achieved (Fig. 14.30). Frequently, however, arteriography reveals that such access is not possible. Usually it is unacceptable electively to infarct uninvolved brain tissue in order to achieve tumor devascularization preoperatively. Consultation between the operating surgeon and the interventionist will lead to good decision making.

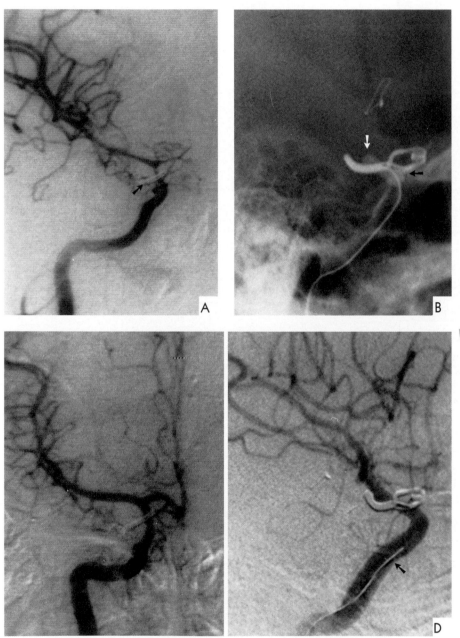

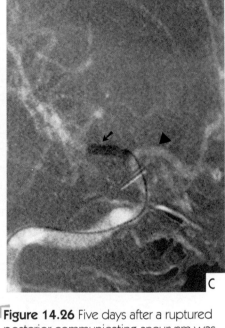

Figure 14.26 Five days after a ruptured posterior communicating aneurysm was clipped in this patient, new drowsiness and hemiparesis were noted, and vasospasm was suspected. (A) Frontal right carotid angiogram. Aneurysm no longer fills; note aneurysm clip (arrow). Severe "proximal" vasospasm of ICA, MCA, and ACA is seen. (B) Lateral spot film with angioplasty balloon (arrows) inflated in ICA across clip site. (C) Frontal roadmap image of angioplasty of MCA (arrow); ACA has already been angioplastied (arrowhead). (D) Postangioplasty appearance (left, right). Vessels now are normal caliber. Arrow points to the shadow of the balloon catheter in ICA.

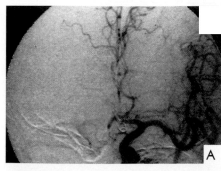
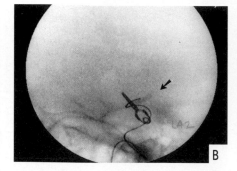
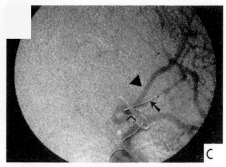

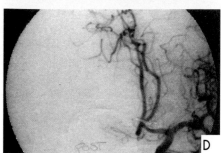

Figure 14.27 After clipping of ruptured anterior communicating artery aneurysm, severe "distal" vasospasm in both ACAs developed. (A) Frontal left carotid angiogram. The aneurysm is well clipped. Spasm is limited to postcommunicating portions of ACAs. (B) Oblique frontal spot film during angioplasty of anterior cerebral artery at clip site. Note contrast-filled balloon (arrow). (C) Roadmap oblique image during angioplasty of left pericallosal artery (arrow). Right pericallosal (arrowhead) and anterior communicating artery (open arrow) already have been dilated. (D) Angioplasty, left carotid oblique angiogram. ACAs are now of normal caliber.

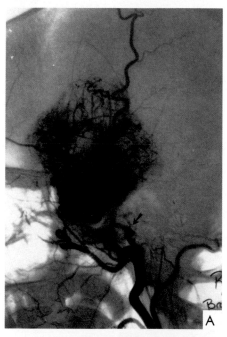
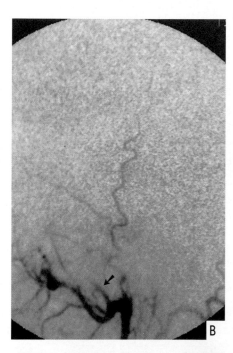

Figure 14.28 (A) Pterional meningioma shows hypervascular blush on preoperative external carotid angiogram. Hypertrophied middle meningeal artery feeds the mass (arrow). (B) After embolization of middle meningeal artery with particles, external carotid angiogram shows no tumor vascularity. Note stump of middle meningeal artery (arrow).

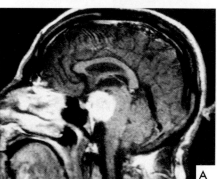
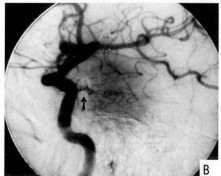
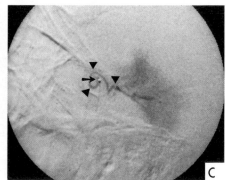

Figure 14.29 Clivus meningioma. (A) Preoperative contrast-enhanced sagittal T1-weighted MR scan. (B) Dominant arterial supply (arrow) was from meningohypophyseal trunk, a branch of the intracavernous ICA. (C) Superselective catheterization of the meningohypophyseal trunk (arrow-heads) was achieved and lateral angiography performed through it. Note radiopaque bead of Tracker catheter tip (arrow). No reflux into ICA occurred. Embolization with particles was performed, without complication in this position.

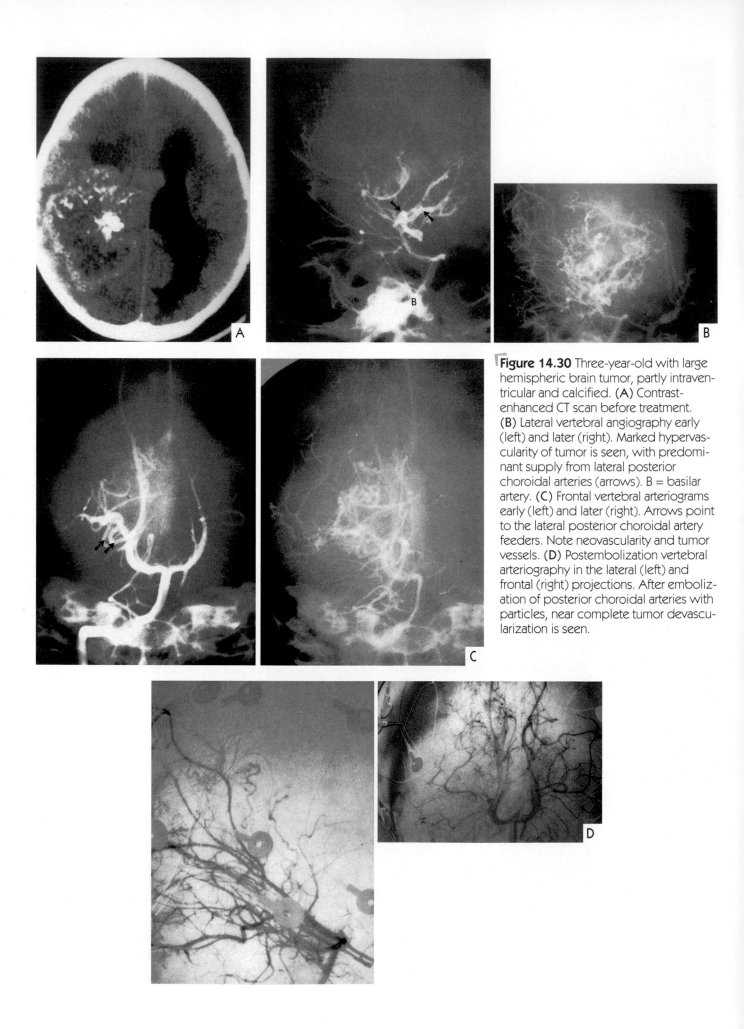

Figure 14.30 Three-year-old with large hemispheric brain tumor, partly intraventricular and calcified. (**A**) Contrast-enhanced CT scan before treatment. (**B**) Lateral vertebral angiography early (left) and later (right). Marked hypervascularity of tumor is seen, with predominant supply from lateral posterior choroidal arteries (arrows). B = basilar artery. (**C**) Frontal vertebral arteriograms early (left) and later (right). Arrows point to the lateral posterior choroidal artery feeders. Note neovascularity and tumor vessels. (**D**) Postembolization vertebral arteriography in the lateral (left) and frontal (right) projections. After embolization of posterior choroidal arteries with particles, near complete tumor devascularization is seen.

REFERENCES

1. Debrun G, Vinuela F, Fox AJ. Aspirin and system heparinization in diagnostic and interventional neuroradiology. *AJNR*. 1982;3:337–349.
2. Halbach W, Higashida RT, Yang P, Barnwell S, Wilson CE, Hieshima GB. Preoperative balloon occlusion of arteriovenous malformations. *Neurosurgery*. 1988;22:301–308.
3. Purdy PD, Samson D, Batjer HH, Rigger RC. Preoperative embolization of cerebral arteriovenous malformations with polyvinyl alcohol particles experience in 51 adults. *AJNR*. 1990;11:501–510.
4. Pelz DM, Fox AJ, Vinuela F, Drake C, Ferguson GG. Preoperative embolization of brain AVMs with isobutyl-2 cyrnoacrylate. *AJNR*. 1988;9:757–764.
5. Vinuela F, Fox AJ, Pelz D. Angiographic followup of large cerebral AVMs incompletely embolized with IBCA. *AJNR*. 1986;7:919–925.
6. Lasjaunias P, Manelfe C, Terbrugge K, Ibor LL. Endovascular treatment of cerebral arteriovenous malformations. *Neurosurg Rev*. 1986;9:265–275.
7. Fox AJ, Pelz DM, Lee DH. Arteriovenous malformation of the brain: recent results of endovascular therapy. *Radiology*. 1990;177:51–57.
8. Spetzler RF, Martin NA, Carter LP, Flom RA, Ravdzens PA, Wilkinson E. Surgical management of large AVMs by staged embolization and operative excision. *J Neurosurg*. 1987;67:17–28.
9. Andrews BT, Wilson CB. Staged treatment of arteriovenous malformations of the brain. *Neurosurgery*. 1987;21:314–323.
10. Dawson RC, Tarr RW, Hecht ST, et al. Treatment of artiovenous malformation of the brain with combined embolization and stereotactic radiosurgery: results after 1 and 2 years. *AJNR*. 1990;11:857–864.
11. Eskridge JM, Hartling RP. Preoperative embolization of brain AVMs using surgical silk and polyvinyl alcohol. *AJNR*. 1989;10:882. Abstract.
12. Fox AJ, Girvin JP, Vinuela F, Drake C. Rolandic arteriovenous malformations: improvement in limb function by IBC embolization. *AJNR*. 1985;6:575–582.
13. Vinuela F, Fox AJ, Debrun G, Pelz D. Preembolization superselective angiography: role in the treatment of brain arteriovenous malformations with isobutyl-2 cyanoacrylate. *AJNR*. 1984;5:765–769.
14. Brothers M, Kaufmann JCE, Fox AJ, Deveikis JP. N-butyl 2-cyanoacrylate—substitute for IBCA in interventional neuroradiology: histopathologic and polymerization time studies. *AJNR*. 1989;10:777–786.
15. Vinuela F, Debrun GM, Fox AJ, Givin JP, Peerless SJ. Dominant hemisphere arteriovenous malformations: therapeutic embolization with isobutyl-2-cyanoacrylate. *AJNR*. 1983;4:959–966.
16. Personal communication with A. Berenstein, MD, 1991.
17. Vinuela F, Fox AJ, Pelz D. Progressive thrombosis of brain arteriovenous malformations after embolization with isobutyl-2-cyanoacrylate. *AJNR*. 1983;4:1233–1238.
18. Vinuela F, Fox AJ. Interventional neuroradiology and the management of arteriovenous malformations and fistulas. *Neurol Clin*. 1983;1:131–154.
19. Lasjaunias P, Manelfe C, Terbrugge K, Ibor LL. Endovascular treatment of cerebral arteriovenous malformations. *Neurosurg Rev*. 1986;9:265–275.
20. Berenstein AB, Choi IS, Kupersmith MJ, Flamm E, Kricheff II, Madrid MM. Complications of endovascular embolization in 202 patients with cerebral AVMs. *AJNR*. 1989;9:876(a).
21. Halbach W, Higashida RT, Dowd CR, Barnwell SL, Hieshima GB. Management of vascular perforations that occur during neurointerventional procedures. *AJNR*. 1991;12:319–327.
22. Bionki A, Merland J, Reizine D, et al. Embolization with particles in thoracic intramedullary arteriovenous malformations. *Radiology*. 1990;177:651–658.
23. Choi IS, Berenstein A. Surgical neuroangiography of the spine and spinal cord. *Radiol Clin North Am*. 1988;26(S):1131–1141.
24. Horton JA, Latchaw RE, Gold L, Pang D. Embolization of intramedullary arteriovenous malformations of the spinal cord. *AJNR*. 1986;7:113–118.
25. Oldfield EH, Doppman JL. Spinal arteriovenous malformations. *Clin Neurosurg*. 1987;34:161–183.
26. Riche MC, Melki JP, Merland JJ. Embolization of spine cord vascular malformations via the anterior spinal artery. *AJNR*. 1983;4:378–381.
27. Kendall B, Logue V. Spinal epidural angiomatous malformations draining into intrathecal veins. *Neuroradiology*. 1977;13:181–189.
28. Hall N, Oldfield EH, Doppman JL. Recanalization of spinal arteriovenous malformations following embolization. *J Neurosurg*. 1989;70:714–720.
29. Theron J, Cosgrave R, Melanson D, Ethier R. Spinal arteriovenous malformations: advances in therapeutic embolization. *Radiology*. 1986;158:163–169.
30. Fox AJ, Vinuela F, Pelz DM, et al. Use of detachable balloons for proximal artery occlusion in the treatment of unclippable cerebral aneurysms. *J Neurosurg*. 1987;66:40–46.
31. Berenstein A, Ransohoff J, Kupersmith M. Transvascular treatment of giant aneurysms of the cavernous carotid and vertebral arteries. *Surg Neurol*. 1984;21:3–12.
32. Erba SM, Horton JA, Latchaw RE, et al. Balloon test occlusion of the internal carotid artery with stable xenon/CT cerebral blood flow imaging. *AJNR*. 1988;9:533–538.

33. Higashida RT, Halbach W, Dowd C, et al. Endovascular detachable balloon embolization therapy of cavernous carotid artery aneurysms: results in 87 cases. *J Neurosurg.* 1990;72:857–863.

34. Heros R, Nelson PB, Ojemann RG, Crowell R, Debrun G. Large and giant paraclinoid aneurysms; surgical techniques, complications and results. *Neurosurgery.* 1983;12:153–163.

35. Spetzler R, Carter LP. Revascularization and aneurysm surgery: current status. *Neurosurgery.* 1985;16:111–116.

36. Higashida RT, Halbach W, Cahan L, Hieshima G, Konish Y. Detachable balloon embolization therapy of posterior circulation aneurysms. *J Neurosurg.* 1989;71:512–519.

37. Romodanov AP, Schehgelov VI. Intravascular occlusion of saccular aneurysms of the cerebral arteries by means of a detachable balloon catheter. *Adv Tech Stand Neurosurg.* 1982;9:25–49.

38. Hooks JE, Fox AJ, Pelz DM, Peerless SJ. Rupture of aneurysms following balloon embolization. *J Neurosurg.* 1990;72:567–571.

39. Strother CM, Lunde S, Graves V, Toutant S, Hieshima GB. Late paraophthalmic aneurysm rupture following endovascular treatment. *J Neurosurg.* 1989;71:777–780.

40. Guglielmi G, Vinuela F, Macellari V, Feliciani M, Dion J, Duckwiler G. Endovascular occlusion by electrothrombosis of experimental small and medium-sized saccular aneurysms. Presented at the Annual Meeting of the American Society of Neuroradiology; 1990; Los Angeles, Calif.

41. Hilal S, Chi LT, Khandji A, Friedman D, Cross D, Solomon R. Preshaped thrombogenic coils for the treatment of intracranial aneurysms. Presented at the Annual Meeting of the American Society of Neuroradiology; 1990; Los Angeles, Calif.

42. Debrun GM, Lacour P, Fox AJ, Vinuela F, Davis KR, Ahn HS. Traumatic carotid cavernous fistulas: etiology, clinical presentation, diagnosis, treatment, result. *Sem Intervent Radiol.* 1987;4:242–248.

43. Lasjaunias P, Berenstein A. *Surgical Neuroangiography.* Berlin: Springer-Verlag; 1987;2:176–211.

44. Halbach W, Hieshima GB, Higashda RT, Reicher M. Carotid-cavernous fistulae: indications for urgent treatment. *AJNR.* 1987;8:627–633.

45. Debrun G. Treatment of traumatic carotid-cavernous fistula using detachable balloon catheters. *AJNR.* 1983;4:355–356.

46. Isamut FI, Ferrer E, Twose J. Direct intracavernous obliteration of high-flow carotid-cavernous fistulas. *J Neurosurg.* 1986;65:770–775.

47. Goto K, Hieshima GB, Higashida RT, et al. Treatment of direct carotid cavernous fistulae. *Acta Radiol Diag Suppl.* 1986;369:576–580.

48. Halbach W, Higashida RT, Hieshima GB, Hardin CW, Yang PS. Transvenous embolization of direct carotid cavernous fistulas. *AJNR.* 1988;9:741–747.

49. Turner DM, Vangilder JC, Maltahedi S, Pierson EW. Instantaneous intracerebral hematoma in carotid-cavernous fistula. *J Neurosurg.* 1983;59:680–686.

50. Kupersmith MJ, Berenstein A, Flamm E, Ransohoff E. Neuro-ophthalmologic abnormalities and intravascular therapy of traumatic carotid cavernous fistulas. *Ophthalmology.* 1986;93:906–912.

51. Tsai F, Hieshima GB, Mehringer CM, Grinnell V, Pribram HW. Delayed effects in the treatment of carotid-cavernous fistulas. *AJNR.* 1983;4:357–361.

52. Halbach W, Higashida RT, Hieshima GB. Treatment of vertebral arteriovenous fistulas. *AJNR.* 1987;8:1121–1128.

53. Lasjaunias P, Berenstein A. *Surgical Neuroangiography.* Berlin: Springer-Verlag; 1987;2:211–223.

54. Bartal AD, Levy M. Excision of a congenital suboccipital vertebral arteriovenous fistula. *J Neurosurg.* 1972;37:452–456.

55. Halbach W, Higashida RT, Hieshima GB, Norman D. Normal perfusion pressure breakthrough occuring during treatment of carotid and vertebral fistulas. *AJNR.* 1987;8:751–756.

56. Vinuela F, Drake CG, Fox AJ, Pelz DM. Giant intracranial varices secondary to high flow arteriovenous fistulae. *J Neurosurg.* 1987;66:198–203.

57. Halbach W, Higashida RT, Hieshima GB, Hardin CW, Dowd CF, Barnwell SL. Transarterial occlusion of solitary intracerebral arteriovenous fistulas. *AJNR.* 1989;10:747–752.

58. Ciricillo SF, Edwards M, Schmidt K, et al. Interventional neuroradiological management of vein of Galen malformations in the neonate. *Neurosurgery.* 1990;27:22–28.

59. Lasjaunias P, Manelfe C, Chiu M. Angiographic architecture of intracranial vascular malformations and fistulas—pretherapeutic aspects. *Neurosurg Rev.* 1986;9:253–263.

60. Halbach W, Higashida RT, Hieshima GB, Goto K, Norman D, Newton TH. Dural fistulas involving the transverse and sigmoid sinuses: results of treatment in 28 patients. *Radiology.* 1987;163:443–447.

61. Halbach W, Higashida RT, Hieshima GB, Mehringer CM, Hardin CW. Transvenous embolization of dural fistulas involving the transverse and sigmoid sinuses. *AJNR.* 1989;10:385–392.

62. Ishii K, Goto K, Ihara K, et al. High risk dural arteriovenous fistulae of the transverse and sigmoid sinuses. *AJNR.* 1987;8:1113–1120.

63. Sundt TM, Piepgras DG. The surgical approach to arteriovenous malformations of the lateral and sigmoid dural sinuses. *J Neurosurg.* 1983;59:32–39.

64. Barnwell SL, Halbach W, Higashida RT, Hieshima G, Wilson CB. Complex dural arteriovenous fistulas: results of combined endovascular and neurosurgical treatment in 16 patients. *J Neurosurg.* 1989;11:352–358.

65. Seiler RW, Reulen HJ, Huber P. Outcome of an-

eurysmal subarachnoid hemorrhage in a hospital population: a prospective study including early operation, intravenous nimodipine, and transcranial doppler ultrasound. *Neurosurgery.* 1988;23:598–604.

66. Newell DW, Eskridge JM, Mayberg MR, Grady MS, Winn HR. Angioplasty for the treatment of symptomatic vasospasm following subarachnoid hemorrhage. *J Neurosurg.* 1989;71:654–660.

67. Brothers M, Holgate RC. Intracranial angioplasty for treatment of vasospasm after subarachnoid hemorrhage: technique and modifications to improve branch access. *AJNR.* 1990;11:239–247.

68. Higashida RT, Halbach W, Cahan LD, et al. Transluminal angioplasty for treatment of intracranial arterial vasospasm. *J Neurosurg.* 1989;71:648–653.

69. Becker GJ, Katzen BT, Dake MD. Noncoronary angioplasty. *Radiology.* 1989;170:921–940.

70. Tsai F, Motovich V, Hieshima G, et al. Percutaneous transluminal angioplasty of the carotid artery. *AJNR.* 1986;7:349–538.

71. Theron J, Raymond J, Casasco A, Courtheoux F. Percutaneous angioplasty of atherosclerotic and postsurgical stenosis of carotid arteries. *AJNR.* 1987;8:495–500.

72. Theron J, Courtheoux P, Alachkar F, Bouvard G, Maiza D. New triple coaxial catheter system for carotid angioplasty with cerebral protection. *AJNR.* 1990;11:869–874.

73. Sundt TM, Smith H, Campbell J, Vlietstra R, Cucchiara R, Stanson A. Transluminal angioplasty for basilar artery stenosis. *Mayo Clin Proc.* 1980;55:673–680.

74. Higashida RT, Hieshima GB, Tsai F, Halbach W, Norman D, Newton TH. Transluminal angioplasty of the vertebral and basilar artery. *AJNR.* 1987;8:745–749.

75. Purdy P, Devous M, Unwin D, Giller C, Batjer H. Angioplasty of an atherosclerotic middle cerebral artery associated with improvement in regional cerebral blood flow. *AJNR.* 1990;11:878–880.

76. del Zoppo G, Ferbert A, Otis S, et al. Local intra-arterial fibrinolytic therapy in acute carotid territory stroke. *Stroke.* 1988;19:307–313.

77. Theron J, Gurtheoux P, Casasco A, et al. Local intra-arterial fibrinolysis in the carotid territory. *AJNR.* 1989;10:753–765.

78. Lasjaunias P, Berenstein A. *Surgical Neuroangiography.* Berlin: Springer-Verlag; 1987;2:57–99.

79. Eskridge J, Scott JA. Preoperative embolization of cerebellar and spinal hemangioblastomas (a). *AJNR.* 1988;9:1030.

80. Halbach W, Higashida RT, Hieshima GB, Hardin CW. Embolization of branches arising from cavernous portion of internal carotid artery. *AJNR.* 1989;10:143–150.

Chapter 15

The Multiply Injured Patient

Jack E. Wilberger

Neurosurgeons are frequently faced with diagnosing and treating head and spine injuries in multitraumatized patients. The neurosurgeon may function as a member of a coordinated trauma team or direct general surgeons and other subspecialists in the management of multitrauma patients. Head and spinal/spinal cord injuries rarely occur in isolation; the incidence of associated injuries is well known (Fig. 15.1).[1-3] In addition, the impact of associated injuries

and subsequent pathophysiologic derangements, such as hypoxia and hypotension, on the morbidity and mortality from head injury have been clearly delineated.

Multitraumatized patients are assessed and treatment priorities established based on the nature of the injuries and the stability of vital signs. Familiarity with assessment and management protocols for multitrauma patients gives the neurosurgeon a better appreciation of the interrela-

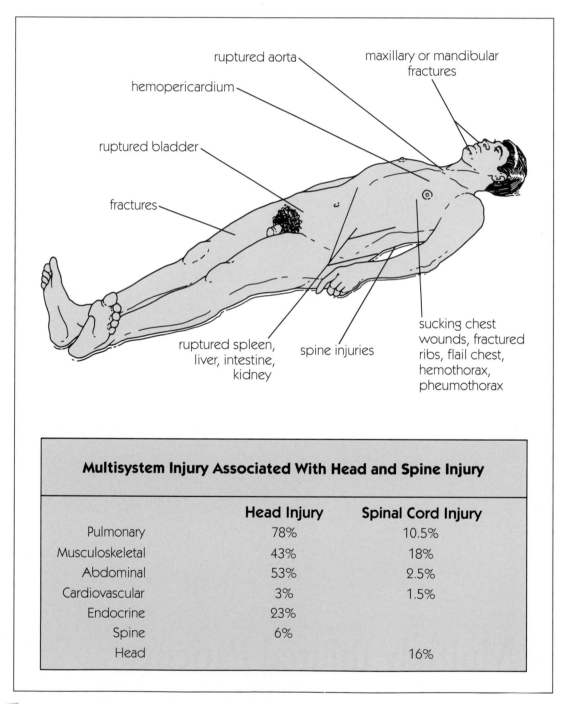

Multisystem Injury Associated With Head and Spine Injury		
	Head Injury	**Spinal Cord Injury**
Pulmonary	78%	10.5%
Musculoskeletal	43%	18%
Abdominal	53%	2.5%
Cardiovascular	3%	1.5%
Endocrine	23%	
Spine	6%	
Head		16%

Figure 15.1 Multiple system injuries associated with head and spinal cord injury.

Principles of Neurosurgery

tionships in multisystem injury, enabling him or her to plan an effective sequence of diagnostic testing and treatment of the associated head and/or spine injury.

ASSESSMENT OF THE MULTITRAUMA PATIENT

Multitraumatized patients require continual reassessment to establish treatment priorities. Most trauma protocols involve a rapid primary assessment of the patient, resuscitation of vital signs, a more detailed secondary assessment, and initiation of definitive care (Fig. 15.2).[4]

The primary assessment of the multitrauma patient has three main goals: establishment and protection of the airway, ventilation, and maintenance or restoration of normal hemodynamic parameters. However, immediately life-threatening injuries—cardiac tamponade, tension pneumothorax, exsanguinating hemorrhage—may require operative intervention after securing airway control but before further assessment.

Airway obstruction may manifest itself in a variety of ways—inability to speak (laryngeal injury), stridor, or abnormal upper airway sounds, such as snoring, gurgling, or gargling. Hypoxia and/or hypercarbia from airway obstruction may result in agitation, combativeness, or obtundation. The most common causes of airway obstruction—prolapse of the tongue, foreign bodies, retained secretions, blood—are easiest to alleviate with such maneuvers as the chin lift, jaw thrust, suctioning, and oropha-

Figure 15.2 Trauma Management Protocol—American College of Surgeons Advanced Trauma Life Support

Primary Survey

Airway
    Airway maintenance
        with C-spine control

Breathing

Circulation
    Hemorrhage control

Disability

Exposure
    Remove all clothes
        for exam

Resuscitation

Ventilate/oxygenate

Shock management

NG/urinary catheters

Operating room

Uncontrollable shock

Life-threatening injuries

Secondary Survey

Complete system by system exam

Radiographs (chest, C-spine)

Peritoneal lavage

CT scan

Complete radiographs

Definitive Care

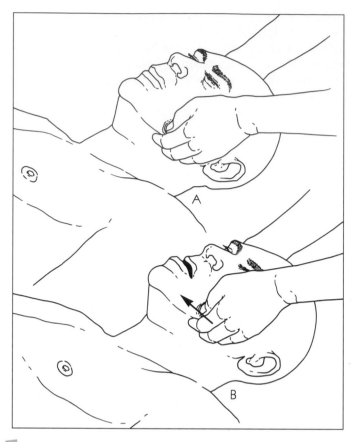

Figure 15.3 Airway management techniques in the unconscious patient. The jaw thrust maneuver is shown.

ryngeal or nasopharyngeal airways (Fig. 15.3). It must be kept in mind that airway obstruction is not only an acute phenomenon but may also be progressive and recurrent. Thus these maneuvers may need to be repeated frequently. If they are primarily or secondarily unsuccessful, airway control must be established by intubation. Endotracheal intubation—orally or nasally—is generally the preferred route. While intubation is being initiated, ventilation of the patient continues to be of paramount importance. Prolonged attempts at intubation should be accompanied by concomitant intermittent ventilation.

In some patients, such as those with massive facial fractures, laryngeal fractures, or tracheal obstruction, endotracheal intubation may be technically impossible. Inability to intubate demands creation of a surgical airway. Surgical cricothyroidotomy appears to provide the quickest and safest route to definitive airway control (Fig. 15.4). Emergency tracheostomy has been largely abandoned because of its time-consuming nature and tendency to cause excessive blood loss. ·

Once the airway is securely established and maintained, adequate ventilation must be provided. Positive pressure breathing techniques supplemented by 100% oxygen are the surest means to this end.

Injured patients who present in shock are near death; thus it is vitally important to recognize shock in the multitrauma patient and rapidly identify its probable cause. Bleeding may be external and controllable by applying direct pressure over lacerations or open extremity fractures.

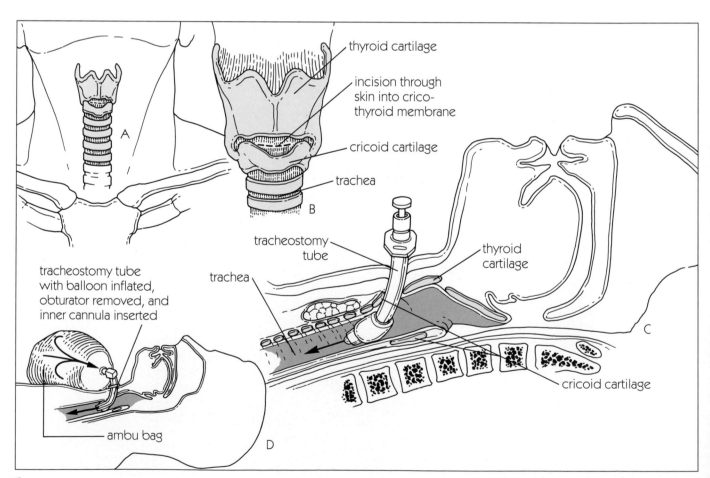

Figure 15.4 (A–D) Surgical technique of cricothyroidotomy. (Modified with permission from the American College of Surgeons Committee on Trauma. *Advanced Trauma Life Support Course Instruction Manual.* 1985:176.)

Principles of Neurosurgery

However, in the blunt trauma victim bleeding is just as likely to be internal, within the retroperitoneum, abdomen, or thorax, and thus occult and not directly controllable.

There is a graded physiologic response to hemorrhage based on the volume of blood loss and compensatory mechanisms that may prevent a significant fall in blood pressure until over 30% of blood volume is lost (Fig. 15.5). The earliest signs of shock are tachycardia and cutaneous vasoconstriction, not hypotension. A mean arterial pressure of 65 to 70 mm Hg (80 to 90 mm Hg systolic) is the goal in maintaining adequate organ perfusion. Palpating the pulse may indicate systolic blood pressure—the presence of a radial pulse indicates a systolic pressure greater than 80, a femoral pulse greater than 70, and a carotid pulse greater than 60.

The first step in fluid resuscitation is establishing vascular access. A large bore 14- to 16-gauge catheter in the peripheral veins is preferable, but saphenous or femoral vein cutdown is an acceptable alternative. Central lines are generally reserved for monitoring rather than initial resuscitation because they are potentially complicated by pneumothorax, hydrothorax, air embolism, or infection.

Fluid resuscitation is generally initiated with isotonic electrolyte solutions (Ringer's lactate, normal saline). Such solutions effectively increase intravascular volume immediately, while over time correcting interstitial fluid deficits.[5] If a 1 to 2 L isotonic fluid bolus (20 mL/kg in children) does not stabilize vital signs, blood replacement should be initiated. Fully crossmatched blood is preferable; however, this is usually too time-consuming in the acute setting. Thus most early transfusions use type-specific or type O packed cells. Recently, considerable interest has arisen over the use of hypertonic solutions (3% saline) in trauma resuscitation because of the small volume required and the rapid restoration of arterial pressure. Holcroft et al. reported significant improvement in patient survival when hypertonic solutions were used in resuscitation during transport.[6]

Isotonic fluid and/or blood may now be replaced at very high infusion rates (up to 1 L/min) using a variety of rapid infusion devices. Such rapid replacement may, however, predispose the patient to problems such as hypothermia, coagulopathy, or fluid overload. Thus all replacement fluids should be warmed prior to administration. If more than 10 units of blood must be replaced, platelets should also be given to reduce the risk of dilutional coagulopathy.

The pneumatic antishock garment (PASG) is frequently used during transport and resuscitation of the multitraumatized patient to assist in blood pressure con-

Figure 15.5 Estimated Fluid and Blood Requirements[1] (Based on Patient's Initial Presentation)

	Class I	Class II	Class III	Class IV
Blood loss (mL)	up to 750	750–1500	1500–2000	2000 or more
Blood loss (%BV)	up to 15%	15%–30%	30%–40%	40% or more
Pulse rate	<100	>100	>120	≥ 140
Blood pressure	normal	normal	decreased	decreased
Pulse pressure (mm Hg)	normal or increased	decreased	decreased	decreased
Capillary blanch test	normal	positive	positive	positive
Respiratory rate	14–20	20–30	30–40	>35
Urine output (mL/hr)	≥ 30	20–30	5–15	negligible
CNS-mental status	slightly anxious	mildly anxious	anxious and confused	confused-lethargic
Fluid replacement (3:1 rule)	crystalloid	crystalloid	crystalloid + blood	crystalloid + blood

[1]For a 70-kg male

Reproduced with permission from the American College of Surgeons Committee on Trauma. *Advanced Trauma Life Support Course Instruction Manual.* 1985:185.

trol (Fig. 15.6). It sustains blood pressure by increasing total peripheral resistance. However, the garment is not a substitute for and should not delay adequate volume replacement. The PASG has been particularly useful in splinting and hemorrhage control for pelvic and multiple lower extremity fractures. It may also help in tamponading soft tissue hemorrhage in the lower half of the body. Because of its effects on the circulatory system, the PASG is contraindicated in patients whose injuries are complicated by myocardial infarction, congestive heart failure, or pulmonary edema.

When there is a transient or minimal response to initial fluid resuscitation a variety of reasons must be considered. The two primary concerns are that fluid loss was greater than initially estimated or that significant blood loss is continuing. The former requires a readjustment in fluid replacement calculations, the latter demands imme-

diate surgical intervention. Other possible etiologies for continued or recurrent hypotension include ventilation problems, cardiogenic shock, acute massive gastric distention, diabetic acidosis, hypoadrenalism, and neurogenic shock.

In neurogenic or vasomotor spinal shock a significant drop in blood pressure is related to an underlying spinal cord injury. The hypotension results from sympathetic vascular denervation with subsequent vasodilatation producing a shock-like picture. In the patient who is multiply injured it is sometimes difficult to determine whether the low blood pressure is secondary to associated blood loss or related to the spinal injury. With spinal vasomotor shock, fluid resuscitation is often ineffective because of the abnormal vascular tone, and vasopressors may be necessary for adequate restoration of normal blood pressure (Fig. 15.7).

The final components of the primary survey are a

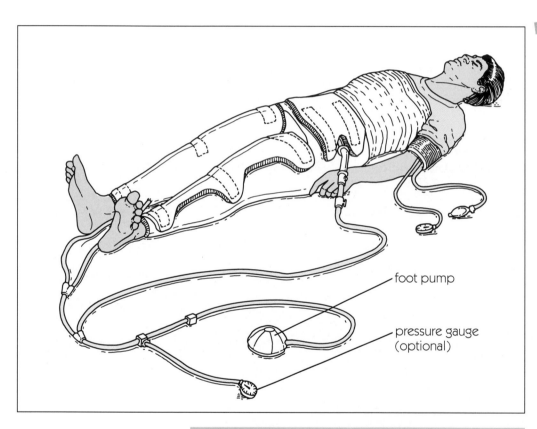

Figure 15.6 Pneumatic antishock garment.

foot pump

pressure gauge (optional)

Figure 15.7 Clinical Differentiation of Hemorrhagic Versus Neurogenic Shock

	Hemorrhagic Shock	Neurogenic Shock
Pulse	tachycardia	bradycardia
Skin	cool, clammy	dry, warm
Mental Status	altered	normal
Urine Output	low	normal

Principles of Neurosurgery

minineurologic examination and complete exposure of the patient to allow adequate examination of all body areas for obvious injury. At this stage the neurologic exam is generally limited to determining if the patient is awake and alert, and appropriately or inappropriately responsive to stimuli or unconscious.

The secondary survey begins when the patient is satisfactorily stabilized, the primary assessment is completed, and fluid resuscitation is progressing. This survey involves an in-depth examination of all body systems—head/neck, chest, abdomen, extremities—as well as important diagnostic studies such as radiographs, peritoneal lavage, and laboratory studies.

Examination of the head and neck aims to clarify intracranial injuries using the Glasgow Coma Score as well as to identify penetrating wounds and closed maxillofacial injuries. The chest is examined visually for penetrating and/or sucking wounds and flail segments and by auscultation for absent or diminished breath sounds and distant heart sounds. Immediate closed tube thoracostomy is indicated for penetrating wounds or pneumo- or hemothorax (Fig. 15.8). For pneumothorax the optimal chest tube is placed in the second intercostal space, midclavicular line, and directed superiorly and anteriorly. For penetrating wounds and hemothorax the tube is placed in the seventh or eighth intercostal space, midaxillary line, and directed posteriorly and inferiorly. Two tubes may be appropriate for combined injuries. After placement the tube must be continually monitored for blood loss. If more than 1500 mL of blood is already in the chest or blood loss continues at a rate exceeding 200 mL/h, thoracotomy is indicated.

Immediate pericardiocentesis is indicated if cardiac tamponade is suspected because the patient has a penetrating injury in the vicinity of the heart, a distended neck vein, and/or muffled heart sounds.

The abdomen is first inspected for evidence of penetrating injury (e.g., gunshot or stab wounds); given the high incidence of associated intraabdominal injury, exploratory laparotomy is virtually always indicated. The traditional findings of intraabdominal injury include pain, guarding, rigidity, and loss of bowel sounds. However, in up to 20% of alert patients the abdominal exam may be misleading after blunt trauma. Thus the ancillary diagnostic tests, such as peritoneal lavage and abdominal CT scanning (discussed later), are often of primary impor-

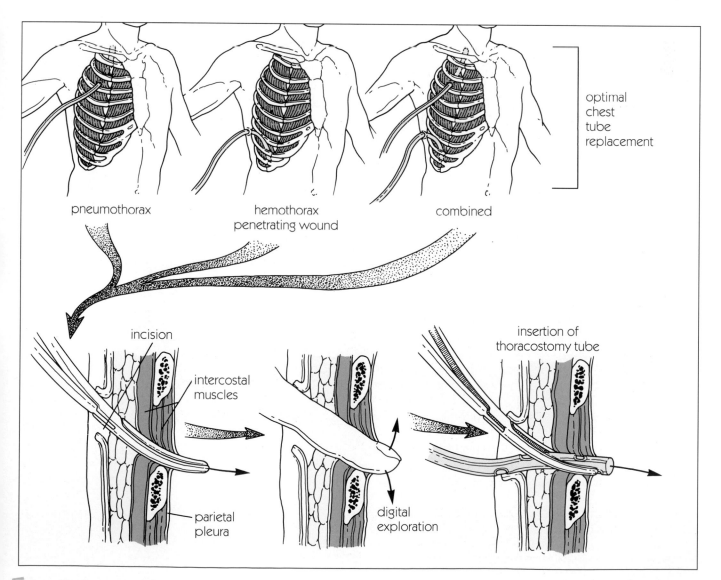

Figure 15.8 Technique of closed tube thoracostomy.

The Multiply Injured Patient

tance in determining the presence or absence of intraabdominal injury.

Extremity trauma is present in up to 80% of multitrauma patients but is rarely life-threatening. Splinting is usually accomplished in the prehospital treatment phase. Examination is directed to identifying and protecting open fractures and dislocations, and determining if there are associated vascular or neurologic injuries. Traumatic amputations, bilateral femoral shaft fractures, and major pelvic fractures demand increased attention and often rapid intervention because they are potentially life-threatening.

The secondary survey is completed with a full neurologic evaluation to determine the degree and extent of any associated head or spinal cord injuries and the necessity for skull x-rays, spine radiographs, CT scan, or MRI studies.

In any multiply injured patient tetanus prophylaxis must be considered. The need for tetanus immunization depends on the patient's immunization status and the risk of the wound. Immunization status is often not elicitable and many patients must be treated prophylactically (Fig. 15.9).

The trauma management protocol is completed when definitive care has been instituted for each organ system injury. However, trauma is not necessarily a static process. As one problem is addressed another may surface, or underlying medical problems may assume increasing importance. As an example, sepsis and organ failure are the most common causes of late death from trauma. Therefore, a high index of suspicion must be maintained, the trauma patient constantly re-evaluated, and diagnostic or treatment approaches readjusted to insure optimal chance for recovery.

TRAUMA SCORING SYSTEMS

A basic understanding of the systems for scoring trauma severity is important when dealing with multitrauma patients. The Glasgow Coma Score is a widely accepted scoring system used to quantify head injury severity, guide treatment, and give preliminary prognostic information. Similar scoring systems have been developed for the multitrauma patient. Most are based on the Abbreviated Injury Scale (AIS), which provides a numerical score to each injured system based on severity. The higher the score, the more likely it is that the patient will die. However, a simple arithmetic relationship does not exist. The

Figure 15.9 Tetanus Prophylaxis of the Injured Patient

History of Tetanus Immunization (doses)	Clean, Minor Wounds		Tetanus Prone Wounds	
	TD[1]	TIG	TD[1]	TIG[2]
Uncertain	yes	no	yes	yes
0–1	yes	no	yes	yes
2	yes	no	yes	no[3]
3 or more	no[4]	no	no[5]	no

[1] For individuals less than 7 years old, DTP (DT, if pertussis vaccine is contraindicated) is preferred to tetanus toxoid alone. For individuals 7 years old and older, TD is preferred to tetanus toxoid alone.

[2] When TIG and TD are given concurrently, separate syringes and separate sites should be used.

[3] Yes, if wound is more than 24 hours old.

[4] Yes, if more than 10 years since last dose.

[5] Yes, if more than 5 years since last dose. (More frequent boosters are not needed and can accentuate side effects.)

Reproduced with permission from the American College of Surgeons Committee on Truama. Advanced Trauma Life Support Course Instruction Manual. 1985:277.

Injury Severity Score (ISS) is derived from the AIS by summing the squares of the AIS values. The ISS has been shown to correlate not only with mortality but also with the length of hospital stay and the degree of permanent disability, provided the patient's age is taken into account.[7] Two major criticisms of the ISS are that it gives inadequate weight to associated head injuries and that it requires detailed identification of anatomic injury, which is usually only accurately determined after definitive management has occurred.

The Trauma Score was developed to overcome these problems by measuring the physiologic state (i.e., the cardiovascular, respiratory, and central nervous systems) of the patient immediately after injury (Fig. 15.10).[8] The

Figure 15.10 Trauma Score

		Points/Score
Respiratory rate	≥36/min	2
	25–35/min	3
	10–24/min	4
	0–9/min	1
	None	0
Respiratory expansion	Normal	1
	Shallow	0
	Retractive	0
Systolic blood pressure	≥ 90 mm Hg	4
	70–89 mm Hg	3
	50–69 mm Hg	2
	0–49 mm Hg	1
	No pulse	0
Capillary return	Normal	2
	Delayed	1
	None	0

Glasgow Coma Score (GCS)

Eye opening	
Spontaneous	4
To voice	3
To pain	2
None	1

Verbal response	
Oriented	5
Confused	4
Inappropriate words	3
Incomprehensible words	2
None	1

Motor response	
Obeys command	6
Localizes pain	5
Withdraw (pain)	4
Flexion (pain)	3
Extension (pain)	2
None	1

Total GCS Points	Score
14–15	5
11–13	4
8–10	3
5–7	2
3–4	1

Total	1–16

Trauma Score is appropriate for both assessment and trauma triage, and can be applied at the scene of the injury. Experience has demonstrated that patients likely to benefit from prompt diagnosis and timely definitive care at a trauma center have scores of twelve or less at the scene of injury.

More recently a system known as ASCOT has been evaluated as a more sensitive descriptor of multisystem injury. ASCOT separates severe head, thoracic, and abdominal injuries from other injuries in an attempt to provide better information for triage, treatment, and prognosis after trauma.

HYPOXIA, HYPOTENSION, AND NEUROLOGIC INJURY

The interrelationships of multisystem and neurologic injury are nowhere more clearly defined than they are regarding hypoxia and/or hypotension (Fig. 15.11). Recognition and prevention or treatment of associated hypoxia and hypotension in the multitraumatized, neurologically injured patient are of paramount importance. Miller et al. in 1978 were among the first to point out the magnitude of the problem.[9] In 100 consecutive severely head-injured patients on initial emergency room evaluation, 13% were hypotensive (systolic blood pressure <95 mm Hg) and 30% were hypoxic (PO_2 <65 mm Hg). Five years later pilot data from 581 comatose head-injured patients in the National Coma Data Bank found almost 20% hypoxic (PO_2 <60 mm Hg) and 31% hypotensive (systolic blood pressure <90 mm Hg) before definitive hospital treatment.

The increased morbidity and mortality in hypoxic/hypotensive head-injured patients has been clearly established. As early as 1977 Rose and coworkers found a 54% incidence of these factors in a group of patients who "talked and died."[10] Gildenberg and Makela found a correlation between time from head injury to intubation and outcome.[11] Similarly, the National Coma Data Bank found a 20% incidence of hypoxia in head-injured patients with a good outcome while 45% of patients with vegetative/dead outcomes were hypoxic.[2] It has also been found that there may be an association between hypoxia and a greater incidence of increased intracranial pressure.[12] Many studies have also shown an association between acute hypotension and poor outcome after head injury.[2,3,10]

The clinical effects of superimposed hypoxia and/or hypotension on the spinal cord injury patient have not been as clearly delineated. However, it is known from research data that hypoxia and ischemia are important in the propagation of further neuronal damage after spinal cord injury.[13]

THE NEUROLOGICALLY INJURED MULTITRAUMATIZED PATIENT

The multitraumatized neurologically injured patient may present particular difficulties in assessment and management. Specific questions often raised in this regard include airway protection and maintenance in association with potential spine injury; fluid resuscitation in the head-injured patient; abdominal evaluation in the unconscious or spinal cord injury patient; and timing of CT/MRI during initial evaluation and resuscitation.

AIRWAY PROTECTION AND MAINTENANCE

Avoiding head/neck hyperextension and hyperflexion is essential to airway control in patients with potential spine injuries. Upper airway obstruction is generally simply relieved by removing foreign debris or using chin lift or jaw thrust maneuvers that do not require any movement of the neck. However, if airway patency cannot be maintained, intubation is necessary. The safest intubation route in this situation is via the nasotracheal route with the neck in a neutral position. Head stabilization with manual in-line traction should be provided by an experienced member of the trauma team. Fiberoptic endotracheal intubation can also be accomplished safely in this setting; however, it may be too time consuming in the multi-

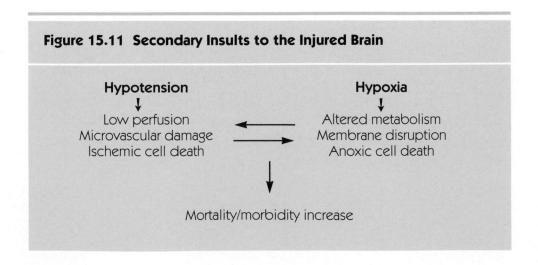

Figure 15.11 Secondary Insults to the Injured Brain

Hypotension → Low perfusion / Microvascular damage / Ischemic cell death

Hypoxia → Altered metabolism / Membrane disruption / Anoxic cell death

→ Mortality/morbidity increase

trauma patient. If a surgical airway must be provided, a cricothyroidotomy is generally the safest and most reliable way to proceed.

An associated issue is that of the risk of passing nasal tubes (nasotracheal or nasogastric) in multitrauma patients suspected of having a significant basilar skull fracture. There have been several dramatic reports of intracranial penetration of such tubes through areas of major bony disruption in the frontal fossa. In patients with routine basilar skull fractures who have either no or minimal evidence of CSF leakage there appears to be negligible risk in passing nasal tubes. However, in those patients with marked CSF rhinorrhea, significant bony disruption should be suspected and strong consideration given to using the oral route for all tubes.

However, with life-threatening airway problems, re-establishment and protection of the airway by any means should take precedence over concerns of spinal alignment or basilar skull disruption.

FLUID RESUSCITATION

There has been longstanding caution over the "excessive" fluid resuscitation of patients with head injury based on concerns about promoting cerebral edema formation and subsequent intracranial hypertension. Hypotension arising from brain injury is a terminal event resulting from brain stem failure. Thus hypotension in the head-injured patient is most often due to volume loss, which requires adequate fluid resuscitation to restore an optimal level of cerebral perfusion. Restoration of adequate cerebral perfusion may in itself result in significant neurologic improvement.

There are few systematic studies of the effects of fluid resuscitation on the outcome of head injury in the multitraumatized patient.[14] One study from Kings County Hospital in New York attempted to correlate intracranial pressure changes with aggressive fluid resuscitation (a mean of 5 L fluid resuscitation per patient) in a consecutive series of multitraumatized patients with associated head injury. No patient had a rise in intracranial pressure greater than 2 mm H_2O or a deterioration in neurologic exam during continuous infusion or bolus fluid therapy.[15] Thus the benefits of adequate fluid resuscitation, regardless of the total volume needed for stable blood pressure, may outweigh the potential disadvantages in the head-injured patient.

There is increasing interest in the use of hypertonic saline and dextran in trauma resuscitation. A 7.5% NaCl/12% dextran-70 solution significantly improved cardiac output over traditional resuscitation fluids.[16] It has been suggested that this regimen has a high plasma oncotic pressure that shifts extracellular fluid into the plasma space. Caution, however, is warranted when using this treatment in head-injured patients. While the 7.5% saline/dextran is superior to Ringer's lactate, with significantly less fluid infused early in resuscitation, the beneficial effects are not sustained and cerebral blood flow decreases 24 hours after injury.[17]

Mannitol is an ancillary method of fluid resuscitation in the head-injured patient. The hyperosmolar effect of osmotic diuretics, such as mannitol, causes transient increases in intravascular volume. However, as diuresis is induced, marked hypotension may be precipitated in the marginally compensated or resuscitated multitrauma victim. Thus osmotic diuretics must be used judiciously in the multitrauma patient lest the potential beneficial effects on lowering ICP be offset by subsequent hypotension and inadequate cerebral perfusion.

ABDOMINAL EVALUATION

Abdominal assessment after blunt trauma may be quite difficult and is often misleading in the multitrauma patient. Signs and symptoms of injury may not become apparent for hours or days. With associated head injury and unconsciousness or spinal cord injury and lack of sensation, the abdominal evaluation becomes treacherous.

Generally the physical examination guides a diagnosis of acute abdominal injury. However, when the physical examination cannot be relied upon, ancillary studies come into play. The two most frequently used are peritoneal lavage and abdominal CT scanning. Such tests are indicated as primary evaluations in unconscious patients, patients with cervical and thoracic spinal cord injury, and patients with unexplained shock.

Peritoneal lavage has proven quite reliable, with a 1% to 2% false negative/false positive rate over a wide variety of published studies.[18-20] There are numerous techniques for peritoneal lavage, but the safest is incising down to the peritoneum and introducing a large lavage catheter into the peritoneal cavity under direct vision (Fig. 15.12). A liter of saline is then introduced and the resultant effluent analyzed. Accepted parameters as heralds of significant intraabdominal injury are a red blood cell count greater than 100,000/mm^3, white blood cell count greater than 500/mm^3, spun hematocrit greater than 2, or the presence of bile, bacteria, or fecal material. A negative peritoneal lavage, however, does not rule out possible retroperitoneal injury.

Abdominal CT scans are becoming popular in the evaluation of stable patients suspected of harboring abdominal injury and may provide more specific and sensitive information regarding the degree and extent of specific organ injury (Fig. 15.13).[21-23]

TIMING OF CT/MRI IN INITIAL EVALUATION AND RESUSCITATION

CT may be critical in managing the head injury patient, and MRI is assuming greater importance in assessing acute spinal cord injury; however, the sequencing of these tests raises difficult questions in the multitrauma patient. Concerns arise over placing the patient in a relatively inaccessible location where vital signs cannot be fully monitored. A trauma-oriented CT scan of the head may take less than 10 minutes, while a spine MRI may take up to 1 hour. During a CT scan it is possible to monitor the ECG and blood pressure; however, during MRI only the ECG can be monitored continuously.

In general a hemodynamically unstable patient should not be subject to CT or MRI. The extreme example of this is patients who require immediate operative intervention—thoracotomy or laparotomy—for uncontrollable shock before assessment or treatment of an associated head or spine injury can be accomplished. Such situations are generally accompanied by marked hypotension that in and of itself renders the neurologic examination invalid. In such a setting, if there is strong suspicion of associated severe head injury based on information from the accident scene, one of two actions may be considered: the making of emergency burr holes or the monitoring and treatment of intracranial pressure during the operation.[24] If the burr holes indicate a significant extraaxial mass, simultaneous craniotomy can be undertaken. However, intracranial surgery in the midst of an emergency thoracotomy or laparotomy may prove technically quite difficult. The alternative, establishing intracranial pressure monitoring, is for the most part more easily accomplished, allowing initiation of appropriate medical therapy as indicated. Regardless of the action chosen, a CT scan can then be performed at the end of the operation or when the patient is felt to be hemodynamically stable.

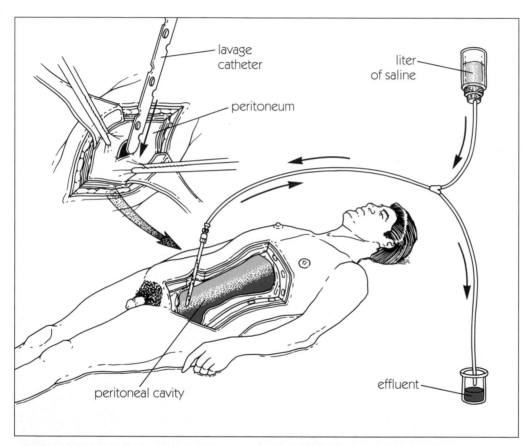

Figure 15.12 Surgical technique of open peritoneal lavage.

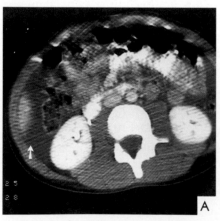

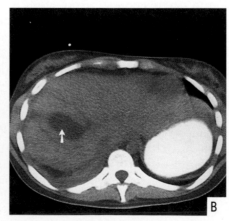

Figure 15.13 Abdominal CT scans posttrauma demonstrating (A) the presence of blood within the peritoneal cavity (arrows) and (B) a liver laceration (arrow).

REFERENCES

1. Bracken MB, Shepard MJ, Collins WF, et al. A randomized, controlled trial of methylprednisolone or naloxane in the treatment of acute spinal cord injury. *N Engl J Med.* 1990;322:1405–1411.
2. Eisenberg HM, Cayard C, Papanicolaou FF, et al. The effects of three potentially preventable complications on outcome after severe closed head injury. In: Ishal S, Nagai H, Brock M, eds. *Intracranial Pressure V.* Tokyo: Springer Verlag; 1983;549–553.
3. Klauber MR, Toutant SM, Marshall LF. A model for predicting delayed intracranial hypertension following severe head injury. *J Neurosurg.* 1984;61:695–699.
4. Commitee on Trauma. *Advanced Trauma Life Support.* Chicago, Ill: American College of Surgeons; 1985.
5. Velanovich V. Crystaloid vs. colloid resuscitation: a meta-analysis of mortality. *Surgery.* 1989;105:65–70.
6. Holcroft J, Vassar M, et al. 3% saline and 7% dextran-70 in the resuscitation of severely injured patients. *Ann Surg.* 1987;206:279–285.
7. Baker SP, O'Neill B, Haddon W, Long WB. The injury severity score: a method for describing patients with multiple injuries and evaluating emergency care. *J Trauma.* 1974;14:187–196.
8. HR, Sacco WJ, Commazzo AJ, et al. Trauma score. *Crit Care Med.* 1981;9:672–676.
9. Miller JD, Corales RL, Sweet RC, et al. Early insults to the injured brain. *JAMA.* 1978;240:439–442.
10. Rosc J, Balronen S, Jennett B. Avoidable factors contributing to death after head injury. *Br Med J.* 1977;21:615–618.
11. Gildenberg PL, Mekela ME. The effect of early intubation and ventilation on outcome following head trauma. In: Dacey RG, Winn RR, et al, eds. *Trauma of the Central Nervous System.* New York, NY: Raven Press; 1985.
12. Harr FL. Incidence and significance of early hypoxia in head-injured patients. *American Association of Neurological Surgery Abstract Book;* 1981.
13. Senter HJ, Venes JL. Altered blood flow and secondary injury in experimental spinal cord trauma. *J Neurosurg.* 1978;49:569–578.
14. Gunnar W, Jonasson O, et al. Head injury and hemorrhagic shock: studies of the blood-brain barrier and intracranial pressure after resuscitation with normal saline solution, 3% saline solution and dextran-40. *Surgery.* 1988;103:398–405.
15. Maltz S, Scalea T, Duncan A, et al. Fluid resuscitation in the head-injured patient. *American Association for the Surgery of Trauma Abstract Book;* 1989.
16. Halvorsen L, Gunther RA, Holcroft JW. Dose-response characteristics of hypertonic saline dextran solutions. *Surg Forum.* 1990;41:30–34.
17. Walsh J, Zhuang J, Shackford SR. Fluid resuscitation of focal brain injury and shock. *Surg Forum.* 1990;41:56–59.
18. Fisher RP, Beverlin BC, Engrav LH, et al. Diagnostic peritoneal lavage: 14 years and 2,568 patients later. *Am J Surg.* 1978;136:701–704.
19. Powell DC, Bivins BA, Bell RM. Diagnostic peritoneal lavage. *Surg Gynecol Obstet.* 1982;155:257–264.
20. Thal ER, Shires GT. Pertoneal lavage in blunt abdominal trauma. *Am J Surg.* 1973;125:64–69.
21. Federle LP, Crass RA, Jeffrey RB, Trunkcy DD. Computed tomography in blunt abdominal trauma. *Arch Surg.* 1982;17:645.
22. Federle MP, Goldberg HI, Kaiser JA, et al. Evaluation of abdominal trauma by computed tomography. *Radiology.* 1981;138:637–644.
23. Marx JA, Moore EE, Jorden RC, Eule J. Limitations of computed tomography in the evaluation of abdominal trauma. *J Trauma.* 1985;25:933–937.
24. Wilberger JE. Emergency burr holes: current role in neurosurgical acute care. In: Mangiardi JR, ed. *Topics in Emergency Medicine.* 1990;11:69-75.

REFERENCES

Chapter 16

Closed Head Injury

Raj K. Narayan

Head injury is arguably the most common cranial condition that neurosurgeons deal with, and unlike certain other clinical entities, it is likely to remain primarily under our purview for the foreseeable future. Contrary to popular belief, major strides have been made over the past three decades in reducing the mortality and morbidity from head injury. While controlled and strictly comparable data are hard to come by, well-documented series have demonstrated declining mortality due to severe head injury: from 50% in 1970 to around 36% in the 1980s. Although this is hard to prove conclusively, the most probable cause for this dramatic improvement in results is the wider availability and better application of emergency medical services and critical care methodologies.

The essential element of such intensive care is to maintain an optimal milieu in the injured brain to facilitate healing and to prevent secondary injury to the damaged neurons (Fig. 16.1). Most importantly, this means providing the brain with adequate oxygen and avoiding hyponatremia and hyperglycemia. Of these, the first priority is the maintenance of oxygenation. Unfortunately, this is also the most difficult to achieve, since several factors conspire against it, including mass lesions with elevated intracranial pressure (ICP), reduced blood pressure, and hypoxia secondary to pulmonary complications. Hence, these occurrences need to be monitored for constantly and treated early.

We are currently experiencing a very exciting period in the field of neurotrauma. The efforts of basic and clinical scientists in the area of CNS protectants are beginning to yield potentially useful drugs, some of which are already undergoing clinical trials.

CLASSIFICATION

While head injuries could be classified in several different ways, the most practical categorizations are based on mechanism, severity, and morphology (Fig. 16.2).

MECHANISM

Although the words "closed" and "penetrating" are widely used to describe types of head injuries, they are not mutually exclusive. For example, a depressed skull fracture could be assigned to either of these two categories, depending on the depth and severity of the bony injury. For practical purposes, the term *closed head injury* is usually associated with auto accidents, falls, and assaults, while *penetrating head injury* is most often associated with gunshot wounds and stab injuries. Penetrating head injuries are dealt with in Chapter 17.

SEVERITY

Prior to 1974, different authors used various terms to describe patients with head injury, making it virtually impossible to compare groups of patients from different centers. In 1974, Teasdale and Jennett,[1] by identifying the clinical signs that predicted outcome most reliably

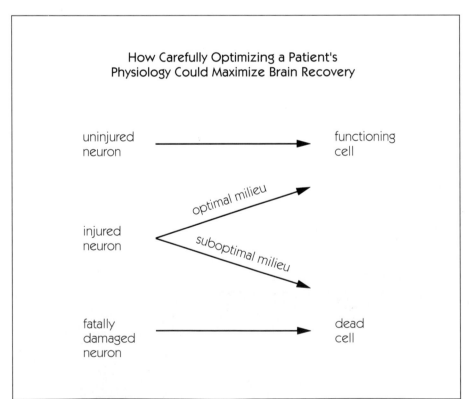

Figure 16.1 An optimal milieu must be maintained for healing in the injured brain.

and seemed to have the least interobserver variation, designed what has come to be known as the Glasgow Coma Scale (GCS). The introduction of the GCS (Fig. 16.3) brought some degree of uniformity into the head injury literature.[1] This scale has achieved widespread use for the description of patients with head injuries and has also been adopted for the description of patients with altered levels of consciousness due to other causes.

Jennett and Teasdale defined coma as the inability to obey commands, to utter words, and to open the eyes.[2] The patient who does not meet all three aspects of this definition is not considered to be comatose. In a series of 2000 patients with severe head injury, these authors observed 4% who did not speak but could obey commands and another 4% who uttered words but did not obey. Among patients who could neither obey nor speak, 16% opened their eyes and were therefore judged not to be in coma. Patients who open their eyes spontaneously, obey commands, and are oriented score a total of 15 points, whereas flaccid patients who do not open their eyes or talk score the minimum of 3 points. No single score within the range of 3 to 15 forms the cut-off point for coma. However, 90% of all patients with a score of 8 or less, and none of those with a score of 9 or more, are found to be in coma according to the preceding definition. Therefore, for all practical purposes, a GCS score of 8 or less has become the generally accepted definition of a comatose patient.

The distinction between patients with severe head injury and those with mild to moderate injury is thus fairly clear. However, distinguishing between mild and moderate head injury is more of a problem.[3] Somewhat arbitrarily, head-injured patients with a GCS score of 9 to 12 have been categorized as "moderate," and those with a GCS score of 13 to 15 have been designated "mild." Eighty percent of head injuries are categorized as mild, 10% as moderate, and 10% as severe. Williams, Levin, and Eisenberg have reported that neurobehavioral deficits in patients with mild head injury (GCS 13 to 15) and an intracranial lesion on initial CT scan were similar to those in patients with moderate head injury

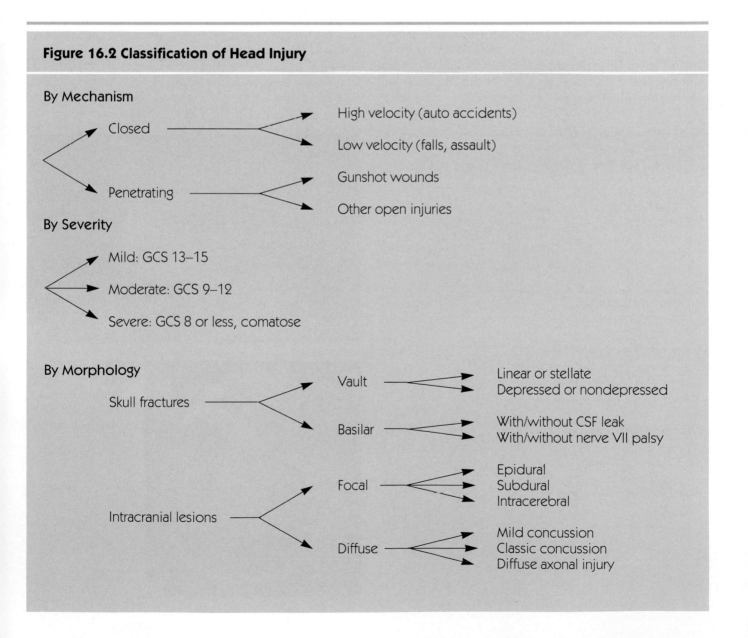

Figure 16.2 Classification of Head Injury

By Mechanism

Closed
- High velocity (auto accidents)
- Low velocity (falls, assault)

Penetrating
- Gunshot wounds
- Other open injuries

By Severity

- Mild: GCS 13–15
- Moderate: GCS 9–12
- Severe: GCS 8 or less, comatose

By Morphology

Skull fractures

Vault
- Linear or stellate
- Depressed or nondepressed

Basilar
- With/without CSF leak
- With/without nerve VII palsy

Intracranial lesions

Focal
- Epidural
- Subdural
- Intracerebral

Diffuse
- Mild concussion
- Classic concussion
- Diffuse axonal injury

(GCS 9 to 12), while patients with mild head injury uncomplicated by an intracranial lesion on CT scan did significantly better.[4]

MORPHOLOGY

The advent of CT scanning has revolutionized the classification and management of head injury. Thus, although certain patients who are rapidly deteriorating may be taken to surgery without a CT scan, the vast majority of severely injured patients should have the benefit of a CT scan before surgical intervention. Furthermore, frequent follow-up CT scans are essential because the morphologic picture in head injury often undergoes a remarkable evolution over the first few hours, days, and even weeks after the injury. Morphologically, head injuries may be broadly classified into two types: skull fractures and intracranial lesions.

Skull Fractures

Skull fractures may be seen in the cranial vault or skull base, may be linear or stellate, and may be depressed or nondepressed (Fig. 16.4). Basal skull fractures are harder to document on plain x-ray films and usually require CT scanning with bone-window settings for identification. The presence of clinical signs of a basal skull fracture should increase the index of suspicion and help in their identification. As a general guideline, frag-

ments depressed more than the thickness of the skull require elevation. Open or compound skull fractures have a direct communication between the scalp laceration and the cerebral surface because the dura is torn. These require early surgical repair.

The frequency of skull fractures varies, with more fractures being found in a population with a preponderance of severe injuries. A linear vault fracture increases the risk of intracranial hematoma by about 400 times in a conscious patient and by 20 times in a comatose patient. For this reason, the detection of a skull fracture generally warrants admission to the hospital for observation.

Intracranial Lesions

Intracranial lesions may be classified as focal or diffuse, although these two forms of injury frequently coexist. Focal lesions include epidural hematomas, subdural hematomas, and contusions (or intracerebral hematomas). Diffuse brain injuries, in general, have normal CT scans (Fig. 16.5A) but demonstrate an altered sensorium or even deep coma. The cellular basis of diffuse brain injury has become much clearer in recent years.

Epidural Hematomas

Epidural hematomas (Fig. 16.5B) are located outside the dura but within the skull. They are most often located in the temporal or temporoparietal region and

Figure 16.3 The Glasgow Coma Scale (GCS)

Eye Opening (E)

Spontaneous	4
To call	3
To pain	2
None	1

Motor Response (M)

Obeys commands	6
Localizes pain	5
Normal flexion (withdrawal)	4
Abnormal flexion (decorticate)	3
Extension (decerebrate)	2
None (flaccid)	1

Verbal Response (V)

Oriented	5
Confused conversation	4
Inappropriate words	3
Incomprehensible sounds	2
None	1

GCS sum score = (E+M+V); best possible score = 15; worst possible score = 3

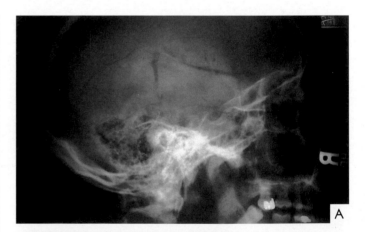

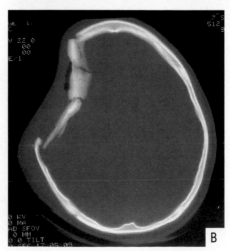

Figure 16.4
(A) Linear skull fracture.
(B) Depressed skull fracture.

often result from tearing of the middle meningeal vessels. While these clots are usually thought to be arterial in origin, they may be secondary to venous bleeding in at least one third of cases. Occasionally, an epidural hematoma may result from torn venous sinuses, particularly in the parietooccipital region or posterior fossa.

Although epidural hematomas are relatively uncommon (0.5% of all head-injured patients and 9% of those who are comatose), they should always be considered in the diagnostic process and treated rapidly. If treated early, the prognosis is usually excellent because the damage to the underlying brain is usually limited. Outcome is directly related to the status of the patient before surgery. For patients not in coma, the mortality from epidural hematoma approximates 0%, for the obtunded patient 9%, and for patients in coma 20%.

Subdural Hematomas

Subdural hematomas (Fig. 16.5C) are much more common than epidural hematomas (approximately 30% of severe head injuries). They occur most frequently from a tearing of bridging veins between the cerebral cortex and the draining sinuses. However, they can also be associated with lacerations of the brain surface or substance. A skull fracture may or may not be present.

The brain damage underlying acute subdural hematomas is usually much more severe and the prognosis is much worse than for epidural hematomas. The mortality in a general series may be around 60% but can be lowered by very rapid surgical intervention and aggressive medical management.[5]

Contusions and Intracerebral Hematomas

Pure cerebral contusions are fairly common. Their frequency has become much more apparent as the quality and number of CT scans have increased. Furthermore, contusions of the brain are almost always seen in association with subdural hematomas. The vast majority of contusions occur in the frontal and temporal lobes, although they can occur at almost any site, including the cerebellum and brain stem. The distinction between contusions and traumatic intracerebral hematomas remains somewhat ill-defined. The classic "salt-and-pepper" lesion is clearly a contusion, while a large hematoma clearly is not (Fig. 16.5D). However, there is a gray zone, and contusions can, over a period of hours or days, evolve into intracerebral hematomas.

Diffuse Injuries

Diffuse brain injuries form a continuum of progressively severe brain damage caused by increasing amounts of acceleration-deceleration injury to the brain. In its pure form, diffuse brain injury is the most common type of head injury.

A mild concussion is an injury in which consciousness is preserved, but there is a noticeable degree of temporary neurologic dysfunction. These injuries are exceedingly common and, because of their mild degree,

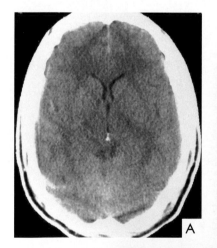
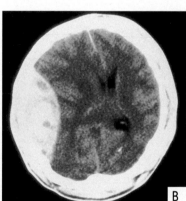
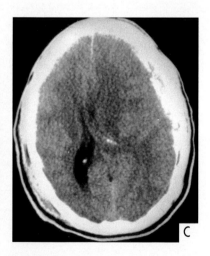

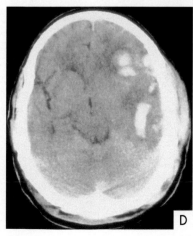

Figure 16.5 (A) Diffuse brain injury. (B) Epidural hematoma. (C) Subdural hematoma. (D) Intracerebral hematoma.

are often not brought to medical attention. The mildest form of concussion results in confusion and disorientation without amnesia. This syndrome is usually completely reversible and is associated with no major sequelae. Slightly more severe head injury causes confusion with both retrograde and posttraumatic amnesia.

A classic cerebral concussion is that posttraumatic state which results in loss of consciousness. This condition is always accompanied by some degree of retrograde and posttraumatic amnesia, and the length of posttraumatic amnesia is a good measure of the severity of the injury. The loss of consciousness is transient and re-versible—in a somewhat arbitrary definition, the patient has returned to full consciousness by 6 hours, although it is usually much sooner. While the great majority of patients with classic cerebral concussion have no sequelae other than amnesia for the events relating to the injury, some patients may have more long-lasting, although sometimes subtle, neurologic deficits.

Diffuse axonal injury (DAI) is the term used to describe prolonged posttraumatic coma that is not due to mass lesions or ischemic insults. There is loss of consciousness from the time of injury that continues beyond 6 hours. This phenomenon may further be broken down

---

Figure 16.6 Algorithm for Management of Mild Head Injury

Definition
The patient is awake, and may be oriented (GCS 13–15).

Initial Work-up
History
    Name, age, sex, race, occupation
    Mechanism of injury
    Time of injury
    Loss of consciousness immediately postinjury
    Subsequent level of alertness
    Amnesia: retrograde, antegrade
    Headache: mild, moderate, severe
    Seizures
General examination, rule out systemic injuries
Limited neurologic examination
Skull radiographs
Cervical spine and other radiographs as indicated
Blood alcohol level and urine toxic screen
CT scan of the head should ideally be obtained in all but the
    completely asymptomatic patient.

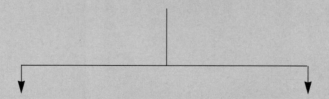

Admit to Hospital if There Is

Significant amnesia
History of loss of consciousness
Deteriorating level of consciousness
Moderate to severe headache
Significant alcoholic/drug-intoxication
Skull fracture
CSF leak—rhinorrhea or otorrhea
Significant associated injuries
No reliable companion at home
Abnormal CT scan

Discharge From ER if

The patient does not meet any of the criteria for
    admission.
Discuss need to return if any problems develop
    and issue a "warning sheet"
Schedule follow-up clinic visit, usually within 1
    week

into mild, moderate, and severe categories.[6] Mild DAI is relatively uncommon and is defined as that group in which coma lasts from 6 to 24 hours, with patients starting to follow commands by 24 hours. Moderate DAI is defined as coma lasting more than 24 hours without prominent brain stem signs. This is the most common form of DAI, comprising 45% of all cases of DAI. Severe DAI usually occurs in vehicular accidents and is the most devastating form. It comprises about 36% of all patients with DAI. These patients are rendered deeply comatose and remain so for prolonged periods of time. They often demonstrate evidence of decortication or decerebration and often remain severely disabled, if they survive. These patients often exhibit autonomic dysfunctions such as hypertension, hyperhidrosis, and hyperpyrexia, and were previously thought to have primary brain stem injury. It is now believed that diffuse axonal injury is the more common pathologic basis.

EVALUATION

MILD HEAD INJURY

Approximately 80% of patients presenting to the emergency room (ER) with head injury fall under the category of mild head injury (Fig. 16.6). These patients are awake but may be amnesic for events surrounding the injury. There may be a history of brief loss of consciousness, which is usually difficult to confirm. The issue is often confounded by alcohol or other intoxicants.

Most patients with mild head injury make uneventful recoveries, albeit with subtle neurologic sequelae. However, about 3% of patients deteriorate unexpectedly, and can become neurologically devastated if the decline in mental status is not noticed early.[7] How can a physician guard against such an occurrence? The classic struggle between "cost-effective" and the "best possible" management is clearly evident here, and practice varies in different centers.

Skull x-ray films may be examined for the following features: linear or depressed skull fractures, position of the pineal gland if calcified, air-fluid levels in the sinuses, pneumocephalus, facial fractures, and foreign bodies. The routine ordering of skull x-rays in patients with minor head injury has come under some criticism, and a multicenter study sponsored by the FDA has recommended guidelines for reducing the number of low-yield studies.[8] Based on an analysis of 7035 head-injured patients at 31 hospitals, the panel defined three levels of risk:

1. Low: Minimal initial signs and symptoms such as headache, dizziness, or scalp lacerations
2. Moderate: Initial signs such as vomiting, alcohol and drug intoxication, posttraumatic amnesia, or signs of a basilar or depressed fracture

3. High: Most serious initial symptoms such as depressed or decreasing level of consciousness, focal neurologic signs or penetrating injuries

In this study, approximately 75% of the 7035 patients would have been assigned to the low-risk group, 23% to the moderate-risk group, and 2% to the high-risk group.

How often does one find a skull fracture? This figure varies with the severity of injury, from 3% of patients with mild head injury (those not admitted) to 65% among those with severe head injuries.[9] The vault is involved three times as often as the base. It should be remembered, however, that basal fractures are often not visualized on initial skull films. Clinical signs of a fractured base—orbital hematoma, CSF rhinorrhea or otorrhea, hemotympanum, or Battle's sign—must be taken as presumptive evidence of a basal fracture and warrant admission for observation.

Ideally, a CT scan should be obtained in all patients with a history of loss of consciousness or amnesia after head injury.[10,11] If the patient is fully awake and alert and can be kept under observation for 12 to 24 hours, this study may be deferred or even canceled. In one study of 658 patients with mild head injury (GCS 13 to 15) who experienced brief loss of consciousness or amnesia, 18% had abnormalities on the initial CT scan and 5% required surgery.[9] Forty percent of patients with a GCS of 13 had abnormal CT scans and 10% required surgery, prompting the authors to suggest that perhaps these patients should be classified with the moderate rather than mild head injury group.[9] None of the 542 patients with normal CT scans on admission showed subsequent deterioration, and none needed surgery. Nevertheless, it is possible for patients with normal early scans to develop mass lesions a few hours later.

The cervical spine and other parts must be x-rayed if there is any pain or tenderness. Nonnarcotic analgesics such as acetaminophen are preferred, although codeine may be used if there is an associated painful injury. Tetanus toxoid must be administered if there are any associated open wounds. Routine blood tests are usually not necessary if there are no systemic injuries. A blood alcohol level and urine toxic screen can be useful both for diagnostic and for medicolegal purposes.

Our practice with a mildly head-injured patient with a normal CT scan is to discharge her or him to the care of a reliable companion, who is instructed according to a "warning sheet" to keep the patient under close observation for at least 12 hours and to bring the patient back if any adverse features develop. If no reliable companion is available, the patient is kept in the emergency room holding area for several hours with frequent neurologic checks and is then discharged if he or she appears stable.

If a lesion is noted on CT scan, the patient must be admitted and managed according to his or her neurologic progress over the next few days. A follow-up CT scan is usually obtained prior to discharge, or sooner in the case of neurologic deterioration. The manage-

that the presence of hypotension (systolic BP <90 mm Hg) in severely head-injured patients increases the mortality rate from 27% to 50%.[20] Furthermore, it was found that 35% of patients arriving at major trauma centers are hypotensive. While the airway is being established, another group of ER personnel should be checking the patient's pulse and blood pressure and taking steps to obtain venous access (see Chapter 15).

If the patient is hypotensive, it is vital to restore normal blood pressure as soon as possible. Hypotension is usually not due to the brain injury itself, except in the terminal stages when medullary failure supervenes. Far more commonly, hypotension is a marker of severe blood loss, which may be either "overt" or "occult," or possibly both (see Chapter 15). One must also consider associated spinal cord injury (with quadriplegia or paraplegia), cardiac contusion or tamponade, and tension pneumothorax as possible causes. While efforts are in progress to determine the cause of the hypotension, volume replacement should be initiated (see Chapter 15). The importance of routine abdominal paracentesis in the hypotensive comatose patient has been demonstrated.[21]

It must be emphasized that *a patient's neurologic examination is meaningless as long as he or she is hypotensive.* Time after time, we have seen hypotensive patients who are unresponsive to any form of stimulation revert to a near-normal neurologic examination soon after normal blood pressure has been restored.

Catheters

A Foley catheter (16 to 18 Fr for average adults) should be carefully inserted and urine sent for urinalysis and toxic screen (when appropriate). Gross hematuria suggests renal injury and is an indication for an emergency intravenous pyelogram. Mild hematuria may be secondary to traumatic catheterization, renal contusion or, rarely, to a dissecting aortic aneurysm. Special attention must be paid to maintaining accurate records of fluid intake and output, especially in children and the elderly. In addition to ensuring fluid balance, such records help assess blood loss and monitor renal perfusion.

A nasogastric tube, preferably a Salem sump (double-lumen plastic catheter), should be inserted and connected to a wall suction unit. Potential complications of this procedure, such as intracranial passage of the tube secondary to a basal skull fracture, must be kept in mind. In patients with anterior basal skull fractures it is probably wise to pass the tube under direct vision with a laryngoscope or to pass it per os.

Diagnostic Radiographs

As soon as the preliminary steps towards cardiopulmonary stabilization have been taken, diagnostic radiographs should be obtained.

Cervical spine films (cross-table lateral and anteroposterior) are the first to be taken in the severely traumatized patient and must be read by a radiologist or neurosurgeon before the patient's neck can be moved. Features to look for in this study are loss of alignment of the vertebral bodies, bony fractures or compressions, loss of alignment of the facet joints, and prevertebral soft tissue swelling (more than 5 mm opposite the C-3 vertebral body is significant). Every effort must be made to visualize the lower cervical levels (C6-T1); these are often obscured by the shoulders, especially in heavy-set patients. Fracture-subluxations at these levels may be overlooked if the films are not repeated with caudal traction on both arms and greater x-ray penetration (Fig. 16.9). If these maneuvers also fail, a "swimmer's view" lateral film can be obtained. If any of these films show any of the abnormalities listed above, the neck must remain immobilized in a hard collar (Philadelphia) pending further studies (high-resolution CT scan or polytomogram).

The chest film is useful in ruling out endotracheal tube malposition, pneumothorax, hemothorax, lung contusion, hemopericardium, rib fractures, thoracic spine fractures, and other thoracic pathology that may have a bearing on patient management.

Although skull films (anteroposterior and lateral) have been somewhat overshadowed by CT scanning, they can help in identifying maxillofacial injuries, depressed skull fractures, and penetrating injuries. The

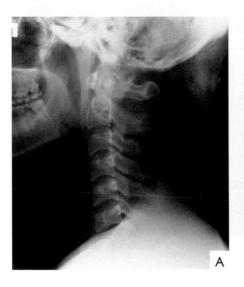
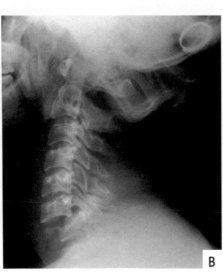

Figure 16.9 (A) The lower cervical spine is obscured by the shoulders. (B) Traction on the shoulders reveals a fracture-subluxation at C6-7.

A

B

presence of intracranial air (pneumocephalus) or of an air-fluid level in one of the sinuses can alert the clinician to a basal skull fracture that might otherwise have gone undetected.

A single anteroposterior abdominal film (KUB) is usually taken in trauma patients. This may help identify large retroperitoneal hematomas, lumbosacral spine fractures, distended viscera, and possibly subdiaphragmatic air.

Anteroposterior and lateral pelvic films are usually obtained, looking for pelvic injuries which may be the site of significant blood loss. The extremities may be studied whenever indicated to rule out fractures or subluxations.

General Examination

During the process of cardiopulmonary stabilization, the clinician conducts a rapid general examination looking for other injuries. In one series of severely head-injured patients, more than 50% had additional major systemic injuries requiring care by other specialists (Fig. 16.10).[17] One must check for head and neck, thoracic, abdominal, pelvic, and spinal injuries, and injuries involving extremities (see Chapter 15).

Neurologic Examination

As soon as the patient's cardiopulmonary status has been stabilized, a rapid and directed neurologic examination is performed (Fig. 16.11). Although various factors may confound an accurate evaluation of the patient's neurologic state (e.g., hypotension, hypoxia, or intoxication), valuable data can nevertheless be obtained. If a patient demonstrates variable responses to stimulation, or if the response on each side is different, the best response appears to be a more accurate prognostic indicator than the worst response. To follow trends in an individual patient's progress, however, it is better to report both the best and the worst responses. In other words, the right-side and left-side motor responses should be recorded separately. As the pain stimuli applied by different examiners are often variable, deep nail-bed pressure may be used as a standard stimulus.

One should not limit the examination to the GCS. Other important data in the initial assessment of patients with impaired consciousness are the patient's age, vital signs, pupillary response, and eye movements.[22] The GCS provides a simple grading of the arousal and functional capacity of the cerebral cortex, while the pupillary responses and eye movements serve as measures of brain stem function. Advanced age, hypotension, and hypoxia all adversely affect outcome. Indeed, there is considerable interplay between all these factors in determining the ultimate outcome in the severely head-injured patient.

Pupils

Careful observation of pupil size and response to light is important during the initial examination (Fig. 16.12). A well-known early sign of temporal lobe herniation is mild dilation of the pupil and a sluggish pupillary light response. Compression or distortion of the oculomotor nerve during tentorial-uncal herniation impairs the function of the parasympathetic axons that transmit efferent signals for pupillary constriction, resulting in mild pupillary dilation. Sometimes, bilateral miotic pupils (1 to 3 mm) can occur in the early stages of central cephalic herniation due to compromise of the pupillomotor sympathetic pathways originating in the hypothalamus, permitting a predominance of parasympathetic tone and pupillary constriction. In either instance, continued herniation causes increasing dilation of the pupil and paralysis of its light response. With full mydriasis (8 to 9 mm pupil), ptosis and paresis of the medial rectus and other ocular muscles innervated by the oculomotor nerve appear. A bright light is always necessary to determine pupillary light responses. A magnifying lens such as the +20-diopter lens on a standard ophthalmoscope is helpful in distinguishing between a weak and an absent pupillary light reaction, especially if the pupil is small.

Figure 16.10 Systemic Injuries in 100 Patients with Severe Head Injury

Type of Injury	Incidence (%)
Long-bone or pelvic fracture	32
Maxillary or mandibular fracture	22
Major chest injury	23
Abdominal visceral injury	7
Spinal injury	2

(Adapted with permission from Miller JD, Sweet RC, Narayan RK, Becker DP. Early insults to the injured brain. JAMA. 1978;240:439–442)

Figure 16.11 Initial Neurologic Examination in Head Injury

Glasgow Coma Score
Pupillary response to light
Eye movements
    Oculocephalic (doll's eye)
    Oculovestibular (caloric)
Motor power
Gross sensory examination

Recognition of additional pupillary disorders that can occur in an unconscious patient is useful in the examination of the patient with head trauma (see Chapter 3). Disruption of the afferent arc of the pupillary light reflex within the optic nerve is detected by the swinging flashlight test. As the flashlight is swung from the normal eye to the injured eye, injury to the optic nerve is indicated by a paradoxic response of the pupil: dilation rather than constriction. This paradoxic pupillary dilation is termed an afferent pupillary defect or Marcus-Gunn pupil, and in the absence of opacification of the ocular media it is unequivocal evidence of optic nerve injury.

Bilaterally small pupils suggest that the patient has used certain drugs, particularly opiates, or has one of several metabolic encephalopathies or a destructive lesion of the pons. In these conditions pupillary light responses can usually be seen with a magnifying lens. Unilateral Horner's pupil is seen occasionally with brain stem lesions, but in the trauma patient attention should be given to the possibility of a disrupted efferent sympathetic pathway at the apex of the lung, base of the neck, or ipsilateral carotid sheath. Midposition pupils with variable light responses can be observed in all stages of coma. Traumatic oculomotor nerve injury is the diagnosis in patients with a history of a dilated pupil from the onset of injury, an improving level of consciousness, and appropriate ocular muscle weakness. A mydriatic pupil (6 mm or more) occurs occasionally with direct trauma to the globe of the eye. This traumatic mydriasis is usually unilateral and is not accompanied by ocular muscle paresis. Finally, bilaterally dilated and fixed pupils in patients with head injury may be the result of inadequate cerebral vascular perfusion caused by hypotension secondary to blood loss or elevation of intracranial pressure to a degree that impairs cerebral blood flow. Return of the pupillary response may occur promptly after the restoration of blood flow, if the period of inadequate perfusion has not been too long.

Eye Movements

Ocular movements are an important index of the functional activity that is present within the brain stem reticular formation. If the patient is sufficiently alert to follow simple commands, a full range of eye movements is easily obtained and the integrity of the entire ocular motor system within the brain stem can be confirmed. In states of depressed consciousness, voluntary eye movement is lost and there may be dysfunction of the neural structures activating eye movements. In these instances, oculocephalic or oculovestibular responses are used to determine the presence or absence of an eye-movement disorder (see Chapter 3). If a neck fracture has been excluded, function of the pontine gaze center is quickly ascertained by the oculocephalic maneuver.

The oculovestibular response can be tested with ice water and only a small expenditure of time. Obstructions within the external auditory canal due to blood or cerumen must be removed, and ocular muscle movement may be limited in patients with orbital edema. In alert patients, cold caloric stimulation causes fast-phase nystagmus in the direction opposite the tonic eye deviation. The mnemonic "COWS" (cold opposite, warm same) refers to this condition. However, in comatose patients, functional suppression of the reticular activating system is reflected by the absence of nystagmus in response to caloric stimulation, so that only the tonic eye deviation is seen (cold same). Thus, irrigation with cold water in a comatose patient causes ipsilateral deviation of the eyes.

While oculocephalic and caloric testing is being performed, infranuclear, internuclear, and supranuclear

Figure 16.12 Interpretation of Pupillary Findings in Head Injury Patients

Pupillary Size	Light Response	Interpretation
Unilaterally dilated	Sluggish or fixed	Nerve III compression secondary to tentorial herniation
Bilaterally dilated	Sluggish or fixed	Inadequate brain perfusion Bilateral nerve III palsy
Unilaterally dilated	Cross-reactive (Marcus-Gunn)	Optic nerve injury
Bilaterally miotic	May be difficult to determine	Drugs (opiates) Metabolic encephalopathy Pontine lesion
Unilaterally miotic	Preserved	Injured sympathetic pathway (e.g., carotid sheath injury)

ocular motility disorders are recognizable. A destructive lesion of a frontal or pontine gaze center results in tonic overaction of the opposite frontal-pontine axis for horizontal eye movement. This overaction results in ipsilateral deviation of the eyes with frontal lobe lesions, and contralateral gaze deviation with pontine lesions.

Third and sixth nerve palsies are generally not difficult to recognize in patients with head injury. Fourth nerve palsies cannot ordinarily be identified in coma because of the select action of the superior oblique muscle. In alert and recovering patients, however, superior oblique paresis causes troublesome double vision, especially with downward and inward gaze. Head tilt opposite the side of the paretic muscle lessens the diplopia, while ipsilateral tilt of the head increases it. Internuclear ophthalmoplegia is suggested by select adduction paresis without additional involvement of the pupil, lid, or vertical muscles innervated by the third nerve. This ophthalmoplegia results from disruption of the ipsilateral medial longitudinal fasciculus that connects the oculomotor subnucleus for medial rectus neurons to the contralateral horizontal gaze center. Either bilateral or unilateral internuclear ophthalmoplegia may be seen, depending on the extent of the brain stem trauma.

Motor Function
The basic examination is completed by a gross test of motor strength, since severely head-injured patients are not sufficiently responsive for such a determination to be reliably made. Each extremity is examined and graded on the internationally used scale shown in Figure 16.13.

Diagnostic Procedures
As soon as a patient's cardiorespiratory condition has been stabilized and a preliminary neurologic examination completed, it behooves the physician to rule out the presence of an intracranial mass lesion. The patient is by this time intubated, often paralyzed with pancuronium (Pavulon) or a similar agent, and on mechanical ventilation. This prevents the patient from straining and moving around, thus avoiding intracranial pressure surges and greatly enhancing the quality of the diagnostic studies. Needless to say, CT scanning has rendered all other diagnostic tests virtually obsolete. However,

other tests have to be used in certain instances either to substitute for CT scanning or, as in the case of angiography, to obtain certain supplemental data.

Computed Tomography
CT scanning is clearly the procedure of choice in the evaluation of the head-injured patient and has probably significantly improved outcome after head injury.[23] It is strongly recommended that an emergency CT scan be obtained as soon as possible (preferably within half an hour) after admission with a severe head injury. Centers dealing with a large number of such patients must make arrangements to have CT technicians in the hospital on a 24-hour basis, or within easy accessibility in an emergency. We also tend to repeat CT scans whenever there is a change in the patient's clinical status or an unexplained rise in intracranial pressure.

In a prospective study of CT scan abnormalities in 207 severely head-injured patients, we found the initial CT scan to be normal in 30% of cases. The remaining 70% of patients had CT scan abnormalities: low-density lesions in 10%, high-density nonsurgical lesions in 19%, and high-density lesions requiring surgery in 41%.[15]

Edema is seen on CT as a zone of low density associated with mass effect on the adjacent ventricles reflected as compression, distortion, and displacement of the ventricular system. The edema may be focal, multifocal, or diffuse. With diffuse cerebral edema it may be hard to appreciate the lower density since no area of normal brain density is available for comparison. In such cases there is usually bilateral ventricular compression which may be so gross that the ventricular system is not seen, especially in children. The picture of diffuse brain swelling on CT can be secondary to edema or vascular engorgement.

Cerebral contusions are seen as nonhomogenous areas of high density often interspersed with areas of low density ("salt and pepper" appearance). The CT appearance results from multiple small areas of hemorrhage within the brain substance, associated with areas of edema (see Fig. 16.5D). The margin is usually poorly defined. A mass effect is often seen, although this may be minimal. Depending on the extent of hemorrhage, the degree of edema, and the time course, a contusion may appear predominantly dense or lucent.

Although it is not always possible to differentiate between subdural and epidural hematomas on CT, the latter are typically biconvex or lenticular in shape, because the close attachment of the dura to the inner table of the skull prevents the hematoma from spreading (see Fig. 16.5B). Approximately 20% of patients with an extracerebral hematoma have blood in both the epidural and subdural spaces at operation or autopsy. Since there is little chance of epidural blood mixing with CSF, these lesions appear as uniformly dense collections and are rarely isodense. However, they may develop in a delayed fashion, especially after evacuation of a contralateral "balancing" lesion.

Figure 16.13 Motor Function Scale	
Normal power	5
Moderate weakness	4
Severe weakness (antigravity)	3
Severe weakness (not antigravity)	2
Trace movement	1
No movement	0

The typical subdural hematoma is more diffuse than an epidural hematoma and has a concave inner margin that follows the surface of the brain (see Fig. 16.5C). The distinction between acute, subacute, and chronic lesions is somewhat arbitrary. However, most acute subdural hematomas are hyperdense, most subacute lesions are isodense or of mixed density, and most chronic hematomas are hypodense as compared with brain tissue. Effacement of the cerebral sulci over the convexity and distortion of the ipsilateral lateral ventricle may suggest the presence of an isodense hematoma.

Traumatic intracerebral hematomas are usually located in the frontal and anterior temporal lobes, although they can occur in virtually any area. The majority of hematomas develop immediately after the injury, but delayed lesions are often noted, usually within the first week. They are high-density lesions and are usually surrounded by zones of low density due to edema. Traumatic hematomas are more often multiple than hematomas from other causes.

Traumatic intraventricular hemorrhage was previously believed to have a uniformly poor prognosis, but this is no longer considered true. It is frequently associated with parenchymal hemorrhage. The blood becomes isodense relatively rapidly and often disappears completely within a couple of weeks. A ventriculostomy is placed in the less bloody ventricle and CSF drainage is used to reduce pressure and drain away the blood.

Acute obstructive hydrocephalus may develop secondary to a posterior fossa hematoma that obstructs the ventricular pathways. However, delayed hydrocephalus is far more common, occurring in about 6% of patients with severe head injury. This communicating hydrocephalus results from blood in the subarachnoid space and is often evident by the 14th day after injury, although it can certainly become evident later.

Acute ischemic infarction appears as a low-density area compared with the adjacent brain. The infarction may be detectable on CT scan within 24 hours of onset and over 60% are clearly seen by 7 days. Contrast enhancement improves the diagnostic yield by nearly 15%, and magnetic resonance imaging (MRI) is even more sensitive.

Ventriculography

Before the advent of CT scanning, air ventriculography and angiography were the most important emergency radiologic tests for evaluating comatose head-injured patients. The former was favored because of the rapidity with which it could be obtained, even though the latter could provide more information. Ventriculography provides two crucial pieces of information: the degree of supratentorial brain shift and the intracranial pressure. If the procedure is performed in a methodical and standardized fashion, the ventricle can usually be cannulated to provide a satisfactory ICP measurement and air study, even when the patient has a major ventricular shift or slit-like ventricles secondary to compression.

Angiography

Angiography may be undertaken in the acutely head-injured patient when CT scanning is not available, when vascular injury is suspected, or when the findings on CT are not consistent with the patient's neurologic status. Traumatic carotid artery dissection may present with Horner's syndrome, dysphasia, hemiparesis, obtundation, and monoparesis. When an isodense subdural hematoma is suspected, its presence can usually be confirmed by altering the CT window setting or with a contrast-enhanced study, before resorting to angiography.

Supratentorial mass lesions usually cause a contralateral shift of the anterior cerebral artery and the internal cerebral vein (Fig. 16.14). The latter, being closer to the midpoint of the cranium, is less affected by rotation of the film—a common problem due to rotation of the head to either side. Although displacement of the vessels does not provide any features differentiating between parenchymal swelling and hematomas, a study of the pattern can help localize the lesion. Frontal lesions cause a bowing of the anterior cerebral artery, the so-called "rounded shift," with limited displacement, if any, of the internal cerebral vein. Parietal lesions tend to cause a "square shift" of the anterior cerebral artery primarily due to widening of the unyielding falx cerebri posteriorly, and the internal cerebral vein is more markedly displaced. Temporal lobe lesions result in medial displacement of the internal carotid artery bifur-

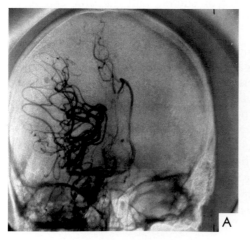 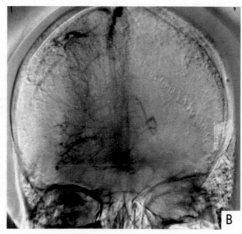

Figure 16.14 Angiograms showing severe mass effect secondary to a right acute subdural hematoma. **(A)** Arterial phase. The middle cerebral branches are displaced towards the midline and the pericallosal artery is markedly shifted across the midline due to subfalcine herniation. **(B)** Venous phase. The internal cerebral vein is shifted 2 cm towards the left.

cation and a characteristic upward displacement of the middle cerebral artery group. Extraaxial mass lesions usually appear as avascular areas on angiography. The classic appearance of an extraaxial hematoma on the AP view consists of a clear gap between the inner table of the skull and the small vessels on the surface of the brain as seen in the venous phase.

Infratentorial mass lesions are difficult to detect angiographically, and vertebral injections are rarely undertaken for this purpose. A posterior fossa mass may be suspected if there is evidence of hydrocephalus on the carotid films, i.e., upward sweep of the pericallosal artery on the lateral film and a lateral bowing of the thalamostriate vessels on the anteroposterior films.

Transtentorial herniation is seen on anteroposterior and lateral carotid angiograms as marked stretching of the anterior choroidal artery as a result of medial uncal displacement. If the posterior communicating arteries are visible, these will also be seen to be stretched and sometimes compressed against the posterior clinoid processes. The posterior cerebral arteries are inferiorly displaced on lateral view and are seen to be medially displaced along with both superior cerebellar arteries on anteroposterior view due to hippocampal gyrus herniation.

SURGICAL THERAPY

INDICATIONS FOR SURGERY

It is difficult to lay down hard and fast rules regarding the management of a disease as diverse as head injury. However, we have arrived at certain guidelines that have proven useful "in the trenches." Some of these practices are based on hard data, some on clinical prejudice, and some on an irresistible desire to simplify a hopelessly complicated problem.

An important reason for operating on a mass lesion is a midline shift of 5 mm or more. Such a shift may be demonstrated by CT scan, angiography, or ventriculography. Most epidural, subdural, or intracerebral hematomas associated with a midline shift of 5 mm or more are surgically evacuated. In a patient who has a small hematoma causing less than 5 mm shift and is alert and neurologically intact, a conservative approach is justified. However, the patient may deteriorate, and very close observation is vital. Should there be any change in mental status, a repeat CT scan should be obtained immediately.

Our policy is to operate on all comatose patients with an intracranial mass lesion and 5 mm or more of midline shift unless they are brain-dead. This policy is based on evidence that some patients with bilaterally nonreactive pupils, impaired oculocephalic responses, and decerebrate posturing can nevertheless make a good recovery. In one series, 3 of 19 such patients who were treated maximally ended up in the "good" or "moderately disabled" category, despite the foreboding constellation of signs.[24]

The management of brain contusions is somewhat less clear-cut. Galbraith and Teasdale,[25] in their series of 26 patients with acute traumatic intracranial hematomas who were managed without surgery, found that all patients with ICP greater than 30 mm Hg eventually deteriorated and required surgery. In contrast, only one patient with ICP less than 20 mm Hg deteriorated. Patients in the 20 to 30 mm Hg range were about evenly divided between the surgical and nonsurgical groups.

We have recently analyzed our experience with 130 head-injured patients with pure contusions who were managed with CT scanning and ICP monitoring as needed.[26] This study showed that patients with brain contusions who could follow commands at admission did not require ICP monitoring and, as a rule, did well with simple observation. However, those who could not follow commands (in the absence of a focal lesion in the speech area) often had intracranial hypertension and needed to have their ICP monitored. The majority of these patients who had a midline shift of 5 mm or more required surgery.

It has been demonstrated conclusively that patients with a large (over 30 mL) temporal lobe hematoma have a much greater risk of developing tentorial herniation than those with a frontal or parietooccipital lesion.[27] The bias should therefore tilt towards early surgery in such cases.

Once a decision has been made as to whether the patient is a surgical candidate or not, he or she is promptly moved to the operating room or to the NICU, respectively. If the patient is harboring a mass lesion, mannitol (1 to 2 g/kg) should be administered en route to the operating room. In addition, the patient should be hyperventilated to achieve an arterial P_{CO_2} of 25 to 30 mm Hg. As in all the maneuvers undertaken thus far, time is of the essence. The sooner the mass lesion is evacuated, the better the possibility of a good recovery.[5] If, on the other hand, no surgical lesion is found, the patient is carefully monitored in the NICU, both clinically and with various physiologic parameters, notably ICP recordings and serial CT scans. Any rise in ICP above 20 mm Hg which cannot be readily explained and reversed or any deterioration in neurologic status warrants prompt repetition of the CT scan followed by appropriate corrective measures.

Since there is great concern about increased intracranial pressure due to a mass lesion, the anesthetic agents that are used in head-injured patients preferably should not increase the ICP. Nitrous oxide has only a slight vasodilatory effect and generally does not cause significant ICP increase. It is therefore considered a good agent for use in the head-injured patient. A commonly used combination is nitrous oxide with oxygen, intravenous muscle relaxant, and thiopental. Hyperventilation and mannitol prior to and during induction can blunt the vasodilatory effect and limit intracranial hypertension to some degree while the cranium is being opened. If, during surgery, malignant brain swelling occurs that is refractory to hyperventilation and mannitol, pentobarbital in large doses (5 to 10 mg/kg) should be used. This agent can cause hypotension, especially in hypovolemic patients, and should therefore be used with caution.

SUBDURAL HEMATOMAS

Acute subdural hematomas may result from bleeding from lacerated brain, ruptured cortical vessels, or an avulsed bridging vein. The most common sites for brain injury are the inferior frontal lobes and the anterior temporal lobes. In the surgical management of subdural hematomas, a large frontotemporoparietal question-mark-shaped incision is recommended. This allows the surgeon to deal with bleeding near the midline as well as to debride effectively parts of the frontal, temporal, and parietal lobes as needed. If the patient is deteriorating rapidly, a quick temporal decompression can be performed via a small craniectomy before opening up the rest of the flap. This maneuver could reduce the probability of tentorial herniation. A generous subtemporal craniectomy may be useful in postoperative intracranial pressure control. Operative ultrasound can be useful in ruling out the presence of an intracerebral hematoma or a growing mass lesion on the opposite side of the brain. If a hematoma cannot be detected with ultrasound but there is evidence of brain swelling, a CT scan of the head is performed immediately after surgery.

EPIDURAL HEMATOMAS

Epidural hematomas are most often located in the temporal region and often result from tearing of the middle meningeal vessels due to a temporal bone fracture. Venous epidural hematomas may occur as a result of a skull fracture or an associated venous sinus injury. These tend to be smaller and usually have a more benign course. Such hematomas often present several hours or days after the initial injury and can be managed nonsurgically. However, usually an epidural hematoma represents a surgical emergency and should be evacuated as rapidly as possible. Every effort should be made to relieve the pressure as soon as possible. A more localized craniotomy flap is warranted for epidural hematomas.

CONTUSIONS/INTRACEREBRAL HEMATOMAS

Contusions are most often located in the anterior and inferior frontal lobes as well as the anterior temporal lobes. Quite commonly, the CT appearance of a contusion evolves over several days so that what are initially small "salt and pepper" lesions coalesce to form hematomas. This phenomenon is also termed delayed traumatic intracerebral hematoma (DTICH). Patients who are awake and alert but demonstrate cerebral contusions can be managed without surgery in the vast majority of cases.[26] However, patients who are comatose and have a significant midline shift usually need surgery. Between these two extremes, there are patients who demonstrate alterations in levels of consciousness or focal neurologic deficits; in these, the decision to undertake surgical debridement is not always easy. As a general rule, debridement of the left frontal and temporal lobes is undertaken more reluctantly because the speech area is on this side.

DEPRESSED SKULL FRACTURES

A skull fracture is considered significantly depressed if the outer table of the skull lies below the level of the inner table of the surrounding bone. Sometimes such depression may not be evident on plain x-rays, but it is usually seen clearly on the CT scan. Most closed depressed fractures occur in young children and may be of the pingpong ball variety. Surgery may be undertaken in such cases for cosmetic reasons or because of brain compression. In compound depressed fractures, the wounds are often dirty and contaminated. Hair, skin, or other foreign debris may be insinuated between the depressed bone fragments. Therefore, except in the simplest of injuries, the use of the operating room for the closure of such wounds is recommended.

VENOUS SINUS INJURIES

Injuries of the major venous sinuses are among the most difficult problems a neurosurgeon has to face. As a general rule, ligation of the anterior third of the superior sagittal sinus is tolerated well; ligation of the posterior third is most likely to produce massive venous infarction of the brain. Ligation of the middle third of the superior sagittal sinus has somewhat unpredictable effects. A dominant transverse sinus usually cannot be safely ligated. While the use of shunts in the repair of these major sinuses has been often described, in our experience simple pressure with the use of hemostatic agents is much more practical in the majority of cases.

POSTERIOR FOSSA HEMATOMAS

Posterior fossa hematomas, fortunately, are less common than supratentorial hematomas. In general, an aggressive surgical approach is recommended for most of these lesions because the patient can deteriorate very rapidly. Because it generally takes longer to expose the posterior fossa and because the brain stem structures are likely to suffer irreversible damage from a shorter period of compression, the surgeon does not have much leeway in terms of time.

INTRACRANIAL PRESSURE

Since the early 1970s, there has been an increasing interest in ICP monitoring and control (see Chapter 2).

This has been associated with progressive evolution of related technology. However, the intraventricular catheter or ventriculostomy remains the most widely used and most useful device for measuring intracranial pressure and helping in its control.[28] Recently, the emphasis has shifted from ICP control per se to maintaining cerebral perfusion pressure.[29]

Cerebral perfusion pressure (CPP) is the mean arterial blood pressure minus intracranial pressure. It is useful to follow cerebral perfusion pressure rather than intracranial pressure alone since there is evidence that suggests that CPPs of less than 60 mm Hg are generally associated with poorer outcomes and pressures of greater than 80 mm Hg are preferable.[29-31] It is certainly possible that too great a CPP may also have a deleterious effect.

Head injury is the most common indication for ICP monitoring. As a general rule, patients who can follow simple commands need not be monitored and may satisfactorily be followed clinically. In patients who are unable to follow commands and have an abnormal CT scan, the incidence of intracranial hypertension is high (53% to 63%), and monitoring is warranted.[18] Severely head-injured patients with normal CT scans generally have a lower incidence of hypertension (approximately 13%) unless they have two or more of the following adverse features at admission: systolic blood pressure less than 90 mm Hg, unilateral or bilateral motor posturing, or age over 40 years. In the presence of these adverse features, the incidence of intracranial hypertension even in patients with normal CT scans is as high as in those with abnormal CT scans on admission.[18] Compression or absence of basal cisterns has also been associated with intracranial hypertension.[32]

Normal ICP in a relaxed or paralyzed patient who is neither hypotensive nor hypercarbic is 10 mm Hg (136 mm H_2O) or less. While pressures in the range of 10 to 20 mm Hg (136 to 272 mm H_2O) may occur with moderate disturbances of intracranial volumes, pressures greater than these herald an intracranial hematoma, diffuse brain swelling, or both.

Most dangerous traumatic, unilateral, intracranial mass lesions shift the midline 5 mm or more. This is invariably associated with an elevated ICP unless a CSF leak is present. Significant temporal lobe lesions may cause only a minimal shift of the midline, but the ICP may be elevated and the third ventricle, if seen, will often be shifted more than the lateral ventricles. If there is little or no midline shift, the ICP is elevated, and the patient is not hypercarbic, then either there are bilateral mass lesions or there is serious diffuse brain swelling.

When intracranial pressure demonstrates an upward trend, certain basic items should be checked. The neck should be in a neutral position to facilitate venous drainage. In most cases, having the head end of the bed elevated approximately 30° is useful.[33] The calibration of the system must be checked, and one should confirm that the transducer is in level with the foramen of Monro. If the patient is fighting the ventilator, he or she should be sedated or chemically paralyzed. If these measures are not adequate, various methods exist to reduce the ICP, including ventricular drainage, mannitol, and hyperventilation (see Chapter 2).

MEDICAL THERAPY

The intensive care approach to severe head injury has been associated with a drop in reported mortality figures from approximately 50% in the 1970s to 36% in the National Traumatic Coma Data Bank.[34,35] The primary aim of these intensive care protocols has been to prevent secondary damage to an already injured brain. Within the last three years, there has been a great deal of excitement over the almost simultaneous arrival of several drugs for neurotrauma that have shown considerable potential in laboratory and early clinical studies. These drugs include tirilizad and superoxide dismutase, amongst others. Some of the more commonly used drugs in head injury are briefly reviewed.

ANTICONVULSANTS

The role of prophylactic anticonvulsants in patients with severe head injury remains somewhat controversial, although they clearly do have a role. The classic studies by Jennett[36] found posttraumatic epilepsy to occur in about 5% of all patients admitted to the hospital with closed head injuries and in 15% of those with severe head injuries. Three main factors were found to be linked to a high incidence of late epilepsy: early seizures occurring within the first week, an intracranial hematoma, or a depressed skull fracture. While certain earlier studies were unable to show significant benefit of prophylactically administered anticonvulsants, a more recent double-blind study of 404 severely head-injured patients, who were randomized to receive phenytoin or placebo beginning within 24 hours of injury and continuing for 1 year, found that phenytoin reduced the incidence of seizures in the first week after injury but not thereafter.[37] This study appears to justify stopping prophylactic convulsants after the first week in most cases. In patients who have had seizures, anticonvulsants are continued for at least a year.

MANNITOL

Mannitol is widely used to reduce intracranial pressure (see Chapter 2). The commonly used preparation is a 20% solution. The most widely accepted regimen is 1 to 2 g/kg given intravenously as a bolus. Serum osmolality should not be allowed to go much above 320 mOsm/L, if possible, in order to avoid systemic acidosis and renal failure. There is clinical and laboratory evidence to suggest that long-term, repeated use of mannitol can worsen brain edema and hence reverse the initial beneficial effect.

FUROSEMIDE

Furosemide (Lasix) has been used alone and in conjunction with mannitol in the treatment of raised intracranial pressure. It has been shown that diuresis can be enhanced by the combined use of these agents with more pronounced and consistent brain shrinkage. A dose of 0.3 to 0.5 mg/kg of furosemide given intravenously is reasonable.

BARBITURATES

Several studies have studied the protective effect of barbiturates on the brain in cerebral anoxia and ischemia. It has also been documented that barbiturates are effective in reducing intracranial pressure.[38] Although it is unclear whether barbiturates improve outcome from severe head injury, it is clear that pentobarbital is one of the few options available in patients with refractory intracranial hypertension (see Chapter 2). This drug should not be used in the presence of hypotension; in fact, the outcome in hypotensive patients who are put into pentobarbital coma is worse than in controls. Furthermore, hypotension is often associated with the use of this agent. Great care should be taken to maintain adequate cerebral perfusion pressure during the use of barbiturates.

STEROIDS

While steroids are clearly useful in reducing the edema associated with brain tumors, their value in head injury is not clear. In fact, most studies to date have not demonstrated any beneficial effect associated with steroids in terms of either ICP control or improved outcome from severe head injury. Furthermore, there is some evidence that steroids may have a deleterious effect on metabolism in these patients. It is possible that very high doses of particular steroids may have a beneficial effect in certain subsets of head-injured patients. However, currently available steroids in standard dose regimens have not proven to be valuable in severe head injury. A new generation of steroid-related agents are currently undergoing clinical trials in various neurologic disorders, including head injury, spinal cord injury, and subarachnoid hemorrhage.

PROGNOSIS

The Glasgow Outcome Scale (GOS) has been widely accepted as a standard means of describing outcome in head injury patients. This is a simple five-point scale (Fig. 16.15).[39] These categories are sometimes lumped together as either favorable outcomes (G, MD) or unfavorable outcomes (SD, V, or D). Several statistical studies have reported the use of various prognostic indicators for predicting outcome in severe head injury. Because of unexpected medical and surgical complications and the inherent unpredictability of disease, there is no absolutely unfailing prediction system. Based on experience with a large group of patients, an algorithm has been developed for approximate expected outcomes associated with certain prognostic features.[40] An attempt to predict mortality with 100% certainty appeared to work in one center.[41] However, when this system was applied to other patient populations, some patients who were predicted to die based on this scale instead survived.[42] This highlights the difficulty in making foolproof predictions of outcome in patients with head injury. Nevertheless, certain broad predictions can be made based on the patient's initial exam and this can be valuable in counseling the family.

Acknowledgment: This author wishes to express his sincere gratitude to Stephanie Goldfield and Roberta Abbott for preparing this manuscript. Some of the material used in the preparation of this chapter has been derived from the author's previous publications, especially from the chapter entitled "Head Injury" in Grossman RG, ed. *Principles of Neurosurgery*. New York, NY: Raven Press; 1991:235–291. All material has been updated.

Figure 16.15 Glasgow Outcome Scale

Good recovery [G]	Patient returns to preinjury level of function
Moderately disabled [MD]	Patient has neurologic deficits but is able to look after self
Severely disabled [SD]	Patient is unable to look after self
Vegetative [V]	No evidence of higher mental function
Dead [D]	

REFERENCES

1. Teasdale G, Jennett B. Assessment of coma and impaired consciousness. *Lancet.* 1974;2:81–84.
2. Jennett B, Teasdale G. Assessment of impaired consciousness. In: *Management of Head Injuries.* Philadelphia, Pa: FA Davis Co; 1981:77–93.
3. Miller JD. Minor, moderate and severe head injury. *Neurosurg Rev.* 1986;9:135–139.
4. Williams DH, Levin HS, Eisenberg HM. Mild head injury classification. *Neurosurgery.* 1990; 27: 422–428.
5. Seelig JM, Becker DP, Miller JD, et al. Traumatic acute subdural hematoma: major mortality reduction in comatose patients treated within four hours. *JAMA.* 1981;304:1511–1518.
6. Gennarelli TA. Cerebral concussion and diffuse brain injuries. In: Cooper PR, ed. *Head Injury.* 2nd ed. Baltimore, Md: Williams & Wilkins; 1987:108–124.
7. Dacey RG, Alves WM, Rimel RW, et al. Neurosurgical complications after apparently minor head injury—assessment of risk in a series of 610 patients. *J Neurosurg.* 1986;65:203–210.
8. Masters SJ, McClean PM, Arcarese JS, et al. Skull x-ray examinations after head trauma: recommendations by a multidisciplinary panel and validation study. *N Engl J Med.* 1987;316:84–91.
9. Jennett B, Teasdale G. Early assessment of the head injured patient. In: *Management of Head Injuries.* Philadelphia, Pa: FA Davis Co; 1981:99.
10. Stein SC, Ross SE. The value of computed tomographic scans in patients with low risk head injuries. *Neurosurgery.* 1990;26:638–640.
11. White RJ, Likavec MJ. The diagnosis and initial management of head injury. *N Engl J Med.* 1992; 327:1507–1511.
12. Bruno LA, Gennarelli TA, Torq JS. Management guidelines for head injuries in athletics. *Clin Sports Med.* 1987;6:17–29.
13. Wilberger JE, Marvon JC. Head injuries in athletes. *Clin Sports Med.* 1989;8:1–9.
14. Stein SC, Ross SE. Moderate head injury: a guide to initial management. *J Neurosurg.* 1992;77: 562–564.
15. Stone JL, Lowe RJ, Jonasson O, et al. Acute subdural hematoma: direct admission to a trauma center yields improved results. *J Trauma.* 1986; 26:445–450.
16. Miller JD, Butterworth JF, Gudeman SK, et al. Further experience in the management of severe head injury. *J Neurosurg.* 1981;54:289–299.
17. Miller JD, Sweet RC, Narayan RK, Becker DP. Early insults to the injured brain. *JAMA.* 1978; 240:439–442.
18. Narayan RK, Kishore PRS, Becker DP, et al. Intracranial pressure: to monitor or not to monitor? A review of our experience with severe head injury. *J Neurosurg.* 1982;56:650–659.
19. Levine JE, Becker DP. Reversal of incipient brain death from head injury apnea at the scene of accidents. *N Engl J Med.* 1979;301:109.
20. Chestnut RM, Marshall LF. Analysis of the role of secondary brain injury in determining outcome from severe head injury. Presented at the Annual Meeting of the American Association of Neurological Surgeons; 1990; Nashville, Tenn.
21. Butterworth JF, Maull KI, Miller JD, et al. Detection of occult abdominal trauma in patients with severe head injuries. *Lancet.* 1980;2:759–762.
22. Narayan RK, Greenberg RP, Miller JD, et al. Improved confidence of outcome prediction in severe head injury: a comparative analysis of the clinical examination, MEPs, CT scanning and ICP. *J Neurosurg.* 1981;54:751–762.
23. Wester K, Aas-Aune G, Skretting P, Syversen A. Management of acute head injuries in a Norwegian county: effects of introducing CT scanning in a local hospital. *J Trauma.* 1989;29:238–241.
24. Becker DP, Miller JD, Ward JD, et al. The outcome from severe head injury with early diagnosis and intensive management. *J Neurosurg.* 1977; 47:491–502.
25. Galbraith S, Teasdale G. Predicting the need for operation in the patient with an occult traumatic intracranial hematoma. *J Neurosurg.* 1981;55: 75–81.
26. Sheinberg MA, Kanter MJ, Kritzer RO, Contant CF, Robertson CS, Narayan RK. Management of cerebral contusions. In press.
27. Andrews BT, Chiles BW, Olsen WL, Pitts LH. The effect of intracerebral hematoma location on the risk of brain-stem compression and on clinical outcome. *J Neurosurg.* 1988;69:518–522.
28. Feldman Z, Narayan RK. Intracranial pressure monitoring: techniques and pitfalls. In: Cooper PR, ed. *Head Injury.* 3rd ed. Philadelphia, Pa: Williams & Wilkins; 1993:247–274.
29. Rosner MJ, Daughton S. Cerebral perfusion pressure management in head injury. *J Trauma.* 1990; 30:933–941.
30. Marmarou AM, Anderson RL, Ward JD, et al. Impact of ICP instability and hypotension on outcome in patients with severe head injury. *J Neurosurg.* 1991;75:559–566.
31. Piek J, Chesnut RM, Marshall LF, et al. Extracranial complications of severe head injury. *J Neurosurg.* 1992;77:901–907.
32. Marshall LF, Marshall SB, Klauber MR, Clark MVB, et al. A new classification of head injury based on computerized tomography. *J Neurosurg.* 1991;75(suppl):S14–S20.

33. Feldman Z, Kanter MJ, Robertson CS, et al. Effect of head elevation on intracranial pressure, cerebral perfusion pressure and cerebral blood flow in head-injured patients. *J Neurosurg.* 1992;76:207–211.

34. Jennett B, Teasdale G, Galbraith S, et al. Severe head injury in three countries. *J Neurol Neurosurg Psychiatry.* 1977;40:291–298.

35. Marshall LF, Gautille T, Klanber MR, et al. The outcome of severe closed head injury. *J Neurosurg.* 1991;75:528–536.

36. Jennett B. *Epilepsy After Nonmissile Head Injuries.* 2nd ed. London: Heinemann; 1975.

37. Temkin NR, Dikmen SS, Wilensky AJ, Keihm J, Chabal S, Winn HR. A randomized, double-blind study of phenytoin for the prevention of post-traumatic seizures. *N Engl J Med.* 1990;323:497–502.

38. Eisenberg HM, Frankowski RF, Contant CF, Marshall LF, Walker MD. High-dose barbiturates control elevated intracranial pressure in patients with severe head injury. *J Neurosurg.* 1988;69:15–23.

39. Jennett B, Bond M. Assessment of outcome after severe brain damage: a practical scale. *Lancet.* 1975;1:480–484.

40. Choi SC, Muizelaar JP, Barnes TY, Young HF. Prediction tree for severely head injured patients. *J Neurosurg.* 1991;75:251–255.

41. Gibson RM, Stephenson GC. Aggressive management of severe closed head trauma: time for reappraisal. *Lancet.* 1989;2(8659):369–371.

42. Feldman Z, Contant CF, Robertson CS, Narayan RK, Grossman RG. Evaluation of the Leeds prognostic score for severe head injury. *Lancet.* 1991;337:1451–1453.

Gunshot Wounds of the Head

Setti S. Rengachary, Derek A. Duke

Firearm-related deaths are the second leading cause of death due to trauma. In the Western world, the United States has the highest frequency of firearm-related deaths. Handguns are the firearms most frequently used in fatal injuries. It is estimated that there are approximately 120 million guns in private hands in the United States; stated differently, about half of all homes in the United States contain one or more firearms. The economic loss from firearm-related injuries is estimated to be nearly 4 billion dollars annually. Around 300,000 missile injuries occur annually in the United States, of which 10% result in mortality. Of these 30,000 deaths, 50% occur from homicide, 42% from suicide, 5% from accidental injuries, 1% by legal action, and 2% from undetermined intent. It is said that since World War II, civilian deaths from gunshot wounds have exceeded the deaths from the Vietnam and Korean Wars combined. Thus it has become very important for surgeons, especially those working in major urban areas, to be familiar with wound ballistics, mechanisms of injury, and current thinking about the management of gunshot wounds to the head.

FIREARMS AND BULLETS

A firearm is any weapon that uses an explosive powder charge to propel a bullet or shell. Firearms generally have the following components (Fig. 17.1): 1) barrel, 2) chamber, 3) breech mechanism, and 4) firing mechanism. The barrel is a long metallic tube whose inner surface may have spiral grooves, such as in a rifle or a pistol, or may be smooth, as in a shotgun. The chamber is an expanded cavity at the rear end of the barrel, which holds the cartridge. The breech mechanism closes the rear end of the barrel. The firing mechanism in most small arms is made of a spring device that drives a pointed firing pin through the breech port against a

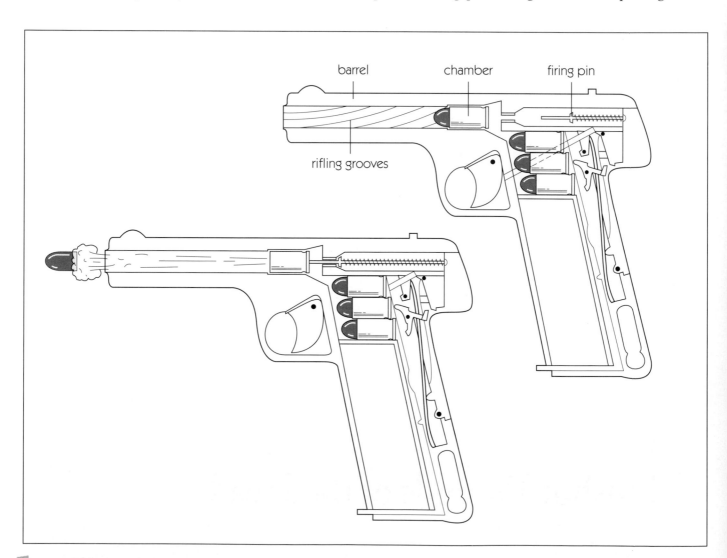

Figure 17.1 Design of a handgun. The major components are the barrel, chamber, breech mechanism, and firing mechanism. Note the rifling grooves within the barrel.

sensitive primer in the cartridge. The firing pin is cocked or drawn back against a hook called the seer. When the trigger is pulled, the seer releases the firing pin, which then leaps forward to strike the primer. A flame from the primer ignites the powder in the cartridge, forming a gas. This explosive gas propels the bullet from the barrel.

CLASSIFICATION OF FIREARMS

There are various classifications of firearms, based on their size, muzzle velocity, and use. Small or light firearms such as handguns, rifles, and shotguns are used in civilian and military settings; heavy firearms used in the military setting are referred to as artillery. Low-velocity firearms have muzzle velocities less than 1000 ft/sec, whereas civilian and military rifles whose bullet speeds exceed 1050 ft/sec (the speed of sound) are considered high-velocity firearms.

Magnum shells are supercharged or overcharged rounds that have extra gunpowder to provide the bullet 20% to 60% more energy than the standard shell of the same caliber. The increased energy is due to increased velocity. Sometimes the shells used by the police may be undercharged so that the bullet will not ricochet and hit an unintended victim nearby.

Handguns, Rifles, and Shotguns

By definition, a handgun is a firearm operated with one hand. Rifles are used in both military and civilian settings. Handguns and rifles may be single-shot, semi-automatic, or fully automatic. Single-shot weapons have to be reloaded after each firing. Semiautomatic weapons fire each time the trigger is pulled. Automatic weapons fire continuously until the trigger is released. Shotguns use multiple missiles or pellets fired from the same shell. The resulting wounds differ from those made by other missiles. Shotguns are designed primarily as sporting guns, and their military use is outlawed.

Shotguns are generally used to kill fast-moving game; the idea is that the numerous pellets within the shell increase the chances of hitting the target. A major determining factor of the wounding capacity of a shotgun is the distance between the target and the weapon. The shotgun is generally classified as a low-velocity firearm. The wound ballistics will vary depending on whether the shotgun is fired from close or long range. At long range, the shotgun pellets scatter and the charge acts as many individual projectiles, with kinetic energy imparted separately by each pellet that hits the target. At close range, the entire charge hits the target as a single missile with kinetic energy equivalent to that of a high-velocity rifle (Fig. 17.2). The smaller lead shot used in shotgun shells are called birdshot, the larger shot are called buckshot. Sawed-off shotguns have a shortened barrel; they are used by criminals for easier concealment. The pellets spread out much more with a sawed-off barrel, so fewer pellets will hit the target at long range. The bore or caliber of a shotgun is stated differently than that of a rifle or handgun. The gauge of a shotgun indicates how many lead balls of the bore size are required to weigh a pound. For example, a 12-gauge weapon originally had a bore enabling a round lead ball weighing 1/12 of a pound to enter its barrel.

BULLETS

Most bullets are made of lead or a lead alloy. Lead is used in the manufacture of bullets almost universally because of its high density. Compared to lighter materials, the small volume relative to mass produces less air drag, and thus the bullet has more kinetic energy at impact. The relatively low melting point of lead causes it to soften, if not melt, in the heat from the explosive gases and from air friction in flight. To overcome this, the bullet is jacketed by a sheath of metal with a higher melting point, such as copper, brass, bronze, aluminum,

Figure 17.2 Shotgun blast at close range.

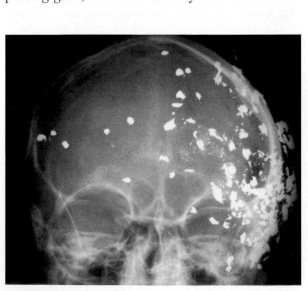

or steel. The jacket maintains the shape of the bullet even at high temperatures. The jacketing may, however, not be complete. The tip of the bullet may be left unjacketed. The purpose of partial jacketing is to permit mushrooming of the bullet tip upon impact. The increased bullet diameter will transfer more kinetic energy to the target as compared to a fully jacketed bullet, which is less likely to deform and more likely to pass completely through the target, thus transferring less kinetic energy to tissues.

Civilian and Military Bullets

Civilian bullets are generally partially jacketed. The rationale is that civilian bullets are usually meant for hunting purposes. To insure quick killing of the game, the bullet is partially jacketed in such manner that on impact the tip will mushroom and impart more kinetic energy, causing more tissue destruction. A partially jacketed bullet, because of its mushrooming effect, produces a wound track three times the original diameter of the bullet. Therefore the Hague Convention of 1899 and the subsequent Geneva Convention required all military bullets to be fully jacketed (Fig. 17.3). This dictate has been followed by all warring parties in major world conflicts since. On the other hand, lower mortality suits present military applications, where the objective is to maim and disable but not kill the soldier. If soldiers are merely incapacitated, the support services of the enemy must be used to care for the wounded, and thus more of the enemy's resources are tied down.

Designs for Deforming the Bullet Tip

Many methods have been used to ensure deformation the shape of the bullet upon impact (Fig. 17.4). The oldest one is called the dumdum bullet, named after a village in India where the arsenal was located that manufactured these bullets.[1] To increase their kill rate in their wars in India, the British scored the surface of the bullet to weaken the jacket, so that the tip would mushroom on impact. In contemporary civilian use, instead of a scored jacket, the bullet is only partially jacketed, leaving the tip uncovered. This has essentially the same effect, in that the soft exposed lead mushrooms upon impact. Hollow-point bullets are not merely unjacketed; the tip of the bullet is also hollow and blunt-nosed. This causes very efficient mushrooming. In an extreme version of this, a powder charge is placed in a small cylindrical canister within the tip of a hollow-point bullet; it explodes upon impact, further insuring expansion of the bullet tip.

BALLISTICS

Ballistics [from Greek *ballein*, to throw] is the study of natural laws governing the motion of projectiles in flight. In this definition, a projectile or missile may be considered as a pointed object or weapon that is ejected, thrown, dropped, fired, or projected at a target. Examples of projectiles are listed in Figure 17.5. Ballistics may be divided into three phases:
1) Interior: study of the projectile as it travels through the barrel of the firearm.
2) Exterior: study of the projectile as it travels during flight through space.
3) Terminal: study of the projectile as it strikes the target.
Wound ballistics is an example of terminal-phase ballistics—studying the projectile when it enters human or animal tissues.

The total kinetic energy of a missile is not as critical a factor in wounding potential as the amount of kinetic energy transferred to the target, which is defined as:

$$\text{Kinetic Energy Transferred} = \frac{\text{Mass} \ (V_i - V_e)^2}{2}$$

where V_i is the initial velocity of the missile when it strikes the target and V_e is the velocity of the missile when it exits the target. Thus, the greater the difference between the initial velocity and the exit velocity, the greater the amount of kinetic energy transferred to the target.

Two major factors tend to retard the speed of the bullet within the tissue. One is the use of hollow-point or soft-point bullets, discussed earlier, and the other is

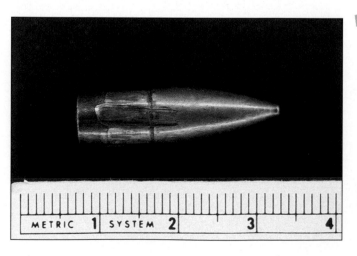

Figure 17.3 Example of a fully jacketed military bullet extracted from the temporal lobe of an Iraqi civilian during Operation Desert Storm by one of the authors (SSR).

the angle of incidence (the angle at which the bullet strikes the target) (Fig. 17.6). If the pointed end of the bullet strikes the target straight on, it imparts less energy than if it strikes the target at an oblique angle, confronting a broader surface area.

Velocity is a more significant factor in wounding potential than the mass of the bullet, but in the design and construction of firearms many manufacturers find it less expensive to increase the mass of the bullet than to increase its velocity. Doubling the mass only doubles the bullet's kinetic energy, whereas doubling the velocity would quadruple the kinetic energy.

BULLET SHAPE AND BALLISTIC COEFFICIENT

Bullet shape is a critical factor in determining the flight of the bullet through both air and tissue. Sharp-nosed, narrow-pointed bullets obviously have a better aerody-

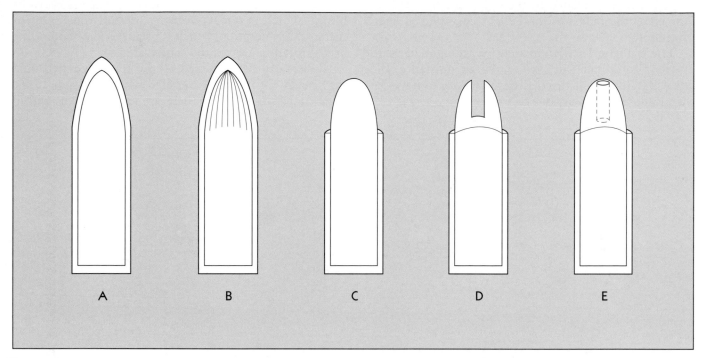

Figure 17.4 Varieties of bullets. **(A)** Fully jacketed military bullet. **(B)** Dumdum bullet, radially scored to weaken the tip so that it will mushroom upon impact. **(C)** Partially jacketed "soft point" bullet. The lead tip is unjacketed so that it will mushroom upon impact. **(D)** Hollow-point bullet. The forward end of the bullet is blunt and hollowed out to facilitate mushrooming. **(E)** Devastator bullet. Like D, but it has a canister filled with an explosive within the hollow tip of the bullet. This explodes upon impact, further increasing damage to the bullet tip. If the canister does not explode, the surgeon or pathologist retrieving the bullet from the tissue is at personal risk.

Figure 17.5 Examples of Missiles

Bullet	Rocket
Shrapnel	Stone and debris
Grenade	Artillery shell
Nail	Cannon ball
Pencil/pen	Torpedo
Screwdriver	Pointed toy

namic profile than hollow-pointed, blunt-ended bullets (Fig. 17.7). This difference can be quantified in the so-called ballistic coefficient,[2,3] defined as:

$$\text{Ballistic Coefficient} = \frac{\text{Sectional Density}}{I}$$

$$\text{where Sectional Density} = \frac{\text{Bullet Weight}}{7000 \times \text{Diameter}^2}$$

and I is inversely related to the ogive number, which is defined as the radius of the bullet's curvature in lateral projection.

The ballistic coefficient may be thought of as the efficiency of a bullet in overcoming air resistance. Bullets with a high ballistic coefficient are able to travel farther, losing less velocity due to friction.

BEHAVIOR OF BULLETS IN FLIGHT

Bullets, even high-velocity bullets, do not follow a perfectly straight trajectory.[4] Because of many physical factors, including the location of the center of mass relative to the geometric center of the bullet, resistance from air, and so on, several destabilizing motions are superimposed on the translational motion of the bullet (Fig. 17.8). They are the following: 1) yaw, which is defined as deviation of the bullet's longitudinal axis from the straight line of flight; 2) tumbling, which is forward rotation around the center of mass; 3) precession (wobbling), which is circular yawing around the center of mass; and 4) nutation, which is oscillatory motion of the axis of rotation around the center of mass.

Bullets can be stabilized by the spin generated during transit through the barrel of the gun (Fig. 17.9). This comes about when there are spiral grooves within

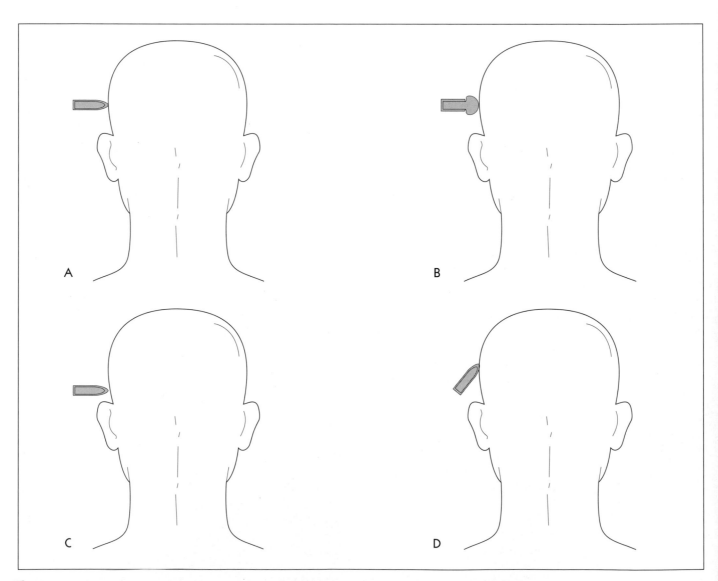

Figure 17.6 Some factors which determine the extent of wounding with bullets. **(A)** A fully jacketed bullet is likely to impart less kinetic energy to tissues than **(B)** a soft-point bullet which mushrooms upon impact. **(C)** A bullet striking the head exactly at a right angle is likely to cause less damage than one striking at an oblique angle **(D)**, which presents a larger surface area against the target.

the barrel, called rifling. Spaces between the grooves are called lands, and the caliber of a gun is defined as the distance between two opposite lands. Generally this is expressed in hundredths of an inch or millimeters. Although the caliber of a gun and the caliber of a bullet are generally stated interchangeably, obviously the bullet must be slightly smaller than the caliber of the gun. As a bullet passes through the barrel of a gun, rotary spin is imparted to the bullet—the longer the barrel, the greater the spin. The angular momentum carried by the bullet also imparts energy to the target; however, there is no definite way experimentally to quantify the energy imparted by spinning separately from the energy imparted by translational motion. The spinning of the bullet lends stability to its flight and increases its total kinetic energy. The rifling process also adds distinctive marks to the bullet sheath, and such marking may be used to identify the weapon by comparing the marks on the bullet retrieved from a wound with those on a test bullet fired from the same weapon.

MECHANISMS OF INJURY

Five of the most common types of missile injuries to the head[5] are discussed in this section (Fig. 17.10), along with some special mechanisms of injury.

VARIETIES OF MISSILE WOUNDS TO THE HEAD

Tangential Wounds
Tangential wounds generally occur when a high-velocity missile strikes the head at an oblique angle and continues to travel under the scalp, but does not pass through the skull (see Fig. 17.10A). After the bullet grazes the skull it generally travels in the subgaleal space and then either exits through the scalp or, if the energy is spent, remains trapped beneath the scalp. In addition to the scalp laceration, the bullet may cause varying degrees of damage to the skull, meninges, and underlying cortex. Linear or depressed skull fractures may be present. If a depressed fracture occurs, the fracture may be confined to the outer table, the inner table, or both tables. Injury to dural vessels can produce either an epidural or a subdural hematoma. The hallmark of this injury is an extensive area of cortical contusion. The clinical presentation may include focal or generalized seizures, or focal sensorimotor deficit. In some situations the neurologic deficit may be much worse than one would expect from the clinical examination of the wound. In most instances, however, the neurologic deficit is minimal; tangential gunshot wounds carry a better prognosis than any other type of gunshot wound to the head. CT will allow a good assessment of the degree of cortical contusion. Surgical management of these patients will depend on whether or not there is an extraaxial hematoma or mass effect and the extent of cortical injury. In the absence of an extracerebral hematoma, conservative treatment is generally followed.

Perforating Wound
With low-velocity missiles the bullet's energy may be spent in penetrating the skull, leaving enough kinetic energy to pass only partially through the brain substance

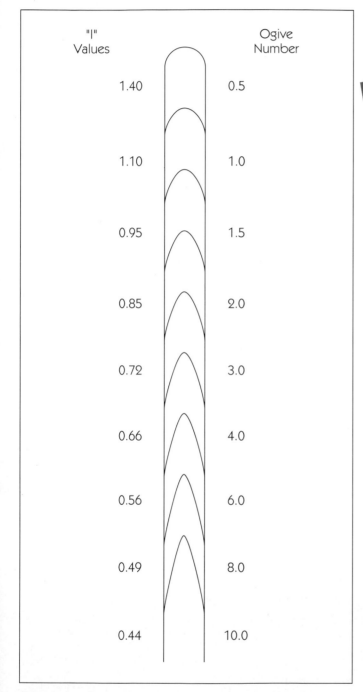

Figure 17.7 Varying bullet shapes. Note that the shape is graded from the most pointed (highest ogive number and lowest I value) to the most blunt (lowest ogive number and highest I value). Bullets with the highest ogive number have the highest ballistic coefficient and thus the least drag.

"I" Values		Ogive Number
1.40		0.5
1.10		1.0
0.95		1.5
0.85		2.0
0.72		3.0
0.66		4.0
0.56		6.0
0.49		8.0
0.44		10.0

(Fig. 17.11; see Fig. 17.10B). The energy absorbed by the skull depends on two factors: whether or not the nose of the bullet mushrooms at impact, and the angle at which the bullet strikes the skull. Bullets striking at exactly 90° are more likely to penetrate the skull and impart less energy to the skull than bullets that strike the skull at an angle because of yaw. Perforating wounds may cause localized brain contusion, laceration, or hematoma. It is not uncommon to find multiple bone or bullet fragments driven into the brain substance. The prognosis in a perforating wound is generally good because of the limited amount of injury to the brain tissue.

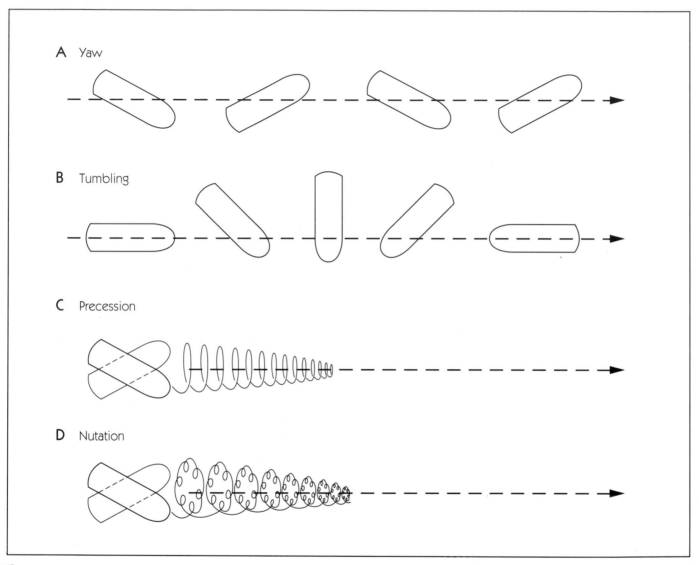

Figure 17.8 Behavior of the bullet in flight. (**A**) Yaw is deviation of the bullet in its longitudinal axis from the straight line of flight. (**B**) Tumbling is forward rotation around the center of mass. (**C**) Precession is circular yawing around the center of mass in a spiral fashion. (**D**) Nutation is rotation in small circles forming a rosette pattern.

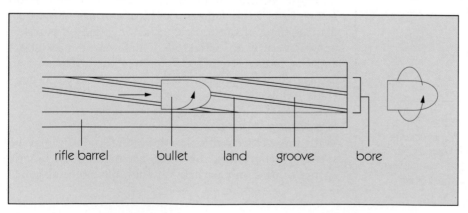

Figure 17.9 Spin stabilization of the bullet. As the bullet passes through the barrel, rifling imparts a rotary spin to the bullet. The spinning of the bullet lends stability to its flight and increases its total energy. The spinning process also adds a distinctive mark to the bullet sheath, which can be used to identify the weapon.

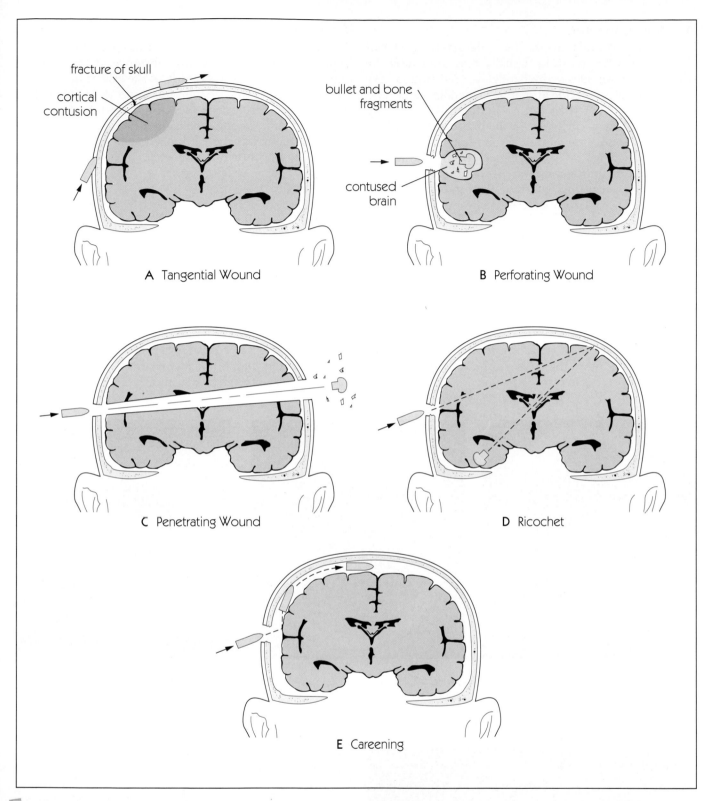

Figure 17.10 Varieties of missile wounds to the head. **(A)** Tangential wound. The bullet grazes the skull but does not penetrate it. There may be a depressed fracture of the skull. Presence of cortical contusion is a hallmark of this type of injury. Tangential wounds carry the best prognosis because they result in limited brain injury. **(B)** Perforating wound. The skull is penetrated, but the bullet does not have enough energy left to penetrate the entire brain. **(C)** Penetrating wound. The bullet goes through the entire head, causing devastating injury due to cavitation. This type of wound carries the worst prognosis. **(D)** Ricochet. The bullet strikes the opposite inner table of the skull and reflects back into the brain causing further damage. **(E)** Careening. The bullet hugs the inner table of the skull and may cause major venous sinus injury.

Penetrating Wounds

Penetrating wounds are the most devastating type of missile injury to the head. Usually they are caused by high-velocity missiles or by handguns fired from a very close range, as in suicide attempts. Generally the wound of entry is smaller than the wound of exit. There are varying degrees of cavitation in the brain along the bullet's path, usually several times larger than the diameter of the bullet (Fig. 17.12; see Fig. 17.10C). During the bullet's transit, a percussion wave is transmitted throughout the brain, causing explosive fractures of the skull (Figs. 17.13, 17.14) and widespread destruction of neuronal cell membranes. The shock wave may propagate as far down as the medulla oblongata, causing transient cardiorespiratory impairment. This may manifest clinically as acute respiratory arrest. Immediately after injury, the intracranial pressure (ICP) rises tremendously because of the transmission of kinetic energy to the brain. The ICP then slowly declines to some extent, only to rise again due to intracranial bleeding from torn blood vessels and to progressive edema. Wounds of this type, especially those that cross in the coronal and midline sagittal planes, are usually fatal.

Ricochet

In some instances, after the bullet has gone through the skull and through the brain substance, it may hit the inner table of the opposite side of the calvarium and ricochet, with re-entry of the bullet into the brain tissue, causing further damage (see Fig. 17.10D). Based on plain x-ray films alone, one cannot be sure that the bullet has actually ricocheted, but CT will show the bullet track and can confirm the ricochet.

Careening

After the bullet has penetrated the outer and inner tables of the skull at the wound of entry, it may change direction after it encounters the dura and travel along the inner table of the skull (see Fig. 17.10E). This is an unusual occurrence. Intracranial hematomas may form, and major venous sinuses are at risk of injury.

SUICIDAL GUNSHOT WOUNDS TO THE HEAD

In the fifth and sixth decades of life, suicidal wounds are more common than homicidal wounds.[6] There are some specific characteristics commonly found with these

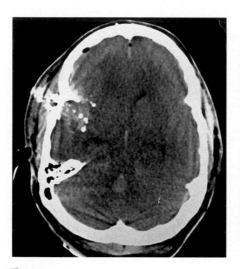

Figure 17.11 Example of a perforating wound.

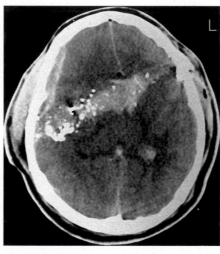

Figure 17.12 Example of a penetrating wound.

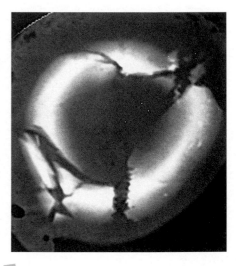

Figure 17.13 CT of the head with bone windows, showing an explosive fracture of the skull caused by a gunshot wound.

Figure 17.14 Intraoperative photograph showing multiple fractures of the skull in a gunshot wound.

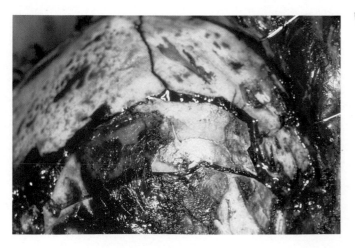

injuries. For instance, in right-handed individuals the wound of entry is generally in the right frontotemporal region (Fig. 17.15). Because the weapon is fired at close range, powder burns are more likely to be apparent with self-inflicted wounds than in those fired by an assailant at a longer range. Another hallmark of close-range injury is dissection of the subgaleal layer by hot exploding gases, which may produce irregular stellate lacerations of the scalp. Because of the invariable involvement of the branches of the middle cerebral arteries in the insula, there is a greater likelihood of major vascular damage. In addition, self-inflicted gunshot wounds that are directed from the frontotemporal region tend to traverse the midline, crossing both hemispheres and the ventricles in the coronal plane. Such a wound carries a very high mortality, greater than 95%. In rare instances when the gun is pointed anteriorly, it may inflict a tangential wound with injury to the nondominant frontal lobe or both frontal lobes. If the patient survives, a frontal lobotomy effect may be manifest, and mental depression that existed before the incident may be cured, but this happens rarely.

Another direction of injury is through the palate, when a person attempts to commit suicide by pointing the gun from the mouth towards the top of the head (Fig. 17.16). There may be a large penetrating wound in the hard palate and, depending on the angle, the clivus may be penetrated and the brain stem or hypothalamus injured. In any event, this also produces catastrophic damage with a through and through injury in the sagittal plane. In rare instances, if the patient did not insert the gun far enough into the mouth, the patient may survive without any significant brain injury but with major tissue loss in the face, requiring protracted and multiple reconstructive efforts.

WOUND CAVITATION WITH HIGH-VELOCITY MISSILES

A high-velocity bullet entering the brain causes a rapid temporary cavitation around its path because of energy imparted to the tissue by the radial velocity of the bullet (Fig. 17.17). This has been shown very clearly by cinephotography of bullets shot through gelatin. This cavitation may cause widespread punctate hemorrhages and rupture of cell membranes far from the bullet track. Even if the primary injury by the missile is to the cerebral hemispheres, temporary cavitation may cause membrane disruptions as far away as the brain stem, causing acute apnea and cardiorespiratory failure. The temporary cavitation then settles down, leaving behind a permanent bullet track lined by necrotic brain tissue.

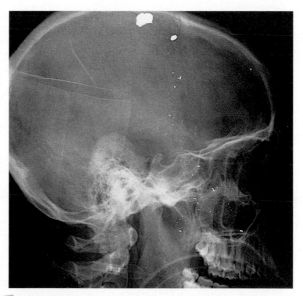

Figure 17.16 Example of a suicidal wound. The patient attempted suicide by placing the gun in the mouth and shooting towards the head. The bullet track is clearly visible due to scattered small bullet fragments.

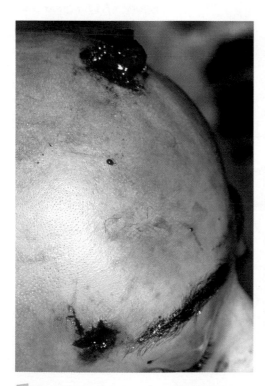

Figure 17.15 Self-inflicted gunshot wound with suicidal intent. The patient was right-handed. The wound of entry is in the right temporal region behind the eye. Note the small area of powder burn immediately below the wound of entry. There is considerable periorbital swelling. The exit wound is near the midline vertex. Note that the wound of exit is much larger than the wound of entry.

The kinetic energy transmitted through the brain by explosive temporary cavitation may be sufficient to cause multiple stellate fractures in the skull.

___ MIGRATION OF BULLETS OR BULLET FRAGMENTS

Occasionally, an entire bullet or major bullet fragments may migrate in a delayed manner within the intracranial cavity (Fig. 17.18). This is a very rare phenomenon,[7] which generally occurs under certain conditions. Fully jacketed bullets, which tend to remain intact after entering the skull, may sink through the substance of the brain because of their mass and because they are not deformed, and thus remain streamlined for motion through the brain substance. Bullets lodged in the ventricular system, especially the lateral ventricles, can migrate within the cavity of the ventricle according to the position of the head. Occasionally such a bullet may block a strategic CSF pathway, such as the foramen of Monro or the aqueduct. Migration is more likely when the bullet is intact than when it is fragmented, because small fragments are not heavy enough to sink through the brain substance. If the initial lodgement of the bullet is in the frontal pole, migration is more likely to occur, because the bullet will tend to gravitate to the

posterior pole if the patient is supine, the position most often assumed by patients with acute gunshot wounds. A bullet contained within necrotic, liquefied brain tissue or an abscess cavity may migrate within the limits of the cavity.

MANAGEMENT OF PATIENTS WITH GUNSHOT WOUNDS TO THE BRAIN

___ INITIAL ASSESSMENT AND CARE

Upon the patient's arrival to the emergency department, initial efforts are directed toward maintaining an adequate airway, especially in patients who have gunshot wounds to the face and mandible in addition to the head. A patent airway is maintained by an oral airway, an endotracheal tube, or a cricothyrotomy, as the clinical situation dictates. Ventilatory support with a respirator may be necessary if the patient has shallow or absent spontaneous respiration. Patients who have lost a considerable amount of blood will require circulatory support as well.

A quick history is obtained from the patient's relatives or law enforcement officers with emphasis on the

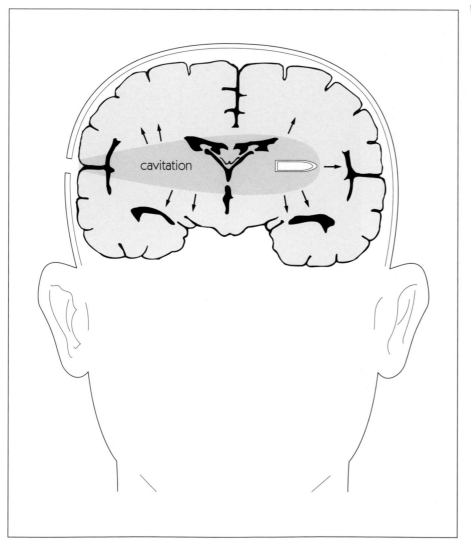

Figure 17.17 Wound cavitation with a high-velocity missile.

cavitation

Principles of Neurosurgery

circumstances of the incident, such as whether the gunshot was suicidal, accidental, or homicidal. Information about the caliber of the weapon and the type of firearm used is also useful. The range at which the patient was shot is an important factor. The information initially obtained may not always be accurate, and indeed may be misleading. Concurrent with obtaining the brief history, a quick clinical assessment is made. The entrance wound (and exit wound, if present) is inspected (Fig. 17.19). Powder stippling near the entrance wound indicates an injury from close range.

Bulky absorptive head dressings are applied as a preliminary measure. A quick neurologic evaluation is made, including assessment of consciousness, pupillary size and reaction to light, and brain stem reflexes, such as doll's eye movements, corneal reflexes, gag and cough reflexes, and the presence of spontaneous respiration. Motor activity is assessed to see whether the patient has spontaneous purposeful movements, decorticate/decerebrate movements, or flaccid limbs.

In addition to the routine work-up, a most useful laboratory test is to screen for disseminated intravascular coagulation (DIC). Because the pulpy, contused brain tissue releases thromboplastin, many patients may manifest features of DIC at some point during their hospital course, if not immediately upon admission. At the end of the clinical assessment, plain radiographs of the skull in the anteroposterior and lateral views are taken as well as a noncontrast CT. The CT is obtained with both soft tissue and bone window settings.

IMAGING

Radiologic imaging of patients with missile wounds of the head is crucial in planning the clinical management and making a prognosis; it is performed soon after a brief clinical assessment is made. Important medicolegal evidence can be obtained from imaging studies as well, which is often necessary in civilian gunshot wounds. The radiographs provide permanent archival evidence of the number of penetrating bullet rounds, the approximate range from which the bullet was shot, and the presence of entry and exit wounds.

Plain Radiographs
Plain radiographs of the skull, usually obtained in the emergency room, often provide considerable basic information about the missile. Most handguns are of a size

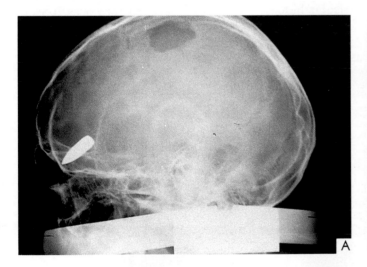
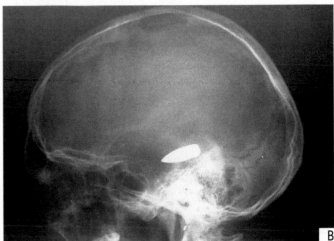

Figure 17.18 Spontaneous migration of an intracranial bullet. (A) A fully jacketed, undeformed bullet is located in the frontal pole of the brain. (B) The bullet has spontaneously migrated to the temporal area, due to gravitational forces causing it to sink within the brain substance.

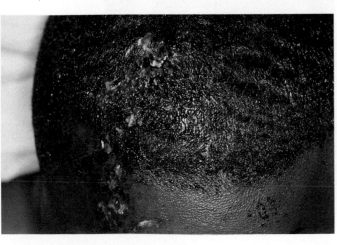

Figure 17.19 Entrance wound of a gunshot, with extruding particulate brain matter.

from .22 to .45 caliber; from the plain films it can usually be determined what caliber of bullet was used. Given that there is some degree of magnification, the true caliber must be determined by the following formula:

$$\text{True Size} = \text{Observed Size} \times \frac{\text{Distance (focal spot to bullet)}}{\text{Distance (focal spot to film)}}$$

It is obvious from this equation that increasing the bullet-to-film distance leads to greater magnification. Magnification is negligible if the distance from the focal spot to the film is 6 feet or more and the part of the body harboring the bullet is positioned closest to the x-ray film. The plain x-ray films will also indicate the degree of bullet fragmentation, and in some cases bullet fragments line the path of the missile and allow the track to be visualized; however, CT is a much more reliable diagnostic modality in this regard. Significant fragmentation of the bullet may prevent precise determination of the caliber of the bullet. The plain radiographs will also allow one to speculate whether the bullet is fully jacketed or not. Jacketed bullets generally stay in a single piece and do not shatter, deforming little, if any. On occasion the jacket may come loose and can be seen clearly as a separate density from the main slug (Fig. 17.20). Unjacketed bullets tend to mushroom readily on impact and to have extensive fragmentation visible on plain radiograph.

Computed Tomography

CT is the mainstay of radiologic assessment in patients with missile wounds to the head. In most instances, a combination of CT with plain radiographs is more useful than either modality alone. CT scans are usually done at the time of emergency evaluation, before admission to the intensive care unit. Noncontrast CT scans with and without bone window settings are generally obtained.

Several important kinds of information can be obtained from CT. The precise location of the bullet or bullet fragments can be determined. On plain x-ray films it is sometimes hard to determine whether the bullet has actually penetrated the skull or is lying just outside of the skull. However, this information can be clearly obtained from CT. One can also detect shattered bone fragments along the bullet track and/or well away from the bullet track. Bone fragments can usually be distinguished from bullet fragments by the lack of scatter on CT in the former (Fig. 17.21). The bullet track itself can be identified on the CT scan, in the form of either a low-density lesion representing edema or a high-density lesion due to bleeding along the track (see Fig. 17.12). Bullet ricochet within the skull can also be assessed on the CT scan. The presence of air within the dural venous sinuses on CT heralds injury to or transection of the major venous sinuses. The greatest advantage of CT is the ability to identify and locate precisely blood collections in various compartments. Intracranial bleeding results from the transection of various dural or parenchymal vessels in the bullet's path. Depending on which vessel is damaged, one may find an epidural hematoma, a subdural hematoma, subarachnoid bleeding, a confluent intracerebral hematoma, or an intraventricular hematoma (Fig. 17.22). On rare occasions, a confluent intracerebral or subdural hematoma may be found far from other damage, in an area opposite the wound of entry (Fig. 17.23). Because no other diagnostic test will give this information, the CT scan assumes a role of primary practical importance.

However, CT does have some limitations. It does not always show the true extent of parenchymal damage. The CT scan is a static image of the brain that does not give information about dynamic events that may have occurred at the time of the bullet's transit through the brain, such as shock waves transmitted to the brain

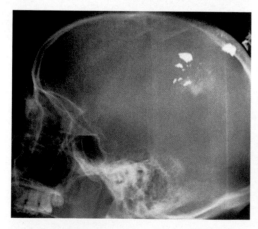

Figure 17.20 Plain x-ray film of the skull showing bullet fragments. Note that the jacket of the bullet has separated (it appears less dense) and is lying just outside the skull (arrow). Dense bullet fragments can be seen within the skull.

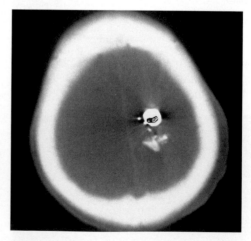

Figure 17.21 CT scan of the head with bone windows in a patient with a gunshot wound. There are indriven bullet *and* bone fragments. The bone fragments can be distinguished from bullet fragments by the lack of scatter.

Principles of Neurosurgery

stem. Thus, the patient may be far more damaged neurologically than the CT scan would indicate. Metallic artifact and scatter may compromise image quality, but with bone windows and thin cuts this can be overcome. If the bullet has gone through the head and exited the skull without leaving metallic fragments within the head, the extent of injury may be concealed.

SURGICAL MANAGEMENT

Surgical planning requires a judicious assessment. Patients should be carefully evaluated with regard to the accepted predictors of outcome. Those whose predicted outcomes are poor should be excluded from consideration for aggressive surgical therapy (Fig. 17.24). The definite indications for surgery are debridement of wounds in patients with a Glasgow Coma Scale score of 8 or higher, presence of an intracranial hematoma, and presence of CSF leak in facioorbital cranial wounds.

Because the extent of brain debridement has been the subject of debate, the history of this issue will be discussed in some detail. In World War I, Cushing meticulously and aggressively debrided all devitalized tissue, removed indriven bone and metal fragments as much as possible, and made a watertight closure of the dura. This gave excellent results with minimal rates of infectious complications. However, in World War II and in the Korean conflict, a less systematic approach was followed, with concomitant increases in the infection and complication rates. This prompted a more aggressive approach in the Vietnam War. Every attempt was made to remove all indriven bone and metal fragments, and all devitalized tissue was removed. If further evaluation at a higher-echelon hospital revealed retained bone or metal fragments, the patient was subjected to a second, and possibly third, operative exploration for their removal. Long-term evaluation of these patients, however, indicated that their rates of infection and posttraumatic seizure disorder were no better than those of patients whose wounds had not been aggressively debrided. This led to a more conservative approach in more recent wars, especially in the Israeli intervention in Lebanon. Systematic analysis of patients who survived gunshot wounds to the head indicated that debridement of the bullet track should consist merely of irrigation, and only fragments freed by gentle irrigation should be removed. No attempt should be made to retract the brain for access to bone or bullet fragments. This conservative approach has yielded results equal to those of any previous tech-

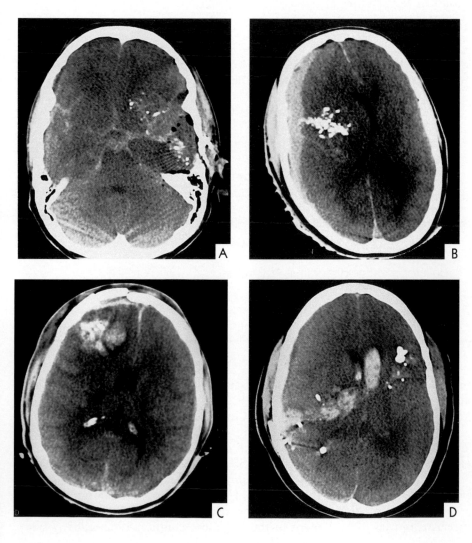

Figure 17.22 Intracranial bleeding from gunshot wounds to the head. **(A)** Subarachnoid hemorrhage. **(B)** Subdural hematoma. **(C)** Confluent intracerebral hematoma. **(D)** Intraventricular hematoma.

nique, with a good survival rate, preservation of neurologic function, and comparable rates of infection and epilepsy.

Thus, the most recent war experience forms the benchmark that is followed in most civilian gunshot wounds today.[8] The primary goal is to remove necrotic brain tissue that is at the surface and remove bone fragments if they are freed by gentle irrigation, but make no attempt to explore the bullet track. The dura and scalp are closed in a watertight fashion and antibiotic therapy is instituted. Prophylactic anticonvulsants are used. Serial follow-up CT scans are made in the immediate postoperative period to make sure that the patient is not developing infectious complications such as cerebritis or abscess. If complications occur, which should only happen in a small fraction of cases, one can reoperate on the patient for drainage of the abscess and removal of necrotic brain tissue.

Patients with orbitofacial cranial wounds have a higher risk of developing cerebrospinal fluid (CSF) fistula. These patients are treated more aggressively, with repair of the floor of the anterior cranial fossa using pericranium, temporalis fascia, or fascia lata graft to achieve primary repair and prevent CSF leakage. Intracranial pressure monitoring should be done in patients with a Glasgow Coma Scale score of 8 or higher.

BACTERIAL CONTAMINATION OF MISSILE WOUNDS

It is commonly believed that because bullets assume high temperatures in the barrel of the firearm and during transit through air, a bullet will be sterile when it strikes the target. Both clinical and experimental observations have indicated that this is not the case. However, the most common source of contamination is the patient's skin, hair, or clothing. In addition, because of negative pressures that develop during cavitation, external air may be sucked into the wound along with dirt, skin flora, and fragments of clothing, and thus bacterial contamination of the depths of the wound may occur. Prophylactic antibiotic therapy is therefore justified in all patients with missile wounds to the head.

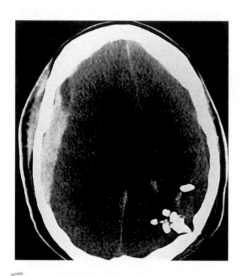

Figure 17.23 Subdural hematoma opposite the entry site of the bullet.

Figure 17.24 Predictors of Poor Outcome

Suicidal wound
Injury with high velocity missile (>1000 ft/sec)
Injury with deforming bullet
Glasgow Coma Scale <5 upon admission
Fixed and dilated pupils
Flaccidity, decerebrate/decorticate rigidity
High ICP (>60 mm Hg)
Bullet track through the entire midsagittal or coronal plane
Transventricular injury
Major arterial injury (e.g., internal carotid, vertebral, basilar, etc.)
Major venous sinus injury (e.g., superior sagittal or transverse sinus)
Injury to posterior fossa structures
Extreme cavitation with explosive deformity of the calvarium
Gunshot wound to the brain in association with other major organ injury
Development of disseminated intravascular coagulopathy

REFERENCES

1. Sykes LN, Champion HR, Fouty WJ. Dumdums, hollow-points, and devastators: techniques designed to increase wounding potential of bullets. *J Trauma.* 1988;28:618–623.
2. Ordog GJ, Wasserberger J, Subramanian B. Wound ballistics: theory and practice. *Ann Emerg Med.* 1984;13:1113–1122.
3. Adams DB. Wound ballistics: a review. *Milit Med.* 1982;147:831–835.
4. Hopkinson DA, Marshall TK. Firearm injuries. *Br J Surg.* 1967;54:344–353.
5. Bakay L. Missile injuries of brain. *NY State J Med.* 1982;313–319.
6. Selden BS, Goodman JM, Cordell W, Rodman GH. Outcome of self-inflicted gunshot wounds of the brain. *Ann Emerg Med.* 1988;17:247–253.
7. Rengachary SS, Carey M, Templer J. The sinking bullet. *Neurosurgery.* 1992;30:291–295.
8. Brandvold B, Levi L, Feinsod M, George E. Penetrating craniocerebral injuries in the Israeli involvement in the Lebanese conflict, 1982–1985. *J Neurosurg.* 1990;72:15–21.

Chapter 18

Traumatic Skull and Facial Fractures

Fred H. Geisler, Paul N. Manson

SKULL FRACTURES

Skull fractures are classified in three ways: by pattern (linear, comminuted, depressed), by anatomic location (convexity, base), and by type (open, closed).

The pattern of a skull fracture is affected by two factors. The first factor is the force of impact. A linear fracture results when the skull structure fails to undergo elastic deformation during impact; the fracture typically starts at the point of maximal stress (often remote from the actual impact) and extends to the point of impact. A comminuted fracture results when the impact force is sufficient to break the bone into multiple pieces under the point of impact. With even larger impact energies, the comminuted pieces can be driven inward and can penetrate the dura and cortical surface of the brain to create a depressed fracture.

The second factor is the ratio of the impact force to the impact area. If the impact, even one of high energy, is dispersed over a large area, as in a head injury to an individual wearing a motorcycle helmet, it often produces no skull fracture, even though the brain may be severely injured. However, if the impact, even one of low energy, is concentrated in a small area, such as from a hammer blow, it often produces multiple linear skull fractures radiating from the site of impact.

The location of a skull fracture is classified to two distinct areas: the skull convexity (generally termed "skull fracture") or the base of the skull (generally termed "basilar fracture"). Any of the three patterns can occur in either area or in both. A skull fracture can be further classified as open or closed by the presence or absence, respectively, of an overlying scalp laceration. In addition, a fracture extending into the skull base with violation of the paranasal sinuses or middle ear structures is also considered an open fracture.

Linear Skull Fractures

A linear skull fracture is a single fracture line that goes through the entire thickness of the skull.

Diagnosis

Although it is generally accepted that clinical indications for radiologic examination include loss of consciousness, retrograde amnesia, discharge from nose or ear, eardrum discoloration, positive Babinski reflex, or cranial nerve abnormalities, controversy exists (based on a cost/benefit analysis) regarding the use of x-rays to diagnose linear skull fractures. The patient's eventual neurologic outcome depends largely on the brain injury, rather than on the fracture. However, for a few patients radiologic examination may make a crucial difference. For example, a linear fracture crossing the path of the middle meningeal artery in even a mild head injury indicates risk for late neurologic deterioration from an epidural hematoma. Furthermore, skull films can detect depressed fractures, puncture wounds, and intracranial foreign objects that might otherwise elude physical examination. If a CT scan is obtained, however, skull radiographs usually add little information.

Management

Linear skull fractures require no stabilization or exploration when the scalp is closed. Even when a scalp laceration is present, very seldom is surgical exploration with bone removal necessary. Exceptions would include a machete injury to the skull producing a linear skull fracture with underlying dural laceration and brain damage. The skull fracture does, however, show that significant head trauma has occurred, and a careful assessment of the brain, facial structures, and cervical spine is required. Open linear fractures are debrided of foreign material and damaged soft tissue at the edges of the laceration and then closed.

Growing Skull Fracture in Children

A rare complication after linear skull fracture in young children (usually less than 2 years) is a growing skull defect at the fracture site. In these cases the dura is torn under the linear skull fracture. The pathogenesis is thought to be an expanding pouch of arachnoid passing through the torn dura and skull fracture, acting as a one-way valve that traps CSF and causes pressure erosion of the fracture edges to enlarge the fracture, or the growth of the brain, which produces spreading tensile forces on the edges of the dural laceration and causes the skull defect to enlarge. The brain may sometimes herniate through the skull defect, causing a new neurologic deficit. These lesions are surgically repaired with closure of the dura.

Comminuted Fractures

A comminuted fracture occurs when multiple linear fractures radiate from the point of impact. Some of the fracture lines may involve the suture lines (diastatic fracture) or stop at them. Around the point of impact there may be free fragments of bone.

Diagnosis

Diagnosis is made on skull radiographs and CT of the head with bone windows.

Management

If the skin is closed and no depression of bone fragments greater than the thickness of the skull is demonstrated on CT, management is as for linear skull fractures. However, in many of these cases surgery is performed for the underlying intracranial pathology, such as an epidural hematoma (Fig. 18.1). After the intracranial pathology has been corrected, the bone fragments are replaced as a cranioplasty. If the skin is open and free bone fragments are present, debridement of the contaminated fragments and soft tissue is performed before dural and scalp closures (Fig. 18.2).

Depressed Skull Fractures

In a depressed skull fracture, the greatest bone depression can occur at the interface of fracture and intact skull or near the center of the fracture if several fragments are displaced inward.

Diagnosis

Many patients with depressed skull fractures experience initial loss of consciousness and neurologic damage. However, 25% of patients experience neither loss of consciousness nor neurologic deficit and another 25% experience only brief loss of consciousness. Although the diagnosis of a depressed skull fracture is often indicated on routine skull radiographs by an area of double density (overlying bone fragments) or by multiple or circular fractures, the full extent and depth of injury are rarely appreciated. Physical examination is difficult because of scalp mobility and swelling. Scalp mobility can result in nonalignment of the scalp laceration and skull fracture; normal skull under a scalp laceration does not exclude a depressed fracture 1 or 2 cm from one edge of the laceration. Furthermore, traumatic swelling of the scalp minimizes the palpable and visual appearance of the step-off at the bony edges, preventing accurate clinical assessment of the extent of skull deformity for the first few days.

CT is the diagnostic method of choice. When image display windows are adjusted to optimize bony detail, they display the position, extent, and number of fractures, as well as the presence and depth of depression. With the imaging windows set to optimize intracranial contents, the same CT scan also allows assessment of the underlying brain for contusion or hematoma, small bone fragments, or foreign bodies, as well as other traumatic intracranial pathology. Occasionally, coronal CT images through fractures near the vertex of the head or extending into the skull base are used to supplement the standard CT images, since the depth of a depression is more accurately measured on CT images perpendicular to the depression.

Management

Combined therapy of depressed fractures of the cranial vault extending to involve the frontal sinus or facial bones is covered in the sections on facial fractures. When a depressed skull fracture on the convexity also includes facial fractures, the intracranial injury is typically repaired first with removal of intracerebral hematoma and repair of dural laceration if present (Figs. 18.3, 18.4).

Although a focal neurologic deficit from the cortex directly under a depressed skull fracture is occasionally improved by elevation of the bone fragments (presumably by increasing local cortical blood flow), this usually produces no neurologic change, implying that impact produces the major cortical damage. The brain dysfunction usually undergoes a neurologic recovery phase of several weeks to months, similar to that after a stroke or a head injury without a depressed fracture. Likewise, the incidence of epilepsy after a depressed skull fracture

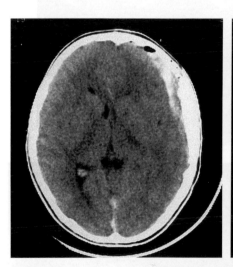
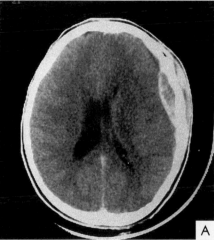

Figure 18.1 Comminuted, minimally depressed open skull fracture with underlying epidural hematoma. **(A)** CT scan through the center of the depressed region. Note the small amount of air at the anterior edge of the epidural hematoma. **(B)** Intraoperative view of the depressed bone before elevation. **(C)** The bone was removed, sutured together, and replaced as a cranioplasty. The epidural hematoma was removed after the bone fragments had been removed.

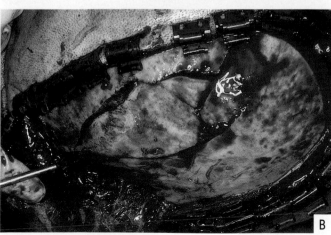
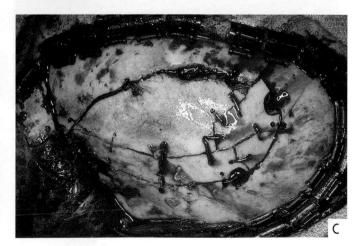

locally and often requires removal of the underlying cranial bone flap, skin debridement/rotation, and delayed cranioplasty.

Depressed Fractures Over Dural Sinuses

Depressed skull fractures over a venous sinus require special handling. Surgical elevation of these fractures may involve massive blood loss if a depressed fragment has been plugging a sinus tear. Unless they are grossly contaminated with foreign material, are a major cosmetic deformity, or cause intracranial hypertension secondary to sinus occlusion, such fractures are managed with scalp debridement and massive irrigation, followed by serial CT scans for signs of brain abscess for at least a year.

Basilar Skull Fractures

Fractures of the base of the skull occur in 3.5% to 24% of head-injured patients. This wide variation results from differences in study populations and the difficulty in obtaining radiographic verification of the fractures. Linear fractures in the skull base carry a risk of meningitis, whereas this risk is extremely low in fractures of the convexity unless the scalp, bone, and dura are all violated. The dura is easily torn in a basal skull fracture; this places the subarachnoid space in direct contact with the paranasal sinuses or middle ear structures, providing a pathway for infection. For example, a persistent fistula allowing a continuous CSF leak and bacterial exposure may develop.

Petrous bone fractures can be either longitudinal or transverse relative to the long axis of the petrous pyramid. Longitudinal fractures are more common and usually involve the tympanic membrane or external ear canal, thereby producing otorrhea. Transverse fractures result from higher-energy impacts and can damage middle ear ossicules or the facial nerve. These fractures occur with or in continuity with linear, comminuted, or depressed skull fractures.

Diagnosis

Clinical signs of basal skull fractures include bilateral periorbital ecchymoses, anosmia, or CSF rhinorrhea for anterior skull base fractures, as well as hemotympanum, blood in the external auditory canal, seventh or eighth nerve palsies, ecchymosis over the mastoids, or CSF otorrhea for temporal bone fractures. Frequently, the CSF leak is first detected several days or weeks after the trauma. This delay often occurs because the CSF leak was hidden in bloody nasal discharge from facial fractures or, less frequently, is due to the delayed development of hydrocephalus with rupture of the arachnoid at the fracture site. A larger clear ring surrounding a central blood-tinged clot when a few drops of bloody discharge are placed on a paper towel indicates that CSF is mixed with the blood. This sign can also be noted on the patient's pillow during morning rounds.

Basal skull fracture with CSF rhinorrhea is common after head injury and has an estimated incidence in the United States of 150,000 cases per year. A clear, watery nasal discharge containing glucose indicates CSF rhinorrhea. An intermittent CSF leak from the paranasal sinuses can often be demonstrated by having the patient sit on the edge of the bed with the head close to the knees for 2 minutes and watching for clear fluid to drip from the nose.

Management

How a basal skull fracture is managed usually depends on whether a CSF leak is present. A patient with a basal skull fracture but no leak is observed for 2 to 3 days. During this time repeated checks for rhinorrhea and otorrhea are made to verify the absence of a CSF leak. Otorrhea is more likely than rhinorrhea to resolve spontaneously. Because antibiotics are not effective in preventing meningitis and may select for resistant organisms if an infection occurs, prophylactic antibiotics are not used in patients with basal skull fractures.

A CSF leak is managed initially by observing the amount of leakage and monitoring for signs of infection: change in temperature, mental status, or white blood cell count. Most traumatic CSF leaks resolve spontaneously within the first week. If the leak persists beyond 5 to 7 days, lumbar taps are performed daily for 3 days, removing 30 to 50 mL of spinal fluid each time.

If spinal taps fail to stop the leak, spinal drainage can be used for 72 hours with the patient in a 30° head-up position. Should pneumocephalus develop during the course of CSF drainage, the drainage procedure is terminated and the dural leak is surgically closed. CSF leaks refractory to spinal fluid drainage require surgical closure; the exact site of the leak is determined preoperatively with a CT scan with water-soluble intrathecal contrast, or with a nuclear cisternogram with nasal pledgets for small or questionable leaks. Tomograms of the base of the skull can provide additional details of the bone spicules of the fracture.

CSF otorrhea usually occurs through a fracture of the petrous bone and perforation of the tympanic membrane, although it can occasionally take place through a laceration of the external canal via fractured mastoid air cells. If the tympanic membrane remains intact, CSF that has gained access to the middle ear can flow through the eustachian tube and present as rhinorrhea. In these cases the CT scan typically images a fracture in the temporal bone and fluid in the mastoid air cells and middle ear.

A patient with CSF otorrhea often presents with hearing loss or blood in the external ear canal. Irrigation and probing of the ear in cases of suspected otorrhea are not indicated initially since they increase the risk of infection. Such a patient is managed by placing a loose-fitting sterile gauze pad over the ear; the pad is changed every nursing shift and saved as an indicator of the amount of drainage from the ear. Most cases of otorrhea stop spontaneously within the first few days. A detailed auditory and vestibular examination is performed 6 to 8 weeks after trauma to diagnose abnormalities and determine treatment.

In patients with basilar skull fracture, immediate complete facial nerve paralysis, and temporal bone fracture, surgical exploration to decompress or graft the nerve is performed. Patients with delayed onset of the facial paralysis or who initially have only facial paresis are followed, because spontaneous recovery usually occurs.

MAXILLOFACIAL INJURIES

Skull and maxillofacial fractures often coexist after head trauma. For instance, fractures of the frontal bone or basilar skull commonly extend into the orbit, and midfacial fractures frequently accompany frontal skull, sinus, or orbital fractures. In addition, fractures through the skull into the nasal sinuses can cause dural lacerations with CSF leak and/or pneumocephalus. When maxillofacial injury is suspected on physical examination, a CT scan of the face is the most useful diagnostic test and should be obtained at the time of initial radiographic survey.

ASSESSMENT

The events of the injury should be ascertained and a complete history of the accident or injury recorded as described by the emergency medical technician, patient, or family members. A thorough facial physical examination is performed, concentrating on areas of injury. Consultations from specific specialists, such as an ophthalmologist, are also obtained. Cranial nerve abnormalities may also accompany facial fractures; oculomotor deficit, facial sensory deficit, or visual deficit are the common ones.

Soft-tissue injury implies the possibility of damage to deeper structures, which should be presumed until appropriate examination rules it out. Localized hematomas can be aspirated and removed to facilitate healing, although they are usually diffuse and not amenable to aspiration.

The facial bones should be examined from top to bottom. Symptoms that imply bony injury include soft-tissue injury (contusion, laceration, hematoma), bone movement, crepitation, localized tenderness, discomfort, numbness in the distribution of a cranial sensory nerve, paralysis in the distribution of a cranial motor nerve, malocclusion, visual acuity disturbance, diplopia, facial deformity or asymmetry, intraoral lacerations, fractured or avulsed teeth, air in soft tissues, and bleeding from the nose or mouth. The examiner should palpate the symmetry of the facial bones, comparing both sides. In some cases reference to old photographs can aid in documenting a preexisting facial deformity. Dental malalignment (malocclusion) is an index of bone or tooth fracture, edema, or temporomandibular joint injury.

Facial sensation is noted in the supraorbital, supratrochlear, infratrochlear, infraorbital, and mental nerve regions of the trigeminal nerve distribution for both pin and light touch sensation. Diminished sensation in the distribution of a specific sensory nerve indicates injury

from transection, impact, or continued compression of the nerve as the result of a fracture. The facial nerve is tested by comparing facial expression bilaterally. Extraocular movements and pupil response are compared, evaluating symmetry, pupil size, and the speed of pupil reaction bilaterally to both direct and consensual responses to light.

Emergency treatment is directed towards immediately life-threatening events such as airway obstruction or major hemorrhage from the scalp or face. During this phase, aspiration is usually prevented and the airway is maintained by orotracheal intubation, although occasionally an emergency tracheostomy is required. The stability of the cervical spine is assessed in every patient with head trauma during this phase.

The early management of maxillofacial injuries is based on clinical examination and facial CT scans (Fig. 18.5). Both soft-tissue and bone windows are necessary on the CT scan to evaluate the brain and orbit fully. Axial (Fig. 18.6) and coronal CT scans (direct or reformatted) are crucial to reveal details of fractures of the middle third of the orbit. Coronal sections (Fig. 18.7) begin with the nasal pyramid and continue posteriorly through the orbital apex. Axial scans begin at the superior aspect of the skull and progress through the brain

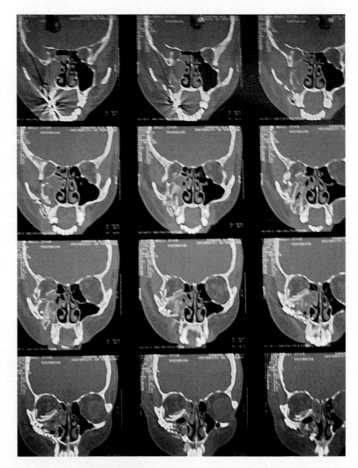

Figure 18.5 Two-dimensional facial CT scans are essential in facial fracture evaluation. They can be obtained rapidly after the CT evaluation of the brain. Axial windows should be obtained through the entire area of injury.

with standard axial brain imaging. The size and spacing of the cuts at the level of the frontal sinus must be reduced to 2 or 3 mm to obtain detail in the frontal sinus and orbit down to the maxillary alveolus. When a mandible fracture is suspected, the axial CT scanning is continued through the mandible, visualizing both its horizontal and vertical portions. Although three-dimensional reconstruction with shading (Fig. 18.8) adds spatial information, it does not provide the detail of two-dimensional axial and coronal images. In some cases, special reconstructions, as in the longitudinal axis of the optic nerve in orbital injury, provide additional information (Fig. 18.9).

Respiratory Obstruction

Facial injuries can impair breathing in several ways. Fractured or avulsed teeth, broken dentures or bridgework, and foreign objects displaced into the airway must be removed. Facial fracture segments may be sufficiently displaced to compromise the airway. In addition, facial bleeding can contribute to aspiration and respiratory obstruction. Patients with combinations of burns and fractures of the upper and lower jaws, fractures of the nose, maxilla, and mandible, or fractures of the mandible that result in significant bleeding into the floor of mouth and neck all may have respiratory obstruction. Noisy res-

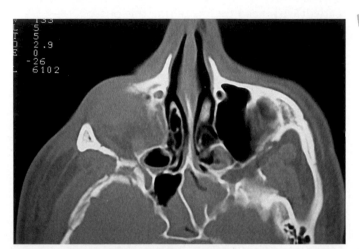

Figure 18.6 Axial window of an orbital fracture.

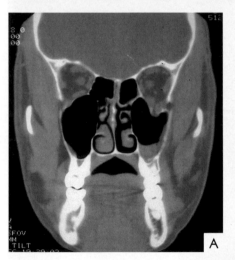

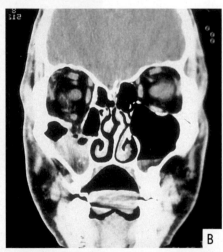

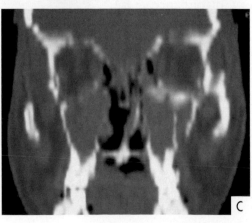

Figure 18.7 Direct coronal windows are preferable for evaluation of the orbit, sinuses, and palate. Both soft-tissue (**A**) and bone (**B**) windows should be obtained for the orbit. (**C**) Reformatted images may be obtained where the direct coronal image is not possible. Their clarity depends on thin axial cuts.

piration, stridor, hoarseness, drooling, inability to swallow or handle oral secretions, sternal retraction, and cyanosis all herald impending death from respiratory obstruction—immediate intubation or tracheostomy is required. The use of plate and screw fixation for facial fracture reduction has allowed intermaxillary fixation to be discontinued postoperatively for many patients. Tracheostomy can often be avoided with the use of rigid fixation.

Profuse Hemorrhage

Bleeding that accompanies facial lacerations is usually controlled with digital pressure, which allows precise identification of the bleeding vessel for control with ligature. Blind probing in facial tissue or unselective ligature placement can damage the facial nerve.

Bleeding from closed maxillofacial injuries usually results from fractures involving the sinuses. Bleeding from the nose (epistaxis) occurs with nasal, zygomatic, orbital, frontal sinus, nasoethmoidal, maxillary, and cranial base fractures. Although the greatest nasopharyngeal hemorrhage usually accompanies Le Fort maxillary fractures, epistaxis is a nonspecific indication. Several maneuvers usually control this hemorrhage, including an anteroposterior nasal pack, manual repositioning and the application of intermaxillary fixation, or an external facial compression dressing.

If profuse hemorrhage from closed fractures does not respond to the above measures, arterial ligation can be performed. An angiogram is usually obtained to determine the major area of bleeding. In Le Fort fractures this usually involves the internal maxillary artery. This artery can be selectively ligated directly through the back wall of the maxillary sinus, or arterial ligations of the external carotid and superficial temporal on the ipsilateral side usually reduce the bleeding substantially. Arterial ligation is rarely necessary.

Because bleeding abnormalities are noted early in patients with concomitant cerebral injuries and facial fractures, replacement of depleted coagulation factors can be based on the hourly assessment of coagulation factors in hemorrhaging patients. Because aspiration of blood, saliva, and gastric contents frequently accompanies maxillofacial injuries and can obstruct respiration, endotracheal intubation or tracheostomy is the definitive treatment.

Coma and Brain Injury

Coma or unconsciousness should not prevent or delay the treatment of facial fractures; many patients with facial fractures are in coma for several weeks before waking up. In patients with maxillofacial fractures, neurologic deficits from frontal lobe symptoms may be subtle or absent despite contusion imaged on brain CT scans. Confusion, somnolence, personality change, irritability, and difficulty in thinking are some of the symptoms of frontal brain contusion.

In patients with Glasgow Coma Scale scores of 14 or less, or when traumatic brain abnormality is visualized on CT scan, an intracranial pressure monitoring device is used in the operating room during the facial repair, thus allowing optimal modification of the anesthesia and surgical time in patients with multiple injuries.

FACIAL FRACTURE CLASSIFICATION BY ANATOMIC REGION

The treatment and thus the description of maxillofacial fractures are organized by anatomic region (Fig. 18.10). The frontal bone region includes the frontal bone, the supraorbital rims bilaterally, and the frontal sinus. The upper midface region includes the zygomas laterally, the internal orbital area, and the nasoethmoidal area cen-

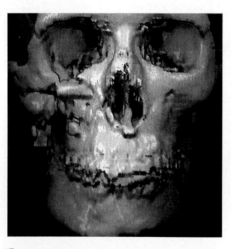

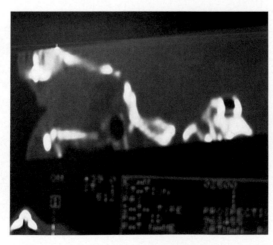

Figure 18.9 CT scans can be taken in the longitudinal axis of the optic nerve. Here, they provide information essential for the reconstruction of the orbital floor. Posteriorly, the intact orbit is visualized. Anteriorly, the broken rim fragments are visualized. Soft tissue may be herniated into the bone gap.

Figure 18.8 Three-dimensional CT scans add spatial perspective, but they do not replace two-dimensional CT scans and are not essential for reconstruction.

trally. The lower midface consists of the maxillary alveolus. The mandible consists of the horizontal portion containing the teeth and the vertical portion that includes the angle, ramus, and coronoid and condylar processes. The pattern and displacement of the fracture in each anatomic region determines treatment. Orbital fractures are classified by their position on the orbital rim and by their involvement of the internal section of the orbit. Orbital rim fractures are divided into the supraorbital region, the nasoethmoidal region medially, and the zygomatic region inferolaterally (Fig. 18.11). The internal orbit consists of the orbital floor, the lateral orbit, the medial (ethmoidal) orbit, and the orbital roof. Maxillary fractures are classified according to the pattern of Le Fort, based on the fracture's location.

Fractures of the Frontal Bone and Supraorbital Area

Fractures of the frontal area frequently extend into the orbit. A fracture in this area implies the possibility of injury to the dura and to the frontal brain. CSF rhinorrhea and pneumocephalus may be present.

Because of its strength the frontal bone is involved in only 5% to 10% of all facial fractures. Fractures that simultaneously involve the cranium and the orbit are high-energy injuries, and soft-tissue damage is more severe. Major injuries to the brain and the cervical spine frequently accompany these fractures, and contusion of the forebrain and orbital contents is routine.

The frontal and ethmoid sinuses render the frontal bone more vulnerable to injury and infection. Each limb of the frontal sinus has a "duct" (usually an ostium) that communicates with the upper portion of the nose. Sinus injury may therefore result in duct obstruction after fracture, mucosal edema, or damage. A cyst-like structure called a *mucocele* (obstructed mucous cyst) sometimes follows mucosal injury; depending on its size, it may erode bone and penetrate into the orbit or intracranial cavity. Surgery at a later time is necessary to remedy either of these conditions, as symptoms of pain and sinusitis will persist. Since the posterior wall of the frontal sinus is in contact with the dura, any infection in that area represents an extradural abscess. Posterior wall fractures of the frontal sinus are often accompanied by dural tears. Many of these tears extend along the anterior basilar frontal region of the skull to cause a CSF leak or pneumocephalus. A small CSF leak is often masked by epistaxis in the early days after facial injury. When fractures in the posterior wall of the frontal sinus

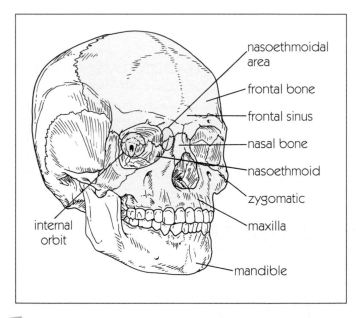

Figure 18.10 The anatomic regions of the face are shown. They include the frontal bone, the frontal sinus, the nose, the nasoethmoidal area, the zygoma, the internal orbit, the maxilla, and the mandible.

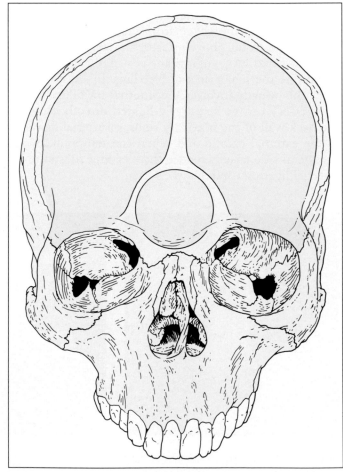

Figure 18.11 The divisions of the frontal bone are shaded. They include the central (frontal sinus) area (blue) and, laterally, the frontotemporoorbital region (green), which extends to the coronal suture. Fractures often involve two of the three areas of the frontal skull.

or the anterior base of the skull are noted, a CSF leak should be suspected.

Fractures of the frontal bone commonly extend to or involve the cranial sutures or other regions. When the fracture extends into the supraorbital region, the bone is usually depressed downward and posteriorly, compressing the orbital contents and producing a downward and forward dislocation of the globe (Fig. 18.12). With more limited injuries, linear frontal skull fractures may extend into the orbit and along the cranial base. These fractures can create a CSF leak or obstruct sinus drainage by virtue of edema or bone displacement. As fracture patterns become more complex and severe, bone displacement occurs. The base of the skull and the roofs of the orbits become comminuted, and linear fractures extend from the anterior into the middle cranial fossa. Again, the anterior and middle sections of the orbit displace, and linear fractures extend from the displaced bone into the posterior portion of the orbit and the middle cranial fossa. These fractures can account for basilar CSF leaks, pituitary disturbances, and dizziness from involvement of the temporal bone and vestibular structures.

Diagnosis

The most common clinical signs of fractures of the frontal bone are an overlying bruise or hematoma and, less often, a laceration of the brow or over the frontal sinus (Fig. 18.13). CT scans occasionally show a posterior wall fracture of the frontal sinus without an accompanying anterior wall fracture. Fractures of the orbit usually result in palpebral and subconjunctival hematomas. A step deformity or irregularity in the orbital rim may be appreciated on palpation, but swelling may obscure the irregularity. If periorbital swelling is severe, complete ptosis exists. If the lid cannot be opened voluntarily, it should be opened manually to inspect the globe for integrity. Visual acuity should be assessed and extraocular muscle motion should be evaluated.

Evaluation of the visual system is critical. Supraorbital fractures, for example, represent 10% of all periorbital fractures but account for 30% of serious eye injuries. The most common serious injuries to the globe are rupture, retinal detachment, and vitreous or anterior chamber hemorrhage. The presence of globe injury modifies fracture treatment by limiting manipulation;

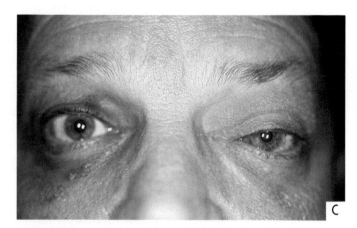

Figure 18.12 In a supraorbital fracture, posterior and inferior displacement of the superior orbital rim produces downward and forward dislocation of the globe. (A) The normal configuration of the superior orbit. (B) Dislocation of the superior orbital rim and globe displacement. (C) A patient with a displaced supraorbital fracture producing inferior globe displacement.

avoidance of pressure on the globe may take precedence over bone reconstruction. Visual acuity and pupil response are documented before and after any surgical treatment using a Rosenbaum pocket visual screening card. If this is not possible, the pupil response to light is evaluated both directly and consensually. Inability to move the globe into a particular field of gaze indicates either a cranial nerve palsy or local interference with an extraocular muscle secondary to contusion, local nerve injury, or incarceration.

Fractures of the roof of the orbit usually produce a temporary paresis of the levator muscle that results in posttraumatic ptosis. This palsy may persist for months; no treatment to elevate the lid further is indicated until all spontaneous activity has returned (at least 6 months). Partial or complete spontaneous recovery usually occurs. The superior rectus muscle is usually undamaged in fractures of the superior orbit, but occasionally paresis occurs and mimics incarceration of the inferior rectus muscle. These conditions are differentiated by the combination of radiographic evaluation, forced-duction testing, and formal eye muscle evaluation. Entrapment of the levator and superior rectus muscles rarely occurs in orbital roof fractures.

Supraorbital fractures are usually displaced inward and downward (see Fig. 18.12), producing a forward and downward displacement of the globe. The globe occasionally bulges forward so that the eyelids cannot close completely. In such cases urgent facial fracture reduction is required to protect the cornea. Fractures of the orbital roof may have a linear extension that enters the superior orbital fissure or optic foramen. Visual acuity is affected if the optic nerve is compressed by a displaced fracture fragment, in which case the direct pupil response to light on the injured side is slower than the direct pupil response on the other side. Superior orbital fissure syndrome may also be present, consisting of palsy of extraocular muscle motion, ptosis, global proptosis, and anesthesia in the first division of the trigeminal nerve (the ipsilateral forehead). Patients may experience numbness in the distribution of the supraorbital or supratrochlear nerves, which is usually transient, although lacerations in the area frequently divide the nerve, producing permanent numbness.

Management
Displacement of more than 4 or 5 mm produces a depression or a change in globe position; release of the pressure on the globe or the nerves may improve function. Open skull fractures require debridement, repair of dural lacerations, evacuation of epidural hematomas, and appropriate surgical procedures for frontal lobe injury. Bone fragments are cleaned of mucosa and debris, and antiseptic irrigation is used. The frontal skull can be reconstructed primarily by linking the bone fragments with interfragment wires and stabilizing the pieces with plate and screw fixation (Fig. 18.14).

Frontal Sinus Fractures
Fractures of the frontal sinus may involve the anterior wall, the posterior wall, or both. Fractures that obstruct the nasofrontal duct must be treated on a functional basis. Fractures that depress only the anterior wall of the frontal sinus are repaired for esthetic reasons. The symptoms of a frontal sinus fracture are usually localized bruising, hematoma, or laceration; the fracture often extends into the orbit, producing both palpebral and subconjunctival hematomas.

Diagnosis
Frontal sinus fractures are diagnosed on CT scan with fracture through the front wall, back wall, or both walls. Displacement of bone at the posterior wall usually indicates an underlying dural laceration.

Management
Localized fractures of the anterior wall are managed by returning the fragments to the proper position and debriding devitalized mucosa. If the nasofrontal duct is intact, fluid will flow freely into the nose; replaced bone

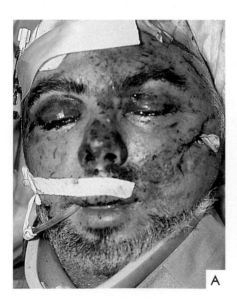
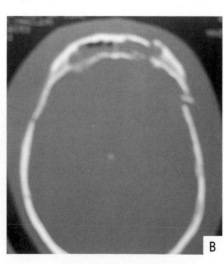

Figure 18.13 (A) A patient with a frontal and supraorbital fracture. (B) CT scan demonstrating fracture displacement.

fragments are stabilized with interfragment wires or plate and screw fixation. If the posterior wall is involved, the integrity of the dura is usually assessed by direct inspection at operation. Significant fractures of the anterior and posterior walls are best managed by intracranial exposure and debridement of small bone fragments. If the posterior wall of the sinus has been removed, the sinus should be "cranialized" by completely removing the mucosa and plugging the naso-frontal duct with several layers of bone grafts. A sheet bone graft is placed over the bone plugs and over involved ethmoid sinuses (Fig. 18.15). Any involved sinus must be debrided to minimize infection and delayed mucocele formation since obstruction of an ethmoid sinus produces an orbital or epidural abscess. The anterior wall of the sinus is then reconstructed. Complete removal of sinus mucosa requires light burring of the bone fragments.

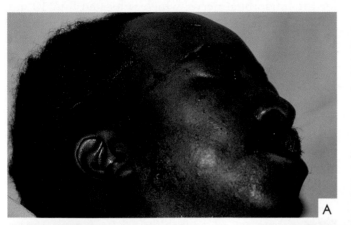
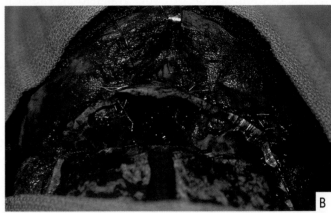

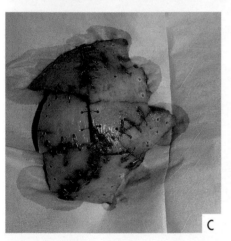
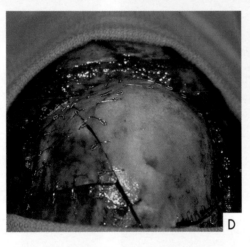
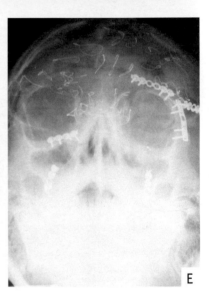

Figure 18.14 (A) A patient with a supraorbital fracture. (B) The defect in the anterior cranial base after removal of fractured bone. (C) The bone has been cleansed and debrided and the small fragments wired together on a back table while neurosurgery was in progress. (D,E) The bone is in place now, linked with interfragment wires. It will be stabilized with rigid fixation to intact bone at its periphery.

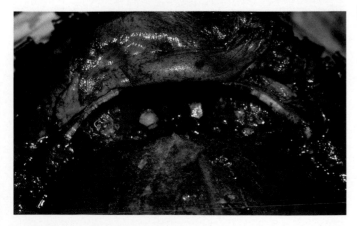

Figure 18.15 The nasofrontal duct should be plugged with several layers of bone graft. Bone provides strong structural material to close the opening between the intracranial cavity and the nose. Muscle and fascia deteriorate rapidly and do not provide stability.

Less involved frontal sinus fractures may be managed by sinus obliteration. When fractures compromise nasal frontal duct function, all sinus mucosa should be removed and the wall of the sinus thoroughly burred to bleeding bone. The nasofrontal duct is then plugged with several layers of bone plugs taken from the calvaria, and the remainder of the sinus is filled with bone shavings (Fig. 18.16). Alternately, the sinus cavity can be left unfilled after the insertion of the bone plugs; obliteration will slowly occur by osteoneogenesis, which consists of proliferation of bone, granulation, and scar tissue. Unfortunately, regrowth of frontal sinus mucosa may occasionally occur, or the development of a cyst in a lacerated area of mucosa may produce a mucocele. Surgical intervention may be required for infection or erosion of the cyst into adjacent structures.

Orbital Fractures

The supraorbital rims are weakened centrally by the presence of the frontal sinus. The supraorbital rim extends to join the temporal bone and the zygoma (see Fig. 18.11). The orbit consists of three sections (Fig. 18.17). The midsection of the orbit can be divided into four regions (Fig. 18.18). Fractures occur first in the thin bone of the middle third of the orbit.

A blow to the lateral aspect of the upper face can fracture both the supraorbital rim and the zygoma. Cranioorbital injuries call for both neurosurgery and orbital reconstruction. Zygomatic fractures usually extend from the junction medially with the maxilla at the infraorbital rim through the inferior and lateral orbit. Medially, the fracture often involves the canal for the infraorbital nerve, which is located 8 to 10 mm inferior to the lower orbital rim parallel to the medial aspect of the cornea. A fracture here produces numbness in the inferior orbital nerve distribution.

The nasoethmoidal orbital region represents the medial rim of the orbit (see Fig. 18.17). Posteriorly, the ethmoid air cells weaken the nasoethmoidal region, one of the thinnest portions of the orbital wall. Fractures involving the medial orbital rim displace the bone bearing the attachment of the medial canthal tendon, which may also block the lacrimal system, resulting in tearing. Displacement of the medial orbital rim or the infraor-

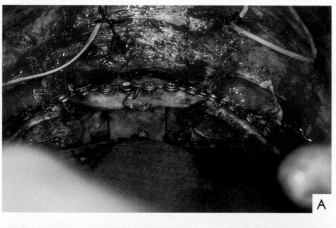
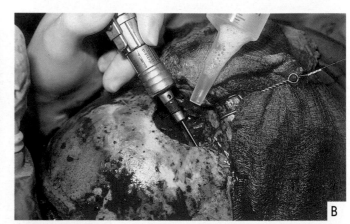
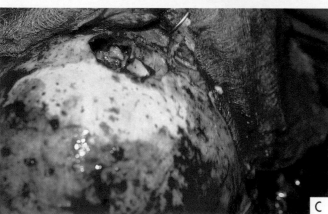
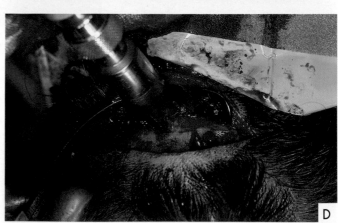

Figure 18.16 (A) A sheet bone graft should be laid across the plugged frontal sinus ducts to cover previously cleansed and debrided fractures involving the cranial base and ethmoidal sinuses. This layer is not watertight but begins to develop its own partition between the intracranial cavity and the nose. (B) In cases where the sinus cavity is to be obliter- ated, the mucosa is thoroughly removed. The walls of the sinus should be burred lightly to eliminate areas where mucosa extends along the veins in the wall of the sinus cavity. After nasofrontal duct obliteration with bone plugs, the sinus cavity can be obliterated with particulate bone graft (C) taken from the parietal area with a craniotome (D).

Principles of Neurosurgery

bital rim and floor of the orbit alters the attachment of the eyelids and the suspensory ligaments of the globe, permitting globe and canthal ligament dystopia, which can be detected on physical examination.

The orbital roof is composed of the greater and lesser wings of the sphenoid. It separates the anterior cranial fossa from the orbital contents. Medially, at the frontal sinus, the orbital roof thins, becoming almost transparent. The attachment of the superior oblique tendon immediately behind the rim is often a separate small fragment in fractures. Diplopia produced by interference with superior oblique function is difficult to remedy. The surgeon must be aware of this attachment and avoid injury by making dissection absolutely subperiosteal. The frontal sinus is extremely variable in size and shape; asymmetry is the rule. It does not develop until the teenage years and thus is absent in the pediatric trauma victim.

The medial wall of the orbit is formed by the thin orbital plate of the ethmoid bone. This bone is reinforced by septa within the ethmoid sinus, which give it some additional strength (Fig. 18.19). The lateral wall of the orbit consists of the orbital process of the malar bone anteriorly and the greater wing of the sphenoid posteriorly (Fig. 18.20). The zygomaticosphenoid suture is involved in all zygoma fractures. Its broad surface forms an excellent area for confirmation of proper zygomatic alignment. With more comminuted orbital fractures, displacement of multiple walls of the orbit contributes to dramatic orbital deformity. Because soft-tissue orbital deformity is not entirely reversible with secondary corrections, the emphasis is on immediate definitive reconstruction.

The lateral canthal ligament attaches with the lateral aspect of the eyelids to the zygoma at Whitnall's tubercle, which is a shallow bulge in the internal aspect of the rim. The anterior limb of the lateral canthal tendon is continuous with the galea, and the posterior limb joins the lateral extension of the levator tendon and Lockwood's suspensory ligament in its attachment to Whitnall's tubercle (Fig. 18.21). The extraocular muscles travel close to the orbital walls in the posterior half of the orbit. In the anterior half, they are protected from orbital wall fractures by a thin cushion of extramuscular cone fat. Thin muscular "check ligaments" extend from the extraocular muscles diffusely to the orbital walls (Fig. 18.22). These ligaments, described by Leo Koorneef, diffusely interconnect the soft tissue of the orbit to provide structural continuity among all the orbital tissues, such as fat, muscle, periosteum, and globe. This interconnection of all orbital soft tissue is why diplopia (extraocular muscle restriction) occurs if a particular section of orbital soft tissue is restricted.

The orbital floor is one of the weakest portions of

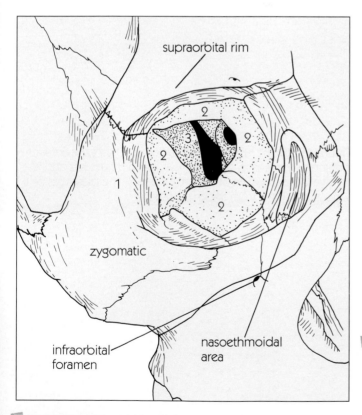

Figure 18.17 The orbit consists of three sections from anterior to posterior: the thick rim anteriorly, the thin middle section, and the thick posterior third of the orbit. The posterior portion of the orbit represents the cranial base. The orbital rim can be conceptualized in three regions: superiorly, the supraorbital rim; inferiorly and laterally, the zygomatic region; medially, the nasoethmoidal area.

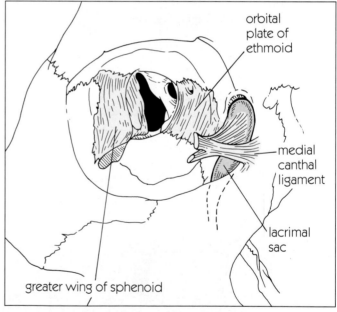

Figure 18.18 The midsection of the orbit is conceptualized in four regions: laterally, the orbital process of the zygoma and the greater wing of the sphenoid; inferiorly, the orbital floor; medially, the lamina papyracea of ethmoid bone; and superiorly, the orbital roof. The posterior third of the orbit contains the superior orbital fissure, the posterior portion of the inferior orbital fissure, and the optic foramen. The medial canthal ligament surrounds the lacrimal sac. A groove for the lacrimal sac is present immediately behind the orbital rim. The medial canthal ligament consists of anterior, superior, and posterior limbs.

the orbit. There is an initial concave section immediately behind the inferior orbital rim, and then a convex constriction. This complex orbital anatomy must be recreated when reconstructing the orbit. Because the complex curves of bone in relation to the soft tissue determine globe position (Fig. 18.23), it is extremely important to mimic the exact curvature of the middle portion of the orbit and the position of the orbital rim. The concave

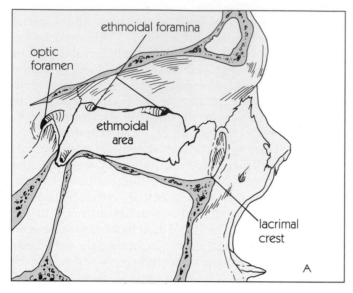

Figure 18.19 (A) The medial wall is the thinnest bone of the orbit but, reinforced by septa within the ethmoid sinus, is strong in comparison to its thickness. The anterior and posterior ethmoidal foramina, located towards the upper portion of the medial orbital wall, are on the same level as the optic canal. These neurovascular foramina can be used as landmarks to direct the surgeon in his protection of the optic nerve. (B) Fractures of the ethmoid frequently show symmetric compression. Reconstruction involves bone grafting to the normal contour.

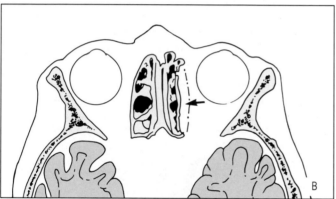

Figure 18.20 The lateral wall of the orbit. Often, the anterior portion of the greater wing of the sphenoid fractures and is involved in expansion of the orbital cavity. The distances of various structures from the rim are shown.

roof must be reconstructed in its exact arching anatomic position or the globe will be displaced inferolaterally.

The posterior third of the orbit contains the optic foramen, the superior orbital fissure, and the posterior aspect of the inferior orbital fissure. The superior orbital fissure is bounded by the greater and lesser wings of the sphenoid (Fig. 18.24). Linear fractures are commonly seen in the posterior portion of the orbit;

however, displacement of bone is less common here. Usually, the anterior and middle sections act as a shock absorber, protecting the posterior portion from severe displacement.

The inferior orbital fissure separates the orbital floor from the lateral orbital wall. It contains veins, the infraorbital artery and nerve, and the zygomaticofacial nerve.

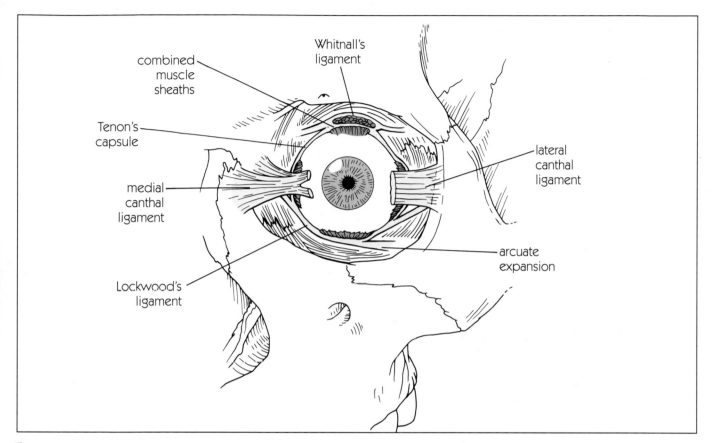

Figure 18.21 The fascial sling for globe support. The globe has been removed. Medially and laterally, the medial and lateral canthal ligaments provide attachments for structures that provide anterior globe support. Indicated are Lockwood's ligament, supporting the globe inferiorly, the medial and lateral canthal ligaments, and behind them, medial and lateral check ligaments. Superiorly, Whitnall's ligament is present. The combined muscle sheaths also attach to the globe and provide a relative sling for fat and globe support. These ligaments and their sheaths join to Tenon's capsule.

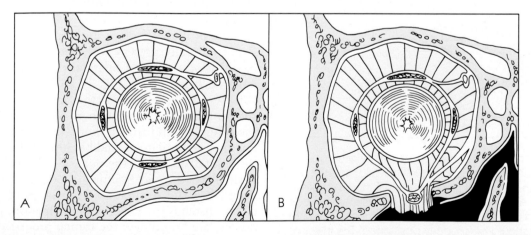

Figure 18.22 Entrapment of the fine ligament system described by Leo Koorneef may produce limitation of extraocular motion. **(A)** The normal system of ligaments that diffusely connect the bony walls of the orbit to the extraocular muscles and the globe. **(B)** An orbital floor fracture has trapped fat and its interconnecting ligaments in the fracture site. Ocular motility may be impaired by impingement of this fine ligament system. (After Koorneef L. Current concepts in the management of blow-out fractures. *Ann Plast Surg.* 1982; 9:185–199)

Diagnosis

A mobile or absent orbital roof may produce a pulsating exophthalmos in which cerebral pulsations are transmitted to the globe and its adnexal structures. This is corrected by reconstruction of the roof, separating the orbit from the intracranial contents with a bone partition.

Fractures involving the orbital roof and middle cranial fossa create a communication (carotid-cavernous sinus fistula) between the carotid artery and the cavernous sinus. A traumatic carotid-cavernous fistula is usually accompanied by severe visual and cranial nerve disturbances. Marked chemosis, globe prominence, extraocular muscle palsy, and blindness are usually present. The fistula is confirmed by arteriography; attempts to obliterate it involve intravascular radiographic techniques.

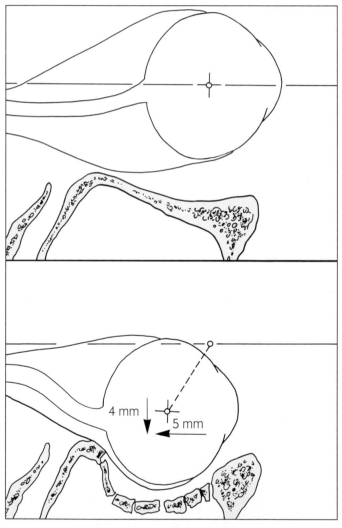

Figure 18.23 The curves of the orbit in the longitudinal axis of the optic nerve. The normal configuration (top) and the usual configuration in enophthalmos (bottom) of the orbital floor are indicated. An intact ledge of bone is present in the posterior orbit and provides a guide for floor reconstruction. First, the orbital rim should be properly positioned. The intact posterior ledge of bone, provides a scaffold for bone support between the rim and posterior orbit. The soft tissue prolapsing into the maxillary sinus must be elevated, restoring globe position.

The most common reason for a visual acuity deficit after trauma is optic nerve injury. Shearing, contusion, or compression may be involved. These injuries may occur with or without demonstrated fractures of the optic canal. If vision is lost at the moment of impact, decompression of an optic canal fracture usually does not increase the chance of visual recovery. However, if bone fragments that compromise the optic canal are demonstrated, or if a fluctuating or partial visual deficit is seen, then decompression should be considered. Immediately after an optic nerve injury the optic disc usually looks normal. A patient may present with a Marcus-Gunn pupil, in which the reaction to consensual constriction is present but the reaction to direct stimulus is reduced. Swinging a light from one globe to the other demonstrates pupillary dilatation in the eye affected (Fig. 18.25).

Atrophy of the optic disk does not appear until 1 month after an optic nerve is injured, so it cannot be used as an acute indication. If vision is initially present after an injury and then deteriorates, swelling from hemorrhage and edema may be compromising the optic canal and compressing the optic nerve. Surgical and/or medical (high-dose steroids) decompression are indicated on an emergency basis.

Management
Specific treatment of the orbital fractures and their interrelation with other facial fractures are covered in other sections.

Nasoethmoid Orbital Fractures

The nasoethmoid orbital fracture consists (in its simplest form) of injury to one or both frontal processes of the maxilla and the nose. The frontal process of the maxilla is the lower two thirds of the medial orbital rim. When this is fractured, the medial canthal ligament is displaced because of its attachment to the fractured bone segment. Nasoethmoid fractures often extend to adjacent areas, including the supraorbital region, the frontal sinus, the inferior orbit, the medial internal orbit, and the floor of the orbit.

These injuries, which may cause significant long-term deformity, are often initially obscured by swelling. Patients usually present with bleeding from the nose, a nasal dislocation, and bilateral periorbital and subconjunctival hematomas (Fig. 18.26). The nasal deformity consists of depression of the nasal dorsum and foreshortening of the nose, with an increased angle between the columella and the lip. Forty percent of nasoethmoid fractures are unilateral, and because of their proximity to the frontal sinus and the dura, a CSF leak may be present. Nasoethmoid fractures produce tearing by compromising the drainage of the lacrimal system as it passes through the maxilla. On palpation, pain and tenderness are found over the frontal process of the maxilla and the palpating finger, inserted deeply over the medial canthal ligament, discloses bony crepitus, movement, and tenderness. Telecanthus may be present if the frac-

Principles of Neurosurgery

ture fragment has been dislocated laterally, in which case the palpebral fissure narrows.

Diagnosis

The presence of a nasoethmoid fracture can be determined by a bimanual examination (Fig. 18.27).

On CT scan, fractures surround the lower two thirds of the medial orbital rim. Medial and inferior internal orbital fractures are present, and the inferior orbital rim, piriform aperture, nose, and internal angular process of the frontal bone at the glabella are fractured.

Lacrimal system injury should be suspected in lacerations of the medial portion of the eyelids. The lacrimal system may also be compromised by fractures involving the bone surrounding the nasolacrimal duct. If the lacrimal system is transected, fluid emerges from a laceration on irrigation of the system with saline.

Management

Nasoethmoid orbital fractures require a definitive open reduction consisting of interfragment wiring and plate and screw fixation of the assembled fragments. In some

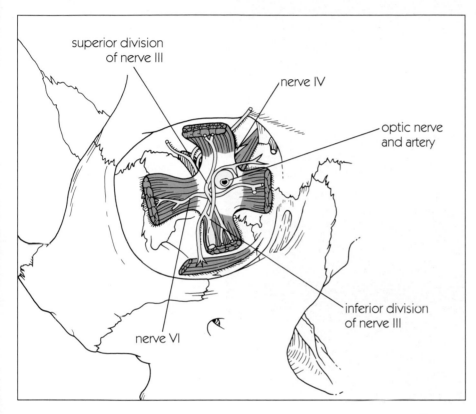

Figure 18.24 The contents of the superior orbital fissure include cranial nerves III, IV, and VI, the ophthalmic division of (trigeminal) cranial nerve V, and vascular structures. The optic foramen is contained within the lesser wings of the sphenoid and admits the optic nerve and ophthalmic artery.

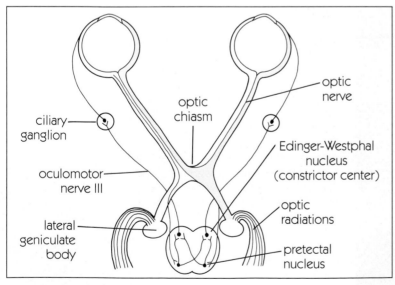

Figure 18.25 The normal pupil reflex pathway and the relation to the Marcus-Gunn pupil. In the normal eye, light striking the retina produces an impulse in the optic nerve that travels to the pretectal nucleus, both Edinger-Westphal nuclei, via nerve III to the ciliary ganglion and pupillary constrictor muscles. In lesions involving the retina or optic nerve back to the chiasm, a light in the unaffected eye produces consensual constriction of the pupil of the affected eye, but a light in the affected eye produces a paradoxic dilatation of the affected pupil. (After Jaboley ME, Lerman M, Saunders HJ. Ocular injuries and orbital fractures: a review of 199 cases. *Plast Reconstr Surg.* 1975;56:410)

situations, this can be accomplished through a laceration or local incision; otherwise, a broad exposure must be provided by a coronal incision (Fig. 18.28). Usually the canthal ligament is not detached from bone during fracture reduction. If the canthal ligament is detached, it must be reattached after assembly of the bone fragments. A separate set of transnasal wires, again passed posterior and superior to the lacrimal fossa through the nose, connects the canal ligament to the bone in its proper position (Fig. 18.29). Contoured bone grafts are used to reconstruct the medial and inferior internal orbit. Long, straight grafts are used to provide contour and to add dorsal height to the nose. These bone grafts are taken from either the calvaria or a split rib.

If a fracture compromises the lacrimal system, replacement of bone into its normal position is the initial

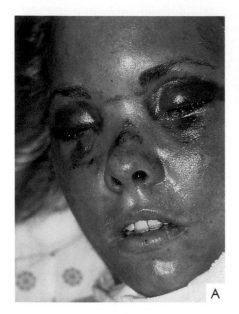

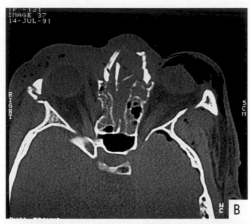

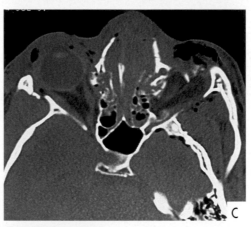

Figure 18.26 (A) In most patients with nasoethmoidal fractures, severe midfacial injury is obvious. Bilateral periorbital hematomas are routine. Here, the nose has literally been driven into the midface and is depressed along its dorsum with foreshortening of the length (increased angle between the lip and columella). (B,C) CT scans of a nasoethmoidal orbital fracture demonstrate comminution of the entire medial orbit and nose.

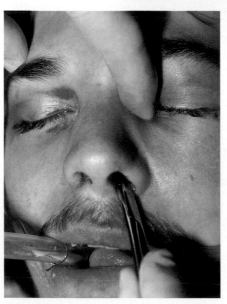

Figure 18.27 The bimanual examination is performed by placing a clamp inside the nose with its tip immediately adjacent to the attachment of the canthal ligament on the frontal process of the maxilla. It is important that the clamp *not* be placed beneath nasal bones or a false-positive diagnosis of a nasoethmoidal fracture will be obtained. A palpating finger is placed externally deeply over the canthal ligament. If the frontal process of the maxilla can be moved between the clamp and the palpating finger, a nasoethmoidal fracture is present. Mobility requires surgical reduction.

treatment. If the lacrimal system is transected, a direct repair of lacrimal canalicular transection is performed with fine sutures under magnification over fine tubes (0.025 inch). Both the upper and lower puncta should be intubated and the tubes brought into the nose through the nasolacrimal canal. They should remain in place for several days to splint the repair.

Fractures of the Orbital Floor

The bony orbital space is a modified cone or pyramid. Fractures of the inferior portion of the orbital floor

often extend 30 to 35 mm behind the rim. The infraorbital nerve weakens the orbital floor. Fractures of the rim and floor damage the function of the nerve, producing hypesthesia of the upper lip, ipsilateral nose, and anterior maxillary teeth.

The most frequent fracture of the internal orbit is the blow-out fracture, which is usually confined to the floor and the lower portion of the medial wall (Fig. 18.30). A depressed fracture of this section of the orbit allows the orbital tissue to be displaced downward into the maxillary and ethmoid sinuses. Medial, inferior,

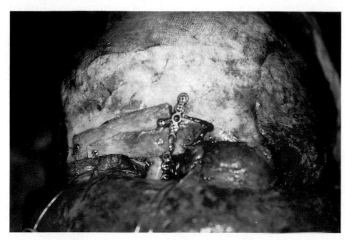

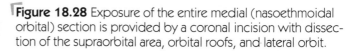

Figure 18.28 Exposure of the entire medial (nasoethmoidal orbital) section is provided by a coronal incision with dissection of the supraorbital area, orbital roofs, and lateral orbit.

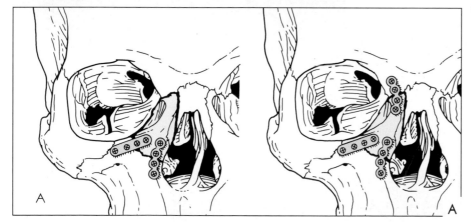

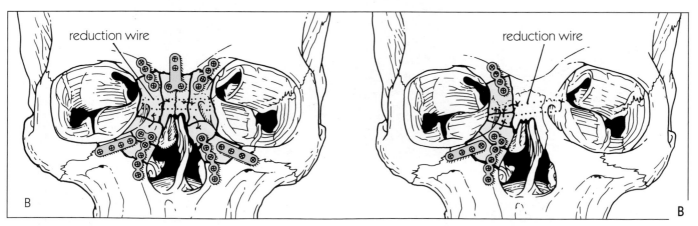

Figure 18.29 (A) Treatment of a simple nasoethmoidal orbital fracture by plate and screw fixation. Noncomminuted fractures can be treated in this fashion. (B) Comminuted fractures require thorough connection of all fragments with interfragment wires. The essential step in the treatment of a nasoethmoidal orbital fracture is to pass a wire between both medial orbital rim segments. This wire is passed transnasally posterior and superior to the lacrimal fossa.

and posterior dislocation of the globe occurs. If fat is trapped in the fracture, it may interfere with the motion of the globe because of the internal ligament system of the orbital soft tissue (Fig. 18.31). Alternatively, the inferior rectus muscle may be directly trapped in a small fracture, leading to restriction of eye movement and possibly incarceration of globe movement.

Patients with orbital fractures usually present with a history of a blunt injury. They may have double vision when looking either upward or downward. Extraocular range of motion may be limited. Periorbital and subconjunctival hematomas are present, as is numbness in the infraorbital nerve distribution. It is imperative that the globe be examined; the possibility of hyphema, retinal detachment, or globe rupture exists with any fracture involving the orbit. The presence of an intraorbital foreign body should always be considered. Orbital fractures are accompanied in 10% to 15% of cases by a globe injury. The visual system and globe are evaluated by visual acuity, visual fields, funduscopic examination, extraocular motion, and intraocular pressure.

Diagnosis

When an inferior orbital floor fracture is accompanied by diplopia, the forced-duction test is used to confirm incarceration of orbital soft tissues in the fracture site. A force generation test provides additional information. Entrapment of soft tissue occurs most frequently with small fractures. Enlargement of the orbital volume is produced by large fractures; globe dystopia and enophthalmos are the results of orbital enlargement.

Enophthalmos denotes the backward dislocation of the globe into the orbit (Fig. 18.32). Large fractures of the orbital floor allow the orbital soft tissue to prolapse backward, downward, and medially, resulting in a loss of globe support and a change in globe position. Anterior globe position, in physical examination, is best compared by assessing the patient from an inferior view (Fig. 18.33). The trauma of the injury may produce fat atrophy, which contributes to globe malposition. Acutely, periorbital injuries produce hemorrhage and edema. Initially, proptosis or exophthalmos appears. Acute enophthalmos is unusual and indicates a dramatic

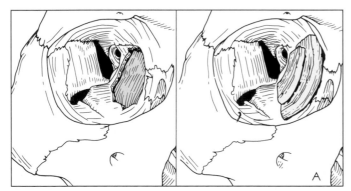 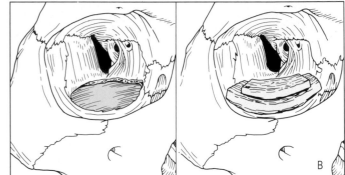

Figure 18.30 (A,B) The usual internal orbital fractures involving the floor and the medial orbital wall. Bone grafts can be used to restore internal orbital integrity.

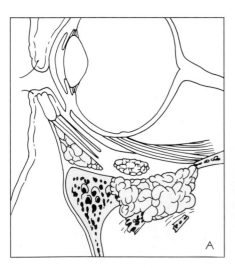 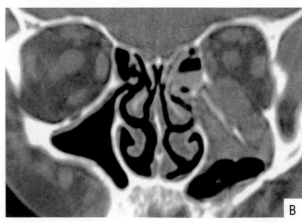

Figure 18.31 (A,B) An orbital blow-out fracture involving the thin portion of the orbital floor. Fat and its interconnecting fascia are trapped among the blow-out fracture fragments and limit the excursion of the inferior oblique and inferior rectus muscles. Diplopia may be present from muscle restriction either in up or down gaze.

Principles of Neurosurgery

enlargement in the orbit. If the globe prolapses away from the lids, lubrication of the cornea cannot be accomplished; this is an urgent indication for repair. Enophthalmos is usually accompanied by inferior displacement (globe dystopia). Posterior displacement of the globe produces a supratarsal hollow and ptosis of the upper eyelid.

Management

In many cases, the symptoms of a small internal orbital fracture resolve substantially within a short period. Frequently, double vision is due to muscular contusion and resolves with observation. Surgery is usually indicated for double vision only when it occurs in a functional field of gaze and is due to incarceration of the muscle or the ligament system. There are thus two indications for surgery for blow-out fractures: muscle or ligament entrapment, confirmed by CT scan and forced-duction examination, and enlargement of the

orbit sufficient to produce enophthalmos. This generally requires more than 2 cm^2 of orbital floor involvement, with displacement of more than 3 to 4 mm. The size of the fracture can be accurately estimated on CT scans.

Le Fort Maxillary Fractures

Fractures of the maxilla involve not only the maxilla but the entire midfacial region. These fractures are termed Le Fort maxillary fractures after the classification used by Rene Le Fort (Fig. 18.34).

Diagnosis

In 10% of Le Fort fractures the maxillary alveolus is split, usually in a sagittal (longitudinal) direction (Fig. 18.35), increasing instability and making preservation of normal occlusion a challenge. Lower maxillary fractures are diagnosed by malocclusion and maxillary mobility. Upper maxillary fractures are diagnosed by

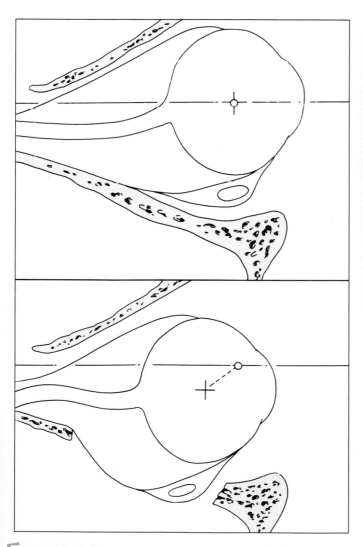

Figure 18.32 The orbit's enlargement allows displacement of the globe backward and downward to produce enophthalmos.

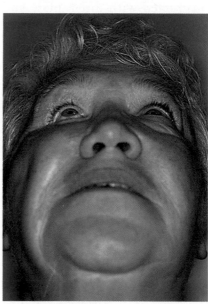

Figure 18.33 Enophthalmos is most accurately assessed by comparison of globe position from an inferior perspective.

maxillary mobility, malocclusion, periorbital hematomas, nasopharyngeal bleeding, pain, and the symptoms of zygomatic, orbital, and nasoethmoidal fractures. Examination for maxillary mobility is essential to confirm the presence of a Le Fort fracture. The maxilla should be grasped with one hand while the head is stabilized with the other. The level at which the mobility occurs indicates the level of the Le Fort fracture. Occasionally, Le Fort fractures are not mobile; they may be either impacted or incomplete.

Management

The principal treatment of Le Fort fractures is intermaxillary fixation with the maxilla in occlusion with the mandible. Initial stabilization is generally accomplished by ligating arch bars to the upper and lower teeth and connecting the maxillary and mandibular arch bars with intermaxillary wires. Fracture sites at the various levels of the midface (as defined by CT scans) are aligned, and then the nasofrontal and zygomaticomaxillary buttresses (Fig. 18.36) are reconstructed with direct plate and screw fixation. This eliminates or decreases the use of intermaxillary fixation postoperatively.

A Le Fort I fracture is treated by placing the patient in intermaxillary fixation, exposing the LeFort I level buttresses, reducing the fracture, and using direct plate and screw fixation (Fig. 18.37).

Le Fort II fractures are treated by placing the patient in intermaxillary fixation. The fracture fragments are aligned with interfragment wires and stabilized with direct plate and screw fixation (Fig. 18.38). Orbital floor defects are spanned with bone grafts, or perhaps with alloplastic implants for smaller defects. If rigid fixation is used, intermaxillary fixation is discontinued postoperatively. Normal occlusion must be confirmed carefully for a 4- to 12-week period postoperatively. Patients with intermaxillary fixation require a liquid diet and should be placed on a soft diet when it is discontinued.

Le Fort III fractures are treated with surgical approaches to zygomatic, nasoethmoidal, and orbital floor fractures and to the Le Fort I level (Fig. 18.39). Again, fragments are initially aligned with interfragment wires and stabilized with plate and screw fixation. A sagittal fracture of the maxilla is directly reduced through the palatal laceration or incision with plate and screw fixation. A small plate is also placed at the piriform aperture

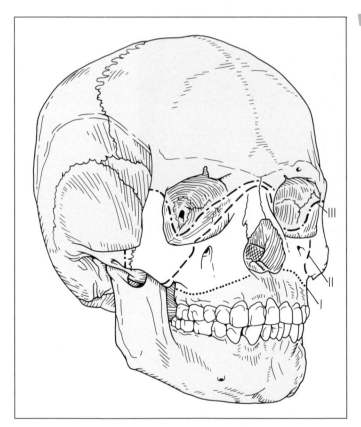

Figure 18.34 Le Fort fractures. Le Fort, on the basis of cadaver experiments, identified thinner areas of the midfacial skeleton that fracture more commonly. Often, combinations of fractures are seen. The Le Fort I fracture travels horizontally across the base of the piriform aperture, separating the lower portion of the maxillary sinuses from the upper midfacial skeleton. In the Le Fort II injury, a pyramidal lower facial segment is separated from the upper cranial facial skeleton. The fracture travels laterally through the Le Fort I, through the inferior orbital rims medially, and through either the cartilaginous portion of the nose or the nasofrontal junction centrally. In the Le Fort III injury, the cranium is separated from the midfacial skeleton through the internal orbital margins of the zygoma. The fracture begins at the zygomaticofrontal suture, extends down the junction of the greater wing of the sphenoid with the orbital process of the zygoma, crosses the orbital floor to travel up the medial orbital wall, comminutes the nasoethmoid region and the nasofrontal junction, and similarly transects the contralateral orbit. In practice, it is usual to see the Le Fort fracture level higher on one side than the other. Commonly, Le Fort III superior level injuries on one side occur with a Le Fort II superior level injury on the other.

to unite the two maxillary segments. In some cases, an acrylic splint is placed in the palatal vault to adjust occlusal relationships further.

Fractures of the Nose

A fracture of the nose may involve the cartilaginous nasal septum, the bony septum, and/or the nasal pyramid.

Diagnosis

Two types of dislocations occur in nasal fractures (Fig. 18.40): posterior dislocation (shortening or flattening of the nose, resulting in a wider nasal bridge) and lateral dislocation. Any patient with a nasal fracture should have the nasal airway inspected. If a significant hematoma exists along the septum, it should be drained to

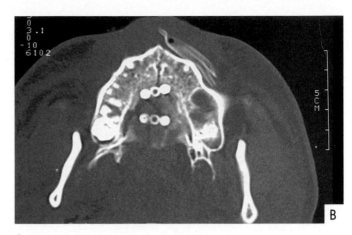

Figure 18.35 (A) Sagittal fracture of the maxilla. (B) Open reduction and internal fixation using small plates and screws is being performed in the roof of the mouth for this sagittal fracture of the palate.

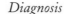

fracture

A

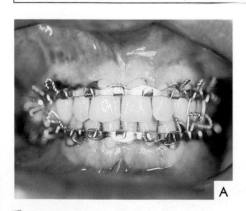

A

Figure 18.36 (A) The treatment of a Le Fort fracture begins with intermaxillary fixation. (B) The internal buttress system of the maxilla must be restored by assembling the fragments and stabilizing them with interfragment plate and screw fixation. Here anterior, middle, and posterior maxillary buttresses are seen.

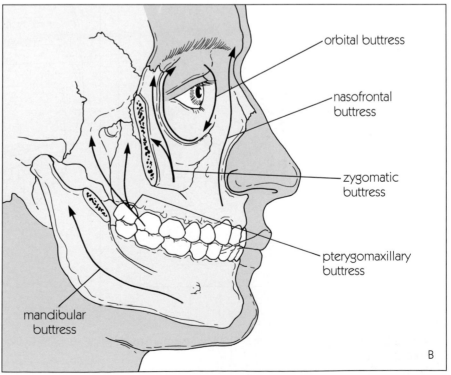

orbital buttress

nasofrontal buttress

zygomatic buttress

pterygomaxillary buttress

mandibular buttress

B

prevent cartilage necrosis. Patients with nasal fractures usually have swelling over the external surface of the nose. A small laceration is often a clue to the presence of a fracture. Pain, crepitation, and periorbital ecchymosis are often present. The most reliable sign of a nasal fracture is epistaxis. Radiographic evaluation of the nose is best performed with a CT scan, which can rule out the possibility of adjacent fractures.

Management
The treatment of nasal fractures involves reduction under local or general anesthesia. The septum is replaced

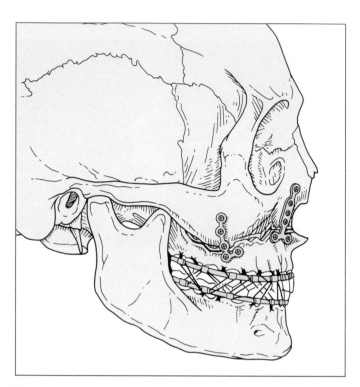

Figure 18.37 Diagram of Le Fort I fracture treatment.

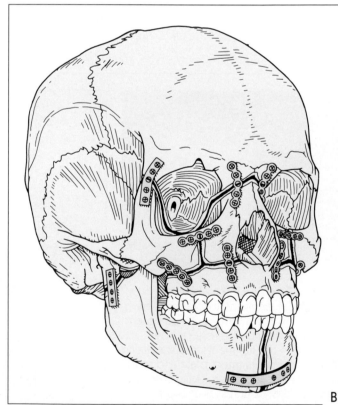

Figure 18.38 Diagram of Le Fort II fracture treatment.

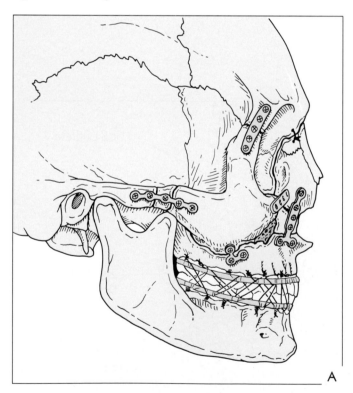

Figure 18.39 (A) Diagram of Le Fort III fracture treatment using plate and screw fixation. (B) Diagram of treatment of panfacial (Le Fort plus mandible) fractures.

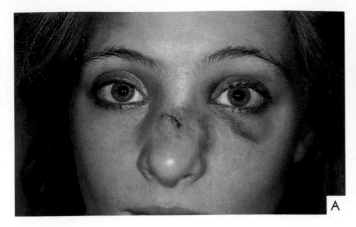

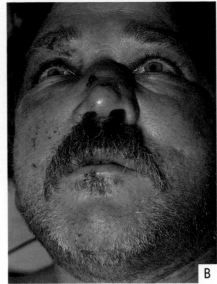

Figure 18.40
Nasal fractures demonstrate either (A) anteroposterior flattening of the nasal bridge or (B) lateral dislocation of the nasal pyramid.

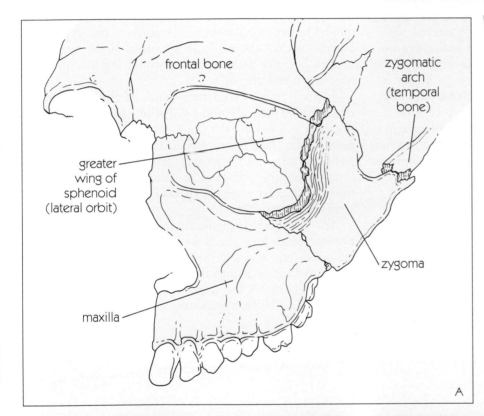

Figure 18.41 Fracture-dislocation of the zygoma. (A) The zygoma attaches to the frontal bone superiorly, to the temporal bone through the zygomatic arch, to the maxilla medially and inferiorly, and to the greater wing of the sphenoid the lateral orbit. All of these surfaces must be aligned in fracture reduction. (B,C) A typical fracture dislocation of the zygoma is seen in these CT scans.

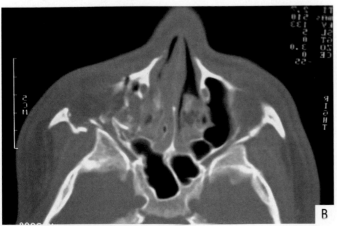

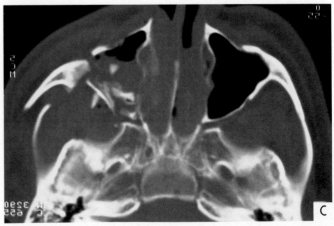

into its proper position with Asch forceps. The nasal bones are first out-fractured, which effectively reconstructs incomplete components of the fracture, and then digitally returned to their proper positions. Antibiotic-impregnated nasal packing supports the reduction of the nasal septum and minimizes bleeding. An external splint is placed over the nasal pyramid to protect it during the healing period. It should be removed at 1 week. Nasal fractures frequently display residual mild deformity after this initial closed management. If the airway remains compromised by a deviated septum, a formal septal resection to improve respiratory symptoms may be performed after 3 to 6 months. Residual deformity of the nasal pyramid requires rhinoplasty.

Fractures of the Zygoma

The zygoma forms the lateral and inferior portion of the orbit and supports the lateral area of the upper midface (Fig. 18.41). The prominent position of the zygoma makes it a frequent recipient of traumatic dislocation. A fracture usually involves the entire zygoma, but may less commonly involve the zygomatic arch alone, which produces a minimal depression in the lateral cheek. Depression of the zygomatic arch may interfere with movement of the coronoid process of the mandible, a symptom requiring reduction. Since zygomatic fractures involve the lateral and inferior internal walls of the orbit, they may produce ocular symptoms that require treatment.

Diagnosis

The symptoms of zygomatic fractures are shown in Figure 18.42. The lateral canthus, which attaches to the frontal process of the zygoma, may be dislocated inferiorly, producing an antimonogoid slant to the palpebral fissure. Either swelling or dislocation of the zygoma may interfere with motion of the coronoid process by producing a mild temporary malocclusion. Hematomas are observed in the cheek, periorbital area, and mouth. Orbital symptoms produced by the fractures include diplopia, ocular dystopia, and eyelid dislocation. Palpation of the orbital rim may demonstrate a step deformity or depression. Palpation of the malar eminence, when compared with the normal side, demonstrates retrusion. With a medially dislocated zygomatic fracture, the orbital volume may be constricted, resulting in exophthalmos. With laterally or inferiorly dislocated zygomatic fractures, the orbital volume increases, and enophthalmos occurs.

Zygomatic fractures should be evaluated with axial and coronal CT scans.

Management

Treatment of fractures of the zygoma involves reduction, accomplished through lower eyelid incisions, and immobilization with interfragment wires stabilized with plate and screw fixation. Thin bone grafts may be required to replace damaged sections of the zygomatic buttress and/or the walls of the orbit. If the zygomatic arch is laterally dislocated, a coronal incision must be used when reducing it.

Initially, dislocated fragments of the zygoma are repositioned and aligned by drilling holes adjacent to fractures and linking the fragments with small interfragment wires. The fracture fragments are held in initial position while rigid internal fixation is performed using small plates and screws (Fig. 18.43). If the lateral canthus is detached in the reduction, it should be replaced after bone assembly.

For an isolated, medially dislocated fracture of the zygomatic arch, a small incision can be made in the temporal hair and the Gilles approach used to elevate the zygomatic arch into its proper position. An elevator is placed beneath the temporal fascia, sliding it under the arch, and the zygomatic arch is pushed into its proper position.

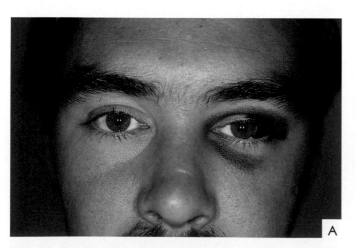
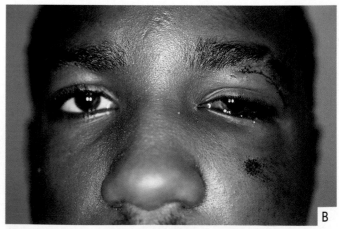

Figure 18.42 (A,B) The symptoms of zygomatic fractures almost always include the combination of periorbital and subconjunctival hematomas. Posterior displacement of the malar eminence, a palpable step deformity in the orbital rim, and numbness in the distribution of the infraorbital nerve are frequently present. Bleeding from the ipsilateral nose occurs if the fracture extends into the ipsilateral maxillary sinus.

Fractures of the Mandible

The mandibular fracture is a common facial injury, because the mandible's prominent position renders it susceptible to trauma. Mandibular fractures are often multiple, and a second mandibular fracture should be suspected if a single fracture is identified. Mandibular fractures may be classified as closed or open; most mandibular fractures are open intraorally. Mandibular fractures frequently occur in structurally weak portions of the mandible, such as the subcondylar region, the region of the angle, or the cuspid region. The edentulous mandible most commonly fractures in the body and angle region.

Diagnosis

The diagnosis of a mandibular fracture is suggested by malocclusion, pain, swelling, tenderness, crepitus, fractured teeth, gaps or discrepancies of level in the dentition, asymmetry of the dental arch, presence of intraoral lacerations, broken or loose teeth, or numbness in the distribution of the mental nerve. Fractured, missing, or dislocated teeth are frequently present. An open bite occurs if the fracture sufficiently dislocates a segment of jaw so that the teeth cannot be brought into occlusion. The open bite may occur anteriorly, laterally, or bilaterally. On opening, the jaw may deviate toward one side because of the fractures. Fractures in the condy-

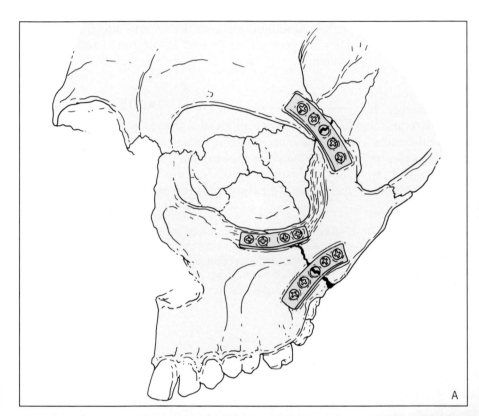
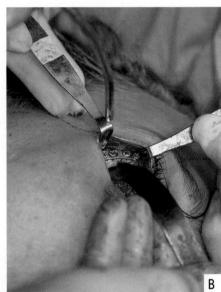
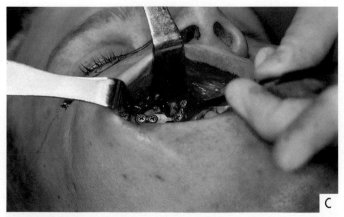
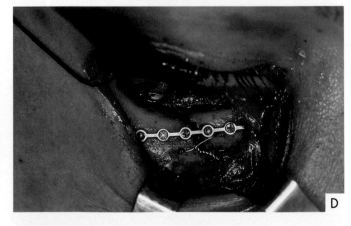

Figure 18.43 (A) Diagram of an open reduction and internal fixation of the zygoma. (B) A strong midface plate is placed at the zygomaticofrontal suture and a thinner microsystem plate at the inferior orbital rim. Depending on the comminution of the fracture, the surgeon may need to plate the zygomaticomaxillary buttress or the zygomatic arch (C,D).

lar and subcondylar area may result in a laceration of the ear canal that produces bleeding. Instability of the alveolar section of the mandible relative to the mandibular body implies the presence of an alveolar fracture. Separation of the alveolar from the basilar bone of the mandible creates dramatic instability.

The mandible has strong muscular attachments that contribute to displacement after injury. The direction of the fracture line may oppose fracture displacement produced by the muscles. The panorex radiograph uses a rotating x-ray tube to obtain a circumferential view for an excellent evaluation of the mandible in a single plane. Lateral oblique, posteroanterior, and Towne's skull views are used to demonstrate the mandible on plain films. A CT scan provides one of the most accurate evaluations of a mandibular fracture but can miss nondisplaced fractures.

Management
The treatment of mandibular fractures depends on the state of the dentition and the location of the fracture. It begins with closure of intraoral and extraoral lacerations and the application of arch bars and intermaxillary fixation to bring the teeth into occlusion. In some cases an acrylic splint can be applied to the teeth temporarily to align them. Some fractures are treated with intermaxil-

lary fixation alone for 4 to 6 weeks after closed reduction. For displaced fractures in both the horizontal and vertical portions of the mandible, direct open reduction of the fracture with plate and screw fixation is the preferred treatment. A plate is placed along the inferior border of the mandible, avoiding the mental nerve and tooth roots (Fig. 18.44). At least two screws are placed to each side of the fracture in stable bone.

The angle region may be treated intraorally, with an intraoral incision, or, for more comminuted fractures, extraorally, with an incision in the upper neck in the hyoid crease or retromandibular area. Fractures of the condyle that require open reduction are treated with a preauricular approach, protecting the facial nerve. Mandibular fractures may be prone to complications such as nonunion, delayed union, and infection. Antibiotics are generally indicated at the time of the fracture reduction.

FACIAL FRACTURES IN CHILDREN
Less than 5% of all facial fractures occur in children; of that 5%, most occur in those over 5 years of age. Children's bones are less brittle than those of adults, and they displace without fracture in many cases. If fractured, bone healing progresses more rapidly than in

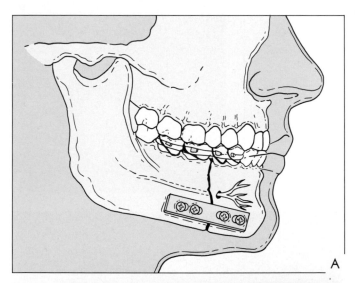

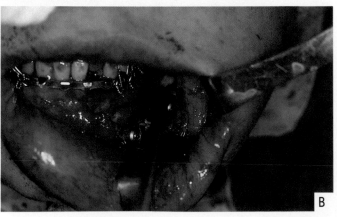

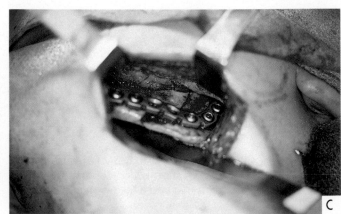

Figure 18.44 (A) A fracture of the body is treated with a compression plate along the inferior border of the mandible. (B) An intraoral exposure is used for plate and screw fixation of a fracture of the mandibular symphysis. (C) Plate and screw fixation of a mandibular angle fracture.

adults. Sinuses are small and therefore do not weaken the bony structure. The treatment of fractures in the upper face of a child follows the same principles described for adults. The emphasis is on early or immediate treatment, since healing occurs rapidly. It may be difficult to reduce a Le Fort fracture after even 1 week. Intermaxillary fixation is often difficult to apply in children because of mixed dentition and inadequate root structure, with difficulty in ligating teeth. Arch bars may have to be supported by the use of piriform aperture wires, circummandibular wires, or suspension wires for stabilization. The application of acrylic splints can facilitate reduction. The use of miniature plate and screw fixation systems in children is preferred.

SUGGESTED READINGS

Skull Fractures

Bakay L, Glasauer FE. *Head Injury.* Boston, Mass: Little, Brown; 1980.

Becker DP, Gade GF, Young HF, Feuerman TF. Diagnosis and treatment of head injury in adults. In: Youmans JR, ed. *Neurological Surgery.* 3rd ed. Philadelphia, Pa: WB Saunders Co; 1990:2017–2148.

Cooper PR. Skull fracture and traumatic cerebrospinal fluid fistulas. In: Cooper PR, ed. *Head Injury.* 2nd ed. Baltimore, Md: Williams & Wilkins; 1987:89–107.

Eisenburg HM, Briner RP. Late complications of head injury. In: McLaurin RL, Venes JL, Schut L, Epstein F, eds. *Pediatric Neurosurgery.* 2nd ed. Philadelphia, Pa: WB Saunders Co; 1989:290–297.

Geisler FH, Greenberg J. Management of the acute head-injury patient. In: Salcman M, ed. *Neurologic Emergencies.* 2nd ed. New York, NY: Raven Press; 1990:135–165.

Geisler FH, Salcman M. The head injury patient. In: Siegel JH, ed. *Trauma—Emergency Surgery & Critical Care.* New York, NY: Churchill Livingstone; 1987:919–946.

Gudeman SK, Young HF, Miller JD, Ward JD, Becker DP. Indications for operative treatment and operative technique in closed head injury. In: Becker DP, Gudeman SK, eds. *Textbook of Head Injury.* Philadelphia, Pa: WB Saunders Co; 1989:138–181.

Jennett B, Teasdale G. *Management of Head Injuries.* Philadelphia, Pa: FA Davis, Co; 1981.

Mealey J Jr. Skull fractures. In: McLaurin RL, Venes JL, Schut L, Epstein F, eds. *Pediatric Neurosurgery.* 2nd ed. Philadelphia, Pa: WB Saunders Co; 1989: 263–270.

Thomas LM. Skull fractures. In: Wilkins RH, Rengachary SS, eds. *Neurosurgery.* New York, NY: McGraw-Hill; 1985;2:1623–1626.

Tyson GW. *Head Injury Management for Providers of Emergency Care.* Baltimore, Md: Williams & Wilkins; 1987.

Wilberger J, Chen DA. The skull and meninges. *Neurosurg Clin North Am.* 1991;2:341–350.

Maxillofacial Fractures

Adekeye EO, Ord RA. Giant frontal sinus mucocele. *J Maxillofac Surg.* 1984;12:184.

Anderson RL. The medial canthal tendon branches out. *Arch Ophthalmol.* 1977;95:2051.

Anderson RL, Panje WR, Gross CE. Optic nerve blindness following blunt forehead traum *Ophthalmology.* 1982;89:445.

Angle EH. Classification of malocclusion. *Dent Cosmos.* 1989;41:240.

Barton FE, Berry WL. Evaluation of the acutely injured orbit. In: Aston SJ, Hornblass A, Meltzer MA, Rees TD, eds. *Third International Symposium of Plastic and Reconstructive Surgery of the Eye and Adnexa.* Baltimore, Md: Williams & Wilkins; 1982:34.

Champy M, Lodde JP, Schmidt R, Jaeger JH, Muster D. Mandibular osteosynthesis by miniature screwed plates via a buccal approach. *J Maxillofac Surg.* 1978;6:14.

Converse JM, Firmin F, Wood-Smith D, Friedland JA. The conjunctival approach in orbital fractures. *Plast Reconstr Surg.* 1973;52:656.

Converse JM, Smith B. Enophthalmos and diplopia in fracture of the orbital floor. *Br J Plast Surg.* 1957; 9:265.

Converse JM, Smith B. Blowout fracture of the floor of the orbit. *Trans Am Acad Ophthalmol Otolaryngol.* 1960; 64:676.

Converse JM, Smith B. Naso-orbital fractures (symposium: midfacial fractures). *Trans Am Acad Ophthalmol Otolaryngol.* 1963;67:622.

Donald PJ, Ettin M. The safety of frontal sinus fat obliteration when sinus walls are missing. *Laryngoscope.* 1986;96:190.

Fujino T. Experimental "blowout fracture" of the orbit. *Plast Reconstr Surg.* 1974;54:81.

Fukado Y. Results in 400 cases of surgical decompression of the optic nerve. In: Bleeker GM, et al, eds. *Proceedings of Second International Symposium on Orbital Disorders.* Basel: Karger; 1975.

Gruss JS, Hurwitz JJ, Nik NA, Kassel EE. The pattern and incidence of nasolacrimal injury in nasoethmoidal orbital fractures: the role of delayed assessment and dacryocystorhinostomy. *Br J Plast Surg.* 1985;38:116.

Gruss JS, MacKinnon SE, Kassel E, Cooper PW. The role of primary bone grafting in complex craniomaxillofacial trauma. *Plast Reconstr Surg.* 1985;75:17.

Hendler N, Viernstein M, Schallenberger C, Long D. Group therapy with chronic pain patients. *Psychosomatics.* 1987;22:333.

Jones LT. An anatomical approach to problems of the "eyelids and lacrimal apparatus." *Arch Ophthalmol.* 1961;66:111.

Koorneef L. *Spatial Aspects of the Orbital Musculofibrous Tissue in Man: A New Anatomical and Histological Approach.* Amsterdam: Swets & Zeitlinger, BV; 1977.

Manson PN. Some thoughts on the classification and treatment of Le Fort fractures. *Ann Plast Surg.* 1986;17:356.

Manson PN, Cifford CM, Su CT, Iliff NT, Morgan R. Mechanisms of global support and post traumatic enophthalmos, I: the anatomy of the ligament sling and its relation to intramuscular cone orbital fat. *Plast Reconstr Surg.* 1986;77:193.

Manson PN, Crawley WA, Yaremchuck MJ, Rochman GM, Hoopes JE, French JH. Midface fractures: advantages of immediate extended open reduction and bone grafting. *Plast Reconstr Surg.* 1985;76:1.

Manson PN, Grivas A, Rosenbaum A, Vannier M, Zinreich J, Iliff N. Studies on enophthalmos, II: the measurement of orbital injuries and their treatment by quantitative computed tomography. *Plast Reconstr Surg.* 1986;77:203.

Manson PN, Shack RB, Leonard LG, Su CT, Hoopes JE. Sagittal fractures of the maxilla and palate. *Plast Reconstr Surg.* 1983;72:484.

Merville L. Multiple dislocations of the facial skeleton. *J Maxillofac Surg.* 1979;2:187.

Milauskas AT, Fueger GF. Serious ocular complications associated with blow-out fractures of the orbit. *Am J Ophthalmol.* 1966;62:670.

Putterman AM, Stevens T, Urist MJ. Nonsurgical management of blow-out fractures of the orbital floor. *Am J Ophthalmol.* 1974;77:232.

Raflo GT. Blow-in and blow-out fractures of the orbit: clinical correlations and proposed mechanisms. *Ophthalmic Surg.* 1984;15:114.

Rumelt MB, Ernest JT. Isolated blowout fracture of the medial orbital wall with medial rectus muscle entrapment. *Am J Ophthalmol.* 1972;73:451.

Sofferman RA, Danielson PA, Quatela V, Reed RR. Retrospective analysis of surgically treated Le Fort fractures. *Arch Otolaryngol.* 1983;109:446.

Stranc MF, Robertson GA. A classification of injuries of the nasal skeleton. *Ann Plast Surg.* 1979;2:468.

Vondra J. *Fractures of the Base of the Skull.* London: Iliffe Books; 1965.

Wolfe SA. Application of craniofacial surgical precepts following trauma and tumour removal. *J Maxillofac Surg.* 1982;10:212.

Zide BM, McCarthy JG. The medial canthus revisited—an anatomical basis for canthopexy. *Ann Plast Surg.* 1983;11:1.

Chapter 19

Traumatic Intracranial Hematomas

Robert H. Wilkins

There are three types of intracranial hematomas based on location. These are the epidural hematoma, subdural hematoma, and intracerebral hematoma.[1-7]

EPIDURAL HEMATOMA

A traumatic intracranial epidural hematoma results when blood collects between the skull and the dura mater as the result of a head injury (Fig. 19.1). The most common location for such a hematoma is along the lateral wall of the middle cranial fossa. The events that cause this classic example are as follows: A blow to the side of the head fractures the squamous portion of the temporal bone (Fig. 19.1B), separates the dura mater from the bone, and produces a tear in the middle meningeal artery, which normally lies against or actually within the bone (Fig.

19.1A). Blood escapes from this vessel under arterial pressure, dissecting the dura inward away from the bone and permitting a hematoma to form (Figs. 19.1B,C). The brain (especially the temporal lobe) is also displaced inward. If the process continues, brain herniation occurs, with caudal displacement of the brain stem and downward herniation of the uncus of the temporal lobe between the edge of the tentorium and the side of the midbrain, and against the ipsilateral oculomotor nerve (Fig. 19.1C). At times a traumatic intracranial epidural hematoma will form in some other location or will result from venous, rather than arterial, bleeding, but these are the exceptions rather than the rule.

In the typical patient with a temporal arterial epidural hematoma, the events progress over hours, with about one third of the treated patients coming to the operating room within 12 hours of injury and between 60% and 75%

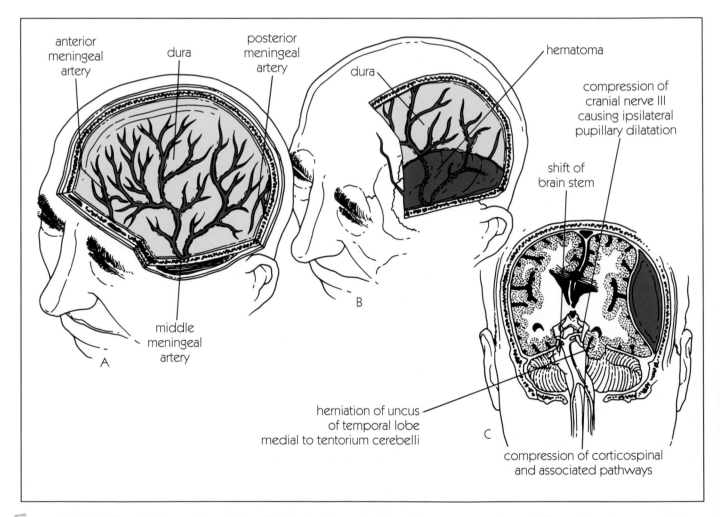

Figure 19.1 (A) The middle meningeal artery. The typical traumatic epidural hematoma is caused by a laceration of this vessel. (B,C) A linear fracture of the squamous portion of the temporal bone has torn the middle meningeal artery, which has resulted in an epidural hematoma.

within 48 hours.[5] If the patient does not have an initial deficit from an associated brain injury, he or she will ordinarily experience a progressive reduction in the level of consciousness as the hematoma enlarges. Symptoms and signs of downward brain stem displacement and uncal herniation may then develop rather rapidly, including the onset of a partial ipsilateral oculomotor palsy (dilated pupil). As the midbrain is displaced to the opposite side by the herniation of the uncus, the contralateral cerebral peduncle may be indented by the adjacent tentorial edge, resulting in a hemiparesis that is ipsilateral to the epidural hematoma, opposite to the effect expected from direct compression of the ipsilateral motor cortex by the hematoma. Thus, the development of a hemiparesis does not necessarily herald the side of the epidural hematoma, and it may be a false localizing sign. The dilated pupil is a better clue to the side of the hematoma that is ipsilateral to the dilated pupil (Fig. 19.1C).

In the unusual cases where an epidural hematoma is venous in origin, for example, arising from a laceration of a middle meningeal vein or a dural venous sinus, the time course is slower, evolving over 2 to 7 days rather than from a few hours to 2 days as with an arterial epidural hematoma. The clinical picture is that of an expanding supratentorial mass, with an alteration in mental status and development of a hemiparesis more likely to appear before the symptoms and signs of brain herniation.

A traumatic intracranial epidural hematoma can be diagnosed by CT or MRI. On axial or coronal views, the hematoma usually has a biconvex lens-shaped appearance (Fig. 19.2). However, if the hematoma is enlarging rapidly and the patient's condition is deteriorating with similar rapidity, the diagnosis is better made by taking the patient directly to the operating room for a procedure that is both diagnostic and therapeutic.

On occasion, an epidural hematoma may achieve only a small size, remain asymptomatic, and not require treatment. However, the usual sequence of events dictates that the hematoma must be evacuated to provide the best chance of preserving or restoring brain function and preventing a fatal outcome. The surgical treatment of a traumatic intracranial epidural hematoma involves making a sufficient opening in the skull (a craniectomy or craniotomy), evacuating the blood, and stopping the source of bleeding. If this is done early enough in the evolution of the hematoma, a complete recovery can be achieved. In contrast, if brain herniation and irreversible secondary brain stem hemorrhages have developed, the evacuation of the epidural hematoma cannot be expected to provide a better result than a persistent vegetative state or death.

SUBDURAL HEMATOMA

In contrast to an epidural hematoma, a traumatic intracranial subdural hematoma usually results from venous bleeding and collects more slowly. In the typical case, the brain moves within the skull at the time of impact, shearing off one or more of the bridging veins that extend

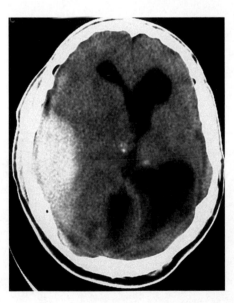

Figure 19.2 Axial CT view of an epidural hematoma showing the associated distortion and shift of the ventricular system.

across the space between the surface of the brain and an adjacent dural venous sinus such as the superior sagittal sinus (Fig. 19.3). The blood then escapes from the venous system, dissects open a space between the dura mater and the arachnoid (the subdural space), and collects over the surface of one cerebral hemisphere. In about 15% to 20% of cases, blood collects over both hemispheres and bilateral subdural hematomas are formed.[5]

Occasionally a subdural hematoma arises from one or two cortical arteries that bleed into the subdural space rather than the subarachnoid space or brain parenchyma. In this case the blood accumulates more rapidly and the

associated symptoms and signs progress more rapidly.

The subdural blood is liquid initially but then clots. With time, it is either reabsorbed or goes on to form an encapsulated and liquefied hematoma that has a propensity to enlarge (Fig. 19.4).

ACUTE SUBDURAL HEMATOMA

The acute traumatic intracranial subdural hematoma is one that is discovered within 2 to 3 days of its onset. The blood appears hyperdense (white) on a CT scan (Fig. 19.5) and its shape resembles the blade of a sickle, with

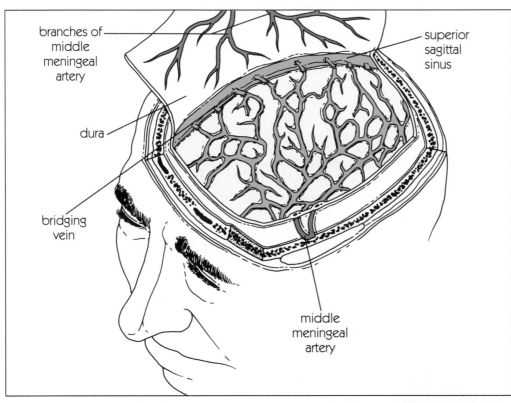

Figure 19.3 Veins are shown extending from the surface of the brain to the superior sagittal sinus. Differential movement of the brain within the skull at the time of head injury may tear one or more of these veins, leading to the formation of a subdural hematoma.

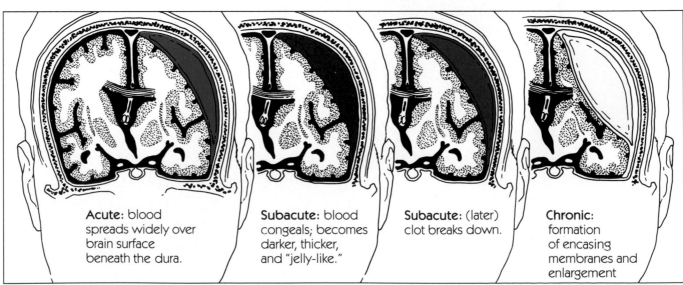

Figure 19.4 A subdural hematoma is liquid at first and subsequently clots. It is then reabsorbed or it develops into a chronic subdural hematoma as a thick vascular outer membrane and a thin inner membrane develop around the liquefying blood, starting about 2 weeks after the injury. The chronic subdural hematoma enlarges as further bleeding occurs within it.

its outer surface lying against the inner surface of the skull (and dura). In the usual setting, the acute subdural hematoma is discovered during the evaluation of a patient with a severe brain injury, and its poor prognosis, without or with treatment, reflects that association. The overall mortality rate of patients with a treated acute subdural hematoma is roughly 50%.[3,5]

The treatment of an acute subdural hematoma involves its surgical evacuation. This is ordinarily best accomplished by creating a large cranial opening via a craniotomy and evacuating the subdural hematoma through various surgically created openings in the dura. Usually, the dura is not opened fully as a flap because the underlying injured brain has a tendency to herniate outward, interfering with the optimal closure of the dura, skull, and scalp.

SUBACUTE SUBDURAL HEMATOMA

The subacute traumatic intracranial subdural hematoma consists of clotted blood that eventually may be lysed and reabsorbed. During this process it becomes isodense in relation to the brain on CT scanning, and it may be difficult to diagnose unless the position of the cortical vessels is shown by the intravenous administration of a contrast agent. Its treatment is essentially the same as that of the acute subdural hematoma, but the patient's prognosis is somewhat better, again primarily related to the degree of the associated brain injury.

CHRONIC SUBDURAL HEMATOMA

The chronic traumatic intracranial subdural hematoma develops insidiously, typically in an elderly or alcoholic individual with some degree of brain atrophy. In this condition the patient may fall or otherwise strike the head and may not remember the blow. The atrophic brain is less likely than a normal brain to tamponade a beginning subdural hematoma, which will then progress, causing symptoms such as an altered mental status, reduced level of consciousness, headaches, or a focal neurologic deficit such as a hemiparesis. After about 2 weeks, membranes begin to form around the hematoma, with the outer membrane being thicker and more vascular than the inner membrane (Fig. 19.6A). The center of the encapsulated hematoma liquefies and becomes hypointense (with respect to the brain) on the CT scan. But instead of being absorbed, the fluid collection enlarges, apparently

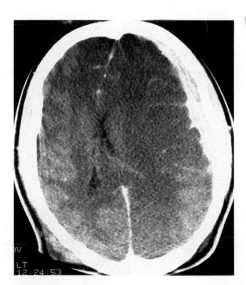

Figure 19.5 Axial CT image of an acute subdural hematoma with associated displacement of the ventricular system.

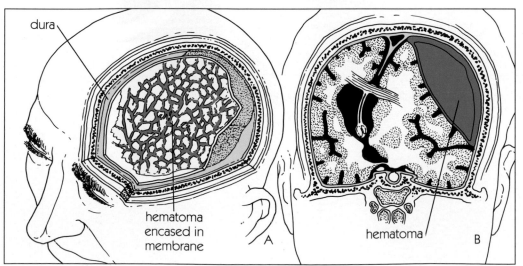

dura

hematoma encased in membrane

A

hematoma

B

Figure 19.6 (A) The thick vascular outer membrane of a chronic subdural hematoma is shown immediately within the dura mater. (B) The liquefied chronic subdural hematoma can be drained through a burr hole or twist drill hole in the skull.

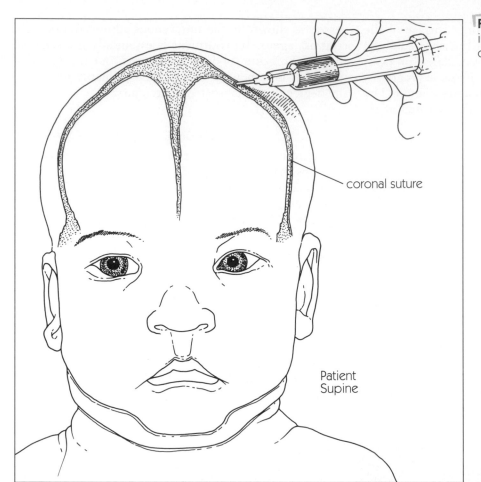

coronal suture

Patient
Supine

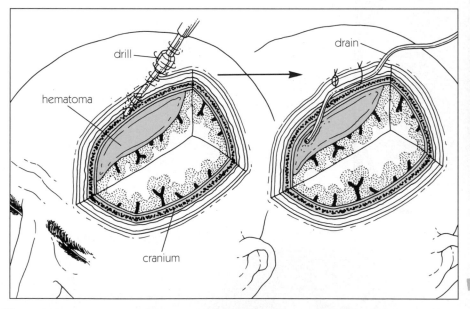

Figure 19.8 A chronic subdural hematoma in an adult can be drained through a twist drill hole in the skull.

drill

hematoma

drain

cranium

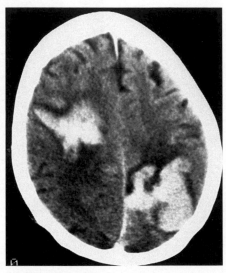

Figure 19.9 Shown on this axial CT scan are two areas of traumatic intracerebral hemorrhage.

Principles of Neurosurgery

from repeated bleeding from the vascular outer membrane. The hematoma thus enlarges, assuming a progressively larger biconvex lens shape (Figs. 19.4, 19.6B).

In an infant, a chronic subdural hematoma may result in head enlargement or the restriction of brain growth. Subdural fluid collections in infants can be evacuated through a needle inserted via the coronal suture (Fig. 19.7). The existence of a subdural hematoma in a child who has not been involved in an accident raises the possibility of child abuse.

The treatment of a chronic subdural hematoma in an adult usually requires less surgery than does the treatment of an acute or subacute subdural hematoma. The contained liquid ordinarily can be evacuated through a small hole in the skull, with or without the insertion of a drain (Figs. 19.6B, 19.8). The main danger of the chronic subdural hematoma is that its existence may not be recognized and it may be left untreated, causing a severe neurologic deficit or death. If the diagnosis is considered, it can be confirmed easily. The treatment is not complicated or associated with much risk, and a satisfactory outcome of the surgical evacuation of a chronic subdural hematoma is usually easier to achieve than with the other two types of subdural hematoma.

INTRACEREBRAL HEMATOMA

A significant intracerebral hematoma resulting from direct nonpenetrating head trauma is unusual (Fig. 19.9). However, cerebral contusions commonly occur, especially in the undersurfaces and tips of the frontal lobes and the tips of the temporal lobes. At times, such contusions will coalesce into a hematoma that reaches a significant size.[8] When this occurs and is the cause of symptoms and signs of cerebral dysfunction, surgical evacuation via a craniotomy may be necessary.

When downward brain stem displacement and uncal herniation occur, secondary brain stem hemorrhages may develop as part of the process. Multiple hemorrhagic areas within the pons and midbrain are commonly found at postmortem examination of a patient who died from a severe head injury that resulted in these types of brain herniation. Secondary brain stem hemorrhages are not amenable to surgical evacuation, and the neurosurgeon's emphasis is on the prevention of brain herniation rather than the treatment of the effects of herniation.

CONCLUSION

A patient who sustains a head injury may develop a hematoma in the epidural space, subdural space, or brain parenchyma. These types of hematomas differ significantly in mechanism and course of development, clinical presentation, and specifics of diagnosis and treatment. But they all may enlarge with time and be visualized by CT scanning. The success of their surgical treatment is in part related to how soon they are treated.[9] Therefore, for optimal results, the physician (e.g., the emergency room physician, the neurosurgeon) must consider the possibility of an intracranial hematoma in any patient with a head injury, especially if the patient was or is unconscious or has a focal neurologic deficit.

REFERENCES

1. Becker DP, Gade GF, Young HF, et al. Diagnosis and treatment of head injury in adults. In: Youmans JR, ed. *Neurological Surgery: A Comprehensive Reference Guide to the Diagnosis and Management of Neurosurgical Problems.* Philadelphia, Pa: WB Saunders & Co; 1990:2017–2148.

2. Becker DP, Gudeman SK, eds. *Textbook of Head Injury.* Philadelphia, Pa: WB Saunders & Co; 1989.

3. Bullock R, Teasdale G. Surgical management of traumatic intracranial haematomas. In: Vinken PJ, Bruyn GW, Klawans HL, et al, eds. *Handbook of Clinical Neurology. Head Injury.* Amsterdam: Elsevier; 1990;57: 249–298.

4. Burger PC, Scheithauer BW, Vogel FS. *Surgical Pathology of the Nervous System and Its Coverings.* 3rd ed. New York, NY: Churchill Livingstone; 1991:453–459.

5. Cooper PR. Traumatic intracranial hematomas. In: Wilkins RH, Rengachary SS, eds. *Neurosurgery.* New York, NY: McGraw-Hill; 1985:1657–1666.

6. Cooper PR, ed. *Head Injury.* 2nd ed. Baltimore, Md: Williams & Wilkins; 1987.

7. McLaurin RL, ed. *Extracerebral Collections.* New York, NY: Springer-Verlag, 1986.

8. Soloniuk D, Pitts LH, Lovely M, et al. Traumatic intracerebral hematomas: timing of appearance and indications for operative removal. *J Trauma.* 1986; 26:787–793.

9. Seelig JM, Becker DP, Miller JD, et al. Traumatic acute subdural hematoma: major mortality reduction in comatose patients treated within four hours. *N Engl J Med.* 1981;304:1511–1518.

Injuries to the Cervical Spine

Mark N. Hadley

An estimated 200,000 traumatic spinal column injuries occur each year in the United States.[1–5] Approximately 10% to 15% of these patients sustain severe neurologic injuries, and an estimated 10,000 patients die as a result of complications of spinal cord injury.[5–9] The vast majority of traumatic vertebral column injuries involve the cervical spine, the most mobile and dynamic portion of the human spinal column. The incidence of cervical spine injuries compared to injuries to the thoracic, lumbar, and sacral spinal segments is depicted in Figure 20.1.

The most common cause of cervical spine injury in the United States is motor vehicle accidents, followed by falls (Fig. 20.2).[1,2,5,10–12] The vast majority of injuries occur in patients 15 to 30 years old.[3,5,12] Males are three to four times as likely to sustain a traumatic vertebral column injury as females. The cause of spine injury varies with age; notably, the very young are most commonly the victims of pedestrian motor vehicle accidents and the very old most commonly suffer falls.

Age is an important determinant of cervical spine injury after trauma.[13,14] The younger pediatric population (less than age 4 years) has significantly fewer vertebral column injuries than the older pediatric population and adults.[13] When spinal column injuries do occur in children 4 years old and younger, the distribution of injuries within the cervical spine is significantly different from that observed among adult spine injury patients. A large proportion of cervical injuries to pediatric patients occur between the occiput and C-2; these represent approximately 40% of all traumatic pediatric spine injuries.[13,14] In contrast, only 20% of adult cervical spine injuries involve the superior cervical spine between the occiput and C-2.[1,3,15,16] Anatomic and physiologic features of the immature spine (Fig. 20.3) contribute to the marked differences in injury types between young pediatric spine-injured patients and adult spine-injured patients.[13,14]

TYPES OF INJURY

The most common types of vertebral column injury following trauma are fractures of the cervical vertebrae and fracture-subluxation injuries (Fig. 20.4).[1–3,5,7,11,12,17] Subluxation injuries without fracture and spinal cord injuries without radiographic abnormality (SCIWORA) are much less common and are more likely to occur in younger patients.[13,14,18] Relatively minor trauma to the cervical spine may result in disc herniation without vertebral fracture or vertebral column instability.

Neurologic injury following cervical spinal column trauma depends on several factors. These include the type and level of injury, the force of the trauma, patient age, and the general condition of the patient both before injury (medical problems or conditions that predispose to abnormal laxity or rigidity of the spinal column) and immediately after injury (hypotension and/or hypoxia).[5,12] Sixty percent of patients who present with cervical spine

Figure 20.1 Incidence of Cervical Spine Injuries

Level of Injury	Pediatric	Adults
All cervical	70%	60%
Occiput–C-2	(40%)	(20%)
All thoracic	15%	8%
Thoracolumbar	10%	20%
All lumbar	4%	10%
All sacral	<1%	2%
Total	100%	100%

Figure 20.2 Etiology of Spine Injuries

Motor vehicle accident (including motorcycle)	50%
Falls	20%
Sports	15%
Violence	12%
Other injuries	3%

Figure 20.3 Characteristics of the Infant Spine

Increased physiologic mobility
Ligamentous laxity
Underdevelopment of neck/paraspinous musculature
Incompletely ossified, wedge-shaped cervical vertebrae
Shallow, horizontally oriented facet joints
Large size of head with respect to torso

Figure 20.4 Types of Spine Injury

Fracture	45%
Fracture-subluxation	35%
Subluxation only (without fracture)	8%
SCIWORA	<2%
Disc herniation (without fracture or subluxation)	>10%
Total	100%

fractures have other major organ system traumatic injuries that may contribute to postinjury hypoxia and/or shock, both of which have deleterious effects on spinal cord function after cervical cord trauma.[3,5,11,12]

Approximately 15% of patients who sustain vertebral column trauma sustain a neurologic injury as a result of that trauma.[5,12] Estimates of neurologic morbidity and mortality following cervical spinal column trauma are considerably higher than those reported for all other spinal column segments combined. Approximately 40% to 60% of all traumatic cervical spine injuries result in neurologic compromise, with a range between 2% and 100% depending on the type and level of the cervical spine injury (Fig. 20.5).[1,2,5–10,17,19] The reported incidence of neurologic mortality after high cervical spinal segment trauma is probably artificially low. Investigators estimate that 25% to 40% of patients with occiput to C-3 level spinal cord injuries die in the field from their neurologic injuries before receiving medical attention (due to high spinal cord compromise and respiratory arrest).[4,5,12]

The unique anatomy, articulations, and physiologic ranges of motion and rotation of the cervical vertebrae, particularly those most cephalad, predispose them to a variety of fracture and dislocation injuries.

ATLANTOOCCIPITAL DISLOCATION

Cranial-cervical disruption injuries are uncommon, the result of massive traumatic flexion and distraction forces, and associated with a 100% neurologic morbidity and/or mortality.[20–23] While most patients with these injuries either die of brain stem disruption or are profoundly neurologically impaired at a mid-to-lower cranial nerve functional level, a small percentage of patients with this type of injury have a favorable functional outcome if prompt medical treatment, rapid diagnosis, and effective cranial-cervical immobilization can be provided (Fig. 20.6).[20–24]

Figure 20.5 Cervical Spine Injury and Neurologic Deficit

Level	Percent of Cervical Spine Injuries	Incidence of Neurologic Deficit
Atlantooccipital dislocation	<1%	100%
Atlas	4%	1%–2%
Axis	3%	10%
C3-T1*	18%	6%
Unilateral cervical facet dislocation	75%	60%
	(4%)	(75%)
Bilateral cervical facet dislocation	(4%)	(100%)

*C-5 is the most common site of vertebral fracture; C5-6 is the most common level of subluxation.

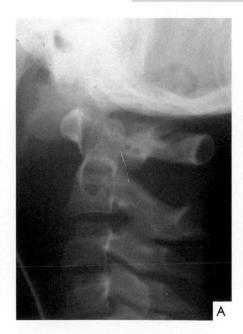 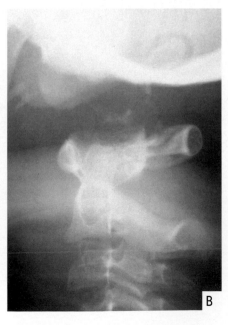

A

B

Figure 20.6 (A,B) Traumatic occipito-cervical dislocation.

Uniquely positioned between the skull and the remainder of the vertebral column, the atlas, a thin bony ring with broad articular surfaces, is vulnerable to a variety of injuries. Fractures of the atlas represent 3% to 13% of all cervical spine fractures reported in the literature.[12,15,16,25–29] Sonntag and Hadley documented a 4.5% incidence of atlas fractures in their review of 1280 acute cervical spine fractures.[4,16]

Atlas fractures may present as isolated injuries after trauma, but frequently (40% of atlas fractures) occur in combination with axis fracture injuries.[12,26,27] The burst or Jefferson fracture is the classic and most frequent atlas fracture identified (Fig. 20.7). Unilateral ring or lateral mass fractures are not uncommon injuries when the traumatic force vectors applied to the C-1 ring are not those of direct axial compression.[4,12,16,28]

Acute fractures of the second cervical vertebra represent approximately 18% of all cervical spine traumatic injuries.[4,10,12,15–17,30] The axis, the largest cervical vertebra and the most irregular in shape, is susceptible to a host of fracture injuries, depending on the force and direction of the traumatic impact. Fractures of the odontoid process are the most common axis fractures and represent 60% of all C-2 injuries. Type I odontoid fractures, those through the tip of the dens, are very uncommon. Type II odontoid fractures, defined as fractures through the base of the dens (Fig. 20.8), are the most common odontoid fracture and the most difficult to treat. Type III odontoid fractures, which occur at the base of the dens, extend into the body of the axis (Fig. 20.9) and represent one third of odontoid fractures and 22% of axis fractures in general.[4,10,12]

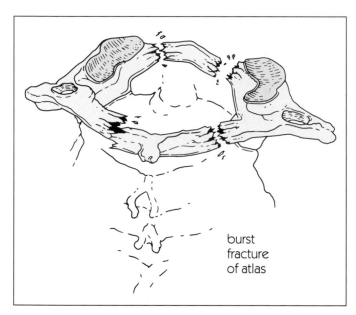

Figure 20.7 Burst fracture of the atlas.

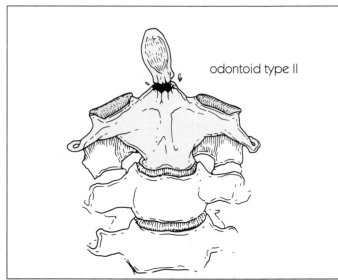

Figure 20.8 Odontoid type II fracture.

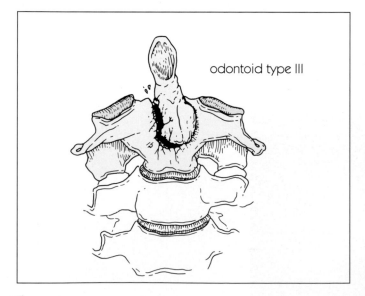

Figure 20.9 Odontoid type III fracture.

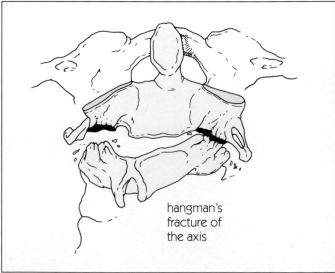

Figure 20.10 Hangman's fracture of the axis.

Hangman's fractures of the axis are a unique C-2 fracture subtype. Defined as bilateral fractures through the pars interarticularis, hangman's fractures represent 20% of all axis fracture injuries (Figs. 20.10, 20.11).[4,10,12,15,16] Variations of hangman's fractures have been described, including bilateral fractures through the lateral masses or pedicles.

Approximately 20% of all axis fractures are non-odontoid, non-hangman's C-2 fractures.[4,10,12,16,31] These have been termed "miscellaneous axis fractures" and include fractures through the body, pedicle, lateral mass, laminae, and spinous process.[12,16,31]

C-3 FRACTURES

Fracture injuries of the third cervical vertebra are distinctly uncommon. Sonntag and Hadley discovered only 12 isolated C-3 fractures among 1280 acute cervical spine injuries they treated.[4] The isolated fracture injuries were primarily chip fractures of the body. Another 11 patients had C-3 fractures in combination with an axis fracture. These were lamina and spinous process fractures and typically were identified in patients with a hangman's fracture. Four other C-3 fractures were identified in association with C-4 and C-5 fracture injuries. The third cervical vertebra appears to be partially protected from injury, positioned between the more vulnerable axis and the more mobile "relative fulcrum" of the cervical spine (the C5-6 level), where the greatest flexion and extension of the cervical spine occurs.[4,16]

C4-T1 FRACTURES AND DISLOCATIONS

A wide variety of fracture and dislocation injuries occur between C-4 and T-1 (Figs. 20.12, 20.13). Bohlman described 300 acute cervical spine fractures, 74% of which occurred between these two levels.[1] Sonntag and Hadley found that 72% of 1280 acute cervical spine fracture-subluxation injuries involved cervical segments C4-T1.[4] The most common level of cervical vertebral fracture is C-5, and the most common level of subluxation injury is the C5-6 interspace, the "relative fulcrum" of the head and neck with respect to the torso in adult patients.[1,4,5]

The most common injury patterns identified at these levels are vertebral body fractures with or without subluxation, subluxation (with or without fracture) of the articular processes (including unilateral and bilateral locked facet dislocations), followed by fractures of the lamina or spinous processes and pedicle or lateral mass fractures. Rarely, ligamentous disruption occurs without fracture or facet dislocation. When subluxation does occur with vertebral body fracture in the lower cervical spine the likelihood of neurologic injury increases dramatically.[5,7,9,17] This is particularly true for facet dislocation injuries. Hadley et al. found an incidence of neurologic injury of 80% for unilateral facet dislocations (29% had root injuries only, 42% had incomplete spinal cord injuries, and 29% suffered complete spinal cord injuries). The neurologic morbidity for patients with bilateral facet dislocations was 100% (16% had incomplete and 84% had complete spinal cord injuries).[17]

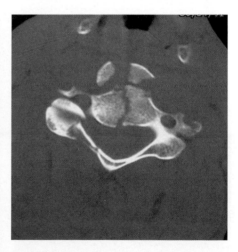

Figure 20.13 CT of C-4 body fracture.

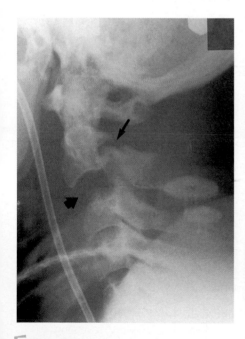

Figure 20.11 Hangman's fracture with marked C2-3 dislocation.

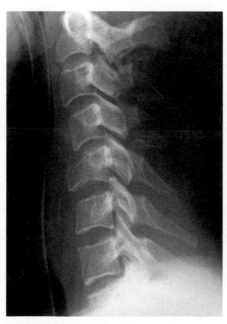

Figure 20.12 Compression fracture of C-4.

GENERAL MANAGEMENT PRINCIPLES

A high index of suspicion of potential spinal injury must be maintained until the presence (or absence) of a cervical vertebral fracture or cervical instability can be determined. Immobilization of the head and neck with respect to the torso is mandatory during the resuscitation, triage, and radiographic evaluation of the trauma patient.[4,12] Roughly half of all patients who sustain cervical spinal column trauma will present without neurologic deficits.[4,5,12] That 10% of patients in one review developed the first onset of neurologic symptoms and signs of cervical spinal cord compromise during their early hospital course (emergency room evaluation or radiographic assessment) underscores the importance of effective head, neck, and torso immobilization until a definitive diagnosis can be made.[4,5]

Sixty percent of patients who have sustained cervical spinal column trauma have head or other major organ system injuries that complicate their initial management.[3,5,11,12] Every effort must be made to resuscitate these patients effectively without compromising cervical spinal alignment or spinal cord function (aggressively treat hypoxia and shock).

The radiographic assessment begins with standard lateral radiographs that show from C-1 to the C7-T1 interspace.[5,12,32] Areas of suspected pathology identified on the plain radiographs should be studied with thin-section CT.[12,32] The levels to be evaluated with CT in potential SCIWORA patients are determined by the level of their neurologic deficits.[13] The exception to early CT after the initial lateral radiographs is the patient with an obvious facet fracture-dislocation injury.[17] These are patients who stand to benefit from early reduction of the fracture-subluxation and realignment of the cervical vertebral column. Early closed reduction of these injuries with cranial-cervical traction offers the possibility of recovery of neurologic function in select patients, particularly those patients with incomplete neurologic injuries.[17]

IMAGING CERVICAL SPINE INJURIES

The radiographic examination of the cervical spine begins with a lateral roentgenographic evaluation of the skull base and the entire cervical spine through the first thoracic vertebra. In many instances this must be accomplished with two lateral radiographs, a routine cross-table lateral and a swimmer's view (Fig. 20.14). This combination of films has been reported to have an 85% sensitivity for fracture and a negative predictive value of 97%.[32,33] To assess the superior cervical spine adequately, particularly if the patient complains of skull base or superior cervical spine pain or if the lateral radiograph is suspicious for a C-1 or C-2 injury, an open-mouth view of the odontoid process and the C1-2 articulations should be obtained. (Figs. 20.15, 20.16). The oblique, pillar view of the odontoid process will reveal the integrity of the dens in patients who will not or cannot cooperate with the open-mouth radiograph. An anteroposterior view of the cervical spine can assist in the identification of a unilateral facet dislocation injury

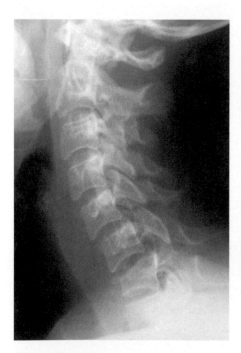

Figure 20.14 Lateral cervical spine radiograph revealing all seven cervical vertebrae and the first thoracic vertebra. Note the C-7 fracture and C6-7 subluxation with unilateral facet dislocation.

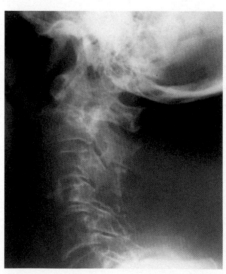

Figure 20.15 Lateral radiograph revealing C-2 fracture with odontoid type II posterior dislocation.

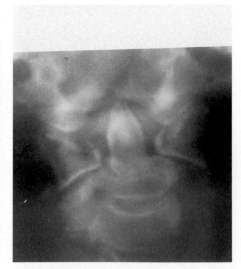

Figure 20.16 AP view of C1-C2 complex (open mouth view) revealing odontoid fracture.

in those instances where there is little or no dislocation identified between the injured vertebrae on the lateral film. The combined use of lateral, anteroposterior, and open-mouth radiographs increases the sensitivity of the radiographic examination to 92% and the negative predictive value for fracture to 99%.[32,33] Approximately 10% of patients with a cervical spine fracture have a second associated, noncontiguous vertebral column fracture, an incidence that warrants a complete spinal column radiographic assessment in selected patients.[5,12]

CT has become an essential component of the radiographic imaging battery for patients who have sustained cervical vertebral column trauma.[5,12,24,32,34,35] CT can identify or more fully characterize fracture injuries of the cervical vertebrae and rule out fracture-subluxation injuries in regions of the cervical spine that are poorly imaged by standard x-ray views of the spine, particularly at the atlas-axis articulations and at the cervico-thoracic junction (Fig. 20.17). To appreciate fully the imaging capabilities of CT, thin-section cuts must be requested and sagittal reconstructions obtained (Fig. 20.18). Thin-section slice acquisition usually prevents "skipping over" a fracture, and sagittal reconstructions assist in indentifying vertebral column subluxation injuries.[32] The CT evaluation of patients with cervical trauma precedes dynamic flexion and extension radiographs (when indicated), myelography, angiography, and MRI (depending on individual patient pathology).

Several adjuncts to routine CT of the cervical spine may help one evaluate selected patients following cervical trauma.[35–37] Water-soluble intrathecal contrast may be used with CT to provide indirect imaging of the thecal sac and neural elements in relation to the bony anatomy. In recent years, however, CT myelography has been reserved for assessment of the spinal canal of patients on whom MR images cannot be obtained. Three-dimensional CT can be useful in the evaluation of complex cervical spine fracture-subluxation injuries or in the identification of occult cervical spine fracture injuries (Fig. 20.19).[37]

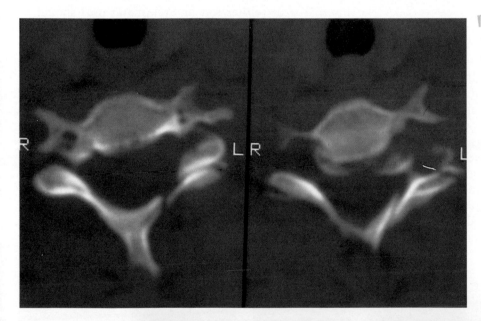

Figure 20.17 CT revealing a multiple fracture of the C-4 body, lateral mass, and lamina.

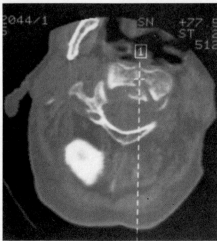

Figure 20.18 Sagittal reconstruction of a CT study depicting a C-2 fracture (arrows).

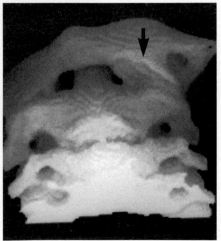

Figure 20.19 Three-dimensional CT study revealing C1-2 rotational subluxation (arrow).

MRI has become a useful radiographic assessment tool for patients who have sustained cervical trauma, particularly those who present with spinal cord injuries, subluxation injuries, disc herniations, and SCIWORA (Fig. 20.20).[5,8,12,25,32,38,39] Relatively long segments of the vertebral column can be imaged at the same setting and multiple image reconstruction planes are routinely provided. While MRI is inadequate for the evaluation of specific bony anatomy, it is an excellent imaging tool for the assessment of vertebral alignment, disc and ligament integrity, soft tissue trauma, and spinal cord injury or compression. MRI is the only radiographic imaging modality that can directly identify hematomas within the confines of the cervical spinal canal[8,20,38]

The use of MRI for acute traumatic injuries of the spine requires a cooperative patient and nonferromagnetic cervical spine immobilization devices.[17,32] Even with MR-compatible halo immobilization and skeletal traction devices, MRI is often difficult, if not impossible, to perform on combative patients and on those who require mechanical ventilation or close hemodynamic or cardiac monitoring.

Flexion and extension lateral cervical spine radiographs are important additions to the radiographic assessment of patients who have sustained cervical trauma but no demonstrable fracture or dislocation injury on the initial standard cervical spine x-rays and CT studies. Dynamic flexion-extension views of the cervical spine can determine the presence of subtle subluxation injuries or abnormal ligamentous laxity in patients who have persistent posttraumatic neck pain yet relatively normal plain x-rays of the cervical spine.[5,12] MRI can be performed in flexion and extension, a technique that may be useful in identifying intermittent or positional compression of the cervical spinal cord.[32,38,39]

TREATMENT OF CERVICAL VERTEBRAL TRAUMA

ATLANTOOCCIPITAL DISLOCATION

Patients who survive cranial-cervical dislocation injuries, like all patients who sustain neurologic deficits from cervical spine trauma, must be evaluated for potential compression of the brain stem and/or superior cervical spinal cord, the relief of which might contribute to the patient's neurologic recovery. This evaluation is best accomplished with myelography/CT or MRI. These patients must then be internally stabilized and fused from the cranial base through the first three or four cervical vertebrae.[20-23] Typically this is accomplished by segmental fixation (wire or braided cable) of an angulated, contoured support loop (either a modified doubled rod or a Steinmann pin) to the skull base and to the posterior elements of each of the first three or four cervical vertebrae, bilaterally (Fig. 20.21). Allograft or autogenic iliac crest strips and cancellous bone make up the fusion mass for long-term stability. The metallic internal strut (either rod or Steinmann pin) should be titanium to allow postoperative MRI evaluation and follow-up.

ATLAS FRACTURES

Historically, isolated atlas fractures have been treated nonoperatively, the form and duration of external stabilization necessary to treat the fracture determined by the degree of dislocation of the atlas fracture.[12,15,25-27,29] Spence suggested guidelines that might help determine therapy.[29] He showed that if the sum (bilateral) of the lateral mass displacement of C-1 over C-2 on an anteroposterior open mouth radiograph is 6.9 mm or

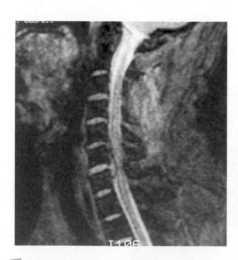

Figure 20.20 MRI revealing a fracture-dislocation injury at C6-7 with large traumatic disc herniation.

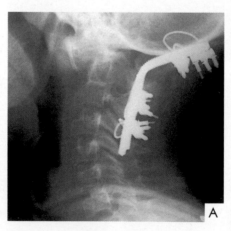

Figure 20.21 Lateral (A) and anteroposterior (B) views of cranial-cervical stabilization utilizing a Steinmann pin and fusion.

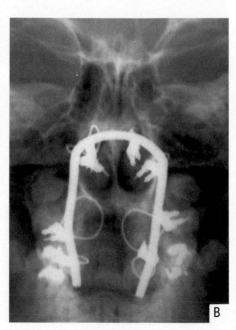

greater, the likelihood is great that the transverse atlantal ligament is disrupted, and thus the atlas fracture is unstable. Hadley et al. used these principles in their management of 32 isolated C-1 fractures, treating patients with atlas fractures displaced more than 6.9 mm with rigid immobilization.[27] Isolated atlas fractures displaced less than 6.9 mm were effectively treated with a collar, preferably a Philadelphia collar. This management scheme appears to work for all but a small percentage of atlas fractures, which fail to fuse or heal despite halo vest immobilization. Dickman et al. hypothesize that C-1 fractures that fail to heal with rigid external immobilization are atlas fractures with transverse atlantal ligament disruption.[25] These authors use MRI to assess the integrity of the ligament, irrespective of the degree of initial C1-2 dislocation. They advocate internal fixation and fusion for patients with ligament disruption.

_____ AXIS FRACTURES

The treatment of axis fractures is based on the specific features of the C-2 fracture and the presence of C2-3 subluxation or a "combination" injury type, typically C1-C2.[4,10,12,15,16,26,30,31,40–42] Odontoid type I and type III fractures are typically effectively treated with rigid external immobilization. Type III fractures have a 97% fusion rate when anatomic alignment can be restored at the fracture site and maintained in a halo immobilization device.[4,10,12,16,30]

Odontoid type II fractures are more difficult to treat and are associated with a 26% to 40% nonunion rate despite attempts at effective external stabilization.[4,10,12,15,30] Several investigators have identified features that assist the surgeon in determining their optimal management.[4,10,12,30] In general, type II odontoid fractures dis-

placed less than 5.0 mm (irrespective of the direction of the dens displacement, the degree of the associated neurologic deficit, or the age of the injured patient) will heal with nonoperative therapy (rigid external stabilization in a halo). Type II dens fracture-dislocations of more than 5.0 mm are associated with a 70% failure-of-fusion rate and deserve early operative reduction and internal fixation (ORIF) (Fig. 20.22).[4,10,12,30] Type IIA odontoid fractures, type II injuries with multiple bone chips at the base of the dens fracture site, should be treated with early ORIF as well.[12,42]

Hangman's fracture and miscellaneous fractures of the axis are uniformly treated effectively with rigid external immobilization.[4,10,12,31] Halo immobilization vests appear to provide the best rates of union and healing, but other braces and collars have been effectively used depending on individual fracture characteristics.[10,12]

Axis fractures (of any subtype) in association with C2-3 subluxation and instability have a high nonunion rate with nonoperative therapy and are best treated with ORIF.[4,10] Axis fractures in combination with atlas fractures are not uncommon.[12,26,27] Treatment of combination C1-C2 injuries is based on the subtype of C-2 fracture present. If surgical stabilization and fusion of the C-2 fracture is necessary, the type of C1-2 arthrodesis to be performed is influenced by the type of atlas fracture.[12,26]

Surgical options for ORIF of C-1, C-2, and C1-C2 combination fractures center on bilateral C1-C2 transarticular screw fixation supplemented by C1-2 posterior intraspinous arthrodesis (Fig. 20.23) (many variations have been described).[4,10,30,43] C1-2 intralaminar clamps, sublaminar wires, or a combination of sublaminar and spinous process wires or braided cables have been advocated as the internal stabilization hardware in addition to the bilateral C1-C2 transarticular

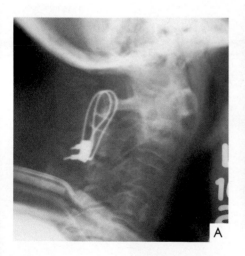
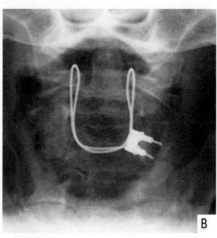

Figure 20.22 Lateral (A) and anteroposterior (B) views of C1-2 wiring and fusion.

screws. Fusion is accomplished by bony healing of the fracture sites and union of the additional fusion mass of autograft or allograft bone placed over the decorticated bony surfaces of the vertebral bodies to be fused. Patients with marked C2-3 instability can be treated via the posterior approach with sublaminar wire or braided cable, or clamp fixation, or lateral mass fixation, in conjunction with bone graft fusion. Lateral mass fixation can be accomplished with wire or braided cable as the internal construct or with lateral mass plates and screws.[26,35,38,44]

Ventral approaches to C-1 and C-2 include odontoid screw fixation for odontoid fractures and C2-3 intervertebral fusion with ventral plating (Fig. 20.24).[4,41,45] The optimal surgical approach for any of these injury types must be dictated by the unique features of the fracture and by the capabilities and experience of the surgeon and the institution.

C3-T1 INJURIES

The wide spectrum of injury types that occur between C-3 and T-1 requires careful consideration and individualization of treatment. The specifics of the mechanism of injury, the fracture-dislocation injury type, the presence (and extent) of a neurologic deficit, and the presence of spinal cord compressive pathology or other associated vertebral body fractures will dictate whether operative or nonoperative management is appropriate for a given patient.[4,5,12,16,29,35,46] General management principles for acute traumatic C3-T1 fracture or subluxation injuries include: 1) early reduction and realignment of the fracture-dislocation injuries, 2) urgent decompression of fracture-dislocation injuries that result in persistent distortion and compression of the cervical spinal cord (despite attempts at closed reduction), particularly among patients with incomplete neurologic injuries, 3) external stabilization of C3-T1 traumatic injuries that have a high likelihood of healing with immobilization alone (nondisplaced vertebral body or posterior element fractures without marked vertebral body collapse, and facet dislocation injuries that have been realigned via closed means and are associated with facet fractures), 4) early ORIF of patients with fracture-dislocation injuries that cannot be reduced by closed means (particularly for patients with incomplete neurologic injuries), and injuries that, once reduced, cannot be effectively immobilized by external means, and 5) nonurgent stabilization and fusion of fracture-dislocation injuries that either cannot be reduced or effectively stabilized in patients who present neurologically intact or in patients with complete neurologic injuries who present more than 24 hours postinjury. Nonurgent operative stabilization is also recommended for the relatively small subset

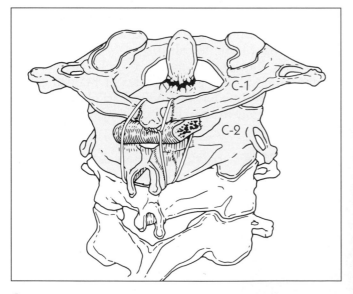

Figure 20.23 C1-2 fusion construct with interposition graft between the dorsal arches of atlas and axis.

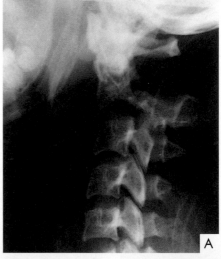

Figure 20.24 (A) Hangman's fracture with marked C2-3 instability and dislocation. (B) The same patient status post ventral C2-3 interbody fusion and internal bicortical screw-plate fixation.

of patients with spinal instability due to traumatic ligament disruption only, without fracture, including facet dislocation without fracture injury.

The surgical approach for patients with C3-T1 acute traumatic fracture-dislocation injuries is dictated by the need to decompress neural elements and the need to provide internal vertebral column stabilization with fusion. The operative approach (ventral or dorsal) should be that which directly and most effectively accomplishes these goals.[4,5,12,16,29,35,46] Posterior decompression and/or stabilization can be accomplished with laminar clamps, sublaminar wires, or lateral mass plates, all in conjunction with bony fusion.[4,35,44,47] Ventral stabilization can be achieved following disc space or vertebral body decompression (corpectomy) with a bony intervertebral strut graft fusion, with or without ventral cervical stabilization plates and bicortical vertebral body screw fixation (Fig. 20.25).[4,46]

CERVICAL SPINAL CORD INJURIES

Patients who present with spinal cord neurologic deficits secondary to acute cervical spine trauma have a variable likelihood of neurologic recovery.[1,2,5,6,9,13,17,48,49] Factors that affect recovery include: 1) the nature and force of the initial fracture-dislocation injury, 2) the depth and extent of the initial neurologic deficit, 3) the ability to reduce cord compression and realign the cervical vertebral column, 4) the presence of irreducible spinal cord compression by bone, disc, or hematoma, often in spite of satisfactory vertebral column realignment, 5) the presence of persistent spinal column instability, 6) the ability to treat associated systemic hypoxia and shock, and, presumably, 7) the time between injury and spinal column realignment/spinal cord decompression.

Some patients who suffer spinal cord injuries are ruined at the time of initial impact (physiologic spinal cord transection). These are patients who, despite early reduction and aggressive early treatment of shock and hypoxia, will have fixed neurologic deficits (usually complete spinal cord injuries). Hadley et al. have observed that signs of cervical spinal cord transection, that is, complete neurologic deficits and neurogenic "spinal shock" (hypotension with bradycardia), herald a poor prognosis for recovery of neurologic function.[17] Other patients, including some with complete neurologic injuries, have their potential for neurologic recovery maximized by treatment of systemic hypoxia and shock and early realignment and decompression of the vertebral column and cervical spinal cord. One large multicenter clinical trial indicates that in addition to the above key treatment principles, the administration of high dose methylprednisolone immediately after severe spinal cord injury can have positive effects on subsequent neurologic recovery.[48] Further clinical investigation is underway.

It has been suggested that patients with neurologic deficits from cervical spinal fracture-dislocation injuries can best be treated with early aggressive attempts at closed reduction followed by rigid external immobilization.[12,17] These patients, including those who have injuries that cannot be reduced by closed means, should be assessed radiographically for persistent spinal cord compression by bone, disc, or hematoma. Early spinal cord decompression and/or vertebral column realignment should then be accomplished surgically, followed by vertebral column stabilization, to provide optimal therapy. Hadley et al. documented significant neurologic recovery in only 10 of 68 patients who presented with profound neurologic deficits from cervical facet dislocation injuries.[17] All 10 patients had their injuries reduced

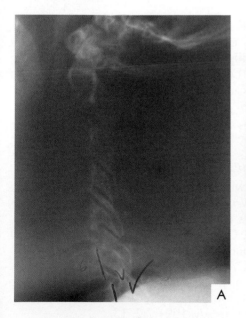 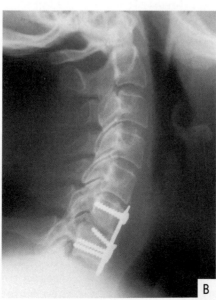

Figure 20.25 (A) Fracture dislocation injury at C6-7. (B) The same patient status post C6-7 discectomy, interbody fusion, and internal bicortical screw-plate fixation.

and/or decompressed (by closed or operative means) within 8 hours of injury. The timing of cervical spinal cord decompression, like documented that for intracranial traumatic injuries, appears to be important with respect to subsequent recovery of neurologic function.

SCIWORA patients are those who, by definition, present with neurologic deficits without radiographic abnormality (fracture or subluxation). These patients must be properly immobilized and studied extensively with CT, MRI, and delayed flexion-extension x-rays. Some advocate somatosensory evoked potential recordings (SSEPs) as well.[13,14,18] As with most spinal cord injuries, patients with incomplete SCIWORA injuries have a higher likelihood of recovery of function than those who present with complete neurologic injuries. Younger patients (less than 4 years) tend to have a worse outcome after SCIWORA than older children.[13,18] Patients with SCIWORA must be rigidly immobilized, restricted from activities that might reproduce their injury, and must be followed closely in the outpatient setting. Several investigators have described delayed SCIWORA injuries and/or recurrent spinal cord injuries among patients who presented with SCIWORA injuries but recovered and were cleared of vertebral column pathology on their initial hospital evaluation.[14,18]

In summary, the vast majority of traumatic vertebral column injuries involve the cervical spinal segment. The level and extent of the vertebral column injury will determine the likelihood of underlying neurologic deficit. Specific injury types have been reviewed and their optimal treatment outlined. General management principles of acute cervical spinal column injury have been discussed and include rigid immobilization, detailed radiographic assessment, aggressive treatment of hypoxia and shock when present, and early reduction of vertebral column fracture-dislocation and spinal cord compression injuries. Adherence to these principles appears to maximize the patient's potential for neurologic recovery following acute cervical spinal column/cord injury.

REFERENCES

1. Bohlman HH. Acute fractures and dislocations of the cervical spine: an analysis of three hundred hospitalized patients and review of the literature. *J Bone Joint Surg (Am)*. 1979;61A:1119–1142.

2. Bohlman HH, Boada E. Fractures and dislocations of the lower cervical spine. In: Cervical Spine Research Society, ed. *The Cervical Spines*. Philadelphia, Pa: JB Lippincott. 1983;232–267.

3. Heiden JS, Weiss MH, Rosenberg AW, Apuzzo MLJ, Kurze T. Management of cervical spinal cord trauma in southern California. *J Neurosurg*. 1975;43:732–736.

4. Sonntag VKH, Hadley MN. Management of nonodontoid upper cervical spine injuries. In: Cooper P, ed. *Management of Posttraumatic Spinal Instability: Neurosurgical Topics*. AANS Publications; 1990;7:99–109.

5. Weiss J. Mid- and lower cervical spine injuries. In: Wilkins R, ed. *Neurosurgery*. New York, NY: McGraw-Hill; 1985;2:211:1708–1715.

6. Harris P, Karmi MZ, McClemont E, Matlhoko D, Paul KS. The prognosis of patients sustaining severe cervical spine injury (C2-C7 inclusive). *Paraplegia*. 1980;18:324–330.

7. Heiden JS, Weiss MH. Cervical spine injuries with and without neurological deficit, I. *Contemp Neurosurg*. 1980;2:1–6.

8. Mesard L, Carmody A, Mannarino E, Ruge D. Survival after spinal cord trauma: a life table analysis. *Arch Neurol*. 1978;35:78–83.

9. Riggins RS, Kraus JF. The risk of neurologic damage with fractures of the vertebrae. *J Trauma*. 1977;17:126–133.

10. Hadley MN, Dickman CA, Browner CM, Sonntag VKH. Acute axis fractures: a review of 229 cases. *J Neurosurg*. 1989;71:642–647.

11. Reiss SJ, Raque GH Jr, Shields CB, Garretson HD. Cervical spine fractures with major associated trauma. *Neurosurgery*. 1986;18:327–330.

12. Sonntag VKH, Hadley MN. Management of upper cervical spinal instability. In: Wilkins R, ed. *Neurosurgery Update*. New York, NY: McGraw-Hill; 1991;82:222–223.

13. Hadley MN, Zabramski JM, Browner CM, Rekate H, Sonntag VKH. Pediatric spinal trauma: a review of 122 cases of spinal cord and vertebral column injuries. *J Neurosurg*. 1988;68:18–24.

14. Ruge JR, Sinson GP, McLone DG, Cerullo LJ. Pediatric spinal injury: the very young. *J Neurosurg*. 1988;68:25–30.

15. Schneider R. High cervical spine injuries. In: Wilkins R, ed. *Neurosurgery*. New York, NY: McGraw-Hill; 1985;2:211:1701–1708.

16. Spence KF, Decker S, Sell KW. Bursting atlantal fracture associated with rupture of the transverse ligament. *J Bone Joint Surg (Am)*. 1970;52A:543–549.

17. Hadley MN, Fitzpatrick B, Browner C, Sonntag VKH. Facet fracture-dislocation injuries of the cervical spine. *Neurosurgery*. 1992;30:661–666.

18. Pollack IF, Pang D, Sclabassi R. Recurrent spinal cord injury without radiographic abnormalities in children. *J Neurosurg*. 1988;69:177–182.

19. Gehweiler JA Jr, Clark WM, Schaaf RE, Powers B, Miller MD. Cervical spine trauma: the common combined conditions. *Radiology*. 1979;130:77–86.

20. Dickman CA, Douglas RA, Sonntag VKH. Occipitocervical fusion: posterior stabilization of the craniovertebral junction and upper cervical spine. *BNI Quarterly*. 1991;7:2–13.

21. Bools JC, Rose BS. Traumatic atlantoccipital dislocation: two cases with survival. *AJNR*. 1986; 7:901–904.

22. Menezes AH, VanGilder JC, Graf CJ, et al. Craniocervical abnormalities: a comprehensive surgical approach. *J Neurosurg.* 1980;53:444–445.

23. Ransford AO, Crockard HA, Pozo JL, et al. Craniocervical instability treated by contoured loop fixation. *J Bone Joint Surg.* 1986;68B:173–177.

24. Menezes AH, Muhonen M. Management of occipito-cervical instability. In: Cooper P, ed. *Management of Posttraumatic Spinal Instability: Neurosurgical Topics.* AANS Publications. 1990;5:65–74.

25. Dickman CA, Mamourian A, Sonntag VKH, Drayer BP. Magnetic resonance imaging of the transverse atlantal ligament for the evaluation of atlantoaxial instability. *J Neurosurg.* 1991;75:221–227.

26. Dickman CA, Hadley MN, Browner C, Sonntag VKH. Neurosurgical management of acute atlas-axis combination fractures: a review of 25 cases. *J Neurosurg.* 1989;70:45–49.

27. Hadley MN, Dickman CA, Browner CM, Sonntag VKH. Acute traumatic atlas fractures: management and long-term outcome. *Neurosurgery.* 1988;23:31–35.

28. Keene GCR, Hone MR, Sage MR. Atlas fracture: demonstration using computerized tomography. *J Bone Joint Surg (Am).* 1978;60A:1106–1107.

29. Sonntag VKH, Hadley MN. Nonoperative management of cervical spine injuries. *Clin Neurosurg.* 1988;34:630–649.

30. Clark CT, Apuzzo ML. The evaluation and management of trauma to the odontoid process. In: Cooper P, ed. *Management of Posttraumatic Spinal Instability: Neurosurgical Topics.* AANS Publications. 1990;6:77–94.

31. Hadley MN, Browner CM, Sonntag VKH. Miscellaneous fractures of the second cervical vertebra. *BNI Quarterly.* 1985;1:34–39.

32. Cohen W. Imaging and determination of posttraumatic spinal instability. In: Cooper P, ed. *Management of Posttraumatic Spinal Instability: Neurosurgical Topics.* AANS Publications. 1990;2:19–35.

33. Ross SE, Schwab CW, David ET, Delong WG, Born CT. Clearing the cervical spine: initial radiologic evaluation. *J Trauma.* 1987;27:1055–1060.

34. Cooper PR, Cohen W. Evaluation of cervical spinal cord injuries with metrizamide myelography-CT scanning. *J Neurosurg.* 1984;61:281–289.

35. Cooper PR, Cohen W, Rosiello A, et al. Posterior stabilization of cervical spine fractures and subluxations using plates and screws. *Neurosurgery.* 1988; 23:300–306.

36. Allen RL, Perot PL Jr, Gudemna SK. Evaluation of acute nonpenetrating cervical spinal cord injuries with CT metrizamide myelography. *J Neurosurg.* 1985;63:510–520.

37. Hadley MN, Sonntag VKH, Amos MR, Hodak JA, Lopez LJ. Three-dimensional computed tomography in the diagnosis of vertebral column pathological conditions. *Neurosurgery.* 1987;21:186–192.

38. Chakers DW, Flickinger F, Bresnahan JC, Beattie MS, Weiss KL, Miller C. MR imaging of acute spinal cord trauma. *AJNR.* 1987;8:5–10.

39. Pech P, Kilgore DP, Pojunas KW, Haughton VM. Cervical spine fractures: CT detection. *Radiology.* 1985;63:510–520.

40. Borne GM, Bedou GL, Pinaudeau M, Cristino G, Huessin A. Odontoid process fracture osteosynthesis with a direct screw fixation technique in nine consecutive cases. *J Neurosurg.* 1967;27:462–465.

41. Geisler FH, Cheng C, Poka A, Brumback RJ. Anterior screw fixation of posteriorly displaced type II odontoid fractures. *Neurosurgery.* 1989;25:130–136.

42. Hadley MN, Browner CM, Liu SS, Sonntag VKH. New subtype of acute odontoid fractures (type IIA). *Neurosurgery.* 1988;22:67–71.

43. Dickman CA, Papadopoulos SM, Hadley MN, Sonntag VKH. The interspinous method of posterior atlantoaxial arthodesis: technical consideration and clinical results. *J Neurosurg.* 1991;74:190–198.

44. Roy-Camille R, Saillant G, Mazel C. Internal fixation of the unstable cervical spine by a posterior osteosynthesis with plates and screws. In: Cervical Spine Research Society, ed. *The Cervical Spine.* 2nd ed. Philadelphia, Pa: JB Lippincott; 1989:390–396.

45. Brant-Zawadzki M, Miller EM, Federle MP. CT in the elevation of spine trauma. *AJR.* 1981;136:369–375.

46. Caspar W, Barbier DD, Klara PM. Anterior cervical fusion and Caspar plate stabilization for cervical trauma. *Neurosurgery.* 1989;25:491–502.

47. Cherney WB, Sonntag VKH, Douglas RA. Lateral mass posterior plating and facet fusion for cervical spine instability. *BNI Quarterly.* 1991;7:2–11.

48. Bracken MB, Shepard MJ, Collins WF, Holford TR, Young W, Baskin OS, Eisenberg HM, Flamm ES, Leo-Summers L, Maroon J, National Acute Spinal Cord Injury Study Group. A randomized, controlled trial of methylprednisolone or naloxone in the treatment of acute spinal cord injury: results of the second national acute spinal cord injury study. *N Engl J Med.* 1990;322:1405–1411.

49. Reid DC, Henderson R, Saboe L, Miller JDR. Etiology and clinical course of missed spine fractures. *J Trauma.* 1987;27:980–986.

Chapter 21

Thoracolumbar Spine Fractures

Setti S. Rengachary, Eric S. Nussbaum

It has been estimated that there are as many as 60,000 spinal column injuries annually in the United States.[1] The thoracolumbar junction appears to be the second most commonly involved region, preceded only by mid to lower cervical injuries. Thoracolumbar fractures generally result from major trauma such as a motor vehicle accident or a fall from significant height. The incidence of reported neurologic deficit associated with thoracolumbar fractures varies greatly between series. Of all patients with thoracolumbar fractures, approximately 35% suffer a complete neurologic deficit, 40% a partial injury, and 25% are neurologically intact.[2–4]

The thoracolumbar junction is a zone of structural and functional transition, which makes it vulnerable to injury.[6] At this level the normal thoracic kyphosis joins the lumbar lordosis. The lever arm of the thoracic spine, which is rigid with regard to flexion and extension, meets the lumbar spine, which allows flexion and extension but lacks the support of the thoracic cage and lower lumbar elements. The thoracolumbar junction may therefore be viewed as a fulcrum for spinal motion between the inflexible thoracic region and the more resilient lumbar levels. Rotation, a movement allowed by the thoracic spine, is abruptly interrupted by the more vertically oriented articular processes of the lumbar region.

BIOMECHANICAL CONSIDERATIONS

Denis[5] described a three-column concept of spinal support involving the anterior longitudinal ligament/anterior vertebral body complex (anterior column); the posterior longitudinal ligament, annulus, and posterior vertebral body (middle column); and the facet joints, ligamentum flavum, laminae, posterior spinous processes, and interspinous ligaments (posterior column) (Fig. 21.1). Fractures may then be considered in the context of failure of one or more columns. It is generally accepted that disruption of more than one column heralds an unstable injury. Injuries involving all three columns are unequivocally unstable and thus require internal stabilization.

TYPES OF FRACTURES

Thoracolumbar fractures may be classified into three broad classes. The specific deformity produced depends on the amount and direction of force applied to the spine. Axial loading with flexion produces an *anterior wedge compression* injury (Fig. 21.2). True vertical axial compression transmits the force directly to the vertebral bodies, causing a *bursting* injury (Fig. 21.3). Distraction applied in flexion, as may be caused by a seat belt, results in a *splitting* injury (Chance fracture), beginning posteriorly and proceeding anteriorly through the vertebral body or intervertebral disc. A number of subtypes for each class have been described (Fig. 21.4).

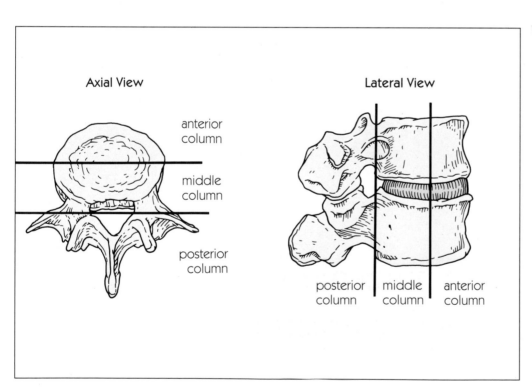

Figure 21.1 The three columns of the thoracolumbar spine. The anterior column consists of the anterior longitudinal ligament and the anterior halves of the annulus and vertebral body. The middle column consists of the posterior longitudinal ligament and the posterior halves of the annulus and vertebral body. The posterior column consists of the laminae, ligamentum flavum, facet joints, pedicles, spinous processes, and interspinal and supraspinal ligaments.

CLINICAL ASSESSMENT

The thoracolumbar region includes elements of the spinal cord, the conus medullaris, and the roots of the cauda equina. Injury to this region may therefore produce a confusing clinical picture of mixed upper and lower motor neuron deficits. A detailed neurologic examination is important to assess the degree of injury to these structures and to plan treatment appropriately. This should include assessment of rectal tone and urinary postvoiding residual measurement. The conus medullaris, like the spinal cord, is relatively "unforgiving" in response to injury. The nerve roots of the cauda equina, in contrast, have a greater capacity for neurologic recovery.

RADIOLOGIC ASSESSMENT

The specific radiologic studies performed will depend on the details of a given case. Plain lateral radiographs will reveal the anterior wedge compression fracture of an axial loading flexion injury or the gross loss of vertebral height with anterior and posterior bone propulsion in a burst fracture. Anteroposterior views may show an increased interpedicular distance.

CT scanning is particularly useful for demonstrating bony detail. It is an excellent study for determining the degree of canal compromise. The horizontal fracture line of a seat-belt-type injury, however, may yield misleading results on CT. Plain tomography may be a better tool for assessing this injury.[5,7]

MANAGEMENT PRINCIPLES

The most important concern with any spinal fracture is the potential for injury to neural elements. Immediate stability as well as long-term potential for healing must be considered in each individual case. The general aim of treatment is the improvement and preservation of neurologic function as well as the prevention of progressive deformity and pain. This may require aggressive operative intervention in some cases but only external immobilization in others.

SPECIFIC INJURIES

FLEXION-COMPRESSION FRACTURES

Flexion-compression injuries generally result in anterior wedge compression fractures with disruption of Denis's anterior column. These fractures are typically stable, since the middle and posterior columns remain intact. Not surprisingly, the vast majority of these patients are neurologically unaffected. In this setting the patient may be treated with bed rest until free of pain, followed by mobilization in a rigid external orthosis.

BURST FRACTURES

Axial compressive forces may also result in severe vertebral body fractures involving the anterior and middle columns, with collapse of the entire vertebral body. These fractures are potentially unstable, with a notable potential for compromise of the spinal canal by retropulsed bone or disc fragments. Of 59 patients with burst fractures seen by Denis, about one half had neurologic dysfunction. No correlation, however, has been demonstrated between the degree of canal compromise and the severity of neurologic deficit.[8] This suggests that neural injury occurs at the time of the accident and may not be related to ongoing neural compression.

Significant controversy exists regarding appropriate treatment of burst fractures in the thoracolumbar re-

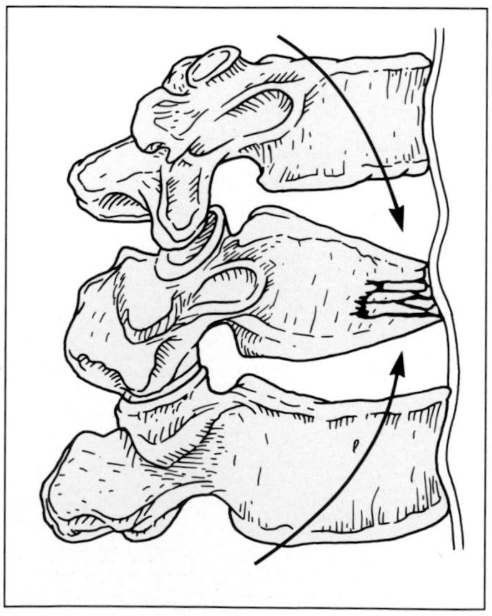

Figure 21.2
Anterior wedge compression fracture.

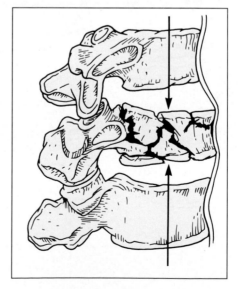

Figure 21.3
Burst fracture.

gion. Indications for operative intervention which have generally been associated with an increased risk of instability include 1) reduction of anterior vertebral body height by more than 50%, 2) kyphotic angulation greater than 20% to 25%, or 3) retropulsed fragments that compromise at least 50% of the spinal canal.

Treatment options range from conservative measures to aggressive operative intervention. Nonoperative treatment generally consists of postural reduction followed by application of a rigid external thoracolumbar orthosis or cast.[9] This may be considered in patients who are neurologically intact and do not meet the above indications for surgery. Nonoperative management relies on Wolf's law, which posits that without continued axial force, the bone will resorb and the spinal canal will remodel.

In the past, operative treatment was advocated in patients with burst fractures who did not have a neurologic deficit, in order to prevent progressive kyphotic deformity, pain, and delayed neurologic deficit from retropulsed bony fragments within the neural canal.[10] However, recent experience, based on careful, long-term follow-up, suggests that nonoperative management consisting of a brief period of bed rest followed by application of a rigid external orthosis is recommended in patients who are neurologically intact.[11,12] Late complications do not occur, contrary to the conventional prediction.

Operative stabilization consists of segmental distraction with pedicle screw fixation one level above and one level below the injured segment. By applying distraction, annulotaxis is exploited to aid in reduction of

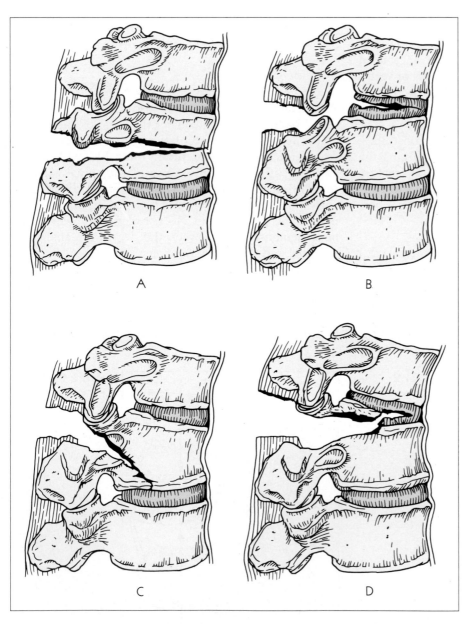

A

B

C

D

Figure 21.4 Subtypes of flexion-distraction (Chance) fractures. **(A)** Disruption entirely through the bony elements. **(B)** Disruption entirely through ligamentous elements. **(C,D)** Disruption through bony and ligamentous elements.

retropulsed bone and disk fragments.[13] Once reduction with distraction has been applied, intraoperative ultrasound may be used to check the position of fragments within the canal. If significant compromise remains, a number of surgical options are available, including transpedicular decompression (Fig. 21.5) or corpectomy followed by strut grafting through a posterolateral extracavitary, retroperitoneal, or thoracoabdominal approach (Fig. 21.6). Laminectomy alone is contraindicated in burst fractures: Holdsworth and Hardy have shown that simple laminectomy may increase instability as well as the incidence of early and late neurologic deficit.[14]

When performing a laminectomy after a burst fracture, it is important to remember that during injury the pedicles widen, allowing retropulsed bone to displace the dural sac posteriorly. An associated laminar fracture may trap the sac as it closes down, allowing inadvertent injury to the dura and underlying nerve roots upon laminectomy.[15]

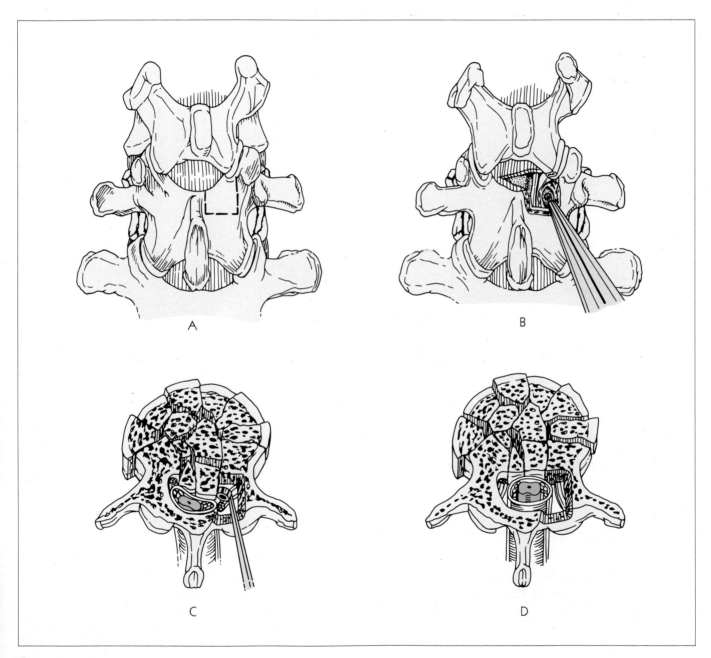

A

B

C

D

Figure 21.5 Technique of removing retropulsed fragments from the spinal canal through pediculotomy. **(A)** A small laminotomy is made. **(B)** The pedicle is exposed and drilled. **(C)** Using an angled curette, the retropulsed fragments are either removed or tapped back in place. **(D)** View after clearance of retropulsed fragments from the canal.

FLEXION-DISTRACTION (CHANCE) FRACTURES

When distraction forces are applied to the spine in flexion, the posterior ligamentous structures may be disrupted. This type of injury was first described by Chance.[16] There may be major ligamentous disruption with associated instability and potential for serious subluxation. Various subtypes of Chance fracture are shown in Figure 21.4.

In contrast to burst fractures, which are treated with distraction, Chance fractures require internal fixation with compression. Segmental compression with pedicle screws one level above and one level below provides adequate stability to allow proper healing of these injuries.

CONCLUSIONS

The management of fractures in the thoracolumbar region remains controversial. Recognition of the mechanisms of injury, the biomechanical forces at play, and the potential for healing with or without operative intervention allows rational planning of treatment.

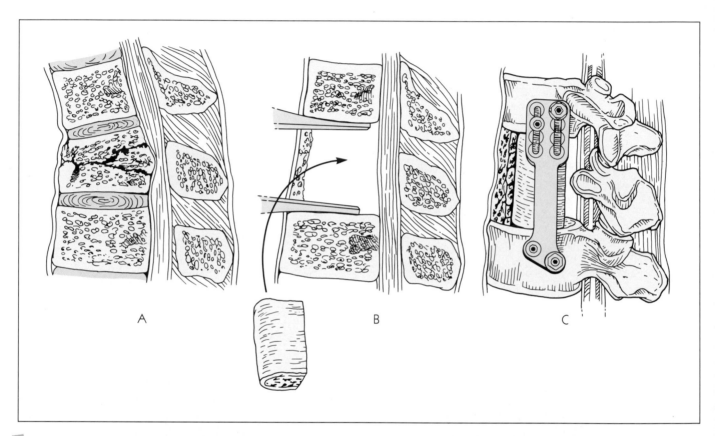

Figure 21.6 Corpectomy, strut grafting, and stabilization through an anterior approach. (**A**) L-1 burst fracture with retropulsed fragments. (**B**) Damaged L-1 body has been removed and a tricortical iliac graft is impacted under distraction. (**C**) A plate is anchored to the normal vertebral bodies above and below.

REFERENCES

1. Riggins RS, Kraus JF. The risk of neurologic damage with fractures of the vertebrae. *J Trauma.* 1977;17:126–133.
2. Convey FR, Minteer MA, Smith RW, et al. Fracture-dislocation of the dorsal-lumbar spine. *Spine.* 1978;3:160–166.
3. Jacobs RR, Asher MA, Snider RK. Thoracolumbar spinal injuries: a comparative study of recumbent and operative treatment in 100 patients. *Spine.* 1980;5:463–477.
4. Schmidek HH, Gomes FB, Seligson D, McSherry JW. Management of acute unstable thoracolumbar fractures with and without neurological deficit. *Neurosurgery.* 1980;7:3035.
5. Denis F. The three column spine and its significance in the classification of acute thoracolumbar spine injuries. *Spine.* 1983;8:817–821.
6. Larson SJ. The thoracolumbar junction. In: Dunsker SB, Schmidek HH, Frymoyer J, et al, eds. *The Unstable Spine.* Philadelphia, Pa: WB Saunders Co; 1986:127–152.
7. McAfee PC, Yuan HA, Frederickson BE, Lubicky

JP. The value of computed tomography in thoracolumbar fractures: an analysis of 100 consecutive cases and a new classification. *J Bone Joint Surg.* 1983;65A:461–473.

8. Shuman WP, Rogers JV, Sickler ME, Hanson JA, Crutcher JP, King HA, Mack LA. Thoracolumbar burst fractures: CT dimensions of the spinal canal relative to postsurgical improvement. *Am J Neuroradiol.* 1985;6:337–341.

9. Frankel HL, Hancock DO, Hyslop G. The value of postural reduction in the initial management of closed injuries to the spine with paraplegia and tetraplegia. *Paraplegia.* 1969;7:179–182.

10. Bergman TA, Seljeskog EL. Management of thoracolumbar and lumbar spine injuries. In: Youmans JR, ed. *Neurological Surgery.* Philadelphia, Pa: WB Saunders Co; 1990:2411–2422.

11. Mumford J, Weinstein JN, Spratt KF, Goel VK. Thoracolumbar burst fractures. The clinical efficacy and outcome of nonoperative management. *Spine.* 1993;18:955–970.

12. Cantor JB, Lebwohl NH, Garvey T, Eismont FJ. Non-operative management of stable thoracolumbar burst fractures with early ambulation and bracing. *Spine.* 1993;18:971–979.

13. Zou D, You JU, Edwards T, Yuan HA. Mechanics of anatomic reduction of thoracolumbar burst fractures. *Spine.* 1993;18:195–203.

14. Holdsworth FW, Hardy A. Early treatment of paraplegia from fractures of the thoracolumbar spine *J Bone Joint Surg.* 1953;35B:540–550.

15. Camissa FP, Eismont FJ, Green BA, Yuan HA. Dural laceration occurring with burst fractures and associated laminar fractures. *J Bone Joint Surg.* 1989;71A:1044–1052.

16. Chance GQ. Note on a type of flexion fracture of the spine. *Br J Radiol.* 1948;21:452–453.

Chapter 22

Acute Nerve Injuries

Allan J. Belzberg, James N. Campbell

Much of the knowledge for the managment of periph-eral nerve injuries has come from treating war injuries. Recent advances in instrumentation and microscopic surgical technique have improved the prognosis of major peripheral nerve injuries. Challenges for the neurosurgeon in managing peripheral nerve injuries include deciding whether surgery is required, when to operate, and which injuries to repair for the best functional outcome.

It is useful to review the meaning of certain terms. *Neurotization* refers to the ingrowth of axons into tissue such as a distal nerve stump or a motor end plate in a muscle, which can occur spontaneously after injury to or surgical repair of a nerve. A *neurorrhaphy* is the joining together, usually by suture, of the two parts of a divided nerve to enable neurotization; if the nerve ends do not easily come together interpositional nerve grafts may be required. *Nerve transfer* refers to the transposition of freshly cut normal nerve to the distal stump of the injured nerve; it is used when the proximal stump of the injured nerve can no longer provide useful re-innervation (e.g., nerve root avulsion from the spinal cord). The term *anastomosis* should not be used for nerve repair since it refers to the union of hollow tubes.

ANATOMY

The structure of a peripheral nerve is constant regardless of the location in the body. It consists of nerve fibers, fasciculi, connective tissue, blood vessels, lymphatics, and nervi nervorum (Fig. 22.1). Within an individual peripheral nerve the fascicular pattern changes along its course due to plexus formation along the course of the nerve and fibers coursing between fascicles. In a proximal nerve, fibers destined for skin are mixed with fibers destined for muscle. More distally, the sensory and motor fibers are segregated into separate fascicles.

RESPONSE TO INJURY

A peripheral nerve responds to injury in a predictable manner regardless of the etiology of the injury.

NEURONAL RESPONSE

Nerve injury leads to chromatolysis—swelling and displacement of the Nissl substance to the periphery of the cell—in the cell body. The closer the injury is to the spinal cord, the more hypertrophic the changes. Specific molecules help the neurons that have sustained an injury to survive. Trophic factors, such as nerve growth factor, are taken from the terminal target tissue by the axon and transported retrograde to the neuronal cell body where they support gene regulation and promote survival of the neuron. The regenerating axons seek out sources of growth factors. Chemotactic factors may guide the growing axon sprouts for re-innervation of their target.

AXONAL RESPONSE

When an axon is divided, wallerian degeneration (changes in the distal nerve) occurs. The axon and myelin

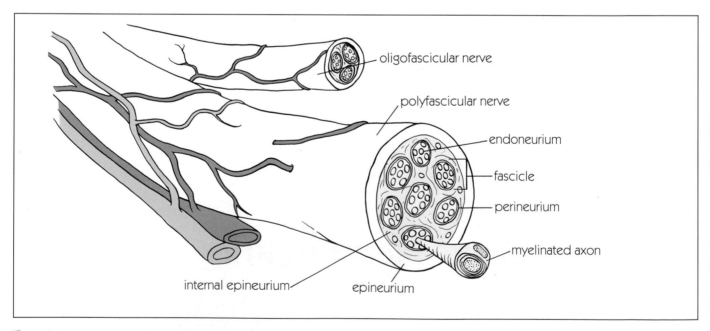

Figure 22.1 Peripheral nerve anatomy: epineurium, perineurium, endoneurium, oligofascicular nerve, polyfascicular nerve.

distal to the injury degenerate and are removed by phagocytic cells. Empty endoneurial tubes within the perineurium of the distal nerve remain. The proximal axons sprout new branches that, in the right environment, grow across the area of damage and enter the distal endoneurial tubes. The endoneurial tubes then direct the growing axons to peripheral targets. Schwann cells eventually move into the tubes to remyelinate the sprouting axons. If the sprouting axons do not reach a distal endoneurial tube or the tube has been replaced by fibrosis, the sprouts will form a local tangle or neuroma.

MUSCLE RESPONSE

When a muscle loses its nervous innervation it degenerates. By three weeks postinjury, the beginnings of muscle fibrosis are reflected in histologic changes in the muscle. The fibrosis will gradually replace the muscle and by 2 years often only scar tissue is present. The muscle must be re-innervated within approximately 18 months of the injury to provide a functional outcome. Proximal nerve lesions are therefore at more risk of poor outcome because of the increased time required for axonal regeneration to reach target muscle.

Signs of acute muscle degeneration on EMG examination include spontaneous muscle activity, fibrillations, and denervation potentials. The EMG changes occur only after wallerian degeneration and therefore take 1 to 2 weeks from the time of injury to appear. The first EMG is most often performed between 10 days and 2 weeks from the time of injury. An EMG performed within days of an injury will be normal, even if a severe injury to the nerve has occurred.

Figure 22.2 Sunderland Classification of Nerve Injury

Classification	Description
Grade I	Loss of axonal conduction
Grade II	Loss of axonal continuity
Grade III	Loss of axonal and endoneurial continuity
Grade IV	Loss of perineurial continuity with fascicular disruption
Grade V	Loss of continuity of entire nerve trunk

CLASSIFICATION OF INJURIES

In 1943 Seddon introduced a classification of nerve injury based on three types of nerve fiber injury. Physiologic disruption is termed *neuropraxia*, axonal disruption is termed *axonotemesis*, and division of the nerve trunk is termed *neuronotemesis*. This was followed by the Sunderland classification based on five degrees of increasing anatomic severity of injury (Fig. 22.2). Pure grades of injury probably do not exist; the severity of most injuries occurs along a continuum.

SUNDERLAND CLASSIFICATION

First-Degree Injury
A grade I injury represents a reversible local conduction block at the site of injury. Symptoms and signs are variable and when mild may consist of paresis or sensory disturbance. A more severe injury may produce paralysis and/or complete sensory loss. Electrical studies demonstrate local conduction block abnormalities only at the site of injury. The pathology, consisting of local demyelination, is reversible. The injury does not require surgical intervention. Signs of recovery can begin within hours but may require several weeks.

Second-Degree Injury
In a grade II injury, there is loss of continuity of the axons. Symptoms and signs consist of a dense sensory and motor loss distal to the lesion. The myelin, which is axon-dependent, degenerates but the endoneurial sheath and supporting elements, including perineurium, are preserved. The intact endoneurial tubes provide a guide for axonal regeneration, and the prognosis for a functional recovery is excellent. The axons can be expected to regenerate at a rate of approximately 1 mm/d.

After sufficient time for axonal growth to occur across the lesion, electrical studies can be used to confirm action potential conduction across the lesion. This is most accurate when performed intraoperatively. If a second-degree injury is confirmed, the lesion should not be surgically resected. An external neurolysis may be indicated to remove extensive scarring, but internal neurolysis is avoided as it will lessen the chance of a functional recovery.

Third-Degree Injury
In a grade III injury, there is damage to the axons, degeneration of myelin, and loss of endoneurial tubes. Symptoms and signs consist of a dense sensory and motor loss. The perineurium is preserved, but because of the loss of the endoneurial tubes there is no guidance for regenerating axons. There is often intrafascicular bleeding, edema, and ischemia leading to fibrosis.

Recovery depends on the degree to which intrafascicular fibrosis prevents axonal regeneration into distal endoneurial tubes. When severe, little recovery can be expected. Spontaneous recovery of some function occurs if axons are able to cross the lesion and re-innervate distal targets. A third-degree injury will rarely recover to more than 60% to 80% of normal function. Surgical intervention such as nerve grafting is required only in severe third-degree injuries.

Fourth-Degree Injury

In a grade IV injury, the epineurium holds the nerve together but the internal anatomy, including the axon, endoneurial tube, and perineurium, is disrupted. The fascicular pattern is lost and regenerating axons cannot reach their targets. Electrical studies show no evidence of conduction across the lesion even after several months. Surgical intervention with nerve grafting is required for a functional recovery.

Fifth-Degree Injury

In a grade V lesion, there is loss of continuity of the nerve trunk. A grade V injury is commonly seen in laceration injuries but can also occur with severe stretch injury. The proximal nerve sprouts axons, but because of the discontinuity with the distal nerve, the sprouts tangle and form a neuroma. This injury requires surgical repair for a functional recovery.

MECHANISM OF INJURY

LACERATION

Common causes of nerve lacerations are knife and glass injuries. The lesion may be a complete transection (grade V) or a partial laceration. In clean, sharp lacerations, the nerve should be repaired acutely. The surgery

Figure 22.3 Stretch Injuries

Nerve	Etiology
Brachial plexus	Motorcycle accident
Upper or lower brachial plexus	Birth injury
Axillary nerve	Shoulder dislocation
Radial nerve	Humerus fracture
Common peroneal nerve	Head of fibula fracture

should be performed by an experienced surgeon with the patient's other injuries stabilized. Waiting a few days to perform the repair while stabilizing other injuries or assembling a skilled surgical team will not affect the outcome.

FOCAL CONTUSION

A focal contusion can produce a variety of injuries often within the same nerve. It is commonly seen in missile injuries such as gunshot wounds. Symptoms and signs are variable depending on the degree of injury. When contusion to the nerve occurs, often some resection of the two ends for a variable distance is required to allow a neurorrhaphy of viable nerve. If a large gap is produced, nerve grafting will be required. When a contusion to the nerve is suspected, repair should be delayed, allowing the extent of pathology to become apparent.

STRETCH/TRACTION INJURY

Traction is a common mechanism of injury in which the nerve may remain in continuity, but severe internal disruption occurs. The area of pathology can be local or spread over a large distance. Focal traction injuries, such as intraoperative retraction injury, have a good prognosis for functional recovery. Severe traction injuries, such as brachial plexus injury secondary to motorcycle injury, often require extensive nerve grafting. Common traction injuries are outlined in Figure 22.3.

Measurement is made beginning at the injury site and moving distal to the first muscle innervated by the nerve. The time required for re-innervation is predicted using an estimated axonal regeneration rate of 1 mm/d. If there is failure to show evidence of re-innervation of the most proximal muscle at the expected time, either by clinical exam or by electrical examination, surgical exploration is indicated. In most instances surgery should not be delayed beyond 3 to 4 months.

COMPRESSION

The extent of nerve damage in compression injuries correlates with the duration and degree of nerve compression. Compressing a nerve also compromises blood flow; therefore it is unclear to what extent physical deformation versus local ischemia forms the basis of the pathology.

Mild compression is associated with changes in paranodal myelin, invagination of myelin, and segmental demyelination. More severe compression produces wallerian degeneration. The symptoms and signs, and the need for surgical intervention, will depend on the severity of injury.

Common acute nerve injuries secondary to compression ischemia include "Saturday night palsy," which involves the radial nerve, nerve injury secondary to compression from a plaster cast, and compression from increased pressure in a fascial compartment.

DRUG INJECTION INJURY

Nearly any drug injected into a nerve can cause damage. The pathology often involves intraneural neuritis. The sciatic and radial nerves are the most commonly involved, often with iatrogenic injury. If there is no evidence of recovery at the predicted time, given the axonal regeneration rate of 1 mm/d, surgical intervention is indicated. A neuroma in continuity is a common finding at surgery. Determining the need for resection and grafting of a neuroma in continuity requires the skills of an experienced peripheral nerve surgeon.

ELECTRICAL INJURY

This injury occurs on contact with high-tension wire. Diffuse muscle and nerve damage is common, often requiring extensive resection and nerve grafting for functional recovery.

CLINICAL ASSESSMENT

To manage a peripheral nerve injury the physician must first determine the location and extent of nerve injury. The clinical history, physical examination, and laboratory investigations often allow an accurate assessment of the peripheral nerve injury. The physical examination includes testing of all muscles innervated by the injured nerve. All modalities of sensory function are tested, with special attention to the area supplied solely by the injured nerve (autonomous zone). An EMG is first performed 2 weeks after injury. If the EMG is normal 2 weeks after injury, a Sunderland grade I lesion is present and full recovery can be expected. The EMG is more sensitive than physical examination for signs of muscle re-innervation, and it should be repeated when axonal regeneration is expected to have reached the most proximal muscle, to confirm spontaneous regeneration of the nerve. A general approach to management of a peripheral nerve injury is seen in Figure 22.4.

The neurosurgeon must determine if there is avulsion of the roots from the spinal cord. This is important because with avulsion there is no spontaneous recovery. Physical examination shows decreased or absent power in all muscles innervated by the avulsed root. If only one root is avulsed, some power is often present, as most muscles are supplied by more than one root. Sensory loss occurs in a dermatomal distribution. Dense sensory loss occurs only in the autonomous zone, which may be quite small if only one root is avulsed. The presence of a Horner's syndrome often indicates avulsion of

T-1 in brachial plexus injury. A myelogram followed by CT scan or an MRI that demonstrates the presence of pseudomeningoceles suggests that root avulsion has occurred.

The presence or absence of a sensory nerve conduction potential can be used to determine if a lesion is likely proximal or distal to the dorsal root ganglion (DRG). The peripheral sensory nerve cell body is located in the DRG. A lesion proximal to the DRG, such as a brachial plexus avulsion from the spinal cord, will usually not disconnect the peripheral axon from the cell body. No wallerian degeneration occurs in the sensory portion of the peripheral nerve and the sensory conduction potential remains intact. If, however, the lesion is distal to the DRG, there is sensory axonal wallerian degeneration and loss of the sensory conduction action potential.

Ectopic mechanosensitivity can be used to assess growth of a nerve. Tapping the regenerating axons of the nerve will produce a paresthesia felt in the distribution normally innervated by the nerve (Tinel's sign). The Tinel's sign should move distally 1 mm/d in accordance with the advancing axonal growth cone. Failure of the Tinel's sign to progress at the expected rate suggests the need for surgical exploration.

Some injuries can progress during the initial 12 hours after injury. Loss of function after 24 hours requires immediate assessment. Pathology such as a hematoma, compartment syndrome, or pseudoaneurysm may require urgent surgical intervention.

SURGICAL REPAIR

Surgical repair is used to restore continuity between proximal and distal axons, without which functional recovery will not occur. A direct suture repair using an epineurally placed suture is the preferred method. Under certain circumstances, such as a very distal lesion with separation of sensory and motor fascicles, a fascicular repair is indicated. If a gap occurs between the nerve ends it may not be possible to bring the nerve ends into close proximity for repair without undue tension at the suture site. An interpositional graft using harvested peripheral nerve from the patient is then used to bridge the gap.

TECHNICAL CONSIDERATIONS

The goals of surgical repair are to appose healthy nerve ends with minimal tension on the suture line and to align the fascicles, allowing appropriate re-innervation of target organs. Failure to achieve either goal leads to a nonfunctional outcome. If more than two 10-0 nylon epineural sutures are required to maintain approximation of the nerve ends, unacceptable tension is present.

A nerve injury often extends for a variable distance proximal and distal along the nerve. Once the nerve ends have been trimmed back to a normal-appearing fascicular pattern, a gap may occur that necessitates grafting (Fig. 22.8). A nerve graft is the preferred method for avoiding tension on the suture line of a repair. Common donor nerves include sural nerves, medial cutaneous antebrachial nerves, and the superficial radial nerve of the arm (Fig. 22.9). Heterogenous grafts and freeze-dried homografts have no role at this time in nerve grafting.

Grafts are revascularized from the recipient bed by small vessels. Small-diameter grafts are preferred because they are quickly revascularized. The center of a thick graft will be revascularized more slowly than the center of a thin graft and is a limiting factor on graft diameter. Several grafts may be required to form a cable whose cross-sectional area is equal to that of the nerve to be grafted (Fig. 22.10).

In certain instances, interfascicular grafting is performed (Fig. 22.11). This technique is often used to repair distal injuries in which motor and sensory fascicles have separated. Performing interfascicular grafting is time-consuming and has not been associated with a significantly better outcome in most situations.

Nerve transfers are performed to restore lost function when suture or nerve graft is not possible. An uninjured nerve is divided, and the proximal stump is used to supply the damaged distal stump of another nerve. The conversion of the donor nerve to a new function depends on its capacity to integrate the proprioceptive messages from the re-innervated area. Some refer to this form of repair as neurotization. An example of nerve transfer is the use of the distal spinal accessory nerve to re-innervate the musculocutaneous nerve. Intercostal nerve transfer to the musculocutaneous nerve is commonly done in cases of brachial plexus avulsion. The seventh cranial nerve can be used to re-innervate an injured twelfth cranial nerve. More recently, the transfer of the contralateral C-7 root to an injured ipsilateral brachial plexus has been considered.

When a surgical repair is performed, the extremity is casted for 3 to 6 weeks, which allows sufficient healing at the suture site to tolerate tension. Once the cast is removed, the patient undergoes aggressive physical therapy to regain full range of motion in the extremity.

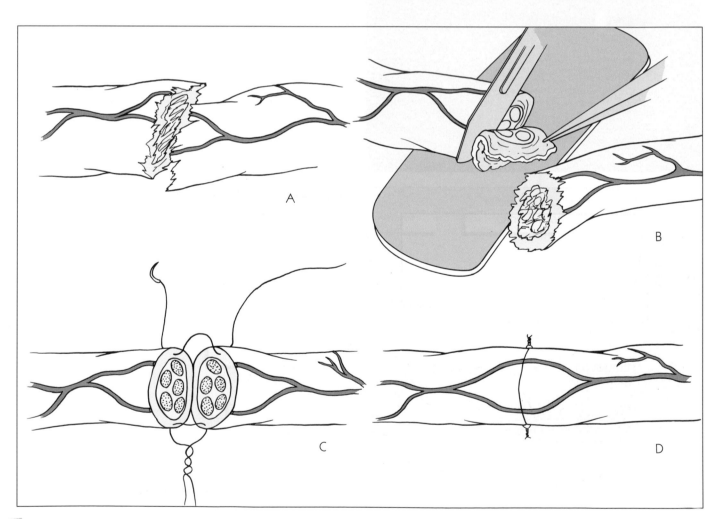

Figure 22.7 End-to-end nerve repair. **(A)** Laceration often results in minimal damage at the severed nerve edges. **(B)** The nerve end is resected back until a healthy fascicular pattern is seen. **(C)** One or two epineurial sutures are used to secure the ends. Visual clues such as surface vessels are used to allow accurate alignment

OUTCOME

Several factors influence the potential for recovery of function after peripheral nerve injury. Recovery of function after injury tends to be more complete in juveniles than in adults. Re-innervation of target organs is more complete in distal than in proximal lesions, which is related to the separation of motor and sensory fibers into fascicles in distal nerves. Recovery is better when end-to-end neurorrhaphy can be performed rather than when grafting is required. Underlying systemic disorders may affect regeneration. For example, regeneration can be severely hampered if alcoholic neuropathy exists.

Evidence of recovery can be found by clinical and laboratory examination. The absence of an advancing Tinel's sign at 8 weeks is evidence that regeneration is not occurring. Evidence for muscle re-innervation can be seen with an EMG weeks or months prior to the onset of voluntary contraction. The first heralds of re-innervation are small-amplitude action potentials. With progressive re-innervation the amplitude of the action potentials increases.

Although it is imperative to provide muscle with re-innervation by 18 months, no such time limit exists for sensory re-innervation. Surgical repair to regain sensory function performed many years after injury often provides a functional outcome (for example, repair of a median nerve many years after injury provides sensation to the palm of the hand).

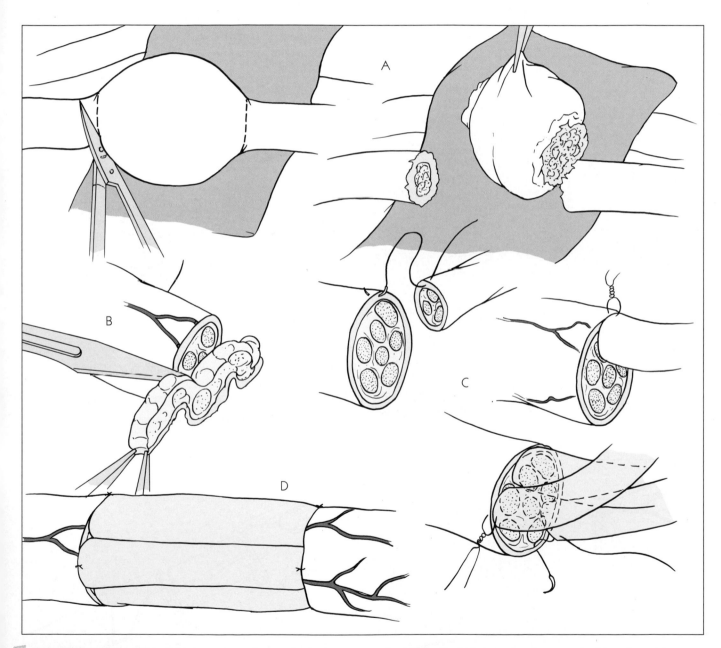

Figure 22.8 Nerve grafting. (A) A neuroma in continuity is resected. (B) The nerve ends are resected back to a healthy appearing fascicular pattern, leaving a large gap between the ends. (C) Grafts are placed and secured with epineurial sutures. (D) Grafting is completed.

Repair of proximal severe injury to nerves that innervate the distal extremity muscles often leads to a nonfunctional outcome. For example, repair of a proximal brachial plexus injury to achieve ulnar re-innervation is generally unrewarding and not warranted.

REHABILITATION

After a nerve repair, the appropriate joints are immobilized for approximately 6 weeks to allow the neural suture line to heal. Aggressive mobilization of the joints is then required to prevent contractures and pain. Although some patients may complain of painful paresthesias during growth of the regenerating axons, joint contractures also produce formidable pain. Immobilization should not exceed 8 weeks, and aggressive physical therapy with passive and active range-of-motion exercises should follow removal of splints.

If there is failure of nervous re-innervation of muscle, other measures can be used to provide some function. Tendon transfers enable functioning muscle to provide joint movement. The transfer is designed to make maximal use of functioning muscle. For example, in a patient with a radial nerve injury, transfer of a wrist flexor to afford wrist extension produces significantly increased function in the hand. If the lack of muscle function produces an unstable joint, fusion to stabilize the joint can also be performed. When there is extensive nerve damage to a limb an experienced surgeon will plan the repair to take advantage of later tendon transfer. This may require nerve transfer for a functional result.

Electrical stimulation of muscles to prevent degeneration prior to nervous re-innervation has been used extensively but is of debated usefulness. There has also been experimentation with electrical stimulation to enhance nerve regeneration. These techniques await scientific validation.

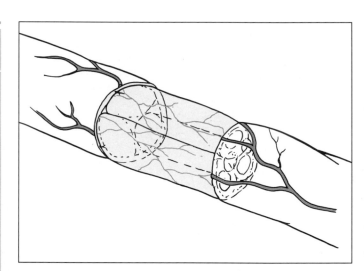

Figure 22.10 The graft covers the entire face of the nerve in an attempt to capture all the sprouting axons. Sutures are only placed in the epineurium to avoid internal scarring.

Figure 22.9 Donor Nerve Graft

Donor Nerve	Length
Medial cutaneous antebrachial	8–10 cm
Lateral cutaneous antebrachial	10–12 cm
Superficial radial sensory	10–12 cm
Dorsal cutaneous branch of ulnar	4–6 cm
Sural	20–35 cm

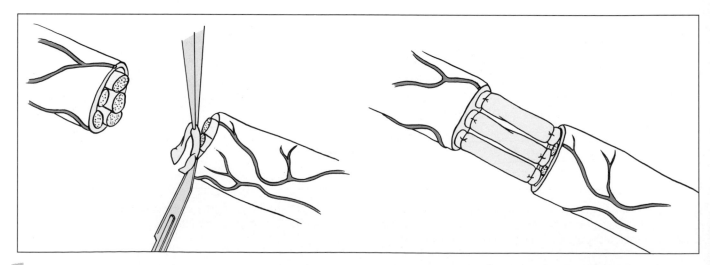

Figure 22.11 Interfascicular grafting. **(A)** Epineurial tissue is resected exposing fascicles and perineurium. **(B)** Grafts are placed between individual fascicles or small group of fascicles. The sutures are placed in the perineurium.

Chapter 23

Entrapment Neuropathies

Setti S. Rengachary

Certain peripheral nerves, whether they are motor, sensory, or of mixed type, as they pass through their normal anatomic path in the extremities, course through narrow constrained areas. Under certain circumstances, the nerves are susceptible to extrinsic compression at these sites. Such a phenomenon is generically termed *entrapment neuropathy*. Entrapment of nerves generally occurs as they pass beside a joint, such as the elbow, wrist, or hip. Although compression may occur elsewhere, it is uncommon in other areas of the extremities. This, along with the fact that entrapment neuropathy seldom occurs in the head or trunk, suggests that repetitive motion is a major factor that precipitates entrapment in an anatomically constrained segment.

Two types of anatomic constraints predispose to entrapment neuropathy. The first type (Fig. 23.1A) is a fibroosseous tunnel. The space available for the nerve within the tunnel becomes constricted because 1) the contents of the tunnel become larger or hypertrophic, as when a patient with tenosynovitis has carpal tunnel syndrome, and 2) the walls of the tunnel encroach upon the tunnel, as when fractured fragments of a carpal bone displace into the carpal canal. Compression of a nerve in a tunnel is an example of *static* compression. The second type (Fig. 23.1B) involves *dynamic* compression of the nerve as it passes through a fibrotendinous arcade. The nerve is flanked by two bellies of a muscle that under static conditions do not compress the nerve. When they contract, however, they cause a shutter-like closure of the arcade, compressing the nerve. For exam-

ple, this can occur at the arcade of Frohse in the supinator muscle, the two heads of the flexor carpi ulnaris at the entrance to the cubital tunnel, or the two heads of flexor digitorum sublimis forming the "sublimis bridge."

PATHOLOGY OF NERVE COMPRESSION

The pathophysiologic changes following nerve compression[1-22] are dependent on the degree, rate, and duration of compression. Loss of function of the nerve due to compression is manifested clinically by motor paralysis, paresthesia, or numbness. In physiologic terms, mild and brief compression produces a transient and reversible conduction block within the nerve. Sustained compression over a long period causes structural changes. Not all components of the nerve are equally susceptible to a given degree of compression. Nerve fibers having a greater amount of epineurium compared to the nerve fascicles are less susceptible to compression than those with larger fascicles and scanty epineurium (Fig. 23.2). Also, within a given nerve, not all fibers undergo degenerative changes to the same extent. The superficially located fibers tend to bear the brunt of the compression, while the central fibers are relatively spared. Large, heavily myelinated fibers subserving light touch and motor function are more sensitive to compressive changes than unmyelinated fibers subserving pain sensation.

Impediment to microvascular flow appears to be a major factor in the pathophysiology of nerve impinge-

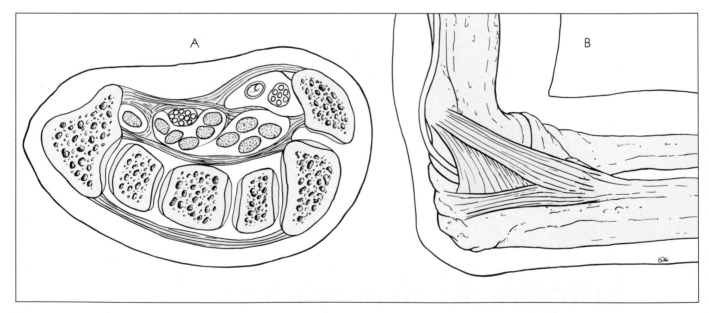

Figure 23.1 (A) Example of a fibroosseous tunnel—the carpal tunnel at the wrist. The median nerve and the tendons of the long flexor muscles are the main contents of the tunnel.

(B) Example of a fibrotendinous arcade—the cubital canal at the elbow. The ulnar nerve enters the fibroaponeurotic arcade formed by the two heads of the flexor carpi ulnaris.

ment. Capillary blanching and venular obstruction herald progressive compression. This leads to nerve ischemia, which in turn leads to endothelial impairment and progressive edema; the edema compounds the ischemia and swelling of the nerve. Critical swelling of a nerve within the constraints of its surroundings may lead to further nerve compression, a phenomenon that can be called a *minicompartmental syndrome.*

Nerve compression blocks axonal transport. The antegrade transport from the nerve cell to the axon towards the synapse can be divided into fast and slow components—the fast component carries the membrane-associated materials and the slow component the cytoskeletal proteins. Nerve compression impedes both the fast and slow components of the antegrade flow, resulting in a swelling of the nerve proximal to the compression due to damming up of the moving axoplasm within the fibers. Thus the distribution of cytoskeletal elements, axolemma constituents, and the transmitter substances required for synaptic conduction are all impaired by a block of antegrade flow. Retrograde axonal flow from the synaptic level to the cell body of the nerve is similarly blocked by compression of the nerve. This results in loss of transfer of neuronotrophic factors to the nerve cell body. The impairment of retrograde axonal transport results in certain changes in the nerve cell body comparable to those that occur after peripheral nerve section (wallerian degeneration). The changes noted in the cell body are eccentric nucleus, dispersion of Nissl substance (chromatolysis), and decrease in nuclear and whole cell volumes. The overall result of the impediment to axoplasmic flow is impaired membrane permeability and conduction block.

With acute and severe compression one observes a characteristic sequential invagination or telescoping of myelin sheath (Fig. 23.3). The polarity of invagination is reversed at the edges of the compression. With chronic compression, segmental demyelination occurs within the compressed segments, accounting for the slowing of conduction velocity of the nerve. In the early phases, the nerve fibers distal to the compression show normal morphology. With sustained compression, axolysis occurs within the compressed segment, leading to distal wallerian degeneration.

DOUBLE CRUSH SYNDROME

If a nerve is compressed proximally, its distal part is more susceptible to compression than a normal nerve would be, because the antegrade axonal flow is blocked by the first compression. In a similar manner, if there is distal compression, the nerve cell body undergoes degeneration more quickly if a second compression is present proximally, because of impediment of retrograde flow. This latter syndrome is called a reverse double crush syndrome.

NERVE COMPRESSION SYNDROME IN DIABETICS

Patients with diabetic neuropathy are more susceptible to compression, presumably because of accumulation of sorbitol, a metabolite of glucose, and the formation of endoneurial edema.

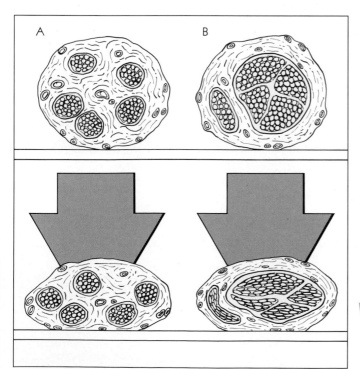

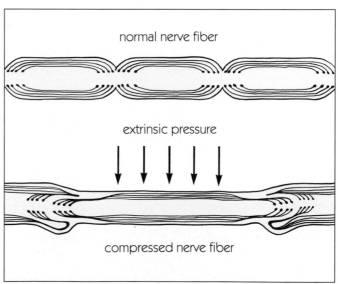

Figure 23.3 Telescoping of myelin sheath with acute and severe nerve compression.

Figure 23.2 Nerves having a greater amount of epineurium (**A**) are less susceptible to compression than those having scanty epineurium (**B**).

The entrapment sites, the nerves involved at each site, and the corresponding syndromes are listed in Figure 23.4. I will discuss in this chapter the three most common entrapment syndromes: carpal tunnel syndrome, cubital tunnel syndrome, and meralgia paresthetica.

The carpal tunnel syndrome[23-47] is the most common entrapment neuropathy encountered in clinical practice. It results from compression of the distal median nerve within the carpal tunnel, located in the proximal part of the palm of the hand. The carpal tunnel is bounded

Figure 23.4 Entrapment Syndromes

Location	Nerve Entrapped	Compressing Element	Clinical Syndrome
Supracondylar region	Median nerve	Ligament of Struthers or supracondylar spur	High median entrapment neuropathy
Elbow	Median nerve	Bicipital aponeurosis (lacertus fibrosus), hypertrophic pronator teres muscle, or tendinous arch of flexor digitorum sublimis (the "sublimis bridge")	Pronator syndrome
Forearm	Anterior interosseous nerve	Variable: anatomic abnormalities such as fibrous bands arising from pronator teres or flexor digitorum sublimis muscles; often no anatomic abnormalities may be demonstrated	Anterior interosseous nerve syndrome
Wrist	Median nerve	Carpal canal or element of its contents	Carpal tunnel syndrome
Elbow	Ulnar nerve	Variable: most commonly the fascial band binding the two heads of the flexor carpi ulnaris	Cubital tunnel syndrome, tardy ulnar palsy
Wrist	Ulnar nerve	Guyon's canal	Guyon's canal syndrome
Forearm	Posterior interosseous nerve	Arcade of Frohse	Posterior interosseous nerve entrapment syndrome
Forearm	Posterior interosseous nerve	Variable	Resistant "tennis elbow," radial tunnel syndrome
Forearm	Superficial radial nerve	Variable: commonly extrinsic compression or trauma; sometimes the deep fascia of the forearm between the extensor carpi radialis longus and brevis	Superficial radial nerve syndrome
Neck	Brachial plexus	Cervical rib or fibrous band or scalenus anterior muscle	Thoracic outlet syndrome
Hip	Lateral femoral cutaneous nerve	Inguinal ligament and associated fasciae	Meralgia paresthetica
Knee	Peroneal nerve	Variable	Peroneal neuropathy
Ankle	Posterior tibial nerve	Tarsal tunnel	Tarsal tunnel syndrome
Shoulder	Suprascapular nerve	Suprascapular notch/foramen	Suprascapular nerve entrapment
Thigh	Saphenous nerve	Deep fascia roofing Hunter's canal	Saphenous nerve entrapment

dorsally by the carpal bones and ventrally by the transverse carpal ligament. The carpal bones form a shallow trough that is converted into a tunnel by the carpal ligament. The contents of the tunnel are the median nerve and tendons of the long flexor muscles (see Fig. 23.1A). Any lesion affecting the synovial sheath tends to compromise the cross-sectional diameter of the carpal canal and may induce compressive neuropathy. Recent studies that include MRI and CT scans show that individuals who are predisposed to be afflicted by the carpal tunnel syndrome tend to have small carpal canals. The small size of the carpal canal, as evidenced by the decrease in its cross-sectional diameter, is a congenital or a developmental phenomenon. The smaller size in women may account for their higher incidence of carpal tunnel syndrome.

Clinical Features

Women are more commonly affected than men by a ratio of seven to three. Most patients are middle-aged at the onset of symptoms. The predominant symptom is an aching, burning, tingling, numb sensation in the hand, ordinarily in the lateral half of the hand and the outer three or four digits. Frequently there may be an aching pain in the proximal forearm or even in the arm up to the shoulder. Typically patients wake up at night with increased pain, and they may shake their hand to obtain relief. Very frequently the symptoms are bilateral. In late stages patients complain of a weakness in the grip and tend to drop things.

In the early stages of the syndrome, at which time most patients are seen in contemporary practice, there are few objective findings. Two mechanical tests can be done: A Tinel's sign may be elicited by lightly tapping over the median nerve at the wrist crease, which results in a tingling in the distribution of the median nerve if positive; the Phalen's test consists of asking the patient to flex the wrist to 90° for about 60 seconds, which will precipitate paresthesia in the distribution of the median nerve if positive. Neither of these tests is conclusive. Perception of light touch or pin prick in the tips of the fingers in the median nerve distribution may be impaired. In advanced cases there may be atrophy of the thenar muscles, especially in the abductor pollicis brevis.

There are several local and systemic risk factors that precipitate the symptoms of carpal tunnel syndrome (Fig. 23.5).

Diagnosis

The most important diagnostic tests are electromyography and study of nerve conduction velocity. The earliest and most significant finding is the prolongation of sensory latency. The sensory evoked response will show a diminution of amplitude and may even be absent. Motor latency abnormalities occur late in the course of the disease. Needle electromyography may show loss of motor unit potentials and the presence of denervation potentials in the median-innervated muscles in the thenar eminence.

Treatment

In early cases with minimal symptoms or in individuals in whom the syndrome is expected to be transient, conservative treatment should be instituted. This consists of a wrist splint at night and antiinflammatory drugs. Injection of local anesthesia and steroids around the median nerve may be beneficial, but accidental injection directly into the nerve may result in annoying paresthesias in the distribution of the median nerve.

Surgical therapy is indicated when conservative measures fail. The surgical procedure can be done by either the open method or endoscopic technique. The steps in the surgical sectioning of the transverse carpal ligament are shown in Figure 23.6. Usually local or regional anesthesia (Bier block) is used. General anesthesia may be used if the patient is extremely nervous.

Endoscopic section of the carpal ligament has recently been introduced. The advantages are that the postoperative recovery period is shorter, a sensitive scar in the palm of the hand is avoided, and the structural integrity of the carpal tunnel mechanism is minimally disturbed. However, there is a greater risk of injury to the ulnar artery and to the sensory branch of the median nerve serving the middle and ring fingers.

CUBITAL TUNNEL SYNDROME

The cubital tunnel syndrome[48-71] results from entrapment of the ulnar nerve at the elbow. The cubital tunnel is located on the medial side of the elbow joint. It is a fibroosseous tunnel that is roofed by the aponeurotic attachment of the two heads of the flexor carpi ulnaris and a tough fascial band that bridges these two heads (see Fig. 23.1B). The floor is formed by the medial ligament of the elbow joint. During flexion of the elbow, the volume of cubital tunnel decreases; the reverse happens in extension. This is because the points of attachment of the flexor carpi ulnaris, that is, the medial epicondyle and the olecranon process, are farthest apart during flexion. Thus, there is more tension on the fascial band between these two heads, which increases the pressure on the cubital tunnel.

Clinical Features

The major presenting symptoms are weakness and atrophy of the intrinsic muscles of the hand and tingling and numbness in the medial two fingers. The onset of symptoms is generally insidious. Men are affected three times more commonly than women. An obvious etiologic factor, such as an old healed supracondylar fracture, a ganglion cyst of the elbow, or synovitis, is sometimes evident. In the majority of instances, however, there is no apparent cause. The presence of a rare anomalous muscle, anconeus epitrochlearis, is an uncommon cause.

On objective testing there is weakness of the ulnar-innervated muscles in the hand, including the palmaris brevis, abductor digiti quinti, opponens digiti quinti, flexor digiti quinti, adductor pollicis, the medial two lumbricals, and all of the interossei. The flexor carpi ulnaris is generally not affected, because the fibers that subserve the motor innervation are thought to be very deep within the nerve and thus less susceptible to compression than the more superficial fibers to the intrinsic muscles.

Froment's sign is elicited by asking the patient to grasp a piece of cardboard between the index finger and thumb against resistance. In patients with weakness of the adductor pollicis there will be flexion of the first interphalangeal joint and the thumb.

Diagnosis

The characteristic electrodiagnostic finding is a delay in the conduction velocity in the ulnar nerve across the elbow. The sensory latency is prolonged, and the amplitude of the motor response in the abductor digiti minimi is decreased. A needle examination of the ulnar-innervated muscles may show denervation potentials.

Tardy ulnar paralysis should be differentiated from lesions in the spinal cord affecting the C-8, T-1 segments,

Figure 23.5 Risk Factors in the Pathogenesis of Carpal Tunnel Syndrome

Local Factors

Increased Volume of the Contents of the Carpal Canal
Hypertrophic tenosynovitis
Masses: neurofibroma, hemangioma, lipoma, ganglion cyst, gouty tophus, xanthoma
Anomalous muscles and tendons
Persistent median artery with or without thrombosis, aneurysm, arteriovenous malformation
Acute palmar space infections
Hemorrhage

Reduction in the Capacity of the Carpal Canal
Congenitally small carpal canal
Idiopathic or familial thickening of the transverse carpal ligament
Malunion or callus following Colles' fracture or fracture of the carpal bones
Unreduced dislocations of the wrist or intercarpal joints
Improper immobilization of the wrist ("cotton loader position")
Compression by cast
Exostoses

Other Local Factors
Burns at the wrist
Long-term hemodialysis

Systemic Factors

Increased Susceptibility of Nerves to Pressure
Alcoholic or diabetic polyneuropathy
Hereditary neuropathy with liability to pressure palsies
Amyloidosis
Proximal lesions of the median nerve ("double crush" syndrome)
Other polyneuropathies

Factors Unique to Women
Pregnancy and lactation
Menstrual cycles
Contraceptive pills
Menopause
Toxic shock syndrome
Eclampsia

Other Hormonal Factors
Myxedema
Acromegaly

Other Systemic Factors
Obesity
Raynaud's disease
Athetoid-dystonic cerebral palsy

Inflammatory and Autoimmune Disorders
Rheumatoid arthritis
Dermatomyositis
Scleroderma
Polymyalgia rheumatica

Metabolic Disorders
Mucopolysaccharidoses
Mucolipodoses
Amyloidosis
Chondrocalcinosis
Gout

Principles of Neurosurgery

such as syringomyelia, spinal cord tumor, or amyotrophic lateral sclerosis, and the extradural spinal lesions, such as cervical disc disease or spondylosis, neurofibroma, or meningioma. Lesions of the brachial plexus involving the lower trunk or the medial cord (Pancoast tumor), entrapment of the ulnar nerve distally at the wrist (Guyon's canal), and polyneuropathy should be ruled out as well.

Treatment

In early, minimally symptomatic cases, a conservative approach is recommended. The patient should wear an elbow pad for protection against direct pressure to the nerve and avoid excessive flexion of the elbow and strenuous exercise for some time, especially sports maneu-

vers that involve vigorous throwing, such as baseball. In persistent or highly symptomatic cases, surgical options should be considered. There is no other entrapment neuropathy for which the surgical options are more controversial than cubital tunnel syndrome. The available surgical methods are listed in Figure 23.7. The simplest and most satisfactory procedure for uncomplicated cases is cubital tunnel release. (The steps of the procedure are shown in Figure 23.8.) In more involved cases complicated by elbow joint abnormality or malunited fractures or other abnormalities, the nerve may be transposed anterior to the elbow joint, into the subcutaneous, intramuscular, or submuscular planes. Randomized prospective trials comparing these surgical options

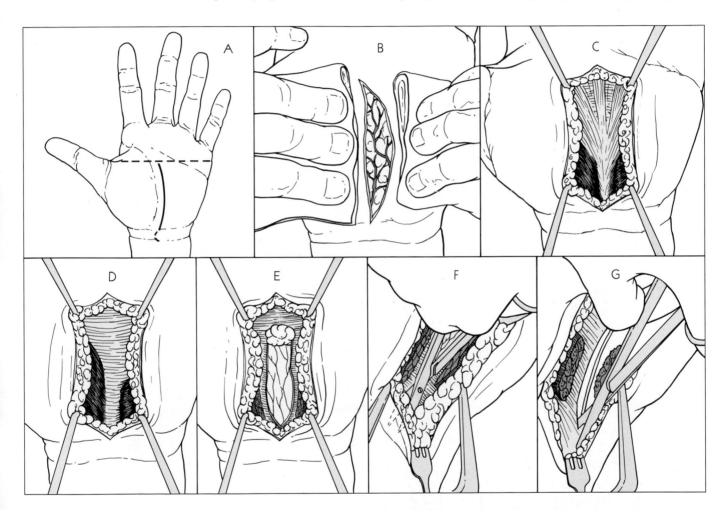

Figure 23.6 (A) The skin incision extends from the wrist crease to a point in the midpalm in line with the fully extended thumb (horizontal interrupted line). An optional extension may be carried out in the distal forearm (curvilinear interrupted line) to facilitate exposure of the proximal part of transverse carpal ligament and the distal part of the deep fascia of the forearm. Note that the main skin incision is not in the palmar skin crease but just medial to it. (B) Protrusion of exuberant palmar subcutaneous fat after the skin incision is made. (C) Exposure of the palmar aponeurosis. (D) Exposure of the transverse carpal ligament after midline section and retraction of the palmar aponeurosis. The distal margin of the transverse carpal ligament can

faintly be seen blending with the deep fascia of the palm. The proximal part of the transverse carpal ligament is covered by the hypothenar and thenar muscles. In many instances (not shown in this illustration) they may meet and interdigitate in the midline, blocking the transverse carpal ligament from view. (E) About 80% of the transverse carpal ligament has been divided, exposing the median nerve. Note the constant fat globule superficial to the median nerve at the distal end of the exposure. (F) Proximal skin is undermined with retraction to facilitate exposure of the proximal part of the transverse carpal ligament. (G) Section of the most proximal part of the transverse carpal ligament and the distal deep fascia of the forearm.

Figure 23.7 Surgical Options for Treating Cubital Tunnel Syndrome

Simple decompression

Medial epicondylectomy

Subcutaneous anterior transposition

Intramuscular anterior transposition

Submuscular anterior transposition

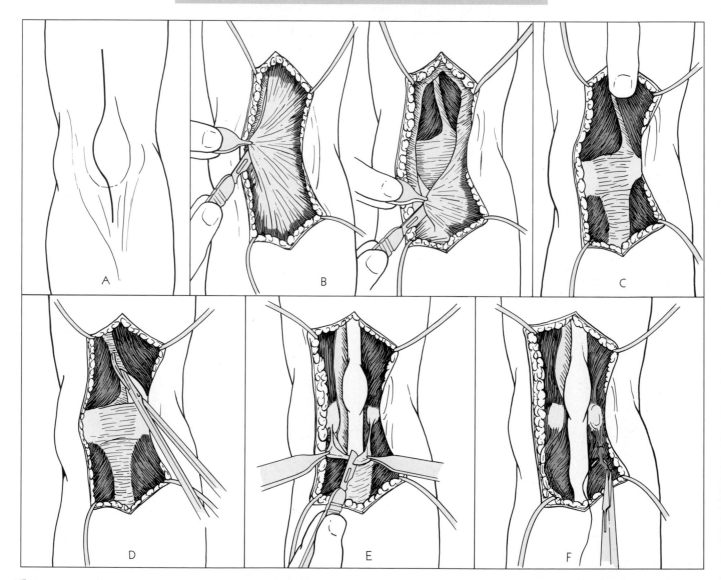

Figure 23.8 (A) Skin incision for decompression of the ulnar nerve. Note that the incision stops short of the basilic vein. (B) Incision of the deep fascia of the arm and forearm. (C) Digital palpation of the medial intermuscular septum and the ulnar nerve in the arm. (D) Section of the fascia over the ulnar nerve. (E) Section of the dense fascia spanning the two heads of the flexor carpi ulnaris; a bulbous enlargement of the ulnar nerve is noticeable. (F) The cut edges of the fascia are sewn over the flexor muscle on either side to prevent reformation of the cubital tunnel.

are not available at present, and the published results are tainted by considerable personal bias.

MERALGIA PARESTHETICA

Meralgia paresthetica[72-74] is a syndrome caused by the entrapment of the lateral femoral cutaneous nerve of the thigh in the inguinal region. The name refers to the burning sensation that affected individuals complain of in the anterolateral thigh (*meros*, thigh; *algos*, pain).

The lateral femoral cutaneous nerve of the thigh arises from the lumbar plexus, emerges at the lateral margin of psoas major muscle, descends obliquely downward and forward under the iliac fascia, pierces the inguinal ligament near the anterior superior iliac spine, courses under the fascia lata for about 5 cm, and then becomes subcutaneous by piercing the fascia lata (Fig. 23.9A). It innervates the skin of the anterolateral aspect of the thigh and the gluteal region (Fig. 23.9B,C).

Entrapment of the nerve occurs in the inguinal region at the point where it pierces the inguinal ligament. Obese individuals with a pendulous, flabby anterior abdominal wall are more prone to this disorder. Persons who are on their feet a lot, such as patrolmen, postal workers, and traveling salesmen, are also more susceptible. Patients complain of a tingling, crawling, pricking, "pins and needles" sensation in the anterolateral thigh. Varying degrees of sensory loss may be pre-

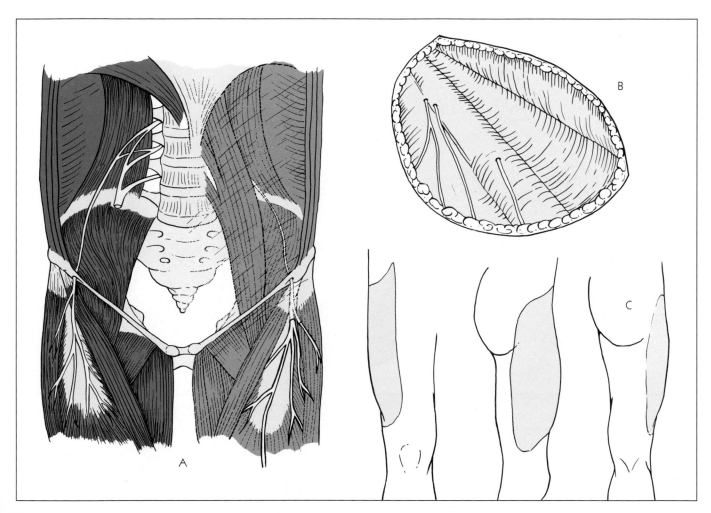

Figure 23.9 (A) Origin, course, and distribution of the lateral femoral cutaneous nerve of the thigh. On the right side of the specimen, the psoas major muscle and the fasciae have been removed. Not all branches of the lumbar plexus are shown. (B) Anatomy of the lateral femoral cutaneous nerve in the thigh. (C) Distribution of the lateral femoral cutaneous nerve in the thigh.

sent in the anterolateral thigh. Because the affected nerve is strictly a cutaneous nerve, there are no motor abnormalities or reflex changes. Indeed, if they are present an alternative diagnosis should be entertained.

Electrodiagnostic tests are generally not helpful in establishing the diagnosis of meralgia paresthetica. Rather they are used to exclude other disorders that involve the lumbosacral plexus or the cauda equina.

The best test for confirmation of the clinical impression is a diagnostic nerve block done by injecting 5 mL of 0.5% lidocaine with epinephrine just medial to the anterior superior iliac spine. Complete relief of symptoms is generally predictive of good operative result.

The technique of section of the inguinal ligament and decompression is shown in Figure 23.10.

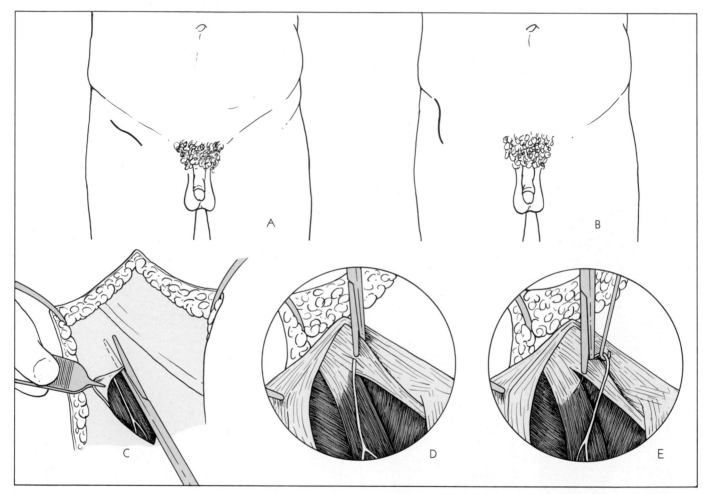

Figure 23.10 (A) Skin incision conventionally used to expose the lateral femoral cutaneous nerve. (B) Skin incision that I prefer. (C) Section of the fascia lata at the anterior border of the sartorius. (D) Section of the superficial portion of the inguinal ligament. (E) Section of the fascial bands posterior to the nerve.

REFERENCES

1. Aguayo A, Nair CPV, Midgely R. Experimental progressive compression neuropathy in the rabbit. *Arch Neurol.* 1971;24:358.

2. Bentley FH, Schlapp W. The effects of pressure on conduction in peripheral nerve. *J Physiol.* 1943; 102:72.

3. Dahlin LB, McLean WG. Effects of graded experimental compression on slow and fast axonal transport in rabbit vagus nerve. *J Neurol Sci.* 1986; 72:19–30.

4. Dahlin LB, Lundborg G. The neurone and its response to peripheral nerve compression. *J Hand Surg.* 1990;15B:5–10.

5. Dahlin LB, Rydevik B, McLean WG, et al. Changes in fast axonal transport during experimental nerve compression at low pressures. *Exp Neurol.* 1984;84:29–36.

6. Dahlin LB, Sjorstrand J, McLean WG. Graded inhibition of retrograde axonal transport by compression of rabbit vagus nerve. *J Neurol Sci.* 1986; 76:221–230.

7. Dahlin LB, Nordborg C, Lundborg G. Morphologic changes in nerve cell bodies induced by experimental graded nerve compression. *Exp Neurol.* 1986;95:611–621.

8. Dahlin LB, Shyu BC, Danielsen N, et al. Effects of nerve compress or ischemia on conduction properties of myelinated and non-myelinated nerve fibers: an experimental study in the rabbit peroneal nerve. *Acta Physiol Scand.* 1989;136:97–105.

9. Denny-Brown D, Brenner C. Paralysis of nerve induced by direct pressure and by tourniquet. *Arch Neurol Psychiatry.* 1944;51:1–26.

10. Duncan D. Alterations in the structure of nerves caused by restricting their growth with ligatures. *J Neuropathol Exp Neurol.* 1948;7:261–273.

11. Fowler TJ, Ochoa J. Unmyelinated fibers in normal and compressed peripheral nerves of the baboon: a quantitative electron microscopic study. *Neuropathol Appl Neurobiol.* 1975;1:247.

12. Fullerton PM, Gilliatt RW. Pressure neuropathy in the hindfoot of the guinea-pig. *J Neurol Neurosurg Psychiatry.* 1967;30:18–25.

13. Fullerton PM, Gilliatt RW. Median and ulnar neuropathy in the guinea-pig. *J Neurol Neurosurg Psychiatry.* 1967;30:393–402.

14. Lundborg G, Myers R, Powell H. Nerve compression injury and increase in endoneurial fluid pressure: a "miniature compartment syndrome." *J Neurosurg Psychiatry.* 1983;46:1119.

15. Neary D, Eames RA. The pathology of ulnar nerve compression in man. *Neuropathol Appl Neurobiol.* 1975;1:69–88.

16. Ochoa J. Nerve fiber pathology in acute and chronic compression. In: Omer GE Jr, Spinner M, eds. *Management of Peripheral Nerve Problems.* Philadelphia, Pa: WB Saunders Co; 1980:487–501.

17. Ochoa J, Marotte L. The nature of the nerve lesion caused by chronic entrapment in the guinea-pig. *J Neurol Sci.* 1973;19:491.

18. Ochoa J, Fowler TJ, Gilliatt RW. Anatomical changes in peripheral nerves compressed by a pneumatic tourniquet. *J Anat.* 1972;113:433.

19. Ogatta K, Naito M. Blood flow of peripheral nerve: effects of dissection, stretching and compression. *J Hand Surg.* 1986;11B:10.

20. Rydevik B, Lundborg G. Permeability of intraneural microvessels and perineurium following acute, graded experimental nerve compression. *Scand J Plast Reconstr Surg.* 1977;11:179.

21. Rydevik B, Nordborg C. Changes in nerve function and nerve fiber structure induced by acute, graded compression. *J Neurol Neurosurg Psychiatry.* 1980;43:1070.

22. Upton ARM, McComas AJ. The double crush in nerve entrapment syndromes. *Lancet.* 1973;2:359.

23. Barnes CG, Currey HLF. Carpal tunnel syndrome in rheumatoid arthritis: a clinical and electrodiagnostic survey. *Ann Rheum Dis.* 1967;26:226–233.

24. Bauman TD, Gelbermann RH, Mubarak SJ, et al. The acute carpal tunnel syndrome. *Clin Orthop.* 1981;156:151–156.

25. Bendler EM, Greenspun B, Yu J, et al. The bilaterality of carpal tunnel syndrome. *Arch Phys Med Rehabil.* 1967;58:363–364.

26. Bradish CF. Carpal tunnel syndrome in patients on haemodialysis. *J Bone Joint Surg.* 1985;67B:130–132.

27. Brain WR, Wright AD, Wilkinson M. Spontaneous compression of both median nerves in the carpal tunnel. *Lancet.* 1947;1:277–282.

28. Carroll MP, Montero C. Rare anomalous muscle cause of carpal tunnel syndrome. *Orthop Rev.* 1980; 9:83–85.

29. Cseuz KA, Thomas JE, Lambert EH, et al. Long-term results of operation for carpal tunnel syndrome. *Mayo Clin Proc.* 1966;41:232–241.

30. Dekel S, Papaioannou T, Rushworth G, et al. Idiopathic carpal tunnel syndrome caused by carpal stenosis. *Br Med J.* 1980;280:1297–1299.

31. Gelberman RH, Hergenroeder PT, Hargens AR, et al. The carpal tunnel syndrome. *J Bone Joint Surg.* 1981;63A:380–383.

32. Goodman HV, Foster JB. Effect of local corticosteroid injection on median nerve conduction in carpal tunnel syndrome. *Ann Phys Med.* 1962;6:287–294.

33. Gould JS, Wissinger HA. Carpal tunnel syndrome in pregnancy. *South Med J.* 1978;71:144–145.

34. Green DP. Diagnostic and therapeutic value of carpal tunnel injection. *J Hand Surg.* 1984;9A:850–854.

35. Halter SK, DeLisa JA, Stolov WC, et al. Carpal tunnel syndrome in chronic renal dialysis patients. *Muscle Nerve.* 1980;3:438A.

36. Karpati G, Carpenter S, Eisen AA, et al. Multiple peripheral nerve entrapments: an unusual phenotypical variant of the Hunter syndrome (mucopolysaccharidosis II) in a family. *Arch Neurol.* 1974;31: 418–422.

37. Hartwell SW, Kurtay M. Carpal tunnel compression caused by hematoma associated with anticoagulant therapy. *Cleve Clin.* 1966;33:127–129.

38. Kremer M, Gilliatt RW, Golding JSR, et al. Acroparaesthesiae in the carpal-tunnel syndrome. *Lancet.* 1953;2:590–595.

39. Phalen GS. Reflections on 21 years' experience with the carpal-tunnel syndrome. *JAMA.* 1970; 212:1365–1367.

40. Phalen GS. The carpal-tunnel syndrome. *J Bone Joint Surg.* 1966;48A:211–228.

41. Phalen GS, Kendrick JI. Compression neuropathy of the median nerve in the carpal tunnel. *JAMA.* 1953;164:524–595.

42. Smith EM, Sonstegard DA, Anderson WH. Carpal tunnel syndrome: contribution of flexor tendons. *Arch Phys Med Rehabil.* 1977;58:379–385.

43. Spinner M, ed. *Management of Peripheral Nerve Problems.* Philadelphia, Pa: WB Saunders Co; 1980:487–501.

44. Spinner M, Spencer PS. Nerve compression lesions of the upper extremity. *Clin Orthop.* 1974;104: 46–67.

45. Tanzer RC. The carpal-tunnel syndrome: a clinical and anatomical study. *J Bone Joint Surg.* 1959;41A: 626–634.

46. Thomas JE, Lambert EH, Czeuz KA. Electrodiagnostic aspects of the carpal tunnel syndrome. *Arch Phys Med Rehabil.* 1980;16:635–641.

47. Votik AJ, Mueller JC, Farlinger DE, Johnston RU. Carpal tunnel syndrome in pregnancy. *Can Med Assoc J.* 1983;128:277–281.

48. Adelarr RS, Foster WC, McDowell C. The treatment of the cubital tunnel syndrome. *J Hand Surg.* 1984;9A:90–95.

49. Apfelberg DB, Larson SJ. Dynamic anatomy of the ulnar nerve at the elbow. *Plast Reconstr Surg.* 1973;51:76–81.

50. Broudy AS, Leffert RD, Smith RJ. Technical problems with ulnar nerves by Learmonth technique. *J Hand Surg.* 1982;7:147–155.

51. Chan RC, Paine KWE, Varughese G. Ulnar neuropathy at the elbow: comparison of simple decompression and anterior transposition. *Neurosurgery.* 1980;7:545–550.

52. Craven PR, Green DP. Cubital tunnel syndrome: treatment by medial epicondylectomy. *J Bone Joint Surg.* 1980;62A:986–989.

53. Dahners LE, Wood FM. Aconeus epitrochlearis, a rare cause of cubital tunnel syndrome: a case report. *J Hand Surg.* 1984;9A:579–580.

54. Eisen A. Early diagnosis of ulnar nerve palsy. *Neurology.* 1974;24:256–262.

55. Eisen A, Danon J. The mild cubital tunnel syndrome: its natural history and indications for surgical intervention. *Neurology.* 1974;24:608–613.

56. Feindel W, Stratford J. The role of the cubital tunnel in tardy ulnar palsy. *Can J Surg.* 1958;1: 287–300.

57. Harrison MJG, Nurick S. Results of anterior transposition of the ulnar nerve for ulnar neuritis. *Br Med J.* 1970;1:27–29.

58. Jabre JF, Wilbourn AJ. The EMG findings in 100 consecutive ulnar neuropathies. *Acta Neurol Scand.* 1979;60(suppl):73–91.

59. Laha RK, Panchal PD. Surgical treatment of ulnar neuropathy. *Surg Neurol.* 1979;11:393–398.

60. Leffert RD. Anterior submuscular transposition of the ulnar nerves by the Learmonth technique. *J Hand Surg.* 1982;7:147–155.

61. Levy DM, Apfelberg DB. Results of anterior transposition for ulnar neuropathy at the elbow. *Am J Surg.* 1972;123:304–308.

62. McGowan AJ. The results of transposition of the ulnar nerve for traumatic ulnar neuritis. *J Bone Joint Surg.* 1950;32B:293–301.

63. Miller RG. The cubital tunnel syndrome: diagnosis and precise localization. *Ann Neurol.* 1979;6: 56–59.

64. Miller RG, Hummel EE. The cubital tunnel syndrome: treatment with simple decompression. *Ann Neurol.* 1980;7:567–569.

65. Osborne G. Compression neuritis of the ulnar nerve at the elbow. *Hand.* 1970;2:10–13.

66. Osborne GV. The surgical treatment of the tardy ulnar neuritis. *J Bone Joint Surg.* 1957;39B:782.

67. Paine KWE. Tardy ulnar palsy. *Can J Surg.* 1970; 13:255–261.

68. Payan J. Cubital tunnel syndrome. *Br Med J.* 1979; 2:868.

69. Payan J. Electrophysiological localization of ulnar nerve lesions. *J Neurol Neurosurg Psychiatry.* 1960; 32:208–220.

70. Wadsworth TG, Williams JR. Cubital tunnel external compression syndrome. *Br Med J.* 1973; 1:662–666.

71. Wilson DH, Krout R. Surgery of ulnar neuropathy at the elbow: 16 cases treated by decompression without transposition. *J Neurosurg.* 1973; 38:780–785.

72. Ecker AD, Woltman HW. Meralgia paraesthetica. *JAMA.* 1938;110:1650–1652.

73. Stevens H. Meralgia paresthetica. *Arch Neurol Psychiatry.* 1957;77:557–574.

74. Stookey B. Meralgia paresthetica. *JAMA.* 1928; 90:1705–1707.

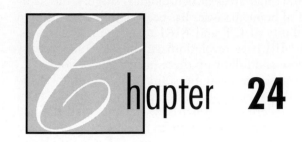

Brain Abscess

Christopher M. Loftus, José Biller

Like many other areas of neurological surgery, the management of brain abscesses has been significantly affected by the ability of CT and MRI to image the abscesses. CT and MRI have revolutionized the surgeon's capacity to diagnose and follow up these intracranial lesions.

Brain abscesses may be solitary or multiple. Radiographically, they appear as a spectrum, ranging from areas of ill-defined cerebritis to mature, well-defined focal suppurative lesions with an enhancing capsule and lucent center (Fig. 24.1). In the pre-CT era only larger lesions could be identified, but CT and MRI have facilitated the diagnosis of both single and multiple small lesions. Whereas the incidence of multiple brain abscesses was originally thought to be 1% to 15% of abscess patients[1,2] it is now recognized that as many as 50% of these patients harbor multiple lesions. Concurrent with improved imaging capabilities is a reduced morbidity and mortality rate due to significant improvements in management techniques (for example, broad spectrum antibiotics that have high brain penetration) as well as computer-assisted stereotactic surgery or ultrasound-guided aspirations, which have in some cases replaced open biopsy techniques.

PRESENTATION AND ETIOLOGY

The presentation of patients with brain abscess has not changed appreciably from classical descriptions, and the clinical findings vary little whether there are solitary or multiple lesions. Most clinical signs and symptoms, which include seizures, altered mental function, focal neurologic deficits, or signs of increased intracranial pressure, indicate the presence of an intracranial mass lesion. About half of the patients have a low grade fever. Patients at risk for brain abscess may be identified because of the presence of hereditary hemorrhagic telangiectasia[3]; known systemic illnesses; sepsis; altered states of immunity; otic, mastoid, paranasal, or odontogenic infections; or fresh intracranial wounds.

The pathogenesis of solitary brain abscess differs somewhat from multiple lesions. It is thought that solitary lesions are often the result of an infected parameningeal focus (paranasal sinuses, middle ear, or thrombosed venous sinuses). A solitary lesion may also arise from direct inoculation of the brain in trauma cases or from infected fluid collections in intracranial operative sites (see Case Histories Two and Three, page 24.7). In contrast, multiple brain abscesses (Case History One, page 24.6) are more common with systemic infections, which are often spread hematogenously. The infective agents in solitary and multiple brain abscesses differ somewhat, depending on the immune status of the host. In otherwise normal hosts, anaerobic or microaerophilic streptococci, staphylococci, enterobacteria, *Haemophilus*, or anaerobes may originate from dental abscesses; cutaneous, bony, pulmonary, intra-abdominal, or renal infections; or infective endocarditis.[4] Parasitic disease in normal hosts most often results from gastrointestinal infection. Infectious agents in abnormal hosts, who may be immunosuppressed either by systemic illness or iatrogenically, may be indolent. These include *Nocardia asteroides* (see Case History Four, page 24.7),[5] *Listeria monocytogenes*, *Aspergillus*, Mucoraceae, *Candida*, *Cryptococcus neoformans*, *Toxoplasma gondii*, and *Strongyloides stercoralis*.

The propensity for hematogenous inoculation of brain abscesses is increased in patients with abnormal intracranial circulation because of potential ischemia or frank brain infarction with subsequent lowered infectious thresholds. This can be recognized in patients who have congenital cyanotic heart disease with or without polycythemia. However, brain abscesses associated with congenital cyanotic heart disease with right-to-left shunt are usually solitary lesions.

EVALUATION AND DIAGNOSIS

Diagnosing single and multiple brain abscesses is essentially the same; in fact, the distinction is not often known until radiographic studies are complete. Most patients presenting with signs of intracranial mass are diagnosed by CT or MRI as showing space-occupying single or multiple lesions. In patients with solitary lesions the primary differential diagnoses are brain abscess, primary or metastatic brain tumor, and infarction, the latter particularly in cases of early abscess because its appearance is similar to cerebritis. The diagnosis of brain abscess is facilitated by associated systemic illnesses or toxic findings, if present. When multifocal intracranial lesions are seen in patients with known systemic disease, a diagnosis of multiple brain abscesses is most likely. In patients without other evidence of infection, the primary differential diagnoses are multiple abscesses and multiple metastases. All patients with such lesions identified on CT should undergo a complete systemic evaluation, including chest, spine, and skull roentgenograms; a complete blood count with differential white blood cell count; serum glucose, blood urea nitrogen, creatinine, and electrolyte determinations; erythrocyte sedimentation rate; urinalysis; multiple blood cultures, human immunodefi-

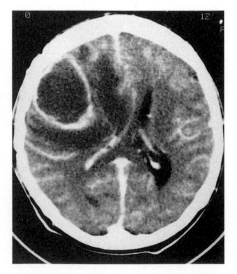

Figure 24.1 Two months after evacuation of a hematoma in the right frontal lobe, this patient presented with mass effect and a large well-defined abscess in the resection bed. A single operation with excision of the abscess and total removal of the capsule was possible in this clearly quite mature lesion.

ciency virus testing; toxoplasma serology; and cultures of obvious sources of infection where these are indicated.

Both enhanced and nonenhanced CT scanning should be performed. MRI with gadolinium enhancement, which is highly sensitive, may be useful in delineating small multicentric lesions that might otherwise be missed. It should be noted, however, that nothing specific about the MR image permits a histologic diagnosis. Arteriography is of no benefit, particularly since MRI can now clearly establish the nonvascular nature of solitary or multiple intracranial lesions. Likewise a lumbar puncture is contraindicated in patients with suspected or proven brain abscesses. Even in the absence of known increased intracranial pressure or mass effect, there is a serious risk of cerebral herniation if a lumbar puncture is attempted in patients with brain abscesses.[6] Furthermore, the information provided by the CSF examination is often nonspecific.

TREATMENT

Management strategies for patients with a brain abscess depend on several important factors, including how the lesion appears on the CT or MRI scan (ill-defined versus mature), the location of the lesion, the number of lesions,

and the clinical circumstances of the patient's illness, if any. As previously mentioned, treatment of brain abscess has been significantly enhanced by improved diagnostic techniques and the availability of high dose broad spectrum antibiotics that attain significant levels of intracranial tissue penetration. Currently, therapeutic controversies center primarily on issues of initial medical therapy versus early surgical intervention, issues particularly salient in patients with multiple lesions or deep-seated, surgically inaccessible solitary lesions. A management scheme for brain abscess is suggested in Figure 24.2.

Primary medical therapy of intracranial abscesses in normal hosts includes the initiation of broad spectrum high dose parenteral antibiotic therapy with a combination of penicillin G or a semisynthetic penicillin, trimethoprim-sulfamethoxazole, and, in many cases, concurrent aminoglycoside therapy.[13] Other alternatives are 1) penicillin G and chloramphenicol with or without gentamicin, 2) cefotaxime and metronidazole, 3) penicillin G, metronidazole and trimethoprim-sulfamethoxazole. If the organism can be isolated from any peripheral source, therapeutic recommendations may be more specific. *Staphylococcus epidermidis* infections are treated with vancomycin with or without rifampin. For abscesses caused by *Staphylococcus aureus*, a semisyn-

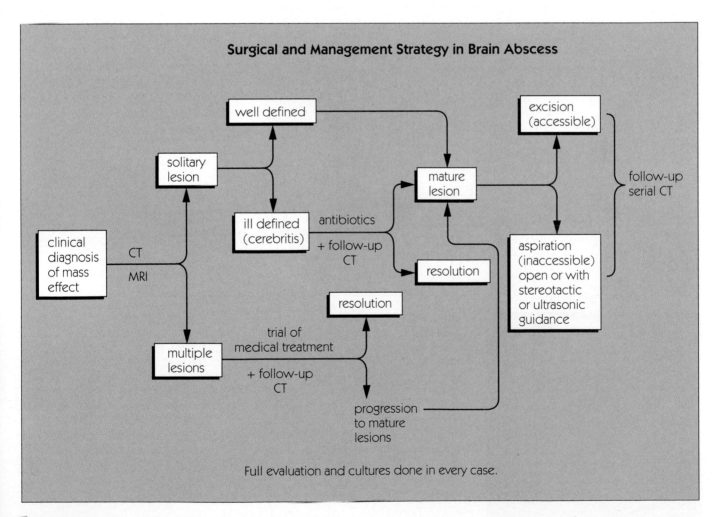

Figure 24.2 Proposed management scheme for new cases of brain abscess.

thetic penicillinase-resistant penicillin (nafcillin) is used unless a resistant isolate is obtained, in which case vancomycin is the drug of choice. Most mouth flora anaerobes (usually Gram-positive) are penicillin-sensitive, whereas metronidazole is the most effective antimicrobial for Gram-negative anaerobes, and especially so for *Bacteroides fragilis* (which is common with chronic otitis, sinusitis, and intraabdominal sepsis).

Brain abscesses in the immunocompromised patient are usually caused by different organisms than those found in the general population. It is important to recognize that one is able to predict broadly the responsible organisms depending on the nature of the underlying anatomic defect and the problem with host defenses. Patients with impaired function of the lymphocyte-directed cellular immune system are prone to develop brain abscesses with *Nocardia asteroides* or *Toxoplasma gondii*. Trimethoprim-sulfamethoxazole, or sulfonamides, are generally regarded as the most effective agents against *N asteroides*. Pyrimethamine plus a short-acting sulfonamide in combination with folinic acid are the cornerstones of treatment of toxoplasmosis of the CNS. In patients allergic to sulfadiazine, clindamycin is the alternative choice. Fungal CNS infections are also common among patients who have a T-lymphocyte, mononuclear phagocyte defect. Recommended therapy for *C neoformans* infections includes amphotericin B and 5-fluorocytosine (not beneficial in patients with AIDS). Infections due to Mucoraceae and *Aspergillus* require amphotericin B alone or in conjunction with 5-fluorocytosine. Immunocompromised patients with *S stercoralis* infection are treated with thiobendazole. Ampicillin remains the first line of attack for *L monocytogenes*, commonly seen in renal transplant patients, patients with hematologic malignancies, or those receiving high-dose corticosteroid therapy. Infection with *Pseudomonas aeruginosa* is often seen in patients with acute leukemia or lymphoma and is usually sensitive to a combination of gentamicin, tobramycin, or amikacin, and an anti-pseudomonas penicillin or certain of the third generation cephalosporins such as ceftazidime. Anaerobic and mixed aerobic/anaerobic infections are less common among immunocompromised patients, except perhaps for patients with Hodgkin's or other lymphomas. A combination of penicillin G, a third generation cephalosporin, and metronidazole is a favored empiric therapeutic approach for those infected with *Bacteroides*, anaerobic streptococci, or Enterobacteriaceae.

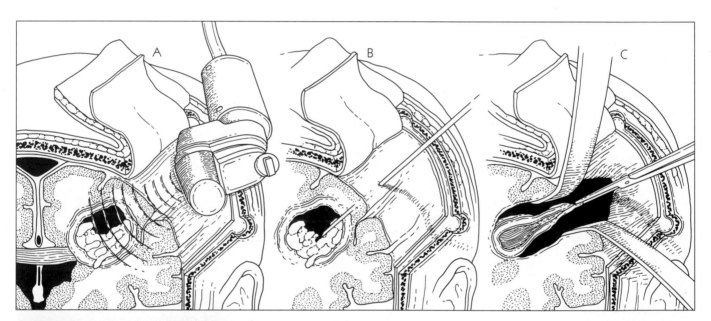

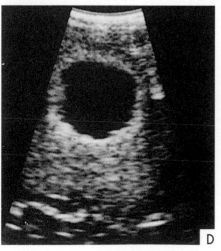

Figure 24.3 (A) Direct application of ultrasound probe to localize a solitary brain abscess through the surface of the brain. (B) Aspiration of pus from the brain abscess via a Scoville cannula. This is often done as a preliminary step once a lesion has been localized and prior to definitive excision of the capsule through cortical incision. (C) Formal removal of the capsule of the brain abscess in a case of solitary mature brain abscess. When the capsule is well developed as is shown here, it is possible to dissect it from the surrounding white matter and remove it in its entirety, particularly in silent areas of the brain. This technique may have to be modified or abandoned in eloquent brain locations. (D) Typical appearance of a mature brain abscess imaged with intraoperative ultrasound.

Principles of Neurosurgery

MEDICAL VERSUS SURGICAL TREATMENT

Perhaps the most difficult management decision in many brain abscess cases is when or if to intervene surgically. Although these questions arise in cases of solitary lesions, they assume much greater importance in patients harboring multiple neuroimaging abnormalities. The respective strategies for solitary and multiple lesions differ enough to be discussed individually (see Fig. 24.2).

Solitary Lesions

In early cases of solitary brain abscess, the CT or MRI image will be of an ill-defined area known as cerebritis. This represents an early stage of infection in which a well-defined capsule has not formed and there is no specific lesion amenable to either Scoville cannula aspiration or direct surgical attack. In such cases, careful attempts must be made to isolate the causative organism from peripheral sources. If this is unsuccessful, it is acceptable to institute broad spectrum antibiotic therapy and follow the patient with serial CT scans until the area of cerebritis either resolves radiographically or matures into a lesion that is amenable to surgery.

The differential diagnoses for a solitary mature lesion within the brain are the same as for multiple lesions, and the patient is subjected to the full battery of diagnostic evaluations prior to considering surgery. One exception is a patient whose intracranial pressure is so high that herniation is incipient and emergency evacuation of the contents of the abscess must be performed. A solitary mature lesion in a superficial location is best treated by open craniotomy, localization of the lesion by surface landmarks or ultrasonic guidance, and preliminary needle aspiration followed by corticotomy and removal of the mature capsule in its entirety. Surgical strategies are outlined in Figure 24.3. Complete excision of the capsule, while ideal, may not be feasible in less mature lesions, thus aspirating the contents of the abscess and openly irrigating all purulent material may suffice. A drain can be left in place at the surgeon's discretion.

Deep seated solitary abscesses or solitary lesions located in eloquent areas of the brain require a different technique. For these abscesses, some form of intraoperative localization is required. This can be either free hand ultrasonic guidance with needle aspiration of the contents of the abscess (see Fig. 24.3B) or a formal stereotactic procedure. With either technique, Scoville cannula aspiration and irrigation of the cyst cavity not only yields diagnostic material but, in conjunction with antibiotic therapy, relieves mass effect and facilitates recovery in most cases. Of course, frequent follow-up CT scans are necessary to evaluate the progression or regression of solitary brain abscesses treated in any fashion.

Few solitary lesions are not amenable to one of these forms of surgical treatment, and the option of empirical medical therapy without bacteriologic diagnosis is probably more relevant in cases of multiple brain abscess.

Multiple Lesions

Multiple lesions, particularly ill defined ones, require a somewhat different medical/surgical management plan (see Fig. 24.2). Although in some cases it is possible to identify causal organisms by peripheral cultures, most authors who advocate primary medical therapy recognize that infectious agents are not identified in the majority of cases.[2,7,8] This form of treatment introduces significant potential for diagnostic error because without direct biopsy or aspiration, multiple brain metastases can be erroneously treated with antibiotics. If the patient fails to improve clinically and radiographically with antibiotics alone, this possibility is reinforced; nonetheless several authors have reported good results after treating multiple intracranial lesions by antibiotics alone.[2,7,8]

Several factors have been identified that appear to predict success with antibiotic treatment alone. Rosenblum et al. report success with small lesions (less than 1.7 cm in average diameter), and lesions treated early, perhaps before the development of a necrotic center, are more likely to be ameliorated with medical treatment only.[8] In the recent series of Dyste et al., cortical abscesses at the gray-white junction were far more likely to resolve than those located in deep intracranial structures; these authors believe that abscess depth was the primary determinant of the success of medical therapy alone.[4] As for solitary lesions, all advocates of antibiotic therapy for multiple abscesses stress the importance of weekly CT evaluations and clear signs of clinical and radiographic improvement when continuing medical therapy alone. Clinical improvement, however, may predate radiographic resolution.[7,9]

Primary surgical treatment of multiple abscesses is often difficult, particularly with bilateral and/or deep lesions, and is not a high-priority approach in the initial management of these lesions, with the exception of life-threatening symptomatic abscesses. Surgical therapy is unquestionably indicated in cases that have mass effect with herniation, fail to resolve, or in which follow-up examinations reveal that the abscesses have progressed.[10] The role of primary surgical biopsy, open or stereotactic, in affording a bacterial diagnosis and thereby facilitating antibiotic choice remains controversial. Good results have been reported with open aspiration of a superficial or accessible lesion followed by appropriate antibiotic treatment.[9,11-13] On the other hand, general anesthesia poses a high risk for many patients with severe systemic disease. The recent technical advances in both ultrasonic imaging and stereotactic technique for aspiration of single or multiple brain abscesses make this a more favorable choice for patients who are at high anesthetic risk and/or have ill-defined or inaccessible lesions (see Fig. 24.3A). Dyste et al. have reported excellent results with stereotactic aspiration of multiple and deep seated abscesses in patients who are poor operative risks and as secondary therapy in patients with abscesses for which medical management has failed.[1]

Empirical medical management is clearly an appropriate consideration for patients with multiple brain abscesses. Single or multiple aspirations, whether open for superficial lesions or guided for deeper lesions, are more common in patients with multiple abscesses, and when done in conjunction with appropriate antibiotic treatment may be curative (see Case History One, page 24.6). Large, mature, superficial lesions in easily accessible areas of the brain are still best treated by evacuation and capsule excision (see Fig. 24.3C). Likewise, life-threatening lesions demand emergency evacuation whether or not multiple lesions are present.

CORTICOSTEROIDS

The role of systemic corticosteroid therapy in the management of brain abscess is another point of controversy. Experimental evidence has suggested that corticosteroids retard the encapsulation process and may decrease the efficacy of antibiotic treatment.[14] Boom and Tuazon reported excellent results with combined antibiotic and dexamethasone therapy in all cases,[7] but most others reserve steroids for patients with clear CT evidence of edema or mass effect.[2,8] Dexamethasone may decrease enhancement on CT scanning, compromising the ability of CT to effectively follow intracranial lesions. At present there is no indication for corticosteroids in the absence of mass effect or surrounding edema, but patients with these findings are placed on dexamethasone at the onset of antibiotic therapy. Where necessary, intracranial pressure monitoring and standard therapeutic regimens designed to lower intracranial pressure, such as intermittent mannitol administration, hyperventilation, and/or ventricular drainage may also be employed in managing these patients.

CASE HISTORIES

CASE ONE

A 5-week-old girl was transferred from another hospital in September, 1987. She had been treated with amoxicillin and erythromycin for presumed right otitis media, but she had become increasingly irritable and was transported to our hospital because meningitis was suspected. Spinal fluid showed 31,000 white cells, all polymorphonuclear. Gram stain showed Gram-negative rods

and the culture was positive for *Citrobacter*. She was initially managed with a combination of ampicillin, gentamicin, and cefotaxime. CT scan showed three areas of low attenuation consistent with brain abscess (Fig. 24.4A).

Antibiotics were continued for a 35 day course with rapid clinical improvement; however, follow-up CT scans showed no change in the character of the abscesses. Because of this the abscesses were tapped percutaneously with ultrasound guidance. The right frontal abscess was aspirated through the anterior fontanelle and the occipital abscess was tapped by translambdoid approach. No organisms were cultured at this time.

The patient had an unremarkable course following aspiration and was discharged on the sixth postoperative day. Follow-up CT scan in 1 month showed good resolution of all three abscesses although hydrocephalus (clinically silent) was present (Fig. 24.4B). She has continued to do well.

Discussion

In this infant the evidence for cerebrospinal fluid infection was clear and her initial evaluation showed multiple brain abscesses with a known organism from spinal fluid analysis. This spinal fluid had been obtained before there was suspicion of brain abscess and prior to obtaining a tomographic study. Although there were no untoward results from lumbar puncture, this diagnostic sequence is not one we consider ideal. In this case, after the initiation of antibiotic treatment clinical improvement ensued but, unfortunately, follow-up CT scan showed that the features of the abscesses remained unchanged. Because of the multiplicity of lesions, ultrasonically guided abscess aspirations were the treatments of choice and this led to complete resolution of the abscesses. No organisms were cultured, indicating that the abscesses were at least partially sterilized by the long course of antibiotic treatment. An alternative choice for an older patient in this situation might be stereotactic aspiration without an open fontanelle. Because the lesions were bilateral and multiple, open craniotomies and capsule excision were contraindicated—at least until less invasive methods were attempted. This case documents a failure of empirical medical therapy, even in the presence of a known

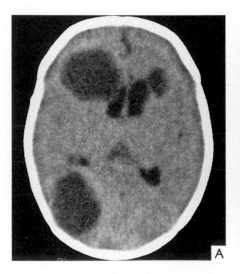
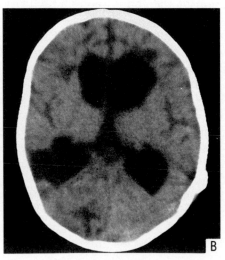

Figure 24.4 (A) CT after 1 1/2 weeks of antibiotics confirms the continued presence of three lesions consistent with brain abscess. (B) CT axial projection following ultrasound-guided aspiration of these three abscesses and a "protracted period" of antibiotics. No further evidence of space-occupying lesions can be seen. The patient had made a complete clinical recovery.

organism, to cure multiple brain abscesses completely; it emphasizes the need for eventual surgical intervention in many such cases.

CASE TWO

A 37-year-old woman had a known history of von Hippel-Lindau disease. She had presented on July 17, 1987 with unsteady gait and was found to have a left cerebellar hemangioblastoma that was resected without complications. She had been discharged but on August 30, 1987, had high fever, nausea, and became unresponsive. CT scan showed acute hydrocephalus and the presence of an enhancing area in the resection bed consistent with a forming cerebellar abscess. She had emergency ventriculostomy placement followed by suboccipital craniectomy and resection of this cerebritic portion of the lateral left cerebellar hemisphere. Blood cultures were positive for *Staphylococcus epidermidis* but wound and cerebellar cultures were entirely negative. She was begun on a 6-week course of vancomycin and made a complete clinical recovery. Follow-up scan 2 weeks following surgery showed good resolution of the abscess with no residual enhancement.

Discussion

This is a classic case of cerebritis and abscess formation in a surgical bed. One month following uneventful craniectomy and tumor removal, this patient presented with mass effect and an ill-defined enhancing lesion in the resection bed. Although the lesion (Fig. 24.5A) was somewhat irregular and not as round as other well-defined solitary abscesses, it was amenable to primary surgical excision because of its location in the cerebellum. In this case, the lateral portion of the cerebellum was removed in an attempt to remove all infected tissue (Fig. 24.5B). In more eloquent areas of the brain, cerebritis must be dealt with in a different fashion, customarily with empirical antibiotic therapy awaiting maturation of a capsule or CT evidence of resolution of the region of cerebritis.

CASE THREE

A 41-year-old man had evacuation of a right frontal-parietal hematoma in another hospital on August 17, 1987. He presented to our hospital on October 11, 1987 with several weeks history of increasing bifrontal headache and leftsided weakness. There were no fevers, chills, or other systemic manifestations. On examination he had bilateral papilledema, left central facial weakness, and a dense left hemiparesis. CT scan demonstrated a 4×5 cm ring enhancing lesion in the right frontal lobe with significant surrounding edema and midline shift. The patient underwent emergency craniotomy, drainage of the abscess, and total excision of the mature abscess capsule. Intraoperative specimens grew *Staphylococcus epidermidis* and anaerobes. The patient was treated with vancomycin, metronidazole, and rifampin, and he had progressive resolution of his residual enhancement on follow-up CT scans. Unfortunately, he succumbed to cardiorespiratory arrest on the 34th postoperative day.

Discussion

This is another example of abscess formation in an operative resection bed, albeit somewhat more delayed. This patient presented 2 months following craniotomy with a large well defined solitary enhancing lesion. In this case, because of the location and the maturity of the lesion, a complete excision of the lesion and capsule was possible at one operative session, which would have represented a good surgical result had it not been for his untimely demise.

CASE FOUR

A 56-year-old man had a 1 month history of a right chest wall mass measuring 5 cm in diameter. He also reported new onset of malaise, low-grade fever, weight loss, and mental status changes with memory loss and disorientation. Past medical history was remarkable for an 80 pack/year smoking history and alcoholism. On October 7, 1985, he had axillary lymph node excision and drainage

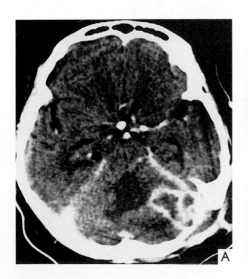
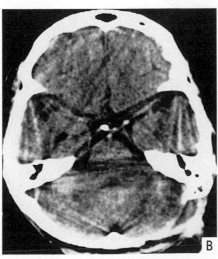

Figure 24.5 (A) A moderately defined lesion in the left cerebellar hemisphere can be seen in this patient with acute hydrocephalus and signs of posterior fossa mass effect. This represents an area of cerebritis and early abscess formation in a postoperative resection bed.
(B) Following resection of the lateral portion of the cerebellum and antibiotic treatment, hydrocephalus has resolved and there is no longer any enhancement in the resection bed. This patient made a complete recovery.

of the chest wall abscess, which contained *Nocardia asteroides*. While the patient was on the surgery service, he became increasingly disoriented and developed a left hemiparesis. CT scan on October 10, 1985, revealed a large mature abscess with significant edema in the right frontal lobe (Fig. 24.6A). He was taken immediately to surgery where the abscess was drained and the capsule was excised through a right frontal craniotomy. Intraoperative cultures grew *N asteroides* from the brain abscess cavity.

This patient had a prolonged but full recovery with 6 weeks of intravenous trimethoprim-sulfamethoxazole. His course was complicated by leukopenia thought to be a direct effect of the antibiotic, but it was ameliorated by decreasing the dose. Following completion of the IV therapy course, he was discharged with an additional 12 months of PO trimethoprim-sulfamethoxazole therapy. Follow-up CT scan 3 years later (Fig. 24.6B) shows complete resolution in the region of the abscess with no evidence of recurrence.

Discussion

Aside from his history of alcoholism, this patient was not known to be immunocompromised. This case clearly represents hematogenous inoculation of brain tissue from a primary abscess in the chest. The maturity of the capsule at first presentation allowed complete excision at one operative setting.

COURSE AND PROGNOSIS

Patients with brain abscess, with or without bacteriological diagnosis and with or without surgery, usually require 3 months of systemic antibiotic therapy, which may be of high dose initially followed by a tapered maintenance dosage. Attention to underlying systemic infections, anatomical defects, and purulent foci must also be scrupulous. Progression or resolution of intracranial lesions can readily be followed by weekly CT scanning, which should be continued throughout the initial treatment period. When the clinical course of the intracranial lesions becomes clear, a biweekly CT interval may be more appropriate. CT scans at 2 to 4 month intervals should be obtained even after therapy has been concluded because of the documented lag between clinical and CT improvement and because of the propensity for lesions to recur, particularly when there is an underlying systemic infection or structural abnormality.[8]

CONCLUSION

The prognosis for patients with brain abscess has been significantly improved by several advances in diagnostic and therapeutic techniques. These include the advent of CT and MRI, the availability of antibiotics with superior brain penetration, improved understanding of the immunocompromised host, and advanced techniques for surgical localization, including ultrasonic guidance and stereotactic systems. Whereas direct surgical attack will continue to be the mainstay in patients with solitary brain abscess, the availability of these alternative strategies facilitates treatment of patients with deep-seated or inaccessible solitary lesions. Alternative strategies assume a more important role in managing patients with multiple lesions who represent a higher percentage of the brain abscess population than was previously recognized. In cases of multiple lesions in particularly ill patients, empirical treatment alone may play a role, although the ability to aspirate such lesions stereotactically for diagnostic purposes will most likely diminish the need for empirical treatment. Meticulous attention to the first principles of clinical diagnosis, thorough evaluation of the patient for sources of infection and anatomical defects, and scrupulous follow up with repeated imaging studies will continue to improve the survival rate and prognosis for these unfortunate patients.

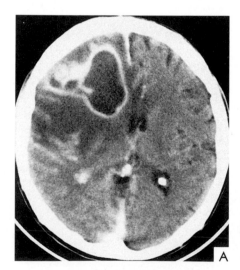
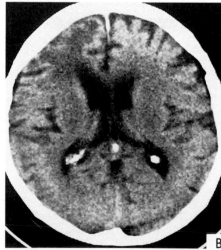

Figure 24.6 (A) This patient, with a chest wall mass that proved to be a *Nocardia asteroides* infection, had a single hematogenously mediated frontal lobe abscess with surrounding edema and mass effect. It was possible to excise this at a single sitting because of the well-developed wall and mature capsule. (B) Follow-up CT scan 3 years later shows no evidence of residual or recurrent lesion in this patient. There is a discrete low attenuation area in the left frontal lobe with slight enlargement of the ipsilateral frontal horn.

REFERENCES

1. Dyste GN, Hitchon PW, Menezes AH, et al. Stereotaxic surgery in the treatment of multiple brain abscesses. *J Neurosurg.* 1988;69:188–194.

2. Rousseaux M, Lesoin F, Destee A, et al. Developments in the treatment and prognosis of multiple cerebral abscesses. *Neurosurgery.* 1985;16:304–308.

3. Press OW, Ramsey PG. Central nervous system infections associated with hereditary hemorrhagic telangiectasia. *Am J Med.* 1984;77:86–92.

4. De Louvois J, Gortvai P, Hurley R. Bacteriology of abscesses of the central nervous system: a multicentre prospective study. *Br Med J (Clin Res).* 1977;2: 981–984.

5. Rosenblum ML, Rosegay H. Resection of multiple nocardial brain abscesses: diagnostic role of computerized tomography. *Neurosurgery.* 1979;4:315–318.

6. Samson DS, Clark K. A current review of brain abscesses. *Am J Med.* 1973;54:201–210.

7. Boom WH, Tuazon CU. Successful treatment of multiple brain abscesses with antibiotics alone. *Rev Infect Dis.* 1985;7:189–199.

8. Rosenblum ML, Hoff JT, Norman D, et al. Nonoperative treatment of brain abscesses in selected high-risk patients. *J Neurosurg.* 1980;52:217–225.

9. Burke LP, Ho SU, Cerullo LJ, et al. Multiple brain abscesses. *Surg Neurol.* 1981;16:452–454.

10. Kobrine AI, Davis DO, Rizzoli HV. Multiple abscesses of the brain. *J Neurosurg.* 1981;54:93–97.

11. George B. Antibiotic therapy for multiple abscesses. *J Neurosurg.* 1981;55:153–154. Letter.

12. George B, Roux F, Pillon M, et al. Relevance of antibiotics in the treatment of brain abscesses: report of a case with eight simultaneous brain abscesses treated and cured medically. *Acta Neurochir (Wien).* 1979;47: 285–291.

13. Hubschmann OR, Wiesbrot FJ, Smith LG. Multiple streptococcal brain abscesses successfully treated by craniotomy and needle aspiration. *Surg Neurol.* 1982;17:57–61.

14. Quartey GRC, Johnston JA, Rozdilsky B. Decadron in the treatment of cerebral abscess: an experimental study. *J Neurosurg.* 1976;45:301–310.

Neuro-Oncology: Overview

Griffith R. Harsh IV

Neuro-oncology is the study of tumors of the nervous system. A brain tumor can be defined at several levels (Fig. 25.1).
(A) Clinical: an intracranial neoplastic mass that because of size or location causes symptoms of mass effect or neurologic deficit.
(B) Tissue: a group of cells and associated extracellular matrix whose growth exceeds and is uncoordinated with that of normal tissue[1]; as a result, tumors are often highly cellular and disrupt normal tissue architecture.
(C) Cellular: individual cells altered in size, shape, nuclear to cytoplasmic ratio, nuclear appearance, and cytoplasmic organelles; as tumors become more malignant, features of cellular anaplasia become more pronounced and those of differentiation less apparent.
(D) Biochemical: an altered assortment of regulatory and functional proteins that causes changes of cell structure and metabolism.
(E) Immunologic: a set of epitopes that distinguishes neoplastic from normal cells.
(F) Chromosomal: karyotypes that may appear normal or may have either aneuploid or polyploid abnormalities; integral changes in the number of chromosomes may be accompanied by amplification, deletion, and translocation of certain chromosomal segments.
(G) Genetic: a constellation of alterations in DNA base sequence that changes either the expression of genes that normally regulate cell proliferation or the structure of the proteins these genes encode.

Primary intracranial tumors may arise from cells of the brain parenchyma or from its intracranial linings. Secondary intracranial tumors may arise in the skull or neighboring structures and extend through the skull or cranial foramina, or they may arise at distant sites and spread hematogenously to the brain or dura; both primary and metastatic tumors may be intraaxial, extraaxial, or both (Fig. 25.2). Intraaxial tumors are located primarily within the brain parenchyma or ventricular system, whereas extraaxial tumors are located in the subarachnoid space or meninges. Unlike most systemic malignancies, primary brain tumors rarely metastasize to other regions of the body.

CLASSIFICATION OF BRAIN TUMORS

A classification scheme is valuable to the extent that it permits accurate predictions regarding the natural history of the disease and the response to therapy. Grouping together tumors with similar etiologies and neoplastic mechanisms is fundamental to both preventive and therapeutic efforts. Ideally, a classification scheme should integrate clinical, tissue, cellular, biochemical, immunologic, chromosomal, and genetic criteria.

CLASSIFICATION BY CELL TYPE

Traditional classifications of brain tumors are based on the premise that each type of tumor results from the abnormal growth of a specific cell type. This is the basis of the original classification of brain tumors by Bailey and Cushing[2] and is fundamental to the widely used World Health Organization system (Fig. 25.3).[3] The nomenclature of these systems reflects this choice (e.g., astrocytomas are tumors of astrocytes). Categorization relies primarily on patterns of tissue and cellular histology identified by light microscopy.[3] Immunohistochemistry using monoclonal antibodies against structural proteins that serve as markers for specialized cell types has increased the specificity. Electron microscopy has also proven a valuable adjunct in cases where the basic cell type can be more accurately identified by the presence of specialized organelles (e.g., secretory granules in pituitary tumors).[4]

Difficulties with these classification systems arise when the tumor consists of more than one cell type or when the predominant cell type cannot easily be related to a normal adult cell type.[4] Cellular heterogeneity can occur to various degrees and may manifest a variety of mechanisms. The two cell types may be derived from different germ layers; this may occur as a result of differentiation within a germ cell tumor or after transformation of the stromal element of a glioma in the genesis of a gliosarcoma. The two cell types may be derived from a common precursor of the same germ layer (mixed malignant gliomas have both astrocytic and oligodendroglial elements). Multiple cell types may

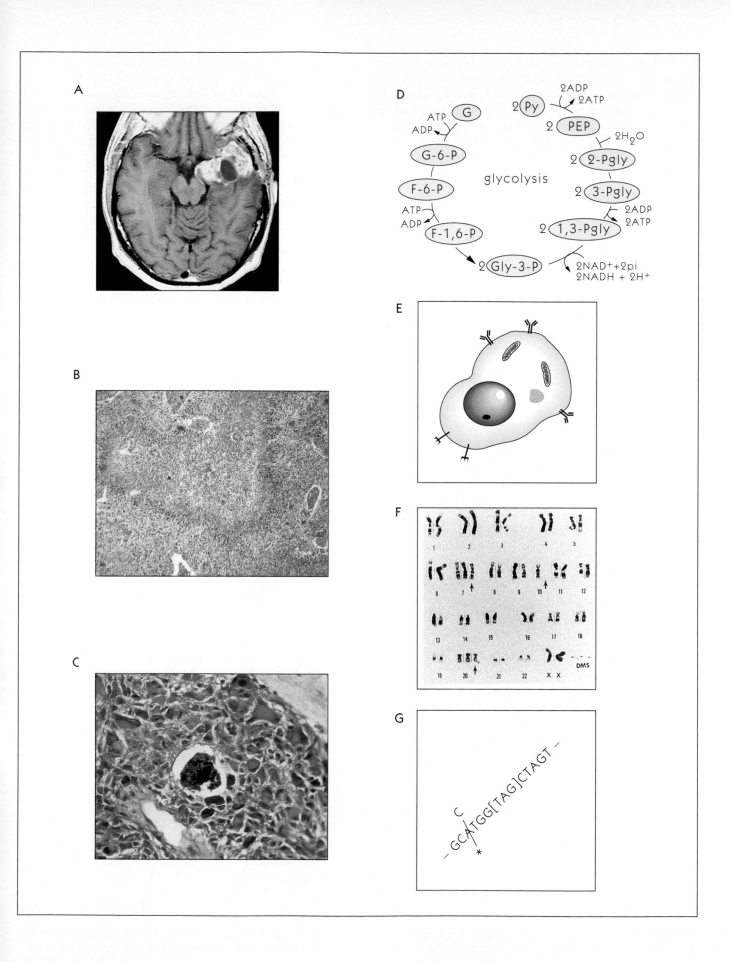

D

glycolysis

result from genotypic and consequent phenotypic evolution within the tumor (a glioblastoma may contain areas of lower degrees of malignancy).[4] Difficulties in relating the predominant cell type of a tumor to a normal cell type most commonly occur when the tumor consists of relatively primitive or undifferentiated cells (e.g., primitive neuroectodermal and embryonal cell tumors).

_____ GRADING THE DEGREE OF MALIGNANCY

Tumors associated with a particular cell type can differ remarkably in their histologic and cytologic characteristics and in their clinical behavior. Clinically malignant CNS tumors grow rapidly; they invade and destroy surrounding normal tissue but, unlike most systemic malignancies, seldom metastasize. They often induce the formation of new blood vessels and produce areas of

necrosis. Such changes are called tissue anaplasia. Cellular abnormalities, such as hypercellularity and an increased number of mitotic figures, also correlate with rapid growth. These and other cytologic features of rapid growth, including variability in cell size and shape, relative lack of cytoplasmic differentiation, and hyperchromatic, pleomorphic nuclei, are called cellular anaplasia.[4]

The correspondence between tissue and cellular anaplasia and malignant clinical behavior has led some classification systems to use the terms interchangeably. The strength of the correlation between histology and clinical behavior varies among tumor types. For ependymomas, the distinction between histologically benign and histologically malignant tumor has little prognostic value. For meningiomas, the critical determinants for malignant behavior are the mitotic index and invasion of brain cortex. For astrocytomas, however, histologic

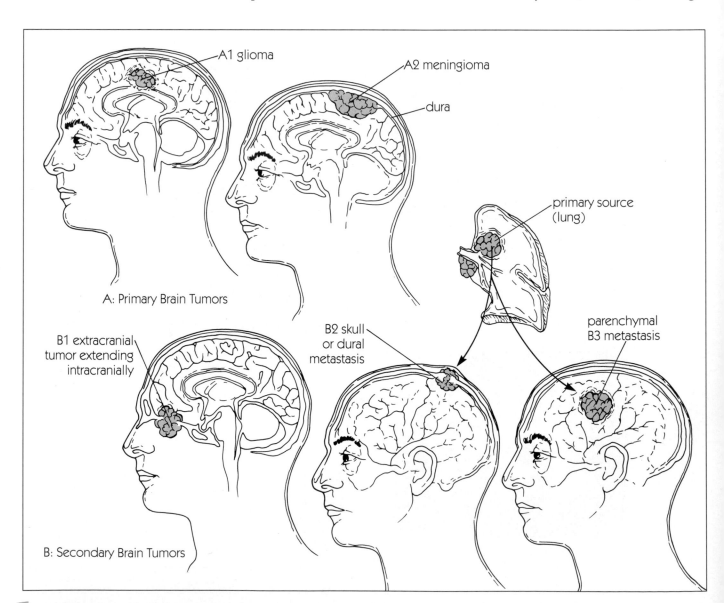

Figure 25.2 Primary or secondary, intraaxial or extraaxial brain tumors. Primary brain tumors, arising from cells of the brain parenchyma (e.g., gliomas, A1) or its meninges (e.g., meningiomas, A2), may be intraaxial or extraaxial respectively. Secondary brain tumors that spread to the brain by local extension (e.g., esthesioneuroblastomas, B1, or skull metastasis) are extraaxial; those that spread hematogenously may be either extraaxial (e.g., dural-based metastasis, B2) or intraaxial (e.g., parenchymal metastasis, B3).

Figure 25.3 WHO Histologic Classification of Tumors of the Central Nervous System

I. Tumors of Neuroepithelial Tissue
  A. Astrocytic tumors
    1. Astrocytoma
      a. Fibrillary
      b. Protoplasmic
      c. Gemistocytic
    2. Pilocytic astrocytoma
    3. Subependymal giant cell astrocytoma
      (ventricular, tumor of tuberous sclerosis)
    4. Astroblastoma
    5. Anaplastic (malignant) astrocytoma
  B. Oligodendroglial tumors
    1. Oligodendroglioma
    2. Mixed oligoastrocytoma
    3. Anaplastic (malignant) oligodendroglioma
  C. Ependymal and choroid plexus tumors
    1. Ependymoma
      a. Myxopapillary ependymoma
      b. Papillary ependymoma
      c. Subependymoma
    2. Anaplastic (malignant) ependymoma
    3. Choroid plexus papilloma
    4. Anaplastic (malignant) choroid plexus
      papilloma
  D. Pineal cell tumors
    1. Pineocytoma (pinealocytoma)
    2. Pineoblastoma (pinealoblastoma)
  E. Neuronal tumors
    1. Gangliocytoma
    2. Ganglioglioma
    3. Ganglioneuroblastoma
    4. Anaplastic (malignant) gangliocytoma
      and ganglioglioma
    5. Neuroblastoma
  F. Poorly differentiated and embryonal tumors
    1. Glioblastoma
      Variants
      a. Glioblastoma with sarcomatous
        component (mixed glioblastoma
        and sarcoma)
      b. Giant cell glioblastoma
    2. Medulloblastoma
      Variants
      a. Desmoplastic medulloblastoma
      b. Medullomyoblastoma
    3. Medulloepithelioma
    4. Primitive polar spongioblastoma
    5. Gliomatosis cerebri

II. Tumors of Nerve Sheath Cells
  A. Neurilemoma (schwannoma, neurinoma)
  B. Anaplastic (malignant) neurilemoma
  C. Neurofibroma

  D. Anaplastic (malignant) neurofibroma
    (neurofibrosarcoma, neurogenic sarcoma)

III. Tumors of the Meninges and Related Tissues
  A. Meningioma
    1. Meningotheliomatous (endotheliomatous,
      syncytial arachnotheliomatous)
    2. Fibrous (fibroblastic)
    3. Transitional (mixed)
    4. Psammomatous
    5. Angiomatous
    6. Hemangioblastic
    7. Hemangiopericytic
    8. Papillary
    9. Anaplastic (malignant) meningioma
  B. Meningeal sarcomas
    1. Fibrosarcoma
    2. Polymorphic cell sarcoma
    3. Primary meningeal sarcomatosis
  C. Xanthomatous tumors
    1. Fibroxanthoma
    2. Xanthosarcoma (malignant fibroxanthoma)
  D. Primary melanotic tumors
    1. Melanoma
    2. Meningeal melanomatosis
  E. Others

IV. Primary Malignant Lymphomas

V. Tumors of Blood Vessel Origin
  A. Hemangioblastoma (capillary
    hemangioblastoma)
  B. Monstrocellular sarcoma

VI. Germ Cell Tumors
  A. Germinoma
  B. Embryonal carcinoma
  C. Choriocarcinoma
  D. Teratoma

VII. Other Malformative Tumors and Tumor-like
    Lesions
  A. Craniopharyngioma
  B. Rathke's cleft cyst
  C. Epidermoid cyst
  D. Dermoid cyst
  E. Colloid cyst of the third ventricle
  F. Enterogenous cyst
  G. Other cysts
  H. Lipoma
  I. Choristoma (pituicytoma, granular cell
    "myoblastoma")
  J. Hypothalamic neuronal hamartoma
  K. Nasal glial heterotopia (nasal glioma)

features influence prognosis so strongly that multilevel grading schemes are used. The four-level grading system of Kernohan et al.,[5] Burger's[6] modification of the three-level (astrocytoma, anaplastic astrocytoma, and glioblastoma multiforme) WHO system, Davis's[7] four-tiered scheme of anaplasia, and Daumas-Duport's[8] quantitative system based on the presence of coagulative necrosis, endothelial proliferation, nuclear atypia, and mitotic figures have all shown predictive value for patient outcome.

MOLECULAR NEUROPATHOLOGY

The details of these multilevel grading schemes have proven controversial. The current trend in neuropathology is to use highly objective indices of tumor biology. The development of indices that register neoplastic changes at the molecular level heralds the arrival of molecular neuropathology.

Indices of Proliferation

The first major advance in molecular neuropathology was in measurement of the rate of tumor cell prolifera-

---

Figure 25.3 (continued)

VIII. Vascular Malformations
   A. Capillary telangiectasia
   B. Cavernous angioma
   C. Arteriovenous malformation
   D. Venous malformation
   E. Sturge-Weber disease (cerebrofacial or cerebrotrigeminal angiomatosis)

IX. Tumors of the Anterior Pituitary
   A. Pituitary adenomas
      1. Acidophil
      2. Basophil (mucoid cell)
      3. Mixed acidophil-basophil
      4. Chromophobe

X. Local Extensions From Regional Tumors
   A. Glomus jugular tumor (chemodectoma, paraganglioma)
   B. Chordoma
   C. Chondroma
   D. Chondrosarcoma
   E. Olfactory neuroblastoma (esthesioneuroblastoma)
   F. Adenoid cystic carcinoma (cylindroma)
   G. Others

XI. Metastatic Tumors

XII. Unclassified Tumors

---

tion. Counting of mitotic figures has been superseded by bromodeoxyuridine and Ki-67 labeling indices. The frequency of incorporation of the bromine analogue of deoxyuridine (a marker for cells in the DNA synthesis phase of the cell cycle) in tumor cell DNA or of immunostaining for Ki-67 (a marker for cycling cells) provides an estimate of the portion of cells in a tumor that are actively dividing (Fig. 25.4).[9,10] The mean bromodeoxyuridine labeling index is less than 1% in astrocytomas, 2.7% in anaplastic astrocytomas, and 7.3% in glioblastomas. It is higher in tumors with necrosis, vascular proliferation, high invasiveness, and absence of differentiation. These estimates of the growth fraction of brain tumors have predictive value for both tumor growth rate and clinical outcome that may exceed the predictive value of tumor histopathology.

Immunohistochemical Markers

The second major advance in molecular neuropathology was the use of immunologic staining to characterize the assortment of structural and functional proteins produced in neoplastic cells. Immunohistochemical identification of marker proteins and glycolipids clarifies a tumor's cell type and degree of differentiation (Fig. 25.5).[11] Expression of intermediate filaments, such as glial fibrillary acidic protein (GFAP) in glial tumors and neurofilaments in neuroepithelial tumors, has been studied extensively. GFAP is produced in normal astrocytes and various tumors derived from astroglial cells: astrocytomas, some glioblastomas, mixed gliomas (oligodendroglioma-astrocytoma), and some ependymomas.[11] In many of these tumor types, the level of expression varies inversely with the degree of anaplasia. Neurofilaments are found in neurons and neural tumors, such as gangliocytomas, neuroblastomas, pineoblastomas, gangliogliomas, and some medulloblastomas.[11]

Panels of monoclonal antibodies against tumor-specific antigens on gliomas, melanomas, and neuroblastomas can be used to study the patterns of antigen expression in neuroepithelial tumors. The findings of such studies may prove valuable in selecting specific therapies. Tumor expression of other molecules commonly found in neuroglial cells, such as neuron-specific enolase, carbonic anhydrase isoenzymes, myelin basic protein, neuroendocrine proteins (e.g., neuropeptides, synaptophysin, and chromogranin), and a variety of glycolipids (e.g., 3′ iso-LM-1 ganglioside) can also be characterized, although their prognostic value has not yet been defined.[11]

Genetic Markers

The third major advance in molecular neuropathology was in describing changes in the nucleic acids of tumor cells. Analysis of tumor DNA by flow cytometry is of little value in neuropathology. The degree of aneuploidy correlates poorly with clinical behavior; even highly malignant brain tumors can have a nearly diploid DNA content. Although karyotyping by itself adds little to a neuropathologic diagnosis, it can provide clues to genetic alterations of fundamental importance. Cytogenetic abnormalities, such as chromosomal deletions, translocations, and amplifications (evident as homogeneously staining regions and double minute chromatin bodies), may signal the loss of tumor suppressor genes or the amplification of oncogenes. Because genetic changes underlie the phenotypic progression of tumors to malignancy, these genetic markers should correlate well with the clinical behavior. Studies of the nature and consequences of primary and secondary genetic changes and the resulting alterations in the number, type, and immunologic structure of cell proteins should also suggest possibilities of therapeutic intervention.

EPIDEMIOLOGY

Epidemiologists attempt to identify patterns of disease in populations.[12] The frequency and distribution of brain tumors in a population and their change over time may provide clues to etiology.

PREVALENCE, INCIDENCE, AND MORTALITY RATE

The prevalence of brain tumors at autopsy is 1% to 2%.[13] The annual incidence of newly diagnosed brain tumors in the United States is approximately 18 per 100,000 persons; one third (14,000) are primary and two thirds are metastatic.[14] The mortality rate for primary brain tumors in North America averages about 5 per 100,000 per year.[15] Less developed regions of the world report lower age-adjusted rates; this difference may reflect less accurate premortem diagnosis or autopsy analysis.[16] The mortality rate from primary brain tumors varies with sex, race, and age. In the United States, it is higher for males than for females, is higher for whites than for blacks, and rises with age until 70 years and then declines.[15]

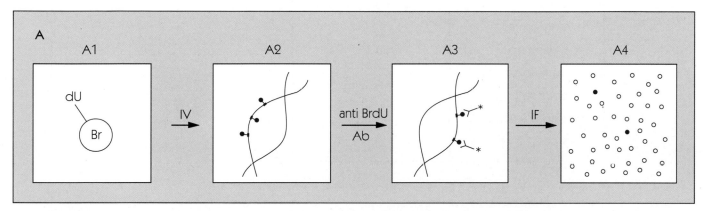

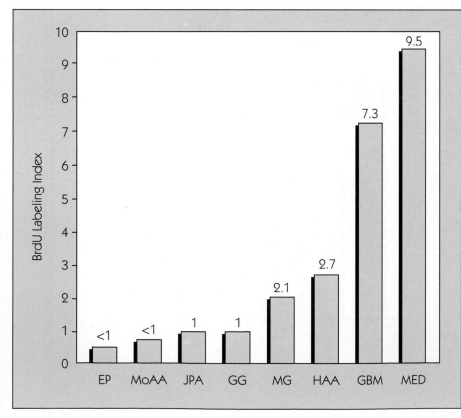

Figure 25.4 Indices of proliferation. (A) Immunofluorescent histochemical analysis of tumors exposed preoperatively to analogues of DNA bases can yield estimates of the rate of cell division. (A1) During the initial stages of surgery, BUdR is administered intravenously. (A2) Cells actively synthesizing DNA incorporate this thymidine analogue. (A3) Incubation of a histologic section of the tumor specimen with antibody specific for BUdR labels cells that have incorporated the marker in their DNA. (A4) The percentage of cells that are labeled provides an estimate of the proliferative fraction, i.e., the portion of the tumor cells that are actively dividing. (B) These estimates of proliferation rate correlate highly with tumor recurrence rate and clinical outcome.[9] EP=ependymoma; MoAA=moderately anaplastic astrocytoma; JPA=juvenile pilocytic astrocytoma; GG=ganglioglioma; MG=mixed glioma; HAA=highly anaplastic astrocytoma; GBM=glioblastoma multiforme; MED=medulloblastoma.

The incidence of primary brain tumors of all histologic types varies with age: There is a small peak at 2 years, a decline for the rest of the first decade, and a slow increase from 2 per 100,000 per year at age 10 to 8 per 100,000 per year at age 40. During late adulthood the incidence doubles to a peak of 20 per 100,000 per year at age 70 before a final decline (Fig. 25.6).[14] This pattern is essentially identical to that for malignant gliomas, reflecting the high proportion of primary brain tumors that are of this pathologic type (Fig. 25.7).

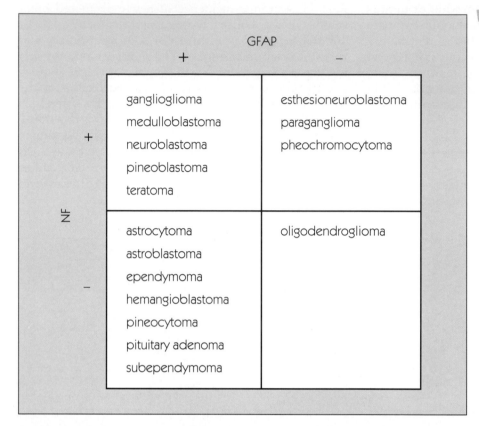

Figure 25.5 Markers of cellular differentiation. Immunohistochemical analysis with panels of monoclonal antibodies specific for glial or neuronal proteins helps classify tumors according to the predominant cell type.

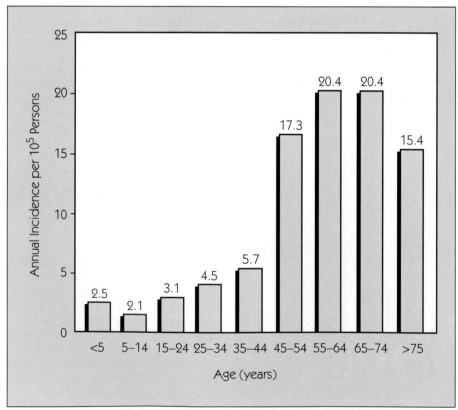

Figure 25.6 Incidence of brain tumors as a function of age. The average annual incidence of primary intracranial neoplasms in the United States, 1973–1974, was 8.2/100,000.

DETERMINANTS OF THE INCIDENCE OF SPECIFIC TUMOR TYPES

The incidence of different types of primary brain tumor varies with age.[17] In adults, malignant gliomas and meningiomas are the most common primary brain tumors, but in children, medulloblastomas and less malignant astrocytomas are most likely to be found (Fig. 25.8).[18] Sex and race are also influential. Unlike most types of gliomas, meningiomas and pituitary adenomas are more likely to occur in women than in men and are more frequent in blacks than in whites.[19] Analysis of recent trends suggests a steady increase in the incidence of malignant brain tumors in various ethnic and sex groups (Fig. 25.9), especially in persons over 70 years of age.[20,21]

FAMILIAL BRAIN TUMORS

An increased incidence of brain tumors within a single family can usually be attributed to one of the phakomatoses (Fig. 25.10). These dominantly inherited predispositions to the development of nervous system tumors include neurofibromatosis types 1 and 2 (NF-1 and NF-2), tuberous sclerosis, and von Hippel-Lindau disease.[22] Neurofibromatosis is the most common. In NF-1, nerve sheath tumors and optic, brain stem, and cerebellar gliomas are associated with café au lait spots, cutaneous neurofibromas, plexiform neurofibromas of peripheral nerves, and Lisch nodules (hamartomas of the iris). In NF-2, bilateral acoustic neuromas, astrocytomas, meningiomas, and spinal nerve root schwannomas occur. Families with von Hippel-Lindau disease have a high incidence of hemangioblastomas, most commonly in the cerebellum, brain stem, and spinal cord, and may also have retinal angiomas, pancreatic cysts and adenocarcinomas, renal cysts, and hypernephromas. In tuberous sclerosis, subependymal giant cell astrocytomas and tuberous hamartomas of the cerebral cortex are associated with mental retardation and epilepsy. Cutaneous stigmata include depigmented lesions (ash leaf spots), angiofibromas of the face (adenoma sebaceum), fingers, and toes, and subepidermal fibrosis (shagreen patches). Rhabdomyomas of the heart and retinal, lung, and renal hamartomas are also found.[22] The occurrence of the same type of brain tumor in members of the same family has prompted speculation regarding familial syndromes of gliomas, medulloblastomas, and meningiomas. Such occurrences are extremely rare, and the patterns of inheritance have not been conclusively established.

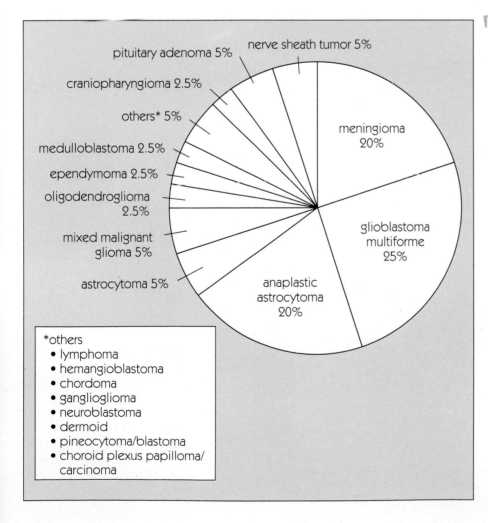

Figure 25.7 Proportions of brain tumors of various pathologic types. The majority of primary brain tumors are gliomas, most of which are malignant.

pituitary adenoma 5%
nerve sheath tumor 5%
craniopharyngioma 2.5%
others* 5%
medulloblastoma 2.5%
ependymoma 2.5%
oligodendroglioma 2.5%
mixed malignant glioma 5%
astrocytoma 5%
meningioma 20%
glioblastoma multiforme 25%
anaplastic astrocytoma 20%

*others
• lymphoma
• hemangioblastoma
• chordoma
• ganglioglioma
• neuroblastoma
• dermoid
• pineocytoma/blastoma
• choroid plexus papilloma/ carcinoma

MULTICENTRIC BRAIN TUMORS

Multicentricity of extraaxial tumors, such as meningiomas and neurofibromas, or the occurrence of different types of tumors in the same person, such as an optic nerve glioma in a patient with a neurofibroma, is readily documented and usually indicates a phakomatosis. Multicentricity of an intraaxial, highly invasive tumor, such as a malignant glioma, is much more difficult to establish. In all but about 5% of cases, careful pathologic analysis of purportedly multicentric gliomas will demonstrate contiguity between lesions, and molecular studies will demonstrate a shared clonal origin. In verified cases of multicentricity, however, an inherited predisposition to brain tumors or evidence of a tumor-inducing environmental exposure should be sought. This applies as well to patients with tumors of both the brain and another organ, which might reflect a germ line genetic defect (e.g., Turcot's syndrome of intestinal polyposis, adenocarcinomas of the colon, and malignant glial tumors) or common exposure of the meninges and breasts to abnormally elevated hormone levels (e.g., the association between meningiomas and breast cancer).[23]

ETIOLOGY

The etiology of brain tumors is essentially a genetic question consisting of three parts: 1) What fundamental genetic alterations underlie the development of the tumor? 2) What causes these genetic alterations? 3) What host factors allow these genetic alterations to be manifested as tumors? The last decade has brought tremendous progress in understanding of the genetic basis of tumorigenesis. Two types of changes in genetic expression have been identified as primary events: the loss of expression of tumor suppressor genes (TSGs)

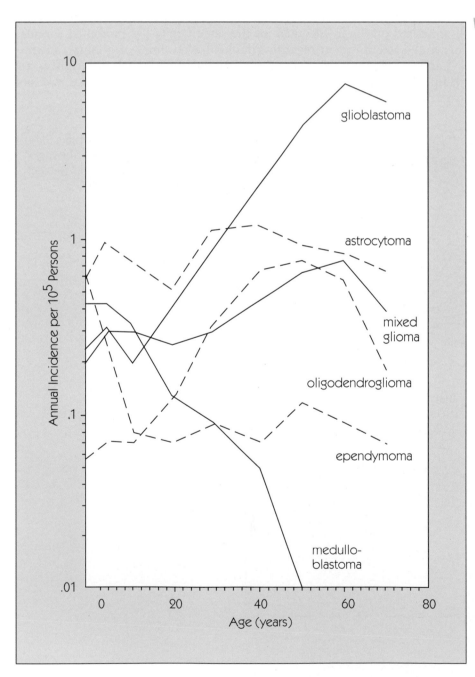

Figure 25.8 Incidences of types of malignant gliomas as a function of age. The incidence of a glioma of a particular histologic type varies with age. This variation is particularly large for medulloblastomas and glioblastomas.[17]

and the overexpression of oncogenes or the expression of altered forms of oncogenes. These changes result from genetic defects in the form of chromosomal loss or DNA injury, which can be inherited or acquired.

ALTERATIONS OF GENETIC EXPRESSION

Tumor Suppressor Genes

The term *TSG* describes genes whose loss or inactivation is associated with tumorigenesis. Most inherited genetic defects that predispose to the development of brain tumors involve the loss or inactivation of a TSG. At the level of the individual cell, the loss of a TSG is recessive; both alleles must be lost or inactivated for this gene locus to contribute to tumorigenesis. (Fig. 25.11). At the level of the organism, however, the number of cells at risk and the frequency of acquired loss or inactivation of the normal allele are high enough that inherited loss or inactivation of even one allele of a TSG

greatly increases the chance that a tumor will form; thus, the trait of tumor development appears to be inherited in dominant fashion.

Identification
Genes such as TSGs may be lost through deletions or inactivated by mutations. Restriction fragment length polymorphism (RFLP) analysis can identify deletions too small to be seen by cytogenetic studies through changes in the pattern of DNA cleavage by restriction enzymes (Fig. 25.12). DNA is cut by a restriction enzyme into fragments whose length depends on the separation of enzyme recognition sites; the presence of a particular base sequence (marker) within any of the fragments can be determined by hybridizing the fragments with a labeled probe specific for that sequence. The DNA sequences of a person's maternal and paternal chromosomes are sufficiently divergent that some restriction enzyme sites occurring on one chromosome

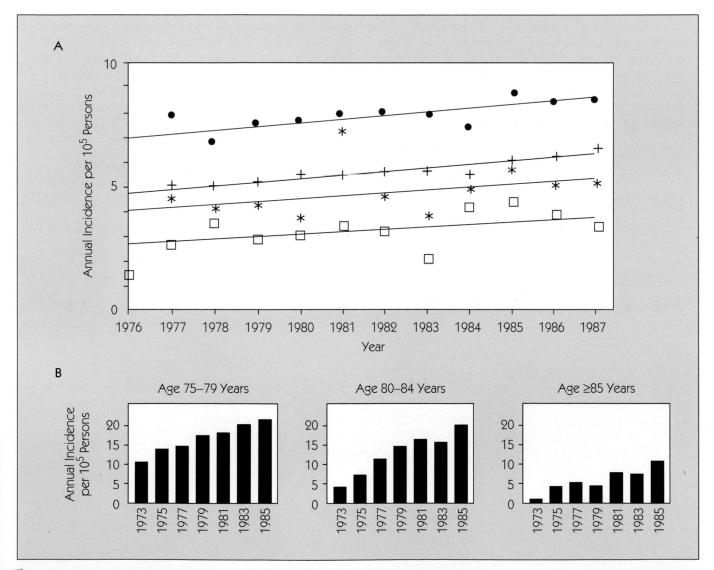

Figure 25.9 Incidence of malignant brain tumors. (A) Recently, there has been a steady increase in the age-adjusted incidence of malignant central nervous system tumors.[21] (B) This increased incidence is particularly prominent in the elderly.[20]

do not occur on the other; sequences with such disparity are termed polymorphic. These polymorphic loci are helpful in two ways. First, the pattern of restriction fragment lengths can distinguish maternal and paternal chromosomes. Second, changes in these patterns can signal that a deletion encompassing the restriction enzyme site has occurred. Informative loci give marked restriction fragments of two different lengths, and the DNA is said to be heterozygous at this locus. When a deletion is large enough to remove both the restriction site and enough surrounding DNA that one chromosome fails to contribute a marked fragment to the digestion products, only one pattern of restriction fragment lengths is obtained, and the DNA is said to be hemizygous at this locus.[22,24]

TSGs in Retinoblastoma

The existence of TSGs was first suggested by studies of familial retinoblastoma, which showed that the tendency to develop retinoblastomas is inherited in dominant fashion.[25] Cytogenetic studies subsequently identified a chromosomal marker, the deletion of the long arm of Ch 13 (13q–), in retinoblastomas. The association between this deletion and tumor development sug-

gested that a gene located on the missing chromosome segment, called the retinoblastoma (Rb) gene, normally suppresses tumor growth. Subsequent studies of retinoblastoma showed that 1) loss of both Rb alleles is necessary for loss of tumor suppressor function, 2) families with inherited retinoblastomas have an inactivating Rb mutation in their germ line, 3) familial tumors occur when the chromosome containing a normal Rb allele suffers a deletion, and 4) sporadically occurring tumors arise only after two genetic insults have been sustained; they are thus less likely to be bilateral or multiple and usually occur later in life than familial tumors.[25]

TSGs in Neurofibromatosis Type 2

Among CNS tumors, those occurring in patients with NF-2 most closely follow the retinoblastoma model. The tendency to develop NF-2 is inherited in dominant fashion and is associated with deletions of the long arm of Ch 22.[26] This suggests the presence of a TSG for NF-2. RFLP studies and genetic linkage analysis have narrowed the search for the NF-2 gene to a sufficiently small area of Ch 22 that genetic testing can now determine if the gene has been lost. Like familial retinoblastomas, tumors in patients with NF-2 are more fre-

Figure 25.10 Phakomatoses

Name	Hallmark Tumor	Other Nervous System Tumors, Abnormalities	Systemic Tumors, Abnormalities	Dermatologic Abnormalities	Frequency (live births)	Gene Locus
NF-1	Cranial, spinal neurofibromas, schwannomas	Optic, brain stem, cerebellar gliomas	Lisch nodules (iris hamartomas)	Café au lait spots, cutaneous neurofibromas	$1/4 \times 10^4$	Dom 17
NF-2	Bilateral acoustic neurinomas	Cerebellar, spinal astrocytomas, meningiomas, and schwannomas	—	—	$1/10^5$	Dom 21
TS	Subependymal giant-cell astrocytoma	Cerebellar, cortical tuberous hamartoma	Retinal, lung, renal hamartomas, cardiac rhabdomyomas	Ash leaf spots, adenoma sebaceum, shagreen patches	$1/10^4$	Dom ?
VHL	Cerebellar, brain stem, spinal cord hemangioblastomas		Retinal angiomas		$1/10^4$	Dom 3

NF=neurofibromatosis; TS=tuberous sclerosis; VHL=von Hippel-Lindau Disease; Dom=dominant.

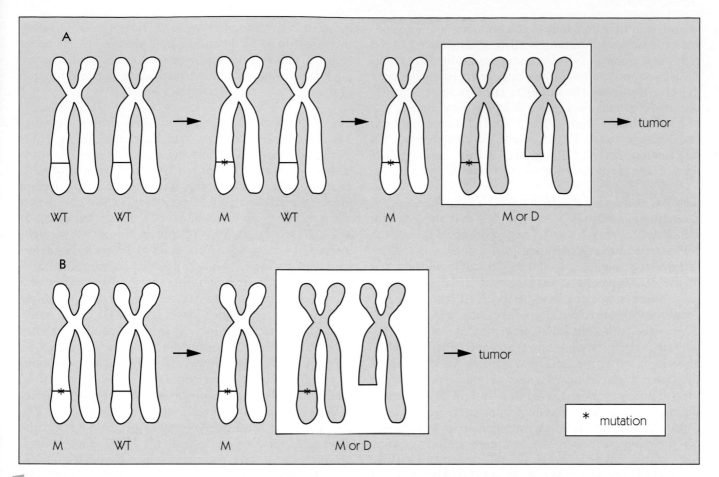

Figure 25.11 Tumor suppressor genes. Tumor suppressor genes are genes whose loss or inactivating mutation (*) contributes to tumorigenesis. (A) Persons with a normal pair of tumor suppressor genes must sustain injury to both genes before tumor suppression is lost. (B) Persons who inherit a mutation in one gene of the pair need only sustain injury to the other gene for tumor suppression to be lost. WT=wild type (normal); M=mutated; D=deleted.

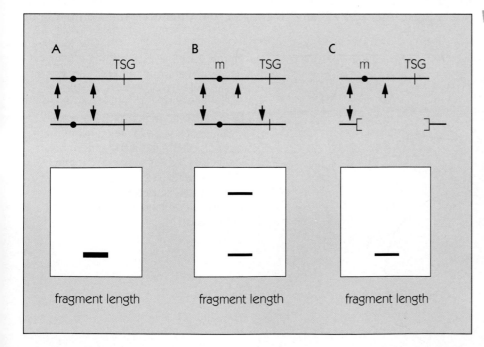

Figure 25.12 Restriction fragment length polymorphism. (A) The genetic locus that contains both the marker gene (m) and the tumor suppressor gene (TSG) is homozygous with respect to the restriction enzyme site (vertical arrow) near the marker gene. Digestion of DNA by the enzyme yields fragments (containing the marker gene) of identical length. A single band of double intensity results. The DNA is homozygous at this locus.
(B) The genetic locus is polymorphic with respect to the restriction enzyme site (vertical arrows). Digestion yields fragments of two different lengths, each of unitary intensity, and the chromosome is heterozygous at this locus.
(C) When a deletion removes the marker gene (as well as the neighboring TSG) from a polymorphic site, digestion yields a single fragment of unitary intensity. The deletion has reduced the previously heterozygous site to hemizygosity.

quently multiple and appear at a younger age than sporadically occurring tumors.[27] Also, when tumors of the types that occur in NF-2 occur sporadically, like nonfamilial retinoblastomas, they appear to have the same genetic lesion as the familial tumors. Sporadically occurring meningiomas have deletions or complete loss of Ch 22. In one study, 43% (17/40) of tumors containing informative Ch 22 loci showed evidence of lost Ch 22 sequences by RFLP analysis, and the karyotypes of 43% (6/14) of tumors showed loss of one Ch 22.[28]

Chromosomal Loss in Neurofibromatosis Type 1

Genetic linkage studies have shown that the gene for NF-1 resides on Ch 17.[29] The hypothetical role of the NF-1 gene in the development of the tumors that characterize this disease is less clearly understood than that of the NF-2 gene. Karyotyping and RFLP analysis of these tumors from patients with NF-1 have failed to show the expected deletions of the long arm of Ch 17. This suggests that the NF-1 gene is not a TSG.

The NF-1 gene may, however, contribute to tumorigenesis by other mechanisms, such as involvement in the signal transduction system of an oncogene similar to ras.[27] The ras oncogene, a 21-kD protein that becomes oncogenic when mutated at particular amino acid residues, is thought to be an intermediary in growth factor signaling pathways. The ras protein binds guanine nucleotides; it is active when GTP is bound and inactive when GTP has been hydrolyzed to GDP. Hydrolysis of ras-bound GTP to GDP is catalyzed by GTPase activating protein (GAP). The NF-1 gene has a 360-bp region that is highly homologous to the catalytic region of GAP.[27] This suggests that a mutation in the NF-1 gene may contribute to tumorigenesis because the

mutated NF-1 protein cannot catalyze the inactivating hydrolysis of GTP bound to a G protein similar to ras (Fig. 25.13). A persistently active protein similar to ras might result in an uninterrupted signal for proliferation of the cell types characteristic of NF-1.

Loss of Chromosomes 10 and 17 in Gliomas

Molecular genetic studies have implicated other TSGs in the development of astrocytomas. Cytogenetic studies have shown the loss of Ch 10 in the majority (19/32) of malignant astrocytomas with nearly diploid stem lines.[30] RFLP analysis of various gliomas has shown that a higher grade of malignancy is associated with loss of Ch 10 sequences. Loss of constitutional heterozygosity for Ch 10 loci was found in 28 of 29 grade IV malignant astrocytomas.[31] Dosage analysis showed that chromosomal nondisjunction rather than recombination was the mechanism of loss. Eleven astrocytomas of lower grade failed to show such loss (Fig. 25.14).

RFLP analysis of loci on other chromosomes has detected losses at nonrandom frequencies of Ch 17 (22%), Ch 22 (19%), and Ch 13 (14%). Allelic deletions of Ch 17 (17p11.2–pter) occur in astrocytomas of all grades of malignancy, but not in nonastrocytic gliomas, such as oligodendrogliomas and ependymomas (see Fig. 25.14).[32] The implicated segment of Ch 17 is on the short arm and does not include the NF-1 gene. It does, however, include the p53 gene, which encodes a nuclear phosphoprotein involved in regulating cell division. The p53 gene appears to be a TSG whose loss or inactivation contributes to the development of colon, breast, and lung carcinomas.[33,34] The wild-type p53 protein binds tumor-promoting viral proteins, such as adenovirus E1B and SV40 large T antigen, and suppresses transformation of

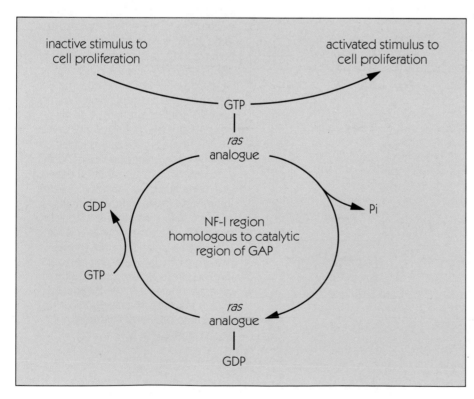

Figure 25.13 Hypothetical tumorigenetic mechanism of neurofibromatosis type 1 (NF-1) mutation. A mutation in the region of NF-1 protein homologous to the catalytic region of GTPase activating protein (GAP) may prevent the catalysis of GTP to GDP that normally inactivates the ras analogue protein. This would result in constitutive activation of a ras-like protein that could provide a continuous stimulus to cell proliferation.[27]

cells by *myc* and *ras* oncogenes.[35] Point mutations in the p53 gene are found more frequently than any other class of genetic changes in human malignancies. These mutations almost always occur at certain "hot spots" in exons 5 through 8. The mutated bases lie within highly conserved sequences of the gene, suggesting that these sequences code for regions of the p53 protein that are critical to its function.[33] Point mutations in exons 5, 7, or 8 that inactivate p53 as a tumor suppressor have been found in astrocytomas (Fig. 25.15).[33]

The short arm of Ch 17 has also been implicated in the development of medulloblastomas and primitive neuroectodermal tumors of the brain, but the role of p53 in these tumors is unknown. Preliminary data suggest that some other locus may be involved.[36]

Oncogenes

The second type of altered genetic expression that leads to tumor development involves oncogenes. Oncogenes are genes whose expression contributes to the origin and maintenance of the transformed state. They have been identified by isolating, from acutely transforming retroviruses and from transfected tumor DNA, the responsible genes.[37] Their oncogenicity is evident in their ability to transform cells in culture into more neoplastic phenotypes and in their capacity when inappropriately expressed in transgenic animals to produce tumors.[38] Many oncogenes are highly homologous or identical to normal cellular genes called proto-oncogenes. Most proto-oncogenes encode proteins involved in the transduction of signals for growth-factor-medi-

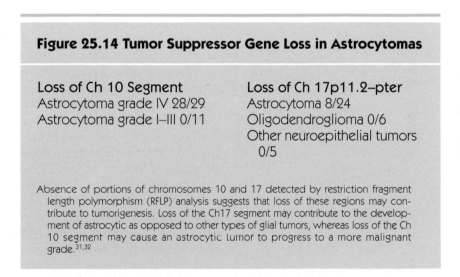

Figure 25.14 Tumor Suppressor Gene Loss in Astrocytomas

Loss of Ch 10 Segment	Loss of Ch 17p11.2–pter
Astrocytoma grade IV 28/29	Astrocytoma 8/24
Astrocytoma grade I–III 0/11	Oligodendroglioma 0/6
	Other neuroepithelial tumors 0/5

Absence of portions of chromosomes 10 and 17 detected by restriction fragment length polymorphism (RFLP) analysis suggests that loss of these regions may contribute to tumorigenesis. Loss of the Ch17 segment may contribute to the development of astrocytic as opposed to other types of glial tumors, whereas loss of the Ch 10 segment may cause an astrocytic tumor to progress to a more malignant grade.[31,32]

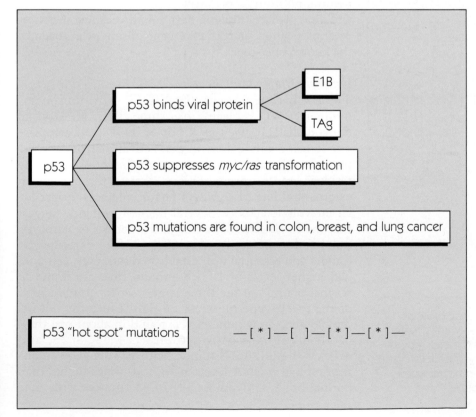

Figure 25.15 The role of the p53 gene in brain tumor development. The p53 gene encodes a protein involved in the control of transcription of genes directing cell division. p53 protein binds to certain transforming viral proteins and suppresses cell transformation by *myc* and *ras* oncogenes. Loss or inactivation of the p53 gene contributes to the development of various carcinomas, and mutations at structurally significant "hot spots" of the p53 gene have been found in astrocytomas.

ated control of cell differentiation and division (Fig. 25.16). Growth factors are small polypeptides that bind to transmembrane receptor molecules, initiating a cascade of biochemical and transcriptional events leading to cell division. Oncogene activation involves genetic changes that lead to increased expression of a proto-oncogene or to expression of a modified proto-oncogene product. The identity of proto-oncogenes and the genes controlling cell division suggests that oncogenes disrupt normal cellular maturation and induce rapid proliferation of tumor cells by coding at inappropriate times for excessive quantities or altered forms of growth factors, growth factor receptors, or related proteins.

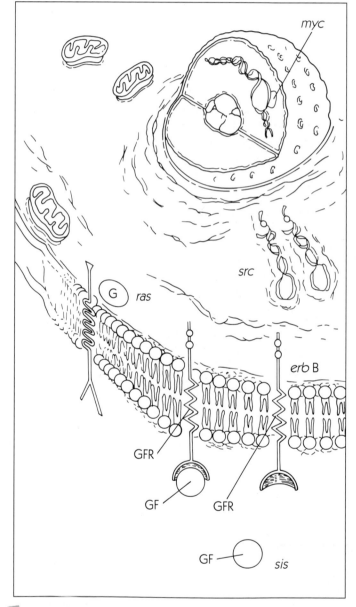

Figure 25.16 Oncogenes. Oncogenes encode proteins involved in growth-factor-mediated control of cell proliferation. Oncoproteins include growth factors (GF-*sis*), growth factor receptors (GFR-*erb*-B), intermediate intracellular signals such as receptor-linked G proteins (*ras*) and nonreceptor tyrosine kinase (*src*), and DNA binding proteins (*myc*).

Oncogenes in Brain Tumors

Evidence of oncogene involvement in the genesis of CNS tumors comes from three types of studies: 1) Southern blotting of tumor DNA to identify amplification or rearrangement of proto-oncogenes; 2) screening of tumor mRNA by Northern blotting, RNA protection assays, or in situ hybridization to identify oncogene expression and increased expression of proto-oncogenes and related genes that might underlie autocrine stimulation; and 3) immunohistochemical studies to identify oncoproteins. Three sets of growth factors and their tyrosine kinase receptors are particularly important to the growth of glial cells and glial tumors: epidermal growth factor (EGF) and transforming growth factor alpha (TGF-α) and their common receptor, EGFR; platelet-derived growth factor (PDGF-α and PDGF-β and their receptors, PDGFR-α and PDGFR-β); and basic fibroblast growth factor (bFGF) and the FGF receptors. Amplification, rearrangement, and overexpression of *erb*-B have been reported in glioblastomas as well as expression of c-*sis* and PDGFRs in anaplastic astrocytomas and glioblastomas and expression of bFGF in malignant gliomas. In addition, amplification and elevated expression of *gli*, *ras*, and N-*myc* proto-oncogenes has been observed in some malignant astrocytomas; such findings are rare, however. Although the c-*myc* proto-oncogene is located on Ch 22, which is altered in many acoustic neuromas, meningiomas, and astrocytomas, it is not in the region of the chromosome usually affected; amplification and rearrangement of the c-*myc* gene has been found in isolated cases of these tumor types as well as in medulloblastomas and primitive neuroectodermal tumors, but such occurrences are rare. Larger surveys of medulloblastomas, primitive neuroectodermal tumors, and glial pediatric tumors have found very few instances of amplification or rearrangement of any of a dozen of the known oncogenes.[39]

Erb-B in Malignant Gliomas

The *erb*-B gene encodes the EGFR. This transmembrane, 170-kD molecule has three parts: an external domain that binds either EGF or TGF-α, a cytoplasmic tyrosine kinase domain that activates secondary signaling molecules by phosphorylating their tyrosine residues, and a transmembrane domain through which external binding of a growth factor enhances intracellular enzymatic activity. Several lines of evidence suggest that the *erb*-B gene has a role in the genesis of astrocytic tumors. In one study, over 80% (25/31) of astrocytic tumors and essentially all established astrocytic cell lines had higher levels of EGFR protein than are found in normal brain.[40] In the three largest series, amplification of the *erb*-B gene in excess of eight times the normal diploid gene copy number was found in about one third of all malignant astrocytomas (24/63, 4/23, and 4/10).[41–43] All (24/24) tumors with EGFR gene amplification had mRNA levels at least 10 times higher than normal brain, and almost all (14/15) tumors with gene amplification had at least twice normal levels of EGFR protein.[41] Many tumors without amplification nevertheless have high levels of mRNA and detectable protein. When the amount of EGFR protein is elevated, enhanced tumor cell proliferation could occur if either ligand were present, and, in fact, expression of EGF or TGF-α or both ligands has been found in all tumors tested.[44]

Rearrangement of the EGFR gene has been observed both with and without amplification.[41–43] Three different rearrangements are commonly found: 1) an internal deletion in the 3′ region similar to that of v-erb-B that lacks sequences essential for down-regulation and, thus, attenuation; 2) a deletion of 248 bp in domain IV that results in an EGFR with elevated basal auto-phosphorylating activity; and 3) an 801-bp deletion in the 5′ region that produces transcripts lacking 267 amino acids of extracellular domains.[41–45] Mutant proteins resulting from these deletions may be abnormally active and provide an unmodulated stimulus to cell proliferation. They may also be good targets for specific immunotherapy; ligand-blocking antibodies to EGFR inhibit proliferation in some malignant glioma cell lines.[46]

C-sis in Malignant Gliomas

The c-sis gene encodes the B chain of PDGF. PDGF, like EGF, stimulates cell proliferation by binding to a transmembrane receptor that has tyrosine kinase activity. PDGF is an important regulator of glial proliferation and differentiation in the optic nerve and cerebrum. In the embryonic optic nerve, type 1 astrocytes, which proliferate in response to EGF, FGF, or trauma, secrete PDGF.[47] This PDGF delays the differentiation and sustains the proliferation of O-2A precursor cells, which occupy a critical branch point in the differentiation of oligodendrocytes and type 2 astrocytes. Many astrocytic tumors have cells that produce both PDGF and PDGFRs; autocrine and paracrine PDGF-induced delay of differentiation and stimulation of proliferation are thus possible.[48,49]

Several other findings suggest a role for c-sis in astrocytic oncogenesis. Simian sarcoma virus (SSV) and its transforming gene, v-sis (a derivative of c-sis), produce glial tumors in animals and transform astrocytes in culture by inducing production of the v-sis protein in cells that have PDGFRs. c-sis DNA, cloned from a human glioma, is transforming when linked to an appropriate upstream transcription initiation site and retroviral LTR promoter. Glial cells transformed in vitro by chemical carcinogens differ from premalignant cells by containing high levels of c-sis mRNA and producing large quantities of PDGF. Antagonists of PDGF (e.g., trapidil) decrease the rate of astrocytoma cell division in vitro.[50–52]

Studies of gene expression in brain tumor specimens have substantiated a role for PDGF A and B and their receptors in the development of glial tumors. Both A and B chains of PDGF are expressed at high levels in most high-grade gliomas but in very few low-grade tumors. In situ hybridization and immunohistochemical studies have shown that the PDGF A chain is commonly produced by tumor cells, and the α receptor is found on tumor cells. The PDGF B chain is produced predominantly by the endothelium of hyperproliferative tumor vessels, and β receptors are highly concentrated in tumor vasculature. These findings suggest that the PDGF A-α receptor pair may be predominant in tumor cell division, whereas the PDGF B-β receptor pair may be more important to vascular proliferation.[53]

The mechanisms underlying the high levels of expression of PDGF and PDGFR in astrocytomas are unknown; searches for rearrangement or amplification of the relevant genes have found only a few cases of amplification of the PDGF-α gene. Thus, although in vitro studies have shown the oncogenicity of alteration or overexpression of the c-sis gene, and analysis of tumor specimens has shown high levels of expression of PDGF and PDGFR genes, it remains to be established whether this expression is a fundamental etiologic feature of tumorigenesis or merely an epiphenomenon of rapid cell division.

Fibroblast Growth Factors in Brain Tumors

FGFs are another class of glial mitogens produced by normal and malignant astrocytes.[54,55] FGF receptors also have tyrosine kinase activity. Although both FGF genes share homology with the int-2 and hst oncogenes, an oncogenic function in brain tumors has not yet been ascribed to either gene. The angiogenic potency of bFGF, its mitogenicity for glial cells, and its omnipresence in astrocytic tumors suggest that bFGF has a role in the development of astrocytomas. In fact, bFGF mRNA transcripts and bFGF protein have been found in virtually all CNS tumors tested: mRNA in 17 of 18 gliomas and 20 of 22 meningiomas; protein in 11 of 12 glioblastomas, 16 of 16 astrocytomas, 5 of 5 ependymomas, 11 of 11 meningiomas, and 6 of 6 nerve sheath tumors.[54,55] Originally isolated from gliomas as a tumor angiogenesis factor, bFGF, like PDGF B, is more common in endothelial cells than in astrocytic cells of a tumor. Other growth factors and growth-factor-related oncogenes implicated in the development of some gliomas are insulin-like growth factor I, a glial mitogen, and its tyrosine kinase receptor and the ros oncogene, another receptor with tyrosine kinase activity.

CAUSES OF GENETIC DAMAGE

The alterations in genetic expression discussed above result from deletions or mutations of DNA. Such changes can occur as a result of errors in normal endogenous cellular processes—nondisjunction during mitosis can result in the absence of an entire chromosome, and infidelity of DNA replication or repair can result in base substitutions. Many, however, are caused by exogenous mutagens. An agent is mutagenic if it induces permanent alterations in a cell's DNA; it is carcinogenic if a tumor results from these alterations. There are three main types of mutagens: radiation, chemical, and viral. Each type has been implicated in the etiology of brain tumors.

Radiation

Three types of radiation have been mentioned as possible mutagens: sparsely ionizing (low linear energy transfer) radiation in the form of gamma photons, x-rays, or electron beams; densely ionizing (high linear energy transfer) radiation, such as neutrons or heavy ions; and nonionizing electromagnetic field (EMF) radiation. Mutations from ionizing radiation result from modification of DNA bases (e.g., dimerization of adjacent pyrimidine bases that interferes with DNA replication by blocking DNA polymerase) or the induction of strand breaks that undergo faulty repair.[56] Ionizing radiation in the form of therapeutic photons, diagnostic or therapeutic x-rays, therapeutic heavy-particle irradiation, or residential or occupational exposure to nuclear facilities is a risk factor for the development of brain tumors. An increased incidence of meningiomas is seen in adults who underwent scalp irradiation for ringworm as children, and there are numerous reports of malignant gliomas, meningiomas, and sarcomas arising 5 to 30 years after brain irradiation in the treatment of childhood tumors. The mechanisms by which EMF radiation might be mutagenic are unknown. The case for EMF as a mutagen is based on increased incidences of brain tumors in children and adults who had residential and occupational exposure.[57] These preliminary observations have not yet been substantiated by rigorous epidemiologic studies.

Chemical

Chemical mutagens include both endogenous and exogenous agents, which may react directly with DNA or exert their effect through a metabolite. Animal studies have demonstrated the mutagenicity of chemicals such as polycyclic aromatic hydrocarbons and nitroso compounds. These agents cause structural DNA damage by altering DNA bases.[58] N-alkyl nitrosoureas (MNU and ENU) alter bases by transferring their electrophilic alkyl group to the O-4 of thymine or the O-6 of guanine. Hydrolysis of altered bases from the DNA promotes mispairing that results in a point mutation. When applied to fetal mice transplacentally, ENU produces multiple types of malignant gliomas in the adult animals.

Epidemiologic studies have confirmed these findings.[58] Nitroso compounds are probably responsible for the increased risk of brain tumors among workers in the rubber industry. Organic chlorides are most likely involved in the increased risk of tumors in agricultural workers. Vinyl chloride and various petrochemicals have also been implicated.

Viral

The case for the oncogenicity of viruses in animals is quite strong. Inoculation of fetal brains with simian sarcoma virus produces glioblastomas. JC human polyoma virus induces medulloblastomas. There are two hypothetical mechanisms of viral oncogenicity: The virus carries an oncogene in its own genome, which, when expressed in the host cell, stimulates cell proliferation, or viral insertion into the host genome changes the expression or structure of a gene involved in the control of cell proliferation. Although highly plausible, the role of viruses in the etiology of human brain tumors has not been substantiated by epidemiologic or clinicopathologic studies.

HOST FACTORS

The susceptibility of animals to tumorigenesis depends on a number of conditions that vary among individuals. Two host factors, one cellular and one systemic, deserve mention. The first is the proliferative state of the cell. An actively dividing cell is much more likely to sustain DNA damage than a quiescent cell. This is due to the increased vulnerability of unraveled DNA to mutagens, the lower fidelity of repair of DNA strand breaks during the S phase of the cell cycle, and the increased likelihood of chromosomal loss during mitosis. This factor explains why many tumors arise from the germinal layers of the brain (e.g., astrocytomas from the subependymal layer and medulloblastomas from the external granular layer), where most cell division occurs; why the brain, most of whose cells are quiescent, has a relatively low incidence of tumors; and why conditions that cause brain cells to re-enter the cell cycle may increase the risk of tumor (e.g., injury to the brain from trauma or multiple sclerosis).[59]

Anecdotal evidence of an association between brain injury and tumor development abounds, but epidemiologic and experimental support is deficient. Reports of meningiomas arising at the site of previous trauma (e.g., dural injury from depressed skull fractures, gunshot wounds, and other in-driven metal fragments) are common. Gliomas have developed at the site of cerebral contusions, abscesses, bullet wounds, and surgical incisions. Most retrospective and prospective studies, however, have found no association.[59] Animal studies have shown that unilateral trauma can increase the incidence and bias the laterality of tumor development in rats treated transplacentally with ENU.[60] This suggests that the role of brain injury in tumorigenesis is to stimulate proliferation with its concomitant vulnerability to mutagens.

Other causes of brain injury (e.g., multiple sclerosis, amyotrophic lateral sclerosis, and progressive multifocal leukoencephalopathy) that induce quiescent glial cells to re-enter the cell cycle may also increase the likelihood of developing a glial tumor. Over 20 cases of brain tumors in patients with multiple sclerosis have been reported.[61] In some cases, the tumor was contiguous with a plaque of demyelination or with plaque and astrocytic hyperplasia in some cases, but in others, no plaque could be seen at the tumor site. The slight female preponderance, the predominance of malignant astrocytomas, and the frequency of tumors arising from the subependymal region in this series of cases have been taken as evidence of a causal relation,[61] but the same findings would be predicted in the case of random co-occurrence. The relatively high incidence of multiple gliomas in this group of patients (25% versus 5% in most unselected series of gliomas) suggests a nonrandom association between multiple sclerosis and brain tumors.

The second host factor that determines susceptibility to tumorigenesis is the immune status of the patient. Iatrogenic immunosuppression by oncologic chemotherapy or drugs given to prevent transplant rejection, inherited immunodeficiency disorders, and acquired conditions such as AIDS can predispose patients to the development of tumors, including those of the brain. The recent rise in the incidence of primary CNS lymphoma that has accompanied the AIDS epidemic is a dramatic example of this phenomenon.[62]

PATHOGENESIS

The mutagenic agents described above are carcinogenic by virtue of their ability to change the structure or expression of oncogenes and TSGs. An individual cell that accumulates several of these changes acquires a growth advantage over surrounding untransformed cells such that subsequent rounds of cell division occur more frequently. The rate of cell division escapes normal controls; proliferation of the transformed cell and its progeny becomes partially autonomous, independent of the requirement for growth factor stimulation to divide, and the neoplastic process is initiated.[63] Tumor initiation usually occurs in a single cell; most tumors are therefore clonally derived from a single precursor.

THE VULNERABILITY OF CLONOGENIC CELLS

Actively dividing cells are more likely than quiescent cells to initiate tumors because they are more likely to sustain transforming DNA injury. Furthermore, for this DNA injury to be tumorigenic, the affected cell must be in or capable of re-entering the cell cycle. Each cell type thus has a "window of vulnerability," during which the cell can sustain DNA injury yet still be able to divide.[63] The types of tumors that arise in the brain and the relative frequencies with which they occur depend on the histologic types of cells that are vulnerable, the quantity of each type, and the duration of the vulnerable period. In animal models, the type of tumor induced by transplacental exposure to carcinogens is highly dependent on the gestational age at exposure; the histology of the tumor reflects the stage of neuroglial differentiation during which exposure occurs.[63]

In humans, environmental factors that may predispose to the development of astrocytomas (e.g., multiple sclerosis and brain trauma) are those which re-open the window of vulnerability by inducing reactive astrocytes to proliferate.[64]

Most neurons and glia have limited proliferative capacity postnatally. Tumors of the CNS are therefore less common than tumors of such tissues as the respiratory or intestinal epithelium. Among CNS tumors, cerebral astrocytomas are relatively common because of the large number of glial cells, some of which can re-enter the cell cycle even in adulthood. Medulloblastomas are also relatively common because primitive medulloblasts continue to divide until several weeks after birth.[64] The spatial distribution of CNS tumors reflects the same factors. Cerebral astrocytomas tend to arise from the subependymal germinal layer, the molecular layer of the cerebral cortex, or the dentate gyrus; cerebral oligodendrogliomas arise from white matter tracts undergoing myelination; and medulloblastomas commonly arise from the outer granular layer of the cerebellar cortex.[63]

TUMOR PROGRESSION

Through repeated cycles of division, a clonogenic cell produces a mass of similar cells that displaces surrounding tissues. At this stage, the tumor is homogeneous; its cells are similar in size and shape to one another and resemble normal cells in their degree of differentiation; necrosis is uncommon and vascularity is usually limited.[64] The tumor expands slowly in a noninvasive fashion and is considered benign. As tumor cells repeatedly re-enter the cell cycle, however, their DNA is highly vulnerable to additional mutagens. Further genetic damage is incurred, and clonogenic subpopulations of cells with greater growth advantage emerge.[63] Proliferation is faster; the growth fraction increases as more tumor cells proliferate rather than remain quiescent. Tumor growth is less respectful of normal tissue boundaries and becomes infiltrative. The tumor's cells become less similar to one another and less differentiated. Mitotic figures abound, vascularity increases, and necrosis occurs. This rapid, more invasive tumor growth indicates progression to a higher grade of malignancy.[64]

TUMOR-HOST INTERACTION

Tumor Heterogeneity

The genetic instability of rapidly dividing tumor cells results in a phenotypic heterogeneity that is of fundamental importance to the interaction of the tumor and the host. Heterogeneous tumor cells constitute the substrate for selection of progressively more malignant tumor subclones and, in turn, the more rapidly proliferating malignant cells have greater genetic lability.[63] The heterogeneity of malignant cells is evident at many levels. Tumor tissue has different degrees of cellularity, vascularity, and necrosis; cells differ in size and shape, as do their nuclei; cytoplasmic differentiation varies but tends to be limited; DNA ploidy varies (from 2C to 8C in some malignant gliomas), and karyotypes may show various patterns of chromosomal loss, gain, and rearrangement.[30] This heterogeneity also hampers therapeutic efforts: Division between well-oxygenated proliferating cells and poorly-oxygenated nonproliferating cells limits the efficacy of radiation therapy, differences in metabolic profiles and enzyme complements hasten the development of drug resistance, and heterogeneity of surface antigens facilitates invasiveness and hinders immunologic defenses.[63]

Invasiveness

Invasiveness is the critical deterrent to cure for most malignant CNS tumors. In malignant gliomas, invasion is achieved by the motility of individual cells, which are usually small, round, and mitotically active and have dark, oval nuclei.[63] These cells often migrate along fiber tracts and cortical and ventricular surfaces; the migration is directed by the interaction of cell surface receptors and extracellular matrix and is facilitated by tumor cell secretion of metallinoproteases and plasminogen activators that promote degradation of the basement membrane. Normal tissue is destroyed by proteolytic activity and phagocytosis.[64]

Immune Suppression

The immune response to brain tumors is hindered by several factors. The blood-brain barrier and the absence of a lymphatic system in the brain confer partial protection from immune surveillance. CNS tumors do not express the major histocompatibility complex antigens or tumor-specific antigens necessary to provoke an immune response; antigens that are expressed in a tumor are heterogeneous and change rapidly. Also, tumor cells produce immuno suppressive factors.[65,66] Both the humoral antibody and cell-mediated immune responses are depressed in patients with malignant gliomas. Antiglioma antibodies are rarely produced, are nonspecific, and are often incapable of mediating cytotoxicity.

Clinical studies of patients with malignant gliomas have demonstrated reduction in delayed hypersensitivity reaction to skin antigens, in the numbers of peripheral blood lymphocytes, in lymphocytic blastogenic responses, in natural killer cell activity, and in the production of interleukin-2 and its receptors by activated T cells.[65] The number of lymphocytes that infiltrate a tumor and the extent of the infiltration are more limited in gliomas than in tumors of other organs. This suppression of the immune response may be mediated by factors secreted by or expressed on the surface of tumor cells. Secreted antigens may activate suppressor T cells or block the cytotoxic T-lymphocyte response by binding to a specific immune receptor.[65] Cytokines such as TGF-β2 and PGE$_2$ secreted by tumor cells may inhibit the generation of cytotoxic lymphocytes and activated natural killer cells.[65-67]

CONCLUSION

Three features—heterogeneity, invasiveness, and immunosuppression—act to give malignant tumors a significant advantage in host-tumor interaction. Once a benign tumor sustains sufficient genetic damage to progress to a more malignant phenotype, the all-too-frequent outcome is progressive tumor growth, clinical deterioration, and death. Additional research into the basic causes of tumor initiation and progression as well as the phenomena of genetic instability, phenotypic heterogeneity, invasiveness, and immunosuppression offers the best hope of altering this prognosis.

REFERENCES

1. Willis RA. *The Spread of Tumors in the Human Body.* 2nd ed. London: Butterworth; 1952.
2. Bailey P, Cushing H. *Classification of the Tumors of the Glioma Group on a Histogenetic Basis with a Correlated Study of Prognosis.* Philadelphia, Pa: JB Lippincott; 1926.
3. Zulch KJ. *Histological Typing of Tumors of the Central Nervous System.* Geneva: World Health Organization; 1979. International Histological Classification of Tumors, 21.
4. Garcia J. Classification of brain tumors. In: Salcman M, ed. *Neurobiology of Brain Tumors: Concepts in Neurosurgery.* Baltimore, Md: Williams & Wilkins; 1991;4:19–32.
5. Kernohan JW, Mabon RF, Svien JH, et al. Symposium on a new and simplified concept of gliomas. *Proc Mayo Clin.* 1949;24:71–75.
6. Burger PC. The grading of astrocytomas and oligodendrogliomas. In: Fields WS, ed. *Primary Brain Tumors: A Review of Histologic Classification.* New York, NY: Springer-Verlag; 1989:171–180.
7. Davis RL. Grading of gliomas. In: Fields WS, ed. *Primary Brain Tumors: A Review of Histologic Classification.* New York, NY: Springer-Verlag; 1989: 150–158.
8. Daumas-Duport C. A new uniform grading system. In: Fields WS, ed. *Primary Brain Tumors: A Review of Histologic Classification.* New York, NY: Springer-Verlag; 1989:159–170.
9. Hoshino T. Cell kinetics of brain tumors. In: Salcman M, ed. *Neurobiology of Brain Tumors: Concepts in Neurosurgery.* Baltimore, Md: Williams & Wilkins; 1991;4:19–32.
10. Zuber P, Hamou M, de Tribolet N. Identification

of proliferating cells in human gliomas using the monoclonal antibody Ki-67. *Neurosurgery.* 1988; 22:364–368.

11. Molenaar WM, Trojanowski JQ. Biological markers of glial and primitive tumors. In: Salcman M, ed. *Neurobiology of Brain Tumors: Concepts in Neurosurgery.* Baltimore, Md: Williams & Wilkins; 1991;4:185–210.

12. Schoenberg BS. Epidemiology of primary intracranial neoplasms: disease distribution and risk factors. In: Salcman M, ed. *Neurobiology of Brain Tumors: Concepts in Neurosurgery.* Baltimore, Md: Williams and Wilkins; 1991;4:3–18.

13. Green JR, Waggener JD, Kriesgsfield BA. Classification and incidence of neoplasms of the central nervous system. *Adv Neurol.* 1976;15:51–55.

14. Walker AE, Robins M, Weinfield FD. Epidemiology of brain tumors: the national survey of intracranial neoplasms. *Neurology.* 1985;35: 219–226.

15. Chandra V, Bharucha NE, Schoenburg BS. Mortality data for the U.S. for death due to and related to twenty neurological diseases. *Neuroepidemiology.* 1984;3:149–168.

16. Bahemuka M, Massey EW, Schoenberg BS. International mortality from primary nervous system neoplasms: distribution and trends. *Neuroepidemiology.* 1983;2:196–205.

17. Helseth A, Mork SJ. Neoplasms of the central nervous system in Normal, III: epidemiological characteristics of intracranial gliomas according to histology. *APMIS.* 1989;97:547–555.

18. Schoenberg BS, Christine BW, Whisnant JP. The descriptive epidemiology of primary intracranial neoplasms—the Connecticut experience. *Am J Epidemiol.* 1976;104:499–510.

19. Heshmat MY, Kovi J, Simpson, et al. Neoplasms of the central nervous system: incidence and population selectivity in the Washington, DC, metropolitan area. *Cancer.* 1979;38:2135–2142.

20. Greig NH, Reis LG, Yancik R, Paroport SI. Increasing annual incidence of primary malignant brain tumors in the elderly. *J Natl Cancer Inst.* 1990;82:1621–1624.

21. *Annual Cancer Statistic Review.* Bethesda, Md: National Cancer Institute; 1989. NIH publication 90-2789.

22. Martuza RL. Neurofibromatosis as a model for tumor formation in the human nervous system. In: Salcman M, ed. *Neurobiology of Brain Tumors: Concepts in Neurosurgery.* Baltimore, Md: Williams & Wilkins; 1991;4:53–62.

23. Shoenberg B, Christine B, Whisnant J. Nervous system neoplasms and primary malignancies of other sites: the unique association between meningiomas and breast cancer. *Neurology.* 1975;25: 705–712.

24. McDonald J, Dohrmann G. Molecular biology of brain tumors. *Neurosurgery.* 1988;23:537–544.

25. Knudson AG. Hereditary cancer, oncogenes, and antioncogenes. *Cancer Res.* 1985;45:1437–1443.

26. Seizinger BR, Rouleau G, Ozelius LJ, et al. Common pathogenetic mechanism for three tumor types in bilateral acoustic neurofibromatosis. *Science.* 1987;236:317–319.

27. Xu G, O'Connell P, Viskochill D, et al. The neurofibromatosis type 1 gene encodes a protein related to GAP. *Cell.* 1990;62:599–608.

28. Seizinger BR, de la Monte S, Atkins L, et al. Molecular genetic approach to human meningioma: loss of genes of Ch 22. *Proc Natl Acad Sci USA.* 1987;84:5419–5423.

29. Barker D, Wright E, Nguyen K, et al. Gene for von Recklinghausen neurofibromatosis is in the pericentric region of Ch 17. *Science.* 1987;236: 1100–1102.

30. Bigner SJ, Mark J, Burger PC, et al. Specific chromosomal abnormalities in malignant human gliomas. *Cancer Res.* 1988;48:405–411.

31. James CD, Carlbom E, Nordenskjold M, et al. Mitotic recombination of Ch 17 in astrocytomas. *Proc Natl Acad Sci USA.* 1989;86:2858–2862.

32. James CD, Carlbom E, Dumanski J, et al. Clonal genomic alterations in glioma malignancy stages. *Cancer Res.* 1988;48:5546–5551.

33. Hollstein M, Sidransky D, Volgestein B, Harris C. p53 mutations in human cancers. *Science.* 1991; 253:49–53.

34. Bruner J, Saya H, Moser R. Immunocytochemical detection of p53 in human gliomas. *Mod Pathol.* 1991;4:671–677.

35. Levine A. p53 tumor suppressor gene and gene product. *International Symposium of Princess Takamatsu Cancer Research Fund.* 1989;20:221–230.

36. Thomas GA, Raffel C. Loss of heterozygosity on 6q, 16q, and 17p in human CNS primitive neuroectodermal tumors. *Cancer Res.* 1991;51:639–643.

37. Bishop JM. The molecular genetics of cancer. *Science.* 1987;235:305–311

38. Weinberg RA. Oncogenes of spontaneous and induced tumors. *Adv Cancer Res.* 1982;37:33–73.

39. Wasson JC, Saylors RL, Zeltzer P, et al. Oncogene amplification in pediatric brain tumors. *Cancer Res.* 1990;50:2987–2900.

40. Bigner SJ, Burger PC, Wong AJ, et al. Gene amplification in malignant human gliomas: clinical and histopathological aspects. *J Neuropathol Exp Neurol.* 1988;47:191–205.

41. Malden LT, Novak U, Kaye AH, Burgess QW. Selective amplification of the cytoplasmic domain of the EGFR gene in primary human brain tumors of glial origin. *Cancer Res.* 1988;48:2711–2714.

42. Libermann TA, Nusbaum HR, Razon N, et al. Amplification, enhanced expression, and possible rearrangement of EGFR gene in primary human tumors of glial origin. *Nature.* 1985;313:144–147.

43. Wong A, Bigner S, Bigner D, Kinzler K, Hamil-

ton S, Vogelstein B. Increased expression of the EGFR gene in malignant gliomas is invariably associated with gene amplification. *Proc Natl Acad Sci USA.* 1988;84:6899–6903.

44. Ekstrand AJ, James CD, Cavanee WK, et al. Genes for EGFR, TGF-α and EGF and their expression in human gliomas in vivo. *Cancer Res.* 1991;51:2643–2172.

45. Walton G, Chen W, Rosenfeld M, et al. Analysis of deletions of the carboxyl terminus of the EGFR reveals self phosphorylation at tyrosine 992 and enhanced in vivo tyrosine phosphorylation of cell substrates. *J Biol Chem.* 1990;265:1750–1754.

46. Humphrey P, Wong A, Vogelstein B, et al. Antisynthetic peptide antibody reacting at the fusion junction of deletion mutant EGFR in human glioblastoma. *Proc Natl Acad Sci USA.* 1990;87:4207–4211.

47. Raff M. Glial cell diversification in the rat optic nerve. *Science.* 1989;242:1450–1455.

48. Nister M, Heldin CH, Westermark B. Clonal variation in the production of a PDGF-like protein and expression of corresponding receptors in a human malignant glioma. *Cancer Res.* 1988;46:332–340.

49. Harsh G, Keating M Escobedo J, et al. Platelet-derived growth factor (PDGF) autocrine component in human tumor cell lines. *J Neurooncol.* 1990;8:1–12.

50. Gazit A, Igarishi H, Ciu IM, et al. Expression of the normal human *sis*/PDGF-2 coding sequence induces cellular transformation. *Cell.* 1984;39:89–97.

51. Lens P, Altena B, Nusse R. Expression of C-*sis* and PDGF in in vitro transformed glioma cells from rat brain tissue transplacentally treated with ethyl nitrosourea. *Mol Cell Biol.* 1986;6:3537–3540.

52. Kuratsu J, Ushio Y. Antiproliferative effects of trapidil, a PDGF antagonist in a glioma cell in vitro. *J Neurosurg.* 1990;73:436–440.

53. Hermansson M, Nister M, Betsholtz C, et al. Endothelial cell hyperplasia in human glioblastoma: co-expression of mRNA for PDGF B chain and PDGF receptor suggests autocrine growth stimulation. *Proc Natl Acad Sci USA.* 1988;85:7748–7752.

54. Paulus W, Grothe C, Sensenbrenner M, et al. Localization of bFGF, a mitogen and angiogenic factor in human brain tumors. *Acta Neuropathol.* 1990;79:418–423.

55. Takahashi JA, Mori H, Fukumoto M, et al. Gene expresson of FGF in human gliomas and meningiomas: demonstration of cellular source of bFGF mRNA and peptide in tumor tissue. *Proc Natl Acad Sci USA.* 1990;87:5710–5714.

56. Marks J. Ionizing radiation. In: Salcman M, ed. *Neurobiology of Brain Tumors: Concepts in Neurosurgery.* Baltimore Md: Williams & Wilkins; 1991;4:299–320.

57. Nasca P, Baptiste M, MacLubbing P, et al. An epidemiologic case-control study of CNS tumors in children and parental occupational exposures. *Am J Epidemiol.* 1988;128:1256–1265.

58. Berger M, Ali-Osman F. Mutagenesis and DNA repair mechanisms. In: Salcman M, ed. *Neurobiology of Brain Tumors: Concepts in Neurosurgery.* Baltimore, Md: Williams & Wilkins; 1991;4:63–72.

59. Morantz RA. Trauma and demyelination as etiologic factors in the development of brain tumor. In: Salcman M, ed. *Neurobiology of Brain Tumors: Concepts in Neurosurgery.* Baltimore, Md: Williams & Wilkins; 1991;4:73–84.

60. Morantz RA, Shain W. Trauma and brain tumors: an experimental study. *Neurosurgery.* 1978;3:181–186.

61. Hochberg F, Gabbai A. Risk factors in the development of glioblastoma and other brain tumors. In: Williams R, Rengachary S, eds. *Neurosurgery Update I.* New York, NY: McGraw-Hill;1990:233–244.

62. So Y, Beckstead J, Davis R. Primary central nervous system lymphoma in acquired immune deficiency syndrome: a clinical and pathological study. *Ann Neurol.* 1986;20:566–572.

63. Rubinstein L. Glioma cytogeny and differentiation viewed through the window of neoplastic vulnerability. In: Salcman M, ed. *Neurobiology of Brain Tumors: Concepts in Neurosurgery.* Baltimore, Md: Williams & Wilkins; 1991;4:35–52.

64. Schiffer O. Patterns of tumor growth. In: Salcman M, ed. *Neurobiology of Brain Tumors: Concepts in Neurosurgery.* Baltimore, Md: Williams & Wilkins; 1991;4:85–136.

65. Couldwell W, Mitchell M, Mazumder A, et al. Immunology and immunotherapy of intrinsic glial tumors. In: Apuzzo M, ed. *Malignant Cerebral Glioma.* Chicago, Ill: American Association of Neurological Surgeons; 1990:41–58.

66. Young H, Merchant R, Apuzzo M. Immunocompetence of patients with malignant giomas. In: Salcman M, ed. *Neurobiology of Brain Tumors: Concepts in Neurosurgery.* Baltimore, Md: Williams & Wilkins; 1991;4:211–228.

67. Sawamura Y, de Tribolet N. Immunology of brain tumors. *Adv Tech Stand Neurosurg.* 1990;17:3–64.

Chapter 26

Gliomas

Jeffrey D. McDonald, Mark L. Rosenblum

Gliomas are central nervous system (CNS) tumors derived from cells believed to be of glial origin. Constituting 45% to 55% of intracranial tumors in most hospital-based series,[1,2] gliomas are the most common of the CNS tumors. In one large population-based survey,[3] it was estimated that as many as 62% of all intracranial tumors, excluding pituitary adenomas, were gliomas. In common usage, the term *glioma* comprises a heterogeneous mixture of tumors whose biology, treatment, and prognosis vary tremendously. Pilocytic astrocytomas, for example, a tumor found in young patients, can often be cured by surgery alone, whereas glioblastoma multiforme, a relentlessly aggressive tumor of older adults, is rapidly fatal despite multimodality therapy. The tumors discussed in this chapter are pilocytic, low-grade, and anaplastic astrocytomas, glioblastoma multiforme, oligodendroglioma, and ependymoma, which constitute a subset of neuroepithelial tumors as defined by the World Health Organization (WHO) (Fig. 26.1).[4]

CLASSIFICATION OF GLIOMAS

Surprisingly little agreement exists as to the classification of glial tumors. For a variety of historical and political reasons, it has been difficult to establish a uniform set of histologic criteria and a common nomenclature. Indeed, many classification systems have been used, and it can be difficult to compare prognoses and treatment outcomes reported in the literature. Therefore, it is important to understand the similarities and differences of the various systems used to classify gliomas.

HISTOLOGIC CLASSIFICATION OF ASTROCYTOMAS

The major systems currently used to classify astrocytomas are summarized in Figure 26.2.

The first widely influential system for classifying gliomas was devised in 1926 by Bailey and Cushing.[5] Based on a perceived histologic resemblance of many

---

Figure 26.1 World Health Organization Classification of Tumors of Neuroepithelial Tissue

Astrocytic Tumors
1. Pilocytic astrocytoma
2. Astrocytoma (fibrillary, protoplasmic, gemistocytic subtypes)
3. Anaplastic astrocytoma
4. Others, including subependymal giant cell astrocytoma and astroblastoma

Oligodendroglial Tumors
1. Oligodendroglioma
2. Mixed oligoastrocytoma
3. Anaplastic oligodendroglioma

Ependymal and Choroid Plexus Tumors
1. Ependymoma (including myxopapillary, papillary, and subependymoma subtypes)
2. Anaplastic ependymoma
3. Choroid plexus papilloma
4. Anaplastic choroid plexus papilloma

Poorly Differentiated and Embryonal Tumors
1. Glioblastoma (including sarcomatous and giant cell variants)
2. Medulloblastoma (including desmoplastic and medullomyoblastoma variants)
3. Gliomatosis cerebri
4. Others (including medulloepithelioma and primitive polar spongioblastoma)

Pineal Cell Tumors (including pineocytoma and pineoblastoma)

Neuronal Tumors (including gangliocytoma and ganglioglioma with anaplastic variants, ganglioneuroblastoma, neuroblastoma)

Tumors commonly designated as gliomas include the astrocytic tumors, oligodendrogliomas, ependymomas, and glioblastoma multiforme (here classified with other poorly differentiated tumors).

---

tumor cells to various types of developing cells in the embryonic brain, this "histogenetic" classification incorporated ideas about the cells of origin of the tumors and yielded prognostic information derived from the presumed proliferative potential of those cells. In practice, the intermediate forms of astrocytomas were difficult to classify with this system.

In 1949, Kernohan et al.[6] proposed a four-tiered system based on the degree of anaplasia. Astrocytomas, as well as ependymomas and oligodendrogliomas, are examined for cellularity, nuclear and cellular morphology, vascular proliferation, mitotic figures, and necrosis, as well as the amount of normal-appearing tissue. The tumors are graded I to IV, from the highest to lowest percentage of normal-appearing tissue, with a corresponding increase in the prominence of anaplastic features in higher-grade tumors. Grade III and grade IV tumors are both considered glioblastoma multiforme, and it has proven difficult to distinguish between them.

For many years, the Kernohan system was the mainstay of pathologic classification of glial tumors, and it remains influential today because of its widespread use in the training of pathologists and neuropathologists.[7] The system has been criticized, however, because well-differentiated low-grade astrocytomas and pilocytic astrocytomas are included in the same category (grade I). Today, these tumors are generally considered separate entities based on biologic and prognostic variables. Furthermore, in some series, little difference in survival was seen between grade II and grade III tumors. Other studies suggested that grade I and grade II tumors behaved similarly, as did tumors in grades III and IV. Thus, the Kernohan classification is effectively a two-tiered system.[8]

In 1950, Ringertz[9] proposed a three-tiered system that was later popularized by Burger et al.[10,11] and used in many cooperative brain tumor clinical trials. In this system, pilocytic astrocytomas are considered a separate group; the other astrocytomas are classified into three types based on the presence of histologic characteristics of anaplasia. Necrosis is a particularly important feature in this scheme because it distinguishes anaplastic astrocytoma from glioblastoma. This system yields useful prognostic information and distinct survival curves for patients in each category.

The persistent lack of agreement concerning classification and nomenclature, especially in international discussions of cancer studies and prognosis, prompted an effort by the WHO to establish uniform criteria to classify brain tumors. As reported by Zulch,[4,12] the WHO classification categorizes neuroepithelial tumors based on the principal cell type and the degree of anaplasia. It further distinguishes tumor grade and hence prognosis based on predicted biologic behavior. Necrosis is not the crucial, or most important, criterion that separates anaplastic astrocytoma from glioblastoma multiforme, as in the Ringertz and Burger scheme. Glioblastoma is classified as a poorly differentiated or embryonal tumor,

a broad category that also includes medulloblastomas (see Fig. 26.1); the WHO scheme is the only one in which glioblastoma is classified separately from the other gliomas. In practice, it is essentially a three-tier system: Nonpilocytic astrocytomas are classified as astrocytoma, anaplastic astrocytoma, and glioblastoma multiforme. (This system will be adhered to as much as possible throughout this chapter.)

In 1988, Daumas-Duport et al.[8] proposed a simple, easily reproducible scheme to classify astrocytomas. Four histologic criteria of anaplasia are defined, and the tumor grade equals the number of criteria present. Tumors with one feature are grade I, those with two features are grade II, and so on. When this system was applied to the Mayo Clinic and Massachusetts General Hospital series, grade I tumors were extremely rare.[8,13] Thus, the vast majority of tumors will fall into one of three categories. This system generates clearly distinct survival curves for patients with grade II to IV tumors. However, when patients over 50 years of age in the Massachusetts General Hospital series were examined separately, the survival curves were essentially the same regardless of tumor grade.[13]

The classification used at our institution divides nonpilocytic astrocytomas into four categories: mildly, moderately, and highly anaplastic astrocytomas and glioblastoma multiforme.[14] Mildly anaplastic astrocytomas are very rare; moderately and highly anaplastic astrocytomas correspond approximately to grades II and III, respectively, of other systems (excluding Kernohan), and glioblastoma multiforme corresponds to grade IV.

HISTOLOGIC CLASSIFICATION OF OLIGODENDROGLIOMAS AND EPENDYMOMAS

In the Kernohan system, oligodendrogliomas and ependymomas, like the astrocytomas, are each classified into four grades.[6] Another four-tiered classification scheme based on the degree of anaplasia has been proposed by Ludwig and coworkers.[15] Neither system consistently generates distinct survival curves for patients in each tier,[4,15,16] and therefore simpler approaches have been advocated. The WHO system identifies three types of oligodendrogliomas: a "pure" type, a mixed type containing oligodendroglial and astrocytic components, and a malignant type.[4] The malignant form, characterized by anaplastic changes in cells and tissue, has a worse prognosis and is considered a grade III lesion. Several studies have shown that the presence of well-differentiated astrocytic elements in an oligodendroglioma has no prognostic significance.[17,18] In mixed tumors with anaplastic astrocytic components, however, the clinical behavior corresponds most closely to the degree of malignancy of the astrocytic component.[19]

The WHO system classifies ependymomas as ordinary (with three histologic variants) or anaplastic. These tumors are grouped with tumors of choroid plexus origin, but in common usage only the ependymal tumors are included with other gliomas. Although most

Figure 26.2 Comparison of the Major Classification Schemes of Astrocytic Tumors

Classification Scheme	Kernohan[7] (Mayo)	Ringertz/Burger[10,11] (Stockholm/Duke)	Zulch[4] (WHO)
Least Malignant	Astrocytomas		Astrocytic Tumors
	Grade I 1. Increased cellularity 2. Otherwise essentially normal cytology 3. Pilocytic astrocytoma included here	Pilocytic Astrocytomas	Pilocytic Astrocytoma (Grade I)
		Fibrillary Astrocytomas Astrocytoma 1. Slight hypercellularity 2. Slight pleomorphism 3. No necrosis 4. No vascular proliferation	Astrocytoma (Grade II) 1. Predominance of astrocytes 2. No areas of anaplasia (see below) 3. Includes fibrillary, protoplasmic, and gemistocytic types
	Grade II 1. Increased cellularity, but majority of cells clearly astrocytic 2. Hyperchromatic nuclei 3. No mitoses or necrosis 4. Some "thickened" vessels		
		Anaplastic Astrocytoma 1. Moderate hypercellularity 2. Moderate pleomorphism 3. No necrosis 4. Vascular proliferation permitted	Anaplastic Astrocytoma (Grade III) 1. Recognizable astrocytic cells present 2. At least focally anaplastic including: hypercellularity nuclear or cellular pleomorphism numerous, sometimes bizarre mitoses vascular proliferation necrosis
	Grade III (GBM) 1. Many cells appear astrocytic 2. Pleomorphism present 3. Few mitotic figures 4. Necrosis common 5. Some vascular endothelial proliferation		
	Grade IV (GBM) 1. Few normal appearing astrocytes 2. Pleomorphism prominent 3. Numerous bizarre mitoses 4. Necrosis common 5. Prominent vascular endothelial proliferation	Glioblastoma Multiforme 1. Moderate to marked hypercellularity 2. Moderate to marked pleomorphism 3. Necrosis required 4. Often vascular proliferation (not required)	**Poorly Differentiated and Embryonal Tumors** Glioblastoma Multiforme (Grade IV) 1. Predominantly anaplastic cells, some with glial processes 2. Hemorrhage frequent 3. May have focal areas of recognizable astrocytoma, oligodendroglioma, or ependymoma
Most Malignant			

Figure 26.2 Comparison of the Major Classification Schemes of Astrocytic Tumors (cont.)

Daumas-DuPort[3] (Paris)	Davis[14] (UCSF)
Pilocytic Astrocytomas	**Pilocytic Astrocytomas**
Astrocytomas	**Infiltrating Astrocytomas**
Grade I Requires any one of the 　features below	Mildly Anaplastic Astrocytoma 1. Mild hypercellularity 2. Enlarged, uniform nuclei
Grade II Requires any two of the 　features below	Moderately Anaplastic Astrocytoma (MoAA) 1. Moderate hypercellularity 2. Enlarged nuclei 3. Uniform cytoplasm
Grade III Requires any three of the 　features below	Highly Anaplastic Astrocytoma (HAA) 1. At least focally hypercellular 2. At least two of the following: 　Increased nuclear to 　　cytoplasmic ratio 　Coarse chromatin 　High mitotic activity 　Nuclear pleomorphism 　Cytoplasmic pleomorphism 3. Does not meet criteria for GBM 　designation
Grade IV Requires all four of the following: 1. Nuclear atypia 2. Mitotic figures 3. Endothelial proliferation 4. Necrosis	Glioblastoma Multiforme (GBM) 1. At least focally highly cellular 2. Nuclear pleomorphism 3. Cytoplasmic pleomorphism 4. Vascular endothelial proliferation 5. Necrosis may or may not 　be present

ordinary ependymomas are classified as grade I, and the anaplastic forms as grade II or III, there does not appear to be a clear correlation between tumor histology and patient survival. The biology of ependymomas is complicated by different sites of occurrence, a broad age spectrum, and great histologic variability. Given this biologic and histologic heterogeneity, it is perhaps not surprising that ependymomas do not readily lend themselves to a simple four-tiered classification, as in the Kernohan system.

RADIOLOGIC CLASSIFICATION

Attempts have been made to classify gliomas on the basis of their appearance on CT scans [20] or MR images.[21] Although the radiologic findings frequently correlate with the pathologic findings, they are no substitute for definitive pathologic diagnosis if tissue can be obtained.

CLASSIFICATION BASED ON PROLIFERATIVE POTENTIAL

The proliferative potential of a tumor can be estimated in vivo by determining the fraction of tumor cells in DNA synthesis. One method of accomplishing this is to administer an intravenous infusion of bromodeoxyuridine (BUdR), a thymidine analogue, shortly before resection of the tumor. BUdR is incorporated into the nucleus of S-phase cells, which can then be identified immunohistochemically in excised tumor specimens. The BUdR labeling index (LI), or percentage of S-phase cells, reflects the proliferative potential. The BUdR LIs of gliomas range from 0% to more than

38%.[22] The higher the BUdR LI, the faster the tumor is considered to be growing. Recent studies suggest that the BUdR LI determined by exposing tumor specimens to BUdR in vitro shortly after their removal also correlates with the tumor growth rate.[23]

In general, the BUdR LI of a glioma correlates with the histologic diagnosis. Most tumors with a BUdR LI less than 1% show a moderate degree of anaplasia, those with BUdR LIs of 1% to 5% are usually more anaplastic, and those with BUdR LIs more than 5% are most commonly glioblastomas. In certain tumors, the BUdR LI correlates better with survival than does the histopathologic diagnosis.[22] In one study of low-grade astrocytomas, for example, the 3-year survival rates for patients whose tumors had BUdR LIs less than 1% and more than 1% were 85% and 10%, respectively, and the difference was statistically significant.[24] Although tumors with a high BUdR LI are not necessarily histologically anaplastic, in a recent study of ependymomas, the BUdR LI correlated better with tumor recurrence after surgical resection than did the pathologic criteria.[25] The BUdR LI did not predict CSF seeding, however. A study of intracranial gliomas showed a good correlation between the BUdR LI, presence of tumor necrosis, vascular proliferation, and abnormal mitotic figures.[26] As an indicator of the biologic activity of gliomas based on their proliferative potential, the BUdR LI appears to be a very useful adjunct to the histologic diagnosis in the management of patients with gliomas.

The proliferative potential can also be estimated with Ki-67, a monoclonal antibody that binds to a nuclear antigen found only in cells that are in the G1, S, G2, and M phase cells. Thus, Ki-67 identifies all cells that are not

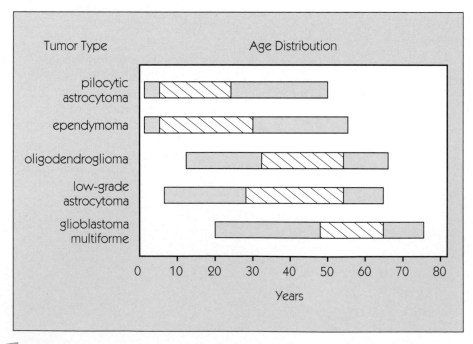

Figure 26.3 The incidence of gliomas plotted against age at diagnosis, based on data from the large series of Zulch.[29] Each bar represents approximately 95% of reported patients; the central hatched areas span approximately one standard deviation on either side of the mean.

in the resting phase (G0). The proliferative potential determined by this in vitro test correlates with both the histologic classification [27] and the BUdR LI [28] of gliomas.

ASTROCYTIC TUMORS

The astrocytic tumors are of four broad types: pilocytic astrocytoma, low-grade astrocytoma, anaplastic astrocytoma, and glioblastoma multiforme. The diagnosis and treatment of each of these will be discussed.

PILOCYTIC ASTROCYTOMAS

Pilocytic astrocytomas are tumors of the young (Fig. 26.3).[29] Because they typically arise in one of three locations and follow a benign course, they are considered a distinct biologic entity.[30,31] Nearly two thirds of pilocytic astrocytomas occur in the cerebellum, 25% to 30% in the region of the optic nerves/chiasm and hypothalamus, and the remainder in the cerebral hemispheres.[30] The CT[32] and MRI[33] findings for each are characteristic (Figs. 26.4–26.6).

These tumors can be cured by complete resection, which is frequently possible, depending on their location. The postoperative treatment of residual tumor is controversial. Some authors[30] advocate radiation therapy for patients over 3 years of age and chemotherapy or radiation therapy for younger patients if progression is noted. Others point to cases of long-term tumor stabilization without adjuvant therapy after resection.[34,35] In any event, the prognosis is relatively good: The 2-year survival rate is more than 50%, even after subtotal resection.[30] Pilocytic astrocytomas rarely spread to other locations and malignant transformation is very rare.[36]

Cerebellar tumors, like most posterior fossa tumors, typically cause signs and symptoms of raised intracranial pressure, including headache, nausea and vomiting, and sixth cranial nerve dysfunction[37]; cerebellar dysfunction is also common. These tumors are usually cystic and have a mural nodule of solid tumor tissue (see Fig. 26.4); they can usually be resected completely unless the brain stem is involved. If the cyst wall does not enhance on CT scans or MR images, removal of the mural nodule alone is usually curative. The tumor cyst capsule sometimes enhances on the preoperative MR image[33]; if the capsule is also thickened, many neurosurgeons believe the likelihood is high that tumor involves the capsule wall, and both the capsule and the mural nodule should be resected if possible.[38]

Pilocytic astrocytomas in the cerebral hemispheres typically occur in young adults, causing seizures, headache, or weakness.[34,39] These tumors may be cystic or solid; their radiologic appearance is typically that of a well-demarcated, inhomogenous, enhancing mass with little surrounding edema (see Fig. 26.5). Except for the lower likelihood of hydrocephalus and the higher risk of seizures, the management and outcome of these tumors are similar to those of cerebellar pilocytic astrocytomas.

Tumors in the chiasm and hypothalamus are the most difficult to treat. Their radiologic appearance is shown in Figure 26.6. They usually cause visual loss, endocrine dysfunction (especially diabetes insipidus, diencephalic syndrome, or precocious puberty), or raised intracranial pressure from obstructive hydrocephalus due to obstruction of the foramen of Monro.[40] At least 40% of optic nerve and chiasmal tumors are associated with neurofibromatosis,[41] and may in fact be the first evidence of that disease. Complete resection is rarely possible, and the management of residual tumor is controversial given the risk of radiation damage to the developing brain.[42]

ASTROCYTOMAS

The astrocytoma of the WHO classification corresponds to the "low-grade," moderately anaplastic, or grade II astrocytoma of other schemes. These tumors constitute 5% to 25% of gliomas in most series.[43] The median age at diagnosis is in the fifth decade (see Fig. 26.3), and the most common location is the cerebral hemispheres. Astrocytomas grow slowly, and seizures,[44] occasionally of several years' duration, are the most common presenting symptom.

Diagnosis by CT scan[45] can be difficult. On T2-weighted MR images[21] the tumor is usually seen as a sharply defined area of homogeneously increased signal; there is little or only modest mass effect, and contrast enhancement is rare (Fig. 26.7).

Surgical resection is the primary treatment. Radiation therapy is generally indicated after subtotal resection.[46] However, because this treatment has not been evaluated in a prospective, randomized study, definitive conclusions about its efficacy cannot be drawn.[47] Several studies have shown only a slight improvement in outcome after radiation therapy,[48–50] while at least one center advocates such treatment even after apparent gross total resection.[35] Recently, Morantz[47] reviewed the literature on radiation therapy for low-grade gliomas and concluded that it probably has some value. Approximately 50% to 80% of recurrent tumors show evidence of progression to a higher grade.[49,51,52] Chemotherapy does not appear to be indicated for low-grade astrocytomas. The median duration of survival ranges from 3 years to more than 5 years in most series. Age, preoperative status, and extent of resection are the prognostic variables.

ANAPLASTIC ASTROCYTOMAS

Anaplastic astrocytomas arise most commonly in the fifth or sixth decade of life (see Fig. 26.3), either de novo or as a result of malignant transformation. These tumors represent approximately 30% of gliomas,[43] but the incidence figures vary widely (Fig. 26.8). They display histologic evidence of anaplasia, are biologically aggressive, and are considered malignant. Compared with low-grade astrocytomas, anaplastic astrocytomas grow faster, more often cause evidence of increased intracranial pressure and neurologic deficit at presentation, and typically have a shorter course before the diagnosis is established. The tumor cells are infiltrative, and neuroimaging studies show mass effect and surrounding edema in which infiltrating tumor cells have been documented.[53] The great majority of the tumors enhance on contrast studies. Therapy consists of surgical resection followed by radiation therapy with or without chemotherapy.

Variations in the classification of anaplastic astrocytomas make it especially difficult to compare the outcome of therapy and the duration of patient survival with these tumors. Recent clinical trials[11,54] using principally postoperative radiation therapy followed by a nitrosourea have yielded 2-year survival rates of 40% to 60% for anaplastic astrocytomas as defined by the Ringertz and Burger classification. The 5-year survival rate after surgery and radiation therapy is about 20%.[31,55,56]

Additional treatment options include reoperation for recurrent tumors and interstitial radiation therapy at the time of tumor recurrence or as part of a multimodality treatment after the initial diagnosis. In selected patients, reoperation extends the median survival times by 14 to 21 months, producing a median survival of almost 5 years after the initial operation.[57,58] In patients whose recurrent tumors are suitable for interstitial brachytherapy,

---

Figure 26.4 Pilocytic Astrocytoma—Clinical Summary

CT Appearance: Cerebellar Location (A)
- Slightly hypodense to isodense
- Well-defined macrocystic hypodense core in >50%[32]
- Calcification seen in 22%
- Displaces/compresses fourth ventricle
- Mural nodule strongly contrast-enhancing, may display mixed densities
- At right, a contrast-enhanced CT scan of a 22-year-old man who presented with headache and decreased balance

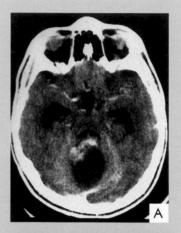

MRI Appearance: Cerebellar Location (B)
- Sharply defined macrocystic mass
- Prolonged T1 and T2 relaxation times
- Mural nodule usually identifiable
- Pronounced contrast-enhancement of nodule; cyst wall enhances variably[33]
- At right, a gadolinium-enhanced axial T1-weighted image of a 15-year-old boy who presented with headache and ataxia

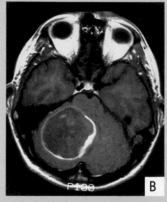

Histologic Appearance[29] (C)
- Fusiform cells with wavy fibrillary processes
- Rosenthal fibers common but not invariable
- Eosinophilic granular bodies common
- Microcystic areas with stellate astrocytes alternate with pilocytic areas (biphasic pattern)
- May form macrocysts, especially in cerebral hemispheres

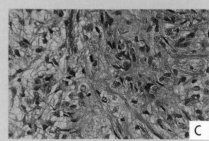

Figure 26.4 Pilocytic Astrocytoma—Clinical Summary (cont.)

Median Age: 13 years[31]

Incidence: 2% of gliomas[31]

Location
- Cerebellum/brain stem (61%)[30]
- Optic chiasm/hypothalamus (28%)
- Cerebral hemispheres (11%)

Presentation
- Cerebellar tumors: symptoms of increased intracranial pressure from hydrocephalus (headache, vomiting, and papilledema), cerebellar dysfunction (gait disturbance, ataxia, nystagmus), or sixth cranial nerve palsy
- Chiasmatic tumors: visual deficit, endocrine dysfunction, or symptoms of hydrocephalus
- Hemispheric lesions: headache, seizures, or focal weakness

Treatment
- Resect if possible
- Radiation therapy (RT) is controversial[30,34,35]; some recommend after subtotal resection (STR) and if patient is at least 3 years old
- Anecdotal reports of chemotherapy in younger patients

Outcome
- Complete resection yields 100% recurrence-free survival without adjuvant therapy[30]
- 10- and 20-year freedom-from-progression rates are 74% and 41% after STR/RT
- 10- and 20-year survival rates are 81% and 54% after STR/RT

Comment
- Incidence of neurofibromatosis with gliomas of optic nerve and chiasm ≥40%[41]
- CSF seeding or anaplastic transformation is rare[36]

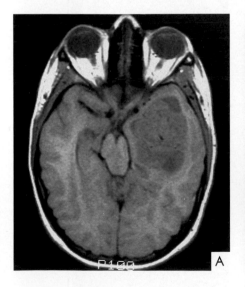

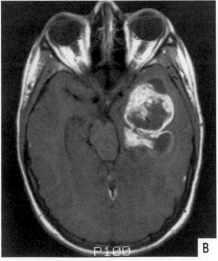

Figure 26.5 Pilocytic astrocytoma of the cerebral hemisphere in a 15-year-old girl with complex partial seizures. **(A)** Axial T1-weighted MR image shows prolonged relaxation time and inhomogeneous signal intensity of a fairly well demarcated tumor in the left temporal lobe. There is little surrounding edema. **(B)** Axial T1-weighted MR image obtained after administration of contrast material shows characteristic pattern of inhomogeneous enhancement and macrocystic appearance of this tumor.

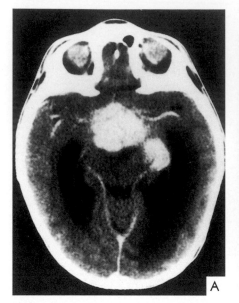
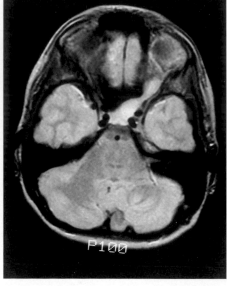
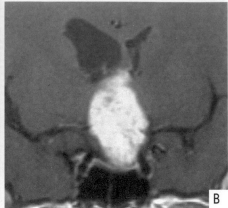

Figure 26.6 Pilocytic astrocytoma of the optic nerve, chiasm, and hypothalamus. **(A)** Contrast-enhanced CT scan shows a brightly enhancing mass in the region of the anterior third ventricle with parasellar extension in a 4-year-old boy with precocious puberty, failure to thrive, and developmental delay. Significant ventriculomegaly is apparent. **(B)** Gadolinium-enhanced T1-weighted MR images from a 13-year-old girl with headache and visual loss show fusiform enlargement of the left optic nerve along with chiasmatic involvement (left); a coronal section through the anterior third ventricle shows a brightly enhancing mass and obstructive hydrocephalus at the foramen of Monro (right).

Figure 26.7 Astrocytoma—Clinical Summary

CT Appearance (A)
- Hypodense or occasionally isodense[45]
- No significant mass effect or edema
- Contrast enhancement rare
- At right, contrast-enhanced CT scan of a low-grade astrocytoma in a 4-year-old girl who presented with a generalized seizure

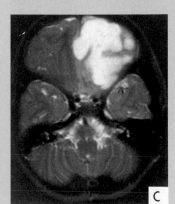

MRI Appearance (B,C)
- Lesion is usually well defined
- Normal to slightly prolonged T1 relaxation time[21]
- Prolonged T2 relaxation time
- Homogeneous signal
- Little mass effect or edema
- Contrast enhancement similar to that seen on CT scans
- At right, axial T1-weighted gadolinium-enhanced image **(B)** and axial T2-weighted image **(C)** of the tumor in Figure 26.7A

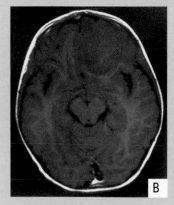

the median survival time after treatment is more than 19 months. In one study, patients treated with interstitial brachytherapy after craniotomy and external beam radiation therapy for primary anaplastic astrocytoma had a median survival time of 4.5 years.[59]

GLIOBLASTOMA MULTIFORME

One of the most discouraging diagnoses in all of neurosurgery is that of glioblastoma multiforme. It is, unfortunately, a common one, as glioblastomas constitute at least 30% of all primary brain tumors and approximately 50%

of gliomas in most series.[2,31] These tumors usually occur in the sixth or seventh decade (see Fig. 26.3). Although its likely site of origin is similar to that of low-grade and anaplastic astrocytomas, glioblastoma may arise anywhere in the CNS, including the cerebral hemispheres, the corpus callosum (the classic "butterfly glioma"), and, more rarely, in the deep gray nuclei, brain stem, cerebellum, and spinal cord.[29] Symptoms of increased intracranial pressure or mass effect, typically of short duration, are more common at presentation in patients with glioblastomas than in those with slower-growing tumors.[11] Headache, mental status changes, and focal weakness are

Figure 26.7 Astrocytoma—Clinical Summary (cont.)

Histologic Appearance (D; see also Fig. 26.2)
- Mild hypercellularity
- Nuclei may be enlarged but no significant pleomorphism
- No vascular proliferation
- No necrosis

Median Age: 35 to 45 years[29]

Incidence: 5% to 25% of gliomas[2,29,43]

Location
- Cerebral hemispheres, especially frontal (40%), temporal (25%), and parietal (25%) lobes[31,44]
- Others (10%) include thalamus, midbrain, pons

Presentation
- Seizures are most common (65%), duration may be years[39]
- Symptoms of increased intracranial pressure (40%), mental status changes (15%), or focal deficits (10%) are less common

Treatment
- Surgical resection
- Postoperative radiation therapy controversial[47,49,50]
- Chemotherapy not indicated

Outcome
- Median survival approximately 3 1/2 years; 5-year survival rate 26% to 33%[31,49]
- Radiation therapy increases 1- and 3-year survival rates but not beyond[48,49]

Comment
- Progression to anaplasia in up to 86% of recurring tumors[52]
- Prognostic factors include patient age, functional status, and extent of resection
- Incidence varies widely, partly because of differences in classification schemes

the most common symptoms at the time of diagnosis; seizures are much rarer (Fig. 26.9).[60]

The characteristic radiologic appearance of glioblastoma is an inhomogeneous area of enhancement surrounding a low-attenuation core of cystic or necrotic tissue. The tumor edges are indistinct, and edema and mass effect are usually present. Glioblastomas originating near the midline readily cross the corpus callosum. Hemosiderin or evidence of acute hemorrhage may be seen.

Although minimal resection has occasionally been advocated for these aggressive, infiltrative tumors,[61,62] radical resection has shown to be beneficial.[63–65] Adjuvant therapy with external beam radiation therapy and chemotherapy, usually with a nitrosourea-based regimen, is standard. In early reviews, median survival times after resection, resection plus radiation, and these combined with chemotherapy were approximately 4 months, 9 months, and 10 months, respectively.[66] With aggressive,

Figure 26.8 Anaplastic Astrocytoma—Clinical Summary

CT Appearance (A)
- Low or mixed attenuation
- Margins frequently ill-defined
- Mass effect and edema
- Contrast enhancement in 80% to 90%[45]
- At right, a contrast-enhanced CT scan of a 36-year-old woman who presented with a dysphasia after a generalized seizure

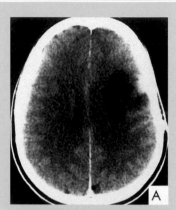

MRI Appearance (B)
- Prolonged T1 and T2 relaxation times
- Less distinct margins than ordinary astrocytomas
- Moderate mass effect and edema
- More heterogeneous signal than lower-grade tumors[21]
- Enhancement may be variable but usually parallels CT pattern
- Minimal hemosiderin
- At right, a gadolinium-enhanced T1-weighted coronal image of a 31-year-old woman who had headache and right-side weakness

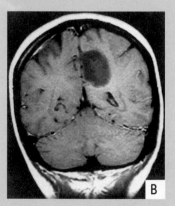

Histologic Appearance (C; see also Fig. 26.2)
- Moderate hypercellularity
- Moderate pleomorphism of cells and nuclei
- At least focal anaplastic changes
- Necrosis allowed in some classification schemes

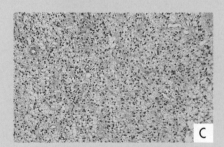

multimodality therapy, including sequential chemo-therapeutic regimens, median survival may be 12 to 15 months. The 5-year survival rate is less than 5%.[31,66]

The tendency of glioblastoma to metastasize to the CSF is well documented, reaching approximately 25% in one autopsy series,[2] but clinically evident CNS metastases occur in only 5% to 10% of such cases. Although primary CNS tumors very rarely metastasize to remote extraneural sites, glioblastoma is among the most likely to do so.[67] As with other nonpilocytic astrocytomas, favorable prognostic indicators include a young age, a good functional status at diagnosis, and a small amount of residual tumor after surgery or radiation therapy.[68–70] The prognosis for patients over 65 years old is extremely poor.[31]

Intensive efforts are underway to increase the duration of survival by additional modalities of treatment. In suitable candidates with recurrent tumors, reoperation and/or

---

Figure 26.8 Anaplastic Astrocytoma—Clinical Summary (cont.)

Median Age: 46 years[11]

Incidence: 10% to 30% of gliomas[2,43]

Location
- Cerebral hemispheres, especially frontal, temporal, and parietal lobes in approximately the same percentages as for low-grade tumors (Fig. 26.7)[31,44]
- Thalamus, midbrain, or pons less likely

Presentation
- Seizures are the initial symptom in at least 50% of patients[44]
- Other symptoms include those due to increased intracranial pressure (40%), mental status changes (15% to 20%), or focal deficit (10% to 15%)
- Mean duration of symptoms 16 months[11]

Treatment
- Surgical resection
- Postoperative radiation therapy regardless of the extent of resection
- Treatment options at recurrence are repeat resection, chemotherapy, interstitial brachytherapy, and radiosurgery

Outcome
- Approximately 40% to 50% 2-year survival[11] and 18% 5-year survival[31] after surgery plus radiation and chemotherapy

Comment
- Prognostic indicators include age, functional status, residual tumor size
- Up to 45% of recurrent tumors show progression to higher grades[52]
- Incidence varies, partly because of differences in classification schemes

interstitial brachytherapy have increased median survival by 9 to 12 months.[58,59] In one recent study, a boost of interstitial brachytherapy after resection and external beam radiation therapy for primary tumor resulted in a median survival time of 23 months after diagnosis.[59] Despite this significant increase in survival, the outcome is still poor. Immunotherapeutic intervention is another treatment option and may hold promise for the future.

OLIGODENDROGLIOMAS

Oligodendrogliomas, like low-grade astrocytomas, arise most often in the fifth or sixth decade (see Fig. 26.3), most commonly in the cerebral hemispheres.[71] The most characteristic presentation is seizures of long duration, although other symptoms of an intracranial mass, including headache, visual changes, and focal deficit, are also possible.[15,71,72]

Figure 26.9 Glioblastoma Multiforme—Clinical Summary

CT Appearance (A)
- Inhomogeneous region of high signal attenuation consisting of necrotic or cystic core
- Significant mass effect and surrounding edema
- Indistinct margins
- At least 95% of tumors enhance after administration of contrast material,[45] characteristically in an irregular, ring-shaped pattern near tumor periphery
- May cross the midline
- At right, contrast-enhanced CT scan of a 30-year-old man who had headache and mental status changes; there is evidence of tumor dissemination.

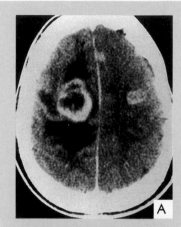

MRI Appearance (B)
- Prolonged T1 and T2 relaxation times
- Tumor margins may be poorly defined
- Significant mass effect and surrounding edema
- Heterogeneous signal within tumor
- Enhancement similar to CT pattern
- Hemorrhage more common and hemosiderin may be observed[21]
- At right, T1-weighted gadolinium-enhanced axial image of a 34-year-old man with headache and dysphasia

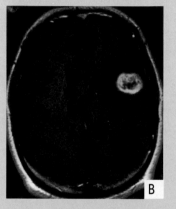

Histologic Appearance (C; see also Fig. 26.2)
- Hypercellular
- Nuclear and/or cytoplasmic pleomorphism
- Often vascular endothelial proliferation
- Necrosis common (required in some classification schemes)

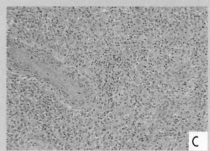

The radiologic appearance is fairly characteristic (Fig. 26.10). CT scans show an irregular area of calcification in a region of tumor that may be hypo- or isodense compared with adjacent brain.[45] Contrast enhancement and peritumoral edema are common only with anaplastic forms, which represent fewer than 10% of the oligodendrogliomas.[31]

Therapy usually consists of surgery followed by radiation therapy in the event of subtotal resection. The value of radiation therapy after subtotal resection is controversial. Some authors have found that it increases median survival after subtotal resection by less than 1 year and does not affect the 10-year survival rate.[73,74] Others have found significant increases in both 5- and 10-year survival rates[17] and, because anaplastic changes are frequent in recurrent tumors, advocate irradiation regardless of the extent of resection. No randomized trials have been undertaken to evaluate the role of radia-

---

Figure 26.9 Glioblastoma Multiforme—Clinical Summary (cont.)

Median Age: 50 to 60 years[11,29,31]

Incidence: 45% to 50% of gliomas[2,31]

Location
- Any region of CNS possible; cerebral hemispheres predominate (40% frontal, 25% temporal, 25% parietal)[31,44]
- Occasionally in corpus callosum (butterfly glioma)
- Deep gray nuclei and brain stem less likely

Presentation
- Symptoms of increased intracranial pressure (86% headaches, 45% nausea and vomiting) more common than with lower-grade tumors
- Mental status changes (47%) and motor deficit (44%) also common
- Seizures at presentation in approximately 32%[60]

Treatment
- Surgical resection
- Postoperative radiation therapy (RT) regardless of extent of resection
- Chemotherapy, reoperation at recurrence, interstitial brachytherapy, and RT are treatment options

Outcome
- Median survival after surgery, surgery plus RT, and surgery plus RT and chemotherapy is 4, 9.25, and 10 months, respectively[66]
- Reoperation and/or interstitial brachytherapy can increase survival by 9 to 12 months in selected patients[58,59]
- 10% 2-year survival[11] and 5.5% 5-year survival[31]

Comment
- Prognostic factors include patient age, functional status, and tumor size after resection and after RT[69]
- Some authors advocate only biopsy and adjuvant therapy for high-grade supratentorial tumors[61,62]

tion therapy. Reports of chemotherapy are only anecdotal and restricted primarily to the treatment of recurrent or malignant tumors.[17,72,75,76] Median survival ranges from 35 to 60 months. Favorable prognostic factors include the absence of anaplastic changes, the presence of calcification, and good preoperative functional status.[18,73,76] Age and extent of resection seem to be less important to the outcome of oligodendrogliomas than of astrocytomas. The presence of low-grade astrocytic elements does not affect the outcome,[18,76] but if a malignant astrocytic component is present, the prognosis is similar to that of malignant astrocytomas.

Figure 26.10 Oligodendroglioma—Clinical Summary

CT Appearance (A)
- Tumor tissue is hypodense or isodense
- Irregular areas of calcification in more than 70%[45]
- Cystic changes and hemorrhage rare
- With anaplastic changes, calcification less common
- Edema and contrast enhancement common only with anaplastic tumors
- At right, CT scan of a 12-year-old girl with a several-year history of complex partial seizures

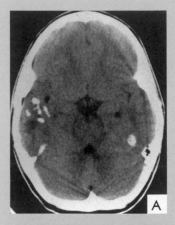

MRI Appearance (B)
- Prolonged T1 and T2 relaxation times
- Absent to slight enhancement typical[33]
- Heterogeneous signal with areas of low intensity due to calcification
- At right, gadolinium-enhanced, T1-weighted axial image of the patient in Figure 26.8A showing patchy foci of enhancement

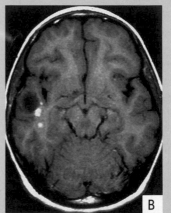

Histologic Appearance[29] (C)
- Uniform cells with oval nuclei, clear cytoplasm, and defined cell membranes
- Mineralization in 70% to 90%
- May have conspicuous astrocytic areas (mixed oligoastrocytoma)
- May show changes typical of anaplasia (anaplastic oligodendroglioma)

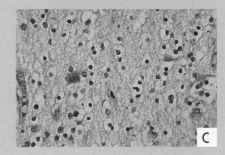

EPENDYMOMAS

Although ependymomas have been diagnosed in patients as old as 81 years,[29] they occur mostly in young patients (see Fig. 26.3) and are the third most common intracranial tumor in children.[77] Ependymomas most often arise in the posterior fossa and cause evidence of increased intracranial pressure due to hydrocephalus; supratentorial and spinal axis tumors are also observed. In general, infratentorial lesions are more common in younger patients, and supratentorial lesions are more common in adults[78,79]; however, earlier studies by Zulch[29] and Ringertz and Reymond[80] were unable to

Figure 26.10 Oligodendroglioma—Clinical Summary (cont.)

Median Age: 43 years[31]

Incidence: 4% to 6% of gliomas[31,43]

Location
- Cerebral hemispheres: frontal (50%), temporal and parietal (15% to 25%) each, most common[71,72,76]
- Occipital (5%) rare

Presentation
- Seizures in >50%; median duration, 48 months[66]
- Headache in 30% to 78%[15,71]
- Others include mental status changes, visual complaints, focal weakness; median duration of symptoms is 20 months in the absence of seizures

Treatment
- Surgical resection
- Radiation therapy after subtotal resection; some authors recommend regardless of extent of resection[17]
- Anecdotal reports of chemotherapy and/or repeat resection for treatment failure

Outcome
- Median survival 35 to 60 months[18,71]
- 5-year survival 35% to 60%; 10-year survival 25% to 30%[17,31,71,73]
- Radiation therapy increases median survival by 12 months or less after subtotal resection; does not affect survival after gross total resection[73,74]

Comment
- No randomized trials of role of radiation therapy
- Progression to anaplastic oligodendroglioma in up to 50% of recurrent tumors[17]
- Low-grade astrocytic elements do not worsen prognosis[17,18]
- Prognosis of a mixed oligoastrocytoma with anaplastic astrocytic elements parallels that of the astrocytic component[19]
- Favorable prognostic factors include preoperative functional status, presence of calcification, and lack of anaplasia[18,73,76]

reach consensus on this point. Ependymomas and astrocytomas occur with approximately equal frequency as the two most common intramedullary tumors of the spinal cord. The conus medullaris is a classic location for myxopapillary ependymomas (see Chapter 39). The subependymoma is an unusual, very slow-growing lobulated mass found in the ventricular system.[29] A papillary variant of ependymoma exists but is very rare.

Neuroimaging studies (Fig. 26.11) demonstrate a heterogeneous mass that usually enhances after the administration of contrast material and often is finely calcified.[32,33] Extension of a fourth ventricular tumor through the foramen of Luschka into the cerebellopontine angle suggests an ependymoma but is not diagnostic. Supratentorial tumors arise in relation to the wall of the ventricular system, commonly in the trigonal region.[29]

Intracranial ependymomas are treated with resection followed in most cases by radiation therapy. They are relatively sensitive to radiation, but the dose and delivery appear critical to a successful outcome. The extent of irradiation depends on the tumor location, grade, and whether or not tumor cells are found in spinal CSF.[81,82] For low-grade, supratentorial lesions, whole-brain or focal irradiation alone is recommended; for low-grade, infratentorial lesions, whole-brain or focal irradiation is supplemented with craniospinal axis therapy only if tumor cells are found in the CSF. All high-grade lesions are treated by irradiating the craniospinal axis.

Figure 26.11 Intracranial Ependymoma—Clinical Summary

CT Appearance (A)

- Mixed density, isodense, or slightly hyperdense tumor tissue
- Fine calcification seen in approximately 50% of tumors[32]
- May have cystic areas, especially in cerebral locations
- More than 80% enhance
- At right, contrast-enhanced CT scan of a 2-year-old child with a posterior fossa ependymoma who presented with vomiting and lethargy; noncontrast scan demonstrated a few fine calcifications (this tumor was recurrent after surgical resection)

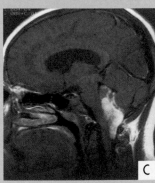

MRI Appearance (B,C)

- Heterogeneous signal intensities; prolonged T1 and T2 relaxation times
- Punctate, markedly hypointense areas on T1-weighted images due to calcification or cystic changes
- Inhomogeneous enhancement with gadolinium
- At right, axial (B) and sagittal (C) gadolinium-enhanced T1-weighted images of a 12-year-old girl with headache and ataxia

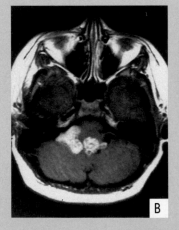
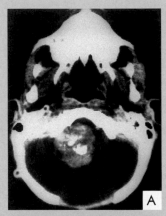

Histologic Appearance[29] (D)

- Uniform ependymal cells in pattern of rosettes, canals, or perivascular pseudorosettes
- Variants include myxopapillary (cauda equina location), papillary, subependymoma (fourth or lateral ventricles usually), and anaplastic (fourth ventricle or cerebrum usually) types

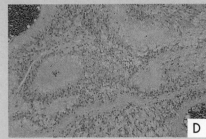

The 5-year survival rate is 35% to 60%.[78,81,82] The outcome for ependymomas, in contrast to astrocytomas, does not seem to correlate with tumor grade, location, or extent of resection.[79,81,83] Although a recurrent tumor may show increased anaplasia,[82] this is rarer than with astrocytomas.[79] Older patients do somewhat better overall,[78,82] despite a slightly greater incidence of higher-grade lesions.[78,79] One third to two thirds of the tumors recur after primary therapy, usually within 2 years, and the great majority of recurrences are local. The likelihood of recurrence correlates with tumor grade. Spinal CSF seeding has been reported in one third to one half of patients in some series,[79] but symptomatic spinal metastasis occurs in only about 10% of adequately irradiated patients.[81,84] High-grade lesions rarely metastasize extracranially.[81] Chemotherapy, particularly with the nitrosoureas, has yielded encouraging results in the treatment of recurrent ependymomas.[85,86]

DIAGNOSIS AND TREATMENT: OVERVIEW

APPROACH TO THE PATIENT WITH CNS SYMPTOMS OR SIGNS

A patient with an intracranial glioma may have CNS symptoms or complaints such as headache, vomiting, confusion, decreased memory, visual changes, weakness, and sensory alteration, to name but a few possibilities. The history and physical examination are key elements in establishing the diagnosis.

The history often provides clues about the type of lesion and its location. The patient with a brain tumor usually has noticed symptoms for months to years before diagnosis. Although a precipitous decline is possible, perhaps due to a hemorrhage into the tumor bed, this is an uncharacteristic presentation, which usually heralds a condition other than a tumor. A short dura-

Figure 26.11 Intracranial Ependymoma—Clinical Summary (cont.)

Median Age: 25 years[31]

Incidence: 3% to 4% of gliomas[31,13]

Location
- Fourth ventricle, including floor and lateral recess; may extend into cerebellopontine angle
- In or near third and lateral ventricles
- 2/3 are posterior fossa (more common in the young), while 1/3 are supratentorial (more common in adults)

Presentation
- Headache in over 80%[78,82]
- Nausea and vomiting in 50% to 80%
- Others include cerebellar dysfunction and papilledema on exam
- Median duration of symptoms 4 months

Treatment
- Surgical resection
- Radiation therapy critical; dosing depends on tumor location, grade, and surgical outcome
- Repeat resection and/or chemotherapy are options at recurrence

Outcome
- Overall survival 35% to 60% at 5 years[29,78,81,82]
- 1/3 to 2/3 will recur, with increased incidence if anaplastic changes are present
- Most treatment failures are apparent within 2 years of therapy, and more than 90% of these are local recurrences

Comment
- Increased incidence of anaplastic changes in supratentorial lesions[78,79,82]
- No clear relationship between anaplastic changes and patient outcome[79,81,83]
- Rare to absent tumor progression to increased anaplasia on recurrence[79,82]

tion of symptoms is associated with high-grade lesions, especially glioblastoma multiforme, or with the development of hydrocephalus in patients with lesions near the fourth ventricle. The new onset of seizures, especially in an adult, suggests the possibility of a mass lesion. Seizures are a common presentation of supratentorial lesions, but are especially characteristic of low-grade astrocytomas and oligodendrogliomas. A focal deficit, particularly of subacute onset, should also raise the suspicion of an intracranial mass lesion. A history compatible with endocrine dysfunction suggests a lesion near the anterior third ventricle. The age of the patient is clearly important in establishing the diagnosis of a suspected mass lesion. Pediatric patients are more likely to have pilocytic astrocytomas, low-grade astrocytomas, or ependymomas (among the tumors discussed in this chapter), whereas older adults are much more likely to have high-grade astrocytomas. The transmission of CNS tumors with diseases such as neurofibromatosis, Li-Fraumeni syndrome,[87] and others is well established[29]; in rare cases, familial tumors may occur in the absence of hereditary diseases.[88] In the great majority of cases, however, CNS tumors and lesions arise spontaneously without known risk factors (see Chapter 25), and family history is less helpful.

The physical examination emphasizes the functional status of the patient and localizing neurologic deficits. Decreased mental status is common in patients with frontal lobe tumors—particularly those of higher grade— or hydrocephalus. Cranial nerve deficits, especially of the sixth nerve, are common symptoms of pilocytic astrocytomas of the fourth ventricle or cerebellum that cause increased intracranial pressure. An ependymoma that extends into the cerebellopontine angle may cause lower cranial nerve deficits at presentation. Optic nerve gliomas usually cause visual field defects. Weakness of the upper or lower extremities is particularly associated with gliomas near the parietal lobes.

MAKING THE DIAGNOSIS

A diagnostic algorithm for evaluating patients with CNS signs or symptoms is shown in Figure 26.12. After the patient has been stabilized, neuroimaging studies are performed. Usually, the first study is a CT scan of the head, which is superior at showing bony anatomy or tumor calcification; mass effect is easily detected from displacement or distortion of the normally symmetric anatomy of the brain and ventricular system. The CT scan may not show the rare low-grade astrocytoma that is isodense and nonenhancing or a small non-mass-producing lesion in the inferior temporal lobe, high on the vertex, in the brain stem, or in the cerebellum. If the CT scan is normal and a mass lesion is still suspected, MRI may be performed. MRI is more sensitive than CT for demonstrating abnormalities in the brain stem and around the skull base. If both CT and MR studies are normal, a neoplastic lesion is extremely unlikely. If a mass lesion is demon-

strated, biopsy or surgery for diagnosis or treatment is warranted in the great majority of cases.

Hydrocephalus may be associated with a mass lesion, especially one in the ventricular system, or may occur in the absence of a mass lesion. Although shunting or drainage may be performed first, if a tumor is present many surgeons initially attempt to resect it and thereby eliminate the cause of the hydrocephalus.

Cerebral angiography is rarely useful in the diagnosis or management of intracranial gliomas. With knowledge of normal cerebrovascular anatomy, one can predict the vascular supply to the tumor based on its location. Because gliomas are usually intraparenchymal and are often invasive, preoperative embolization to reduce their blood supply is seldom possible.

SURGICAL MANAGEMENT OF GLIOMAS

After the radiologic demonstration of a mass lesion, a biopsy or a surgical resection is usually indicated to obtain a definitive diagnosis. Except for pilocytic astrocytomas, gliomas cannot in most instances be cured by surgery alone. The goal of the neurosurgeon is to preserve and improve the quality of life and prolong survival of the patient. Only rarely should a nonsurgical approach be considered. For example, a small nonenhancing, non-mass-producing lesion that does not cause symptoms and that has demonstrated no growth in the past could be followed radiographically. In addition, a large tumor in a very old, debilitated patient who would not be treated even if a definitive diagnosis were made should probably not be operated upon. In most other cases, a definitive diagnosis should be made.

Many factors relating to the tumor must be considered in planning a neurosurgical procedure (Fig. 26.13).[89] A large tumor or one that has a significant mass effect frequently causes neurologic impairment, which may improve dramatically after reduction of the tumor mass. Infiltrating tumor cells may also cause edema and mass effect, but attempted resection of these cells from functional cortex would probably increase the neurologic deficit. Tumor location, composition, estimated vascularity, and multiplicity are also important in planning a neurosurgical approach.

As in other types of surgery, factors related to the patient must also be considered (Fig. 26.13). The patient's ability to tolerate the stress of an operation is important. Therefore, unless the operation is emergent (e.g., for imminent brain herniation from a tumor causing significant mass effect), it should be delayed to allow the patient's medical condition to be optimized. Bleeding diatheses, infections, and anesthetic risks (pulmonary, cardiac, or metabolic) should be diagnosed and treated appropriately. An older patient at high risk for general anesthesia, infection, or poor healing postoperatively would be approached in a less aggressive manner than a younger, healthier patient. Age and preoperative functional status are also independent predictors of the

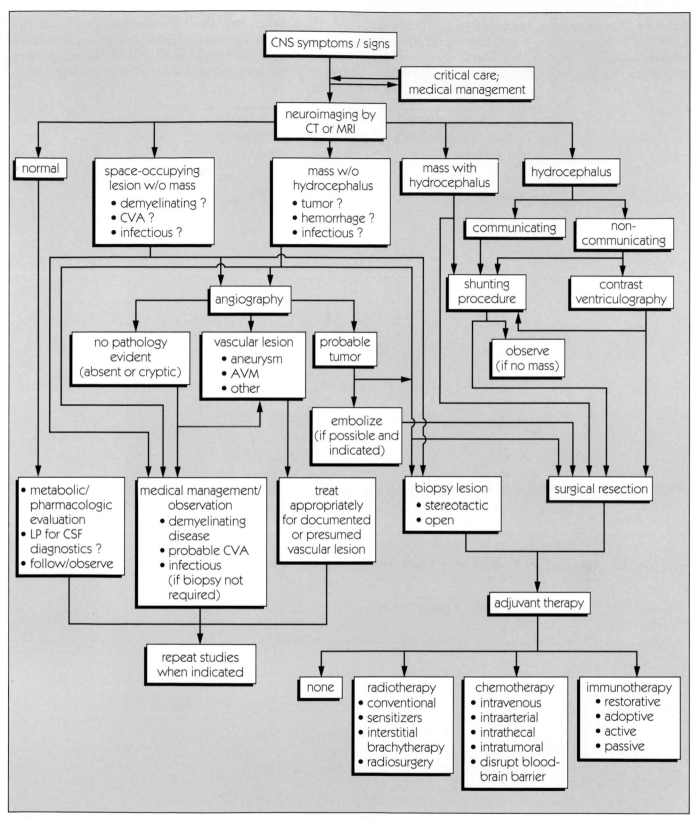

Figure 26.12 Diagnostic algorithm for suspected intracranial tumor or other mass lesion. After acute care and stabilization, the initial diagnostic test is usually CT scanning of the head. MR imaging is more sensitive for evaluating the brain stem and skull base. Cerebral angiography is rarely of value in the treatment of glioma patients but may provide important information, particularly if a vascular lesion is suspected or if preoperative tumor embolization is required. If a mass lesion is demonstrated, biopsy or surgical resection is recommended in almost all cases. Hydrocephalus is either managed with a shunting procedure or is relieved by resection of the tumor. Adjuvant treatment is frequently beneficial to the patient with a glioma. CVA=cerebrovascular accident; AVM=arteriovenous malformation; LP=lumbar puncture.

duration of survival postoperatively in patients with nonpilocytic astrocytomas. Survival rates are more than twice as high in patients with a Karnofsky score[90] of 70 as they are in those with lower scores[31] (Fig. 26.14).

Prior therapy may also influence management choices. A patient with a recurrent tumor after surgical resection and radiation therapy may be offered chemotherapy, reoperation, interstitial brachytherapy, or other adju-

Figure 26.13 Factors to Consider When Planning Brain Tumor Surgery

Tumor Factors	Patient Factors
Mass effect	Neurologic status (Karnofsky score)
Location (deep vs. superficial, eloquent vs. silent)	Age
Size	Surgical risks (bleeding, healing, infection)
Vascularity	Anesthesia risks (pulmonary, cardiac, metabolic)
Composition (solid vs. cystic)	Prior therapy
Multiplicity	Patient's and family's desires

Adapted with permission from Rosenblum ML, 1990

Figure 26.14 Karnofsky Performance Scale for Assessment of Functional Status and Quality of Life

Score	Functional Status Characteristics
100	Normal; no complaints and no evidence of disease
90	Able to carry on normal activity with only minor symptoms
80	Normal activity with effort; some moderate symptoms from disease
70	Cares for self but unable to carry on normal activities
60	Cares for most needs but requires occasional assistance
50	Requires considerable assistance to carry on activities of daily living; frequent medical care
40	Disabled; requires special assistance and care
30	Severely disabled; hospitalized, but death not imminent
20	Very sick; requires active supportive treatment
10	Moribund; death threatened or imminent

Principles of Neurosurgery

vant therapy. The possibility of anemia or bone marrow compromise must be considered in patients who have recently received chemotherapy. The indications for reoperation or brachytherapy are discussed below, but in most centers a severely debilitated patient would not be judged a suitable candidate for such aggressive approaches.

Finally, the wishes and concerns of patients and their families must be addressed. In most cases, thorough preoperative counseling and frank discussions allow the family to make appropriate decisions and prepare them for the risks and anticipated outcome of surgical intervention; preoperative review of the neuroradiologic studies is especially helpful. Poor communication between the doctor and the patient and family is possibly the single most important factor contributing to postoperative misunderstanding and litigation.

BIOPSY VERSUS RESECTION

In most cases of glioma, the surgeon's goal is to remove all apparent tumor tissue (gross total resection), but in some instances a biopsy is preferable (Fig. 26.15). A closed, stereotactic biopsy is usually indicated for small, deep lesions that cause minimal mass effect; this is particularly true if the patient is neurologically intact or nearly so, given the potential morbidity from attempted resection. If a significant cyst is present, drainage by needle aspira-

tion frequently alleviates neurologic deficits. Finally, a biopsy performed under local anesthesia avoids the risks of general anesthesia in older or medically ill patients.

Because brain tumors are often heterogeneous, there has been some concern that tissue obtained by needle biopsy may not be representative. Many glioblastomas, for example, contain large areas of tissue that have the histologic characteristics of anaplastic astrocytoma.[91] Nevertheless, with appropriate stereotactic biopsy technique, an accurate, or at least clinically appropriate, diagnosis can be made in 93% of brain tumor patients.[92]

Although a biopsy can provide an accurate pathologic diagnosis, surgical resection usually offers the best chance of improved survival. Debulking large tumors and those that cause mass effect can reduce intracranial pressure and lead to marked improvement in neurologically impaired patients. Superficial lesions are especially amenable to resection. Electrocorticography and other intraoperative mapping techniques, which are used to determine the potential extent of resection of tumors located near highly functional ("eloquent") cortex, require an open procedure. This may be an attempted resection or limited biopsy, depending on the mapping results. Highly vascular lesions cannot be approached safely by stereotaxy, and therefore a craniotomy should be performed for either biopsy or resection.

The mortality rate from craniotomy in most large series is 1% to 2%.[93,94] Surgical morbidity[31] includes

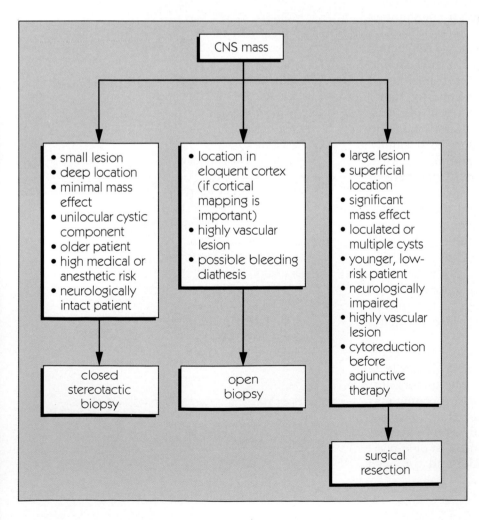

Figure 26.15 Biopsy versus surgical resection in the treatment of the glioma patient. Open biopsy may be advisable if mapping is required, if the lesion is vascular (increasing the risk of hemorrhage after biopsy), or if the patient has a bleeding diathesis. In most cases, resection offers the best chance for short-term improvement of neurologic deficits and improved long-term survival.

increased neurologic deficit from tumor resection or swelling (11% in the first 24 hours), hemorrhage at the operative site (4% to 5%), and wound infection (1% to 2%). Medical complications such as deep vein thrombosis, myocardial infarction, and pneumonia occur in 8% to 9% of patients.[63] Older, neurologically impaired patients with deep-seated, midline, or bilateral lesions are at relatively increased risk. Total resection does not increase the risks of surgery and offers improved survival for most glioma patients, and should therefore be attempted if it is safe to do so.

OUTLINE OF SURGICAL TECHNIQUE

The general outline of an intracranial neurosurgical procedure is shown in Figure 26.16.[89] Many of the points are self-explanatory and will not be repeated here. Proper scheduling is vital not only to insure the fitness of the surgeons, but also to guarantee the availability of experienced operating room personnel, neuroanesthesia, and needed equipment. Because neurosurgical procedures are usually elective, scheduling should not be a problem at most institutions. The preoperative availability of blood is of paramount importance because of the risk of blood transfusions. Some states, in fact, by law require that the family and patient be informed of the advantages and availability of donor-designated or autologous blood. The use of perioperative steroids, anticonvulsants (for supratentorial lesions), antibiotics, and sequential compression stockings has become routine for craniotomies (see also Chapter 4).

Equipment for bipolar electrocautery and for suction to achieve hemostasis and field visualization should always be available; microneurosurgical instruments and an ultrasonic aspirator are frequently helpful for tumor debulking. Lasers are rarely used to resect gliomas. With every maneuver of the surgeon, care is taken to protect adjacent normal brain and its vascular supply. Traction on the brain itself must be minimized; when needed, a self-retaining retractor of the Greenberg or Yasargil type is used.

Preoperative patient positioning and incision planning are particularly important in neurosurgery, perhaps more so than in other fields, because of the small cranial opening and operative field and the risks of retracting adjacent neural and vascular structures to gain access to tumors within, behind, or beneath functioning brain. Descriptive anatomic names are given to the various surgical approaches (Fig. 26.17). Each approach requires a particular craniotomy "opening."

For intracranial gliomas, there are four basic craniotomy openings. The pterional approach (Fig. 26.18A) allows access to frontal and temporal lobe tumors near the sylvian fissure and skull base; the basic opening may be extended posteriorly or toward the vertex to expose the temporoparietal or lateral frontal regions, respectively. The patient is usually placed in the supine position with a bump under one shoulder and the head

Figure 26.16 General Outline for Planning a Brain Tumor Operation

A. Preoperative
  1. Review presentation and studies
  2. Informed consent
  3. Optimal scheduling
B. Anesthesia
C. Intraoperative Preparation
  1. Radiographic studies selected
  2. Stereotactic target acquisition
  3. Blood available
  4. Corticosteroids
  5. Anticonvulsants
  6. Antibiotics
  7. Minimize venous stagnation
  8. Urinary catheter
  9. Intravenous access
  10. Monitors (anesthesia and neurophysiologic)
  11. Intraoperative adjuncts available
    a. Microscope, ultrasound, x-ray equipment
    b. Surgical tools
    c. Anatomic aids
  12. Prepare operative field
  13. Plan incision
    a. Scalp flap
    b. Cranial opening
  14. Position patient
    a. Head fixation
    b. Avoid pressure points
  15. Draping
  16. Minimize exposure of personnel to blood
  17. Operating room decorum
D. Surgical Removal
  1. Approach
  2. Removal
  3. Avoid complications
E. Postoperative
  1. Immediate concerns
    a. General clinical status
    b. Bleeding in operative site
    c. Brain swelling
    d. Neurologic deficits
  2. Delayed concerns
    a. Hydrocephalus
    b. Infection
    c. Phlebitis and pulmonary emboli
    d. Wound healing
  3. Patient and family support

The order of presentation is roughly chronologic and is for a typical craniotomy. Not all steps are required for every operation.

Adapted with permission from Rosenblum ML, 1990

tilted 30° to 90° away from the involved side. The incision follows a gentle curve in the shape of a reverse question mark, usually starting just anterior to the tragus of the ear and posterior to the palpable pulse of the superficial temporal artery at the level of the zygomatic process and ending behind the hairline at the midpupillary line or near the midline superiorly. Care must be taken to preserve the frontotemporal branch of the facial nerve.[95] The temporalis muscle is either cleared off the bone with the scalp itself ("free-flap" opening) or split for placement of the burr holes and left on the bone ("osteoplastic" opening) after elevation of the scalp in the subgaleal plane. Four burr holes are traditionally placed, and the bone flap is elevated carefully so as not to allow the sphenoid ridge to impale the dura or brain.

The Sutar or bicoronal incision (Fig. 26.18B) is used to approach the frontal region more anteriorly or medially than is suitable from a pterional craniotomy. This allows access to a frontal tip or medial frontal lobe lesion and, via a subfrontal approach, to the chiasm or anterior hypothalamic region. The patient is usually supine with the head in the neutral position. The skin incision may extend from one zygomatic process to the other if needed (though this is rarely the case if a unilateral skull opening is planned), approximately 1 cm posterior to the hairline. The forehead tissues are reflected forward in the subgaleal/supraperiosteal plane, and care is taken to preserve both the superficial temporal artery laterally and the supraorbital branch of the ophthalmic nerve as it exits the supraorbital foramen. A minimum of four burr

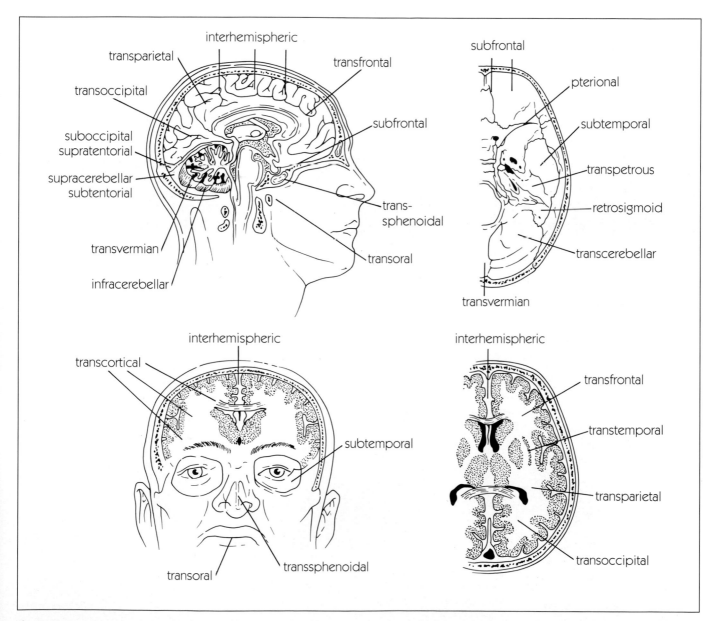

Figure 26.17 The various surgical approaches to brain tumors. Schematic anatomic drawings of the cranium and its contents in the midsagittal (upper left), axial skull base (upper right), coronal frontotemporal (lower left), and axial midcortical (lower right) planes. (Adapted with permission from Rosenblum ML, 1990)

holes (but occasionally six or even eight if a bilateral opening is needed) are placed, usually with two or more medial holes directly over or on both sides of the sagittal sinus. The anterior third of the sinus may be sacrificed, but care should taken not to violate it inadvertently when the bone flap is elevated. If the frontal air sinus is entered during the craniotomy, it should be exenterated of mucosal lining and packed with fat or muscle.

The corpus callosum and interhemispheric fissure are approached through a laterally based horseshoe-shaped incision extending at least 1 cm over the vertex medially (Fig. 26.18C). If positioned anteriorly over the coronal suture, this opening also allows transcallosal access to the anterior third ventricle through the foramen of Monro. The horseshoe opening is suitable for gliomas near the midline of the frontal lobe, ependymomas near the lateral ventricles, and hypothalamic astrocytomas. The patient is supine with the head in the neutral position and slightly flexed forward. Tumors of the parietal and occipital lobes can be approached through a more posterior opening. The patient can be positioned laterally for

parietal tumors and prone or sitting for occipital tumors. Four burr holes, the medial pair directly over the sagittal sinus, are usually placed; great care should be taken to protect the sinus during the opening.

The suboccipital craniectomy (Fig. 26.18D) is used to expose infratentorial lesions, such as cerebellar pilocytic astrocytomas or ependymomas. It may be located either in the midline, as shown, or in a paramedian position. For a midline opening, the patient is usually placed in the prone, sitting, or Concorde position. If the sitting position is used, care is required to prevent an air embolism, and both the surgical and anesthetic teams must be prepared to act promptly in the event of an embolus. Preoperative preparation for this position includes placement of an intracardiac catheter to withdraw air and preoperative cardiac echocardiography to rule out cardiac septal defects that could allow right-to-left air passage. For more lateral openings, such as the retromastoid suboccipital craniectomy, the patient is placed in the lateral decubitus position with the head rotated away from the lesion toward the floor and the

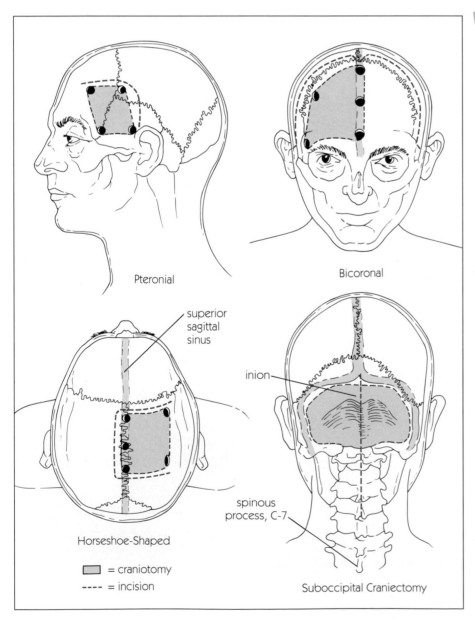

Pteronial

Bicoronal

superior sagittal sinus

inion

spinous process, C-7

Horseshoe-Shaped

▭ = craniotomy
---- = incision

Suboccipital Craniectomy

Figure 26.18 The four major types of craniotomy incisions and skull openings. The pterional opening (**A**) is useful for tumors of the frontal or temporal lobes near the sylvian fissure or skull base. The bicoronal opening (**B**) allows access to the anterior frontal lobes or subfrontal regions. The horseshoe-shaped opening (**C**) is appropriate for parietal or occipital lobe tumors, or for transcallosal access to the anterior third ventricle. The suboccipital craniectomy (**D**) allows access to tumors of the posterior fossa.

vertex tilted downward. The midline opening requires a linear incision from the inion to the third or fourth cervical spinous process. The incision is carried down to the bone of the occiput, and the semispinalis capitis and associated muscles are split and reflected laterally. In the region of the foramen magnum, the vertebral arteries must be carefully preserved as they loop over the lateral arches of the atlas toward the midline before they enter the dura. One to three burr holes are placed, and the craniectomy is enlarged, typically until the transverse sinuses, transverse-sigmoid junctions, and the margin of the foramen magnum are exposed.

RADIATION THERAPY OF GLIOMAS

Radiation therapy is the primary adjuvant treatment after surgical resection of most gliomas. Irradiation increases long-term survival of patients with anaplastic astrocytomas and glioblastoma multiforme, especially those younger than 65 years, regardless of the extent of resection. Ependymomas are particularly radiosensitive, and the duration of survival after resection depends on proper dosage and delivery of radiation. Although patients with low-grade astrocytomas and oligodendrogliomas also benefit in the short term from irradiation, particularly

after subtotal resection, it is unclear whether this leads to improvement in long-term survival.[17,47–50,73,74] Part of the rationale for irradiating these tumors is the likelihood of progression of tumor grade in the event of recurrence. Irradiation of incompletely resected pilocytic astrocytomas is controversial. The great majority of studies upon which these conclusions are based are retrospective and nonrandomized. The only prospective, randomized studies of the efficacy of radiation therapy were conducted in patients with high-grade astrocytomas.[47,50,96]

The side effects of radiation therapy have been divided into three categories.[50] Acute side effects, including reversible neurologic deficits due to tissue swelling that is responsive to steroid administration, occur during treatment. Early-delayed side effects, such as self-limited nausea, vomiting, dysphagia, or cerebral and cerebellar dysfunction presumably due to transient demyelination, occur weeks to months after treatment. Late-delayed side effects, principally radiation necrosis, occur months to years later. The brain, especially the developing brain, is sensitive to the effects of ionizing radiation on higher mental function.[42,97,98] Traditional methods of limiting the deleterious effects of ionizing radiation include careful fractionation and focal, rather than whole-brain, irradiation (Fig. 26.19).

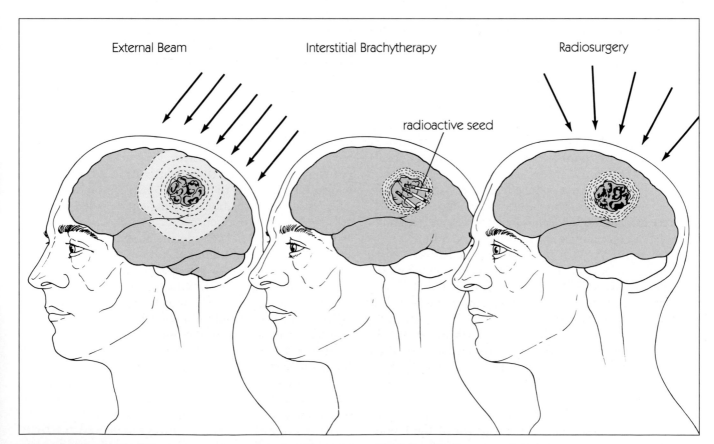

Figure 26.19 Radiation therapy for gliomas. The standard method of delivery is by external beam irradiation, either to the whole brain or a selective regional port (at left). Interstitial brachytherapy (center) uses implantable stereotactically placed radioactive seeds (usually iodine-125) for direct treatment to the region of the tumor bed. Focused external beam irradiation, or radiosurgery, delivers radiation to a narrowly defined region of the brain (at right) either by a calculated arc of a linear accelerator or by focused external cobalt sources.

The primary limitation of radiation therapy is the ability of normal surrounding brain to tolerate irradiation. Experimental efforts to circumvent this problem include novel methods of delivering ionizing radiation to the tumor bed, sensitizing the tumor cells to the effects of the radiation either chemically or thermally, and alternative sources of radiating particles, such as neutrons or heavy ions.[99] These topics are explored in more detail in Chapter 41.

Stereotactic implantation of iodine-125 seeds directly into the tumor bed (brachytherapy) has prolonged survival times in patients with recurrent and primary anaplastic astrocytomas and glioblastomas.[59] Similar results have been obtained by combining brachytherapy with hyperthermia to sensitize tumor cells to radiation.[100] Brachytherapy has been used primarily to treat patients in good functional classes who have relatively discrete tumors less than 5 cm in diameter that are not near midline or dural structures. More than 40% of such patients require reoperation for persistent tumor or radiation necrosis within 18 months after brachytherapy.

Stereotactic radiotherapy in the form of focused photons from a linear accelerator or targeted multiple cobalt sources is another method of directing high doses of radiation to the tumor while minimizing the exposure of adjacent normal brain. Experience with this approach in the treatment of malignant gliomas is extremely limited, and it is unlikely that it will be useful for large tumors. Additional information on this topic is reviewed in Chapter 42.

CHEMOTHERAPY OF GLIOMAS

Chemotherapy combined with surgical resection and postoperative radiation therapy is moderately effective in the treatment of anaplastic astrocytomas and glioblastomas.[101] Anecdotal and case reports suggest that chemotherapy may have some effectiveness against unresectable pilocytic astrocytomas in very young children[30,36] and recurrent oligodendrogliomas[17,72,75,76] and ependymomas,[85,86] especially those with anaplastic features.

One of the first drugs used successfully to treat malignant astrocytomas was 1,3-bis(2-chloroethyl)-1-nitrosourea (BCNU).[96] Despite enormous effort to improve upon the early results, BCNU remains the standard against which other regimens are frequently judged.[101] Another drug in this class is 1-(2-chloroethyl)-3-cyclohexyl-1-nitrosourea (CCNU), which has been used in many trials because it can be administered orally. Procarbazine is another oral agent with significant activity against brain tumors.

Multidrug regimens, intrathecal or intraarterial injection with or without transient disruption of the blood-brain barrier, and even intratumoral delivery of drugs are all being tested. Clinical trials have been undertaken to increase the efficacy of chemotherapy by manipulating cell sensitivity or enhancing drug delivery to tumor cells, while decreasing toxicity to normal tissues. A review of these efforts and future directions is presented in Chapter 43.

Immunotherapy for gliomas has been the focus of a great deal of investigation in recent years. There has been an exponential increase in basic knowledge of the intricate interplay and balance of the numerous cells and humoral factors of the immune system. So far, however, there is little evidence that immunotherapy improves survival in glioma patients. Four broad classes of immunotherapy—restorative, adoptive, active, and passive—are currently under investigation.[102]

Restorative immunotherapy seeks to stimulate the immune system of the cancer patient nonspecifically by administering agents that enhance immune function or remove immunosuppressive factors. Cytokines, including tumor necrosis factor, interferons, and interleukins, are molecules with immunomodulatory properties. Tumor necrosis factor is active against tumors, but its usefulness in the treatment of gliomas appears to be limited.[103,104] The interferons are glycoproteins produced by lymphocytes, fibroblasts, or epithelial cells in response to viral or antigenic stimulation. At least three families (alpha, beta, and gamma), each with different properties of production, regulation, and function, have been identified. Only interferon alpha has shown any effectiveness in clinical trials of patients with recurrent gliomas.[105] Interleukins stimulate cells of the immune system in a specific manner to enhance or amplify an immune response. The number of known interleukin molecules increases yearly, but to date most glioma work has centered on the first two. IL-1 has powerful and wide-ranging stimulatory properties, but side effects limit its usefulness. IL-2 has been principally used as an adjunct to adoptive immunotherapy.

Adoptive immunotherapy attempts to convey immunoreactivity by administering immune cells that have been activated in vitro. This activation may be either specific, as in the sensitization of a patient's pooled immune cells to his or her own tumor, or nonspecific, as in the activation of a patient's pooled immune cells by exposure to a nonspecific immunostimulant such as IL-2. Clinical trials of specific adoptive immunotherapy are still pending, although promise has been shown with in vitro testing.[106] Nonspecific adoptive immunotherapy in which lymphokine-activated killer (LAK) cells and IL-2 are injected into the bed of a malignant glioma have shown only limited efficacy and significant side effects, including local brain edema.[107,108]

Active immunotherapy attempts to stimulate the immune response by immunizing the patient with tumor-specific antigens. A recent prospective randomized trial of this therapy did not demonstrate improved survival in patients with malignant gliomas.[109]

Passive immunotherapy conveys enhanced reactivity to the tumor cells by the administration of specific antitumor antibodies. These antibodies either stimulate the patient's own immune defense against the tumor or are used to deliver radioactive or chemotherapeutic ligands to kill tumor cells.[102] Recent reports of monoclonal antibody production against tumor-specific antigens make this a promising field of immunotherapy research.[110,111]

The only glioma that can be cured by surgery alone is the pilocytic astrocytoma. Long-term survival is common in patients with low-grade astrocytomas, oligodendrogliomas, and occasionally, with appropriate adjuvant therapy, even ependymomas. Malignant astrocytomas are usually rapidly fatal despite multimodality therapy. One treatment option for tumor recurrence or progression is reoperation to resect additional tumor tissue. In cases of recurrent nonanaplastic lesions in otherwise healthy patients, reoperation is seldom questioned, given the likelihood of additional survival, and few studies have addressed this issue.[112]

Reoperation for malignant astrocytoma is more controversial, and the indications have been the subject of many reports. To those who believe a primary mass with the radiologic appearance of a high-grade glioma may be appropriately managed with biopsy and/or supportive care,[61,62] reoperation after failure of maximal multimodality therapy may appear inappropriate. Others have shown that the morbidity and mortality rates are no higher after reoperation than after the initial operation.[63] In selected patients with recurrent anaplastic astrocytoma or glioblastoma multiforme,[57,58] reoperation for tumor recurrence significantly improved median survival by 88 and 36 weeks, respectively. In one study, the proportion of additional survival time that was judged of high quality was substantially greater for anaplastic astrocytomas than for glioblastoma (90% versus less than one third).[58]

The prognostic variables associated with a good outcome after reoperation for tumor recurrence are essentially the same as for the initial operation: young age, good functional status, and apparent gross total resection. Age is a good predictor of total survival in patients undergoing reoperation, at least in part because of the interval between operation and reoperation,[113] but it does not correlate with survival after reoperation.[57,58,113] The importance of preoperative functional status of the patient is demonstrated by the two and one half times greater length of survival of patients with Karnofsky performance scores of 70 or greater compared with those with lower scores.[57] In this same study, complete resection at reoperation resulted in survival after the second surgery more than twice that after partial resection. Thus, in selected patients with tumor recurrence or progression despite multimodality therapy, reoperation can be performed safely and with improved overall survival.

Acknowledgement: The authors thank Stephen Ordway for editorial assistance.

REFERENCES

1. Berens ME, Rutka JT, Rosenblum ML. Brain tumor epidemiology, growth, and invasion. *Neurosurg Clin North Am.* 1990;1:1–18.

2. Jellinger K. Pathology of human intracranial neoplasia. In: Jellinger K, ed. *Therapy of Malignant Brain Tumors.* Berlin: Springer-Verlag; 1987:23–27.

3. Schoenberg BS, Cristine BW, Whisnant JP. The descriptive epidemiology of primary intracranial neoplasms: the Connecticut experience. *Am J Epidemiol.* 1976;104:499–510.

4. Zulch KJ. *Histological Typing of Tumors of the Central Nervous System.* Geneva: World Health Organization; 1979.

5. Bailey P, Cushing H. *A Classification of the Glioma Group on a Histogenetic Basis With a Correlated Study of Prognosis.* Philadelphia, Pa: JB Lippincott; 1926.

6. Kernohan JW, Mabon RF, Svien HJ, et al. A simplified classification of the gliomas. *Proc Staff Meeting Mayo Clin.* 1949;24:71–75.

7. Kernohan JW, Sayre GP. Atlas of Tumor Pathology, Section X, Fascicles 35, 37: *Tumors of the Central Nervous System.* Washington DC: Armed Forces Institute of Pathology; 1952:22–42.

8. Daumas-Duport C, Scheithauer B, O'Fallon J, et al. Grading of astrocytomas: a simple and reproducible method. *Cancer.* 1988;62:2152–2165.

9. Ringertz N. Grading of gliomas. *Acta Pathol Microbiol Scand.* 1950;27:51–64.

10. Burger PC, Vogel FS. *Surgical Pathology of the Nervous System and Its Coverings.* 2nd ed. New York, NY: John Wiley and Sons; 1982:226–266.

11. Burger PC, Vogel S, Green SB, et al. Glioblastoma multiforme and anaplastic astrocytoma: pathologic criteria and prognostic implications. *Cancer.* 1985; 56:1106–1111.

12. Zulch KJ. Principles of the new World Health Organization (WHO) classification of brain tumors. *Neuroradiology.* 1980;19:59–66.

13. Kim TS, Halliday AL, Hedley-Whyte ET, et al. Correlates of survival and the Daumas-Duport grading system for astrocytomas. *J Neurosurg.* 1991; 74:27–37.

14. Davis RL, Liu HC, Vestnys P, et al. Correlation of survival and diagnosis in supratentorial malignant gliomas. *J Neurooncol.* 1984;2:267. Abstract.

15. Ludwig CL, Smith MT, Godfrey AD, et al. A clinicopathological study of 323 patients with oligodendrogliomas. *Ann Neurol.* 1986;19:15–21.

16. Müller W, Afra D, Schröder R. Supratentorial recurrences of gliomas morphological studies in relation to time intervals with oligodendrolioma. *Acta Neurochir.* 1977;39:15–25.

17. Wallner KE, Gonzales M, Sheline GE. Treatment of oligodendrogliomas with or without postoperative irradiation. *J Neurosurg.* 1988;68:684–688.

18. Burger PC, Rawlings CE, Cox EB, et al. Clinico-

pathologic correlations in the oligodendroglioma. *Cancer.* 1987;59:1345–1352.

19. Hart MN, Petito CK, Earle KM. Mixed gliomas. *Cancer.* 1974;33:134–140.

20. Tchang S, Scotti G, Terbrugge K, et al. Computerized tomography as a possible aid to histological grading of supratentorial gliomas. *J Neurosurg.* 1977;46:735–739

21. Dean BL, Drayer BP, Bird CR, et al. Gliomas: classification with MR imaging. *Radiology.* 1990; 174:411–415.

22. Hoshino T, Prados M, Wilson CB, et al. Prognostic implications of the bromodeoxyuridine labeling index of human gliomas. *J Neurosurg.* 1989; 71:335–341.

23. Nishizaki T, Orita T, Saiki M, et al. Cell kinetics studies of human brain tumors by in vitro labeling using anti-BUdR monoclonal antibody. *J Neurosurg.* 1988;69:371–374.

24. Hoshino T, Rodriguez LA, Cho KG, et al. Prognostic implications of the proliferative potential of low-grade astrocytomas. *J Neurosurg.* 1988; 69:839–842.

25. Nagashima T, Hoshino T, Cho KG, et al. The proliferative potential of human ependymomas measured by in situ bromodeoxyuridine labeling. *Cancer.* 1988;61:2433–2438.

26. Germano IM, Ito M, Cho KG, et al. Correlation of histopathological features and proliferative potential of gliomas. *J Neurosurg.* 1989;70:701–706.

27. Zuber P, Hamou M-F, de Tribolet N. Identification of proliferating cells in human gliomas using the monoclonal antibody Ki-67. *Neurosurgery.* 1988;22:364–368.

28. Nishizaki T, Orita T, Furutani Y, et al. Flow-cytometric DNA analysis and immunohistochemical measurement of Ki-67 and BUdR labeling indices in human brain tumors. *J Neurosurg.* 1989;70:379–384.

29. Zulch KJ. *Brain Tumors: Their Biology and Pathology.* Berlin: Springer-Verlag; 1986.

30. Wallner KE, Gonzales MF, Edwards MSB, et al. Treatment results of juvenile pilocytic astrocytoma. *J Neurosurg.* 1988;69:171–176.

31. Mahaley MS, Mettlin C, Natarajan N, et al. National survey of patterns of care for brain-tumor patients. *J Neurosurg.* 1989;71:826–836.

32. Naidich TP, Lin JP, Leeds NE, et al. Primary tumors and other masses of the cerebellum and fourth ventricle: differential diagnosis by computed tomography. *Neuroradiology.* 1977;14:153–174.

33. Barkovich AJ. *Pediatric Neuroimaging.* New York, NY: Raven Press; 1990:151–175.

34. Palma L Guidetti B. Cystic pilocytic astrocytomas of the cerebral hemispheres. *J Neurosurg.* 1985; 62:811–815.

35. Shaw EG, Daumas-Duport C, Scheithauer BW, et al. Radiation therapy in the management of low-grade supratentorial astrocytomas. *J Neurosurg.* 1989;70:853–861

36. Civitello LA, Packer RJ, Rorke LB, et al. Leptomeningeal dissemination of low-grade gliomas in childhood. *Neurology.* 1988;38:562–566.

37. Gol A, McKissock W. The cerebellar astrocytomas: a report on verified cases. *J Neurosurg.* 1959; 16:287–296.

38. Michael Edwards, MD. Personal communication.

39. Garcia DM, Fulling KH. Juvenile pilocytic astrocytoma of the cerebrum in adults: a distinctive neoplasm with favorable prognosis. *J Neurosurg.* 1985;63:382–386

40. Oxenhandler DC, Sayers MP. The dilemma of childhood optic gliomas. *J Neurosurg.* 1978;48: 34–41.

41. Imes RK, Hoyt WF. Childhood chiasmal gliomas: update on the fate of patients in the 1969 San Francisco study. *Br J Ophthalmol.* 1986;70: 179–182.

42. Danoff BF, Cowchock FS, Marquette C, et al. Assessment of the long-term effects of primary radiation therapy for brain tumors in children. *Cancer.* 1982;49:1580–1586.

43. Harsh GR IV, Wilson CB. Neuroepithelial tumors of the adult brain. In: Youmans JR, ed. *Neurological Surgery,* 3rd ed. Philadelphia, Pa: WB Saunders Co; 1990:3041.

44. McKernan RO, Thomas DGT. The clinical study of gliomas. In: Thomas DGT, Graham DI, eds. *Brain Tumors: Scientific Basis, Clinical Investigation, and Current Therapy.* London: Butterworths; 1980: 197–215.

45. Kazner E, Wende S, Grumme T, et al, eds. *Computed Tomography in Intracranial Tumors.* Berlin: Springer-Verlag; 1982.

46. Leibel SA, Sheline GE, Wara WM, et al. The role of radiation therapy in the treatment of astrocytomas. *Cancer.* 1975;35:1551–1557.

47. Morantz RA. Radiation therapy in the treatment of cerebral astrocytoma. *Neurosurgery.* 1987;20: 975–982.

48. Weir B, Grace M. The relative significance of factors affecting postoperative survival in astrocytomas, grades one and two. *Can J Neurol Sci.* 1976; 3:47–50

49. Soffietti R, Chio A, Giordana MT, et al. Prognostic factors in well-differentiated cerebral astrocytomas in the adult. *Neurosurgery.* 1989;24:686 692.

50. Leibel SA, Sheline GE. Radiation therapy for neoplasms of the brain. J Neurosurg. 1987;66:1–22.

51. Laws ER, Taylor WF, Clifton MB, et al. Neurosurgical management of low-grade astrocytoma of the cerebral hemispheres. *J Neurosurg.* 1984; 61:665–673.

52. Muller W, Afra D, Schroeder R. Supratentorial recurrences of gliomas: morphological studies in relation to time intervals with astrocytomas. *Acta Neurochir (Wien).* 1977;37:75–91.

53. Kelly PJ, Daumas-Duport C, Scheithauer BW, et al. Stereotactic histologic correlations of computed

tomography- and magnetic resonance imaging-defined abnormalities in patients with glial neoplasms. *Mayo Clin Proc.* 1987;62:450–459.

54. Shapiro WR, Green SB, Burger PC, et al. Randomized trial of three chemotherapy regimens and two radiotherapy regimens in postoperative treatment of malignant glioma: Brain Tumor Cooperative Group trial 8001. *J Neurosurg.* 1989;71:1–9.

55. Marsa GW, Goffinet DR, Rubinstein LJ, et al. Megavoltage irradiation in the treatment of gliomas of the brain and spinal cord. *Cancer.* 1975; 36:1681–1689.

56. Kramer S. Radiation therapy in the management of malignant gliomas. In: *Cancer of the Central Nervous System. Proceedings of the Seventh National Cancer Conference.* Philadelphia, Pa: JB Lippincott; 1983:823–826.

57. Ammirati M, Galicich JH, Arbit E, et al. Reoperation in the treatment of recurrent intracranial malignant gliomas. *Neurosurgery.* 1987;21:607–614.

58. Harsh GR IV, Levin VA, Gutin PH, et al. Reoperation for recurrent glioblastoma and anaplastic astrocytoma. *Neurosurgery.* 1987;21:615–621.

59. Larson DA, Gutin PH, Leibel SA, et al. Stereotactic irradiation of brain tumors. *Cancer.* 1990; 65:792–799.

60. Frankel SA, German WJ. Glioblastoma multiforme: review of 219 cases with regard to natural history, pathology, diagnostic methods, and treatment. *J Neurosurg.* 1958;15:489–503.

61. Newelt EA, Nazarro JM, Gumerlock MK. Is there a role for biopsy in the treatment of supratentorial high grade glioma? *Clin Neurosurg.* 1990; 36:384–407.

62. Wroe SJ, Foy PM, Shaw MDM, et al. Differences between neurological and neurosurgical approaches in the management of malignant brain tumors. *Br Med J.* 1986;293:1015–1018.

63. Fadul C, Wood J, Thaler H, et al. Morbidity and mortality of craniotomy for excision of supratentorial gliomas. *Neurology.* 1988;38:1374–1379.

64. Ciric I, Ammirati M, Vick N, et al. Supratentorial gliomas: surgical considerations and immediate postoperative results. *Neurosurgery.* 1987;21:21–26.

65. Ammirati M, Vick N, Liao Y, et al. Effect of the extent of surgical resection on survival and quality of life in patients with supratentorial glioblastomas and anaplastic astrocytomas. *Neurosurgery.* 1987; 21:201–206.

66. Salcman M. Survival in glioblastoma: historical perspective. *Neurosurgery.* 1980;7:435–439.

67. Hoffman HJ, Duffner KP. Extraneural metastases of central nervous system tumors. *Cancer.* 1985; 56:1778–1782.

68. Burger PC, Green SB. Patient age, histologic features, and length of survival in patients with glioblastoma multiforme. *Cancer.* 1987;59:1617–1625.

69. Wood JR, Green SB, Shapiro WR. The prognostic importance of tumor size in malignant gliomas: a computed tomographic scan study by the Brain Tumor Cooperative Group. *J Clin Oncol.* 1988; 6:338–343.

70. Stenning SP, Freedman LS, Bleehen NM. Prognostic factors for high-grade malignant glioma: development of a prognostic index. *J Neurooncol.* 1990;9:47–55.

71. Mørk SJ, Lindegaard K-F, Halvorsen TB, et al. Oligodendroglioma: incidence and biological behavior in a defined population. *J Neurosurg.* 1985; 63:881–889.

72. Chin HW, Hazel JJ, Kim TH, et al. Oligodendrogliomas, I: a clinical study of cerebral oligodendrogliomas. *Cancer.* 1980;45:1458–1466.

73. Sun ZM, Genka S, Shitara N, et al. Factors possibly influencing the prognosis of oligodendroglioma. *Neurosurgery.* 1988;22:886–891.

74. Lindegaard K-F, Mørk SJ, Eide GE, et al. Statistical analysis of clinicopathological features, radiotherapy, and survival in 170 cases of oligodendroglioma. *J Neurosurg.* 1987;67:224–230.

75. Saarinen UM, Pihko H, Makipernaa A. High-dose thiotepa with autologous bone marrow rescue in recurrent malignant oligodendroglioma: a case report. *J Neurooncol.* 1990;9:57–61.

76. Smith MT, Ludwig CL, Godfrey AD, et al. Grading of oligodendrogliomas. *Cancer.* 1983;52: 2107–2114.

77. Wallner KE, Wara WM, Sheline GE, et al. Intracranial ependymomas: results of treatment with partial or whole brain irradiation without spinal irradiation. *Int J Radiat Oncol Biol Phys.* 1986;12:1937–1941.

78. Barone BM, Elvidge AR. Ependymomas: a clinical survey. *J Neurosurg.* 1970;33:428–438.

79. Fokes EC Jr, Earle KM. Ependymomas: clinical and pathologic aspects. *J Neurosurg.*1969;30:585–594.

80. Ringertz N, Reymond A. Ependymomas and choroid plexus papillomas. *J Neuropathol Exp Neurol.* 1949;8:355–380.

81. Salazar OM, Castro-Vita H, Van Houtte P, et al. Improved survival in cases of intracranial ependymoma after radiation therapy. *J Neurosurg.* 1983; 59:652–659.

82. Shaw EG, Evans RG, Scheithauer BW, et al. Postoperative radiotherapy of intracranial ependymoma in pediatric and adult patients. *Int J Radiat Oncol Biol Phys.* 1987;13:1457–1462.

83. Ross GW, Rubinstein LJ. Lack of histopathological correlation of malignant ependymomas with postoperative survival. *J Neurosurg.* 1989;70:31–36.

84. Marks JE, Adler SJ. A comparative study of ependymomas by site of origin. *Int J Radiat Oncol Biol Phys.* 1982;8:37–43.

85. Kahn AB, D'Souza BJ, Wharam MD, et al. Cisplatin therapy in recurrent childhood brain tumors. *Cancer Treat Rep.* 1982;66:2013–2020.

86. Levin VA, Edwards MSB, Gutin PH, et al. Phase II evaluation of dibromodulcitol in the treatment of

recurrent medulloblastoma, ependymoma, and malignant astrocytoma. *J Neurosurg.* 1984;61: 1063–1068.

87. Li FP, Fraumeni JF. Soft-tissue sarcomas, breast cancer, and other neoplasms: a familial syndrome? *Ann Intern Med.* 1969;71:747–749.

88. Lossignol D, Grossman SA, Scheidler VR, et al. Familial clustering of malignant astrocytomas. *J Neurooncol.* 1990;9:139–145.

89. Rosenblum ML. General surgical principles, alternatives, and limitations. *Neurosurg Clin North Am.* 1990;1:19–36.

90. Karnofsky DA, Abelmann WH, Craver LF, et al. The use of the nitrogen mustards in the palliative treatment of carcinoma: with particular reference to bronchogenic carcinoma. *Cancer.* 1948; 1:634–656.

91. Burger PC, Kleihues P. Cytologic composition of the untreated glioblastoma with implications for evaluation of needle biopsies. *Cancer.* 1989; 63:2014–2023.

92. Chandrasoma PT, Smith MM, Apuzzo MLJ. Stereotactic biopsy in the diagnosis of brain masses: comparison of results of biopsy and resected surgical specimen. *Neurosurgery.* 1989; 24:160–165.

93. Salcman M. Resection and reoperation in neurooncology: rationale and approach. *Neurol Clin.* 1985;3:831–842.

94. Ciric I, Vick NA, Mikhael MA, et al. Aggressive surgery for malignant supratentorial gliomas. *Clin Neurosurg.* 1990;36:375–383.

95. Yasargil MG, Reichman MV, Kubik S. Preservation of the frontotemporal branch of the facial nerve using the interfascial temporalis flap for pterional craniotomy: technical note. *J Neurosurg.* 1987; 67:463–466.

96. Walker MD, Alexander E Jr, Hunt WE, et al. Evaluation of BCNU and/or radiotherapy in the treatment of anaplastic gliomas: a cooperative clinical trial. *J Neurosurg.* 1978;49:333–343.

97. Al-Mefty O, Kersh JE, Routh A, et al. The long-term side effects of radiation therapy for benign brain tumors in adults. *J Neurosurg.* 1990;73: 502–512.

98. Martins AN, Johnston JS, Henry JM, et al. Delayed radiation necrosis of the brain. *J Neurosurg.* 1977;47:336–345.

99. Woo SY, Maor MH. Improving radiotherapy for brain tumors. *Oncology.* 1990;4:41–45.

100. Sneed PK, Stauffer PR, Gutin PH, et al. Interstitial irradiation and hyperthermia for the treatment of recurrent malignant brain tumors. *Neurosurgery.* 1991;28:206–215.

101. Kornblith PL, Walker M. Chemotherapy for malignant gliomas. *J Neurosurg.* 1988;68:1–17.

102. Gillespie GY, Mahaley MS. Biological response modifier therapies for patients with malignant gliomas. In: Thomas DGT, ed. *Neuro-oncology: Primary Malignant Brain Tumors.* Baltimore, Md: Johns Hopkins University Press; 1990:242–282.

103. Barna BP, Estes ML, Jacobs BS, et al. Human astrocytes proliferate in response to tumor necrosis factor alpha. *J Neuroimmunol.* 1990;30:239–243.

104. Bethea JR, Gillespie CY, Chung IY, et al. Tumor necrosis factor production and receptor expression by a human malignant glioma cell line, D54-MG. *J Neuroimmunol.* 1990;30:1–13.

105. Mahaley MS Jr, Urso MB, Whaley RA, et al. Immunobiology of primary intracranial tumors, 10: therapeutic efficacy of interferon in the treatment of recurrent gliomas. *J Neurosurg.* 1985; 63:719–725.

106. Miyatake S, Handa H, Yamashita J, et al. Induction of human glioma specific cytotoxic T-lymphocyte lines by autologous tumour stimulation and interleukin-2. *J Neurooncol.* 1986;4:55–64.

107. Barba D, Saris SC, Holder C, et al. Intratumoral LAK cell and interleukin-2 therapy of human gliomas. *J Neurosurg.* 1989;70:175–182.

108. Merchant RE, Ellison MD, Young HF. Immunotherapy for malignant glioma using human recombinant interleukin-2 and activated autologous lymphocytes: a review of pre-clinical and clinical investigations. *J Neurooncol.* 1990; 8:173–188.

109. Mahaley MS, Gillespie GY, Bertsch L, et al. Active immunotherapy of patients with malignant gliomas: a prospective randomized study. Manuscript in preparation.

110. Nanda A, Liwnicz B, Atkinson BF, et al. Monoclonal antibodies with cytotoxic reactivities against human gliomas. *J Neurosurg.* 1989;71:892–897.

111. Kokunai T, Tamaki N, Matsumoto S. Antigen related to cell proliferation in malignant gliomas recognized by a human monoclonal antibody. *J Neurosurg.* 1990;73:901–908.

112. Pool JL. The management of recurrent gliomas. *Clin Neurosurg.* 1968;15:265–287.

113. Salcman M, Kaplan RS, Ducker TB, et al. Effect of age and reoperation on survival in the combined modality treatment of malignant astrocytoma. *Neurosurgery.* 1982;10:454–463.

Chapter 27

Metastatic Tumors

Byron Young, Roy A. Patchell

A recent randomized study showed that surgical excision of a single cerebral metastasis followed by whole-brain radiation therapy provides significantly longer survival, higher quality of life, and fewer local brain recurrences than treatment with whole-brain radiotherapy alone. Death and impairment in this study of patients with systemic cancer and a brain metastasis were more often due to the cerebral metastasis than to the systemic cancer. Surgical excision of the cerebral metastasis consequently accounted for the better survival rate achieved in this group of patients. This series of patients had a 4% death rate within the first 30 days following the surgery; this mortality rate was identical to that of patients receiving radiation therapy alone. Operative morbidity was 8%, whereas the morbidity rate was 17% in the group treated by radiation alone. Eleven percent of the patients with presumed single metastasis have had a nonmetastatic lesion.[1]

INDICATIONS FOR SURGERY

Based upon the findings of the study cited above, I recommend surgical excision when the cerebral metastasis is single, the systemic disease is either controlled or presumed eradicated, and the metastasis can most likely be removed without increasing the neurologic deficit (Fig. 27.1).

Although nearly 25% of patients with systemic cancer develop brain metastasis, only approximately 50% of these cerebral metastases are single at the time of their diagnosis. Approximately one half of the patients with a single metastasis should not be considered for surgical excision of the cerebral lesion because of the presence of uncontrolled systemic disease or because the location of the metastasis makes the risk of a postoperative neurologic deficit too great. Thus, only approximately 25% of all patients with solitary cerebral metastasis remain as potential candidates for surgical excision of the brain metastasis.[1]

To establish a histologic diagnosis of the cerebral lesion, surgical excision or stereotactic biopsy should be performed in patients with a single lesion thought to be metastatic from known systemic cancer. Because approximately 10% of these single lesions will not be metastases from the systemic disease, a definitive diagnosis often changes the subsequent treatment. Approximately one half of the single lesions are inflammatory in nature and can be treated with antibiotics.

Patients with lymphoma, leukemia, and other exquisitely radiosensitive lesions who develop multiple intracranial lesions should undergo radiation therapy

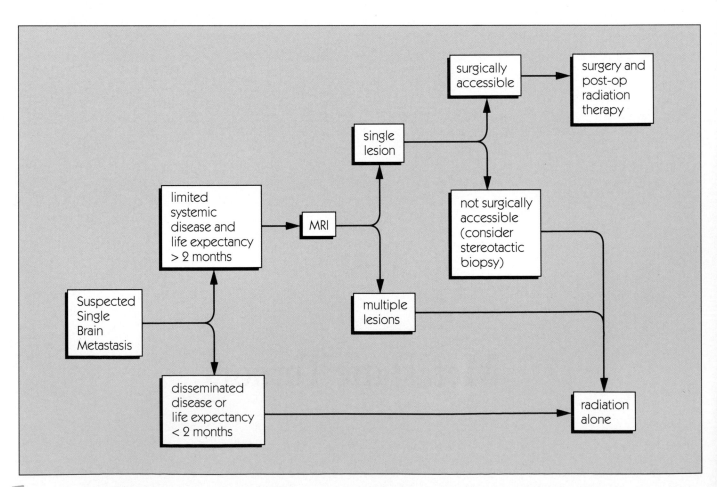

Figure 27.1 Therapeutic approach to brain metastasis. (Adapted with permission from Young B, Patchell R. Surgery for a single brain metastasis. In: Wilkins RH, Rengachary SS, eds. *Neurosurgery Update I: Diagnosis, Operative Technique and Neuro-Oncology.* New York, NY: McGraw-Hill; 1990:474)

rather than surgery. In this setting, stereotactic biopsy is not necessary prior to beginning therapy. Stereotactic biopsy should be performed, however, in patients with highly radiosensitive lesions who develop a single lesion, to prove that the new lesion is in fact metastatic.

Treatment with radiosurgery has been advocated by some for treatment of brain metastasis, but the efficacy of this method compared to that of surgery plus radiation remains unproven.

PREOPERATIVE PLANNING

The first month mortality rate for patients with metastatic lesions treated with radiation therapy alone is 5% or less.[1] To be considered as an option, surgery to remove a metastatic tumor must have a similarly low mortality rate and must result only infrequently in neurologic deficits.

In the study by Patchell et al. the median survival of patients treated with surgical excision was only 40 weeks. The median hospital stay for these patients was 3 to 4 weeks, with much of this time devoted to the work-up and treatment of the primary tumor.[1] Because long survival times are unlikely following surgery for metastatic brain tumors, the highest possible postoperative quality of life must be achieved if surgery is to be considered worthwhile. Consequently, neurologic deficits due to surgical manipulation should occur in less than 10% of cases.

Except in emergency situations, preoperative steroids should be given to decrease cerebral edema and mass effect associated with the cerebral metastasis, in order to prevent herniation through the opening in the dura at the time of the craniotomy. Even when they cause symptoms, very small lesions will not be demonstrated by CT scans and MRI studies in patients receiving steroids. Consequently, when possible, steroids should not be administered until the cranial MRI or CT scan is obtained.

Prior to operative intervention, an MRI or a double-dose CT scan should be performed in patients with systemic disease and presumed single metastasis to the brain. These studies are more likely than the conventional scanning to pick up additional lesions that may contraindicate intracranial surgery. An MRI that demonstrates surface anatomy should be obtained and carefully studied to plan the safest operative avenue to the tumor. Precise localization of the central sulcus is necessary for lesions in the motor strip.

SURGICAL TECHNIQUE

A stereotactic frame is placed on the patient preoperatively in the CT or MRI suite. The stereotactic probe is used to determine the position of the scalp incision (Fig. 27.2). Because most of these patients will receive postoperative radiation therapy, wound healing is impaired and delayed. I consequently make a linear incision centered over the tumor rather than a U- or question mark-shaped incision.

Cerebral metastases are frequently associated with a large amount of cerebral edema. Often the lesion to be

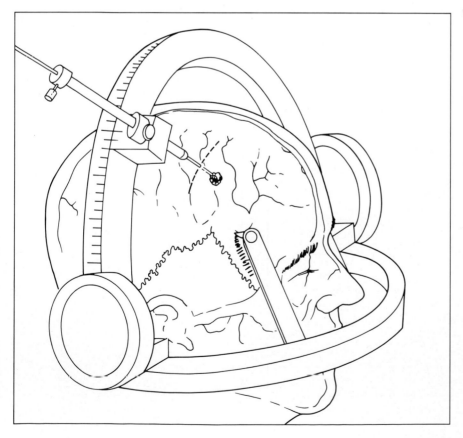

Figure 27.2 A small intracranial lesion is localized with a stereotactic frame in place. The dotted line marks the scalp incision. The probe is touching the surface of the tumor. (After R. Gersony)

resected is quite small, frequently only 1 cm in diameter. The symptoms or signs that herald the tumor are largely due to the mass effect of the edema. Many small, asymptomatic lesions are discovered as a part of a complete survey to detect the presence of metastasis from a primary systemic site.

Subcortical tumors, even when small, may be associated with a large amount of surrounding edema and difficult to locate. Additionally, the presence of a small lesion and the administration of preparatory steroids can cause the overlying cortical surface to appear normal. An extensive search for these elusive lesions may result in injury to functioning brain. A single direct approach to the lesion must be undertaken, however, to lessen the chances of a postoperative neurologic deficit. We always use stereotactic techniques to localize small lesions (Fig. 27.3).

Cerebral metastases should be removed using microsurgical techniques. Occasionally, the plane between a tumor and normal brain tissue is unclear. Meticulous hemostasis is critical to preserve visualization in the plane of demarcation between tumor and compressed and/or edematous normal brain. Even the slightest bleeding should be immediately controlled. Such control is only possible with the magnification and illumination provided by the microscope. Use of the microscope allows gentler handling of tissues, which lessens the chance of damage to contiguous functioning brain tissue. Self-retaining brain retractors should be used to minimize the manipulation of tissues necessary for gaining exposure of the tumor.

Prolonged searching for a small elusive lesion is probably the major cause of postoperative neurologic deficits. For deep lesions we use the technique described by Kelly[2] to develop a dissection plane through the sulcus rather than the gyrus. A gyral incision should only be made when the lesion is very superficial and more dissection would be required through a sulcal than through a gyral approach. The stereotactic probe is used as a guide to locate the tumor directly (Fig. 27.4).

Many cerebral metastases occur in the distribution of the middle cerebral artery. As such, many are located in or near eloquent areas of the brain. Surgical injury to these areas results in a deficit in speech, vision, or sensorimotor function. Lesions located under the precentral gyrus usually should not be directly approached through the gyrus but should be approached either through the precentral or postcentral sulcus. An approach through the sylvian fissure is often preferred for tumors deep and medial to the middle cerebral artery.[2] When the lesion is in the speech area, consideration should be given to performing the surgery with the patient awake, using cortical mapping and cortical stimulation to identify speech and motor areas. If the decision is made to remove a deeply located lesion, stereotactic localization and careful planning of the surgical approach are essential. For deep midline lesions, a computer-assisted system is helpful in planning the trajectory so as to avoid important vascular and neural structures.[2]

Intraoperative ultrasound can be used to identify the lesion, but I prefer stereotactic localization because of its greater precision. This enables the craniotomy to be smaller than the opening needed for adequate exposure for ultrasonographic localization. Another reason for preferring stereotactic localization rather than ultrasonography is that a larger craniotomy is necessary with ultrasonography to insure that the bony opening is over the tumor. Placing markers on the scalp with either CT or plain film localization is not as accurate as stereotactic localization. Superficial lesions in the prefrontal and occipital areas may be treated without stereotactic localization.

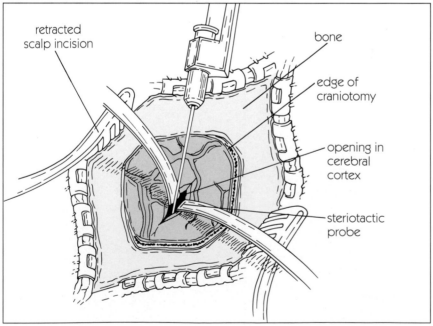

Figure 27.3 The linear scalp incision and small craniotomy are illustrated. The opening in the brain has been localized with the stereotactic probe, and the approach to the tumor is guided by the probe in place.

retracted scalp incision

bone

edge of craniotomy

opening in cerebral cortex

steriotactic probe

Every effort should be made to excise the lesion completely, because complete removal appears related to both the length and the quality of postoperative survival.[1-3] Metastatic lesions are usually very well circumscribed; in the vast majority of cases, therefore, complete excision should be achievable. Some series report that a complete excision is obtained in only about two thirds of cases. More recent series show that complete excision is possible in almost 100% of cases, at least as judged by early postoperative CT scan or MRI.[2,3]

If there is any question of residual or metastatic tumor after resection, a frozen section of the tumor bed should be performed so that an intraoperative decision can be made about complete resection of the lesion. Complete resection with tumor-free margins should be accomplished.

TREATMENT FOR PERSISTENT NEW CEREBRAL METASTASIS

After the immediate postoperative period, the patient should be followed at least every 2 months. The reap-

pearance of a persisting lesion in the surgical site could be treated with re-excision, additional stereotactic radiosurgery, or interstitial brachytherapy. The appearance of a second, single lesion in a remote site can be treated with surgical excision, brachytherapy, or radiosurgery. I am much more likely to operate for a second lesion occurring serially, particularly after an interval of several months, than if two lesions occur simultaneously.

SURGERY FOR MULTIPLE METASTASES

Patients with more than one intracranial lesion are not ordinarily considered surgical candidates. On the rare occasions that a patient has one or more additional lesions in silent areas, excision of a life-threatening lesion should be undertaken. An example of such an occasion is a large metastasis to the cerebellum causing brain stem compression; such a lesion must be excised to preserve life even when several small, asymptomatic, intracranial supratentorial lesions are coexistent. The supratentorial lesions can then be irradiated postoperatively. This approach is more likely to be helpful in the

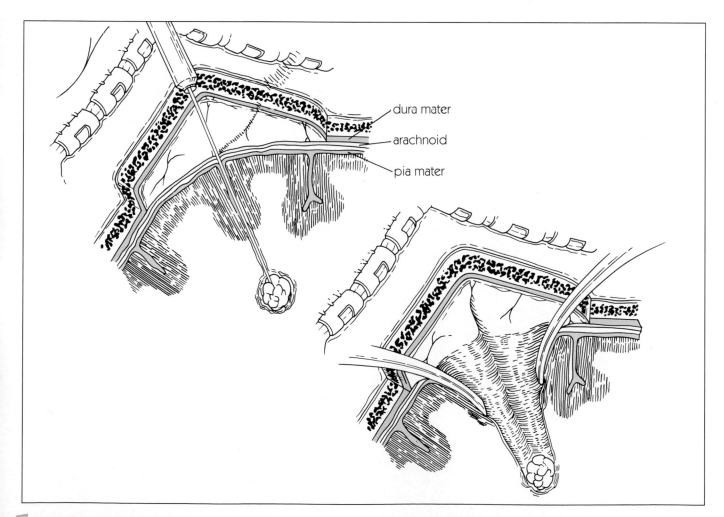

dura mater
arachnoid
pia mater

Figure 27.4 (A) The stereotactic probe precisely locates the tumor. (B) The tumor is exposed with minimal brain retraction.

treatment of lesions that are relatively radiosensitive, such as breast carcinoma and small cell lung metastasis than in the treatment of radioresistant lesions, such as melanomas.

On unusual occasions, we recommend excision of one or more intracranial lesions. When one lesion is life-threatening, the systemic disease is controlled, and the patient is expected to return to a Karnofsky rating score of 70 or more after excision of the single lesion, I recommend surgery. When multiple lesions have failed to respond to radiotherapy or chemotherapy, and subsequently one lesion becomes life-threatening, emergency surgery is not usually performed.

POSTOPERATIVE CARE

Whether or not patients should have postoperative radiation therapy is a matter of debate when the CT scan or MRI shows no residual tumor and the surgeon's opinion is that total excision of the tumor has been accomplished. The standard treatment in the United States is to administer whole-brain radiation therapy with 30 to 36 Gy. A national randomized trial is now being conducted to compare the results of surgical excision alone in patients with no postoperative residual tumor proven by CT or MRI to those achieved by surgical excision plus postoperative radiation therapy. We usually maintain steroid administration until radiotherapy is completed.

REFERENCES

1. Patchell RA, Tibbs PA, Walsh JW, et al. A randomized trial of surgery in the treatment of single metastases to the brain. *N Engl J Med.* 1990; 322:494–500.
2. Kelly PJ. *Tumor Stereotaxis.* Philadelphia, Pa: WB Saunders Co; 1991:358–369.
3. Kelly PJ, Kall BA, Goerss SJ. Results of computed tomography-based computer-assisted resection of metastatic intracranial tumors. *Neurosurgery.* 1988;22:7–17.

Chapter 28

Meningiomas

Ossama Al-Mefty, T.C. Origitano

The term *meningioma* is the noncommittal, all-encompassing name coined by Harvey Cushing for this tumor of the meninges, which is usually benign.[1] Meningiomas are discrete and vary from a few millimeters to many centimeters in diameter. Symptoms are caused by compression. Meningiomas are particularly dear to the neurosurgeon because they can often be totally surgically removed.

EPIDEMIOLOGY

Meningiomas account for 15% of intracranial tumors. They commonly occur in the fourth through sixth decades of life, with a peak incidence at age 45 years. Females have meningiomas more often than males, but this varies according to site from a ratio of 3:2 in the supratentorial area to a ratio of 5:1 in the intraspinal area. They are rare in children; only about 1.5% of all meningiomas occur in childhood, but these tumors are more aggressive. Meningiomas strike both sexes equally

in this age group. Ninety percent of meningiomas are intracranial; of these about 90% are supratentorial. Meningiomas outside the central nervous system are rare and are believed to result from ectopic rests of meningeal cells. The frequency of tumors and their most common sites are shown in Figure 28.1.[2-4]

ETIOLOGY

As with virtually all other brain tumors, the etiology of meningiomas is unknown. Cases exist, however, in which the tumor has arisen under a fracture, from an area of scarred dura, or around a retained foreign body.[5] Conceivably, these factors contributed to the formation of the meningiomas. Low- and high-dose radiation has been implicated in meningioma formation, especially during childhood.[6] These tumors have been induced in laboratory animals with oncogenic viruses. Antigens from both DNA and RNA viruses have been recovered from a significant number of human meningiomas.

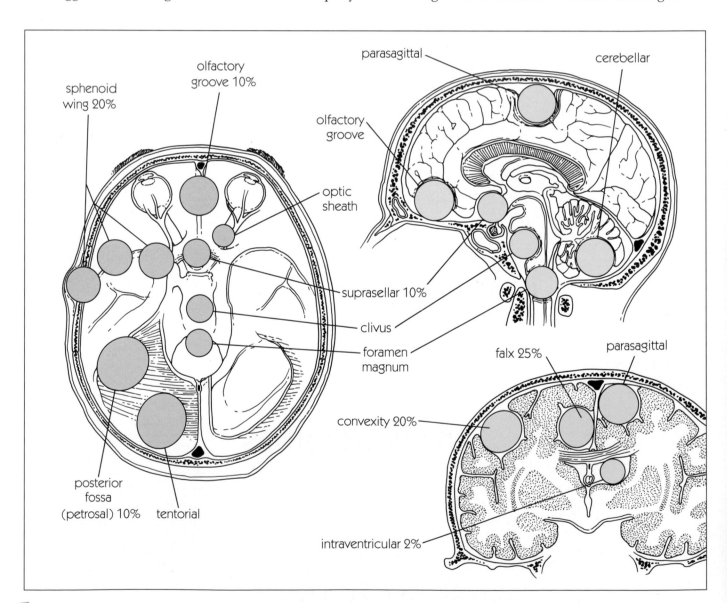

Figure 28.1 Three views of the skull and brain demonstrate the various locations of tumors and their relative occurrence at these sites.

Patients with von Recklinghausen's disease tend to develop multiple meningiomas at a young age in association with other central nervous system tumors. Chromosomal aberrations are regularly seen in the tumor; meningioma cells often lose one copy of chromosome 22. In 75% of cases, the tumors show hypoploidy. A significant number of meningiomas in males lose the Y chromosome. Hormonal factors may play a role in the genesis of meningiomas; both estrogen and progesterone receptors have been found in meningioma preparations. These steroid receptors are perhaps related to the genesis of the neoplasm, thus explaining the higher incidence of these tumors in women than in men.

HISTOGENESIS

Meningiomas are thought to originate from arachnoid cap cells, which form the outer lining of the arachnoid granulations, a theory supported by the similar ultrastructural features in normal meningeal cap cells and the cells of meningiomas, as well as the tendency of both to form whorls. These cells are most prevalent near collections of arachnoid villi at the dural-venous sinuses and their large tributary veins, and meningiomas may arise anywhere the cells are located. Arachnoid cell clusters at the cranial base, studied as early as 1912, are usually found at the cribriform plate, the medial region of the middle fossa, and at the foramina where the cranial nerves exit. Ventricular meningiomas appear to arise from arachnoid cell rests within the choroid plexus. Spinal meningiomas probably arise from arachnoid villi in the vicinity of existing nerve roots. Figure 28.2 demonstrates the arachnoid villi with the cap cells as they relate to the origin of meningiomas.[7]

PATHOLOGY

GROSS PATHOLOGY

A meningioma is usually a globular tumor arising from a small attachment to the dura, although more extensive secondary dural attachments may develop. Meningiomas are well-demarcated, round or oval, and frequently mul-

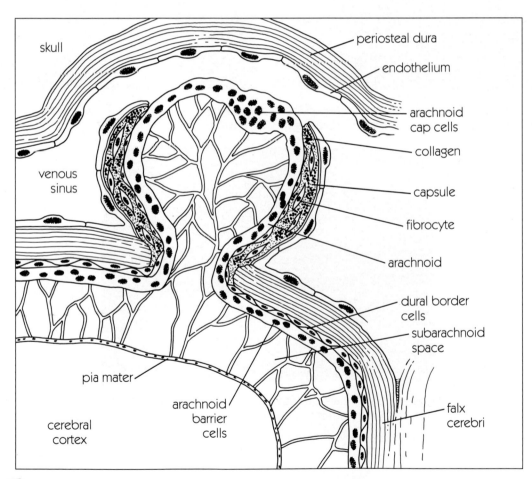

Figure 28.2 The architecture of the arachnoid villi, depicting arachnoid cap cells, the origin of meningiomas.

tilobulated (Fig. 28.3).[3,8] They are firm and pink, and vary in consistency from easily suckable to rock hard (Fig. 28.4). Their vascularity varies greatly, as does the degree of edema around the tumor. Edema might be massive despite the small size of the tumor.[2] An *en plaque* meningioma, which has a flat pancake appearance under a thickened area of involved bone (Fig. 28.5), occasionally occurs, usually in the area of the sphenoid ridge. Multiple meningiomas occur in 5% to 15% of patients, particularly in association with von Recklinghausen's disease (Fig. 28.6).

The histologic hallmark of meningiomas is whorls that form around a central hyaline material, which eventually calcify and form psammoma bodies or interlacing bundles of elongated fibroblasts with narrow nuclei (Fig. 28.7). The microscopic appearances of meningiomas fall into a variety of patterns that have led to a multiplicity of classifications and a variety of terms. Five categories of meningiomas have been designated: syncytial, transitional, fibrous, angioblastic, and malignant. Aside from the latter two categories, the histologic patterns do not predict tumor behavior. Malignant tumors are

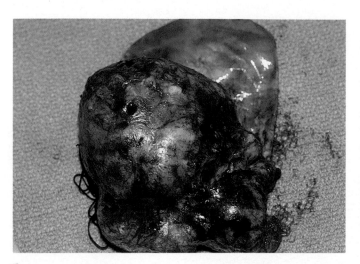

Figure 28.3 Surgical specimen of a meningioma demonstrating a well-demarcated multilobulated tumor on a dural base.

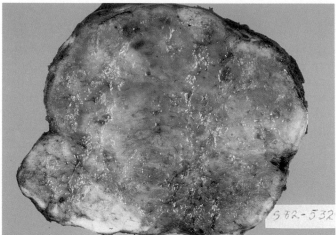

Figure 28.4 Cut surface of a meningioma demonstrating its firm character and pinkish color.

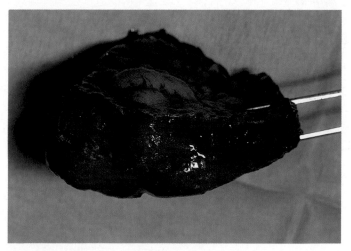

Figure 28.5 Operative photograph of *en plaque* meningioma with bony involvement.

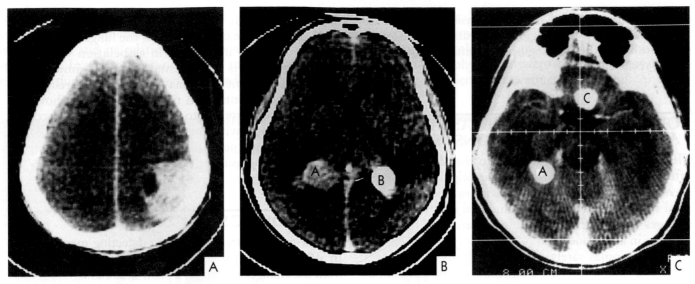

Figure 28.6 CT scan studies of multiple meningiomas in a patient with neurofibromatosis type II. (**A**) Left convexity meningioma. (**B**) A,B=bilateral intraventricular meningiomas. (**C**) A,C=tuberculum sellae meningioma. (**D**) Bilateral acoustic neurofibromas (arrows).

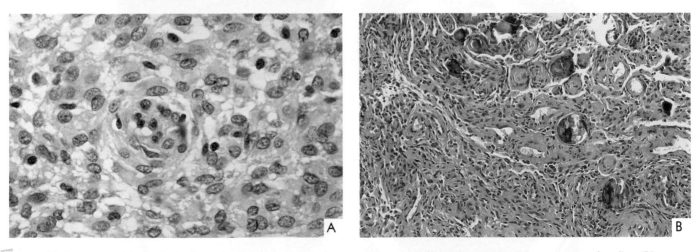

Figure 28.7 H & E stain of a typical meningioma showing characteristic whorl formations (**A**) and psammoma bodies (**B**).

graphy demonstrates the tumor's vascularity and its feeders in preparation for preoperative embolization. It shows adjacent venous drainage and the patency of major venous sinuses, and it helps the neurosurgeon evaluate the cerebral circulation for collateral vessels. A typical angiographic finding is a tumor supplied by a hypertrophied meningeal vessel, depicted by a prolonged homogenous vascular blush in the late venous phase. The vessels entering the tumor show a sunburst pattern (Fig. 28.12). Preoperative embolization of meningiomas can greatly ease their surgical resection.

CLINICAL PRESENTATION

The clinical symptoms and signs of meningiomas are related to those of an intracranial mass lesion or seizure.

The tumor has a predilection for certain regions and a tendency to produce hyperostosis of the skull, and some symptoms and signs are specific to the tumor's location. The clinical course of a meningioma characteristically spans a period of years. Depending on the location, the tumor may be giant before it becomes symptomatic, it may be discovered only after death because the patient was asymptomatic, or the patient may have a typical neurologic syndrome because adjacent neural structures are compressed (Fig. 28.13).

CONVEXITY

More than 70% of convexity meningiomas are frontal and anterior to the central sulcus. If located anteriorly, they may remain asymptomatic while growing to a large size. These tumors are usually concentrated around the

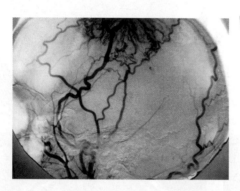

Figure 28.12 External carotid angiogram of a meningioma. Note the sunburst pattern.

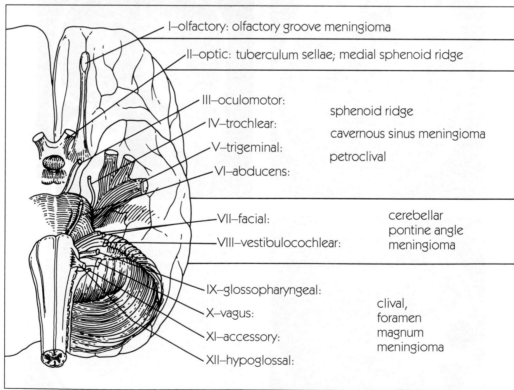

I–olfactory: olfactory groove meningioma

II–optic: tuberculum sellae; medial sphenoid ridge

III–oculomotor:
IV–trochlear:
V–trigeminal:
VI–abducens:
  sphenoid ridge
  cavernous sinus meningioma
  petroclival

VII–facial:
VIII–vestibulocochlear:
  cerebellar
  pontine angle
  meningioma

IX–glossopharyngeal:
X–vagus:
XI–accessory:
XII–hypoglossal:
  clival,
  foramen
  magnum
  meningioma

Figure 28.13 Involvement of the cranial nerves at the base of the brain with meningiomas at different sites in the skull base.

coronal suture. Epilepsy and focal neurologic signs are common. These meningiomas have the best potential for total removal (Fig. 28.14).

PARASAGITTAL

Parasagittal meningiomas arise in relation to the superior sagittal sinus, frequently in its middle third. They often cause focal epilepsy and later paralysis, particularly of the lower extremities. Hyperostosis often accompanies this tumor. The distinguishing feature of these meningiomas is that they involve the superior sagittal sinus and have an intimate relationship to the cortical vein draining into the sinus (Fig. 28.15).

FALX

Tumors arising from the falx also favor the anterior third and tend to be bilateral. Both falcine and sagittal meningiomas that involve the posterior part of the sagittal sinus or peritorcular area present a formidable surgical challenge and are likely to recur. The final outcome is guarded.

OLFACTORY GROOVE

Olfactory groove meningiomas arise from the cribriform plate. They grow bilaterally and become large without causing significant neurologic deficits or evidence of increased intracranial pressure. Anosmia, which is rarely

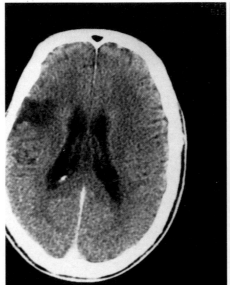
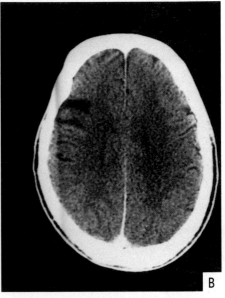

Figure 28.14 Preoperative (A) and postoperative (B) CT scans of a patient with a large convexity meningioma.

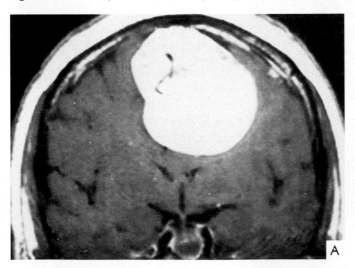

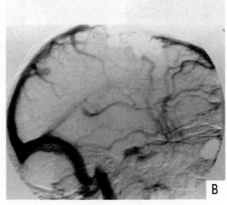

Figure 28.15 Parasagittal meningioma involving the sagittal sinus. MR image (A) of the tumor and angiogram (B) demonstrating sagittal sinus occlusion.

noticed, can be the only localizing sign. Changes in mental status are seldom striking until a tumor reaches an advanced stage. Once the tumor becomes large, it impinges on the optic nerves and chiasm, producing visual loss. These meningiomas may extend through the cribriform plate into the nasal cavity (Fig. 28.16). The prognosis is excellent after surgical removal.

TUBERCULUM SELLAE

Tuberculum sellae meningiomas arise from the planum sphenoidal tuberculum sellae or the diaphragm sellae (Fig. 28.17). They cause early and characteristic visual failure. Typically, loss of visual acuity and field is progressive and asymmetric, although it can be sudden. These tumors often show hyperostosis over the planum sphenoidale.

SPHENOID RIDGE

Meningiomas of the sphenoid ridge are traditionally divided into three types: outer, middle, and medial. The outer sphenoid ridge usually harbors a large globoid tumor, accompanied by epilepsy, focal weakness, and dysphasia on the left side. The *en plaque* variety is rare and is associated with hyperostosis, exophthalmos, and obvious swelling in the temporal region. Tumors of the inner sphenoid ridge of the clinoidal type usually compress the optic nerve and present with early unilateral visual loss. They involve the cavernous sinus and may produce oculomotor palsies and facial hypesthesia. When the tumor becomes large, Foster-Kennedy syndrome with optic atrophy on one side and contralateral papilledema is seen (Fig. 28.18). Meningiomas in the medial part of the sphenoid ridge (Fig. 28.19) present a

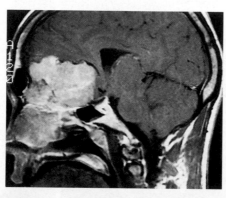

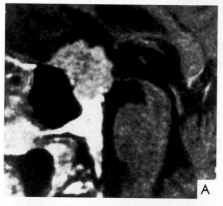

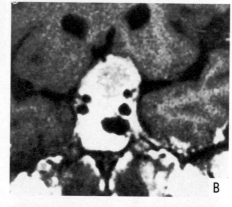

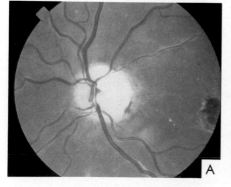

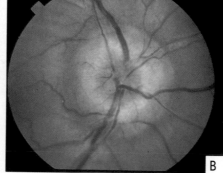

Figure 28.16 An olfactory groove meningioma extending through the cribriform plate into the nasal cavity.

Figure 28.17 Sagittal (A) and coronal (B) MR image of a tuberculum sellae meningioma.

Figure 28.18 Fundoscopic examination demonstrating optic atrophy (A) and papilledema (B), the findings in Foster-Kennedy syndrome.

surgical challenge because they adhere to and encase the carotid artery (Fig. 28.20).

POSTERIOR FOSSA

Posterior fossa meningiomas constitute about 10% of all meningiomas. They frequently arise from the posterior surface of the petrous bone and are divided into four areas: petrosal, clival, foramen magnum, and the convexity of the cerebellar hemispheres (see Fig. 28.1). When they arise from the tentorium, they can grow in both the infratentorial and supratentorial spaces (Fig. 28.21). The neurologic findings in these tumors might be confusing because they are a combination of posterior fossa deficits associated with hemanopia and epilepsy. Meningiomas arising from the petrous bone usually involve the cranial nerves, especially the eighth nerve, producing a loss of hearing mimicking that caused by acoustic nerve tumors (Fig. 28.22). Trigeminal neuralgia and hemifacial spasm sometimes herald petroclival meningiomas. Tumors arising from the foramen magnum cause cervical and occipital pain and involve the cervical cord, causing spasticity and paresis.

INTRAVENTRICULAR

Intraventricular meningiomas that arise wholly within the ventricle originate from arachnoid cluster cells, which presumably accompany the tela choroidea or choroid plexus. They most commonly occur in the atrium of the left lateral ventricle and the posterior part of the third ventricle. They are usually associated with a long-standing increase in intracranial pressure and focal dilation of the ventricle.

INTRAORBITAL

Intraorbital meningiomas present with a loss in visual acuity and optic atrophy. They may be primary, arising from the meningeal extension surrounding the optic nerve, or secondary, originating in the adjacent dura and invading the orbit by local extension. Meningiomas of the orbit, both primary and secondary, occur more often in females. The two major presenting symptoms and signs are progressive, painless visual loss and proptosis. MR images or CT scans are the current mode of evaluation (Fig. 28.23).

SPINAL

Most spinal meningiomas are intradural extramedullary masses. They arise from mesothelial cell rests found where the arachnoid joins the dura of the nerve root sheath, creating signs and symptoms of a dermatomal pattern. As they progress, these tumors produce signs of spinal cord compression often associated with the Brown-Séquard syndrome. Their distribution in the spinal canal is thoracic, followed by cervical, and, rarely, lumbar-sacral. These tumors occur more often in women than men, with a ratio of 5:1, usually between the ages of 40 and 70. Pain is the most common symptom, followed by motor weakness and sensory distur-

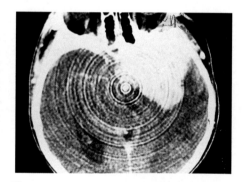

Figure 28.19 CT scan of a sphenoid ridge meningioma.

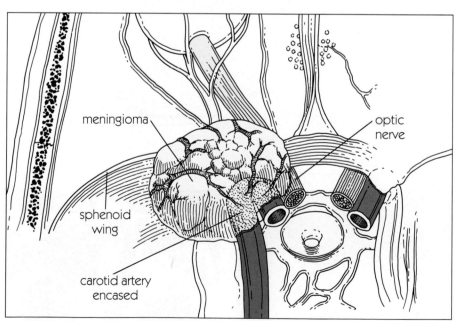

meningioma

optic nerve

sphenoid wing

carotid artery encased

Figure 28.20 Encasement of the carotid artery by a medial sphenoid wing meningioma.

bances. Symptoms can often be related to the level at which they occur (Fig. 28.24).

TREATMENT

Meningiomas are generally thought to be slow-growing and benign, and every effort is aimed at total removal. Certain tumors, however, present a formidable technical challenge because they adhere to vital neural and vascular structures at the base of the brain. The microscope and microdissection have significantly improved the surgeon's ability to remove these tumors completely (Fig. 28.25). The results of radiation therapy in the treatment of meningiomas are difficult to assess. Radiation for malignant meningiomas and hemangiopericytomas seems beneficial and is usually prescribed. For benign meningiomas, radiation is thought to be helpful in palliating inoperable

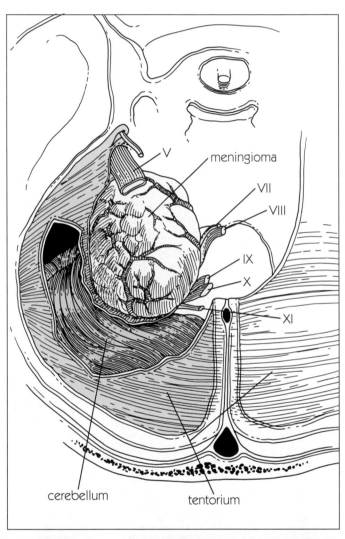

Figure 28.21 Tentorial meningioma growing above and below the tentorium and involving multiple cranial nerves.

V

meningioma

VII

VIII

IX

X

XI

cerebellum

tentorium

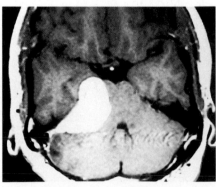

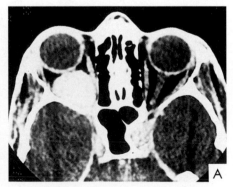

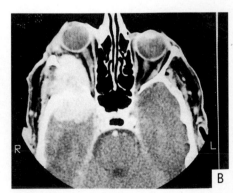

Figure 28.22 Contrast-enhanced MR image of a meningioma of the posterior fossa originating from the petrous portion of the temporal bone and filling the cerebellopontine angle.

Figure 28.23 Primary (A) and secondary (B) orbital meningioma.

Principles of Neurosurgery

tumors, residual nonresectable tumors, and recurrent nonresectable tumors. Benign meningiomas should not be irradiated, however, unless they are deemed unresectable after surgery. Stereotactic radiation and hormonal manipulation of meningiomas might play a larger role in the future.

RECURRENCE

Meningiomas are known to recur. Many factors relate to recurrence, the most important of which is the extent of the original removal. If the tumor has been totally removed, including the margin of the dura and involved bone, recurrence is thought to be from a multicentric focus. Naturally, malignant and atypical tumors are associated with a higher incidence of recurrence, and radiation therapy is recommended for these tumors. Symptomatic recurrence usually occurs within 5 years but can be detected in 2 1/2 years with the newest methods of neurological imaging. Reasons for incomplete tumor removal include venous sinus invasion, investment of vital structures, and bone involvement.

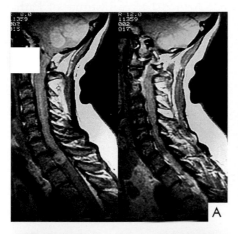
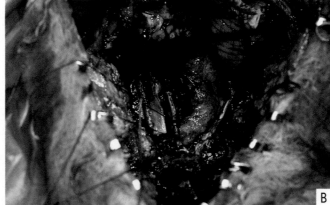

Figure 28.24 MR image (A) and intraoperative photo (B) of a spinal cord meningioma.

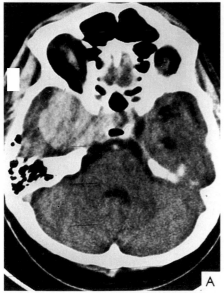
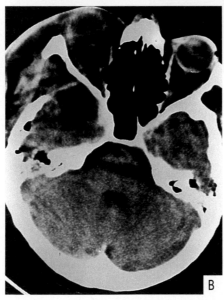

Figure 28.25 Original CT scan (A) and postoperative study (B) of a medial sphenoid meningioma.

REFERENCES

1. Cushing H, Eisenhardt L. *Meningiomas: Their Classification, Regional Behaviour, Life History, and Surgical End Results.* Springfield, Ill: Charles C Thomas Publisher; 1938.
2. Al-Mefty O, ed. *Meningiomas.* New York, NY: Raven Press; 1991.
3. Kepes JJ. *Meningiomas: Biology, Pathology, and Differential Diagnosis.* New York, NY: Masson Publishing; 1982.
4. MacCarty CS. *The Surgical Treatment of Intracranial Meningiomas.* Springfield, Ill: Charles C Thomas Publisher; 1961.
5. Barnett GH, Chou SM, Bay JW. Posttraumatic intracranial meningioma: a case report and review of the literature. *Neurosurgery.* 1986;18:75–78.
6. Al-Mefty O, Kersh JE, Routh A, Smith RR. The long-term side effects of radiation therapy for benign brain tumors in adults. *J Neurosurg.* 1990;73: 502–512.
7. Kida S, Yamashima T, Kubota T, Ito H, Yamamoto S. A light and electron microscopic and immunohistochemical study of human arachnoid villi. *J Neurosurg.* 1988;69:429–435.
8. Rubinstein LJ. *Tumors of the Central Nervous System.* Washington, DC: Armed Forces Institute of Pathology; 1982.

Chapter 29

Tumors of the Pineal Region

Konstantin V. Slavin, James I. Ausman

Tumors of the pineal region account for just 0.5% to 1.6% of human brain tumors, but they present a challenge to any neurosurgeon. Problems associated with the management of these tumors include the choice of operative approach, the use of additional treatment modalities, and preoperative diagnostic strategies.

The physiologic role of the pineal gland itself is not completely understood. In the seventeenth century, Descartes thought that the pineal body (epiphysis cerebri) served as a valve that regulated the passage of spirits between the ventricles; thus the organ was thought to be the "seat of the soul." Now the pineal gland, which is a major photoreceptive organ in some vertebrates, is known to have a neurotransmitter secretory function in mammals. Light stimuli reach the pineal gland from the retina by a polysynaptic pathway and affect the production of the neuroendocrine substance melatonin. Melatonin, a derivative of serotonin, is essential in regulating circadian rhythms in endocrine gland activity and produces an antigonadal effect through the hypothalamic-hypophyseal axis. The production of melatonin is inhibited by light. Apparently in many animals the major function of the pineal gland is to regulate the reproductive cycle; in fall and winter when days are short more melatonin is produced, causing the gonad-suppressive effect. The exact function of the pineal gland in humans remains unclear. However, the absence of production of melatonin, as after pinealectomy, causes a "jet-lag"-like syndrome consisting of a complete disturbance of circadian rhythms.[1]

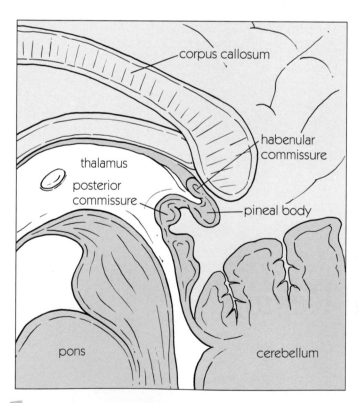

Figure 29.1 Anatomy of the pineal gland and related structures.

ANATOMY

Topographically, the pineal body (epiphysis), which is part of the interbrain, or diencephalon,[2,3] lies on the superior surface of the midbrain (mesencephalon) within the quadrigeminal cistern and forms part of the posterior border of the third ventricle (Fig. 29.1). Some authors include the pineal body in the mesencephalon, considering it to be the posterosuperior part of the midbrain.[4]

The pineal body itself has an average length of 7 mm (±2 mm). It is oval in shape and its dimensions in a transverse section are 7.7 mm (±2 mm) in transverse diameter and 3 mm (±1.5 mm) in vertical diameter.[5] It projects posteriorly into the quadrigeminal cistern and is concealed by the splenium of the corpus callosum above, the thalamus laterally, and the quadrigeminal plate and vermis of the cerebellum inferiorly.[6]

This location determines the neurosurgical definition of the pineal region, which is limited dorsally by the splenium of the corpus callosum and the tela choroidea, ventrally by quadrigeminal plate, rostrally by the posterior part of the third ventricle, and caudally by the vermis of the cerebellum.[7] Tumors in the pineal region include tumors of the midbrain and posterior part of the third ventricle, on the basis of surgical or radiologic considerations.

Forming the posterior wall of the third ventricle, the pineal body and pineal recess are located between the suprapineal recess and habenular commissure above and the posterior commissure and the aqueduct of Sylvius below. The suprapineal recess projects posteriorly between the upper surface of the pineal gland and the lower layer of tela choroidea in the roof. The stalk of the pineal body, from which the gland extends into the quadrigeminal cistern, has a cranial lamina and a caudal lamina. The habenular commissure, which connects the habenulae, crosses the midline over the cranial lamina, and the posterior commissure crosses the caudal lamina. The pineal recess projects posteriorly from the third ventricle into the pineal body between the two laminae. The posterior commissure forms the base of the triangular orifice of the aqueduct of Sylvius; the other two limbs are formed by the central gray matter of the midbrain.[8]

The quadrigeminal cistern—the subarachnoid space of the pineal region, which bathes the pineal body—provides protection of the midbrain from the sharp edge of the tentorial notch. The arteries and veins inside the cistern are embedded in the firm arachnoidal septa (Fig. 29.2). The quadrigeminal cistern communicates anteriorly with the cistern of the tela choroidea of the third ventricle, dorsally along the great vein of Galen with the dorsal cistern of the corpus callosum, laterally into the alae, caudally into the superior cistern of the cerebellum, which is formed by the medullary velum and the vermis, and anterodorsally into the ambient cistern. Through the latter cistern the large arteries, the posterior cerebral artery and its branches, and the superior cerebellar artery approach the dorsal surface of the brain stem along the edge of the tentorium.[5]

The posterior border of the quadrigeminal cistern is formed by thickened opalescent arachnoid.[9] Care must be taken when dissecting this area, because the vein of Galen and its tributaries lie immediately rostral.

The mesencephalon with the pineal body has its arterial blood supply from various sources. Small vessels supplying the parenchyma of the cerebral peduncles and the rest of the midbrain arise from the posterior communicating artery as perforating branches forming an internal or direct system. Another source of arterial blood for the midbrain consists of the medial peduncular arteries, short and long branches of the posterior cerebral artery. The crura cerebri are also supplied by branches of the posterior communicating, quadrigeminal, and anterior choroidal arteries. All these arteries widely anastomose with each other, which explains the rarity of infarcts in the mesencephalon and the relative tolerance of the midbrain to direct surgical intervention.[5]

The pineal body is supplied by the pineal artery, which originates from the medial posterior choroidal artery and enters the gland through its lateral portion from both sides. The medial posterior choroidal artery arises usually from the posterior cerebral artery, lies lateral to the pineal body after entering the quadrigeminal cistern, and courses anteriorly in the roof of the third ventricle. This artery supplies the tegmentum, lateral geniculate body, quadrigeminal plate, pulvinar, pineal body, medial thalamus, and choroid plexus of the third ventricle.[6]

The great vein of Galen and its tributaries form a rooflike dense venous network above the pineal body and the quadrigeminal plate. The pessimistic attitude of

neurosurgeons toward lesions in the pineal region is caused mainly by venous vulnerability in this area. Anatomic studies[5,6] show that the venous system of the midbrain-quadrigeminal region is the mainstream flow to the great vein of Galen and the straight sinus. The great vein of Galen is formed from the internal cerebral veins after they pass posteriorly through the tela choroidea and unite with the basal veins of Rosenthal.[10] Other tributaries of the vein of Galen include the precentral cerebellar vein, internal occipital vein, posterior pericallosal vein, pineal vein, posterior mesencephalic vein, and posterior ventricular vein.[6] This large venous confluence is located dorsal to the pineal gland and ventral to the overlying splenium of the corpus callosum. The straight sinus is formed by the joining of the great vein of Galen with the inferior sagittal sinus.

PATHOLOGY

The pathologic classification of pineal region tumors[11] divides them into several different groups, including germ cell tumors, pineal parenchymal tumors, tumors of supporting and adjacent structures, and nonneoplastic tumor-like conditions (Fig. 29.3).

GERM CELL TUMORS

Germ cell tumors account for more than half of all pineal region tumors. These tumors have their origin, hypothetically,[12] in primordial germ cells that failed to migrate properly during the first few weeks of embryonic development (Fig. 29.4). This hypothesis also explains why these neoplasms are found at other intracranial sites, most often in the suprasellar region, and extracranially elsewhere in the midline of the body (e.g., the mediastinum and the retroperitoneum).

The International Histologic Classification of Tumors No. 16 (1977) divides this germ cell group into two subgroups: tumors of one histologic type and tumors of more than one histologic type. In turn, the first subgroup consists of germinomas, embryonal carcinomas, endodermal sinus tumors (yolk sac tumors), choriocarcinomas, and teratomas (mature, immature, and malignantly transformed); the second subgroup includes embryonal carcinoma and teratoma (teratocarcinoma), choriocarcinoma with any other type, and other combinations.[10,13]

Pure germinomas account for 65% to 72% of all intracranial germ cell tumors.[14] They usually are poorly circumscribed, light gray, granular, solid neoplasms that destroy the pineal gland and early seed the ventricular system and subarachnoid space (Fig. 29.5).[11] Hemorrhage into the tumor and necrosis or cystic degeneration are not found. Histologically, the tumor is composed of lobules of large cells with a centrally placed round vesicular nucleus, one or more prominent nucleoli, and abundant clear cytoplasm with distinct cytoplasmic borders. The lobules are separated by loose

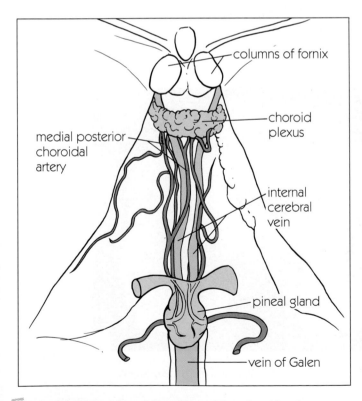

Figure 29.2 Vascular relationships of the pineal body.

Labels in figure: columns of fornix; medial posterior choroidal artery; choroid plexus; internal cerebral vein; pineal gland; vein of Galen

Figure 29.3 Classification of Pineal Region Masses

Germ Cell Tumors
Pure germinoma
Embryonal cell carcinoma
Endodermal sinus tumor
Choriocarcinoma
Immature teratoma
Mature teratoma

Pineal Parenchymal Tumors
Pineoblastoma
Pineocytoma

**Tumors of Supportive Tissues
and Adjacent Structures**
Astrocytomas
Ependymomas
Meningiomas
Hemangiopericytomas

Metastatic Tumors to the Pineal Gland

**Nonneoplastic Mass Lesions in the
Pineal Region**
Pineal cysts
Arachnoid cysts
Cysticercus cysts
Vein of Galen malformations

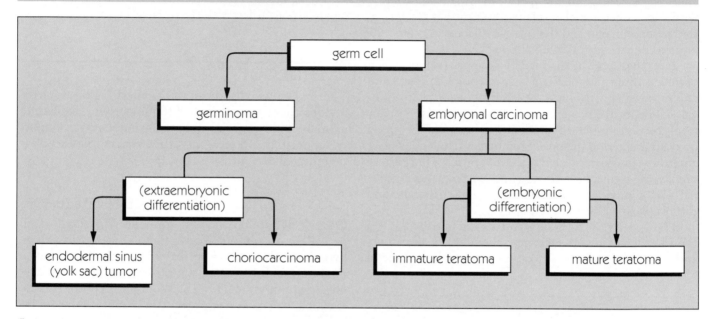

Figure 29.4 Histogenetic relations of germ cell tumors. (Adapted from Fig. 3.300 from Okazaki H, Scheithauer BW. *Atlas of Neuropathology*. New York, NY: Gower Medical Publishing; 1988)

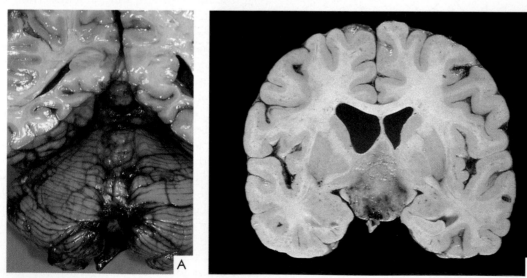

Figure 29.5 (A,B) Gross appearance of pineal germinoma. (Figs. 3.302, 3.303 from Okazaki H, Scheithauer BW, 1988)

connective tissue strands that are focally infiltrated by clusters of lymphocytes (Fig. 29.6).

The embryonal cell carcinoma, which is the least frequently reported intracranial germ cell tumor, is a primitive neoplasm composed of pluripotential epithelial cells. This tumor, rarely found in its pure form, is usually highly malignant and is composed of sheets of cuboidal to columnar cells with large vesicular nuclei and distinct nucleoli (Figs. 29.7, 29.8).[15]

The histologic appearance of endodermal sinus tumors classically features Schiller-Duval bodies, which resemble the yolk sac or endodermal sinus, an extra-embryonic endodermal derivative in lower animals. These bodies are composed of a blood vessel invaginating a space, with both being covered by a layer of cuboidal tumor cells with clear cytoplasm, small dark nuclei, and prominent nucleoli (Fig. 29.9). Endodermal sinus tumors are usually highly invasive.[15]

Choriocarcinomas rarely arise extragenitally. Histologically, these tumors are characterized by two cell types: uniform cytotrophoblastic cells of medium size, with clear cytoplasm, vesicular nucleus, and distinct cell

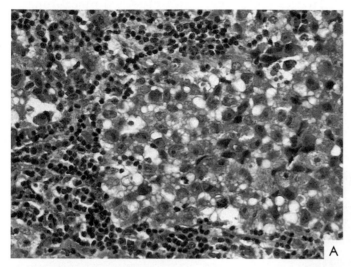

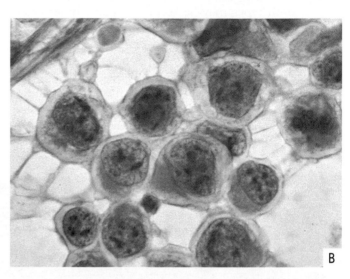

Figure 29.6 (A) Histologic appearance of germinoma showing monomorphous proliferation of germ cells arranged in a lobular pattern separated by a delicate lymphocyte-rich stroma. (B) Touch preparation showing cytologic features of a germinoma. (Figs. 3.304, 3.305 from Okazaki H, Scheithauer BW, 1988)

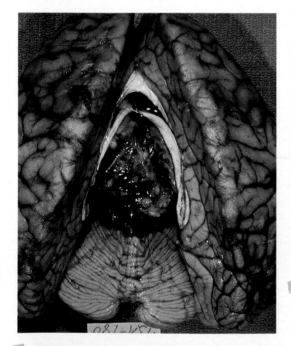

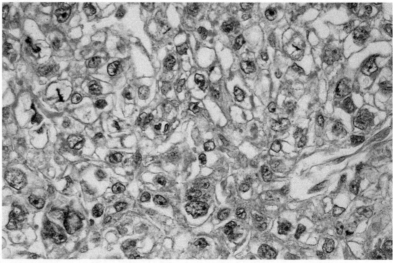

Figure 29.8 Microscopic appearance of embryonal carcinoma. It consists of primitive epithelium growing in patternless sheets. (Fig. 3.308 from Okazaki H, Scheithauer BW, 1988)

Figure 29.7 Gross appearance of an embryonal carcinoma of the pineal region viewed from above; the corpus callosum has been split. (Fig. 3.307 from Okazaki H, Scheithauer BW, 1988)

borders, and syncytiotrophoblastic cells, which are larger and multinucleated. The gross appearance of choriocarcinoma is a granular, reddish brown mass, almost always with hemorrhage and necrosis (Fig. 29.10).[12] As all other tumors of germ cell origin, choriocarcinoma is usually accompanied by elements of other tumors of this group.

According to Scheithauer,[15] teratomas represent the expression of embryonic differentiation in germ cell tumors. Teratomas can be either immature or mature, the former resembling embryonic or fetal tissues and the latter resembling mature or adult tissue (Figs. 29.11, 29.12). Both types may be accompanied by other germ cell elements. By definition, the term teratoma can be used only in cases where tumor elements derive from two or three germ layers. These tumors are usually well-circumscribed, round or lobulated, and multicystic, and compress the surrounding structures. The cystic component of the tumor may be watery, mucoid, or sebaceous. Sometimes bone, cartilage, hair, or teeth are present.[12] Immature tumors are more frequently associated with a

malignant course, but malignant potential may be explained by the presence of other germ cell tumor elements, such as choriocarcinoma or germinoma.

PINEAL PARENCHYMAL TUMORS

Tumors of the pineal parenchymal cells comprise the second major group of pineal region tumors, accounting for 20% to 30% of all neoplasms of this location. These tumors consist of two types—pineoblastoma and pineocytoma—which differ from one another by histologic appearance, level of differentiation, and degree of malignancy.

Herrick and Rubinstein[16] classified pineal tumors according to their histologic type and biologic behavior. They stated that pineoblastoma without special differentiation, pineoblastoma with pineocytic or retinoblastomatous differentiation, and pineocytoma without special differentiation are malignant; pineocytoma with astrocytic differentiation may be malignant or benign; and pineocytomas with neuronal or with neuronal and astrocytic differentiation are benign.

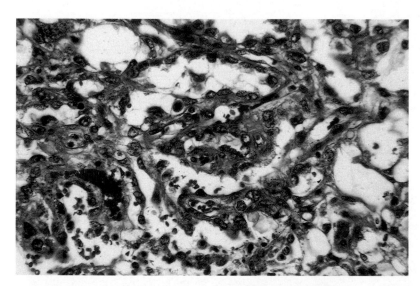

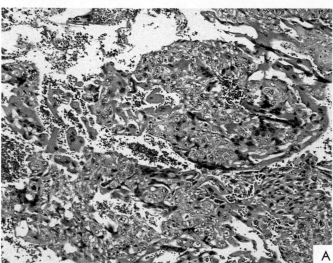

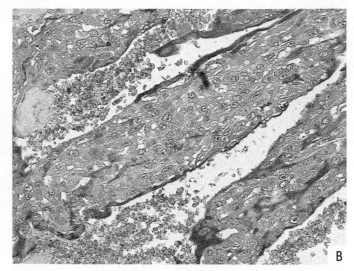

Figure 29.9 Endodermal sinus tumor showing typical Schiller-Duval body. (Fig. 3.309 from Okazaki H, Scheithauer BW, 1988)

Figure 29.10 (A) Histologic appearance of choriocarcinoma consisting of multinucleate syncytiotrophoblastic and cytotrophoblastic cells arranged in bilayer fashion surrounding vascular spaces. (B) Syncytiotrophoblasts in choriocarcinoma staining positively for human chorionic gonadotropin (HCG). (Figs. 3.319, 3.320 from Okazaki H, Scheithauer BW, 1988)

Pineoblastomas are the least differentiated pineal parenchymal neoplasms and may constitute up to one half of all pineal parenchymal tumors. They are highly malignant and represent true primitive neuroectodermal tumors (PNET).[17] Tumor usually replaces the tissue of the pineal gland. It is pink, white, or gray; smooth or granular when cut; sometimes cystic; and frequently hemorrhagic or necrotic. The neoplasm itself is highly cellular, containing sheets of small, primitive cells that resemble medulloblastoma (Fig. 29.13), cerebral neuroblastoma, or primitive cerebral neuroectodermal tumor.[12] Retinoblastomatous differentiation of pineoblastomas sometimes occurs and supports the theory of photoreceptive origin of pineal gland cells. Pineoblastomas may accompany bilateral retinoblastomas, in which case together they are called trilateral retinoblastoma. Pineoblastomas sometimes contain melanin pigment.

Pineocytomas are a better-differentiated variant of pineal parenchymal tumors and occur mostly in adult life, in contrast to pineoblastomas, which tend to occur during the first or second decades of life. Pineocytomas are usually well circumscribed, but may disseminate widely along the CSF pathways. Histologically, the tumors are characterized by the formation of clusters and strands of cells resembling normal pineocytes; frequently, however, areas of pineoblastomatous change are seen (Fig. 29.14).[15] Pineocytomas may contain astrocytic or neuronal components or both (so-called ganglioglioma of the pineal). Such tumors are the most benign of the pineal parenchymal neoplasms.

TUMORS OF SUPPORTIVE AND ADJACENT STRUCTURES

Astrocytomas, ependymomas, and other less frequently occurring gliomas can also be considered pineal parenchymal tumors,[11] because theoretically, they arise from the pluripotential pineal parenchymal cells.[15]

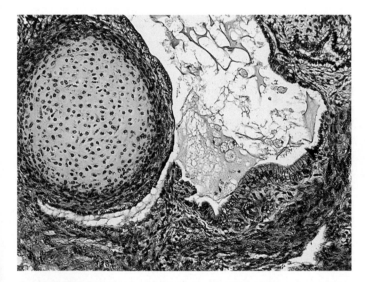

Figure 29.11 Immature teratoma containing cartilage, mucin-producing epithelium, and an immature spindle cell stroma. (Fig. 3.314 from Okazaki H, Scheithauer BW, 1988)

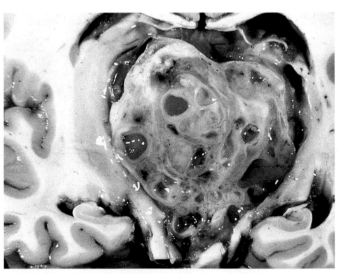

Figure 29.12 Mature cystic teratoma. Note that the tumor is discrete and noninvasive. (Fig. 3.317 from Okazaki H, Scheithauer BW, 1988)

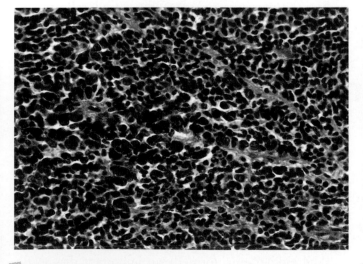

Figure 29.13 Histologic appearance of pineoblastoma. Pineoblastomas resemble medulloblastomas. (Fig. 3.188 from Okazaki H, Scheithauer BW, 1988)

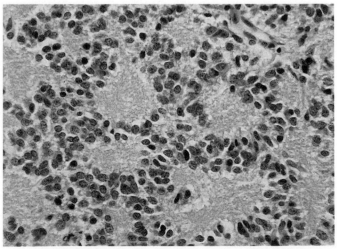

Figure 29.14 Histologic appearance of pineocytoma. (Fig. 3.185 (left) from Okazaki H, Scheithauer BW, 1988)

However, some authors[12] believe that these tumors originate from structures in the vicinity of the pineal gland and should be grouped with tumors of the supporting and surrounding tissues. These tumors also include meningiomas and hemangiopericytomas, which arise mostly from the falx and tentorium near their junction or from the velum interpositum at the roof of the third ventricle, as well as unique cases of chemodectoma and craniopharyngioma of the pineal region.

NONNEOPLASTIC TUMOR-LIKE CONDITIONS

The last group in DeGirolamo's classification of pineal region tumors[11] consists of nonneoplastic conditions of neurosurgical importance. Included in this group are arachnoid cysts and "degenerative" cysts lined by fibrillary astrocytes (so-called pineal cysts). Cysticercosis and vascular lesions, such as arteriovenous malformations and aneurysms of the vein of Galen, can also be included.

METASTASES TO THE PINEAL REGION

Metastatic tumors of the pineal region are extremely rare; the total number of cases recorded is about 75.[18,19] The most common site of origin for metastases to the pineal region is the lung, followed by breast and some other organs, such as stomach and kidney.

SYMPTOMS

The clinical presentation of tumors of the pineal region varies as much as the pathology. Symptoms arise when tumor invades or compresses adjacent structures, producing local effects, or when tumor cells spread to distant sites. The manifestations depend on the size of the lesion and whether it is an invasive tumor, which infiltrates surrounding neural structures, or an expanding mass, which grows into the ventricular cavity.[20]

Involvement of the cerebral aqueduct causes hydrocephalus and intracranial hypertension, which also can be caused by tumor growth into the third ventricle and are manifested in headaches, vomiting, lethargy, and alteration of mental status. Headache and papilledema are the most common heralds of pineal tumor.[21]

Involvement (infiltration or compression) of the superior colliculus and pretegmental area causes visual disturbance with characteristic ocular signs.[22] The most common ocular movement disorder is Parinaud's syndrome,[23] which includes paralysis of upward gaze, convergence or retraction nystagmus, and light-near dissociation. Direct pressure of the tumor on the tectum or dilatation of the proximal aqueduct causes the less common sylvian aqueduct syndrome, which includes paralysis of downgaze or horizontal gaze superimposed on Parinaud's syndrome. Convergent nystagmus may be present when upward gaze is attempted.[22,24] The anatomic substrate of these ocular functions is located below the posterior part of the third ventricle and anterior to the aqueduct.[20] Lid

retraction (Collier's sign) is quite rare; it is caused by compression of levator inhibitory fibers in the posterior commissure.

Invasion of the thalamus by the tumor may cause contralateral hemihypesthesia or hemianesthesia and sometimes paresthesias and intermittent pain. Hemiparesis or hemiplegia may result from invasion of the internal capsule, and extrapyramidal syndromes and movement disorders may be caused by involvement of the basal ganglia. Invasion of the hypothalamus may cause disturbances in body temperature and water regulation (such as diabetes insipidus), somnolence, and weight gain. Defects of the visual fields indicate involvement of the posterior capsule. Memory problems, especially short-term memory loss, may be caused not only by hydrocephalus but also by direct tumor invasion of the fornices (mamillothalamic pathway).[10] Dysmetria, hypotonia, and intentional tremor may result from compression or invasion of the cerebellum.

A commonly described endocrine disturbance in pineal region tumors is precocious puberty, which occurs in 10% of male patients with these lesions and has been attributed to three hypothetical causes. One hypothesis connects the development of precocious puberty with ectopic secretion of beta human chorionic gonadotropin by choriocarcinoma or germinoma and thus explains the absence of precocious puberty in girls with pineal region tumors. Another hypothesis links precocious puberty with mass effect in the region of the posterior diencephalon, which blocks its inhibitory effect on the median eminence of the hypothalamus, thereby augmenting secretion of gonadotropins. This hypothesis explains the association of precocious puberty with other symptoms of hypothalamic dysfunction (e.g., diabetes insipidus and polyphagia). According to a third hypothesis, the growth of a tumor in the pineal region causes a decrease in the secretion by the pineal gland of a substance (or substances) with antigonadotropic effect. If a pineal parenchymal tumor causes hypersecretion of such an agent, isolated hypogonadism may occur.[25]

Another group of symptoms is caused by tumor seeding the meninges or spreading intradurally to the spinal cord or cauda equina or by hematogenous metastases of tumor to structures outside the nervous system.

IMAGING

The radiologic assessment of pineal region tumors has changed dramatically in the past 15 years. In the past, ventriculography with air or a positive contrast agent was used to define the anatomy of the posterior third ventricle and cerebral aqueduct in patients with obstructive hydrocephalus. Pneumoencephalography with lumbar air injection was used to outline the position of the cerebral aqueduct, the configuration of the third ventricle, and the anatomy of the quadrigeminal cistern.[26]

Skull radiography, formerly an important diagnostic study for pineal neoplasms, has fallen into disuse because of its low sensitivity in detecting tumors.[26] Some diagnostic criteria, however, should be mentioned in the discussion of current techniques. On plain roentgenogram the normal pineal gland is seen as a calcified mass in 60% of the population over 20 years of age; however, this is very rare in children before 6 years.[27] The normal pineal gland is 5 to 9 mm in length, and any calcified pineal gland that is larger than 1 cm in any dimension should be looked upon with suspicion. The appearance of a calcified pineal gland in early childhood is usually abnormal, although in up to 5% of cases it is physiologic.[26] In patients with pineal tumors conventional skull radiography may show premature calcification, irregular or amorphous calcifications, or an abnormally large pineal gland. A low position of the pineal calcification may be a sign of increased intracranial pressure due to hydrocephalus.[27]

In the early 1980s, CT superseded all other radiologic imaging methods for detection of pineal region tumors.[28] High-resolution CT with or without intravenous contrast administration and metrizamide CT-ventriculography and cisternography[29] are currently used to examine the pineal region. MRI has markedly improved the localization and characterization of tumors by means of its unique features: increased sensitivity and tissue discrimination compared to CT, direct multiplanar (e.g., axial, sagittal, coronal) imaging capability, and lack of the beam-hardening artifact encountered with posterior fossa CT (Fig. 29.15).[29,30]

Carotid and vertebral arteriography are quite helpful in demonstrating the nature or lack of vascularity of a mass in the posterior third ventricular location. Vascular displacement helps to localize lesions. However, CT and MRI usually suffice for making a diagnosis of mass lesion in the region of the pineal gland and for assessing its size. Cerebral angiography has a role in evaluating pineal neoplasms and defining arterial and venous anatomy, but its use is limited to cases in which surgical resection is contemplated.[27]

Myelography and CT myelography and/or spinal MRI are strongly indicated in all cases of pineal region tumors, especially in those with positive CSF cytology.[28]

IMAGING CHARACTERISTICS OF TUMORS

On a CT scan, a germinoma typically appears as a well-defined, hyperdense, occasionally calcified tumor that engulfs the pineal gland and enhances homogeneously.[31,32] On an MR image, the tumor mass is isodense relative to normal white matter on T1-weighted images and slightly hyperdense relative to white matter on T2-weighted images. In some cases, small cystic areas can be noted.[30]

Teratomas usually exhibit fat densities and calcification. Unlike the coarse stippled calcification of germinomas, teratomas have a mixture of linear and nodular calcifications.[31] This tumor has heterogeneous high signal intensity on T1-weighted and T2-weighted MR images.[30]

In embryonal cell carcinoma, CT without contrast demonstrates a slightly hyperdense mass, often containing calcium. Diffuse enhancement after contrast is the usual pattern. The lesion may infiltrate surrounding structures or be well circumscribed.[29] Such a tumor is

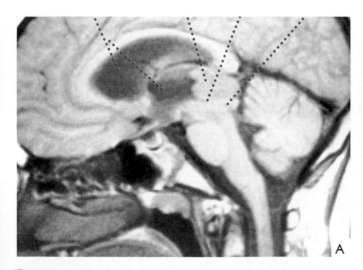
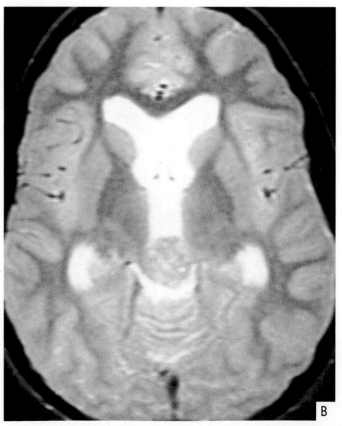

Figure 29.15 (A) T1-weighted sagittal image showing a well-defined ovoid tumor in the pineal gland. It is compressing the cerebral aqueduct, causing obstructive hydrocephalus. (B) T2-weighted axial image showing a tumor in the pineal gland. The tumor is slightly hyperintense relative to white matter with some heterogeneous internal signal. (Fig. 1.90A,B from Kucharczyk W. *MRI: Central Nervous System.* New York, NY: Gower Medical Publishing; 1990)

isodense relative to white matter on T1-weighted MR images and has heterogeneous high signal intensity on T2-weighted images.[30]

Choriocarcinomas on CT scan are indistinctly marginated and usually enhance intensely, showing spread into adjacent tissues.[10] On MRI the tumorous mass is heterogeneous with a hemorrhagic component on T1- and T2-weighted images.[30]

Pineal cell tumors are slightly hyperdense on plain CT scans and generally enhance strongly following intravenous contrast infusion.[33] The enhancement of tumor is homogeneous, without breakdown or necrosis, in the case of pineocytoma. Pineoblastoma, in contrast, is characterized by a lucent center.[31] On MR images of pineoblastoma some cystic/necrotic areas can be seen. On T1- and T2-weighted images the solid portions of the tumors are nearly isointense relative to gray matter and they invade surrounding structures.[30]

The precontrast CT is helpful in diagnosing gliomas, since these tumors are hypodense relative to brain.[26,31] Prominent enhancement is encountered occasionally in exophytic components.[29] On the T1-weighted MR images pineal region astrocytomas are hypointense relative to gray matter. On T2-weighted images they are hyperintense, invading the tectum and/or tegmentum.[30]

Meningiomas in the pineal area are hyperdense in most cases on unenhanced CT scan and enhanced in a nodular fashion after contrast injection.[29,31] The tumor usually has a very sharp, distinct margin.[10] The tumor tissue is isointense relative to gray matter on T1-weighted MR images and isointense or hyperintense on T2-weighted images.[30]

The CT and MRI appearance of pineal region metastases is variable—multiple lesions are the only distinguishing radiologic feature. Individual metastases may be isodense or slightly hyperdense, with variable degrees of edema and enhancement on CT, hypointense relative to gray matter on T1-weighted MR images, and isointense on T2-weighted MR images.[19,29,30]

An aneurysm of the vein of Galen should be suspected in cases of intensely enhancing mass in the posterior third ventricular region in an adult.[10] The venous phase of cerebral angiography is very informative in such cases.

It must be remembered that the histologic diagnosis cannot be made with certainty from imaging methods. The value of MRI is its definition of the anatomy of the tissues surrounding the tumor. Because of the inherent variability in the pathology of the pineal region lesions, surgical diagnosis and removal provides the only means of establishing the diagnosis with certainty.

TUMOR MARKERS

Understanding of the pathology of pineal region tumors has increased in recent years as a result of the discovery of biochemical markers, which can be demonstrated in the patient's serum and CSF and in biopsy specimens by different immunohistochemical techniques.[33]

The most useful and specific markers for pineal region tumors are the beta-subunit of human chorionic gonadotropin (β-HCG) and the alpha-fetoprotein (AFP). β-HCG is produced by syncytiotrophoblastic cells of choriocarcinoma or germinoma and can be found in serum and CSF. Elevated CSF or serum levels of AFP with normal β-HCG suggest a malignant germ cell tumor, most often endodermal sinus tumor ("yolk-sac" tumor). Elevation of both markers can be found in embryonal cell carcinomas, malignant teratomas, or mixed germ cell tumors.[30,34,35] The levels of both markers in serum and CSF have been found to be extremely useful in assessment of the efficacy of various treatment modalities and as an indicator of the recurrence of tumors.

Diagnostically, the most important clinical discrimination is between the highly radiosensitive germinomas and the less radiosensitive malignant tumors.[10] Sano[36] proposed an algorithm for treatment of pineal region tumors (both germ cell and pineal parenchymal cell in origin) according to the presence of tumor markers, CT appearance, and biopsy results. He also recommended examining tumor markers in every patient suspected of having pinealoma or any of the germ cell tumors. Not just the presence but the level of tumor markers may be of some prognostic value: All patients with serum β-HCG level more than 1000 IU/L or serum AFP level more than 10 ng/mL died within 4 years, while 14 of 16 (87.5%) with levels lower than this survived.[37]

Until recently, a specific biochemical marker for germinomas had not been found. However, recent studies have suggested levels of placental alkaline phosphatase in serum and CSF as specific tumor markers for germinomas.[38] Although there is no biologic tumor marker for pineal parenchymal cell tumors, measurement of melatonin may be useful, because pineal tumors may interfere with its production. Before surgery, serum deficiency of melatonin may be used as a nonspecific marker for tumors that destroy the pineal gland. The absence of melatonin in serum after surgery indicates complete pinealectomy.[39] Elevation of the polyamines putrescine and spermidine in CSF has been reported in malignant brain tumors of childhood, especially PNETs.[40]

Again, tumor markers alone do not yield a definite histologic diagnosis—pineal tumors can contain multiple histologic types. Although both neuroimaging (CT and MRI) and tumor marker evaluation improve diagnostic accuracy, a combination of CT, MRI, biopsy, and assay for tumor markers is necessary for optimal diagnosis and treatment.[30]

CHOICE OF TREATMENT

The treatment of tumors of the pineal region has been intensively debated for the past 40 years. Although the first attempt to remove a pineal tumor by direct surgical attack was made by Horsley in 1905,[41] the first successful extirpation of a tumor from the pineal region was reported by Oppenheim and Krause in 1913.[42] It was Dandy (1921)[43] who first proposed a transcallosal approach for tumors of the pineal area. This approach was used by several other surgeons with some limited success. Van Wagenen (1931)[44] was the next to operate successfully in the pineal region. However, the operative mortality in other series using his transventricular approach remained high.

Until the mid 1970s, the therapy of pineal region tumors consisted of ventricular shunting and radiation therapy, with 5-year survival rates of 60% to 80%.[45] Today, however, the treatment of pineal region tumors, according to Stein,[45] should involve three principles: 1) control of hydrocephalus, which is always associated with tumors in this region; 2) total resection of benign encapsulated tumors of the pineal region; and 3) histologic identification of nonresectable tumors and adjunctive treatment with radiation and chemotherapy. The surgical exploration and identification of the nature of the tumors is considered to be the foundation of therapy. This approach to pineal region tumors has resulted in a much higher cure rate, decreased surgical mortality and morbidity, and increased longevity for those individuals who have recurrence of tumor at a distance from therapy.[45]

SURGICAL APPROACHES

The pineal region and the third ventricle are located in the geometrical center of the intracranial cavity, so operative approaches from every conceivable angle have been developed.[10] The five most common surgical approaches include 1) posterior transcallosal approach by Dandy; 2) transventricular approach by Van Wagenen; 3) occipital transtentorial approach by Heppner-Poppen, 4) infratentorial-supracerebellar approach by Krause, and 5) the three-quarter-prone, operated side down, occipital transtentorial approach by Ausman. Other approaches include resection of the occipital lobe by Horrax, which is not used anymore because of its high traumaticity, the frontal (anterior) transcallosal transventricular transvelum-interpositum approach by Sano,[36,46] which is useful for large pineal tumors with anterior extension into the third ventricle, and many technical modifications of the first four approaches.

The transcallosal approach as proposed by Dandy (1921)[43] is performed along the falx at the level of the parietooccipital junction. This is posteriorly free of veins to the superior sagittal sinus, but anteriorly the parietal bridging veins are often encountered and could be damaged by excessive retraction. Preservation of these veins is important because dividing them always initiates a mild hemiparesis or a contralateral astereognosia.[47] After retraction of the parietal lobe away from the falx, a 1 cm incision of the corpus callosum just in front of the splenium is carefully performed. After this callosal incision, the internal cerebral veins can usually be seen capping the tumor. These veins can be retracted to one side off the dome of the tumor, and then the tumor can be dissected from surrounding structures. The ultrasonic aspirator can be useful in debulking the tumor.[32]

With the superior approach, arteries coming from the medial branches of the posterior choroidal arteries are seen at the end of procedure.[47] Pineal tumors are often tightly adherent to or embedded in the quadrigeminal plate, making the dissection in this area a most dangerous step of the operation.[48] It is also important to know precisely whether the tumor invades brain structures, because the brain stem cannot be seen well in the transcallosal approach until most of the tumor has been removed.[32]

The posterior transcallosal approach had been widely used in the past[49,50] but was replaced in most cases by the occipital transtentorial or the infratentorial supracerebellar approach. Now its use is limited by tumors that expand anteriorly into the third ventricle as well as those extending upward into the corpus callosum.[32,48]

The transcortical transventricular approach, described by Van Wagenen in 1931,[44] has the disadvantage of being too lateral. Surgery is performed after entering the posterior part of the lateral ventricle, usually dilated due to hydrocephalus, through a cortical incision located in the parietal region. This approach is limited to the nondominant hemisphere. The route is direct and medial behind the hilum of the choroid plexus and tangential to the posterior thalamic mass.[47] This approach provides wide exposure of the atrium and the posterior portions of the body of the lateral ventricle. It may be preferred for pineal tumors that grow into the third ventricle and extend from it into the posterior part of the lateral ventricle or lesions that predominantly involve the atrium or the glomus of the choroid plexus.[48] However, in approaching the pineal region, the thalamic mass is restricting, and it is difficult to work on the midline and more difficult beyond it.

The occipital transtentorial approach was proposed by Foerster in 1928,[41,42] and it was described in detail by Poppen in 1966.[51] The pole of the occipital lobe is retracted superolaterally. Then the tentorium is divided parallel and lateral to the straight sinus from the point anterior to the transverse sinus to the free edge, partially removing the tentorial wedge for better exposure of the tumor.[17,48,51] The main disadvantage of this approach is that the vein of Galen with its tributaries usually obstructs the approach to the pineal region.[48] The internal occipital vein, which crosses the field to the occipital lobe, can be sacrificed, but neither the internal cerebral vein nor the basal vein of Rosenthal can be transected.[52]

The occipital transtentorial approach allowed a decrease in mortality and morbidity and achieved quite good results: 60% of patients have a normal life after surgery and 40% are free of any symptoms or signs.[23]

The infratentorial supracerebellar approach was first described by Krause in 1913 and revived by Stein in 1971 (Fig. 29.16).[53] In this approach gravity assists the cerebellum in falling away from the tentorium. The wide suboccipital craniotomy with opening of the torcula and transverse sinuses is made with the patient in a sitting position.[48,54,55] After one opens the dura and sacrifices the bridging veins from the cerebellum to the tentorium, the cerebellum sinks down and reveals a wide gap under the tentorium to the quadrigeminal cistern.[55]

The main advantage of the supracerebellar infratentorial approach is that with retraction of the upper cerebellum the surgical corridor is free of delicate nervous structures. The venous structures are well exposed above the surgical field, and the precentral cerebellar vein can be sacrificed without any adverse effects. The main disadvantage of this approach is the presence of tentorium, which is restricting, giving two lateral blind corners. Limited visualization on each side by the slope of the tentorium restricts the use of this approach to resection of small tumors without lateral extension.[47]

The common disadvantages of these last two approaches, as they were originally described,[51,53] include the sitting position of the patient, which increases the chance of air embolism, and the great degree of discomfort for the surgeon, who is working with the arms extended in a very deep surgical field for a long time. To avoid these disadvantages, Jamieson in 1971[52] proposed a lateral position for the patient with the operative side up for an occipital transtentorial approach. Reid and Clark in 1978[56] reported using this approach with the patient in a semisitting or prone position. However, all these modifications still require retraction of the occipital lobe. Kobayashi et al. in 1983[57] introduced the Concorde position for performing the supracerebellar infratentorial approach, which also diminishes the chance of air embolism. This approach is inconvenient for the surgeon, assistant, and scrub nurse. Ausman et al. in 1984[58] reported the successful use of a three-quarter position, operative side down, which decreases the risk of air embolism and minimizes the occipital lobe retraction. Ausman's approach avoids all the disadvantages of the other approaches (Fig. 29.17).

Stereotactic biopsy of tumors of the pineal region has recently become popular. Stereotactic technique is associated with no mortality and low morbidity and gives satisfactory biopsy samples.[59,60] Successful biopsy also can be performed endoscopically using a flexible ventriculofiberscope.[61] The enthusiasm of neurosurgeons about these procedures is limited, however—different parts of the tumor of this region may show different histology, so that biopsy of a small piece of the tumor may not indicate the true nature of the whole. So unless removal is possible, exploration and debulking of the tumor are preferred.[46]

The ability of pineal cell tumors to metastasize through a diversionary CSF shunt is apparent and requires the incorporation of a filter in the shunting system. A versapore filter, which is malleable and will not fracture, has a built-in bypass system so that if the filter clogs, it can be safely bypassed on the presumption that radiotherapy will have destroyed any CSF-borne cells.[32]

The prognosis of pineal tumors does not change if malignant cells are found in the CSF before operation. Tumors associated with malignant cells are limited and resectable as frequently as others. But postoperative radiation therapy and chemotherapy are indicated if tumor cells were observed before operation.[47]

OTHER THERAPEUTIC MODALITIES

More than 70% of tumors in the pineal region and the posterior third ventricle are highly radiosensitive. They usually respond to adequate courses of radiation therapy within 3 to 6 months.[62]

In the 1960s and 1970s, shunting and irradiation of pineal tumors were the standard approach, primarily because of the unsatisfactory outcome of direct surgery. Reports of impressive results of direct surgery on lesions

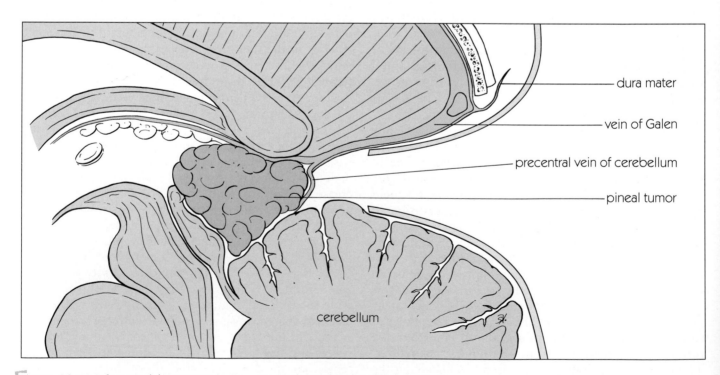

dura mater

vein of Galen

precentral vein of cerebellum

pineal tumor

cerebellum

Figure 29.16 Infratentorial supracerebellar approach to pineal region neoplasms.

Principles of Neurosurgery

of the pineal area during the 1970s have led to a more aggressive surgical approach.

The current neurosurgical concept of the treatment of pineal region tumors consists of the surgical removal of the tumor followed by appropriate CSF shunting and irradiation of the brain locally or the whole neural axis, depending on the histology and the completeness of the resection. Preoperative radiation therapy should be avoided if a direct approach is possible.[23]

It was clinically proved that germinomas, like seminomas, and pineal cell tumors (pineoblastoma and pineocytoma), like medulloblastomas, are highly sensi-

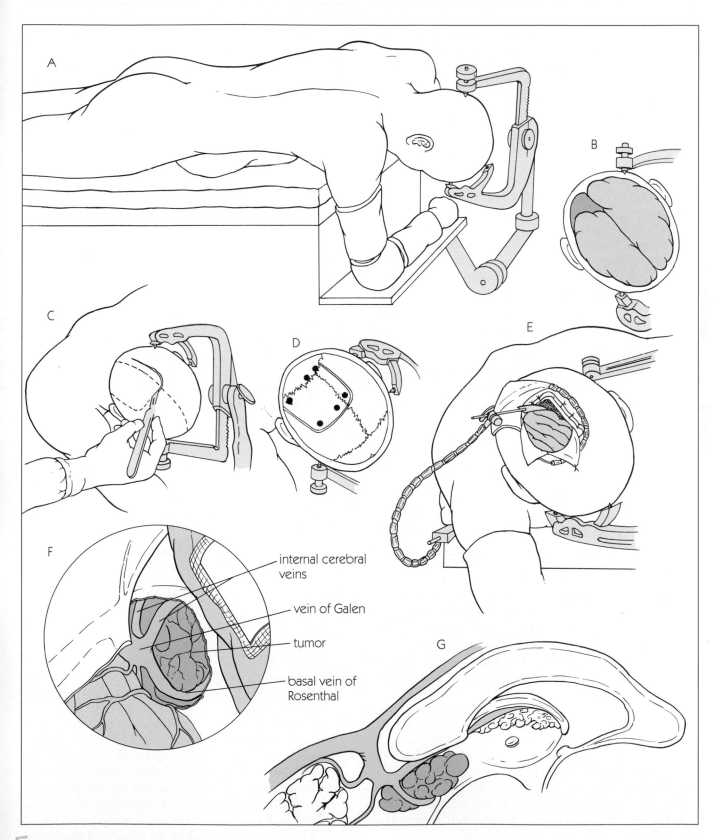

internal cerebral veins

vein of Galen

tumor

basal vein of Rosenthal

Figure 29.17 (A–G) Three-quarter-prone, operated side down, occipitoparietal transtentorial approach to pineal region masses.

tive to radiation therapy.[63] There are some controversies regarding the optimal tumor dose, volume to be irradiated, and role of elective spinal irradiation.

For irradiation of pineal tumor mass, total doses of 45 to 55 Gy are generally employed. The ability of lower doses of 25 to 30 Gy to achieve equal results is questionable.[64,65] Analysis of the dose-response curve for pineal region tumors indicates greater local control with increasing dose. In patients receiving less than 50 Gy there was 63% local control, while in those receiving 50 Gy or more local control was achieved in 87.5%.[66] Doses of 25 to 35 Gy are used for adjuvant radiotherapy to uninvolved areas of the brain and spine.[65]

Spinal irradiation is strongly recommended by some authors if a proven germinoma, malignant germ cell tumor, or pineoblastoma has been found.[32,67,68] Others recommend routine craniospinal axis irradiation for patients with a positive myelogram.[64,65]

Radiotherapy is not a benign form of treatment. Serious consequences of such treatment include gross evidence of cerebral atrophy on CT and, sometimes, marked calcification of cerebral hemispheres; seizure problems; endocrine deficiences; significant mental impairment with low IQ; and severe vasculitis and necrosis of brain, which can be fatal.[32] All this significantly limits the use of radiotherapy in young children.

Other radiotherapeutic modalities are stereotactic radiosurgery[69,70] and interstitial irradiation.[71]

In 1977 de Tribolet and Barrelet[72] reported the successful use of chemotherapy in a patient with a large pineal tumor. The chemotherapeutic regimen included daunorubicin, vincristine, and bleomycin. Later, the combination of cisplatin, bleomycin, and vincristine (PVB therapy) was used for treatment of germ cell tumors in several series with limited success.[73,74] Takakura in 1987[75] recommended the use of ACNU and vincristine together with radiotherapy in cases of immature teratomas and PVB therapy after finishing the whole course of radiotherapy to prevent recurrence.

Despite the high toxicity of chemotherapeutic agents and very limited experience using them, most neurosurgeons believe that chemotherapy will soon have an accepted role in the treatment of pineal region tumors.[10]

CONCLUSION

In the United States, tumors of the pineal region constitute about 1% of all intracranial neoplasms. In Asia, particularly in Japan, all germ cell tumors are more common (for unknown reasons), and pineal region tumors constitute 4% to 7% of all intracranial neoplasms.

Pathologically, primary tumors of the pineal region can be divided into four groups: germ cell tumors, pineal parenchymal tumors, tumors of supportive and adjacent structures, and nonneoplastic tumor-like conditions. The most commonly found histologic groups are germ cell tumors and pineal parenchymal tumors.

Symptoms of tumors in the pineal region are caused either by obstruction of CSF pathways or by local involvement (compression or invasion) of adjacent structures. Characteristic local signs include visual disturbances, the most common being Parinaud's syndrome.

The diagnostic method of choice is MRI. However, imaging techniques cannot give definitive information about the histologic type of the tumor. Qualitative and quantitative assessment of tumor markers is nonspecific in diagnostic evaluation but useful for following the tumor after treatment. It is well documented that there can be a diverse histology in any pineal tumor.

The treatment of tumors of the pineal region depends mostly on their histologic type and may include a combination of surgery, irradiation, and chemotherapy. At the present time, surgery of pineal region tumors is quite safe. The surgical removal of the lesion or its detailed biopsy presents the best way of establishing the histologic diagnosis. Various surgical approaches have been advocated, which have a high degree of success.

REFERENCES

1. Neuwelt EA, Gumerlock MK. The challenge of pineal region tumors. In: Neuwelt EA, ed. *Diagnosis and Treatment of Pineal Region Tumors.* Baltimore, Md: Williams & Wilkins; 1984:1–30.

2. Ranson SW, Clark SL. *The Anatomy of the Nervous System: Its Development and Function.* Philadelphia, Pa: WB Saunders Co; 1959.

3. Williams DL, Warwick R, Dyson M, Bannister LH, eds. *Gray's Anatomy.* 37th ed. Edinburgh: Churchill Livingstone; 1989.

4. Pernkopf E. *Topographische Anatomie des Menschen.* München: Urban und Schwarzenberg; 1960.

5. Pendl G. Microsurgical anatomy of the pineal region. In: Neuwelt EA, ed. *Diagnosis and Treatment of Pineal Region Tumors.* Baltimore, Md: Williams & Wilkins; 1984:155–207.

6. Yamamoto I, Kageyama N. Microsurgical anatomy of the pineal region. *J Neurosurg.* 1980;53:205–221.

7. Ringertz N, Nordenstam H, Flyger G. Tumors of the pineal region. *J Neuropathol Exp Neurol.* 1954; 13:540–561.

8. Yamamoto I, Rhoton AL Jr, Peace DA. Microsurgery of the third ventricle, 1: microsurgical anatomy. *Neurosurgery.* 1981;8:334–356.

9. Quest DO, Kleriga E. Microsurgical anatomy of the pineal region. *Neurosurgery.* 1980;6:385–390.

10. Sawaya R, Hawley DK, Tobler WD, Tew JM Jr, Chambers AA. Pineal and third ventricle tumors. In: Youmans JR, ed. *Neurological Surgery.* 3rd ed. Philadelphia, Pa: WB Saunders Co; 1990: 3171–3203.

11. DeGirolami U. Pathology of tumors of the pineal

region. In: Schmidek HH, ed. *Pineal Tumors*. New York, NY: Masson Publishing USA; 1977:1–19.

12. Herrick MK. Pathology of pineal tumors. In: Neuwelt EA, ed. *Diagnosis and Treatment of Pineal Region Tumors*. Baltimore, Md: Williams & Wilkins; 1984:31–60.

13. Mostofi FK, Sobin LH. Histologic typing of testicular tumors. In: *International Histologic Classification of Tumors, No 16*. Geneva: World Health Organization; 1976.

14. Jennings MT, Gelman R, Hochberg F. Intracranial germ-cell tumors: natural history and pathogenesis. In: Neuwelt EA, ed. *Diagnosis and Treatment of Pineal Region Tumors*. Baltimore, Md: Williams & Wilkins; 1984:116–138.

15. Scheithauer BW. Neuropathology of pineal region tumors. *Clin Neurosurg*. 1985;32:351–383.

16. Herrick MK, Rubinstein LJ. The cytological differentiating potential of pineal parenchymal neoplasms (true pinealomas). *Brain*. 1979;102:289–320.

17. Clark WK. Occipital transtentorial approach. In: Apuzzo MLJ, ed. *Surgery of the Third Ventricle*. Baltimore, Md: Williams & Wilkins; 1987: 591–610.

18. Kashiwagi S, Hatano M, Yokoyama T. Metastatic small cell carcinoma to the pineal body: case report. *Neurosurgery*. 1989;25:810–813.

19. Vaquero J, Martinez R, Magallon R, Ramiro J. Intracranial metastases to the pineal region: report of three cases. *J Neurosurg Sci*. 1991;35:55–57.

20. Schmidek HH, Waters A. Pineal masses: clinical features and management. In: Wilkins RH, Rengachary SS, eds. *Neurosurgery*. New York, NY: McGraw-Hill; 1985:688–693.

21. Jooma R, Kendall BE. Diagnosis and treatment of pineal tumors. *J Neurosurg*. 1983;58:654–665.

22. Wray SH. The neuro-ophthalmic and neurologic manifestations of pinealomas. In: Schmidek HH, ed. *Pineal Tumors*. New York, NY: Masson Publishing USA; 1977:21–59.

23. Lapras C. Surgical therapy of pineal region tumors. In: Neuwelt EA, ed. *Diagnosis and Treatment of Pineal Region Tumors*. Baltimore, Md: Williams & Wilkins; 1984:289–299.

24. Shults WT. Neuro-ophthalmology of pineal tumors. In: Neuwelt EA, ed. *Diagnosis and Treatment of Pineal Region Tumors*. Baltimore, Md: Williams & Wilkins; 1984:108–115.

25. Axelrod L. Endocrine dysfunction in patients with tumors of the pineal region. In: Schmidek HH, ed. *Pineal Tumors*. New York, NY: Masson Publishing USA; 1977:61–77.

26. Zimmerman RA. Pineal region masses: radiology. In: Wilkins RH, Rengachary SS, eds. *Neurosurgery*. New York, NY: McGraw-Hill; 1985: 680–687.

27. Grossman CB, Gonzalez CF. Neuroradiology of the pineal region. In: Schmidek HH, ed. *Pineal Tumors*. New York, NY: Masson Publishing USA; 1977:79–98.

28. Anderson RE. Diagnostic radiology of pineal tumors. In: Neuwelt EA, ed. *Diagnosis and Treatment of Pineal Region Tumors*. Baltimore, Md: Williams & Wilkins; 1984:61–85.

29. Kwan E, Wolpert SM, Smith SP, Modic MT. Radiology of third ventricular lesions. In: Apuzzo MLJ, ed. *Surgery of the Third Ventricle*. Baltimore, Md: Williams & Wilkins; 1987:262–300.

30. Tien RD, Barkovich AJ, Edwards MSB. MR imaging of pineal tumors. *AJNR*. 1990;11: 557–565.

31. Ganti SR, Hilal SK, Stein BM, Silver AJ, Mawad M, Sane P. CT of pineal region tumors. *AJNR*. 1986;7:97–104.

32. Hoffman HJ. Transcallosal approach to pineal tumors and the Hospital for Sick Children series of pineal region tumors. In: Neuwelt EA, ed. *Diagnosis and Treatment of Pineal Region Tumors*. Baltimore, Md: Williams & Wilkins; 1984:223–235.

33. Arita N, Ushio Y, Hayakawa T, et al. Tumor markers: their role and limit for management of pineal tumor. In: Samii M, ed. *Surgery in and Around the Brain Stem and the Third Ventricle*. Berlin: Springer-Verlag; 1986:318–325.

34. Allen JC, Nisselbaum J, Epstein F, Rosen G, Schwartz MK. Alphafetoprotein and human chorionic gonadotropin determination in cerebrospinal fluid: an aid to the diagnosis and management of intracranial germ-cell tumors. *J Neurosurg*. 1979; 51:368–374.

35. Edwards MSB, Levin V. Chemotherapy of tumors of the third ventricular region. In: Apuzzo MLJ, ed. *Surgery of the Third Ventricle*. Baltimore, Md: Williams & Wilkins; 1987:838–842.

36. Sano K. Pineal region tumors: problems in pathology and treatment. *Clin Neurosurg*. 1983;30:59–91.

37. Takakura K. Intracranial germ cell tumors. *Clin Neurosurg*. 1985;32:429–444.

38. Shinoda J, Yamada H, Sakai N, Ando T, Hirata T, Miwa Y. Placental alkaline phosphatase as a tumor marker for primary intracranial germinoma. *J Neurosurg*. 1988;68:710–720.

39. Vorkapic P, Waldhauser F, Bruckner R, Biegelmayer C, Schmidbauer M, Pendl G. Serum melatonin level: a new diagnostic tool in pineal region tumors. *Neurosurgery*. 1987;21:817–824.

40. Phillips PC, Kremzner LT, De Vivo DC. Cerebrospinal fluid polyamines: biochemical markers of malignant childhood brain tumors. *Ann Neurol*. 1986;19:360–364.

41. Pendl G. The surgery of pineal lesions—historical perspective. In: Neuwelt EA, ed. *Diagnosis and Treatment of Pineal Region Tumors*. Baltimore, Md: Williams & Wilkins; 1984:139–154.

42. Zülch KJ. Reflections on the surgery of the pineal gland (a glimpse into the past). *Neurosurg Rev*. 1981;4:159–162.

43. Dandy WE. An operation for the removal of pineal tumors. *Surg Gynecol Obstet*. 1921;33:113–119.

44. Van Wagenen WP. A surgical approach for the removal of certain pineal tumors: report of a case. *Surg Gynecol Obstet.* 1931;53:216–220.

45. Stein BM, Fetell MR. Therapeutic modalities for pineal region tumors. *Clin Neurosurg.* 1985;32:445–455.

46. Sano K. Treatment of tumors in the pineal and posterior third ventricular region. In: Samii M, ed. *Surgery in and Around the Brain Stem and the Third Ventricle.* Berlin: Springer-Verlag; 1986:309–317.

47. Lapras C, Patet JD. Controversies, techniques, and strategies for pineal tumor surgery. In: Apuzzo MLJ, ed. *Surgery of the Third Ventricle.* Baltimore, Md: Williams & Wilkins; 1987:649–662.

48. Rhoton AL Jr, Yamamoto I, Peace DA. Microsurgery of the third ventricle, 2: operative approaches. *Neurosurgery.* 1981;8:357–373.

49. Kunicki A. Operative experiences in 8 cases of pineal tumor. *J Neurosurg.* 1960;17:815–823.

50. Suzuki J, Iwabuchi T. Surgical removal of pineal tumors (pinealomas and teratomas): experience in a series of 19 cases. *J Neurosurg.* 1965;23:565–571.

51. Poppen JL. The right occipital approach to a pinealoma. *J Neurosurg.* 1966;25:706–710.

52. Jamieson KG. Excision of pineal tumors. *J Neurosurg.* 1971;35:550–553.

53. Stein BM. The infratentorial supracerebellar approach to pineal lesions. *J Neurosurg.* 1971;35:197–202.

54. Bruce JN, Stein BM. Infratentorial approach to pineal tumors. In: Wilson CB, ed. *Neurosurgical Procedures: Personal Approaches to Classic Operations.* Baltimore, Md: Williams & Wilkins; 1992:63–76.

55. Pendl G. Microsurgical anatomy of the pineal and midbrain region. In: Samii M, ed. *Surgery in and Around the Brain Stem and the Third Ventricle.* Berlin: Springer-Verlag; 1986:65–76.

56. Reid WS, Clark WK. Comparison of the infratentorial and transtentorial approaches to the pineal region. *Neurosurgery.* 1978;3:1–8.

57. Kobayashi S, Sugita K, Tanaka Y, Kyoshima K. Infratentorial approach to the pineal region in prone position: Concorde position. *J Neurosurg.* 1983;58:141–143.

58. Ausman JI, Malik GM, Pearce J, Rogers JS. A new operative approach to the pineal region. In: Samii M, ed. *Surgery in and Around the Brain Stem and the Third Ventricle.* Berlin: Springer-Verlag; 1986:326–328.

59. Conway LW. Stereotaxic diagnosis and treatment of intracranial tumours including an initial experience with cryosurgery for pinealomas. *J Neurosurg.* 1973;38:453–460.

60. Moser RP, Backlund E-O. Stereotactic techniques in the diagnosis and treatment of pineal region tumors. In: Neuwelt EA, ed. *Diagnosis and Treatment of Pineal Region Tumors.* Baltimore, Md: Williams & Wilkins; 1984:236–253.

61. Fukushima T. Endoscopic biopsy of intraventricular tumors with the use of a ventriculofiberscope. *Neurosurgery.* 1978;2:110–113.

62. Brady LW. The role of radiation therapy. In: Schmidek HH, ed. *Pineal Tumors.* New York, NY: Masson Publishing USA; 1977:127–132.

63. Laws ER Jr, Abay EO III, Forbes GS, Grado GL, Bruckman JE, Scott M. Conservative management of pineal tumors—Mayo Clinic experience. In: Neuwelt EA, ed. *Diagnosis and Treatment of Pineal Region Tumors.* Baltimore, Md: Williams & Wilkins; 1984:323–331.

64. Danoff B, Sheline GE. Radiotherapy of pineal tumors. In: Neuwelt EA, ed. *Diagnosis and Treatment of Pineal Region Tumors.* Baltimore, Md: Williams & Wilkins; 1984:300–308.

65. Wara W, Gutin PH. Radiotherapy of pineal and suprasellar tumors. In: Apuzzo MLJ, ed. *Surgery of the Third Ventricle.* Baltimore, Md: Williams & Wilkins; 1987:831–837.

66. Abay II EO, Laws ER Jr, Grado GL, Bruckman JE, Forbes GS, Gomez MR, Scott M. Pineal tumors in children and adolescents: treatment by CSF shunting and radiotherapy. *J Neurosurg.* 1981;55:889–895.

67. Haimovich IC, Sharer L, Hyman RA, Beresford HR. Metastasis of intracranial germinoma through a ventriculoperitoneal shunt. *Cancer.* 1981;48:1033–1036.

68. Jenkin RDT, Simpson WJK, Keen CW. Pineal and suprasellar germinomas: results of radiation treatment. *J Neurosurg.* 1978;48:99–107.

69. Backlund E-O, Rähn T, Sarby B. Treatment of pinealomas by stereotactic radiation surgery. *Acta Radiol Ther.* 1974;13:368–376.

70. Colombo F, Benedetti A, Pozza F, et al. External stereotaxic irradiation on a linear accelerator. *Neurosurgery.* 1985;16:154–160.

71. Weigel K, Ostertag CB, Mundinger F. Interstitial long-term irradiation of tumors in the pineal region. In: Szikla G, ed. *Stereotactic Cerebral Irradiation.* Amsterdam: Elsevier; 1979:283–292.

72. de Tribolet N, Barrelet L. Successful chemotherapy for pinealoma. *Lancet.* 1977;2:1228–1229.

73. Neuwelt EA, Frenkel EP. Germinomas and other pineal tumors: chemotherapeutic responses. In: Neuwelt EA, ed. *Diagnosis and Treatment of Pineal Region Tumors.* Baltimore, Md: Williams & Wilkins; 1984:332–343.

74. Siegal T, Pfeffer MR, Catane R, Sulkes A, Gomori MJ, Fuks Z. Successful chemotherapy of recurrent intracranial germinoma with spinal metastases. *Neurology.* 1983;33:631–633.

75. Takakura K, Matsutani M. Therapeutic modality selection in management of germ cell tumors. In: Apuzzo MLJ, ed. *Surgery of the Third Ventricle.* Baltimore, Md: Williams & Wilkins; 1987:843–846.

Chapter 30

Cerebellopontine Angle Tumors

Robert H. Wilkins

ANATOMY

The term *cerebellopontine angle* is ordinarily used to denote more than the angle between the cerebellum and the pons. It normally means the space bounded anteromedially by the lower midbrain, pons, and medulla; posteromedially by the cerebellum; and laterally by the petrous portion of the temporal bone (Fig. 30.1). This elongated space, which in cross-section is roughly triangular, is filled with CSF contained within three cisterns: ambient, superior cerebellopontine, and inferior cerebellopontine (lateral cerebellomedullary) (Fig. 30.2).

The cerebellopontine angle (i.e., space) is crossed by

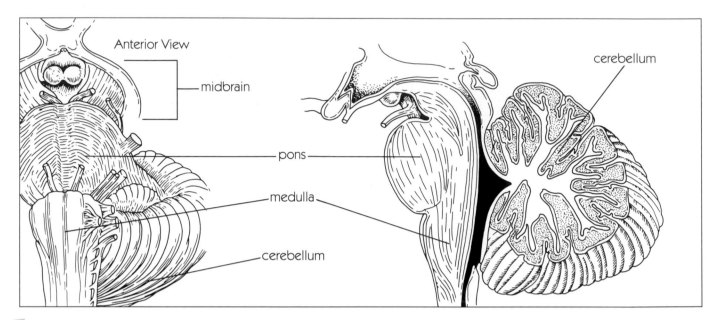

Figure 30.1 Ventral and sagittal views of the brain stem and cerebellum.

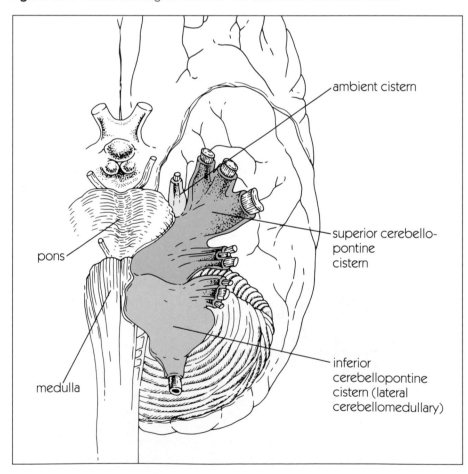

Figure 30.2 Ventral view of the brain showing the cisterns of the cerebello-pontine angle. (Modified from Yasargil MG. *Microneurosurgery: Microsurgical Anatomy of the Basal Cisterns and Vessels of the Brain, Diagnostic Studies, General Operative Techniques and Pathological Considerations of the Intracranial Aneurysms.* Stuttgart: George Thieme Verlag; 1984:1;16)

three groups of structures (Fig. 30.3). Superiorly are the trochlear nerve and superior cerebellar artery, which pass through the ambient cistern, and the superior petrosal vein and trigeminal nerve, which lie in the upper part of the superior cerebellopontine cistern. In the middle are the facial and acoustic nerves and the anterior inferior cerebellar artery, which also course through the superior cerebellopontine cistern. And inferiorly are the glossopharyngeal, vagus, and accessory nerves and the vertebral and posterior inferior cerebellar arteries, which cross the inferior cerebellopontine cistern. The hypoglossal nerve also lies within the inferior cerebellopontine cistern but is located more anteriorly than the other cranial nerves. Likewise, the abducens nerve, which lies within the prepontine cistern, is located anterior to the brain stem.

PATHOLOGY AND CLINICAL PRESENTATION

Various types of tumors can and do grow within the cerebellopontine angle. In general, these are benign tumors that can be cured if they are totally removed. The challenge for the surgeon is to achieve such a cure without injury to the structures within the cerebellopontine angle (listed above).

The tumors that occur within the cerebellopontine angle vary according to the age of the patient.[1] In adulthood, the most common tumors are the acoustic schwannoma (also known as the acoustic neurinoma, neuroma, or neurilemoma), the meningioma, the epidermoid cyst, the glomus jugulare tumor, and the choroid plexus papilloma. In childhood, the most common tumor is the ependymoma.

An *acoustic schwannoma* is a benign tumor that arises from the acoustic nerve (most often from one of the two vestibular nerves).[2] Because the tumor grows slowly, the gradual unilateral loss of vestibular function is compensated and the patient remains asymptomatic in that regard. However, a unilateral diminution in auditory acuity occurs, typically affecting speech discrimination out of proportion to pure tone loss initially, and ipsilateral tinnitus may also develop. Despite the fact that the facial nerve lies immediately adjacent to the acoustic nerve and is progressively distorted by an enlarging acoustic schwannoma, facial weakness does not ordinarily occur, even when the tumor has become large. Typically, the next cranial nerve to be affected is the ipsilateral trigeminal nerve, the earliest sign of which may be diminished corneal sensation. When the tumor reaches a large size, dysfunction of the other cranial nerves of the cerebellopontine angle may occur, and the symptoms and signs of brain stem distortion and hydrocephalus may develop. However, ordinarily the tumor is diagnosed and treated before it reaches this advanced stage.

At the time it is discovered, an acoustic schwannoma may lie wholly within the internal auditory canal or

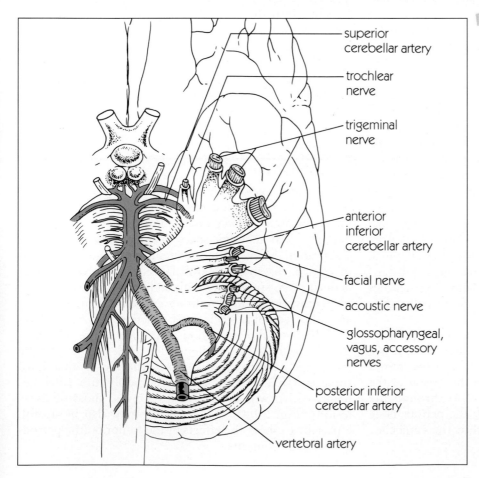

superior cerebellar artery

trochlear nerve

trigeminal nerve

anterior inferior cerebellar artery

facial nerve

acoustic nerve

glossopharyngeal, vagus, accessory nerves

posterior inferior cerebellar artery

vertebral artery

Figure 30.3 Ventral view of the brain showing the main nerves and arteries of the cerebellopontine angle.

wholly within the cerebellopontine angle, but most commonly it has portions in both areas—resembles a mushroom whose "stem" lies within the internal auditory canal and expanded "cap" within the cerebellopontine angle.

A *meningioma* is a benign, slowly-growing tumor that arises from meningothelial cells of the arachnoid membrane.[1] Meningiomas are more common in women than men and typically do not come to medical attention until after the fourth decade of life. Among the several locations in which a meningioma is likely to occur is the posterior slope of the petrous portion of the temporal bone, from which the tumor grows into the cerebellopontine angle.[3] In addition to surrounding the adjacent nerves and blood vessels of the cerebellopontine angle, such a tumor may also penetrate the dura mater and grow into the petrous bone.

Depending on the direction of its growth, such a tumor first interferes with the function of one or more of the cranial nerves and then involves the cerebellum and brain stem. Thus, in a reported series of 30 patients with a meningioma of the cerebellopontine angle,[3] the initial symptoms or manifestations included decreased hearing in 9, vertigo in 9, pain in the face or tongue in 8, occipital headache in 8, facial numbness or paresthesias in 4, imbalance in 2, and hoarseness in 2. By the time of their admission to the hospital, 20 patients had decreased hearing, 17 had decreased corneal sensation, 15 had facial weakness, and 13 had decreased facial sensation; there were 29 examples of other posterior fossa cranial nerve palsies; and 21 patients had gait ataxia, 14 had nystagmus, and 11 had limb ataxia.

An *epidermoid cyst* is a benign neoplasm that arises from embryologically misplaced epithelial cells.[1] The thin generative epithelium produces keratinous debris that fills the cyst; as the epithelium grows and the keratinous debris accumulates, the cyst slowly enlarges. The cerebellopontine angle is the most common location for an epidermoid cyst, and in this location it gradually insinuates itself into every available space, adhering firmly in the process to the nerves and vessels that cross the cerebellopontine angle.[4]

As is true of the acoustic schwannoma and the meningioma, the epidermoid cyst in the cerebellopontine angle may give rise to tic douloureux or hemifacial spasm (or both) as a manifestation of involvement of the trigeminal or facial nerve, respectively. Frank cranial nerve deficits may develop and most frequently involve the trigeminal, facial, and acoustic nerves. As with the acoustic schwannoma and the meningioma, if an epidermoid cyst reaches a large size, evidence of brain stem and cerebellar dysfunction may also occur.

A *glomus jugulare tumor* is a benign tumor of one portion of the extraadrenal paraganglion system (i.e., it is a paraganglioma in a specific location) that arises from a small focus of paraganglionic tissue in the region of the middle ear.[1] As it grows, it may extend through the jugular foramen or may erode through the petrous bone to enlarge in a lobulated fashion within the cerebellopontine angle.

The initial symptoms and signs reflect this growth pattern. For example, in one reported series of 36 patients, the initial symptoms included tinnitus in 24, hearing loss in 20, ear pain in 17, blockage in 12, and dizziness in 5.[5] There were 19 instances of acoustic nerve dysfunction, 8 of vagus nerve dysfunction, 8 of hypoglossal nerve dysfunction, 6 of facial nerve dysfunction, 5 of spinal accessory nerve dysfunction, 3 of glossopharyngeal nerve dysfunction, and 1 of abducens nerve dysfunction.

A *choroid plexus papilloma*, as the name implies, is a papilloma arising from the choroid plexus.[1,6] The choroid plexus of the fourth ventricle extends as a tuft out of each of its two lateral recesses into the ipsilateral cerebellopontine angle between the attachments of the acoustic and glossopharyngeal nerves. A papilloma forming from one of these tufts is ordinarily a benign tumor whose microscopic appearance mimics that of the normal choroid plexus.

In children the choroid plexus papilloma occurs most frequently in a lateral ventricle, but in adults it occurs most frequently in the fourth ventricle or a cerebellopontine angle. In one series of 19 adult patients,[6] 4 tumors were located in the cerebellopontine angle and 15 in the fourth ventricle. Headache is the most common presenting symptom in adults, followed by posterior fossa cranial nerve deficits.

An *ependymoma* arises from the ependyma, cells that normally line the ventricular system.[1] In this circumstance, the tumor probably arises in the fourth ventricle and grows through one of the two lateral foramina of Luschka into the adjacent cerebellopontine angle. The common form of clinical presentation is that of increased intracranial pressure from hydrocephalus (e.g., headache, vomiting, irritability, lethargy, papilledema) perhaps accompanied by cerebellar, brain stem, and/or lower cranial nerve symptoms and signs.[7]

DIAGNOSIS

The initial suspicion that a patient is harboring a cerebellopontine angle tumor comes from the history and physical examination, which indicate involvement of structures unique to that anatomic space. If the patient has a unilateral hearing deficit, with or without tinnitus, or complains of vertigo, dizziness, or imbalance, the problem can be defined more specifically with audiometry, electronystagmography, brain stem auditory evoked potential testing, and other tests of acoustic nerve function.

The most direct method of arriving at the presumptive diagnosis of a cerebellopontine angle tumor is with a radiologic examination. Overall, the most valuable of these is MRI, without and with gadolinium enhancement, which will be expected to reveal most of these lesions (Fig. 30.4). CT scanning may also be useful, especially to show the effects of the tumor on the petrous bone and its contents.

TREATMENT

The main therapeutic consideration for tumors of the cerebellopontine angle is their surgical excision, and ordinarily this is the next step taken after the presumptive diagnosis is made. However, the glomus jugulare tumor is typically very vascular, so consideration is usually given to treating this first by intraarterial embolization to occlude as many of the vascular channels within the tumor as possible before the surgical resection in order to minimize the operative blood loss.[5]

The easiest and most direct surgical approach to the cerebellopontine angle is through an opening made in the occipital bone just inferior to the transverse sinus and just posterior to the sigmoid sinus (Fig. 30.5).[8,9] Based on exactly where and how the bone is removed, this procedure is called a retromastoid, retrosigmoid, or suboccipital craniectomy or craniotomy. The dura mater is opened and the cerebellar hemisphere is retracted medially to provide access into the cerebellopontine angle.

The tumor contained therein is then dealt with according to its nature, exact location, and relationships with the important structures in the area. In general, the tumor is removed piecemeal, with the surgeon first devoting attention to the reduction of its bulk and the interruption of its blood supply. If the tumor being resected is an epidermoid cyst, the surgeon must be careful not to permit the irritating cyst contents to spread within the subarachnoid spaces because such an occurrence would be expected to give rise to aseptic meningitis.[4] As the size of the tumor and its blood supply are reduced, it becomes easier for the surgeon to separate the tumor from the surrounding normal structures such as the cerebellum, brain stem, cranial nerves, and vessels. With two exceptions, the surgeon's eventual goal is the complete removal of the tumor with the preservation of these normal structures.

The two exceptions relate to the surgical treatment of acoustic schwannomas and glomus jugulare tumors. During the resection of an acoustic schwannoma, it is expected that at least the vestibular portions of the acoustic nerve (and often the cochlear portion as well) will have to be sacrificed to accomplish complete tumor removal. Similarly, it is usually necessary to occlude the sigmoid and inferior petrosal venous sinuses to permit the removal of a large glomus jugulare tumor.

In some circumstances, especially for the treatment of acoustic schwannomas, it is advantageous to make a somewhat different surgical approach, either through the

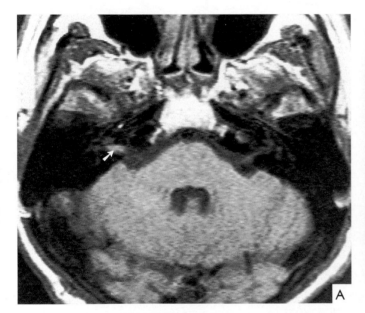
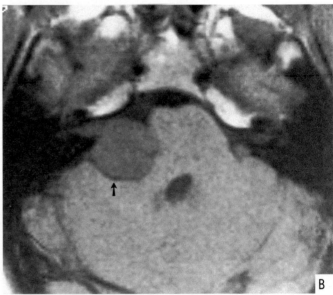

Figure 30.4 MRI is a valuable radiologic examination for detecting a cerebellopontine angle tumor. Shown are two acoustic schwannomas. **(A)** This tiny schwannoma (arrow), located within the internal auditory canal, stands out because of its enhancement by gadolinium. **(B)** This larger tumor (arrow) extends out of the internal auditory canal to form a mass that indents the pons and cerebellum.

mastoid bone and labyrinth (Fig. 30.6) or through the floor of the middle cranial fossa.[2] The translabyrinthine approach ordinarily sacrifices hearing in that ear but provides an increased probability of preserving the facial nerve because that nerve can be identified distal to the tumor, within the temporal bone, before the tumor resection is begun. The middle fossa approach offers the possibility of preserving hearing as well as facial nerve function during the removal of a small tumor that is contained wholly or largely within the internal auditory canal.

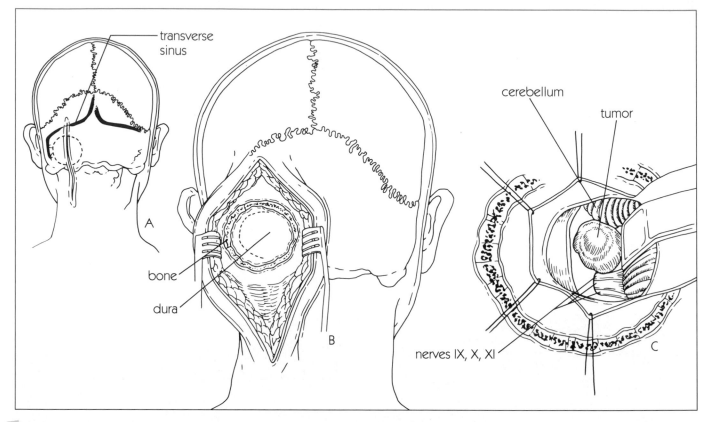

Figure 30.5 Steps in the surgical exposure of an acoustic schwannoma. (**A**) An incision is made over the lateral aspect of the occipital bone and an underlying craniectomy is performed: this bony opening extends to the transverse sinus superiorly and the sigmoid sinus laterally. (**B**) A curved dural incision provides access into the cerebellopontine angle. (**C**) The cerebellum is retracted medially to expose the tumor and the adjacent cranial nerves.

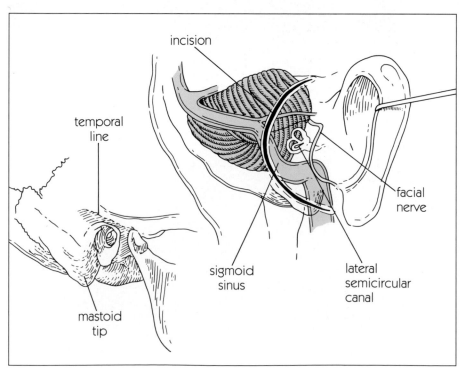

Figure 30.6 The translabyrinthine approach provides an alternative method of exposing the cerebellopontine angle. Shown here are the key anatomic features and the incision used.

For various reasons, such as the extension of a meningioma into the petrous bone or the firm adherence of the wall of an epidermoid cyst to a cranial nerve, it may not be possible to achieve complete tumor removal. However, because of the slow growth of most cerebellopontine angle tumors, it is usually more prudent to leave a small amount of tumor than to sacrifice an important normal structure.

The glomus jugulare tumor is potentially curable by excision, but its location makes this difficult, with risk of injury to the many important surrounding structures, not only within the cerebellopontine angle, but also within the temporal bone and in the neck just below that area of the skull. Furthermore, even with preoperative embolization of the tumor, bleeding during the operative removal of a glomus jugulare tumor may be excessive. Such surgery ordinarily involves the exposure of the tumor within the temporal bone and neck as well as the cerebellopontine angle, and is more extensive than the operative removal of the other cerebellopontine angle tumors.[5,10] Because of these factors, glomus jugulare tumors have also been treated with radiotherapy, either as a sole form of treatment or in combination with surgical resection.[5]

Although choroid plexus papillomas may recur after surgical resection (especially after subtotal resection, even despite postoperative radiotherapy), long-term survival is the rule.[6] In contrast, ependymomas of the posterior fossa, especially in children, do not have a favorable prognosis, even with treatment. For example, in a series of 35 infratentorial ependymomas treated surgically at a large children's hospital during the years from 1970 to 1987, 9 (26%) extended into a cerebellopontine angle.[7] Four of these nine tumors involved both cerebellopontine angles; two tumors were not invasive and could be removed totally, and these two patients survived longer than 5 years without postoperative radiotherapy. Five of the nine tumors extended into one cerebellopontine angle; in all five the tumor invaded into the adjacent parenchyma and in only one could gross total tumor removal be achieved. Considering all 35 patients, 27 received postoperative radiotherapy and 11 received postoperative chemotherapy. The 5-year survival of patients with invasive tumors (31%) was significantly less than the 5-year survival of patients with noninvasive tumors (79%).

A relatively new approach to the treatment of some small intracranial lesions, including acoustic schwannomas, is the use of stereotactically directed high energy radiation. This form of therapy, called stereotactic radiosurgery, can be accomplished in various ways, such as with multiple cobalt-60 sources of gamma radiation that are focused on a small fixed target, or with a photon beam emitted from a single linear accelerator that is rotated in relation to a small fixed target. In contrast to standard radiotherapy, all of the radiation is given in a single session. However, even with precise focusing there may be damage to adjacent tissue such as the facial nerve and the trigeminal nerve. At present, the role of stereotactic radiosurgery in the treatment of acoustic schwannomas is still being defined.

REFERENCES

1. Burger PC, Scheithauer BW, Vogel FS. *Surgical Pathology of the Nervous System and its Coverings.* 3rd ed. New York, NY: Churchill Livingstone, 1991.

2. House WF, Luetje CM. *Acoustic Tumors. Volume I: Diagnosis. Volume II: Management.* Baltimore, Md: University Park Press; 1979.

3. Yasargil MG, Mortara BW, Curcic M. Meningiomas of basal posterior cranial fossa. *Adv Tech Stds Neurosurg.* 1980;7:3–115.

4. Berger MS, Wilson CB. Epidermoid cysts of the posterior fossa. *J Neurosurg.* 1985;62:214–219.

5. Gardner G, Robertson JT, Robertson JH, et al. Glomus jugulare tumors—skull base surgery. In: Schmidek HH, Sweet WH, eds. *Operative Neurosurgical Techniques: Indications, Methods and Results.* 2nd ed. Orlando, Fla: Grune & Stratton; 1988: 739–752.

6. McGirr SJ, Ebersold MJ, Scheithauer BW, et al. Choroid plexus papillomas: long-term follow-up results in a surgically treated series. *J Neurosurg.* 1988,69:843–849.

7. Nazar GB, Hoffman JH, Becker LE, et al. Infratentorial ependymomas in childhood: prognostic factors and treatment. *J Neurosurg.* 1990;72: 408–417.

8. Ojemann RG. Microsurgical suboccipital approach to cerebellopontine angle tumors. *Clin Neurosurg.* 1978;25:461–479.

9. Yasargil MG, Smith RD, Gasser JC. Microsurgical approach to acoustic neurinomas. *Adv Tech Stds Neurosurg.* 1977;4:94–129.

10. Fisch U, Mattox D. *Microsurgery of the Skull Base.* Stuttgart: Georg Thieme Verlag; 1988.

Chapter 31

Posterior Fossa Tumors

Marion L. Walker, Joseph Petronio

For progress to be expedited, it was necessary for some one of the three groups mentioned to assume a more comprehensive role in these matters; and thus it has come about that so-called neurosurgeons have taken upon themselves the quadruple obligation (a) of making the preoperative diagnosis; (b) of conducting the operation; (c) of studying the tissues in detail for purposes of classification; and (d) of following the patient with an unfavorable type of intracranial tumor to the end of his story.—Harvey Cushing, 1929

Considerable progress has been made in the management of tumors of the posterior fossa since Cushing's day. While some lesions, such as the cerebellar astrocytoma, were surgically curable even in the early days of neurosurgery, advances in diagnostic imaging, microsurgical technique, neuroanesthesia, and critical care medicine have reduced the operative mortality and morbidity associated with their removal. Advances in radiation and chemical therapy and an improved understanding of the cellular and molecular biology of brain tumors have resulted in significant improvements in the long-term prognosis for patients with even the most malignant tumors. For example, while the cerebellar medulloblastoma was universally fatal in Cushing's first reported series of 61 patients,[1] current 5-year survival rates exceed 60% for all patients and 80% for certain "good risk" individuals.[2,3]

This chapter focuses on primarily intrinsic tumors occurring in the posterior fossa. We review tumors of the posterior fossa in two general groups, those occurring within the cerebellum and fourth ventricle and those in the brain stem.

INCIDENCE AND EPIDEMIOLOGY

Tumors of the posterior fossa are more common in children than in adults. In fact, between 54% and 70% of all childhood brain tumors originate in the posterior fossa,[4–12] compared with 15% to 20% in adults.[13]

Although most histopathologic varieties of posterior fossa tumor have been reported at any age, certain types (including the primitive neuroectodermal tumors [PNETs] medulloblastoma and pineoblastoma, ependymomas, and astrocytomas of the cerebellum and brainstem[4]) more commonly affect infants and children. Certain types of glial tumors, including mixed gliomas, are unique to children. They are more frequently located in the cerebellum (67%) than the cerebrum and are usually histologically benign. The most common combination is that of neoplastic astrocytes and oligodendroglia.[4] As a rule astrocytic tumors of adults more commonly display the histologic features of malignancy than those of children.[4,14] Certain tumors, including metastatic lesions, hemangioblastoma, and lymphoma, more commonly affect adults than children.

SIGNS AND SYMPTOMS

With most tumors of the posterior fossa the clinical syndrome at presentation is largely determined by the tumor's anatomic site of origin and its rate of growth. Many characteristic signs and symptoms of cerebellar neoplasia are uniformly present in both adults and children and in both benign and malignant lesions. Many symptoms are attributable to increased intracranial pressure rather than focal compression of nuclei, long tracts, or cranial nerves. When the circulation of CSF is compromised at the cerebral aqueduct, fourth ventricle, or its exit foramina, obstructive hydrocephalus occurs. Headache, vomiting, strabismus, papilledema, meningismus, dizziness, and macrocephaly in children may be observed.[12,15] A "vermian" syndrome is distinguished, if only in retrospect, from a "hemicerebellar" syndrome by the presence of truncal ataxia and characteristic eye findings in the former and appendicular ataxia and nystagmus in the latter. In general, signs and symptoms more suggestive of a cerebellar tumor include focal ataxia, dysmetria, nystagmus, and dizziness,[12,15] although it is nearly impossible to make a completely accurate diagnosis based solely on the clinical presentation.

In contrast, tumors of the brain stem usually present with focal signs of cranial nerve dysfunction and/or long tract findings. Truncal ataxia is common in patients with pontine or medullary tumors, while hemiparesis is more common with tumors of the cerebral peduncles. Headache is uncommon unless hydrocephalus is present. Tumors of the tectal plate usually present with hydrocephalus and, occasionally, associated eye findings.

Headache is the most common symptom of patients with a cerebellar mass, occurring in nearly 100% of patients in some series.[16] The headache associated with most cerebellar tumors is generalized or frontal in location.[12,15,17] It ultimately may localize to the occiput in individuals old enough to complain. Associated neck pain, neck stiffness, or a head tilt suggests tonsillar herniation into the foramen magnum.[15] Initially the headache from a posterior fossa mass is insidious and intermittent and can be most severe in the morning or after a nap,[12] presumably because the combination of hypoventilation during sleep and the increased intracranial pressure associated with recumbency serve to provoke a more severe headache on awakening.[15] In infants, headache may manifest itself only as increased irritability and a desire not to be handled. Since it is not a common complaint in early childhood, persistent or recurrent headache in this age group should immediately suggest increased intracranial pressure.[12]

Vomiting is also commonly associated with posterior fossa neoplasms. It may represent a generalized manifestation of increased intracranial pressure or direct compression and irritation of vagal nuclei in the medulla oblongata[12] or area postrema of the fourth ventricle. So-called projectile vomiting rarely occurs.[12] Vomiting is frequently limited to the morning, when intracranial pressure is often highest, while the act of vomiting and its associated hyperventilation may sometimes relieve headache.[15] Since it is nonspecific, vomiting is commonly misinterpreted, especially in pediatric patients, as a symptom of a gastrointestinal ailment or an emotional disturbance.[12] Nevertheless, the work-up for persistent vomiting in a child should include radiographic evaluation for a posterior fossa tumor.[15]

Although ataxia is commonly associated with cerebellar tumors, it can be truncal or appendicular depending on the location of the mass. Midline (vermian) tumors such as medulloblastomas, ependymomas, and vermian astrocytomas tend to produce a truncal ataxia with relative sparing of the extremities. This is characterized in children by a tendency to fall frequently, a lurching, wide-based gait, and an abnormal Romberg maneuver.[12] Patients with tumors of the cerebellar hemisphere such as metastases, cystic hemangioblastomas, and cerebellar astrocytomas often present with a "hemicerebellar" syndrome of unilateral ataxia or dysmetria of the extremities.

Eye findings are common in patients with posterior fossa neoplasms, and include nystagmus, strabismus, and papilledema. While nystagmus is often absent until late in the clinical course, it is useful in localizing the lesion. Lateral nystagmus suggests involvement of the cerebellar hemisphere, whereas vertical nystagmus implies a lesion of the anterior vermis, periaqueductal region, or craniocervical junction.[12]

Strabismus and its associated diplopia are usually secondary to sixth nerve palsies from hydrocephalus,[12,15] although third nerve palsies also may occur. With intrinsic tumors of the brain stem, direct involvement of the nuclei or tracts of the third, fourth, or sixth cranial nerves may result in ocular palsies and diplopia.

Although most of Cushing's patients with cerebellar astrocytomas were blind at diagnosis from long-standing papilledema and optic atrophy, such advanced disease at presentation fortunately has become uncommon.[15] The optic discs are frequently abnormal in patients, especially in children,[12] with posterior fossa tumors, and a careful fundoscopic examination is mandatory.

NEURODIAGNOSTIC EVALUATION

MRI has superseded CT as the optimal imaging modality for nearly all types of posterior fossa tumors.[13,18,19] Obvious advantages of MRI include its superior anatomic resolution, multiplanar imaging capabilities, and the lack of radiation exposure. While recent generation CT is highly sensitive,[20,21] CT imaging in the posterior fossa is still compromised by beam hardening artifact from dense posterior fossa bone.[19]

While neither MRI nor CT can distinguish with certainty one tumor type from another, certain trends exist (Fig. 31.1). Clues about the most likely histologic diagnosis are often obtained from the exact location of the mass (i.e., whether it is entirely intraventricular or arises from the cerebellar vermis or hemisphere), from the signal characteristics on long and short TR images, and from the pattern of enhancement with intravenous contrast administration (gadolinium).

Figure 31.1 Magnetic Resonance Features of Posterior Fossa Tumors

	Juvenile Pilocytic Astrocytoma	PNET	Ependymoma	Brain Stem Astrocytoma
Signal intensity characteristics (on long TR images)	Sharply demarcated; commonly cystic	Homogeneous; low-moderate intensity	Markedly heterogeneous	Ill-defined; high intensity
Contrast enhancement	Common in solid portion (mural module)	Common; dense	Common; irregular	Common
Calcification	Uncommon	Uncommon	Common	Rare
Hemorrhage	Rare	Uncommon	Common	Uncommon
Tendency to seed CSF pathways	Low	High	Moderate	Low

Adapted from Atlas S, 1991

The typical MRI appearance of a cerebellar astrocytoma is that of an intraaxial mass, either midline or hemispheric, often with a prominent cystic component and mural nodule (Figs. 31.2, 31.3). The mass usually displaces or effaces the fourth ventricle, and hydrocephalus is commonly present at the time of diagnosis. While the mural nodule or solid portion of the cyst often enhances with paramagnetic contrast agents, the cyst wall may or may not enhance (see Fig. 31.3). The solid portion of the tumor is usually hyperintense to brain on long TR images while the cystic portion can be slightly hyperintense to CSF because of an increased protein content.[13] As a rule, while both signal heterogeneity and calcification are less prominent with the cerebellar astrocytoma than with the ependymoma, both may occur in the former.[13]

In contrast, the PNET appears as an intraventricular midline or paramedian mass on MRI, often with homogenous signal intensity that is isointense to brain. The PNET usually enhances prominently following intravenous contrast administration (Fig. 31.4). Occasionally PNETs appear heterogenous on MRI, with areas of cystic degeneration and central necrosis, which may portend a poorer prognosis.[13] Other "atypical" features that can be present in up to 10% of PNETs include calcification, an eccentric location, and lack of contrast enhancement.[13]

On gross inspection, ependymomas are commonly multicystic, hemorrhagic, and calcified; not surprisingly, these features are typical of their MRI appearance (Fig. 31.5).[13,22] In the posterior fossa they are commonly intraventricular and, like several other tumors, associated with hydrocephalus. Since calcification occurs more

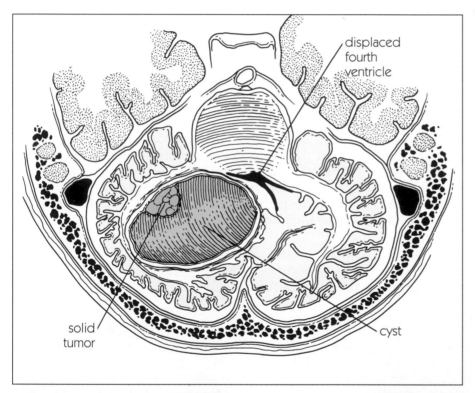

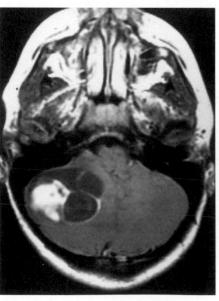

Figure 31.3
Axial MRI appearance of a cystic cerebellar astrocytoma following the administration of paramagnetic contrast material.

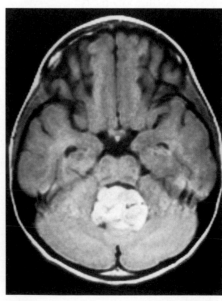

Figure 31.2 Gross appearance of laterally located cystic cerebellar astrocytoma.

Figure 31.4
Axial postcontrast MRI appearance of a cerebellar primitive neuroectodermal tumor (PNET).

commonly in ependymoma (nearly 45%) than in any other posterior fossa tumor,[23] MRI or CT evidence of calcification often supports this diagnosis but does not exclude others. Extension through the foramina of Magendie and Luschka with resultant compression of the craniocervical junction and lateral brain stem has been well reported—the so-called plastic ependymoma.[24] Extension of tumor through the foramen of Luschka into the cerebellopontine angle is essentially pathognomonic of ependymoma (see Fig. 31.5). While nearly all ependymomas enhance with paramagnetic contrast agents, they often appear more heterogenous than the uniformly enhancing PNET.[23]

The availability of MRI has greatly simplified the preoperative management of adults suspected of harboring a cerebellar hemangioblastoma.[25,26] The freedom from beam hardening artifacts, which have plagued CT imaging of the posterior fossa, has improved the accuracy of preoperative diagnoses and facilitated the identification of multiple lesions and a vascular nidus to be

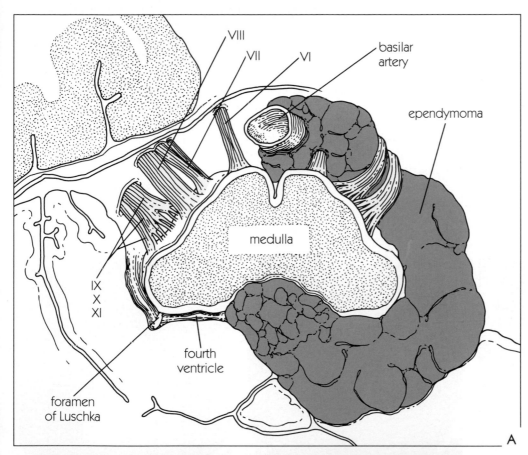

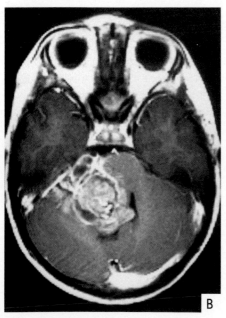

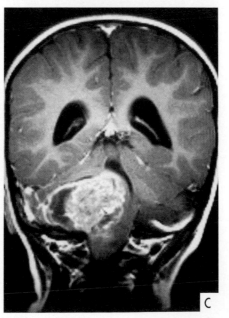

Figure 31.5 Fourth ventricular ependymoma with extension into basal cisterns and subarachnoid spaces, i.e., the so-called plastic ependymoma, shown diagrammatically (**A**) and radiographically following gadolinium administration in the axial (**B**) and coronal (**C**) planes.

resected, often obviating preoperative angiography. The typical MRI features of a posterior fossa hemangioblastoma include a cystic mass with a pial-based mural nodule that enhances prominently with intravenous contrast agents and the presence of abnormally prominent vessels within or adjacent to the tumor (Fig. 31.6). These findings in the setting of an intraaxial mass in an adult are virtually pathognomonic for hemangioblastoma.[13] The MR signal intensity of the cyst fluid varies with its composition and ranges from isointense to CSF on all images to hyperintense on short and long TR sequences.[26] The cyst wall is often sharply delimited.[13] The mural nodule is typically only slightly hyperintense to cerebellar cortex on long TR sequences, and enhances brightly following intravenous contrast administration (see Fig. 31.6B,C). The presence of large tumor-associated vessels, appearing as regions of signal void on spin-echo images, is readily determined on MRI (see Fig. 31.6A).[26] Variations in the MRI appearance include the presence of hemorrhage into the cyst, solid rather than cystic masses, occurring in 30% to 40% of hemangioblastomas, usually in supratentorial lesions,[27] the finding of multiple lesions, and associated syrinx cavities, especially with medullary or cervical tumors.[26]

The MRI appearance of a choroid plexus papilloma is one of an intraventricular mass with a lobulated margin and hypointense signal to gray matter on short TR/TE images. Calcification and hypervascularity may manifest themselves as linear and patchy regions of hypointensity. Long TR/TE sequences may reveal regions of hyperintensity from calcification and old hemorrhage. Choroid plexus papillomas usually enhance prominently with paramagnetic contrast agents (Fig. 31.7), and any heterogeneity to the pattern of enhancement suggests calcification, cyst formation, or old hemorrhage. Tumors of the fourth ventricle may extend out through the foramina of Luschka or Magendie into the basal cisterns. Hydrocephalus is commonly present, sometimes without obvious obstruction of the CSF pathways.[13]

The MRI appearance of a dermoid cyst is usually one of hyperintensity on short TR/TE images and hypointensity on long TR images due to their fat content.[13] Dermoid cysts are most commonly located in the posterior fossa in the midline, although they may also occur in the parasellar region, or intraventricularly in the lateral, third, or fourth ventricles. Rupture of the fatty contents of a dermoid cyst into the subarachnoid space or ventricular system is also visible radiographically.[13]

MRI scans are useful postoperatively for surveillance purposes, as recurrent tumors must usually reach a large size before they become symptomatic[15] and can often be

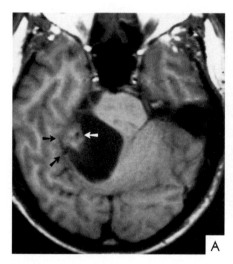
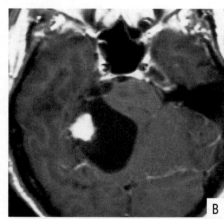
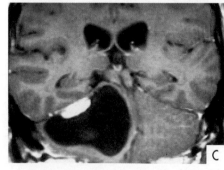
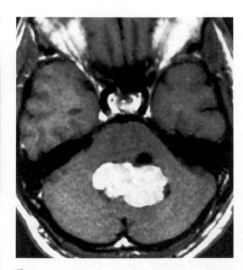

Figure 31.6 MRI appearance of a cystic cerebellar hemangioblastoma in the axial plane before (**A**) and after (**B**) contrast administration and in the coronal plane (**C**), demonstrating pial-based, contrast-enhancing mural nodule. Note the signal voids (arrows) corresponding to flow through feeding vessels.

Figure 31.7 Axial MRI appearance of choroid plexus papilloma of the fourth ventricle following administration of intravenous gadolinium.

detected earlier with MRI.[15,28] The interval for surveillance scans is determined by the histology of the tumor and the duration of freedom from disease progression or recurrence, as patients with malignant lesions and recently diagnosed lesions require more frequent scans. Patients receiving adjuvant chemotherapy for malignant lesions should also be studied between cycles of chemotherapy to assess response. The presence of residual or recurrent contrast enhancement of the tumor bed in a scan done more than 2 months postoperatively[28] or persistent distortion of the fourth ventricle suggests recurrent or residual tumor. In some cases, postradiation changes may mimic recurrent tumor on MRI or CT, requiring repeated scans, or, less commonly, reoperation.

Gadolinium-enhanced MRI has also become the first step in screening patients for leptomeningeal metastases in the spinal and cranial compartments.[29] Recent evidence suggests it is more sensitive than myelography with CT follow up in delineating nodular metastases and "sugar coating" of the spinal cord and nerve rootlets (Fig. 31.8).[29]

OPERATIVE APPROACHES/STRATEGY

INITIAL MANAGEMENT

Frequently children with posterior fossa tumors are very ill at the time of presentation, with severe headache and vomiting, which are usually the result of obstructive hydrocephalus. The initial management is often directed at the secondary effects of tumors and increased intracranial pressure, including headache, nausea, vomiting, and, occasionally, dehydration. Because brain stem compression is often present, rapid and catastrophic deterioration is always a danger. Some controversy still exists as to the most appropriate initial management of the hydrocephalus following diagnosis. While some have advocated initial management of the hydrocephalus alone, either with external ventricular drainage[30] or placement of a CSF shunt prior to tumor removal,[31-37] most advocate preoperative treatment with glucocorticoids followed by tumor removal.[15,38,39] Shunting prior to craniotomy has largely fallen from favor, since most posterior fossa tumors can be excised so the CSF pathways are again open.[37,40,41] Shunting before tumor removal not only takes away the patient's chance to be shunt independent, but exposes the patient to the potential perils of shunt dependency and its attendant risks. At the Primary Children's Medical Center of the University of Utah in Salt Lake City, patients with posterior fossa masses are treated with glucocorticoids, usually dexamethasone (1 mg/kg/d) following admission, and surgery is scheduled for the next elective operating day. If the patient should deteriorate neurologically, the tumor is removed on an emergent basis.

OPERATIVE MANAGEMENT

Virtually all cerebellar and fourth ventricular tumors except those in the cerebellopontine angle and pineal region can be effectively removed with the patient in a

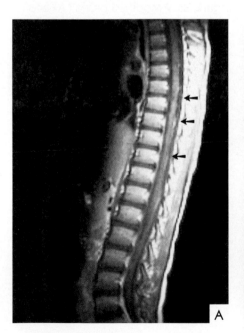 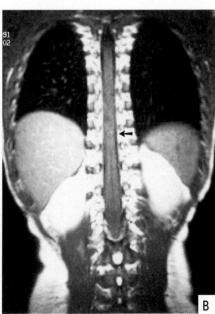

Figure 31.8 Postcontrast spinal MRI in sagittal (**A**) and coronal (**B**) planes, demonstrating subarachnoid metastases (arrows) of a recurrent cerebellar PNET.

prone or modified prone position (Fig. 31.9A). With this position the risk of air emboli is nearly eliminated, and there is less fatigue to the surgeon's arms than with the sitting position. The patient's head is immobilized in three-point head fixation if he or she is over 2 years of age and in a padded Mayfield headrest if below 2 years of age. A moderate amount of cervical flexion is desirable in either the prone or sitting position if access to the superior vermis or aqueduct is needed (Fig. 31.9A,B).

In patients with obstruction or effacement of the fourth ventricle, an occipital burr hole is placed prior to attempted removal of the tumor. In patients with hydrocephalus, the ventricle is cannulated and the catheter is tunneled subcutaneously and connected to an external ventricular drainage system for postoperative management.

Tumors of the vermis, fourth ventricle, and paramedian cerebellar hemisphere can be approached through a midline incision extending from the inion to the upper cervical spine. The paracervical and suboccipital musculature is then elevated with electrocautery in the subperiosteal plane. In children we have advocated a free craniotomy flap in the posterior fossa, extending from the transverse sinus to the area just above the foramen magnum. The foramen magnum is then removed with sharp rongeurs. The arch of C-1 is usually removed for tumors that extend to the inferior fourth ventricle or craniocervical junction. The dura is best opened in a Y-shaped fashion extending below the cerebellar tonsils; care should be taken to keep the dura moist to facilitate

a watertight closure at the conclusion of the case. For midline tumors the cerebellar vermis is opened in the midline using a combination of bipolar electrocautery and gentle suction. Self-retaining retractors are usually employed to facilitate exposure (Fig. 31.10).

Although many techniques can be used for tumor removal, certain general principles apply. The surgical goal for nearly all noninfiltrating tumors should be a complete excision,[15,42] provided the floor of the fourth ventricle or brain stem is not involved. In most cases the initial objective should be decompression of the brain stem and reduction of tumor bulk. Large solid masses with a capsule or pseudocapsule are safely debulked from within the capsule using either gentle suction, the ultrasonic surgical aspirator, or, less commonly, the carbon dioxide laser. The tumor capsule thereby serves to protect adjacent vital elements and limit the resection. It is often safer to remove large tumors in a piecemeal fashion rather than apply needless traction on the brain stem or lower cranial nerves. The mass effect associated with cystic or hemorrhagic lesions can be quickly and effectively reduced by early aspiration of the cyst or clot. Once the tumor has been debulked the capsule or pseudocapsule can often be removed under magnification in an extratumoral plane. Cottonoid patties are used to protect the surrounding nervous structures and preserve the plane of dissection. Attachments of tumor to the brain stem, cerebellar peduncles, or lower cranial nerves are often removed last, using the operating microscope and carbon dioxide (CO_2) or contact neodymium-

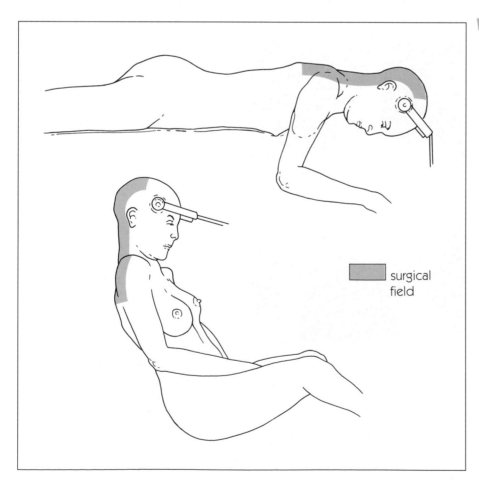

Figure 31.9 Modified prone (A) and sitting (B) positions used for most suboccipital approaches to the posterior fossa.

surgical field

YAG (Nd:YAG) lasers. If possible, all radiographically enhancing tissue, including the cyst wall if it enhances, should be removed.[38,43] Unusually fibrous or tough tumors can be effectively removed with the ultrasonic surgical aspirator (e.g., CUSA).

The dura should be closed in a watertight fashion to reduce the likelihood of cerebellar hernias and CSF fistulas. A variety of substances are available for dural grafting, including pericranium, fascia lata, and freeze-dried cadaver dura. We do not recommend the use of silastic dural substitute. Fibrin glue can be used to facilitate attachment of the graft and repair of small defects. Meticulous attention to proper wound closure is necessary in the posterior fossa, especially when hydrocephalus is present.

Tumors of the cerebellar hemispheres are more effectively approached through a paramedian or retromastoid incision. Care should be taken to avoid injury to the vertebral artery as it traverses from the vertebral canal of C-1 to the foramen magnum. The craniotomy or craniectomy can be extended laterally to the transverse sinus or even past it (transsigmoid approach), if access to the cerebellopontine angle is needed. If the mastoid air cells are entered, they may be occluded with bone wax; larger exposures may require mastoidectomy and obliteration. Laterally located tumors are often approached through the cerebellar hemisphere. The intraoperative ultrasound can be used to locate subcortical tumors and plan the corticectomy, which is usually in the horizontal plane, parallel to the cerebellar folia. Bipolar electrocautery and gentle suction are again used for the cortical

incision, and self-retaining retractors are often required to maintain exposure.

Intrinsic tumors of the cervicomedullary junction can be approached in a similar fashion, using a midline approach with the patient in the prone position. The operating microscope must be used. After exposure of the cerebellum, lower brain stem, and upper cervical spinal cord, a midline or paramedian incision is made in the medulla with either a CO_2 laser or contact Nd:YAG laser. The incision in the medulla begins just below the obex and extends down to the upper cervical region if necessary. The laser is ideal for making this type of opening into the medulla. It allows a precise, sharp incision with little damage to surrounding neural tissue. These tumors are often dorsally exophytic in several areas, allowing easy access into the brain stem. If the tumor is not exophytic, it is always immediately beneath the surface. Operating in the midline causes minimal deficits and is well tolerated in these patients. Once the tumor is identified, removal is accomplished by staying within tumor tissue. The laser and CUSA are especially useful surgical adjuncts. A gross total resection of tumor is often possible. The distinct tumor texture and coloration, as compared with the normal white color of the brain stem, allows for a distinctive plane to be recognized and used by the surgeon. Occasionally the tumor tissue is not distinct from surrounding normal brain. We have found this to be true most often in cases with an associated diagnosis of neurofibromatosis. When this occurs, biopsy only is the appropriate therapeutic choice. Attempts at gross total removal should be limited to

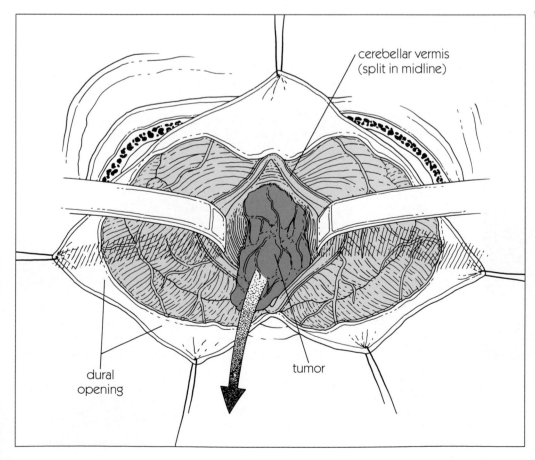

Figure 31.10 Midline, transvermian approach for most tumors of the cerebellar vermis or fourth ventricle.

cerebellar vermis (split in midline)

dural opening

tumor

those tumors that are visually distinct when compared with surrounding normal tissue. Fortunately, this is the usual case.

The operative management of intrinsic tumors of the pons should be limited to CT- or MR-guided stereotactic biopsy, which is accomplished most safely by approaching the lesion from the vertex through the ipsilateral cerebral hemisphere. The biopsy tract passes through the cerebral peduncle and into the tumor within the pons (Fig. 31.11). Adequate tumor sample must be obtained so that an appropriate diagnosis can be made. These patients tolerate CT- or MR-guided stereotactic biopsy with low risk of acute complications.

TUMORS OF THE CEREBELLUM AND FOURTH VENTRICLE

Tumors of the cerebellum and fourth ventricle comprise a diverse group of neoplasms that can occur from infancy through senescence. Although they are more common in children, adults are not spared. Considerable differences, with respect to anatomic location, histology, and prognosis, exist between those tumors that commonly affect children and those that affect adults.

Anatomically, a neoplasm can begin in the cerebellar hemispheres, the cerebellar vermis, or the fourth ventricle. This excludes extraaxial tumors such as neurinomas and the majority of posterior fossa meningiomas.

CEREBELLAR ASTROCYTOMA

The cystic cerebellar astrocytoma comprises between 12% and 28% of all pediatric brain tumors, and represents nearly one third of all posterior fossa tumors in children.[15,40,44] Although cases have been reported in older adults,[40,45] it almost exclusively occurs in children and young adults. In Cushing's original series,[17] the average age at presentation was 13 years, but most of these children had been symptomatic for 2 or more years, and most were blind at the time of presentation from chronic papilledema. By 1971 the average age at the time of admission to the hospital had decreased to 8.9 years.[16]

The cerebellar astrocytoma can be located medially in the vermis or laterally in the hemisphere. It may be solid or cystic. The classical tumor is a laterally located cyst with a well-defined mural nodule and yellow-brown cyst fluid (see Fig. 31.2). Involvement of the cerebellar vermis in cystic astrocytomas occurs in over 40% of cases.[40,41,46]

Histologically the most common subtype is called "juvenile" or, more recently, "pilocytic."[47] While the latter term refers to the elongated "hair-like" bipolar astrocytes,[48] the majority of astrocytes that comprise such tumors in children are typical fibrillary astrocytes with round to oval nuclei, some cytoplasmic pleomorphism, and Rosenthal fibers. The histologic appearance of the pilocytic astrocytoma is one of alternating areas of densely and loosely cellular areas, imparting a characteristic honeycomb pattern (Fig. 31.12). Although some nuclear pleomorphism and hyperchromatism may be seen, malignant transformation is uncommon.[15,49] A minority (11% to 15%) of cerebellar astrocytomas, usually in older children and young adults, are of the infiltrative fibrillary type. These tumors usually display the histologic features of anaplasia.

In a series of 361 pediatric brain tumors over a 10-year period ending in 1986,[15] 43 (11.9%) purely astrocytic cerebellar tumors were reported; of which 61%

Figure 31.11 Coronal MR image showing transfrontal biopsy tract for MR-guided stereotactic biopsy of intrinsic pontine lesions.

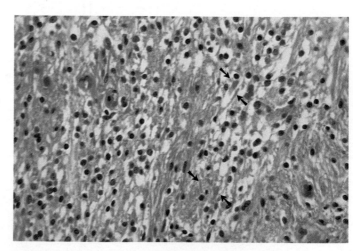

Figure 31.12 Light microscopic appearance of a pilocytic astrocytoma, consisting of alternating areas of densely and loosely packed cells, imparting a "honeycomb" appearance. Note the presence of Rosenthal fibers (arrows). (H&E; ×250)

were "pilocytic," 28% were fibrillary, and 11% were more anaplastic astrocytomas. In this series mixed glial tumors, including astrocytoma-oligodendroglioma, astrocytoma-ependymoma, and ganglioglioma were more common in the cerebellum (12 cases) than in the cerebrum (5 cases).

The surgical ideal in managing patients with newly diagnosed or recurrent cerebellar astrocytomas is that of total resection of all radiographically enhancing tissue, including the cyst wall if it enhances. Sound judgement must temper the resection, especially in cases of recurrent or more anaplastic tumors, where the tumor invades the floor of the fourth ventricle. The prognosis for most patients with cerebellar astrocytoma is the most favorable of nearly all glial tumors, with 25-year survival exceeding 94%.[44] Adjuvant therapy is not indicated unless the lesion is incompletely resected or is malignant.

MEDULLOBLASTOMA

The cerebellar medulloblastoma arises in the inferior medullary velum and grows to fill the fourth ventricle and infiltrate surrounding areas (Fig. 31.13).[3] The name derives from the putative "pluripotential medulloblast," postulated by Bailey and Cushing,[50] which probably does not exist. According to Rorke[51] it is better included in the family of PNETs first described by Hart and Earle.[52] This group includes medulloblastomas, ependymoblastomas, pineoblastomas, cerebral neuroblastomas, medulloepitheliomas, and the so-called pigmented medulloblastomas (or melanotic vermian PNET of infancy). These tumors are believed to arise from a pool of undifferentiated cells in the subependymal region of the fetal brain.[51] This theory explains the observed ability of this class of tumors to differentiate along multiple lines, including neuronal, spongioblastic, glial, and ependymal.

The cerebellar PNET is regarded as second to the cerebellar astrocytoma in frequency of occurrence, comprising approximately 25% of all intracranial tumors of childhood.[53] While over half of these tumors occur in the first decade, usually between ages 5 and 9 years, a second peak in early adulthood (ages 20 to 24 years) has been reported.[53]

Macroscopically the medulloblastoma is soft and friable. Areas of necrosis and focal hemorrhage are sometimes present,[3] while calcification is uncommon. The tumor may be confined to the vermis and fourth ventricle or may infiltrate the brain stem or adjacent cerebellar hemisphere in approximately 30% of cases. Isolated involvement of one cerebellar hemisphere is much less common.[54] Dissemination through the subarachnoid space is common. Between 11% and 43% of patients have myelographic evidence of asymptomatic spinal subarachnoid metastases at the time of diagnosis,[55,56] and metastatic lesions are present in over 50% of patients at autopsy.[57]

Microscopically, the medulloblastoma appears as a highly cellular tumor composed of round to oval cells with scant cytoplasm and hyperchromatic nuclei, giving it the appearance of a "blue tumor" on hematoxylin and

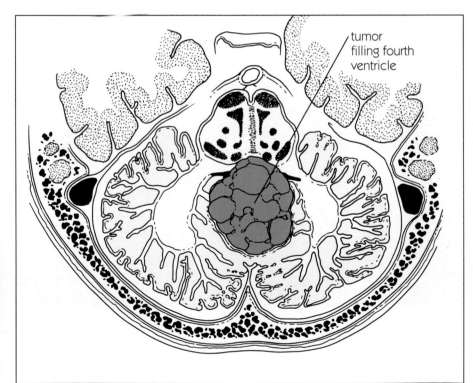

tumor filling fourth ventricle

Figure 31.13 Gross diagrammatic interpretation of common neuroanatomic site of origin and growth pattern of cerebellar primitive neuroectodermal tumor (PNET).

eosin stained slides (Fig. 31.14). Homer-Wright rosettes, which suggest neuronal differentiation, as well as pseudorosettes are commonly present. A desmoplastic variant is well described, and it is more commonly found in young adults, more commonly located in the cerebellar hemisphere, firm, and better demarcated, involving the meninges.[57,58]

The surgical goal in managing patients with a posterior fossa medulloblastoma is again an aggressive but sensible resection. An attempt should be made to remove all grossly visible tumor, although the temptation to attempt removal of tumor that invades the floor of the fourth ventricle should be avoided unless there is a clean anatomic plane of separation. Patients have been separated into two prognostic groups: so-called good-risk and bad-risk based on age at diagnosis, extent of surgical resection, and the presence or absence of leptomeningeal dissemination or metastatic disease.[3] Survival data are significantly worse for children under 2 years of age at the time of diagnosis, for individuals with subtotal (less than 80%) resections or biopsies, for individuals with subarachnoid metastases or brain stem invasion at the time of diagnosis, and for patients with persistently positive CSF cytology more than 2 weeks following surgery.[3]

Adjuvant therapy is universally indicated postoperatively in patients harboring medulloblastomas. Presently at the University of Utah–Primary Children's Medical Center, all patients over 3 years with newly diagnosed medulloblastomas receive adjuvant radiotherapy consisting of 35 to 45 Gy to the whole brain, 30 to 40 Gy to the spinal cord, and a boost to the posterior fossa to 55 Gy. Five-year survival rates of 60% or greater are considered routine for "good-risk" patients. Patients with "poor-risk" tumors are also receiving adjuvant chemotherapy with a variety of regimens, including vincristine-CCNU, or cyclophosphamide-cisplatin-vincristine. The utility of neoadjuvant chemotherapy, that is, prior to craniospinal axis irradiation, in an attempt to reduce or eliminate the

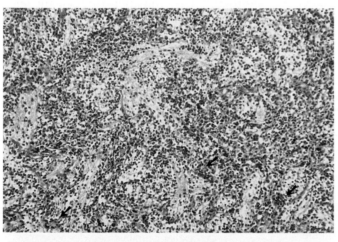

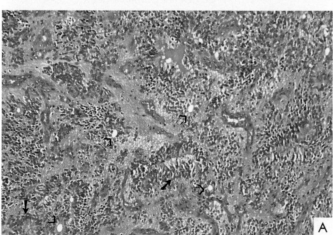

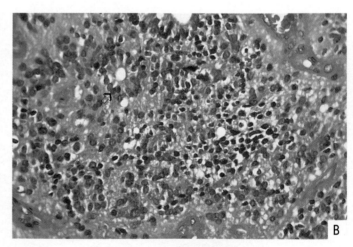

Figure 31.14 Photomicrographs of a cerebellar PNET (medulloblastoma) stained with hematoxylin and eosin. Note Homer-Wright rosettes (arrows). (H&E; ×100)

Figure 31.15 Photomicrograph of an ependymoma of the fourth ventricle, shown at 100× magnification (**A**) and 250× magnification (**B**). (H&E). Note the presence of perivascular pseudorosettes (arrows) and true ependymal rosettes (open arrows).

spinal dose remains under investigation. In addition, the increasing availability of autologous bone marrow transplantation techniques may permit delivery of higher levels of tumoricidal drugs.

EPENDYMOMA/ANAPLASTIC EPENDYMOMA

Ependymomas are derived from and have the appearance of differentiated ependymal cells. They tend to occur in younger patients, with nearly 50% presenting in children less than 3 years,[12,59–62] but they are rarely congenital.[63] There appears to be a slight predilection for females.[4]

Presenting symptoms and signs again relate to the anatomic location and are similar to those for other posterior fossa masses. Because this tumor may occur in very young patients in whom some of the presenting symptoms and signs may be nonspecific, such as developmental delay, irritability, and weight loss,[64] a certain degree of vigilance is warranted.

Most ependymomas are classified histologically as either ependymoma or anaplastic ependymoma (ependymoblastoma). Numerous alternative classification schemes have been proposed.[65–67] Microscopically, ependymomas display three classic histologic features. Rather uniform-appearing cells are arranged around vascular structures and send cell processes to the vessel wall, forming perivascular pseudorosettes (Fig. 31.15). They also may form true ependymal rosettes, in which a group of cells is arranged around a lumen, simulating the central canal of the spinal cord (see Fig. 31.15B). Lastly, the cells contain blepharoplasts, which are the basal bodies of cilia; these structures are best demonstrated with special silver stains or electron microscopy.[57]

Ependymoblastomas display the histologic features of malignancy, namely, cytoplasmic and nuclear pleomorphism, nuclear hyperchromatism, mitoses, necrosis, and cytoarchitectural disorganization. The prognosis for patients harboring an ependymoblastoma is significantly worse than for those with the less malignant phenotype.[64,66,68,69] In a series from the Hospital for Sick Children in Toronto, the 5-year survival rate in patients with ependymoma was 20% compared with 6% in patients with ependymoblastoma.[64]

The surgical approach for ependymomas is identical to that for all other vermian and midline posterior fossa tumors. In the case of ependymoma, tumor can usually be identified in the vallecula; the vermis is split early to provide access to the fourth ventricle. The tumor is usually easily removed as it does not adhere to the walls of the ventricle except at the site of origin. Care must be taken to remove all tumor in the lateral recesses of the ventricle and to follow any extension out the foramina of Luschka. The tumor frequently molds itself to the available spaces without adhering to them, the so-called plastic ependymoma (see Fig. 31.5).[24]

Adjuvant therapy should include irradiation to the posterior fossa, which has been shown to improve the survival rate.[60,62,70,71] The role of craniospinal axis irradiation in the management of patients with ependymoma remains unresolved.[72,73] Subarachnoid seeding of tumor appears to occur more frequently with anaplastic ependymomas, and more commonly with fourth ventricular tumors.[73,74] The exact incidence of subarachnoid metastases remains unclear; it has been reported to range between 0% and 68% of patients in different series.[64] At the Primary Children's Medical Center of the University of Utah, craniospinal axis irradiation is usually reserved for patients over 3 years with anaplastic ependymomas or with subarachnoid seeding on enhanced MRI or CT myelography. Chemotherapy is usually reserved for recurrences; although no large-scale study has reported on effective chemotherapy, anecdotal reports describe responses to BCNU[71,76] and dibromodulcitol.[77]

Reported 5-year survival rates in the literature range from 16% to 58%. Several studies have reported a worse prognosis in children with fourth ventricular tumors as opposed to lateral ventricular tumors,[60,72,73] and in children less than 2 years.[73] Survival may also be related to extent of tumor resection.[78] The histologic presence of anaplasia appears to confer a worse prognosis.[60,68,69,79,80]

CHOROID PLEXUS PAPILLOMA/CARCINOMA

Neoplasms of the choroid plexus are uncommon, accounting for 0.4% to 0.6% of all intracranial tumors[81,82] and 3% of all intracranial tumors in the pediatric age group.[83,84] Forty percent of the tumors of the choroid plexus in children occur in patients less than 1 year of age, and 86% occur in children aged 5 years and younger.[85] In children 60% to 70% of the tumors occur in the lateral ventricles, while only 20% to 30% occur in the fourth ventricle.[84,86] The remainder occur in the third ventricle and cerebellopontine angle. The fourth ventricle is more commonly the site of origin in adults. There is no sex predilection.[83,86]

The majority of choroid plexus papillomas of the fourth ventricle present with the signs and symptoms of hydrocephalus, including headache, nausea, vomiting, irritability, enlargement of the head, and papilledema.[83,84] Overproduction of CSF has been reported to occur at as much as four times the normal rate, and may contribute to the hydrocephalus.[84,87,88] The CSF formula is commonly abnormal, with increased protein, xanthochromia, or both, seen in approximately 60% of cases.[83,89,90]

The gross appearance of a choroid plexus papilloma is that of a reddish tumor with an irregular surface. The histologic features are those of cuboidal epithelial cells arranged in fronds, resembling normal choroid plexus (Fig. 31.16).[91] The malignant counterpart, that is, choroid plexus carcinoma, has been described in older individuals and is associated with a poor prognosis.

The surgical approach is similar to that used for other fourth ventricular and vermian tumors, although the craniectomy/craniotomy need not be extended up to the transverse sinus. The vascular supply to the tumor must be coagulated and divided early on in the resection, including any midline vessels. The tumor does not invade brain parenchyma and should be totally removed.

The long-term survival of patients with choroid plexus papillomas is excellent, approaching 100%. Subarachnoid seeding has been reported even with benign appearing lesions, and is common in cases of choroid plexus carcinoma. Although radiation therapy has been given in cases of subarachnoid dissemination, its efficacy remains unproven.[89,91]

DERMOID TUMORS

Dermoid cysts can occur anywhere in the skull, although they are more common in the posterior fossa, near or at the midline. In the posterior fossa, they may be extradural, vermian, or intraventricular. Many are associated with a complete or incomplete dermal sinus.[92] They are believed to arise as a result of incomplete separation of epithelial ectoderm from neuroectoderm in the region of the anterior neuropore at about the fourth week of gestation. The cyst wall contains both epidermal and dermal elements, the latter including hair follicles, sweat glands, and sebaceous glands. These tumors enlarge slowly and become filled with desquamated epithelium, sweat, and sebaceous materials.[93] They may rupture and give rise to an aseptic meningitis, although patients more commonly present with repeated episodes of bacterial meningitis, most frequently caused by *Staphylococcus epidermidis*. Alternatively, the patient may present with a sinus tract or with hydrocephalus. The former may be quite difficult to identify if the occiput is not shaved or combed. Hydrocephalus may be either obstructive, secondary to occlusion of the fourth ventricle, or communicating, secondary to arachnoidal scarring from recurrent bouts of bacterial or aseptic meningitis.

Dermoid tumors appear as hypodense lesions on precontrast CT scans. The cyst contents have a CT density intermediate between CSF and fat. The capsule may enhance following administration of intravenous contrast.[64] Plain skull films occasionally reveal an occipital bony defect with sclerotic margins in the presence of a sinus tract.[94]

The goal of surgical management is one of total excision, including the sinus tract, if present. Although they are always extrinsic to brain parenchyma, recurrent bouts of bacterial or aseptic meningitis can lead to significant scarring and adhesions. In approaching any child with a sinus tract of the suboccipital region, one should anticipate a posterior fossa exploration, since the entire tract must be removed.[64]

HEMANGIOBLASTOMA

Cerebellar hemangioblastomas represent from 7% to 12% of all posterior fossa tumors.[95] Approximately 1.5% of meningiomas can be classified histologically as hemangioblastomas (angioblastic meningiomas).[95] While they can occur in any part of the brain,[96,97] they occur most commonly in the posterior fossa. The brain stem, especially the area postrema, is the site in approximately 10% of cases.[48,98] Approximately 70% of cerebellar hemangioblastomas are cystic,[99–101] compared with only 20% of cerebral or bulbar lesions.[48,97,102] They are common in middle aged adults, with the mean age in most series between 30 and 40 years. Patients with von Hippel-Lindau disease develop cerebellar hemangioblastomas at a younger age. They are slightly more common in males.[95,103]

Cerebellar hemangioblastoma is the most characteristic lesion in von Hippel-Lindau disease, occurring in 35% to 60% of patients, more commonly in males.[104] This tumor also occurs sporadically, usually in older individuals. When it occurs in young adults, it is usually associated with von Hippel-Lindau disease. Macroscopically, these tumors are pink to yellow, and often abut the pial surface of the cerebellum, where the mural nodule is found.[48,105,106] Dural involvement is present in up to 20% of posterior fossa hemangioblastomas.[107] They may be associated with enlarged arteries and veins on the cere-

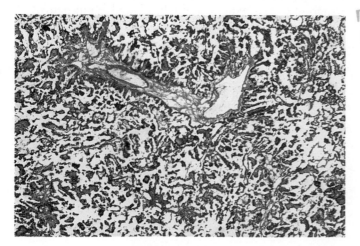

Figure 31.16 Light photomicrograph of choroid plexus papilloma of the fourth ventricle. (H&E; ×25)

bellar surface. The cyst wall, if present, is usually yellow to white with clear to yellow fluid.

Histologically, these are benign tumors, characterized by a proliferation of vascular channels and endothelial cells, a reticulin-rich stromal network and "pseudoxanthoma" (fat-laden) cells (Fig. 31.17). There is little histologic evidence of anaplasia, including an absence of nuclear or cytoplasmic pleomorphism and mitoses.[96] Approximately 60% are cystic. Even those tumors that appear solid may have many small cysts with neoplastic cells forming the walls.[95] In the typical cystic lesions, the cyst wall is usually composed of compressed cerebellum.

The clinical presentation is largely identical to that seen in other cerebellar tumors. Headache is the most common initial symptom. A focal cerebellar deficit (hemicerebellar syndrome) occurs as the presenting symptom in only about 10% of patients, but is present during the course of at least 60%.[95] An erythrocytosis is often seen in patients, presumably caused by some erythropoietic factor secreted by the tumor. Since the erythrocytosis often returns to normal after treatment, it may serve as an indicator of the efficacy of removal or other therapy.

The CT appearance of the hemangioblastoma is that of a cystic or isodense lesion that is well delineated and enhances uniformly in the solid portion following administration of intravenous contrast. Multiple lesions are often present; angiography has been reported to be useful in detecting smaller asymptomatic lesions, some of which can be removed at the same operation for a larger symptomatic mass.[103] Angiography is useful in locating the mural nodule in a cystic tumor or in assessing the vascular supply to a solid mass. Preoperative angiography is no longer routinely necessary, with the availability of MRI.

Complete surgical resection is usually curative for this lesion, and adjuvant therapy is unnecessary following complete removal. Radiation therapy has been reported to be useful in subtotally resected or recurrent lesions.[108]

Hemangioblastomas also may occur in the spinal cord, brain stem, and cerebral hemispheres. Medullary lesions are most common, and may be difficult to remove surgically. Spinal cord lesions are occasionally associated with a syrinx cavity. In a patient undergoing vertebral angiography for a posterior fossa lesion, neck films may reveal cervical hemangioblastomas.[109]

In terms of numbers of affected patients, the problem of metastatic disease to the central nervous system far outweighs that of primary lesions.[110] In fact, an estimated 124,000 patients died of intracranial metastatic disease in 1986—of whom approximately 82,000 had intraparenchymal metastases—compared with an estimated 10,200 patients dying of primary CNS neoplasms.[110,111] In autopsy series nearly 20% of patients dying of cancer have intraparenchymal metastases.[110,112,113] Since they are believed to arise from tumor emboli trapped at sites of acute arterial narrowing,[110] such as the cortical gray-white matter junction, their anatomic distribution in cerebrum, cerebellum, and brain stem roughly corresponds to the relative size and blood flow of these sites.[110] Of all solitary metastases, approximately 80% occur in the cerebral hemispheres, 16% to 18% occur in the cerebellum, and 2% to 3% occur in the brain stem.[112] The most common primary sites of origin include lung, breast, skin (malignant melanoma), and kidney. Surgical removal of metastatic lesions should be considered in cases of solitary lesions, as recent data suggest improvements in survival and functional status in those patients undergoing resection prior to radiation therapy compared with those treated with radiation alone.[113] Consideration should be given to surgical removal when the primary site of origin cannot be established and when lesions are from known radioresistant primary sites such as kidney (renal cell carcinoma) and skin (malignant melanoma).

Brain metastases in children are rare. Compared with adults, where the overall frequency of intracranial metastases reported in autopsy studies is approximately 25%,[110,112,113,115] a study of 217 children dying of cancer[118] reported a 6% incidence of brain metastases. This may reflect, at least in part, the rarity of bronchogenic carcinoma in children. The primary tumors of childhood with a proclivity for brain metastases include Wilms' tumor, rhabdomyosarcoma, osteogenic sarcoma, and germ cell tumors.[112,116–118]

The presenting symptoms in children with metastatic disease to the posterior fossa are usually related to increased intracranial pressure; associated focal deficits, including hemicerebellar symptoms, can occur. The acute onset of focal deficits is more common in children with

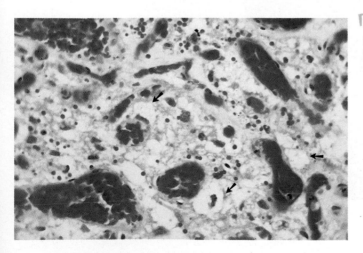

Figure 31.17 Light photomicrograph of a cerebellar hemangioblastoma. Note presence of fat-laden (pseudoxanthomatous) cells (arrows). (H&E; ×250)

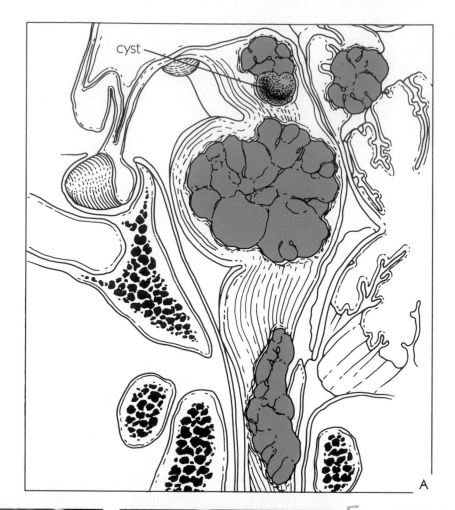

cyst

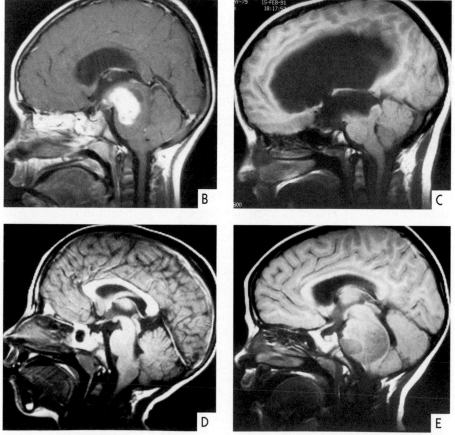

Figure 31.18 Schematic composite representation (**A**) of the common locations and radiographic appearance of commonly seen brain stem tumors: astrocytoma of cerebral peduncle (**B**), tectal plate low-grade astrocytoma (**C**), astrocytoma of medulla oblongata (**D**), pontine glioma (**E**).

metastatic disease than in adults, and may reflect a greater tendency toward intratumoral hemorrhage.[117,119,120]

The CT and MRI appearance of metastatic disease in children differs little from that seen in adults. Since intracranial metastases without pulmonary metastases are rare in children, chest x-ray and chest CT are useful.

Although Wilm's tumor (nephroblastoma) is one of the most common abdominal tumors of childhood,[121] it rarely metastasizes to the brain.[122–124] Vannucci and Baten reported brain metastases in 12.9% of children with Wilms' tumor examined postmortem. While metastases to the brain stem have been reported,[125] the majority of metastatic lesions in Wilms' tumor are supratentorial. Present day use of surgery, radiation, and chemotherapy have resulted in recent improvements in the survival of children with metastatic Wilms' tumor.[55,121,124,126,127]

While neuroblastoma is also one of the most common extracranial solid tumors of childhood, metastatic involvement of the brain is extremely unusual.[128] When it does occur, it usually results from direct invasion of the brain from contiguous structures,[48,129–133] such as the leptomeninges.

Although the rarity of metastatic neuroblastoma precludes large clinical series, therapy should involve surgical removal as well as adjuvant radiotherapy and chemotherapy.[121]

Brain metastases from osteogenic sarcoma are rare but also usually occur together with pulmonary metastases.[134] In one autopsy series, brain metastases were seen in 1.5% of children with osteogenic sarcoma.

BRAIN STEM GLIOMAS

It is unfortunate that one of the more common locations of gliomas in childhood is within the brain stem. Despite the specific histology, they must all be classified as malignant tumors, since their location renders them inoperable.
—Donald Matson, 1969

For many years, the term *brain stem glioma* has signified a tumor that is considered inoperable. Since these tumors may represent 15% of all intracranial tumors and 25% to 30% of posterior fossa tumors in children,[135] it is fortunate that the outlook is changing. Recent experience has shown that the location of a tumor within the brain stem greatly influences not only the histology but whether or not surgical excision can be accomplished.[136–139] Epstein, Hoffman, and Walker have all suggested a scheme for classification of tumors within the brain stem.[138–142] It now appears that astrocytomas within the brain stem may have different potential for malignancy depending on their location. Most brain stem tumors are low-grade astrocytomas, except those that occur within the pons. It is well known that almost all pontine gliomas are malignant both in histologic type and in clinical behavior. Figure 31.18 shows the various locations of tumors that occur within the brain stem and their appearance. Although the overwhelming majority of these tumors are astrocytomas, other tumor types may occur. Particularly noted are the gangliogliomas that may occur within the brain stem parenchyma.[141]

TUMORS OF THE MEDULLA OBLONGATA

Although tumors of the medulla oblongata are somewhat rare, they occur almost exclusively in children. Adults may harbor these lesions, but the diagnosis of neurofibromatosis should be strongly considered in this circumstance. It is curious that many of these children present with small stature, yet this finding has rarely been reported in the literature. These children may be referred to an endocrinologist for "failure to thrive" before eventually having the proper diagnosis made. They all show some degree of ataxia and usually have signs of lower brain stem dysfunction. They commonly present with focal abnormalities. One patient in our series presented with episodic facial pain and was found to have a focal lesion in the medulla adjacent to the descending tract of the fifth cranial nerve (Fig. 31.19). Another patient, presenting with intractable vomiting, was found to have a small lesion just below the obex at the origin of the vagus nerve.

Tumors that occur within the medulla are usually histologically benign.[138–140,142] Exceptions to this rule have been noted, but malignancy is relatively uncommon. In our series we have not yet found a malignant tumor originating within the medulla. Epstein has

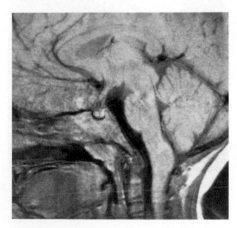

Figure 31.19 Sagittal MRI appearance of a focal intrinsic medullary tumor. Histologically this lesion proved to be a ganglioglioma and was completely excised.

noted a few cases of malignancy in the series that he has reported.[137] These tumors are most often low-grade astrocytomas. The pathology is frequently that of a microcystic astrocytoma (Fig. 31.20). In fact, these lesions may appear identical to the microcystic astrocytomas that occur within the cerebellum. These tumors often extend downward into the upper cervical spinal cord. Many surgeons consider them analogous to intrinsic spinal cord astrocytomas.

Diagnostic tests should include MRI and brain stem auditory evoked responses (BAER). MRI may show a large lesion with significant enhancement following gadolinium injection (Fig. 31.21) or a small focally located lesion with no significant change with gadolinium (Fig. 31.22). CT scans, due to bone hardening artifact in the posterior fossa, are not as helpful as MRI in the neurodiagnostic evaluation of these patients. BAERs, somewhat surprisingly since the lesion is in the medulla, often show changes. We have found BAER monitoring during surgery to be especially helpful. Slowing of the evoked response is often associated with retraction on the brain stem or with heating of the tissue from laser use. This slowing is easily reversed when the retraction is released or the laser use is discontinued temporarily. The evoked responses then return quickly to baseline levels.

Postoperatively most of these children have temporarily increased problems with ataxia and difficulty swallowing. All the children on whom we have operated have had their swallowing mechanism return to normal. Their balance may remain permanently impaired, but only slightly so. All the children have returned to normal activity and have not required assistance for daily living. None of these children have required prolonged ventilation.

We do not feel that either radiation therapy or adjuvant chemotherapy is indicated after surgery if the lesion is benign. If tumor recurrence occurs, consideration for reoperation and/or adjuvant therapy can be given at that time. A prolonged recurrence-free interval can be expected in most of these patients.

PONTINE GLIOMA

When the term *brain stem glioma* is used, the usual image that comes to mind is the patient with a large infiltrative tumor in the pons. Indeed, this is the most common form of tumor occurring within the brain stem. This is unfortunate because pontine gliomas are usually malignant. In our series, all the patients with pontine tumors have had at least an anaplastic astrocytoma on stereotactic biopsy. A few patients have had obvious glioblastomas.

The patient presenting with rapid onset and progression of symptoms and a diffusely enlarged pons usually harbors a malignant astrocytoma. Although the possibility of another disease process, such as encephalitis, must be considered, the usual pontine glioma has a very classic presentation and typical findings on MRI (Fig. 31.23). We have had a policy to perform stereotactic biopsies of all pontine gliomas for the past 8 years. It was a part of our protocol to see if there were differences in the tumors and if these differences were associated with differences in outcome. Unfortunately, it now appears that the clinical course is essentially identical no matter what the findings on biopsy. All lesions have been either anaplastic astrocytomas or glioblastomas. The clinical course, however, is essentially the same. With hyperfractionation radiation therapy these patients may survive 12 to 15 months, but this disease process is essentially universally fatal. Attempts at radical surgical removal appear futile.

We have chosen to treat patients with pontine glioma

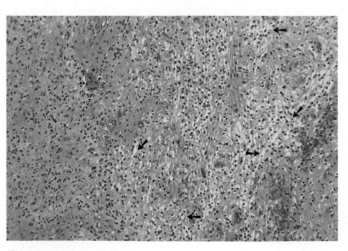

Figure 31.20 Light photomicrograph of a microcystic astrocytoma of the medulla. Note the lack of cellular and nuclear pleomorphism and the appearance of microcysts (arrows). (H&E; ×100)

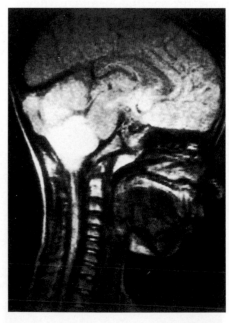

Figure 31.21 Postcontrast sagittal MR image of an intrinsic medullary glioma, with extensive contrast enhancement.

using hyperfractionated radiation therapy. Although this gives good relief of symptoms associated with rapid progression of their disease process, these patients will all eventually have tumor recurrence. In the interim, however, they are functional and essentially resume normal activity. When recurrence occurs there is typically a rapid downward progression in their clinical course.

Only a few of our patients have chosen to have chemotherapy as an adjunctive therapy. Others have had more extensive experience with chemotherapy for pontine gliomas. However, there appears to be little long-term benefit to adjuvant chemotherapy for these highly malignant lesions.[143]

TUMORS OF THE MESENCEPHALON

Tumors of the Cerebral Peduncle

Tumors within the midbrain typically occur either within the cerebral peduncle or the tectal plate. Tumors in these locations are usually low-grade astrocytomas.

Astrocytomas of the cerebral peduncles can often be surgically excised. Frequently a large cyst is associated with these lesions (Fig. 31.24). Evacuation of the cyst and removal of the surrounding tumor tissue often give relief of symptoms to the patient and allow many years of stability before further tumor growth occurs. Some have advocated stereotactic cyst aspiration as the only therapy.[144] Surgical judgement is required, but an attempt at total removal is justified when the patient has progressive symptoms from a mostly solid lesion.

We have chosen to approach these lesions by a subtemporal transtentorial approach. The notch of the tentorium is split, giving excellent exposure to the region of the cerebral peduncle. These lesions will often present to the surface of the peduncle, thus allowing access to the tumor without going through normal neural tissue. These tumors will occasionally extend rostrally toward the thalamus and caudally into the pons. Approaching the tumor subtemporally limits the exposure in the rostral and caudal directions. However, in our experience, many of these lesions will continue to deliver themselves into the operative area despite extensive extension in a rostral or caudal direction. Gross total excision of these tumors is occasionally possible. The surgical approach, however, should consist of decompression and removal of distinct tumor tissue that disengages easily. Removal of much of the mass will give relief of symptoms for many years without further adjunctive therapy.

Many patients will be left with a hemiparesis on the side contralateral to the surgical approach. Although improvement in hemiparesis is expected, many are left with a mild to moderate deficit. This deficit, however, is frequently less than the preoperative hemiparesis.

Tumors of the Tectal Plate

Tumors occurring in the tectal plate are also histologically benign lesions. Since the arrival of MRI many of these lesions have been discovered. If a child presents with hydrocephalus in late childhood or early adolescence there exists the possibility of obstruction at the level of the cerebral aqueduct caused by a tumor in the region of the tectal plate. Many of these tumors have been present for a long time and left alone grow slowly, if at all. These tumors rarely enhance on gad-

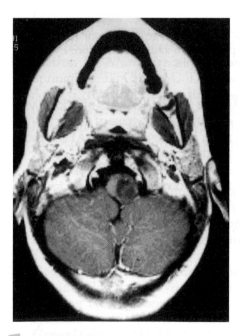

Figure 31.22 Axial postcontrast MR image of a small focal medullary astrocytoma showing little contrast enhancement.

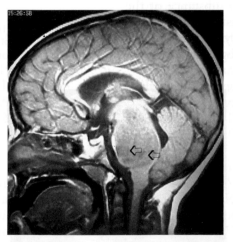

Figure 31.23 Characteristic MRI appearance of a diffuse pontine glioma. Note expanded brain stem with areas of hypointense signal (arrows).

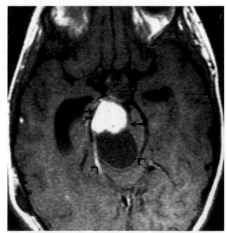

Figure 31.24 Axial MR image of focal tumor of the cerebral peduncle (midbrain) demonstrating intense contrast-enhancement (arrows) and cyst formation (open arrows).

creased intracranial pressure without lateralizing signs: the midline syndrome. *Neurochirurgia.* 1967; 10:197–209.

37. Stein B, Tenner M, Fraser R. Hydrocephalus following removal of cerebellar astrocytomas in children. *J Neurosurg.* 1972;36:763–768.

38. Lapras C, Palet J, Lapras CJ, et al. Cerebellar astrocytomas in childhood. *Childs Nerv Syst.* 1986; 2:55–59.

39. Wilson C. Diagnosis and surgical treatment of childhood brain tumors. *Cancer.* 1975;35:950–956.

40. Gol A, McKissock W. The cerebellar astrocytomas: a report on 98 verified cases. *J Neurosurg.* 1959;16: 287–296.

41. Page L. Astrocytomas involving the cerebellar midline. In: Marlin A, ed. *Concepts in Pediatric Neurosurgery 7.* Basil: Karger; 1987;93–104.

42. Matson D. Surgery of posterior fossa tumors in childhood. *Clin Neurosurg.* 1968;15:247–264.

43. Zimmerman R, Bilaniuk L, Bruno L, et al. Computed tomography of cerebellar astrocytoma. *Am J Roentgenol.* 1978;130:929–933.

44. Gjerris F, Klinken L. Long-term prognosis in children with benign cerebellar astrocytoma. *J Neurosurg.* 1978;49:179–184.

45. Obrador S, Blazquez M. Benign cystic tumors of the cerebellum. *Acta Neurochir (Wien).* 1975;32:55–68.

46. Davis C, Joglekar V. Cerebellar astrocytomas in children and young adults. *J Neurol Neurosurg Psychiatry.* 1981;44:820–828.

47. Russell D, Rubenstein L. *Pathology of Tumours of the Central Nervous System.* 5th ed. Baltimore, Md: Williams & Wilkins; 1989.

48. Russell D, Rubenstein L. *Pathology of Tumours of the Central Nervous System.* 4th ed. Baltimore, Md: Williams & Wilkins; 1977.

49. Raffel C, Edwards M, Davis R, et al. Post-irradiation cerebellar glioma. *J Neurosurg.* 1985;62:300–303.

50. Bailey P, Cushing H. Medulloblastoma cerebelli, a common type of mid-cerebellar glioma of childhood. *Arch Neurol Psychiatry.* 1925;14:192–224.

51. Rorke L. The cerebellar medulloblastoma and its relationship to primitive neuroectodermal tumors. *J Neuropathol Exp Neurol.* 1983;42:1–15.

52. Hart MN, Earle KM. Primitive neuroectodermal tumors of the brain in children. *Cancer.* 1973;32: 890–897.

53. Russell D, Rubenstein L. *Pathology of Tumors of the Nervous System.* Baltimore, Md: Williams & Wilkins; 1989.

54. Park T, Hoffman J, Hendricks E, et al. Medulloblastoma: clinical presentation and management. *J Neurosurg.* 1983;58:543–552.

55. Deutsch M, Reigel D. The value of myelography in the management of childhood medulloblastoma. *Cancer.* 1980;45:2194–2197.

56. Dorwart R, Wara W, Norman D, et al. Complete myelographic evaluation of spinal metastases from medulloblastoma. *Radiology.* 1981;139:403–408.

57. Rubenstein L, ed. *Tumors of the central nervous system, fasc. 6.* Washington, DC: Armed Forces Institute of Pathology; 1972:104–126. Atlas of Tumor Pathology.

58. Hughes P. Cerebellar medulloblastoma in adults. *J Neurosurg.* 1984;60:994–997.

59. Coulon R, Till K. Intracranial ependymomas in children. *Childs Brain.* 1977;3:154–168.

60. Dohrman G, Farwell J, Flannery J. Ependymomas and ependymoblastomas in children. *J Neurosurg.* 1976;45:273–283.

61. Koss W, Miller M. *Intracranial Tumors of Infants and Children.* St. Louis, Mo: CV Mosby Co; 1971.

62. Salazar O, Castro-Vita H, VanHoutte P, et al. Improved survival in cases of intracranial ependymoma after radiation therapy. *J Neurosurg.* 1983;59:652–659.

63. Abbott M, Namiki H. Congenital ependymoma: case report. *J Neurosurg.* 1968;28:162–165.

64. Hendrick E, Raffel C. Tumors of the fourth ventricle: ependymomas, choroid plexus papillomas, and dermoid cysts. In: McLaurin R, Schut L, Venes J, et al, eds. *Pediatric Neurosurgery: Surgery of the Developing Nervous System.* Philadelphia, Pa: WB Saunders Co; 1989:366–372.

65. Kernohan J, Fletcher-Kernohan E. Ependymomas: a study of 109 cases. *Res Publ Assoc Res Nerv Ment Dis.* 1937;16:182.

66. Kernohan J, Sayre G, eds. *Tumors of the central nervous system, fasc. 35.* Washington, DC: Armed Forces Institute of Pathology; 1952;129. Atlas of Tumor Pathology. Sect. X.

67. Ringertz N, Reymond A. Ependymomas and choroid plexus papillomas. *J Neuropathol Exp Neurol.* 1949;8:355–380.

68. Renaudin J, DiTullio M, Brown W. Seeding of intracranial ependymomas in children. *Childs Brain.* 1979;5:408–412.

69. Rubenstein L. The definition of ependymoblastoma. *Arch Pathol.* 1970;90:35–45.

70. Bloom H. Intracranial tumors: response and resistance to therapeutic endeavors, 1970–1980. *Int J Radiat Oncol Biol Phys.* 1982;8:1083–1113.

71. Sheline G. Radiation therapy of tumors of the central nervous system in childhood. *Cancer.* 1975;35: 957–964.

72. Oi S, Raimondi A. Ependymoma in children. In: McLaurin R, Schut L, Venes J, et al, eds. *Pediatric Neurosurgery: Surgery of the Developing Nervous System.* New York, NY: Grune & Stratton; 1982: 419–428.

73. Pierre-Kahn A, Hirsch J, Roux R, et al. Intracranial ependymomas in childhood. Survival and functional results of 47 cases. *Childs Brain.* 1983;10:145–156.

74. Kim Y, Fayos J. Intracranial ependymoma. *Radiology.* 1977;124:805–808.

75. Levin V. Chemotherapy of recurrent brain tumors. In: Prestayko A, Crooke S, eds. *Nitrosoureas: Current Status and New Developments.* New York, NY: Academic Press; 1981:159–167.

76. Wilson C, Gutin P, Boldrey E. Single-agent chemotherapy of brain tumors: a five-year review. *Arch Neurol.* 1976;33:739–744.

77. Levin V, Edwards M, Gutin P, et al. Phase II evaluation of dibromodulcitol in the treatment of recurrent medulloblastoma, ependymoma and malignant astrocytoma. *J Neurosurg.* 1984;61:1063–1068.

78. Tomita T, Raimondi A. Fourth ventricle tumors. In: McLaurin R, Schut L, Venes J, et al, eds. *Pediatric Neurosurgery: Surgery of the Developing Nervous System.* New York, NY: Grune & Stratton; 1982; 383–393.

79. Barone B, Elbidge A. Ependymomas: a clinical survey. *J Neurosurg.* 1970;33:428–438.

80. Fokes E, Earle D. Ependymomas: clinical and pathological aspects. *J Neurosurg.* 1969;30:585–594.

81. Cushing H. *Intracranial Tumors: Notes Upon a Series of Two Thousand Verified Cases With Surgical-Mortality Figures Pertaining Thereto.* Springfield, Ill: Charles C Thomas Publisher; 1932.

82. Russell D, Rubinstein L. Pathology of tumors of the nervous system. London: Edward Arnold; 1959: 139–142.

83. Matson D, Crofton F. Papilloma of the choroid plexus in childhood. *J Neurosurg.* 1960;17:1002–1027.

84. Milhorat T, Hammock M, Davis D, et al. Choroid plexus papilloma, I: proof of cerebrospinal fluid overproduction. *Childs Brain.* 1976;2:273–289.

85. Harwood-Nash D, Fitz C. *Neuroradiology in Infants and Children.* St Louis, Mo: CV Mosby Co; 1976.

86. Raimondi A, Gutierrez F. Diagnosis and surgical treatment of choroid plexus papilloma. *Childs Brain.* 1975;1:81–115.

87. Eisenberg H, McComb J, Lorenzo A. Cerebrospinal fluid overproduction and hydrocephalus associated with choroid plexus papilloma. *J Neurosurg.* 1974;40: 381–385.

88. Fairburn B. Choroid plexus papilloma and its relation to hydrocephalus. *J Neurosurg.* 1960;17:166.

89. Hawkins J. Treatment of choroid plexus papillomas in children: a brief analysis of twenty years' experience. *Neurosurgery.* 1980;6:380–384.

90. May PL, Blaser SI, Hoffman HJ, et al. Benign intrinsic tectal "tumors" in children. *J Neurosurg.* 1991;74:867–871.

91. Nasser S, Mount L. Papillomas of the choroid plexus. *J Neurosurg.* 1968;29:73–77.

92. Logue V, Till K. Posterior fossa dermoid cysts with special reference to intracranial infection. *J Neurol Neurosurg Psychiatry.* 1952;15:1–12.

93. Lekias J, Stokes B. Dermoid lesions of the central nervous system in children. *Aust NZ J Surg.* 1970; 39:335–340.

94. Corkill G, McCullough G, Tonge R. Cranial dermal sinus: value of plain skull x-ray examination and early diagnosis. *Med J Aust.* 1974;1:885–887.

95. Cobb C, Youmans J. Sarcomas and neoplasms of blood vessels. In: Youmans J, ed. *Neurological Surgery.* Philadelphia, Pa: WB Saunders Co; 1990:3152–3170.

96. Horten B, Urich H, Rubinstein L, et al. The angioblastic meningioma: a reappraisal of the nosological problem: light-, electron-microscopic, tissue, and organ culture observations. *J Neurol Sci.* 1977;31: 387–410.

97. Singounas E. Hemangioblastomas of the central nervous system. *Acta Neurochir (Wien).* 1978;44: 107–113.

98. Melmon K, Rosen S. Lindau's disease: review of the literature and study of a large kindred. *Am J Med.* 1964;36:595–617.

99. Jeffreys R. Pathological and haematological aspects of posterior fossa haemangioblastomata. *J Neurol Neurosurg Psychiatry.* 1975;38:112–119.

100. Mondkar V, McKissick W, Russell R. Cerebellar hemangioblastomas. *Br J Surg.* 1967;54:45–49.

101. Obrador S, Martin-Rodriquez J. Biological factors involved in the clinical features and surgical management of cerebellar hemangioblastomas. *Surg Neurol.* 1977;7:79–85.

102. McDonnell D, Pollock P. Cerebral cystic hemangioblastoma. *Surg Neurol.* 1978;10:195–199.

103. Schut L, Duhaime A, Sutton L. Phakomatoses: surgical considerations. In: McLaurin R, Schut L, Venes J, et al, eds. *Pediatric Neurosurgery: Surgery of the Developing Nervous System.* Philadelphia, Pa: WB Saunders Co; 1989:453–462.

104. Hubschmann O, Vijayanathan T, Countee R. Von Hippel-Lindau disease with multiple manifestations: diagnosis and management. *Neurosurgery.* 1981;8:92–95.

105. Olivecrona H. The cerebellar angioreticulomas. *J Neurosurg.* 1952;9:317–330.

106. Rawe S, Gilder JV, Rothman S. Radiographic diagnostic evaluation and surgical treatment of multiple cerebellar, brain stem, and spinal cord hemangioblastomas. *Surg Neurol.* 1978;9:337–341.

107. Silver M, Hennigar G. Cerebellar haemangioma (haemangioblastoma): a clinicopathological review of forty cases. *J Neurosurg.* 1952;9:484–492.

108. Sung D, Chang C, Harisiadis L. Cerebellar hemangioblastoma. *Cancer.* 1982;49:553–555.

109. Seeger J, Burke D, Knake J, et al. Computed tomographic and angiographic evaluation of hemangioblastomas. *Radiology.* 1981;138:65–73.

110. Galicich J, Arbit E. Metastatic brain tumor. In: Youmans J, ed. *Neurological Surgery.* Philadelphia, Pa: WB Saunders Co; 1990:3204–3222.

111. Silverberg E, Lubera J. Cancer statistics. *CA.* 1986;36:9–25.

112. Posner J, Chernik N. Intracranial metastases from systemic cancer. *Adv Neurol.* 1978;19:579–592.

113. Takakura K, Sano K, Hojo S, et al. *Metastatic Tumors of the Central Nervous System.* Tokyo: Igaku-Shoin; 1982.

114. Patchell R, Tibbs P, Walsh J, et al. A randomized

trial of surgery in the treatment of single metastases to the brain. *N Engl J Med.* 1990;322:494–500.

115. Cairncross J, Kim J, Posner J. Radiation therapy for brain metastases. *Ann Neurol.* 1980;7:529–541.

116. Gercovich F, Luna M, Gottlieb J. Increased survival in sarcoma patients. *Cancer.* 1975;36:1843–1851.

117. Graus F, Walker R, Allen J. Brain metastases in children. *J Pediatr.* 1983;103:558–561.

118. Vannucci RC, Baten M. Cerebral metastatic disease in childhood. *Neurology.* 1974;24:981–985.

119. Mandybur T. Intracranial hemorrhage caused by metastatic tumors. *Neurology.* 1977;27:650–655.

120. Takamiya Y, Toya S, Otani M, et al. Wilms' tumor with intracranial metastases presenting with intracranial hemorrhage. *Childs Nerv Syst.* 1985;1: 291–294.

121. Jaffe N. Metastases in malignant childhood tumor—the role of "adjuvant" therapy and the utility of multidisciplinary treatment. *Semin Oncol.* 1977;4:117–126.

122. Bannayan G, Huvos A, D'Angio G. Effect of irradiation on the maturation of Wilms' tumor. *Cancer.* 1971;27:812–818.

123. Klapproth H. Wilms' tumor: a report of 45 cases and an analysis of 1351 cases reported in the world literature from 1940 to 1958. *J Urol.* 1959;81: 633–648.

124. Mohammad A, Meyer J, Hakami N. Long-term survival following brain metastasis of Wilms' tumor. *J Pediatr.* 1977;90:660. Letter.

125. Gandolfi A, Orsoni J. Occult nephroblastoma (Wilms' tumor) presenting with symptoms of central nervous system involvement. *Acta Neurol (Napoli).* 1979;34:424.

126. Kalousek D, deChadarevian J, Mackie G, et al. Metastatic infantile Wilms' tumor and hydrocephalus: a case report with review of the literature. *Cancer.* 1977;39:1312–1316.

127. Morgan S, Buse M. Survival following brain metastases in Wilms' tumor. *Pediatrics.* 1976;58: 130–132.

128. O'Brien M, Prats A. Metastatic tumors. In: McLaurin R, Schut L, Venes J, et al, eds. *Pediatric Neurosurgery: Surgery of the Developing Nervous System.* Philadelphia, Pa: WB Saunders Co; 1989: 417–420.

129. Alpert J, Mones R. Neurologic manifestations of neuroblastoma. *J Mt Sinai Hosp.* 1969;36:37–47.

130. Dresler S, Harvey D, Levisohn P. Retroperitoneal neuroblastoma widely metastatic to the central nervous system. *Ann Neurol.* 1979;5:196–198.

131. Krol G, Horten B. Neuroblastoma metastatic to the meninges. *Clin Bull.* 1978;8:120–122.

132. Normann T, Havnen J, Mjolnerod O. Cushing's syndrome in an infant associated with neuroblastoma in two ectopic adrenal glands. *Pediatr Surg.* 1971;6:169–175.

133. Ringertz N, Lidholm S. Mediastinal tumors and cysts. *J Thorac Surg.* 1956;31:458–487.

134. Danzinger J, Wallace S, Handel S, et al. Metastatic osteogenic sarcoma to the brain. *Cancer.* 1979;43: 707–710.

135. Hoffman H, Becker L, Craven M. A clinically and pathologically distinct group of benign brain stem gliomas. *Neurosurgery.* 1980;7:243–248.

136. Tomita T, Radkowski M, Cheddia A. Brain stem tumors in childhood. In: Marlin A, ed. *Concepts in Pediatric Neurosurgery 10.* Basel: S Karger; 1990: 78–96.

137. Epstein F. Intra-axial tumors of the cervicomedullary junction in children. In: Marlin A, ed. *Concepts in Pediatric Neurosurgery 7.* Basel: S Karger; 1987: 117–133.

138. Walker M, Storrs B. Surgical therapy for intrinsic brain stem gliomas. In: Humphreys R, ed. *Concepts in Pediatric Neurosurgery 5.* Basel: S Karger; 1985: 178–186.

139. Epstein F, McCleary E. Intrinsic brain-stem tumors of childhood: surgical indications. *J Neurosurg.* 1986;64:11–15.

140. Hoffman H, Stroink A, Davidson G, et al. Pediatric brain stem gliomas: evaluation of biopsy. In: Marlin A, ed. *Concepts in Pediatric Neurousurgery 7.* Basel: S Karger; 1987:105–116.

141. Epstein F, Wisoff J. Brainstem tumors in childhood: surgical indications. In: McLaurin R, Schut L, Venes J, et al, eds. *Pediatric Neurosurgery: Surgery of the Developing Nervous System.* Philadelphia, Pa: WB Saunders Co; 1989:357–365.

142. Epstein F. Brain stem tumors in childhood: surgical indications. In: Marlin A, ed. *Concepts in Pediatric Neurosurgery 8.* Basel: S Karger; 1988:165–176.

143. Levin V, Edwards M, Wara W, et al. 5-Fluorouracil and 1-(2-chloroethyl)-3-cyclohexyl-1-nitrosurea (CCNU) followed by hydroxyurea, misonidazole, and irradiation for brain stem gliomas: a pilot study of the Brain Tumor Research Center and the Childrens Cancer Group. *Neurosurgery.* 1984;14: 679–681.

144. Hood T, McKeever P. Stereotactic management of cystic gliomas of the brain stem. *Neurosurgery.* 1989;24:373–378.

Chapter 32

Assessment of
Pituitary Function

Douglas W. Laske, Edward H. Oldfield

The pituitary gland regulates function of the thyroid gland, the adrenal glands, the ovaries, and testes; controls lactation, uterine contraction during labor, and linear growth; and regulates the osmolality and volume of the intravascular fluid by providing resorption of water in the kidney (Fig. 32.1). Symptoms and signs of disorders that affect the pituitary reflect the normal function and anatomy of the pituitary gland.

The pituitary gland rests in the sella turcica, a saddle-shaped concavity of the sphenoid bone. The optic nerves, chiasm, and tracts lie just above the diaphragma sella, a transverse extension of dura that covers the su-

Figure 32.1 Summary of Pituitary Function

Hypothalamus	Pituitary		Endorgan		
Anterior lobe	Pituitary Cell	Pituitary Hormone	Organ	Hormone	Primary Functions
Releasing Factors Corticotropin-releasing hormone (CRH)	Corticotroph	Adrenocorticotropin (corticotropin, ACTH)	Adrenals	Cortisol	General metabolism; required for physiologic adaptation to stress
	Thyrotroph	Thyroid-stimulating hormone (TSH)	Thyroid	Thyroid hormones (T_3, T_4)	General metabolism; influences pace of metabolism
Gonadotropin-releasing hormone (Gn-RH)	Gonadotroph	Follicle-stimulating hormone (FSH)	Ovaries	Estradiol, progesterone	Required for normal female sexual development and fertility
		Luteinizing hormone (LH)	Testes	Testosterone	Required for normal male sexual development and fertility
Growth hormone-releasing hormone (GRF)	Somatotroph	Growth hormone (somatotropin, GH)	Liver and other tissues	Somatomedin (insulin-like growth factor-I, GF-I)	Growth, glucose regulation
Inhibiting Factors Dopamine (PIF)	Lactotroph	Prolactin (PRL)	Breast, gonads		Lactation
Somatostatin	Somatotroph	Growth hormone (GH)	Liver and other tissues	Somatomedin (insulin-like growth factor-I, GF-I)	Growth, glucose regulation
Posterior Lobe Antidiuretic hormone (vasopressin, ADH)	ADH produced in hypothalamus; stored in posterior pituitary		Kidney		Resorption of water in the kidney
Oxytocin	Oxytocin produced in hypothalamus; stored in posterior pituitary		Uterus		Uterine contractions during labor

perior surface of the pituitary, a perforation through which passes the pituitary stalk (Fig. 32.2). The cavernous venous sinuses, the medial walls of which form the lateral walls of the sella, contain the cranial nerves that provide eye movement (the oculomotor, trochlear, and abducens nerves), the ophthalmic and maxillary division of the trigeminal nerves, and the internal carotid arteries.

The pituitary gland controls a diverse group of biochemical and physiological functions by secreting eight peptide hormones, two from the posterior lobe (vasopressin and oxytocin) and six from the anterior lobe (see Fig. 32.1). Disorders that alter pituitary function produce symptoms by 1) intrinsic disorders that cause excess or deficient secretion of the pituitary hormones, 2) extrinsic compression on the pituitary and adjacent structures by mass lesions, or 3) interruption of the blood supply to the pituitary.

Assessment of pituitary function requires clinical evaluation for symptoms and signs of hormonal deficiency or excess and laboratory testing of the various pituitary-target organ axes. Endocrine evaluation confirms the presence or absence of endocrinopathy, defines it, and helps establish the etiology. In addition, endocrine evaluation of patients with tumors in the sellar region is used to document pre- and postoperative hypothalamic-pituitary deficiencies and to assess the effects of treatment, such as surgery and radiation therapy. Advances in endocrine testing in recent years, which include new and more specific radioimmunoassays, new dynamic tests, improved and less invasive computerized imaging techniques, use of new techniques in immunohistochemistry and molecular biology, and refinements in vascular radiology, have resulted in more precise and more reliable endocrine diagnoses.

The pituitary gland is comprised of anterior and posterior lobes, which provide specific functions and have quite different origins. Appropriate evaluation requires a thorough knowledge of pituitary physiology as well as an understanding of the basis of the laboratory tests available.

ANTERIOR PITUITARY HORMONES

The anterior lobe, the adenohypophysis, is a remnant of Rathke's pouch, a diverticulum of the embryonic foregut. The cells of Rathke's pouch migrate dorsally to abut the anterior surface of the posterior lobe in the sella turcica, where they proliferate to form the anterior lobe. The hypothalamus controls function of the adenohypophysis indirectly. Processes of hypothalamic nuclei that surround the inferior aspect of the third ventricle extend inferiorly into the median eminence where they terminate on a cluster of fenestrated vessels. Extensions of these small vessels, the portal venous system, carry hormones (releasing and inhibiting factors) from the hypothalamus to govern the function of the anterior lobe (Fig. 32.3).

In the anterior lobe five distinct types of cells produce and release six different hormones: corticotrophs, adrenocorticotropic hormone (ACTH); somatotrophs,

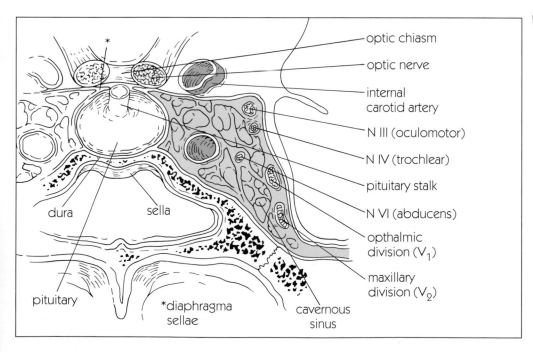

optic chiasm

optic nerve

internal
carotid artery

N III (oculomotor)

N IV (trochlear)

pituitary stalk

N VI (abducens)

opthalmic
division (V_1)

maxillary
division (V_2)

cavernous
sinus

dura   sella

pituitary   *diaphragma
sellae

Figure 32.2 Anatomic relationships of the pituitary gland. A coronal section through the sella turcica shows the pituitary gland in relation to surrounding structures: the cavernous sinuses, carotid arteries, and cranial nerves II, III, IV, V (V_1, V_2), and VI.

growth hormone (GH); lactotrophs, prolactin (PRL); thyrotrophs, thyroid-stimulating hormone (TSH); and gonadotrophs, follicle-stimulating hormone (FSH) and luteinizing hormone (LH). The secretion of these hormones is regulated by the hypothalamus and by negative (inhibitory) feedback regulation by the hormonal product of the target organ (Fig. 32.4). The posterior lobe of the pituitary, the neurohypophysis, secretes antidiuretic hormone (ADH) and oxytocin, which are produced by hypothalamic neurons and released directly from nerve terminals in the posterior pituitary. Derangement of pi-

tuitary function can result from various and disparate causes, including secreting or nonsecreting pituitary adenomas, hypothalamic lesions, or end-organ dysfunction.

Input into the pituitary from the hypothalamus and feedback regulation by the products of the target organs govern production and release of the anterior pituitary hormones. The hypothalamus, which is connected to the pituitary gland by the pituitary stalk, exerts its control over the adenohypophysis by secreting several small peptide hormones. These hypothalamic peptides, releasing or inhibitory factors, reach the cells of the adenohy-

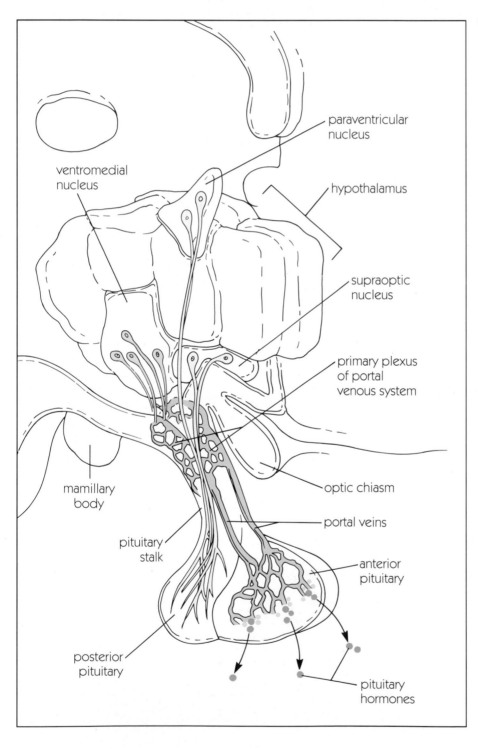

Figure 32.3 Hypothalamic control of the pituitary. Anterior Pituitary: The neural processes of the hypothalamic nuclei (green) terminate on fenestrated vessels of the portal venous system in the median eminence. The portal veins (blue) carry releasing and inhibiting factors to the anterior lobe of the pituitary, where they regulate the release of anterior pituitary hormones (red). Posterior Pituitary: The neural processes of the hypothalamic neurons of the supraoptic and paraventricular nuclei (yellow) carry the posterior pituitary hormones, antidiuretic hormone, and oxytocin, which are released directly from nerve terminals in the posterior pituitary.

pophysis via the portal veins that traverse the pituitary stalk (see Fig. 32.3). For ACTH, TSH, LH, and FSH, the corresponding hypothalamic regulating factors, corticotropin-releasing hormone (CRH), thyrotropin-releasing hormone (TRH), and gonadotropin-releasing hormone (Gn-RH), appear to be exclusively stimulatory. In contrast, GH secretion receives both positive and negative hypothalamic influence, via GH-releasing hormone (GRF) and somatostatin, respectively, and prolactin release is primarily under tonic inhibition by dopamine, also known as prolactin-inhibiting factor, from the hypothalamus. These releasing and inhibitory factors enable the hypothalamus to convert neural and metabolic inputs into signals that control the output of the anterior pituitary hormones. In addition, several of these hypothalamic factors affect more than one type of anterior pituitary cell and influence secretion of more than one anterior pituitary hormone. For instance, TRH, which stimulates TSH production, also stimulates prolactin release.

Additional important regulation of anterior pituitary function occurs as inhibition by hormones secreted from the target organs of the pituitary. This negative feedback occurs at the level of the hypothalamus and at the level of the pituitary (see Fig. 32.4). For example, cortisol inhibits release of CRH by the hypothalamus, suppresses production of ACTH by the pituitary corticotrophs, and blocks the stimulation of ACTH secretion by CRH.

PROLACTIN

Physiology

Prolactin (PRL), a 198-amino-acid peptide (molecular weight 23,000) secreted by the lactotrophs of the adenohypophysis, interacts with receptors in the breast and gonads. PRL acts on the mammary gland to initiate and maintain lactation. Hypothalamic restraint of prolactin secretion occurs by the release of dopamine (prolactin-inhibiting factor, PIF) into the portal circulation from nerve processes that originate in the arcuate nucleus of the hypothalamus (Fig. 32.5). Sleep, TRH, vasoactive intestinal polypeptide (VIP), opiates, and estrogen stimulate prolactin release. During pregnancy, estrogen stimulates lactotroph hyperplasia and hyperprolactinemia, but blocks the action of PRL on the

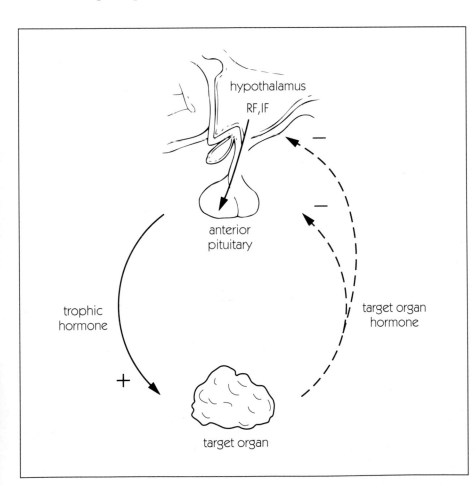

Figure 32.4 Feedback regulation of the anterior pituitary. The production and secretion of anterior pituitary hormones is inhibited by the hormonal products of the target organs (negative feedback).

breast, inhibiting lactation until after delivery. A prolactin-releasing factor seems to be involved in the regulation of normal PRL secretion, but it has not been identified. Therefore, prolactin is unique among the pituitary hormones in that control of its secretion from the hypothalamus is primarily under inhibitory control.

Hyperprolactinemia

Stimulation of prolactin release and increased serum prolactin levels have many causes (Fig. 32.6). Since the influence of the hypothalamus on the pituitary is one of restraint of PRL secretion, hyperprolactinemia can be caused by: 1) excess autonomous production (prolactin-secreting pituitary adenomas) (Fig. 32.7A); 2) diminished hypothalamic production of dopamine or interruption of dopamine delivery to the pituitary (hypothalamic disorders, such as tumors and sarcoidosis; drugs, such as reserpine and methyldopa, which block dopamine production; interruption of the portal venous system in the pituitary stalk by a sellar mass (pituitary tumor, aneurysm); following pituitary irradiation, or in the empty sella syndrome) (Fig. 32.7B); 3) inhibition of

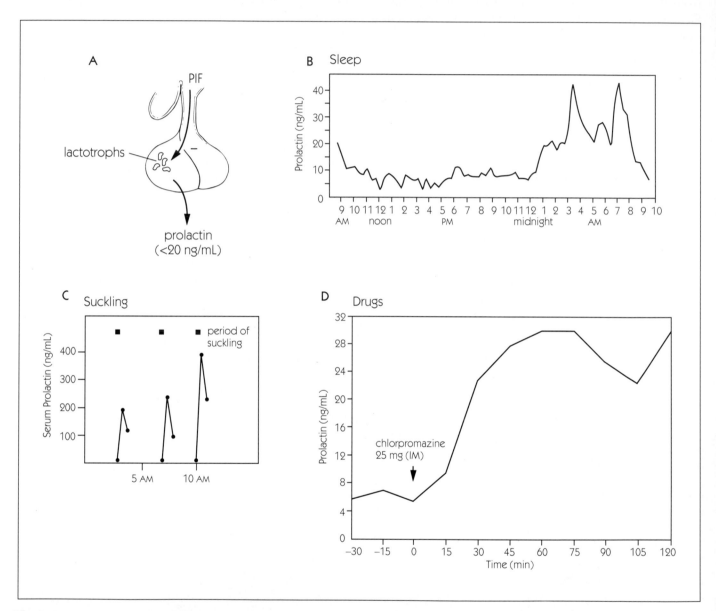

Figure 32.5 Normal control of prolactin secretion. (A) Lactotrophs of the anterior pituitary are primarily under inhibitory control of prolactin-inhibiting factor (PIF; probably dopamine). (B) Serum prolactin levels follow a diurnal pattern with increased levels several hours after the onset of sleep. Elevation in prolactin levels can be caused by a variety of stimuli, including suckling (C) or medications such as chlorpromazine (D). (B: data from Sassin JF, et al., 1972; C: data from Hwang P, et al., 1971; D: data from Sachar EJ, 1980)

dopamine activity on the lactotrophs (drugs that block interaction of dopamine with its receptor; i.e., the phenothiazines, and others); and 4) stimulation of PRL secretion by estrogens, TRH, or opiates. Physiologic stimulation of prolactin secretion and of sporadic hyperprolactinemia occurs with exercise and other forms of stress and with postpartum suckling.

Hyperprolactinemia causes hypogonadism and galactorrhea. The symptoms of hyperprolactinemia in women are amenorrhea and galactorrhea, diminished libido, and infertility. Gonadal deficiency with diminished estrogen secretion leads to osteoporosis in susceptible women. In males, hyperprolactinemia results in diminished libido, impotence, and infertility with decreased sperm counts.

Evaluation and Laboratory Testing

Laboratory testing in patients with suspected hyperprolactinemia consists of repeated measurements of basal, resting serum prolactin levels by radioimmunoassay. Serum prolactin levels in normal subjects range between 5 and 20 ng/mL (Fig. 32.8). A PRL level greater than 200 is nearly always due to a prolactinoma and a value greater than 300 ng/mL is diagnostic of one. Prolactinomas are the most common type of secreting pituitary tumors. They comprise about 30% of all pituitary tumors. In patients with amenorrhea, pregnancy has to be excluded, as it is associated with prolactin levels of 100 to 250 ng/mL by the third trimester (see Fig. 32.8). An intermediate degree of serum prolactin elevation, 20 to 250 ng/mL, can result from several other

Figure 32.6 Causes of Hyperprolactinemia

I. Neurogenic
1. Suckling or nipple stimulation
2. Stress (transient)
II. Hypothalamic and interruption of portal circulation
1. Granulomatous diseases of hypothalamus: sarcoid, histiocytosis
2. Neoplasms: craniopharyngiomas, hypothalamic astrocytomas
3. Stalk section: surgical or traumatic
4. Empty sella
5. Nonlactotropic cell pituitary tumors (which affect portal venous blood flow)
6. Radiation treatment to sella
III. Pituitary
1. Prolactinomas
IV. Endocrine
1. Pregnancy
2. Estrogen administration, contraceptive pills
3. Hypothyroidism
V. Drugs that inhibit dopamine secretion and action
1. Psychotropic (phenothiazines, butyrophenones, thioxanthenes, reserpine)
2. Opiates (morphine)
3. Antiemetics (metoclopramide)
4. Antihypertensives (methyldopa, reserpine)
5. H_2-receptor blockers (cimetidine)

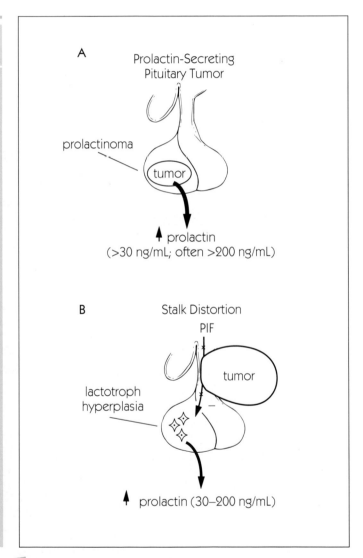

Figure 32.7 (A) Abnormal prolactin regulation. Prolactin-secreting adenomas (prolactinomas) can cause marked elevation of serum prolactin levels. (B) Distortion of the pituitary stalk by pathologic processes, such as tumors arising in the suprasellar region, can cause mild to moderate hyperprolactinemia.

conditions, described above and listed in Figure 32.6. The conditions that inhibit hypothalamic suppression of the lactotrophs by dopamine, such as distortion of the pituitary stalk, rarely cause serum PRL greater than 100 ng/mL, but elevations as high as 250 ng/mL occasionally occur. The phenothiazines also can cause PRL levels greater than 100 ng/mL.

Stimulation of PRL secretion during the TRH-stimulation test is not sufficiently reliable, because of the variability of individual responses, for diagnosing the presence of a PRL-secreting tumor, but can provide information that supports this diagnosis. In normal subjects intravenous administration of TRH (200 to 500 µg) stimulates a three- to fivefold rise in

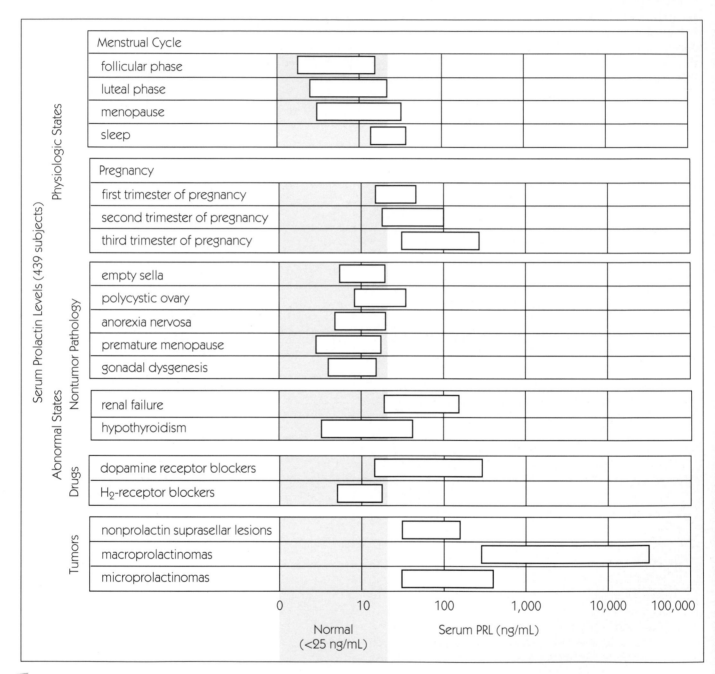

Figure 32.8 Serum prolactin levels in a variety of physiologic states and abnormal states. (Adapted with permission from Tolis G, 1980)

serum prolactin levels within an hour, whereas patients with a prolactinoma usually have a blunted response (less than a twofold increase) (Fig. 32.9). Since the dopaminergic drugs (bromocriptine, intravenous dopamine, oral levodopa) suppress PRL secretion in almost all forms of hyperprolactinemia, use of them as tests for the differential diagnosis of hyperprolactinemia is not helpful.

PRL Deficiency

Deficiency of prolactin can cause failure of lactation, which is often one of the early indications of peripar-

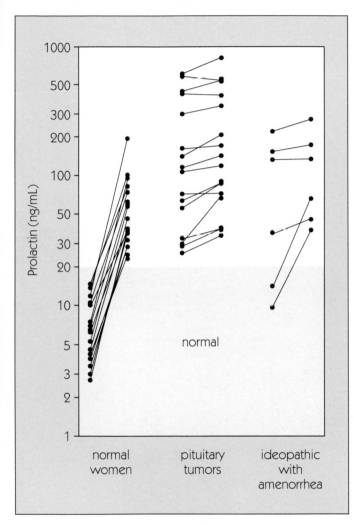

Figure 32.9 Serum prolactin before and after administration of TRH, 500 mg intravenously, in normal subjects and in patients with galactorrhea, either due to a prolactinoma or idiopathic galactorrhea with amenorrhea. (Data from Kleinberg DL, et al., 1977)

tum pituitary necrosis (Sheehan's syndrome). Lymphocytic hypophysitis, an autoimmune pituitary disorder usually associated with hyperprolactinemia during the active phase and usually occuring during or immediately after pregnancy, also produces hypopituitarism. A blunted PRL response (less than a twofold increase in serum PRL over basal values) in the TRH-stimulation test, which heralds an inadequate lactotroph reserve, occurs in hypopituitarism.

GROWTH HORMONE

Physiology

Growth hormone, a 191-amino-acid peptide that is required for normal linear growth, is secreted in pulses by the somatotrophs. Two hypothalamic peptides dually control GH release: 1) GH-releasing hormone (GRF), a 44-amino-acid peptide, which stimulates GH release, and 2) somatostatin, a 14-amino-acid peptide, which inhibits GH secretion (Fig. 32.10A). GH controls growth by stimulating the production and release of somatomedin-C, (also known as insulin-like growth factor I; IGF-I), a 7600-molecular-weight polypeptide that is synthesized in the liver and other tissues. Changes in the serum concentration of somatomedin-C closely parallel GH deficiency or excess. Somatomedin-C exerts negative feedback of GH release at the hypothalamus, where it stimulates somatostatin release, and at the pituitary, where it inhibits GH secretion and suppresses GRF-induced GH release. Hypothalamic control also mediates various neurogenic, metabolic, and hormonal influences on GH secretion. For instance, sleep, stress, and exercise stimulate GH release, as arginine does also, whereas hyperglycemia and obesity inhibit GH secretion (Fig. 32.10B–D).

In normal subjects serum GH is undetectable for most of the day. Although it is secreted in bursts associated with meals, much of the 24 hour secretion of GH occurs during the early stages of sleep. Since GH has a half-life in serum of only 20 to 30 minutes and is secreted in brief pulses, during waking hours serum levels of GH fluctuate greatly (see Fig. 32.10B). In contrast, the serum half-life of soma-tomedin-C (IGF-I) is prolonged (3 to 18 hours) and serum levels of somatomedin-C (IGF-I) are relatively stable. Thus, the serum level of somatomedin-C (IGF-I) provides a more reliable indication of the exposure of the body to GH than does random determination of serum GH.

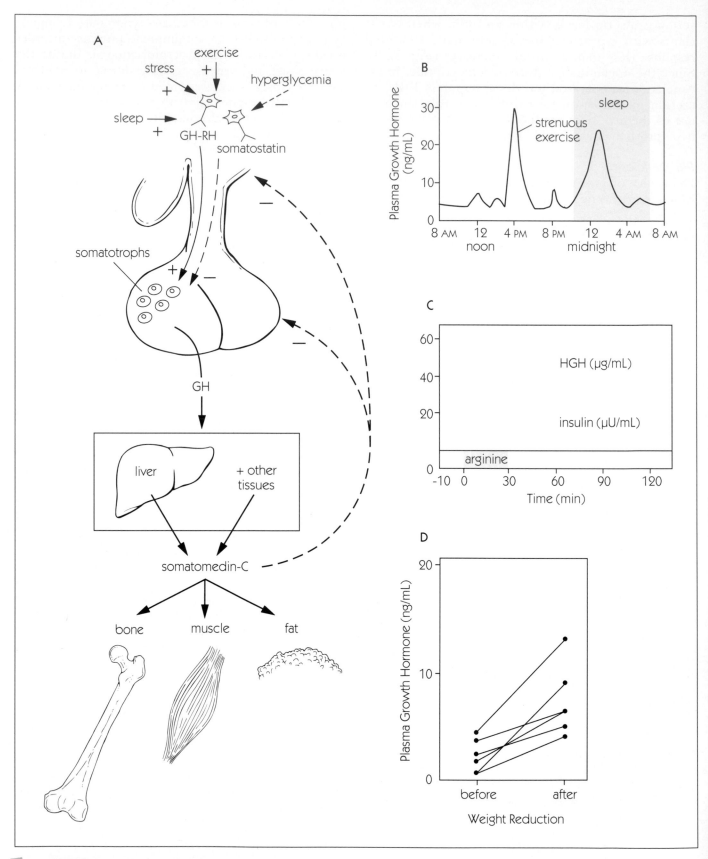

Figure 32.10 Regulation of growth hormone secretion. (**A**) Hypothalamic-pituitary axis. Somatotrophs of the anterior pituitary are stimulated to release GH by GRF and are inhibited by somatostatin. Stress, exercise, sleep rhythms, and hyperglycemia modify GH secretion. Somatomedin-C exerts negative feedback on GH release at the pituitary and hypo-thalamus. (**B**) Plasma GH levels fluctuate during a 24-hour period with peaks related to stress, exercise, and sleep. (**C**) Arginine infusion stimulates GH secretion. (**D**) Obesity suppresses GH secretion. Peak plasma GH levels during arginine infusion are shown for patients before and after weight reduction. (Data from El-Khodary AZ, et al., 1971)

Excess Growth Hormone

Excess GH secretion, which results in excess growth of the soft tissues, bony changes, and various biochemical effects of excess GH and somatomedin-C, produces the syndromes of acromegaly in adults (Fig. 32.11) and gigantism in children who are affected before epiphyseal closure. Evidence of acromegaly includes enlargement of the paranasal sinuses with frontal bossing and deepening of the voice, coarse facial features with prognathism and separation of the teeth with malocclusion, enlargement of the hands and feet requiring a change in shoe, glove, and ring size, increased skin sweating, oiliness and areas of cutaneous pigmentation (acanthosis nigricans), hypertrichosis, and organomegaly. Tongue enlargement produces obstructive sleep apnea. Accu-

mulation of excess soft tissue in the hands results in a wet, doughy handshake and in the feet it produces increased heel pad thickness, which can be detected radiographically. Many patients have headaches. Acromegalics also often present with complaints related to osteoarthritis. Insulin resistance associated with excess GH causes glucose intolerance and diabetes mellitus. Additional common accompaniments of acromegaly are proximal myopathy with weakness, carpal tunnel syndrome with nocturnal paresthesias and pain in the hands, and hypertension and cardiomegaly. The metabolic derangements lead to accelerated atherosclerosis and a shortened life expectancy due to cardiovascular, cerebrovascular, and respiratory causes. Before successful treatment was available as many as

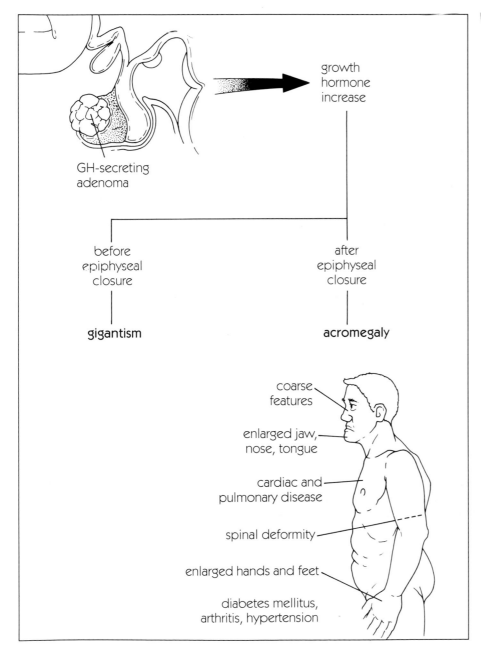

Figure 32.11 Clinical manifestations of acromegaly.

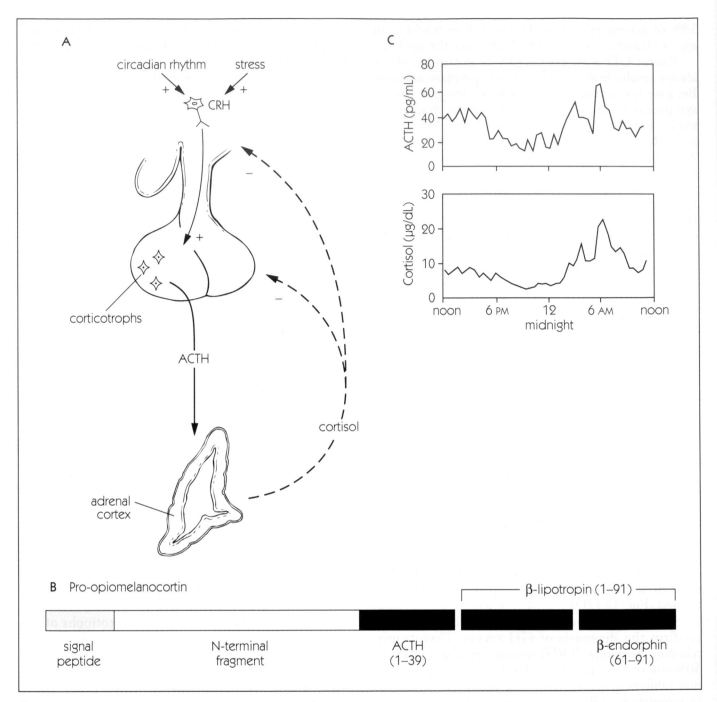

Figure 32.13 Regulation of cortisol secretion. **(A)** Regulation of the hypothalamic-pituitary-adrenal axis. CRH is released by the hypothalamus to stimulate the corticotrophs of the anterior pituitary to secrete adrenocorticotropic hormone (ACTH), which stimulates cortisol secretion from the adrenal cortex. Cortisol exerts negative feedback at the pituitary and hypothalamus. **(B)** Schematic representation of pro-opiomelanocortin, the prohormone from which ACTH is cleaved. **(C)** The circadian rhythm of serum ACTH and cortisol levels. (**C**: data from Tanaka K, et al., 1978)

into the portal venous blood at the median eminence and is carried to the pituitary, where it stimulates pituitary ACTH production and secretion. Hypothalamic secretion of CRH occurs in response to signals from the brain to produce the circadian rhythm of plasma cortisol concentrations (Fig. 32.13C), and in response to emotional, biochemical (hypoglycemia), and physical stress.

The hypothalamic-pituitary-adrenal axis is regulated by the balance between the stimuli for secretion of CRH, ACTH, and cortisol and the inhibition (negative feedback) of cortisol on production and secretion of

CRH and ACTH, and by suppression of CRH-induced ACTH secretion (see Fig. 32.13A).

Hypercortisolism (Cushing's Syndrome)

Prolonged excess exposure to cortisol produces the constellation of signs and symptoms known as Cushing's syndrome (Fig. 32.14). Since several different processes (Figs. 32.15, 32.16) can cause Cushing's syndrome, the diagnostic task for the physician in patients who have Cushing's syndrome (i.e., establishing the specific cause) occasionally can be difficult.

Figure 32.14 Clinical features of Cushing's syndrome.

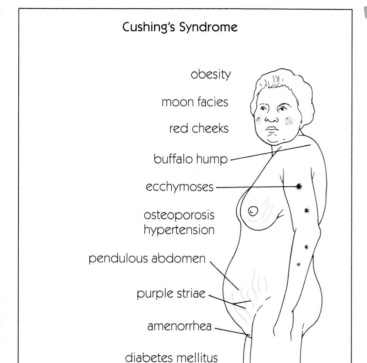

Cushing's Syndrome

obesity
moon facies
red cheeks
buffalo hump
ecchymoses
osteoporosis
hypertension
pendulous abdomen
purple striae
amenorrhea
diabetes mellitus

Figure 32.15 Etiology of Cushing's Syndrome

ACTH-Dependent	85%	ACTH-Independent	15%
Cushing's disease	80–85%	Adrenal adenoma	7%
Ectopic ACTH-secreting tumor	15–20%	Adrenocortical carcinoma	7%
Ectopic CRH-secreting tumor	Rare	Primary adrenal nodular hyperplasia	Rare
Diffuse corticotroph hyperplasia	Rare		

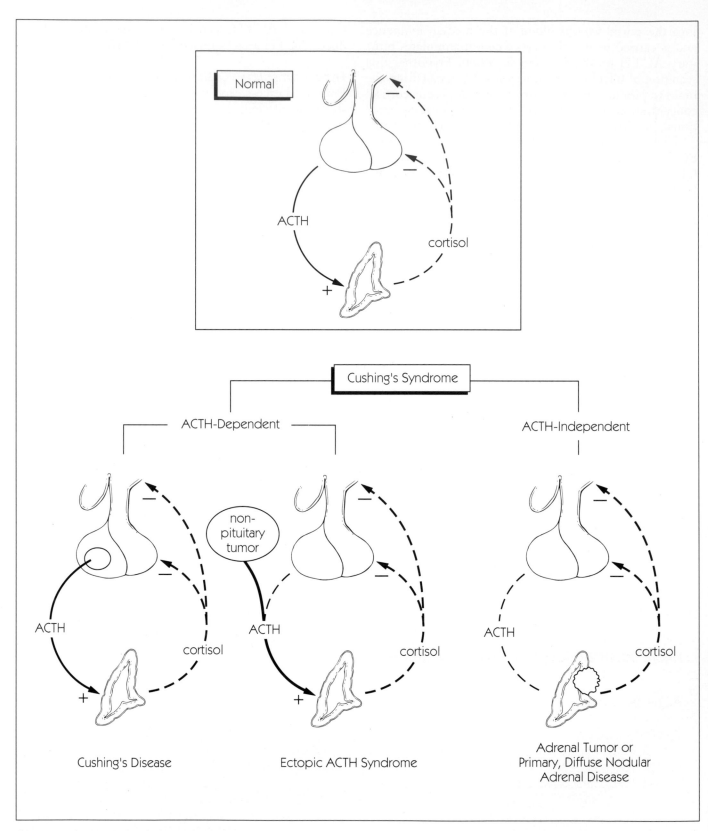

Figure 32.16 Causes of Cushing's syndrome. In ACTH-dependent hypercortisolism, cortisol secretion is excessive in response to ACTH secretion by either a corticotroph pituitary adenoma or a nonpituitary (ectopic) tumor. In ACTH-independent hypercortisolism, there is autonomous overproduction of cortisol because of an adrenal gland abnormality.

Evaluation and Laboratory Testing

The first step in the differential diagnosis of the patient suspected of having hypercortisolism is to confirm the presence of Cushing's syndrome, that is, to establish that the patient has abnormal, excess secretion of cortisol (Fig. 32.17). This is accomplished by tests that 1) directly or indirectly measure cortisol production over 24 hours, by 24-hour urine collection for free cortisol and 17-hydroxyglucocorticoid excretion (Fig. 32.18A,B), and 2) assess whether normal sensitivity of

Figure 32.17 Clinical Approach to Patients Suspected of Having Cushing's

I. Establish Presence of Cushing's Syndrome
A. Establish hypercortisolism
   24-hour urinary free cortisol
      or
   24-hour urinary 17-hydroxysteroid per gram of urinary creatinine
B. Establish resistance to dexamethasone suppression
   Overnight low-dose (1 mg) dexamethasone suppression test

II. Differential Diagnosis of Cushing's Syndrome
A. Distinguish between ACTH-independent and ACTH-dependent types of Cushing's syndrome
   1. Plasma ACTH
B. ACTH-independent Cushing's syndrome (adrenal disease)
   1. Adrenal CT or MRI
C. ACTH-dependent Cushing's syndrome
   1. CRH stimulation test
   2. High-dose dexamethasone suppression test
      a. Overnight high-dose (8 mg)
         or
      b. 6-day low-dose, high-dose test (Liddle)
   3. Bilateral petrosal vein sampling for ACTH (with and without CRH)
D. Confirm diagnosis
   1. If tests indicate Cushing's disease: Pituitary MRI
   2. If tests indicate ectopic ACTH secretion: MRI of chest and abdomen

the hypothalamic-pituitary-adrenal axis to negative feedback by glucocorticoids is present (Fig. 32.18C), using one of the low-dose glucocorticoid tests (the overnight test or the low-dose portion of the 6-day dexamethasone suppression test). Furthermore, since in Cushing's syndrome the diurnal rhythm of the plasma cortisol levels is disturbed, plasma cortisol levels at 6 to 8 AM and 11 PM to 1 AM reveal the loss of the normal circadian rhythm in patients with Cushing's syndrome.

If the results of the tests described above indicate that the patient has Cushing's syndrome, the final portion of the diagnostic assessment—establishing the specific cause of Cushing's syndrome—is performed. For the differential diagnosis of Cushing's syndrome the causes are classified as ACTH-dependent processes, which cause Cushing's syndrome via excess secretion of ACTH (ACTH-secreting pituitary tumors, ectopic ACTH-secreting tumors, diffuse corticotroph hyperplasia, and ectopic CRH secretion), or ACTH-independent processes, which cause Cushing's syndrome by a primary process of excess cortisol secretion (cortisol-secreting adrenal tumors, diffuse multinodular primary adrenal disease) (see Fig. 32.17). Since the hypothalamic and pituitary portions of the adrenal axis are normal with primary adrenal disease, hypercortisolism suppresses pituitary ACTH secretion and *plasma ACTH levels are either undetectable or very low* (Fig. 32.19; see Fig. 32.16). In contrast, since the ACTH-dependent forms of Cushing's syndrome act via excess ACTH secretion, with the ACTH-dependent etiologies the *plasma ACTH levels are inappropriately elevated for the level of cortisol secretion* (see Figs. 32.16, 32.19). Thus, the ACTH-independent and ACTH-dependent forms are distinguished by the level of plasma ACTH in the presence of hypercortisolism.

In almost 100% of patients with adrenal tumors, the most common form of ACTH-independent Cushing's syndrome, adrenal imaging with MRI or CT scanning identifies the adrenal tumor as the source of the excess cortisol secretion. Thus, the combined results of the plasma ACTH levels and adrenal imaging are used either to diagnose a primary adrenal disorder or to eliminate primary adrenal disease as the etiology.

Differential Diagnosis of ACTH-Dependent Cushing's Syndrome

Because of the very small size of most ACTH-secreting pituitary tumors and ectopic ACTH-secreting tumors, the differential diagnosis in patients with ACTH-dependent Cushing's syndrome is often not obvious. The differential diagnosis of patients with ACTH-dependent Cushing's syndrome is based on endocrino-

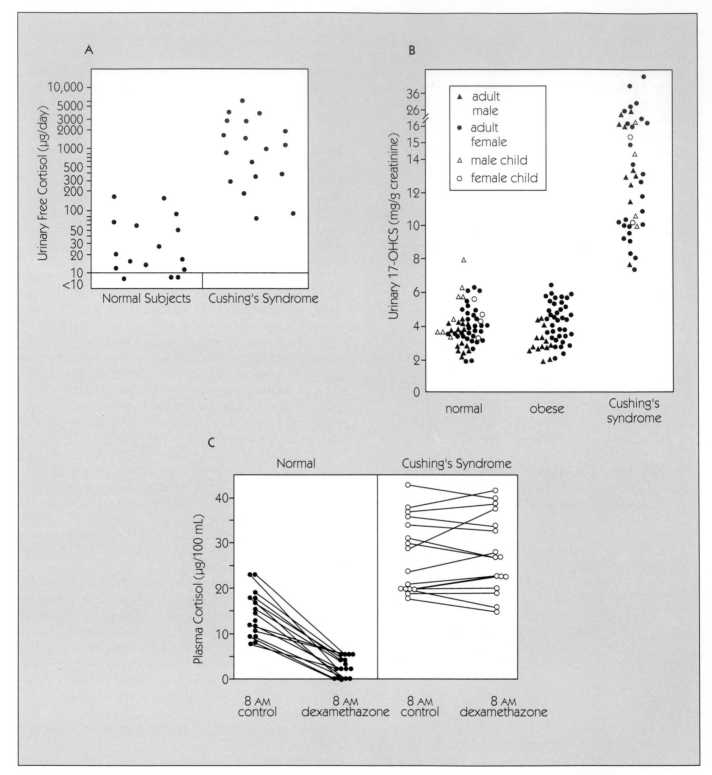

Figure 32.18 In the evaluation of the patient with hypercortisolism the first laboratory procedures are designed to establish the presence of Cushing's syndrome. Cortisol production is measured by 24-hour urinary free cortisol excretion (**A**) and 24-hour urinary 17-hydroxysteroid excretion (**B**), and by dexamethasone suppression testing. (**C**) In the overnight low-dose dexamethasone suppression test, plasma cortisol levels are measured at 8 AM on two successive days before and after 1 mg of dexamethasone is taken orally at 11 PM on the first day. The lack of suppression in patients with Cushing's syndrome contrasts with the response of normal subjects. (**A:** data from Loriaux DL, Cutler GB Jr, 1986; **B:** data from Streeten DHP, et al., 1969; **C:** adapted with permission from Melby JC, 1971)

logic and anatomic principles. 1) ACTH-secreting pituitary adenomas are well-differentiated tumors that originate from pituitary corticotrophs. They are more likely to retain the negative-feedback response to glucocorticoids (dexamethasone suppression) and respond to CRH stimulation than the ectopic ACTH-secreting tumors, which arise from tissues that do not normally secrete ACTH, respond to negative feedback by glucocorticoids, or contain receptors for CRH. 2) The source of excess ACTH secretion must be localized (inferior petrosal sinus sampling and radiographic imaging). Thus, the high-dose 8 mg overnight dexamethasone suppression test (Fig. 32.20A) or the high-dose portion of the 6-day dexamethasone suppression test, the Liddle test (Fig. 32.20B), the CRH stimulation test (Fig. 32.20C), bilateral catheterization and simultaneous sampling of the inferior petrosal sinuses for ACTH concentrations (Fig. 32.20D,E), and high-resolution imaging of the pituitary with MRI before and after contrast enhancement with gadolinium are used today to determine the differential diagnosis of Cushing's syndrome.

Most patients receive a combination of these tests. In addition to being important tests for the differential diagnosis of Cushing's syndrome, in patients with Cushing's disease the inferior petrosal sinus sampling

test and MRI often provide information that localizes a small ACTH-secreting tumor within the pituitary gland. The latter information is helpful during pituitary surgery, since these tumors are often so small that they are difficult to localize during exploratory transsphenoidal procedures.

It is critical to establish the presence of Cushing's syndrome before proceeding with the differential diagnostic portion of the evaluation described above. Since in subjects without Cushing's syndrome ACTH secretion from the pituitary is suppressed by dexamethasone and responds to CRH and the concentration of ACTH is greater in the inferior petrosal sinuses than in peripheral blood, the results of these endocrine tests will suggest, erroneously, Cushing's disease, potentially resulting in pituitary surgery in a normal subject.

In patients with Cushing's disease who are treated by bilateral adrenalectomy, the loss of the suppressive effects of the excess cortisol on tumor ACTH secretion and growth results in very high levels of plasma ACTH, levels frequently sufficient to increase skin pigmentation, and progression of the ACTH-secreting pituitary tumor, which occasionally becomes invasive or even metastatic. This circumstance is known as Nelson's syndrome.

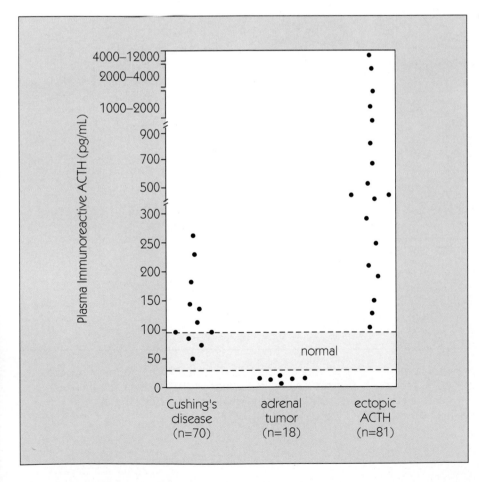

Figure 32.19 If the patient has hypercortisolism, the differential diagnosis of the etiology of Cushing's syndrome must be established. Initially, this is accomplished by distinguishing ACTH-dependent and ACTH-independent causes by measuring plasma ACTH levels and by evaluating the adrenal glands for an adrenal tumor with CT or MRI. (Data from Besser GM, Edwards CRW, 1972)

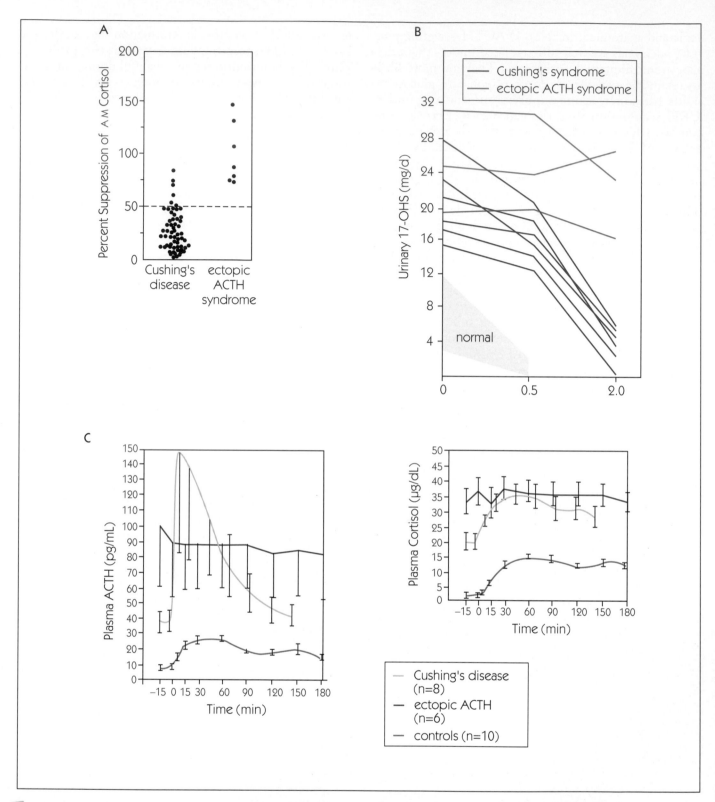

Figure 32.20 With ACTH-dependent Cushing's syndrome, the differential diagnosis of Cushing's disease (ACTH-secreting pituitary adenoma) versus ectopic ACTH syndrome is made with one or more of the following tests: high-dose dex- amethasone suppression test, either the overnight suppression test (**A**) or the Liddle test (**B**); (**C**) the CRH stimulation test. (**A**: data from Tyrrell JB, et al., 1986; **C**: data from Chrousos GP, et al., 1984)

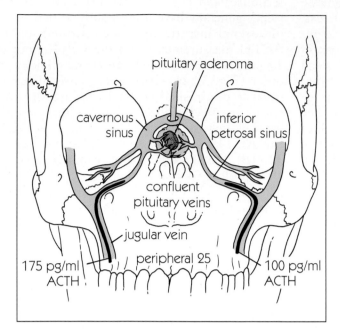

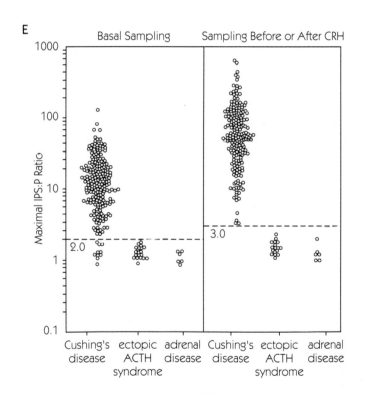

Figure 32.20 continued (D) anatomy and catheter placement in bilateral simultaneous blood sampling of the inferior petrosal sinuses; (E) bilateral inferior petrosal vein sampling in the differential diagnosis of Cushing's syndrome); maximum ratio of ACTH concentration from one of the inferior petrosal sinuses to the simultaneous peripheral venous ACTH concentration in patients with Cushing's syndrome in basal samples (left) and in basal and CRH-stimulated samples (right). (D: adapted with permission from Oldfield EH, et al., 1985; E: adapted with permission from Oldfield EH, et al., 1991)

Hypocortisolism

Adrenocortical insufficiency causes weakness, anorexia, nausea and vomiting, abdominal pain, weight loss, hypotension, hyponatremia, and the incapacity to respond to stressful stimuli. It is classified on the basis of whether it results from a disorder of the adrenal gland (primary adrenocortical insufficiency—Addison's disease) or from a disturbance of the hypothalamic-pituitary axis (secondary adrenocortical insufficiency). The adrenal disorders tend to produce more severe and life-threatening symptoms and are more likely to result in disturbance of salt wasting (hyponatremia, hyperkalemia, and hypovolemia due to absent aldosterone secretion). In the past, tuberculous infection of the adrenals was the most common cause of Addison's disease, but today primary adrenal insufficiency is more likely to result from autoimmune disorders that produce adrenal atrophy (idiopathic adrenal atrophy), other types of granulomatous infection, adrenal hemorrhage associated with severe stress, or after surgical removal of both adrenals.

Although secondary adrenocortical insufficiency occurs with hypothalamic-pituitary disorders that produce panhypopituitarism, ACTH secretion is the most resistant to loss of all the pituitary hormones. Thus, selective pituitary ACTH insufficiency is uncommon. The exception is the selective ACTH deficiency that occurs with prolonged hypercortisolism associated with glucocorticoid administration or with the excess endogenous production of glucocorticoids in Cushing's syndrome. Prolonged hypercortisolism, whether endogenous or exogenous, suppresses hypothalamic CRH secretion and pituitary ACTH secretion such that after the excess exposure to glucocorticoids is eliminated it requires 6 to 24 months for the hypothalamic-pituitary-adrenal axis to resume normal function and for recovery of the normal response to CRH and ACTH. In these circumstances hypocortisolism is only evident after withdrawal of prolonged glucocorticoid therapy or after successful treatment of Cushing's syndrome.

Evaluation and Laboratory Testing

In severe adrenal insufficiency, cortisol secretion, assessed by AM plasma cortisol levels and 24-hour urine collections for free cortisol and 17-hydroxysteroids, is low. However, basal cortisol secretion may be in the low normal range in even moderately severe hypoadrenalism. Thus, dynamic testing is usually required to detect and confirm adrenal insufficiency.

Since the adrenal cortex atrophies without normal ACTH stimulation, the response to ACTH stimulation in primary or secondary adrenal insufficiency is suppressed. In the short ACTH stimulation test 0.25 mg (25 units) of cosyntropin, synthetic short ACTH (α^{1-24}-ACTH), which retains the biological activity of ACTH, is injected intravenously or intramuscularly and plasma cortisol is measured just before and at 30 and 60 minutes after injection. An increment of greater than or equal to 7 µg/dL over basal levels or a peak value greater than or equal to 20 µg/dL is expected in normal subjects. In contrast, patients with longstanding ACTH

deficiency or suppression have a definite, but blunted, response, and patients with primary adrenal insufficiency generally have no response. When the diagnosis of adrenal insufficiency is confirmed, basal plasma ACTH measurements and the CRH stimulation test are used to establish the location and etiology of the disorder (Fig. 32.21). In primary adrenal insufficiency, because diminished cortisol production provides reduced negative feedback of the pituitary corticotrophs, basal plasma ACTH levels are high (Fig. 32.21A) and the ACTH response to CRH is exaggerated (Fig. 32.21B). On the other hand, with pituitary disease, or after prolonged excess glucocorticoid exposure, basal plasma ACTH levels are low and do not respond, or respond minimally, to CRH infusion.

GLYCOPROTEIN HORMONES

The glycoprotein pituitary hormones, thyroid-stimulating hormone (TSH), follicle-stimulating hormone (FSH), and luteinizing hormone (LH) are comprised of two glycopeptide chains, an alpha chain and a beta chain. The alpha chains of these hormones share an entire 96-amino-acid sequence, while the beta chains differ and confer the binding specificity of each hormone with its receptor (Fig. 32.22). The alpha and beta

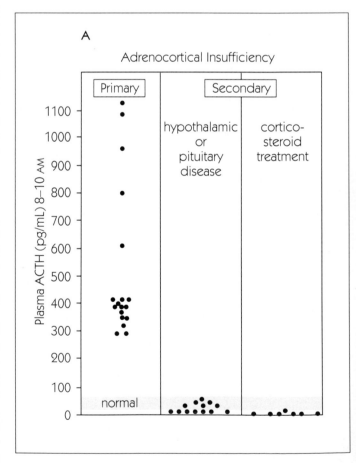

Figure 32.21 (A) Plasma ACTH levels in normal subjects and patients with primary and secondary adrenal cortical insufficiency. (A: data from Rees LH, et al., 1974)

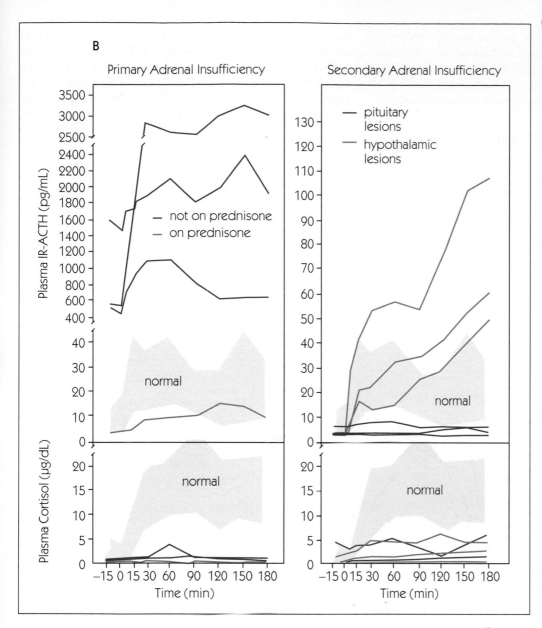

Figure 32.21 continued
(**B**) CRH stimulation test in adrenal insufficiency. Plasma ACTH (top) and cortisol (bottom) responses to oCRH (1 µg/kg UV) in patients with primary (left) and secondary (right) adrenal insufficiency. (**B**: data from Schulte HM, et al., 1984)

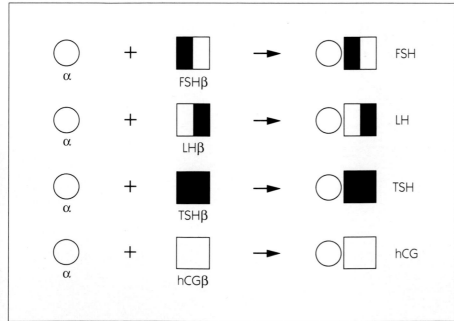

Figure 32.22 Glycoprotein hormones. Follicle-stimulating hormone (FSH), luteinizing hormone (LH), thyroid-stimulating hormone (TSH), and human chorionic gonadotropic hormone (hCG) have a common α subunit but a unique β subunit, which confers binding specificity. The α and β subunits are linked by hydrogen binding.

chains are coded by separate genes, synthesized separately, and joined in the Golgi apparatus into the functional dimer. There is normally slight excess production of the alpha chain, which is secreted alone, and which can be detected in the serum by radioimmunoassay.

PITUITARY-THYROID AXIS

Physiology

Production and secretion of the thyroid hormones, thyroxine (T_4) and triiodothyronine (T_3), are regulated via hypothalamic secretion of thyrotropin (TRH) into the portal venous system. In response to TRH the thyrotropic cells of the adenohypophysis release TSH (molecular weight 28,000), which acts on the thyroid gland to elicit release of T_4 and T_3. Whereas hypothalamic thyrotropin-releasing hormone (TRH) stimulates TSH secretion from the pituitary, T_3 and T_4 inhibit TRH secretion by the hypothalamus and TSH release by the pituitary (Fig. 32.23). Somatostatin, glucocorticoids, and dopamine also act to suppress TRH release and suppress the TSH response to TRH. Assessment of the hypothalamic-pituitary-thyroid axis is performed when hyperthyroidism, hypothyroidism, or hypopituitarism is suspected.

Hyperthyroidism

Hyperthyroidism causes tremulousness, anxiety, heat intolerance, diarrhea, and changes in mental status. The majority of hyperthyroid patients have either a circulating "thyroid-stimulating" antibody, a thyroid adenoma, or thyroiditis. These disturbances elevate serum levels of free T_4, which results in low plasma TSH in screening tests of thyroid function (Fig. 32.24A). Because of the

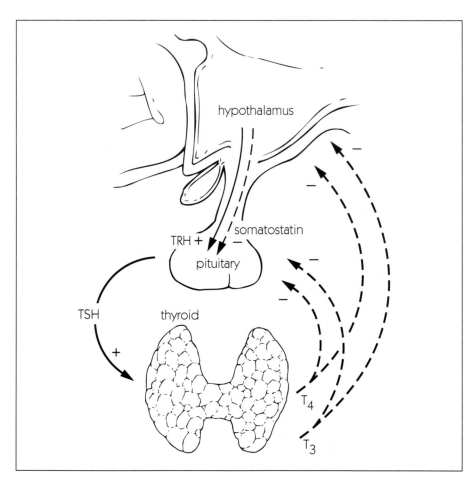

Figure 32.23 Hypothalamic-pituitary-thyroid axis. Thyrotropin-releasing hormone (TRH), released by the hypothalamus, stimulates the thyrotrophs of the anterior pituitary to secrete thyroid-stimulating hormone (TSH), which stimulates T_4 and T_3 secretion from the thyroid gland. Somatostatin suppresses the TSH response to TRH. T_4 and T_3 exert negative feedback at the pituitary and hypothalamic levels.

negative feedback of the excess thyroid hormones on the pituitary thyrotrophs, hyperthyroidism also suppresses the TSH response to TRH stimulation (Fig. 32.24B), a result that helps to confirm hyperthyroidism in a minimally symptomatic patient.

Hypersecretion of TSH by a pituitary adenoma is a rare cause of hyperthyroidism (less than 1% of patients)(Fig. 32.25A). In TSH-secreting tumors the production of alpha and beta subunits is sufficiently imbalanced that excess alpha subunit is secreted, which produces a ratio of plasma alpha subunit (mol/L) to plasma TSH (mol/L) greater than 1.0 (Fig. 32.25B). In

a patient with hyperthyroidism, or a patient with a pituitary tumor who has had thyroid treatment for hyperthyroidism, an elevated TSH level combined with a ratio of the molar concentration of alpha-subunit to TSH greater than 1.0 indicates a TSH-secreting pituitary adenoma and calls for further evaluation of the pituitary. Many TSH-secreting pituitary tumors also secrete GH and/or prolactin. Figure 32.26 summarizes the expected findings on thyroid screening tests.

Since hyperthyroidsim is common and TSH-secreting tumors are very rare, many patients with TSH-secreting pituitary tumors are initially misdiagnosed

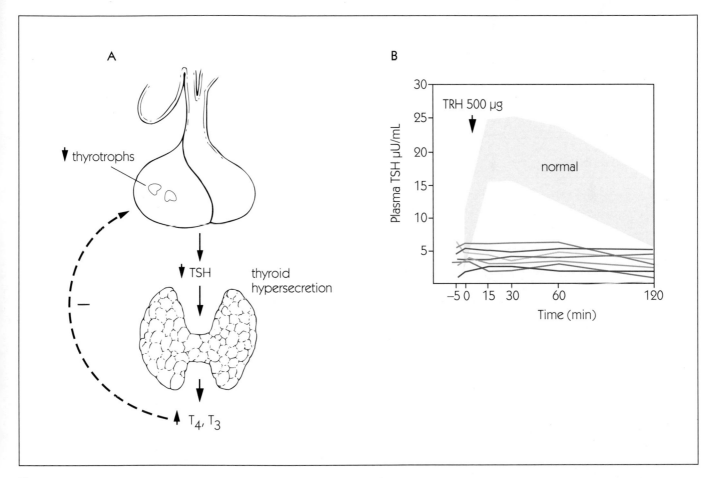

Figure 32.24 Hypothalamic-pituitary-thyroid axis. **(A)** In primary hyperthyroidism, because of thyroid disease excessive secretion of T_4 and T_3 occurs and provides feedback inhibition of the pituitary thyrotrophs (decreased TSH secretion).

(B) The graph depicts the flat response to TRH in patients with hyperthyroidism compared to the range of responses in normal subjects. (Data from Gaul C, et al., 1972)

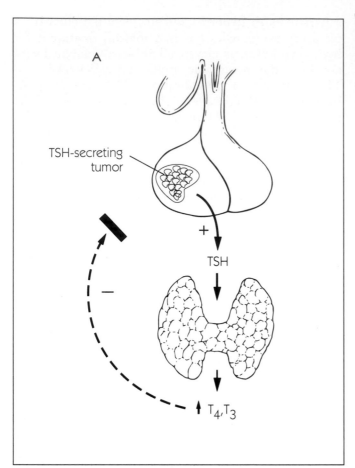

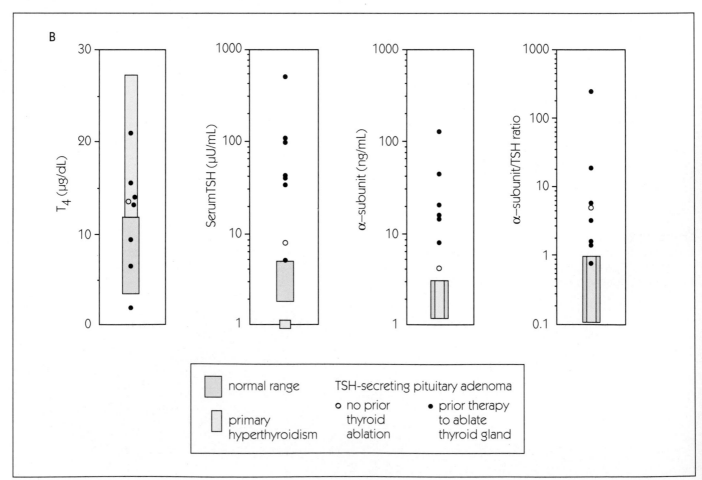

Figure 32.25 (A) In secondary hyperthyroidism, a TSH-secreting thyrotroph adenoma of the pituitary secretes excessive amounts of TSH, which stimulates increased T_4 and T_3 output from the thyroid. **(B)** In contrast to patients with primary hyperthyroidism, who have low serum levels of TSH, α-subunit levels in the normal range, and an α-subunit/TSH molar ratio less than 1.0, patients with TSH-secreting tumors have high serum TSH levels, high α-subunit levels, and an α-subunit/TSH molar ratio greater than 1.0. (Data from McCutcheon IE, et al., 1990)

and receive ablative therapy of the thyroid gland. Thus, they may not have hyperthyroidism when the pituitary tumor is recognized (see Fig. 32.25). In these patients the high plasma TSH levels do not fully suppress when the patient is given thyroid hormone and the TSH response to TRH is blunted. Because of the delay in diagnosis, TSH-secreting pituitary adenomas are often large, invasive tumors by the time they are recognized. In patients who receive thyroid ablation as treatment for hyperthyroidism, the evolution to a large and invasive tumor seems to be analogous to the circumstance that occurs in Nelson's syndrome with the ACTH-secreting tumors after adrenalectomy.

Hypothyroidism

The signs and symptoms of hypothyroidism include fatigue, dry skin, cold intolerance, alopecia, and, in severe cases, progression to myxedema coma. The majority of patients with hypothyroidism have primary hypothyroidism due to failure of function of the thyroid gland. This most often results from autoimmune Hashimoto's thyroiditis or from thyroid destruction after ^{131}I therapy or surgery for hyperthyroidism. In these conditions of primary hypothyroidism, absence of the feedback inhibition of the thyroid hormones on the pituitary and hypothalamus typically results in increased TRH secretion and elevated TSH levels (Fig. 32.27A). In untreated patients the increased TRH secretion stimulates thyrotroph hyperplasia and, in some instances, pituitary enlargement. Since the TRH also stimulates PRL secretion, these patients may be misdiagnosed as having a PRL-secreting or a TSH-secreting tumor and, mistakenly, receive pituitary surgery.

TSH deficiency, which causes secondary hypothyroidism, results from pituitary or hypothalamic disease. Often it accompanies multihormonal pituitary deficiency from large pituitary adenoma or a suprasellar tumor (Fig. 32.27B).

Evaluation and Laboratory Testing

In primary or secondary hypothyroidism, the serum level of free thyroxine (free T_4) is low (see Fig. 32.26).

Figure 32.26 Thyroid Screening Tests

	Free T_4	TSH
Hypothyroidism		
Primary	↓	↑
Secondary (pituitary)	↓	↓
Hyperthyroidism		
Primary	↑	↓
Secondary (pituitary)	↑	↑

Free T_4 can be measured by direct radioimmunoassay of serum dialysate or estimated by the free thyroxine index (FTI = total $T_4 \times T_3$ resin uptake). Although it is usually reliable, the FTI can be misleading in euthyroid "sick" patients in whom prolonged illness causes a low FTI despite clinical euthyroidism and normal serum levels of free T_4. When serum free T_4 is low, measurement of plasma TSH is used to distinguish primary (TSH elevated) from secondary (TSH low) hypothyroidism (Fig. 32.27C). However, various nonthyroidal illnesses (e.g., liver failure, sepsis) also can alter TSH levels. A TRH stimulation test further differentiates primary and secondary hypothyroidism, and in secondary hypothyroidism may distinguish between pituitary and hypothalamic disorders (Fig. 32.27D). TRH (200 to 500 µg) is given intravenously over 30 minutes and serum TSH levels are obtained at −5, 0, 15, 30 and 60 minutes. In primary hypothyroidism basal TSH levels are elevated and respond briskly and excessively to TRH. In normal subjects serum TSH peaks at 15 minutes and increases greater or equal to 6 µU/mL over the basal values, and in subjects with primary hypothyroidism TRH stimulates a rise in plasma TSH levels. Patients with pituitary lesions that destroy the thyrotrophs have no TSH response to TRH, whereas patients with hypothalamic disorders and surviving thyrotrophs have a delayed TSH response which peaks at 60 minutes.

GONADOTROPINS

Physiology

FSH and LH are produced and released by the gonadotrophs of the adenohypophysis to regulate ovarian and testicular function (Fig. 32.28). As indicated above, these glycoprotein hormones are structurally similar to TSH and human chorionic gonadotropin (hCG), in that they are a heterodimer formed by an alpha subunit and a beta subunit. Normally the alpha subunit is produced in slight excess. The plasma levels of FSH, which has a half life of about 3 to 4 hours, are more stable than the levels of LH, which has a half life of 50 minutes.

FSH stimulates growth of the granulosa cells of the ovarian follicle and controls estrogen secretion by them. At the midportion of the menstrual cycle, increasing concentration of estradiol stimulates a surge of LH secretion, which in turn triggers ovulation. After ovulation LH supports the formation of the corpus luteum. Exposure of the ovary to FSH is required for expression of the receptors for LH.

In men LH is responsible for the production of testosterone by the Leydig cell. The combined effects of FSH and testosterone on the seminiferous tubule stimulate sperm production.

FSH and LH secretion is stimulated in a pulsatile fashion in response to pulses of secretion of gonadotropin-releasing hormone (Gn-RH), a decapeptide,

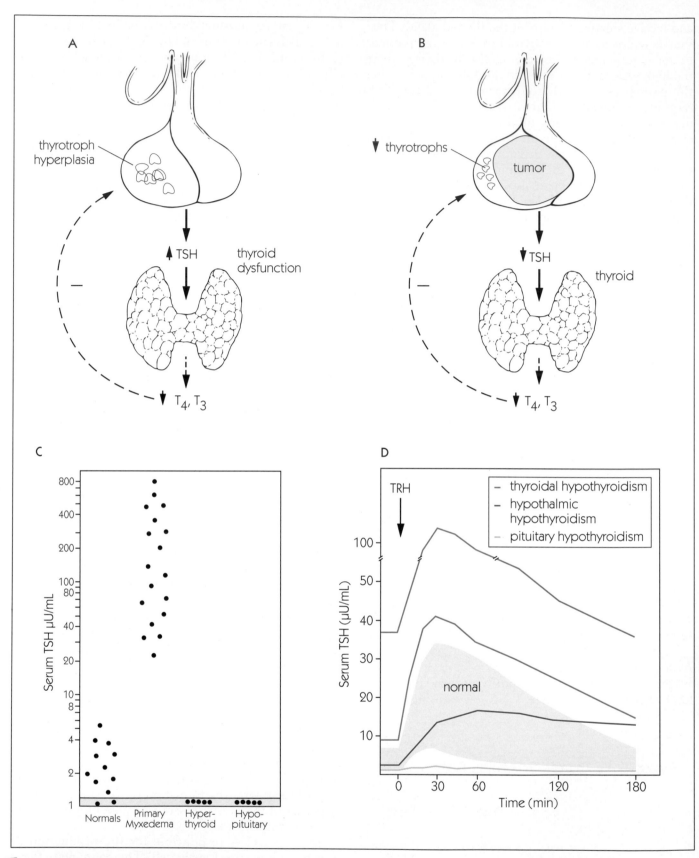

Figure 32.27 (A) In primary hypothyroidism, disease of the thyroid gland results in insufficient secretion of T_4 and T_3 and reduced feedback inhibition, pituitary thyrotroph hyperplasia, and increased TSH secretion. (B) In secondary hypothyroidism, any type of tumor in the sellar region can compress and destroy the pituitary thyrotrophs or distort the pituitary stalk and disrupt delivery of TRH to the pituitary, reducing TSH secretion and leading to decreased T_4 and T_3 output from the thyroid. (C) Serum TSH levels as determined by radioim-munoassay. The shaded area represents levels below the minimum detectable level. (D) Typical changes of serum TSH with TRH-stimulation test. Patients with pituitary (secondary) hypothyroidism have a flat TSH response to TRH in contrast to the excess levels and the rise in serum TSH in patients with thyroidal (primary) hypothyroidism. Patients with hypothalamic hypothyroidism have a delayed and intermediate response. (C: data from Hershman JM, Pittman JA, 1971; D: data from Utiger RD, 1978)

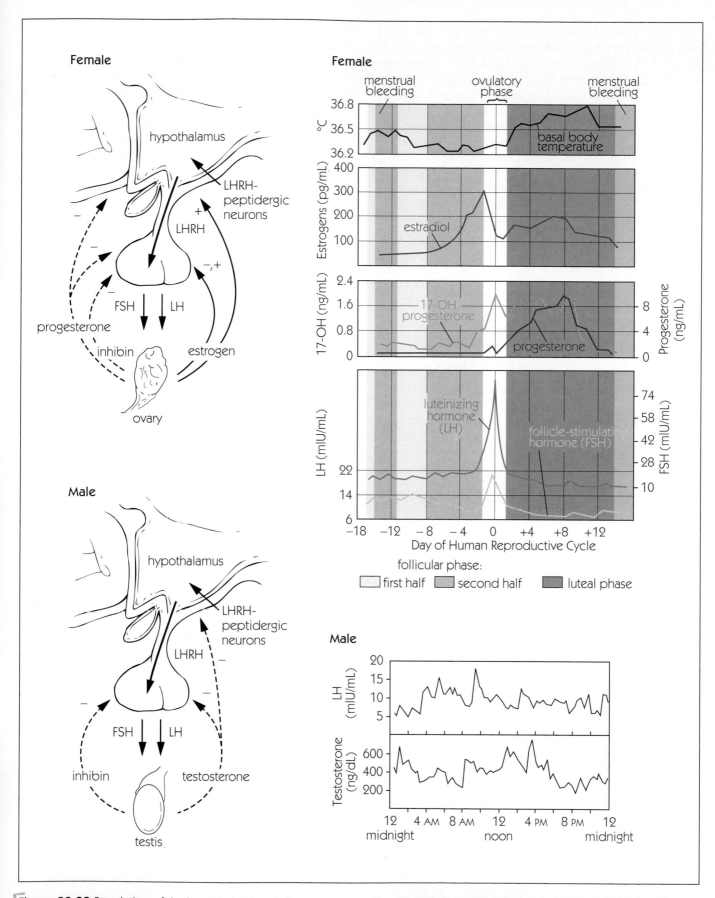

Figure 32.28 Regulation of the hypothalamic-pituitary-gonadal axis. Pulsatile release of LH-RH from the hypothalamus stimulates episodic pituitary release of FSH and LH. Negative feedback regulation is exerted by the sex steroids and the peptide inhibin. (Data from Yen SSC, 1980; Griffin JE, Wilson JD, 1980)

from the hypothalamus. Gn-RH is also known as LH-releasing hormone (LH-RH) because it is a potent stimulator of LH seretion. Levels of FSH and LH are regulated by the balance of Gn-RH stimulation, negative feedback regulation exerted by inhibin, a peptide secreted by the ovaries and the testes, and the effect of the sex steroids on the pituitary and the hypothalamus (see Fig. 32.28). Appropriate levels of FSH and LH are needed for normal sexual development and reproductive function in men and women. Although Gn-RH can stimulate gonadotropin secretion from the pituitary for the first few months of life, the pituitary then becomes unresponsive to Gn-RH until puberty, when pulsatile secretion of FSH and LH occur in response to pulses of Gn-RH. After gonadal failure associated with menopause the negative feedback provided by the hormonal products of the gonads is eliminated and serum levels of FSH and LH increase. Because of the pulsatile nature of serum Gn-RH, LH, and FSH, and their fluctuation during the menstrual cycle, isolated and random FSH and LH levels are of little diagnostic use, but must be correlated with the results of simultaneous levels of estradiol or testosterone and/or the results of dynamic testing.

Excess Gonadotropin Secretion

Although FSH-secreting and LH-secreting pituitary adenomas are rarely recognized clinically, about 5% of pituitary adenomas have immunohistochemical staining for the gonadotropins or their subunits. Nearly all of these tumors are clinically "nonfunctional" pituitary macroadenomas that cause symptoms because of their mass effect on sellar or parasellar structures, as there is no characteristic hypersecretory endocrinopathy, as occurs with the other types of tumors described above. About 20% of these tumors hypersecrete the alpha-subunit, the level of which can be determined by radioimmunoassay. It is not yet known if measurements of FSH, LH, or alpha-subunit will accurately indicate response to therapy or tumor recurrence.

Precocious puberty is often associated with hypothalamic hamartomas, which, by interrupting the normal suppression of pituitary gonadotropin function by higher neural centers in children, lead to pulsatile secretion of Gn-RH and, in turn, secretion of FSH and LH, estrogen, and testosterone and premature sexual development. Sustained, nonpulsatile exposure to Gn-RH desensitizes the gonadotrophs to Gn-RH and inhibits

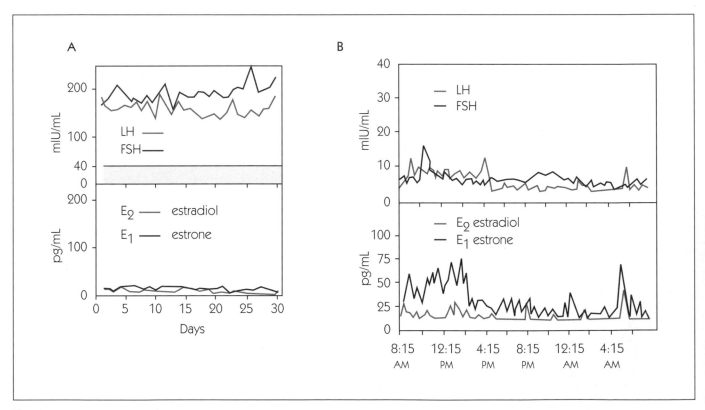

Figure 32.29 Typical pattern of FSH, LH, and corresponding ovarian estrogen and androgen levels in daily samples from a woman with premature ovarian failure. (**A**) Primary hypogonadism. Ovarian failure is associated with low levels of sex steroids and high levels of FSH and LH. The shaded area represents concentrations up to 40 mIU/ml; FSH levels above this are considered to represent ovarian failure. (**B**) Hypogonadotropic hypogonadism. Typical pattern of FSH, LH, and corresponding ovarian estrogen and androgen levels in sam-

ples obtained at 15-minute intervals over a 24-hour period in a woman with hypogonadotropic hypogonadism, in which inadequate secretion of FSH and LH results in decreased levels of the sex steroids. This can result from destruction of pituitary gonadotrophs, distortion of the pituitary stalk and interruption of delivery of LH-RH, or hypothalamic dysfunction with insufficient LH-RH release. (**A**: data from Rebar RW, et al., 1982; **B**: data from Yen SSC, 1978)

FSH and LH release. Knowledge of this phenomenon and the development of a long-acting analogue of Gn-RH is now used to suppress pituitary gonadotropin secretion and reverse sexual development in children with idiopathic precocious puberty and precocious puberty associated with hypothalamic hamartomas. Ectopic production of gonadotropin, usually of human chorionic gonadotropin (which has LH-like activity), by germinomas of the nonseminiferous type, lung carcinomas, and other types of tumors can also cause precocious puberty.

Deficient Gonadotropin Secretion

Hypogonadism is suspected in women who develop loss of libido and amenorrhea associated with uterine and vaginal atrophy. In men, low testosterone results in loss of libido, impotence, decreased body hair (including reduced beard growth), and testicular softening. In patients suspected of having hypogonadism, endocrine evaluation includes measurement of plasma FSH, LH, and the sex steroids, estradiol in women and testosterone in men. Primary hypogonadism due to end-organ failure (e.g., premature ovarian failure) is associated with low levels of sex steroids and high levels of FSH and LH (Fig. 32.29A). If FSH and LH are inappropriately low and are associated with a decreased level of sex steroids, the patient has hypogonadotropic hypogonadism (Fig. 32.29B). This may be primary and result from congenital causes, as in Kallman's syndrome, in which Gn-RH deficiency is associated with anosmia and defective development of the midline structures of the brain. More commonly, hypogonadotropic hypogonadism is a secondary, acquired defect of Gn-RH production associated with hypothalamic dysfunction, as in anorexia nervosa or bulimia, or due to destruction of the pituitary gonadotrophs and/or interruption of function of the pituitary stalk from a sellar mass, or from surgery or radiation therapy used to treat a sellar or parasellar tumor. LH-RH stimulation testing can be used to determine the presence of adequate gonadotroph reserve (Fig. 32.30). If a detectable elevation of FSH and LH levels occurs after LH-RH administration (the response to LH-RH often requires "priming" of the gonadotrophs by repeated injections of LH-RH), functional gonadotropic cells are still present.

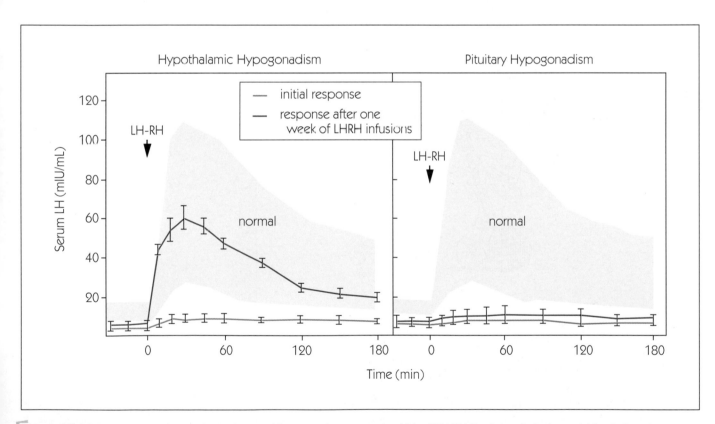

Figure 32.30 Response to LH-RH in patients with secondary hypogonadism. Mean serum LH levels in men with secondary hypogonadism before and after a 250 µg intravenous bolus of LH-RH before and after priming with daily infusions (500 µg over 4 h) of LH-RH for 1 week. Patients with pituitary hypogonadism lack gonadotropin secretion. (Data from Snyder PJ, et al., 1979)

POSTERIOR PITUITARY HORMONES

The posterior lobe, the neurohypophysis, is a direct extension of the neural processes of nerve cells in the supraoptic and paraventricular nuclei of the hypothalamus. The nerve cell bodies in the hypothalamus produce two peptide hormones, antidiuretic hormone (ADH, vasopressin) and oxytocin, which are synthesized in separate neurons and transported down axons in association with carrier proteins, neurophysins, through the pituitary stalk into the posterior lobe, where they are stored and secreted (Fig. 32.31). Although these hormones normally are stored in secretory granules in the nerve termi-

nals of the neurohypophysis and released from the posterior lobe into the systemic circulation in response to various stimuli, if the pituitary is selectively damaged and the median eminence and hypothalamus are intact, they can be secreted from the median eminence.

ADH conserves water. Derangements in ADH secretion can result in severe, potentially lethal, disturbances in plasma osmolality and volume. Oxytocin stimulates uterine contractions at parturition and acts to expel milk from the secretory tissue of the breast to the nipple during suckling. Oxytocin is not routinely assayed in the assessment of pituitary function.

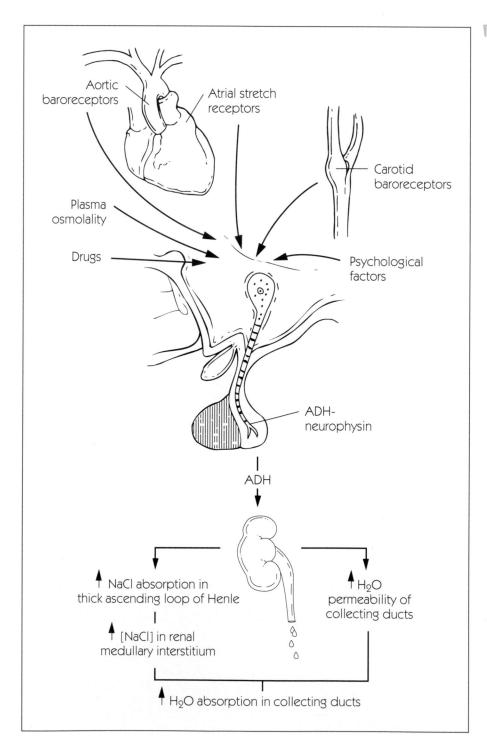

Figure 32.31 Control of antidiuretic hormone (ADH, vasopressin) secretion.

ANTIDIURETIC HORMONE (ADH)

ADH, a nonapeptide, acts on the kidney to conserve water. As with many other peptide hormones, its action is mediated by a second messenger, cyclic AMP (cAMP). ADH binds to specific receptors on cells of the thick ascending loop of Henle and the collecting ducts, which activate adenyl cyclase in the plasma membrane via alteration of a guanine regulatory protein. Activation of adenylate cyclase increases production of cAMP from ATP. Increased cAMP enhances NaCl absorption in the thick ascending loop of Henle and increases permeability to water in the collecting ducts. These effects increase water absorption from the collecting ducts.

Although multiple hypothalamic inputs influence ADH secretion, the primary stimuli for ADH release are an increase in plasma osmolality (Fig. 32.32) or a decrease in plasma volume. As little as a 2% increase in plasma osmolality caused by an impermeable solute, such as NaCl, causes shrinkage of hypothalamic osmoreceptor cells and stimulates ADH release. Thirst is also stimulated. The other major physiologic stimulus to ADH release is decreased intravascular volume. Small decreases stimulate ADH secretion via activation of stretch receptors in the left atrium, whereas decreases in circulating volume of approximately 10% stimulate ADH release via baroreceptors in the carotid arteries and the aortic arch. Higher neural centers also influence ADH release. Beta-adrenergic and cholinergic agonists stimulate ADH release, while alpha-adrenergic agonists and atropine inhibit release. Thus, psychological factors, pain, and stress increase ADH release. Various drugs also influence ADH release; nicotine, morphine, and the barbiturates stimulate, while alcohol, phenytoin, and narcotic antagonists inhibit ADH secretion.

Excess ADH (Syndrome of Inappropriate ADH Secretion, SIADH)

The syndrome of inappropriate ADH secretion results from excess ADH secretion, either from the hypothalamus or from an ectopic source. Excess ADH secretion stimulates excess retention of free water associated with the inability to excrete dilute urine and results in hyponatremia and hypotonicity of the plasma. Continued nonsuppressible ADH release in association with elevated urine osmolality above plasma osmolality is considered inappropriate in patients with low plasma osmolality and hyponatremia. The many causes of SIADH include ectopic production of ADH by tumors (especially oat cell carcinoma) or by lung tissue during inflammatory diseases (tuberculosis), excessive neurohypophyseal release of ADH caused by a variety of intracranial disorders (head trauma, subarachnoid hemorrhage, meningitis, etc.), or by drugs that stimulate ADH release (e.g., chlorpropamide, carbamazepine, tricyclic antidepressants). SIADH also can occur after transsphenoidal surgery or pituitary apoplexy.

The clinical features of SIADH include weight gain, weakness, lethargy, and mental confusion. As the serum sodium drops below 120 mEq/L seizures and coma ultimately occur.

Evaluation and Laboratory Testing

The characteristic laboratory features of SIADH include hyponatremia, hypotonicity of plasma, urine osmolality that is hypertonic to plasma, and urinary sodium concentration greater than or equal to 20 mEq/L (except in patients who are chronically depleted of sodium). The diagnosis of SIADH is made when these features are present and adrenal, thyroid, renal, or hepatic dysfunction and prior diuretic use have been excluded as possible etiologies. Measurement of plasma

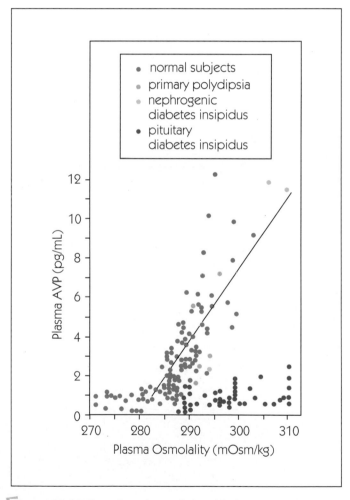

Figure 32.32 There is a close relationship between plasma osmolality and plasma arginine vasopressin (AVP) in normal subjects, patients with nephrogenic diabetes insipidus, and primary polydipsia, but not with pituitary diabetes insipidus. (Data from Robertson GL, 1981)

ADH reveals inappropriately elevated levels despite low plasma osmolality (Fig. 32.33) and confirms, but is not essential for, the diagnosis.

Deficient ADH (Diabetes Insipidus)

Deficient ADH secretion in response to physiological stimuli, pituitary diabetes insipidus, impairs renal conservation of water. Causes of diabetes insipidus include sellar and parasellar tumors (especially craniopharyngiomas, large nonfunctional pituitary adenomas, germinomas, and metastatic tumors), infiltrative processes (hypothalamic sarcoidosis and histiocytosis X), pituitary or hypothalamic surgery, head trauma, ruptured intracranial aneurysms, and idiopathic causes. The typical clinical features include polyuria, excessive thirst and polydipsia, and nocturia (Fig. 32.34). Urine volumes can vary from a few liters a day to more than 15 liters per day. If access to water is restricted or interrupted, dehydration can rapidly become severe and result in altered mentation, fever, hypotension, and death.

Evaluation and Laboratory Testing

The characteristic laboratory findings of diabetes insipidus include persistent urine osmolality of less than 300 mOsm/kg H_2O associated with urine specific gravity of 1.005 or less and plasma osmolality greater than

the normal 287 mOsm/kg H_2O (Fig. 32.35A; see Fig. 32.32). To confirm the diagnosis, patients are tested to document that there is inadequate release of ADH to an osmotic stimulus. The simplest, safest, and most widely used test to raise plasma osmolality is the water deprivation test (Fig. 32.35B,C).

In the water deprivation test all oral intake is stopped after obtaining baseline body weight, urine and plasma osmolality, and vital signs. Water deprivation begins the night before the test in patients with mild polyuria, and early on the day of the test in patients with severe polyuria. Hourly measurements of urine osmolality and weight are obtained. Dehydration continues until either two sequential urine osmolalities vary by less than 30 mOsm/kg H_2O or loss of greater than 3% of body weight occurs. Subjects then receive 5 units of aqueous vasopressin subcutaneously and a final urine osmolality is measured 1 hour later. In normal subjects endogenous ADH secretion concentrates the urine and preserves normal plasma osmolality. Thus, urine osmolality normally exceeds 500 mOsm/kg H_2O and plateaus, and plasma osmolality remains below 300 mOsm/kg H_2O before vasopressin injection, and urine osmolality rises less than 5% after injection. In patients with central (pituitary or hypothalamic) diabetes insipidus, urine osmolality usually plateaus at 300 to 500

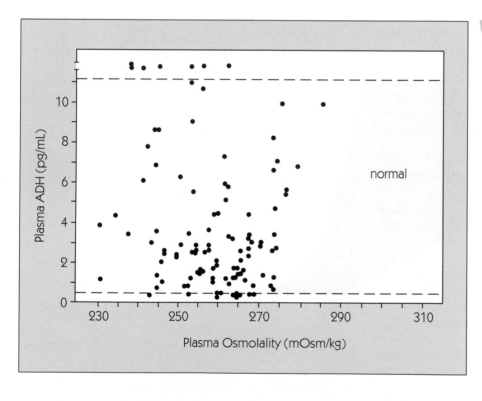

Figure 32.33 Levels of plasma vasopressin (ADH) as a function of plasma osmolality are inappropriately high in patients with the syndrome of inappropriate ADH secretion (SIADH). (Adapted with permission from Martin JB, Reichlin S, 1987)

mOsm/kg H$_2$O, plasma osmolality may exceed 300 mOsm/kg H$_2$O, and urine osmolality rises greater than 9% after vasopressin injection. This test not only establishes whether or not diabetes insipidus is present, it also distinguishes central diabetes insipidus from other causes of polyuria. In patients with polyuria from renal disease or nephrogenic diabetes insipidus (renal tubular insensitivity to ADH), the rise in urine osmolality with dehydration is limited and does not increase after vasopressin administration. In patients with primary poly-dipsia (compulsive water drinking), water deprivation has to be prolonged for urine osmolality to plateau and urine osmolality does not increase after the dose of vasopressin.

Plasma ADH measurements by RIA also can be used during or as an adjunctive test to the water deprivation test (see Fig. 32.33), but because of the simplicity and reliability of the measurements of plasma and urine osmolality, ADH determinations are rarely required.

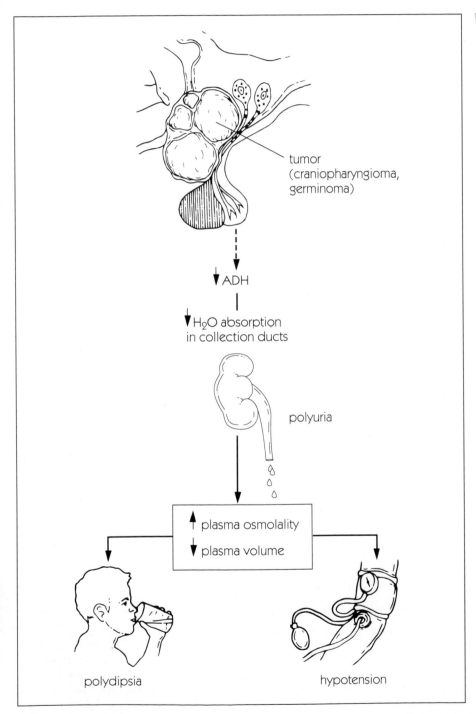

Figure 32.34 Deficient ADH secretion. Destruction of hypothalamic neurons by hypothalamic masses or injury, including surgery, produces pituitary diabetes insipidus.

tumor (craniopharyngioma, germinoma)

↓ ADH

↓ H$_2$O absorption in collection ducts

polyuria

↑ plasma osmolality
↓ plasma volume

polydipsia

hypotension

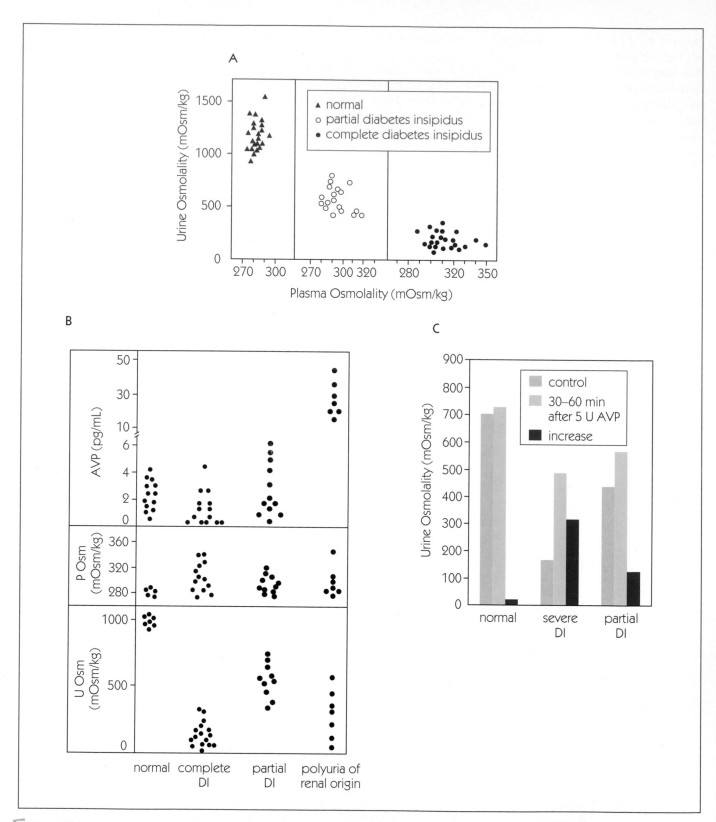

Figure 32.35 Characteristic laboratory findings with diabetes insipidus. **(A)** Typical plasma and urine osmolalities in patients with diabetes insipidus compared to normal subjects. **(B)** Characteristic plasma and urine osmolality and plasma AVP level after water deprivation in patients with diabetes insipidus, normal subjects, and patients with polyuria of renal origin. **(C)** The differences in the increase in urine osmolality after 5 units of subcutaneous vasopressin in patients with central (hypothalamic-pituitary) diabetes insipidus compared to normal subjects after water deprivation. Urine osmolality rises less than 5% in normal subjects but more than 9% in patients with central diabetes insipidus. (Data from Verbalis J, et al., 1985)

SUGGESTED READINGS

General

Bennett JC, Smith LH, Wyngaarden JB, eds. *Cecil Textbook of Medicine*. 19th ed. Philadelphia, Pa: WB Saunders Co; 1992.

Cooper PR, ed. *Contemporary Diagnosis and Management of Pituitary Adenomas*. Park Ridge: American Association of Neurological Surgeons; 1991.

Gilman AG. Guanine nucleotide-binding regulatory proteins and dual control of adenylate cyclase. *J Clin Invest*. 1984;73:1–4.

Kannan CR. *The Pituitary Gland*. New York, NY: Plenum Publishing Corp; 1987.

Klibanski A, Zervas NT. Diagnosis and management of hormone-secreting pituitary adenomas. *N Engl J Med*. 1991;324:822–831.

Martin JB, Reichlin S. *Clinical Neuroendocrinology*. 2nd ed. Philadelphia, Pa: FA Davis Co; 1987.

Reeves WB, Andreoli TE. The posterior pituitary and water metabolism. In: Foster DW, Wilson JD, eds. *Williams Textbook of Endocrinology*. 8th ed. Philadelphia, Pa: WB Saunders Co; 1992.

Reichlin S. Neuroendocrinology. In: Foster DW, Wilson JD, eds. *Williams Textbook of Endocrinology*. 8th ed. Philadelphia, Pa: WB Saunders Co; 1992.

Thorner MO, Vance ML, Horvath E, Kovacs K. The anterior pituitary. In: Foster DW, Wilson JD, eds. *Williams Textbook of Endocrinology*. 8th ed. Philadelphia, Pa: WB Saunders Co; 1992.

Prolactin

Boyd AE III, Reichlin S, Turksoy RN. Galactorrhea-amenorrhea syndrome: diagnosis and therapy. *Ann Intern Med*. 1977;87:165–175.

Frantz AG. Prolactin. *N Engl J Med*. 1978;298:201.

Hwang P, Guyda H, Friesen II. A radioimmunoassay for human prolactin. *Proc Natl Acad Sci USA*. 1971; 68:1902–1906.

Kleinberg DL, Noel GL, Frantz AG. *N Engl J Med*. 1977;296:589–600.

Sachar EJ. Hormonal changes in stress and mental illness. In: Krieger DT, Hughes JC, eds. *Neuroendocrinology*. Sunderland, Mass: Sinauer Associates; 1980:177–183.

Sassin JF, Frantz AG, Weitzman ED, Kapen S. Human prolactin: 24-hour pattern with increased release during sleep. *Science*. 1972;177:1205–1207.

Tolis G. Prolactin: physiology and pathology. In: Krieger DT, Hughes JC, eds. *Neuroendocrinology*. Sunderland, Mass: Sinauer Associates, 1980: 321–330.

Growth Hormone

Barkan AL, Beitins IZ, Kelch RP. Plasma insulin-like growth factor-I/somatomedin-C in acromegaly: correlation with the degree of growth hormone hypersecretion. *J Clin Endocrinol Metab*. 1988;67:69–73.

Carlson HE. The diagnosis of acromegaly. In: Robbins RJ, Melmed S, eds. *Acromegaly: A Century of Scientific and Clinical Progress*. New York, NY: Plenum Press; 1987:197–208.

Clemmons DR, Van Wyk JJ, Ridgeway EC, et al. Evaluation of acromegaly by radioimmunoassay of somatomedin C. *N Engl J Med*. 1979;301:1138–1142.

El-Khodary AZ, Ball MF, Stein B, et al. Effect of weight loss on the growth hormone response to arginine infusion in obesity. *J Clin Endocrinol Metab*. 1971;32:42–51.

Melmed S. Acromegaly. *N Engl J Med*. 1990;322: 966–977.

Melmed S, Braunstein GD, Horvath E, et al. Pathophysiology of acromegaly. *Endocr Rev*. 1983;4: 271–290.

Raiti S, Tolman RA, eds. *Human Growth Hormone*. New York, NY: Plenum Medical Book Co; 1986.

Van Wyk JJ, Underwood LE. Growth hormone, somatomedins and growth failure. In: Krieger DT, Hughes JC, eds. *Neuroendocrinology*. Sunderland, Mass: Sinauer Associates; 1980:299–309.

Pituitary-Adrenal Axis

Besser GM, Edwards CRW. Cushing's syndrome. *Clin Endocrinol Metab*. 1972;1:451–490.

Chrousos GP, Schulte HM, Oldfield EH, Gold PW, Cutler GB Jr, Loriaux DL. The corticotropin-releasing factor stimulation test: an aid in the evaluation of patients with Cushing's syndrome. *N Engl J Med*. 1984;310:622–626.

Kaye TB, Crapo L. The Cushing syndrome: an update on diagnostic tests. *Ann Intern Med*. 1990;112:434–444.

Liddle GW. Tests of pituitary-adrenal suppressibility in the diagnosis of Cushing's syndrome. *J Clin Endocrinol Metab*. 1960;20:1539–1560.

Loriaux DL, Cutler GB Jr. Disease of the adrenal glands. In: Kohler PO, ed. *Clinical Endocrinology*. New York, NY: John Wiley & Sons; 1986.

Melby JC. Assessment of adrenocortical function. *N Engl J Med*. 1971;285:735–739.

Nieman LK, Loriaux DL. Corticotropin-releasing hormone: clinical applications. *Annu Rev Med*. 1989; 40:331–339.

Oldfield EH, Chrousos GP, Schulte HM, et al. Preoperative lateralization of ACTH-secreting microadenomas by bilateral and simultaneous inferior petrosal sinus sampling. *N Engl J Med*. 1985;312: 100–103.

Oldfield EH, Doppman JL, Nieman LK, et al. Bilateral petrosal sinus sampling with and without corticotropin-releasing hormone for the differential diagnosis of Cushing's syndrome. *N Engl J Med*. 1991;325:897–905.

Rees LH, Holdaway IM, Phenekos C, et al. ACTH secretion and clinical investigations. In: *Some*

Aspects of Hypothalamic Regulation of Endocrine Functions: Symposium, Vienna, June 3–6, 1973. Stuttgart: F Schattaur Verlag; 1974.

Schulte HM, Chrousos GP, Avgerinos PC, Oldfield EH, Gold PW, Cutler GB Jr, Loriaux DL. The corticotropin-releasing factor stimulation test: an aid in the evaluation of patients with adrenal insufficiency. *J Clin Endocrinol Metab.* 1984;58: 1064–1067.

Streeten DHP, Stevenson CT, Dalakos TG, et al. The diagnosis of hypercortisolism: biochemical criteria differentiating patients from lean and obese normal subjects and from females on oral contraceptives. *J Clin Endocrinol Metab.* 1969;29:1191–1211.

Tanaka K, Nicholson WE, Orth DN. Diurnal rhythm and disappearance half-time of endogenous plasma immunoreactive B-MSH (LPH) and ACTH in man. *J Clin Endocrinol Metab.* 1978;46:883–890.

Tyrrell JB, Findling JW, Aron DC, Fitzgerald PA, Forsham PH. An overnight high-dose dexamethasone suppression test for rapid differential diagnosis of Cushing's syndromes. *Ann Intern Med.* 1986;104: 180–186.

Glycoprotein Hormones

Demura R, Kubo O, Demura H, et al. FSH and LH secreting pituitary adenoma. *J Clin Endocrinol Metab.* 1977;45:653–657.

Gaul C, et al. Administration of thyrotropin release hormone (TRH) as a clinical test for pituitary thyrotropin reserve. *Rev Invest Clin.* 1972;24:35.

Gesundheit N, Petrick PA, Nissim M, et al. Thyrotropin-secreting pituitary adenomas: clinical and biochemical heterogeneity. *Ann Intern Med.* 1989; 111:827–835.

Gharib H, Carpenter PC, Scheithauer BW, et al. The spectrum of inappropriate pituitary thyrotropin secretion associated with hyperthyroidism. *Mayo Clin Proc.* 1982;57:556–563.

Griffin JE, Wilson JD. The testis. In: Bondy PK, Rosenberg LE, eds. *Metabolic Control and Disease.* 8th ed. Philadelphia, Pa: WB Saunders Co; 1980:1535.

Hershman JM, Pittman JA. Utility of the radioimmunoassay of serum thyrotropin in man. *Ann Intern Med.* 1971;74:481–490.

Ishibashi M, Yamaji T, Takaku F, et al. Secretion of glycoprotein hormone alpha-subunit by pituitary tumors. *J Clin Endocrinol Metab.* 1987;64:1187–1193.

Jackson, IMD. Thyrotropin-releasing hormone. *N Engl J Med.* 1982;306:145–155.

Klibanski A. Nonsecreting pituitary tumors. *Endocrinol Metab Clin North Am.* 1987;16:793–804.

Kourides IA, Weintraub BD, Rosen SW, Ridgeway EC, Kliman B, Maloof F. Secretion of alpha subunit of glycoprotein hormones by pituitary adenomas. *J Clin Endocrinol Metab.* 1976;43:97–106.

McCutcheon IE, Weintraub BD, Oldfield EH. Surgical treatment of thyrotropin-secreting pituitary adenomas. *J Neurosurg.* 1990;73:674–683.

Pierce JG. The subunits of pituitary thyrotropin—their relationship to other glycoprotein hormones. *Endocrinology.* 1971;89:1331–1344.

Rebar RW, Erickson GF, Yen SSC. Idiopathic premature ovarian failure: clinical and endocrine characteristics. *Fertil Steril.* 1982;37:35–41.

Snyder PJ. Gonadotroph cell adenomas of the pituitary. *Endocr Rev.* 1985;6:552–563.

Snyder PJ, Rudenstein RS, Gardner DF, et al. Repetitive infusion of gonadotropin-releasing hormone distinguishes hypothalamic from pituitary hypogonadism. *J Clin Endocrinol Metab.* 1979;48: 864–868.

Utiger RD. Tests of the hypothalamic-pituitary-thyroid axis. In: Werner SC, ed. *The Thyroid.* 4th ed. Hagerstown: Harper & Row; 1978.

Weintraub BD, Gershengorn MC, Kourides IA, et al. Inappropriate secretion of thyroid-stimulating hormone. *Ann Intern Med.* 1981;95:339–351.

Yen SSC. Chronic anovulation due to CNS-hypothalamic-pituitary dysfunction. In: Yen SSC, Jaffe RB, eds. *Reproductive Endocrinology.* Philadelphia, Pa: WB Saunders Co; 1978:341–372.

Yen SSC. Neuroendocrine regulation of the menstrual cycle. In: Krieger DT, Hughes JC, eds. *Neuroendocrinology.* Sunderland, Mass: Sinauer Associates; 1980:259–272.

Posterior Pituitary

Andreoli TE. The polyuric syndromes. In: Andreoli TE, Hoffman JF, Fanestil DD, eds. *Physiology of Membrane Disorders.* New York, NY: Plenum Medical Book Co; 1978:1063–1091.

Brownstein MJ, Russell JT, Gainer H. Synthesis, transport and release of posterior pituitary hormones. *Science.* 1980;207:373–378.

Miller M, Dalakos T, Moses AM, Fellerman H, Streeten DHP. Recognition of partial defects in antidiuretic hormone secretion. *Ann Intern Med.* 1970;73:721–729.

Robertson GL. Diseases of the posterior pituitary in endocrinology and metabolism. In: Felig P, Baxter JD, Broadus AE, Frohman LA. New York, NY: McGraw-Hill; 1981:251–280.

Robertson GL. Thirst and vasopressin function in normal and disordered states of water balance. *J Lab Clin Med.* 1983;101:351–371.

Sklar AH, Schrier RW. Central nervous system mediators of vasopressin release. *Physiol Rev.* 1983;63: 1243–1280.

Verbalis J, Robinson A, Moses S. Postoperative and posttraumatic diabetes insipidus. *Frontiers in Hormone Research.* 1985;13:247–265.

Chapter 33

Nonfunctioning
Pituitary Adenomas

Paul B. Nelson

CLINICAL PRESENTATION

Nonfunctioning pituitary adenomas account for approximately 30% of pituitary tumors. The tumors are usually seen in the fourth and fifth decades and are more common in males than females. Nonfunctioning pituitary adenomas have also been referred to as *null cell tumors, undifferentiated tumors,* and *non-hormone-producing adenomas.*[1] It had been thought that these tumors do not produce hormone units. Recently, however, improved immunoperoxidase staining techniques reveal that some "nonfunctioning adenomas" actually secrete one or more of the glycoprotein hormones follicle-stimulating hormone (FSH), luteinizing hormone (LH), and thyroid-stimulating hormone (TSH) and/or their alpha and beta subunits. Alpha subunit production has been found more commonly than beta subunit production.[2]

Because these hormones often do not produce a functioning hormone that would alert the patient and the physician to the presence of a pituitary adenoma, the tumors are not generally diagnosed until they are very large (Fig. 33.1). The tumors are usually solid (Fig. 33.2), although they may be both solid and cystic (Fig. 33.3).

If an enlarging tumor extends into the suprasellar area, optic chiasmal compression will occur, which may cause bitemporal visual field deficits. Because the inferior nasal fibers located in the inferior aspect of the optic chiasm subserve the superior temporal field, the first visual field deficits are frequently bitemporal superior quadrant defects (Fig. 33.4). Occasionally the tumors extend into the cavernous sinus (Fig. 33.5). Extraocular muscle palsies are extremely rare even if there is cavernous sinus extension, presumably because these tumors grow slowly.

Enlargement of the nonfunctioning adenoma causes progressive loss over months or years of pituitary function.[1,3] Gonadotropin function is usually lost first; followed by loss of growth hormone function, then loss of thyroid function, and finally loss of adrenocorticotropic hormone (ACTH) function. Loss of antidiuretic hormone function is almost never a presenting symptom.

Although progressive bitemporal visual field loss and progressive hypopituitarism are the typical presenting clinical manifestations, occasionally large pituitary adenomas become apparent suddenly, secondary to hemorrhage (apoplexy) or infarction.[4] When there is a large hemorrhage into the pituitary tumor, the patient may have a sudden headache, a decreased level of consciousness, vision loss, and acute adrenal insufficiency (Fig. 33.6). Patients

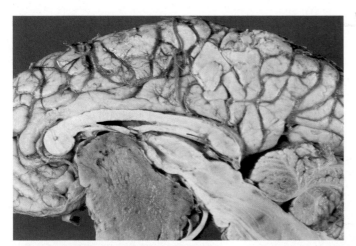

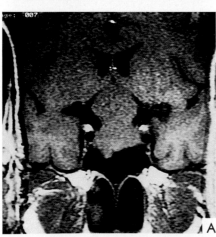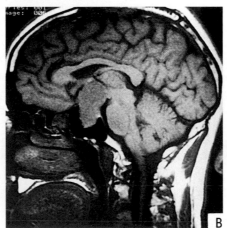

Figure 33.1 Midline sagittal section of the brain of a patient who had an extremely large sellar-suprasellar nonfunctioning pituitary adenoma.

Figure 33.2 Coronal (A) and sagittal (B) MRIs showing a large solid sellar-suprasellar nonfunctioning pituitary adenoma.

Figure 33.3 Coronal MRI showing a large sellar-suprasellar nonfunctioning pituitary adenoma that has a solid inferior portion and a cystic superior portion.

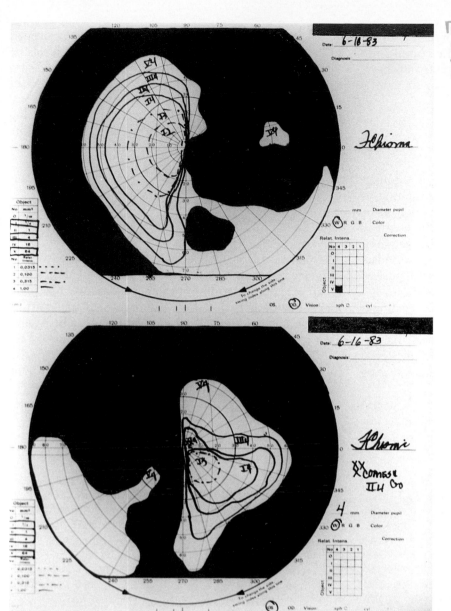

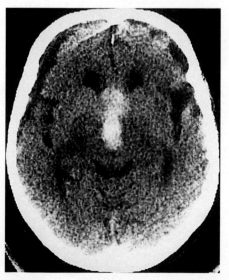

Figure 33.4 Visual field examination on a patient with a pituitary tumor causing inferior chiasmal compression. The largest defects are in the superior temporal fields.

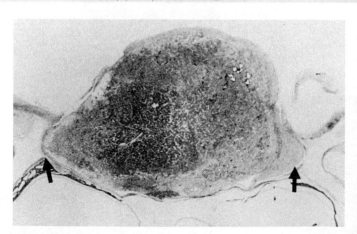

Figure 33.5 Coronal block section through a pathologic specimen of the sella and cavernous sinuses of a patient with a large pituitary adenoma. Arrows show slight extension into the cavernous sinus.

Figure 33.6 Unenhanced CT scan of a patient with pituitary apoplexy showing a hemorrhage that extends into the suprasellar area and third ventricle.

who have abscesses within pituitary tumors have similar symptoms, but they also have fever. The spinal fluid analysis in both pituitary apoplexy and pituitary abscess is generally nonrevealing, except for a possible parameningeal response with increased lymphocytes.

EVALUATION

Lateral radiographs of the skull help diagnose nonfunctioning pituitary adenoma (Fig. 33.7). Since the tumors are large, the sella turcica also enlarges. The floor of the sella (lamina dura) frequently thins, and if the enlarged adenoma is asymmetrical, the lateral radiograph may show a double floor. The sella itself becomes more rounded. Also, the dorsum sellae may be thinned and pushed back, and the anterior clinoids may be undercut.

MRI and CT help show the exact anatomical configuration of the adenoma.[5,6] MRI is preferable to CT because it better demonstrates the carotid arteries and chiasm; however, CT also demonstrates the nonfunctioning adenomas and may be better than MRI for demonstrating the bony anatomy of the sphenoid sinus (Fig. 33.8).

Visual acuity and visual field examinations are necessary. Formal visual fields will be needed to evaluate the patient properly. Gross confrontational visual fields are not adequate alone.

Stimulation testing of endocrine function is needed to determine loss of hormonal function—basal levels by themselves may not reveal hypofunction. Stimulation testing is frequently done in a clinical research unit. LH and follicle-stimulating hormone (FSH) levels are determined both before and after gonadotropin-releasing hormones (Gn-RH) administration. Growth hormone and cortisol levels can be determined both before and after insulin hypoglycemia. TSH and prolactin measurements are made before and after thyrotropin releasing hormone (TRH) administration.

DIFFERENTIAL DIAGNOSIS

The differential diagnosis of the large nonfunctioning pituitary adenoma is quite extensive. Tuberculum sellae meningiomas may mimic pituitary adenoma, but plain x-ray usually does not show significant enlargement of the sella; tuberculum sellae meningiomas may be associated with bony thickening of the tuberculum (Fig. 33.9). A large internal carotid artery aneurysm may also fill the sella turcica (Fig. 33.10). An aneurysm should be able to be diagnosed with the flow void seen on an MRI. Although craniopharyngiomas are generally suprasellar tumors, they may occasionally present within the sella turcica. Patients with metastasis to the sella frequently have associated extraocular muscle palsies

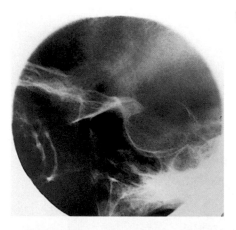

Figure 33.7 Coned down lateral radiograph of the skull of a patient with a large pituitary tumor. The sella is rounded and enlarged and shows thinning of the floor and dorsum.

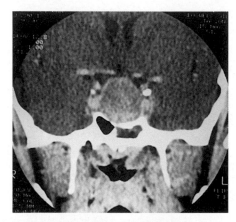

Figure 33.8 Coronal enhanced CT scan of a patient with a large sellar-suprasellar nonfunctioning pituitary adenoma.

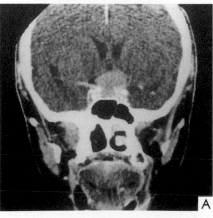

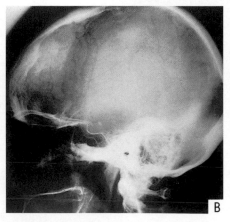

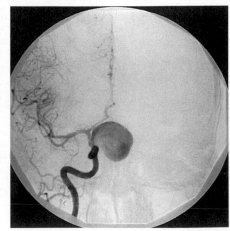

Figure 33.9 (A) Coronal CT of a patient with tuberculum sellae meningioma. The CT scan appearance is similar to that of a patient with a large nonfunctioning adenoma. (B) Skull radiograph shows the sella is not enlarged.

Figure 33.10 An internal carotid aneurysm that filled and enlarged the sella turcica.

Principles of Neurosurgery

and/or diabetes insipidus (Fig. 33.11), findings almost never seen in pituitary adenomas. Rathke's pouch cleft cysts occasionally present as large sellar and suprasellar cystic masses (Fig. 33.12). Tuberculoma, giant cell hypophysitis, and sarcoidosis may mimic nonfunctioning adenoma, but they are seen infrequently.

TREATMENT

The usual treatment of a nonfunctioning pituitary adenoma in a medically stable patient is microscopic transsphenoidal removal of the tumor.[1,7-9] In most cases this is an elective procedure. The typical indications are visual loss or hypopituitarism. If the patient has loss of thyroid or ACTH function preoperatively, surgery is usually delayed 2 to 3 weeks so the patient can begin thyroid and/or hydrocortisone replacement therapy. If vision loss is rapid or the adenoma is associated with hemorrhage or abscess, a more urgent surgical approach is needed. Sellar and suprasellar tumors can be removed from the transsphenoidal approach by either a sublabial or transseptal incision (Fig. 33.13). Some surgeons insert a lumbar drain and instill saline

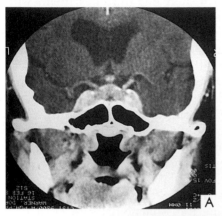
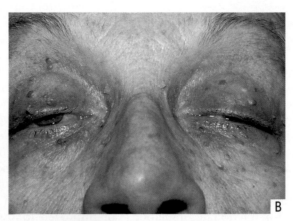

Figure 33.11 (A) Enhanced coronal CT scan of a patient presenting with a metastasis to the sella. There is sellar and suprasellar mass effect and fullness in both cavernous sinuses. (B) This patient presented with bilateral ptosis secondary to bilateral third nerve palsies.

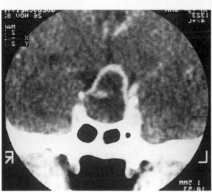

Figure 33.12 Enhanced coronal CT scan of a patient with a large sellar-suprasellar Rathke's pouch cleft cyst.

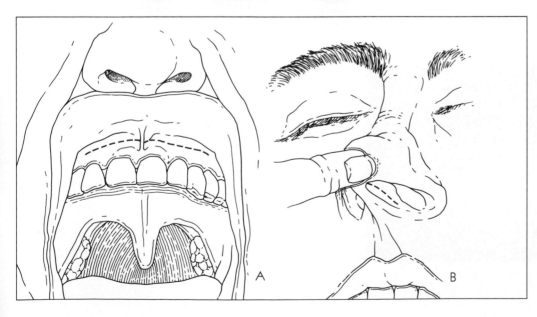

Figure 33.13 (A) Incision used for a sublabial transsphenoidal approach. (B) Incision used for a transseptal transsphenoidal approach.

to help bring down the suprasellar extension. C-arm guidance is often used with (Fig. 33.14) the transsphenoidal approach because it orients the surgeon correctly in the anterior-posterior direction. The surgeon needs a thorough understanding of sphenoid sinus anatomy for correct positioning relative to the midline.

Contraindications to transsphenoidal surgery include a dumbbell tumor, which has an extremely narrow waist at the junction of the sellar and suprasellar portions; a tumor with a large subfrontal or parasellar extension; a tumor with massive suprasellar extension; and, sometimes, an extremely fibrous tumor. Occasionally, craniotomy will be needed in patients who are contraindicated for transsphenoidal surgery.

Significant complications from transsphenoidal surgery are not common. The incidence of rhinorrhea is about 5%. Approximately 20% of patients develop diabetes insipidus; however, permanent diabetes insipidus is uncommon. Approximately 10% of patients have partial worsening of their hormone function. The chances of visual loss, stroke, and death are less than 1%.

Radiation therapy can be used in patients with nonfunctioning pituitary adenomas.[10] If the patient is elderly or medically unstable, radiation therapy may be the only viable treatment. The patient who postoperatively has a significant amount of residual tumor or who shows regrowth may be a candidate for fractionated radiation therapy, generally 4000 to 5000 cGy over 25 treatments.

Although complications from radiation therapy are not common, it may cause radiation necrosis, other benign and malignant tumors, and further loss of visual and endocrine function.[3] Despite the frequent dural invasion of these tumors, many patients do well for long periods of time without radiation therapy.

PATHOLOGY

Pathologic staining with H&E stain usually shows the adenoma arranged in a papillary fashion (Fig. 33.15). A touch preparation done at surgery shows a monolayer of adenomatous cells that sticks well to the slide (Fig.

33.16). In a truly nonfunctioning pituitary adenoma, the immunoperoxidase staining from the pituitary necrosis is negative. Immunoperoxidase staining is done to detect if the tumor is producing any of the six anterior pituitary hormones.

SURGICAL OUTCOME

Following operative decompression of nonfunctioning adenomas, vision improves in approximately 80% of patients.[1] Generally, endocrine function is the same pre- and postoperatively, although transsphenoidal surgery usually stops the progressive loss of hormonal function. Unfortunately, approximately one third of patients with nonfunctioning adenomas are already panhypopituitary before their surgical treatment.

Postoperative evaluation with MRI and CT has several limitations. It is difficult to evaluate the sella immediately after surgery because of postoperative bleeding and intrasellar packing.[6] It is probably best to delay the initial postoperative anatomical study for at least 4 to 6 weeks. In most cases, no suprasellar mass is seen following operative decompression. Persistent mass effect seen in the early postoperative period will generally go away. The gradual resolution of the mass effect can be documented with serial anatomical studies. If vision is stable or improved following transsphenoidal surgery, it may be best simply to follow the patient, even if he or she has persistent suprasellar mass effect.

FOLLOW UP

Most patients with nonfunctioning pituitary adenomas should have annual CT scan or MRI, visual field, and endocrine evaluations whether or not they have had surgical and/or radiation treatment.[1] If these tumors are not treated, they grow slowly over months or years. There is a significant recurrence rate following transsphenoidal surgery (approximately 20%). The recurrence rate following both surgical decompression and radiation therapy is approximately 10%. A significant number of

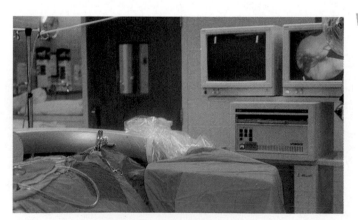

Figure 33.14 The operating room for a transsphenoidal approach in which C-arm radiographic imaging is used.

patients who undergo postoperative radiation therapy develop further hormonal loss that progresses to panhypopituitarism. Replacement hormonal therapy should be monitored by an endocrinologist. Patients must be aware that hydrocortisone replacement doses may need to be increased during illness and/or stressful periods.

CONCLUSION

Nonfunctioning pituitary adenomas comprise a significant portion of patients with pituitary tumors. The tumors are usually large before they are discovered. Bitemporal visual field loss and/or loss of pituitary function is the most common presenting clinical manifestation. Transsphenoidal removal of the adenoma and appropriate replacement therapy is the most common treatment for this disorder. Radiation therapy may be used in selected patients.

In the future, medical therapy may play a more important role in patients with nonfunctioning adenomas. If, in fact, the "nonfunctioning adenoma" is found to be producing a glycoprotein-secreting hormone or a subunit of one of these hormones, treatment with agents such as somatostatin and Gn-RH antagonists may be developed. The role of focused radiation treatment techniques such as gamma knife, proton beam, and the linac accelerator in nonfunctioning adenomas has yet to be determined. The goal of transsphenoidal surgery is to remove the adenomas as completely as possible while leaving any remaining compressed normal gland. However, invasion of the cavernous sinus and frequent invasion of the surrounding dura may limit the ability to remove a large adenoma totally.

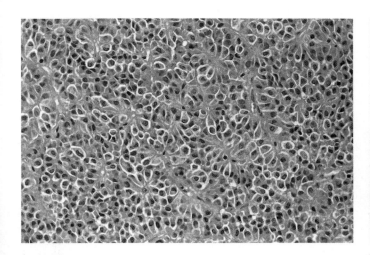

Figure 33.15 A nonfunctional pituitary adenoma arranged mostly in a papillary fashion. (H&E; ×250)

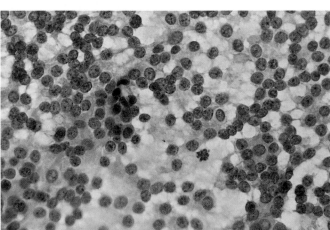

Figure 33.16 Touch preparation of a nonfunctioning pituitary adenoma showing a monolayer of adenomatous cells that stick well to the glass. Some nuclear atypism and prominent nucleoli are noted. The cytoplasm is barely visible. (H&E; ×250)

REFERENCES

1. Nelson PB. Management of large pituitary tumors. *Cont Neurosurg.* 1986;8:16.
2. Black PM, Hsu DW, Klibanski A, et al. Hormone production in clinically nonfunctioning pituitary adenomas. *J Neurosurg.* 1987;66:244–250.
3. Nelson PB, Goodman M, Flickenger JC, et al. Endocrine function in patients with large pituitary tumors treated with operative decompression and radiation therapy. *Neurosurgery.* 1989;24:398–400.
4. Nelson PB, Haverkos H, Martinez AJ, et al. Abscess formation within pituitary tumors. *Neurosurgery.* 1983;12:331–333.
5. Mikhael M, Ciric I. MR imaging of pituitary tumors before and after surgical and/or medical treatment. *JCAT.* 1988;12:441–445.
6. Dolinskas C, Simeone F. Transsphenoidal hypophysectomy: postsurgical CT findings. *AJNR.* 1985; 6:45–50.
7. Ciric I, Mikhael M, Stafford T, et al. Transsphenoidal microsurgery of pituitary macroadenomas with long-term follow-up results. *J Neurosurg.* 1983;59: 395–401.
8. Wilson CB. A decade of pituitary microsurgery. *J Neurosurg.* 1984;61:814.
9. Laws ER Jr. Transsphenoidal tumor surgery for intrasellar pathology. *Clin Neurosurg.* 1979;26:391.
10. Sheline GE. *Conventional Radiotherapy in the Treatment of Pituitary Tumors.* New York, NY: Raven Press; 1979;287–314.

Chapter 34

Functioning Pituitary Tumors

Mark B. Eisenberg, Steven Onesti, Kalmon D. Post

The anterior pituitary gland is responsible for the secretion and regulation of a variety of peptide hormones and stimulating factors. Tumors originating in the anterior pituitary gland may, therefore, produce excess quantities of a particular peptide hormone. When this occurs the resulting adenoma is classified as a functioning or secretory adenoma. Tumors without hormonal activity are logically classified as nonfunctioning or nonsecretory adenomas (see Chapter 33). A brief review of the hypothalamic-pituitary-end organ axis will be helpful in understanding the diagnosis and treatment of patients with functioning pituitary tumors.

The anterior pituitary gland is under predominantly stimulatory control by the hypothalamus. The pituitary hormones adrenocorticotropic hormone (ACTH), growth hormone (GH), prolactin, thyroid-stimulating hormone (TSH), luteinizing hormone (LH), and follicle-stimulating hormone (FSH) are controlled by the hypothalamic hormones corticotropin-releasing hormone (CRH), growth hormone releasing factor (GRF), dopamine (also known as prolactin inhibitory factor [PIF]), thyroid-releasing hormone (TRH), and gonadotropin-releasing hormone (Gn-RH) respectively. This is efficiently accomplished via a portal vascular system connecting the hypothalamus with the anterior pituitary gland. The fact that prolactin is under inhibitory control by the hypothalamus becomes advantageous in the medical treatment of prolactin-secreting tumors. These hypothalamic releasing factors are then under negative feedback control from the end-organ products, i.e., adrenal gland products, thyroid hormone, etc., thereby completing the axis loop.[1]

Anterior pituitary gland adenomas are identified pathologically both by their in vivo endocrine activity and by their in vitro immunohistochemical staining characteristics. The advent of immunohistochemical staining for the various peptide hormones has revealed the fact that many adenomas once thought to be nonsecretory actually secrete endocrinologically inactive peptides.[2] The alpha subunit, which has no known systemic effects, is one of the commonly found peptides.

Adenomas may be further subdivided into micro- or macroadenomas based upon size (Fig. 34.1).[3] Tumors less than 1 cm in diameter are considered microadenomas and are predictably located solely within the sella turcica. They characteristically do not invade neighboring structures such as the sphenoid and cavernous sinuses. Macroadenomas, by definition greater than 1 cm, typically enlarge the sella turcica and frequently invade neighboring structures. Microadenomas usually are discovered because of an endocrinopathy, whereas macroadenomas present with compressive effects of the tumor, i.e., bitemporal hemianopsia, as well as endocrinopathy. The endocrinopathy may be one of either oversecretion or undersecretion.

The evaluation of a patient with a suspected functioning pituitary tumor will be discussed in relation to each tumor type; however, because of the protean and often subtle manifestations of these endocrinopathies, a detailed history and physical examination are mandatory in guiding the rest of the work-up. Subtle changes in hair growth, skin texture or color, and body mass may be the only heralds of early endocrine dysfunction. The radiographic evaluation of patients with pituitary ade-

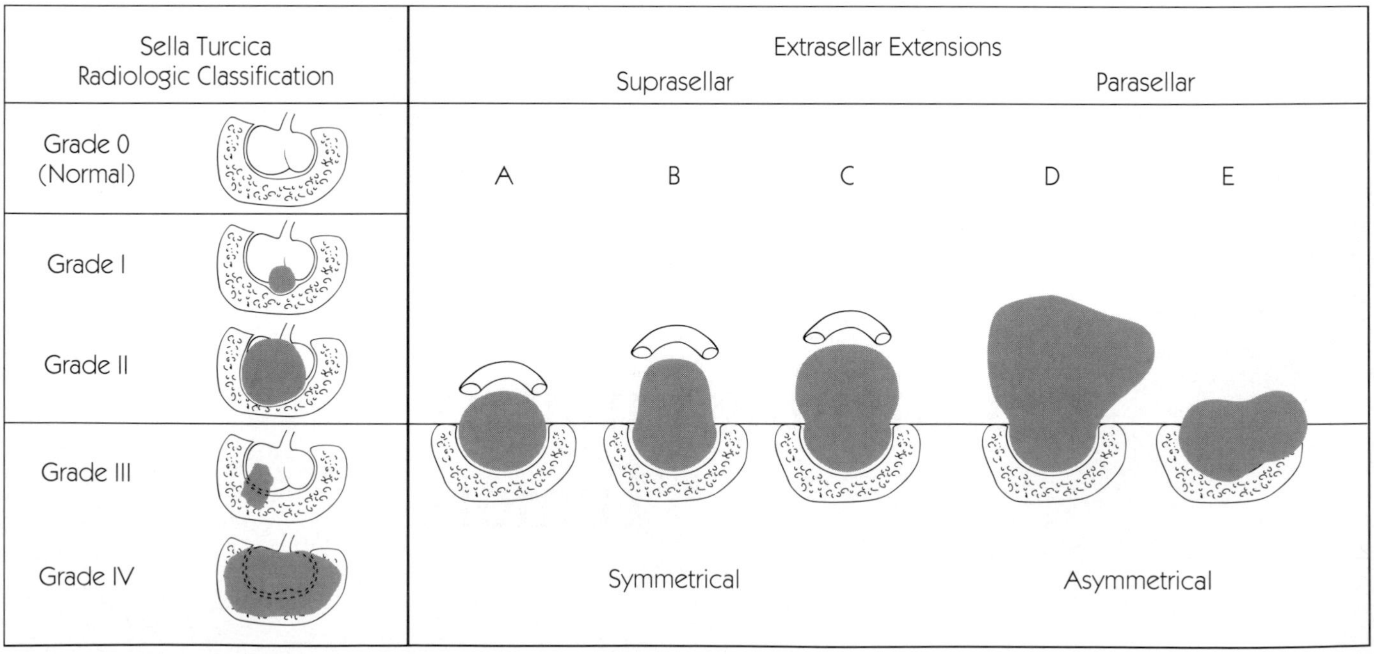

Figure 34.1 Radiographic/imaging classification of pituitary adenomas. Grades I and II are enclosed adenomas. Grades III and IV are invasive adenomas. Extensions A,B,C are directly suprasellar, while D is asymmetric intracranial and E is asymmetric into the cavernous sinus. (Adapted from Hardy J, Somma M, 1979)

nomas has been dramatically changed with the advances of MRI technology. MRI with and without gadolinium enhancement is now considered the study of choice in evaluating patients with suspected pituitary abnormalities (Figs. 34.2–34.4).[4–7] The normal pituitary gland will enhance within 5 minutes of contrast administration, leaving the adenoma hypointense compared to the surrounding pituitary tissue. If the study is performed more than 5 minutes after contrast administration, the tumor will appear enhanced while the nor-

mal gland will appear unenhanced. It is therefore imperative that the neuroradiologist indicate the timing of the study in relation to contrast enhancement. Computed axial tomography (CT) is helpful in evaluating bony changes in the sella and surrounding structures but is much less sensitive than MRI in detecting small adenomas (Fig. 34.5).[8–11] Patients with endocrinologically silent tumors may infrequently require angiography to exclude a carotid artery aneurysm, although MRI has made this very rare.

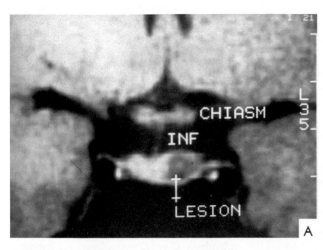
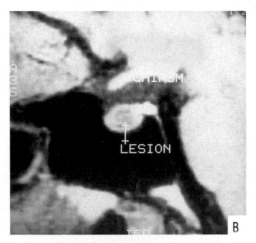

Figure 34.2
(A) Coronal MR image of the pituitary gland. Note the optic chiasm above and the pituitary stalk (infundibulum) deviated from left to right (grade I). (B) Sagittal MR image of the pituitary gland with a central lesion.

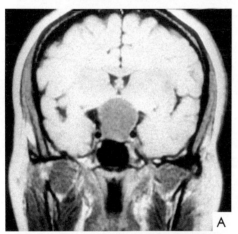
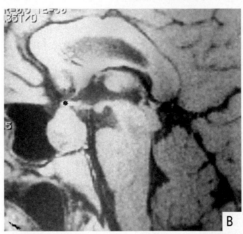

Figure 34.3 (A) Coronal MR image of the sella. Note the large adenoma with suprasellar extension. The optic chiasm is compressed and is not visible (grade IIc). (B) Sagittal MR image of the sella. Adenoma is seen reaching the lower surface of the optic chiasm (asterisk) (grade IIa).

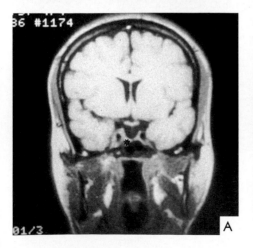
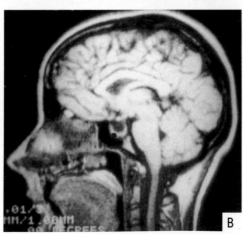

Figure 34.4 (A) Coronal MR image of sella postoperatively. Note the residual gland at the bottom of the sella (asterisk). The stalk is seen midline. (B) Sagittal MR image of the sella postoperatively. The residual gland is seen at the bottom of the sella (asterisk).

Patients with macroadenomas must undergo detailed visual field testing that may reveal previously unnoticed abnormalities. This will also serve as a baseline for comparison to subsequent visual field testing. With all this in mind, it is appropriate to focus on the management of patients with various secretory pituitary adenomas.

PROLACTIN-SECRETING ADENOMAS

Prolactin is classified as a somatomammotropic hormone along with growth hormone and chorionic somatomammotropin.[12] It is a peptide chain 198 amino acids long, necessary for the normal lactation in postpartum women. Prolactin levels begin to rise shortly after conception and reach levels of 150 to 200 ng/mL at term, however it is not until the postpartum decline in estrogen is complete that lactation may occur. Stimulation of tactile receptors on the nipple and areola of the breast leads to prolactin secretion that in the postpartum estrogen-primed breast results in lactation. TRH and vasoactive intestinal peptide (VIP) both appear to have minor prolactin-releasing activity, although their significance is presently unclear. Although the above stimuli lead to increases in prolactin secretion, the overwhelming control of prolactin release is inhibitory in nature, via dopamine. Dopamine, also known as prolactin-inhibiting factor (PIF), is released by the hypothalamus and leads to a decrease in prolactin secretion. As mentioned earlier, this inhibitory control becomes vitally important in the medical management of prolactinomas.[13,14] Normal prolactin levels are less than 15 ng/mL in men and less than 20 ng/mL in nonpregnant women.

Causes of hyperprolactinemia other than a pituitary adenoma include pregnancy, stress, hypoglycemia, renal failure, hypothyroidism, and phenothiazine-like medications. These, as well as several other etiologies, must be considered prior to a detailed investigation of a patient's pituitary gland.[15]

SIGNS AND SYMPTOMS

Prolactin-secreting tumors represent 40% of all pituitary adenomas and are typically more symptomatic in women. Hyperprolactinemia in women leads to amenorrhea, galactorrhea, and osteoporosis, while in men it may result in diminished sexual drive and impotence or it may be asymptomatic. Because of this difference, men are not usually diagnosed until the tumor has reached a size sufficient to cause compressive effects on neighboring structures.[16]

DIAGNOSIS

Random measurements of the serum prolactin level are reliable to establish the diagnosis of hyperprolactinemia (Fig. 34.6). In the absence of the other above-mentioned disorders investigation of the pituitary gland is necessary. This should begin with a gadolinium-enhanced MRI, which will often disclose a pituitary macroadenoma. Hyperprolactinemia in the presence of a macroadenoma does not mean a priori that the tumor is a prolactinoma. The degree of prolactin elevation is directly related to the functionality of the tumor. Serum prolactin levels greater than 150 ng/mL correlate very well with the presence of a prolactinoma; however,

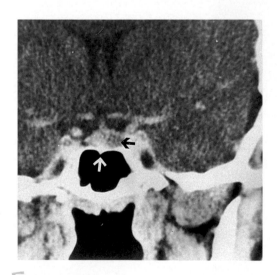

Figure 34.5 Coronal enhanced CT scan of sella. Note the adenoma (dark arrow) in the left side of the pituitary gland. The white arrow points to a bony septation within the sphenoid sinus.

Figure 34.6 Diagnosis of Pituitary Function

1. Thyroid function tests, e.g., T_4, T3RU, TSH

2. Baseline AM plasma cortisol and response to ACTH

3. LH, FSH, and testosterone in men; no tests if menstruating female

4. Prolactin—no stimulation test

5. Growth hormone

milder elevations may be due to stalk compression leading to interference with the inhibitory effects of dopamine (Fig. 34.7).

_____TREATMENT

The dopamine agonist bromocriptine has radically changed the treatment of symptomatic prolactinomas (Fig. 34.8).[17-31] Except for specific situations discussed below, bromocriptine therapy has virtually replaced transsphenoidal resection as the therapy of choice for this group of tumors. Bromocriptine is a dopamine agonist that directly stimulates the dopamine receptors located on lactotrophs (prolactin-secreting cells). Dosages of 2.5 to 7.5 mg/d are usually sufficient to treat most patients. The response to bromocriptine is remarkable. Prolactin levels will begin to decrease in a matter of hours following the first dose and tumor size will often diminish within a few days. Patients with visual field deficits may begin to improve after a few days of treatment. Other than pregnancy or rapidly deteriorating visual function, there are virtually no con-

---

Figure 34.7 Differential Diagnosis of Hyperprolactinemia

Nonpathologic Causes
Pregnancy
Early periods of nursing
Stress

Primary Pituitary Causes
True prolactinomas
Stalk compression secondary to
    nonprolactin-secreting adenomas
Traumatic stalk section
Empty sella syndrome

Systemic Disorders
Hypothyroidism
Renal failure
Liver disease
Chest wall surgery/trauma

Pharmacologic Causes
Dopamine antagonists, e.g.,
    phenothiazine-like drugs
MAO inhibitors
MAO depleters
Opiate derivatives
Oral contraceptives

---

traindications to an initial trial of bromocriptine therapy. Follow-up with periodic serum prolactin measurements and imaging studies of the sella is necessary to insure that therapy is effective. In approximately 66% of patients, tumor size will be reduced by as much as 75%, with the best response seen in patients with large tumors (Figs. 34.9, 34.10).[20] Endocrine function often returns to normal with establishment of cyclic menses in women and return of libido in men. Many previously infertile women have, in fact, been able to conceive while on bromocriptine therapy.

Since bromocriptine is not tumoricidal, it is said that tumor reexpansion will occur as soon as therapy is stopped.[32] There is, however, a small subset of patients in which neither discontinuation of therapy nor microdosage leads to a return of symptoms or hyperprolactinemia.[19,33] Because it is impossible to predict which patients will have such a dramatic response, it is prudent to stop therapy every few years and determine whether there is continued need for treatment. Bromocriptine is clearly the leading medical therapy for prolactinomas; other ergot derivatives show some usefulness in lowering prolactin levels but are not as well tolerated as bromocriptine.[34] A newer nonergot dopamine agonist designated CV 502-205 shows some promise as a once-daily administration.[30]

While bromocriptine appears to be a true panacea, it is not without problems and side effects. Most commonly, patients complain of nausea and vomiting and the need for potential lifelong therapy. Although there are as yet no definite teratogenic effects from bromocriptine, pregnancy is a relative contraindication to bromocriptine therapy. Women harboring tumors larger than 12 mm who wish to conceive are often referred for tumor resection prior to pregnancy to avoid pregnancy-induced enlargement of the tumor and neurologic symptoms. In women with tumors smaller than 12 mm, the risk of neurologic dysfunction during pregnancy is less than 1%.[35]

Bromocriptine has greatly limited the indications for transsphenoidal resection of prolactinomas. Surgery is usually reserved for patients who are either completely intolerant or show zero to minimal response to medical therapy, patients with severe or worsening visual field deficits, and patients with deficits that do not improve after 2 months of medical therapy (Fig. 34.8).[36]

Radiation therapy has a very limited role in the treatment of prolactinomas. Primary radiation therapy is reserved for elderly or debilitated patients who have large tumors that threaten vital neurovascular structures and who are not adequately helped by medical therapy. Secondary radiation therapy as an adjunct to transsphenoidal surgery is indicated in patients with residual tumor who are unresponsive to or intolerant of bromocriptine.

Pretreatment with bromocriptine to "shrink" the tumor has been suggested to increase the surgical cure rate.[37,38] Thus far, there has been no appreciable benefit. If surgery is contemplated, it is best performed within a year of bromocriptine therapy. Long-term bromocriptine use has been associated with tumor fibrosis, making surgical resection more difficult.[39,40]

Do all patients with prolactinomas require treatment of some sort? There is a subset of patients with so-called asymptomatic microprolactinomas whose treatment remains controversial. Both tumor size and serum prolactin levels may remain unchanged or even decrease over many years in some women with microprolactino-

mas who receive no treatment.[41,42] Aside from regular surveillance it would not appear that any treatment is indicated. Some reports favor treatment to normalize prolactin and thereby decrease the future risks of osteoporosis.[43,44] This is still being studied.

GROWTH-HORMONE-SECRETING ADENOMAS (ACROMEGALY)

Acromegaly or gigantism results from the hypersecretion of growth hormone (GH), and although it was described before the turn of the century, Cushing is

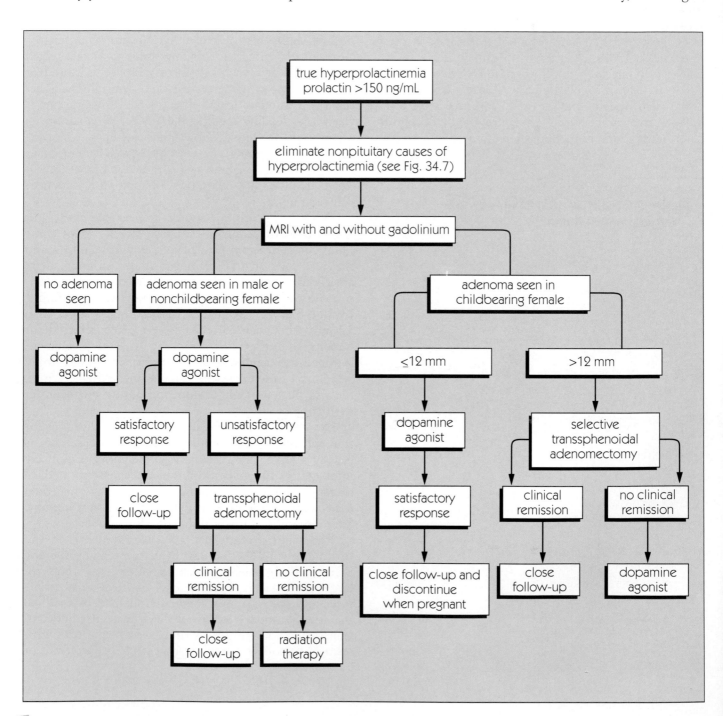

Figure 34.8 Management of prolactinomas.

Principles of Neurosurgery

credited with relating it to the overproduction of growth hormone from a pituitary source.[45] GH is a polypeptide hormone, 191 amino acids long, normally produced and released by the somatotropic cells found in the anterior pituitary in response to hypothalamic GRF.[46] Somatostatin is a 14-amino-acid cyclic peptide-releasing factor that inhibits GH release.[47] Three or four bursts of GH secretion occur per day, punctuating a basal state of minimal activity.[48] Sleep, physical exertion or stress, hyper- and hypoglycemia, and a variety of pharmacologic agents may also precipitate GH release. Circulating GH results in the secretion from the liver of a family of peptides called somatomedins. Somatomedin-C (insulin-like growth factor I) is the most familiar somatomedin measured in clinical practice. These secondary hormones, in turn, produce a variety of anabolic effects throughout the body and mediate the effects of GH at the end-organ level. Unlike GH, the somatomedins do not exhibit significant diurnal variation in serum levels and therefore may be a better means of evaluating patients.[49] To summarize, GH is released in response to GRF from the hypothalamus, leading to increased levels and activity of somatomedin-C (insulin-like growth factor I), which, in turn, negatively feeds back to limit the production of GH. In addition, GH secretion is tightly regulated by somatostatin.

Hypersecretion of growth hormone may result from a number of conditions. The most common, and the focus of this section, is a pituitary adenoma. However, GH may also be produced by ectopic adenomas derived from remnants of the embryonic pituitary diverticulum or from tumors of the breast, lung, or ovary.[50] Acromegaly may rarely be caused by excessive production of GRF by a hypothalamic tumor or from peripheral sources such as carcinoid tumors of the abdomen.[51]

SIGNS AND SYMPTOMS

Acromegaly affects males and females equally, most often in the fifth decade.[52] The effects of chronically elevated growth hormone are gradual and will result either in gigantism in a child whose epiphyseal plates have not yet closed or in classic acromegalic features in an adult. Typically there is an insidious coarsening of the facial features and an increase in the soft tissues. A significant number of patients present, not because of somatic disturbances, but because of local compressive effects of an expanding pituitary mass. The somatic changes may be so insidious as to go unnoticed until old snapshots are used for comparison. Classically patients first note an increase in shoe size or inability to wear rings that previously fit well. Later in the disease process patients may develop visceromegaly, arthralgias, nerve entrapment syndromes, hyperhidrosis, prognathism, and acrochordon (skin tags). The development of skin tags is interesting and deserves some com-

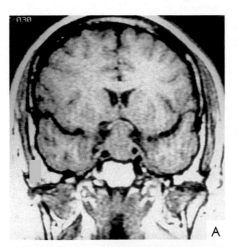
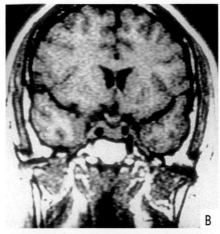

Figure 34.9 (A) Prebromocriptine coronal MRI demonstrating a large prolactin-secreting pituitary adenoma. The chiasm (white arc above tumor) is distorted. (B) Coronal MRI of same patient after 4 months of bromocriptine therapy. Note the dramatic decrease in the size of the tumor. The chiasm is no longer compressed.

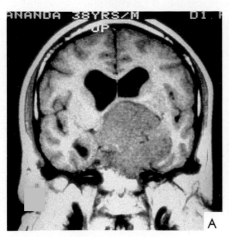
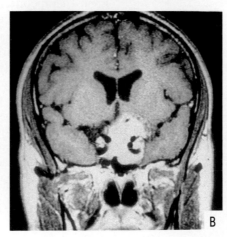

Figure 34.10 (A) Prebromocriptine MRI demonstrating enormous prolactin-secreting pituitary adenoma with hydrocephalus. (B) The same patient 2 years later, treated only with bromocriptine. The tumor is dramatically smaller and the hydrocephalus is resolved.

ment because of its relationship to potentially malignant colonic polyps. It has been noted in several studies that as many as 46% of patients with acromegaly will have colonic polyps, of which more than 50% are adenomatous.[53] Some studies have also shown that the incidence of true colon carcinoma in acromegalics may be higher than in the general population. Because of this relationship it has been recommended that acromegalic patients older than 50 years, patients with more than a 10-year history of acromegaly, or patients with more than three skin tags should have careful screening for colonic disease.[54]

DIAGNOSIS

The laboratory diagnosis of acromegaly is hampered by the normally wide daily variations in serum GH levels. In fact, the daily bursts of secretion are maintained even in the presence of oversecretion of GH from an adenoma. Unlike the other secretory adenomas, static measurements of serum GH are, therefore, unreliable in establishing the diagnosis of acromegaly. Normal basal GH levels are generally below 1 ng/mL, with several secretory bursts seen throughout the day.[55] In acromegaly the basal level is often elevated to levels above 5 ng/mL, although some patients may have normal basal levels with elevations only during the daily secretory bursts (Fig. 34.11).

Fortunately, somatomedin-C levels not only are even throughout the day, but are consistently elevated in acromegaly. Static measurements of somatomedin-C are an effective and reliable method for confirming the diagnosis of acromegaly.[56,57] Alternatively, a glucose tolerance test can be performed. Normally, GH is suppressed to levels below 2 ng/mL after an oral glucose load (100 g). Failure of this normal suppression is consistent with hypersecretion of GH. In addition, infusions of either GRF or TRH will lead to increased GH in affected individuals but not in normal subjects.

Once a patient is confirmed as having a hypersecre-

Figure 34.11 Diagnosis of Acromegaly

Usual Studies
Plasma GH
Response to oral glucose (GTT)
CT or MRI

Other Studies
Somatomedin-C
Response to TRH
GRF

---

tory state, the goal is to discover the source. The overwhelming majority of patients will have an anterior pituitary adenoma and, therefore, the radiographic work-up should begin with a contrast-enhanced MRI. Only in the few cases where no pituitary mass is demonstrated should a search be made for ectopic sources of growth hormone.

TREATMENT

The effects of untreated acromegaly are eventually fatal. Patients will develop cardiac failure, diabetes, disfigurement, and possibly blindness, leading to a markedly shortened life expectancy.[58] The goal of treatment, therefore, is the safe and rapid reduction of GH levels, elimination of any mass effect, and preservation of normal hormonal balance. The type of treatment must be judged on its ability to normalize GH levels and thereby to eliminate the development of the various metabolic derangements associated with hypersecretory states. The criteria for successful treatment of acromegaly are quite controversial. The accepted postoperative levels of GH that are indicative of a cure have declined in recent years. The current standard for cure is clinical remission associated with a postoperative GH level of less than 5 ng/mL with a normal somatomedin-C level.[59] Growth hormone levels may return to normal in hours or days, but it has been our experience that somatomedin-C levels may take weeks or months to normalize. Postoperative adjuvant therapy should be reserved for patients who do not meet these criteria (Fig. 34.12).

Transsphenoidal resection remains the primary treatment modality for acromegaly (Fig. 34.13). Successful resection results in a rapid reduction in GH levels and can be achieved with very low morbidity and mortality, even in older patients.[3,60–65] In addition, the preservation of pituitary function has been reported to be as high as 95%, avoiding the need for lifelong hormone replacement. For larger tumors not amenable to curative resection, surgery still plays a significant role in reducing tumor load prior to any adjuvant therapy.

While transsphenoidal resection of pituitary adenomas is a safe and well tolerated procedure, there are still many patients who simply are not surgical candidates. In those cases medical treatment and radiotherapy have great therapeutic importance. The medical treatment of acromegalics has undergone considerable change in the past 10 to 15 years. Medical therapy, which included estrogens, chlorpromazine, and antiserotonergic agents, had met with only limited success. Bromocriptine therapy, then used for its dopaminergic effects, was able to reduce GH levels to 5 to 10 ng/mL in more than 20% of patients.[66–70] Most patients did achieve some relief of their somatic symptomatology, with reduced soft-tissue swelling and decreased perspiration, even though GH levels were still elevated. The dosages necessary to achieve these effects are much higher than the dosages needed to control a prolactinoma and the consequent incidence of side effects and drug intolerance is much higher.

Since somatostatin naturally suppresses GH production, the ideal would be to give somatostatin; however, this would require multiple administrations each day for life because of somatostatin's short half-life (2 minutes). A recently developed somatostatin analogue named octreotide has a longer half-life and has been shown to be very effective.[71–79] It must be administered three times each day as a subcutaneous injection or as a continuous subcutaneous infusion. The most common side effects reported include diarrhea and cholelithiasis,[80] and the incidence of these side effects increases the

longer the drug is administered. Some recent studies have shown dramatic reductions in GH levels and moderate tumor shrinkage. The perioperative period may be significantly improved by using octreotide for 3 to 4 months preoperatively. The soft-tissue changes about the tongue and throat may lessen the risks of anesthesia.

The only other treatment option for patients is radiation therapy. Not only is this treatment fraught with difficulties such as hypopituitarism in up to 25% and radiation necrosis, but it has not been shown to be uniformly effective.[81] Many patients will have persistently elevated GH levels for years following radiation therapy and may never reach normal levels, resulting in delayed or incomplete remission.[82]

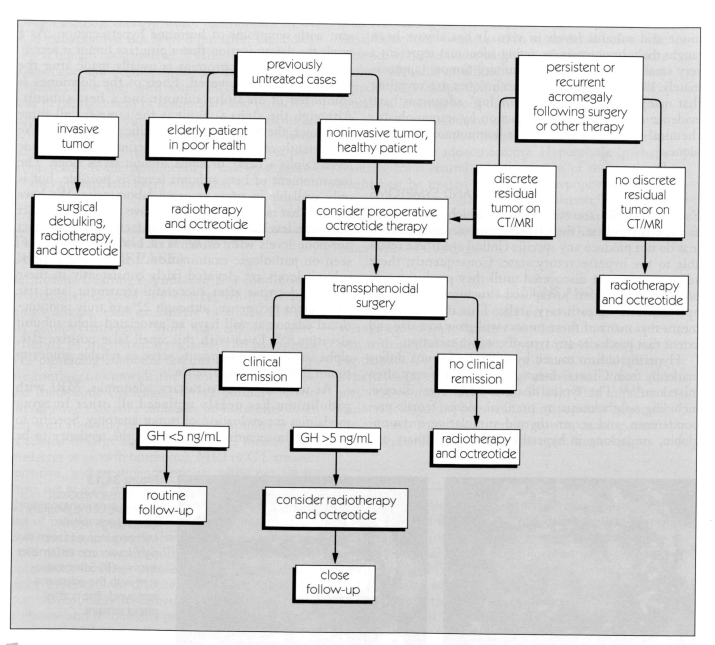

Figure 34.12 Management of acromegaly. (Adapted from Contemporary Neurosurgery)

tion, cortisol levels normally increase any time the body is subjected to stress, either physical or metabolic. Cortisol then negatively feeds back to reduce ACTH secretion. Since ACTH is difficult to measure clinically, circulating levels of cortisol or its urinary metabolites are used to diagnose states of adrenal excess.

While Cushing's syndrome is usually easy to recognize clinically, it is not always so easy to define etiologically. The various diagnostic testing protocols have been extensively reviewed and appear to be always increasing.[102,104,107,111-123] Measurements of plasma and urinary cortisol and cortisol derivatives, basally and in response to dexamethasone or metryapone, as well as determination of plasma ACTH, may suggest either a primary adrenal, pituitary, or ectopic neoplastic source of disease (Fig. 34.15).[118,124] If these data are equivocal, CRH measurements[105,106,114,125] and CRH stimulation testing with measurement of ACTH and/or cortisol[101,111,112,116,117,122] peripherally or in the bilateral venous effluent from the petrosal sinuses,[115,119,121,123] are now frequently employed to provide additional biochemical evidence for the diagnosis of Cushing's disease (Fig. 34.15).

Once it has been determined that a patient has a pituitary source of ACTH hypersecretion (Cushing's disease) it can be extremely difficult to identify the pituitary source. Since most ACTH-producing adenomas are small, their radiographic detection is difficult at best. Improvements in MRI with gadolinium enhancement have identified many microadenomas that would otherwise be radiographically invisible. Because many cases have no evidence of tumor on the MRI, the technique of petrosal sinus sampling has been developed to confirm the diagnosis and guide the surgical resection. The rationale behind this technique, which has been described in detail elsewhere, is quite straightforward (Fig. 34.16).[121] Patients with Cushing's disease should have high (or inappropriately high) levels of ACTH production coming directly from the pituitary gland,[115] and the levels should lateralize[121,123] to the side containing the adenoma. Comparison of pituitary to peripheral ACTH levels should demonstrate a gradient. Those with ectopic ACTH secretion whose pituitary glands are suppressed should have neither an elevated pituitary-to-peripheral gradient nor a difference between sides. Patients without a discrete pituitary tumor (i.e., with hyperplasia of the corticotrophs) may have an increased central level of ACTH that is equal in blood from both sides of the gland. Some have advocated petrosal sinus sampling in all patients with ACTH-dependent disease, either to supplement or to supplant the conventional methods for establishing the etiology of the hypercortisolism.[111,119,124] Published series indicate that the usefulness and reliability of this technique may be variable.

In Mampalam's series,[97] 39 of 116 subjects (34%) had selective venous sampling of ACTH. An inferior petrosal sinus to peripheral gradient was seen in 36. Of these 36, 31 (86%) were found to have adenomas. In 3 patients without a significant gradient, 2 had adenomas. Nine percent had false localization as to the side of the adenoma. In Ludecke's series,[120] 6 of 19 (31%) had incorrect lateralization of the adenoma by inferior petrosal sinus sampling. Ludecke recommended intraoperative measurement of ACTH in the peripituitary blood as a means of lateralizing the adenoma. In our institution, we use the technique in the following situations:

1. Patients with equivocal lab data, if doubt exists as to the source of ACTH overproduction, and radiographic studies are not helpful.
2. Patients with laboratory data clearly pointing to the pituitary gland but with normal radiographic studies. A petrosal-sinus-directed hemihypophysectomy is done if an adenoma is not seen at surgery.
3. Young patients, especially women, for whom preservation of fertility is an important consideration and whose radiologic studies are not grossly abnormal. Even when the lab studies clearly indicate pituitary-dependent disease, we routinely study these patients to lateralize the tumor. If nothing is found at the time of surgery, hemihypophysectomy on the side with the higher CRH-stimulated ACTH levels would then be done.

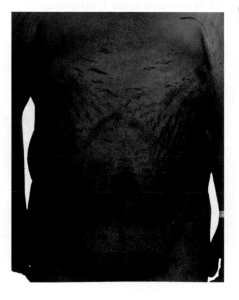

Figure 34.14
Patient demonstrating cushingoid changes.

Figure 34.15 Diagnosis of Cushing's Disease

Usual Studies
Plasma and urinary free cortisol—baseline and response to dexamethasone
Plasma ACTH
MRI

Other Studies
CRH stimulation test
Petrosal sinus ACTH sampling with CRH stimulation

4. Patients who have not been cured following transsphenoidal surgery. In these patients the question to be answered is whether the diagnosis of Cushing's disease, which had obviously been thought sound enough to justify the initial surgery, was truly correct. Lack of a gradient would suggest ectopic production.

In the most skilled hands, this sampling of venous effluent from the petrosal sinuses appears to be reliable and safe. Because of our experience with false lateralization and inability to cannulate both sides simultaneously (problems that are less frequent as we do more procedures), we consider the information gained from the study along with, not in place of, the more conventionally acquired data.

TREATMENT

The treatment of Cushing's disease has been advanced significantly by the development and refinement of transsphenoidal pituitary microsurgery (Fig. 34.17). The dramatic results of selective adenomectomy include immediate reversal of hypercortisolism and eventual return of normal pituitary corticotroph function.

As will be discussed below, most cases of Cushing's disease are caused by isolated adenomas of the anterior gland. In less than 10% of patients with pituitary ACTH excess there occurs basophilic hyperplasia involving the entire gland. The treatment of choice for Cushing's disease advocated by most authorities today is transsphenoidal exploration of the pituitary gland, with either selective adenomectomy or partial or hemihypophysectomy.[94–98,126,127] For those with very large or invasive tumors, most would suggest surgery for diagnosis and debulking, followed by conventional radiation therapy, medications, and, rarely, adrenalectomy. We

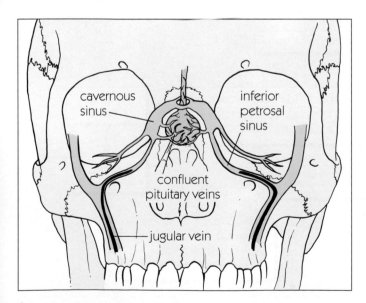

Figure 34.16 Catheter placement for simultaneous blood sampling of the inferior petrosal sinuses. The confluent pituitary veins empty laterally into the cavernous sinuses, which drain into the inferior petrosal sinuses. (Adapted from Oldfield EH et al, 1985)

have reviewed the larger series published to assess the results of pituitary surgery in patients with Cushing's disease.

Probably because there are different etiologic and pathologic subtypes within the category of Cushing's disease (as discussed under the preceding section), the cure rate for this illness in all series remains under 90%. Repeat surgeries and nonselective partial or total hypophysectomies often must be done to attain those cures. Thus, some controversy exists as to what the initial surgical intervention should be. Some suggest visual exploration of the gland, with removal of abnormal tissue for frozen section; if an adenoma is seen, its selective excision would be the only intervention. If permanent disease remission is not achieved, only then would more extensive surgery be suggested.[97] Others feel that petrosal-sinus-directed or blind partial hemihypophysectomy is a more reasonable initial approach. Because incidental (nonfunctioning) adenomas or small inhomogeneities in the gland are common, the surgeon may be guided toward an abnormal part of the gland that is not responsible for the cushingoid state. Since frozen section is not always reliable, some recommend removal of more than just the grossly abnormal tissue identified intraoperatively. That same type of argument, as well as the controversy over whether a higher source of stimulation (e.g., CRH[128]) is responsible for Cushing's disease, has caused others to suggest total hypophysectomy as the surest way of achieving permanent disease remission.

Recurrence rates from 3.7% to 9.3% have been reported[94,96–98,127,129] and some of these patients have been re-explored. According to Nakane et al.,[98] verification of all pituitary adenomas was done by reoperation, during which no corticotroph cell hyperplasia was found. It was concluded that late recurrence of Cushing's disease may follow adenomectomy due to re-growth of adenoma cells not removed from peritumoral tissue during the original surgery. The alternative explanation, of course, is that the primary etiologic event was not an isolated pituitary tumor but rather overstimulation; thus, as remaining pituitary tissue continues to be overstimulated, relapse is inevitable.

Friedman et al.[130] studied the efficacy of repeat surgery for recurrent or persistent Cushing's disease. The incidence of remission of hypercortisolism was greatest if an adenoma was identified at surgery and the patient received selective adenomectomy.

Patients who are not cured by selective resection fall into several groups: 1) those with invasive adenomas, 2) those with unidentified microadenomas, 3) those with corticotroph hyperplasia without a discrete adenoma, and 4) those with ectopic secretion of ACTH or CRH. Those with lateral invasive extension will not be cured by any surgical procedure and, therefore, hypophysectomy is not a consideration. Patients with microadenomas that are unidentified preoperatively are often cured by partial or total hypophysectomy; the microadenomas may be discovered within the excised tissue. If surgery has completely removed the tumor, the patient will be hypocortisolemic for 3 to 6 months. Patients who are eucortisolemic immediately postoperatively have a high incidence of recurrence.[131,132]

While transsphenoidal resection remains the primary procedure of choice, as illustrated above, it does not carry a 100% success rate. There are other treatment modalities available for use as adjuvants for those cases in which initial or repeat surgical therapy has failed.

Stereotactic radiation has been used alone or in combination with surgery for the treatment of Cushing's disease[133,134]; reports on its efficacy (cure rates) vary from 50% to 100%. Because of the length of time needed to effect a cure and because of the high incidence of hypopituitarism, we currently suggest that radiation therapy be used only when pituitary surgery has failed.

In addition to radiotherapy, there are a number of medical therapies available. One immediate drawback to medical therapy for Cushing's disease is that all currently available medications block ACTH or cortisol production; in doing so, however, they treat symptoms rather than abolish the tumor, and often ameliorate them incompletely and at a high price in terms of unpleasant and potentially dangerous side effects.

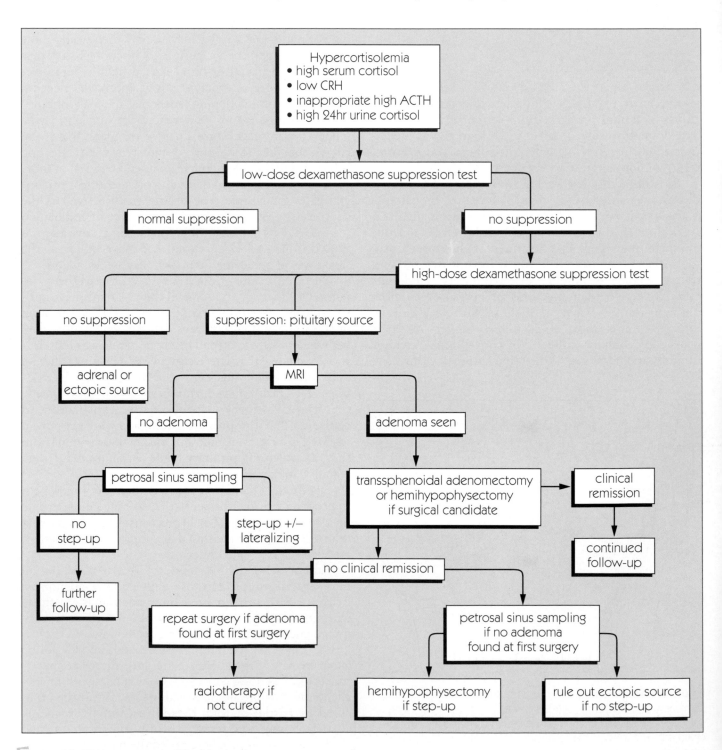

Figure 34.17 Management of Cushing's disease.

Ketoconazole, a potent antifungal agent, inhibits adrenal steroidogenesis by blocking the 11β-hydroxylase (and other enzymes involved in both cortisol and testosterone production as well). It is generally well tolerated, although sedation is not uncommon. While it may be possible to titrate the dose carefully to achieve eucortisolemia, this may be difficult. Often, the aim is to achieve complete adrenal suppression, at which time supplemental steroid treatment is begun.[135,136] Because several steps in steroid production are halted, effects on cholesterol, vitamin D, mineralocorticoid, and estrogen and androgen production need to be evaluated more closely before ketoconazole's use on a long-term basis should be recommended. We often use this drug if there is to be a delay between diagnosis and treatment, or if precise etiologic diagnosis is in doubt (depression versus mild Cushing's) and some interim treatment is desirable.

Cyproheptadine is a drug that has antiserotonin (as well as antihistamine and anticholinergic) effects that Krieger et al.[128] have suggested may make it useful in modulating ACTH release. Experience with this drug has been disappointing.

Bromocriptine, which is very specifically useful in decreasing prolactin production and in shrinking prolactin-producing tumors, has also been given to patients with other pituitary adenomas.[110] Its effectiveness with such tumors is variable but certainly much lower than with prolactinomas. Recent reports suggest that bromocriptine, with or without cyproheptadine, can normalize cortisol production in patients with Cushing's syndrome.[110] In particular, patients with intermediate-lobe Cushing's disease, who often have concomitant elevations of prolactin levels, may do well with bromocriptine treatment. The side effects of the drug, including fatigue, nausea, anorexia, and orthostatic lightheadedness, vary but may be considerable.

Because many of these drugs are quite costly, have significant side effects, and must be taken continuously to be effective, their usefulness in the treatment of a disease that most large centers cure with transsphenoidal adenomectomy in 85% to 90% of patients will likely remain limited.

CONCLUSION

As illustrated above, patients with functioning pituitary adenomas pose very different management problems and decisions than do patients with nonfunctioning adenomas. The issue of medical versus surgical treatment is ever-present in the management of this group of patients. One must weigh all the factors such as age, medical condition, and tumor size before choosing any course of action. The most important thing to remember in the management of these patients is that they require meticulous follow-up for evidence of tumor regrowth regardless of the treatment plan chosen.

REFERENCES

1. Reichlin S. Anatomical and physiological basis of hypothalamic-pituitary regulation. In: Post KD, Jackson IMD, Reichlin S, eds. *The Pituitary Adenoma.* New York, NY: Plenum Medical Book Co, 1980:3–28.

2. Klibanski A. Nonsecreting pituitary tumors. *Endocrinol Metab Clin North Am.* 1987;16:793–804.

3. Hardy J, Somma M. Acromegaly: surgical treatment by transsphenoidal microsurgical removal of the pituitary adenoma. In: Tindall GT, Collins WF, eds. *Clinical Management of Pituitary Disorders.* New York, NY: Raven Press; 1979:209–217.

4. Litt AW, Kricheff II. Magnetic resonance imaging of pituitary tumors. In: Cooper PR, ed. *Contemporary Diagnosis and Management of Pituitary Adenomas.* Illinois: Am Assoc of Neurologic Surgeons; 1991:1–19.

5. Macpherson P, Hadley DM, Teasdale E, et al. Pituitary microadenomas: does gadolinium enhance their demonstration? *Neuroradiology.* 1989; 31:293–298.

6. Kulkarni MV, Lee KF, McArdle CB, et al. 1.5T MR imaging of pituitary microadenomas: technical considerations and CT correlation. *AJNR.* 1988;9:5–11.

7. Doppman JL, Frank JA, Dwyer AJ, et al. Gadolinium DTPA enhanced MR imaging of ACTH-secreting microadenomas of the pituitary gland. *J Comput Assist Tomogr.* 1988;12:728–735.

8. Marcovitz S, Wee R, Chan J, et al. The diagnostic accuracy of preoperative CT scanning in the evaluation of pituitary ACTH-secreting adenomas. *AJR.* 1987;149:803–806.

9. Marcovitz S, Wee R, Chan J, et al. Diagnostic accuracy of preoperative scanning of pituitary prolactinomas. *AJNR.* 1988;9:13–17.

10. Marcovitz S, Wee R, Chan J, et al. Diagnostic accuracy of preoperative CT scanning of pituitary somatotroph adenomas. *AJNR.* 1988;9:19–22.

11. Davis PC, Hoffman JC Jr, Tindall GT, et al. Prolactin-secreting pituitary microadenomas: inaccuracy of high-resolution CT imaging. *AJR.* 1985; 144:1541–156.

12. Frantz AG. Prolactin. *N Engl J Med.* 1978;298: 201–207.

13. Jaquet P, Guibout M, Lucioni J, et al. Hypothalamopituitary regulation of prolactin in hypersecreting prolactinoma. In: Robyn C, Harter M, eds. *Progress in Prolactin, Physiology and Pathology.* New York, NY: Elsevier-North Holland Biochemical Press; 1978:371–382.

14. Boyd AE III, Reichlin S. Neural control of pro-

lactin secretion in man. *Psychoneuroendocrinology.* 1978;3:113–130.

15. Kleinberg DL, Noel GL, Frantz AG. Galactorrhea: a study of 235 cases including 48 with pituitary tumors. *N Engl J Med.* 1977;296:589–600.

16. Goodman RH, Molitch MD, Post KD, Jackson, IMD. Prolactin secreting adenomas in the male. In: Post KD, Jackson IMD, Reichlin S, eds. *The Pituitary Adenoma.* New York, NY: Plenum Press; 1980:91–108.

17. Thorner MO, McNeilly AS, Hagan C, Besser GM. Long-term treatment of galactorrhea and hypogonadism with bromocriptine. *Br Med J.* 1974; 2:419–422.

18. Vance ML, Evans WS, Thorner MO. Bromocriptine. *Ann Intern Med.* 1984;100:78–91.

19. Zarate A, Canales ES, Cano C, Pilonieta CJ. Follow-up of patients with prolactinomas after discontinuation of long-term therapy with bromocriptine. *Acta Endocrinol (Copenh).* 1983;104:139–142.

20. Molitch ME, Elton RL, Blackwell RE, et al. Bromocriptine as primary therapy for prolactin-secreting macroadenomas: results of a prospective multicenter study. *J Clin Endocrinol Metab.* 1985; 60:698–705.

21. Thorner MO, Martin WH, Rogol AD, et al. Rapid regression of pituitary prolactinomas during bromocriptine treatment. *J Clin Endocrinol Metab.* 1980;51:438–445.

22. Tindall GT, Kovacs K, Horvath E, et al. Human prolactin-producing adenomas and bromocriptine: a histological, immunocytochemical, ultrastructural, and morphometric study. *J Clin Endocrinol Metab.* 1982;55:1178–1183.

23. Barrow DL, Tindall GT, Kovacs K, et al. Clinical and pathological effects of bromocriptine on prolactin-secreting and other pituitary tumors. *J Neurosurg.* 1984;60:1–7.

24. Barrow DL, Mizuno J, Tindall GT. Management of prolactinomas associated with very high serum prolactin levels. *J Neurosurg.* 1988;68:554–558.

25. Molitch ME, Reichlin S. Hyperprolactinemic disorders. *Dis Mon.* June 1982;28:1–58.

26. Reichlin S. The prolactinoma problem. *N Engl J Med.* 1979;300:313–315.

27. Thorner MO, Schran HF, Evans WS, et al. A broad spectrum of prolactin suppression by bromocriptine in hyperprolactinemic women: a study of serum prolactin and bromocriptine levels after acute and chronic administration of bromocriptine. *J Clin Endocrinol Metab.* 1980; 50:1026–1033.

28. Thorner MO, Edwards CRW, Charlesworth M, et al. Pregnancy in patients presenting with hyperprolactinemia. *Br Med J.* 1979;2:771–774.

29. Tindall GT, Barrow DL, Tindall SC. Current management of pituitary tumors, II. *Contemp Neurosurg.* 1988;10:1–6.

30. Vance ML, Cragun JR, Reimnitz C, et al. CV 205-502 treatment of hyperprolactinemia. *J Clin Endocrinol Metab.* 1989;68:336–339.

31. Wang C, Lam KSL, Ma JTC, et al. Long-term treatment of hyperprolactinaemia with bromocriptine: effect of drug withdrawal. *Clin Endocrinol (Oxf).* 1987;27:363–371.

32. Thorner MO, Perryman RL, Rogol AD, et al. Rapid changes of prolactinoma volume after withdrawal and reinstitution of bromocriptine. *J Clin Endocrinol Metab.* 1981;53:480–483.

33. Liuzzi A, Dallabonzana D, Oppizzi G, et al. Low doses of dopamine agonists in the long-term treatment of macroprolactinomas. *N Engl J Med.* 1985; 313:656–659.

34. Kleinberg DL, Boyd AE III, Wardlaw S, et al. Pergolide for the treatment of pituitary tumors secreting prolactin or growth hormone. *N Engl J Med.* 1983;309:704–709.

35. Molitch ME. Pregnancy and the hyperprolactinemic woman. *N Engl J Med.* 1985;312:1364–1370.

36. Post KD. Surgical approaches to the treatment of prolactinomas. In: Olefsky JM, Robbins RJ, eds. *Prolactinomas: Practical Diagnosis and Management.* New York, NY: Churchill Livingstone; 1986: 159–194.

37. Fahlbusch R, Buchfelder M, Schrell U. Short-term preoperative treatment of macroprolactinomas by dopamine agonists. *J Neurosurg.* 1987;67:807–815.

38. Hubbard JL, Scheithauer BW, Abboud CF, Laws ER Jr. Prolactin-secreting ademonas: the preoperative response to bromocriptine treatment and surgical outcome. *J Neurosurg.* 1987;67:816–821.

39. Landolt AM, Osterwalder V. Perivascular fibrosis in prolactinomas: is it increased by bromocriptine? *J Clin Endocrinol Metab.* 1984;58:1179–1183.

40. Landolt AM, Keller PJ, Froesch ER, et al. Bromocriptine: does it jeopardize the result of later surgery for prolactinomas? *Lancet.* 1982;2:657.

41. Weiss MH, Teal J, Gott P, et al. Natural history of microprolactinomas: six-year follow-up. *Neurosurgery.* 1983;12:180–183.

42. Sisam DA, Sheehan JP, Sheeler LR. The natural history of untreated microprolactinoma. *Fertil Steril.* 1987;48:67–71.

43. Klibanski A, Greenspan SL. Increase in bone mass after treatment of hyperprolactinemic amenorrhea. *N Engl J Med.* 1986;315:542–546.

44. Klibanski A, Biller BMK, Rosenthal DI, Schoenfeld DA, Saxe V. Effects of prolactin and estrogen deficiency in amenorrheic bone loss. *J Clin Endocrinol Metab.* 1988;67:124–130.

45. Cushing H. Partial hypophysectomy for acromegaly, with remarks on the function of the hypophysis. *Ann Surg.* 1909;50:1002–1017.

46. Lewis UJ, Singh RN, Tutwiler GF, Sigel MB, Vanderlaan EF, Vanderlaan WP. Human growth hormone: a complex of proteins. *Recent Prog Horm Res.* 1980;36:477–508.

47. Reichlin S. Somatostatin. *N Engl J Med.* 1983; 309:1495–1501.

48. Vance ML, Kaiser DL, Evans WS, et al. Pulsatile growth hormone secretion in normal man during a

continuous 24-hour infusion of human growth hormone releasing factor (1-40): evidence for intermittent somatostatin secretion. *J Clin Invest.* 1985; 75:1584–1590.

49. Van Wyk JJ. The somatomedins: biological actions and physiologic control mechanisms. In: Li CH, ed. *Growth Factors.* New York, NY: Academic Press; 1984:81–125. Hormonal proteins and peptides, Vol 12.

50. Frohman LA, Szabo M, Berelowitz, Stachura ME. Partial purification and acharacterization of a peptide with growth hormone-releasing activity from extrapituitary tumors in patients with acromegaly. *J Clin Invest.* 1980;65:43–54.

51. Melmed S, Ziel FH, Braunstein GD, Downs T, Frohman LA. Medical management of acromegaly due to ectopic production of growth hormone-releasing hormone by a carcinoid tumor. *J Clin Endocrinol Metab.* 1988;67:395–399.

52. Melmed S. Acromegaly. *N Engl J Med.* 1990; 322:966–977.

53. Klein I, Parveen G, VanThiel DH. Colonic polyps in patients with acromegaly. *Ann Intern Med.* 1982;97:27–30.

54. Leavitt J, Klein I, Kendricks F, Gavaler J, VanThiel DH. Skin tags: a cutaneous marker for colonic polyps. *Ann Intern Med.* 1983;98:928–930.

55. Thorner MO, Vance ML. Growth hormone, 1988. *J Clin Invest.* 1988;82:745–747.

56. Clemmons DR, Van Wyk JJ, Ridgway EC, Kliman B, Kjellberg RN, Underwood LE. Evaluation of acromegaly by radioimmunoassay of somatomedin-C. *N Engl J Med.* 1979;301:1138–1142.

57. Barkan AI, Beitins IZ, Kelch RP. Plasma insulin-like growth factor-1/somatomedin-C in acromegaly: correlation with the degree of growth hormone hypersecretion. *J Clin Endocrinol Metab.* 1988;67:69–73.

58. Wright AD, Hill DM, Lowy C, Fraser TR. Mortality in acromegaly. *Q J Med.* 1970;39:1–16.

59. Baumann G. Acromegaly. *Endocrinol Metab Clin North Am.* 1987;16:685–703.

60. Ross DA, Wilson CB. Results of transsphenoidal microsurgery for growth hormone-secreting pituitary adenomas in a series of 214 patients. *J Neurosurg.* 1988;68:854–867.

61. Grisoli F, Leclercq T, Jaquet P, et al. Transsphenoidal surgery for acromegaly—long-term results in 100 patients. *Surg Neurol.* 1986;25:513–519.

62. Serri O, Somma M, Comtois R, et al. Acromegaly: biochemical assessment of cure after long-term follow-up of transsphenoidal selective adenomectomy. *J Clin Endocrinol Metab.* 1985;61:1185–1189.

63. Roelfsema F, van Dulken H, Frolich M. Long-term results of transsphenoidal pituitary microsurgery in 60 acromegalic patients. *Clin Endocrinol (Oxf).* 1985;23:555–565.

64. Ludecke DK, Saeger W, William T. Effectiveness of microsurgery in acromegaly: study of 210 cases. *Periodicum Biologorum.* 1983;85:59–66.

65. Laws ER Jr, Randall RV, Abboud CF. Surgical treatment of acromegaly: results in 140 patients. In: Givens J, ed. *Hormone-Secreting Pituitary Tumors.* Chicago, Ill: Year Book Medical Publishers; 1982: 225–228.

66. Liuzzi A, Chiodini PG, Botalla A, Cremascoli G, Muller EE, Silvestrini F. Decreased plasma growth hormone (GH) levels in acromegalics following CB 154 (2-Br-alpha-ergocriptine) administration. *J Clin Endocrinol Metab.* 1974;38:910–912.

67. Lindholm J, Riishede J, Verstergaard S, Hummer L, Faber O, Hagen C. No effect of bromocriptine in acromegaly: a controlled trial. *N Engl J Med.* 1981;304:1450–1454.

68. Wass JAH, Thorner MO, Morris DV, et al. Long-term treatment of acromegaly with bromocriptine. *Br Med J.* 1977;1:875–878.

69. Bell P, Atkinson AB, Hadden DR, et al. Bromocriptine reduces growth hormone in acromegaly. *Arch Intern Med.* 1986;146:1145–1149.

70. Besser GM, Wass JAH, Thorner MO. Acromegaly—results of long-term treatment with bromocriptine. *Acta Endocrinol Suppl (Copenh).* 1978;88(suppl 216):187–198.

71. Lamberts SWJ, Zweens M, Verschoor L, del Pozo E. A comparison among the growth hormone-lowering effects in acromegaly of the somatostatin analog SMS 201-995, bromocriptine, and the combination of both drugs. *J Clin Endocrinol Metab.* 1986;63:16–19.

72. Halse J, Harris AG, Kvistborg A, et al. A randomized study of SMS 201-995 versus bromocriptine treatment in acromegaly: clinical and biochemical effects. *J Clin Endocrinol Metab.* 1990;70: 1254–1261.

73. Chiodini PG, Cozi R, Dallabonzana D, et al. Medical treatment of acromegaly with SMS 201-995, a somatostatin analog: a comparison with bromocriptine. *J Clin Endocrinol Metab.* 1987; 64:447–453.

74. Lamberts SW. The role of somatostatin in the regulation of anterior pituitary hormone secretion and the use of its analogs in the treatment of human pituitary tumors. *Endocr Rev.* 1988; 9:417–436.

75. Kohler PO. Treatment of pituitary adenomas. *N Engl J Med.* 1987;317:45–46.

76. Lamberts SWJ, Uitterlinden P, Verschoor L, van Dongen KJ, del Pozo E. Long-term treatment of acromegaly with the somatostatin analogue SMS 201-995. *N Engl J Med.* 1985;313:1576–1580.

77. Comi RJ, Gorden P. The response of serum growth hormone levels to the long-acting somatostatin analog SMS 201-995 in acromegaly. *J Clin Endocrinol Metab.* 1987;64:37–42.

78. Barnard LB, Grantham WG, Lambewrton P, O'Dorsio TM, Jackson IMD. Treatment of resistant acromegaly with a long-acting somatostatin analogue (SMS 201-995). *Ann Intern Med.* 1986; 105:856–861.

79. Harris AG, Prestele H, Herold K, et al. Long-term efficacy of Sandostatin (SMS 201-995, octreotide) in 178 acromegalic patients: results from the International Multicentre Acromegaly Study Group. In: Lamberts SWJ, ed. *Sandostatin in the Treatment of Acromegaly.* New York, NY: Springer-Verlag; 1988: 117–125.

80. Ho KY, Weissberger AJ, Marbach P, Lazarus L. Therapeutic efficacy of the somatostatin analog SMS 201-995 (octrotide) in acromegaly: effects of dose and frequency and long-term safety. *Ann Intern Med.* 1990;112:173–181.

81. Snyder PJ, Fowble BF, Schatz NJ, Savino PJ, Gennarelli TA. Hypopituitarism following radiation therapy of pituitary adenomas. *Am J Med.* 1986;81:457–462.

82. Eastman RC, Gorden P, Roth J. Conventional supervoltage irradiation is an effective treatment for acromegaly. *J Clin Endocrinol Metab.* 1979; 48:931–940.

83. Smallridge RC. Thyrotropin-secreting pituitary tumors. *Endocrinol Metab Clin North Am.* 1987; 16:765–792.

84. Smallridge RC, Smith CE. Hyperthyroidism due to thyrotropin-secreting pituitary tumors: diagnostic and therapeutic consideration. *Arch Intern Med.* 1983;143:503–507.

85. Snyder PJ, Johnson J, Muzyka R. Abnormal secretion of glycoprotein alpha-subunit and follicle stimulating hormone (FSH) beta-subunit in men with pituitary adenomas and FSH hypersecretion. *J Clin Endocrinol Metab.* 1980;51:579–584.

86. Oppenheim DS, Kana AR, Sangha JS, Klibanski A. Prevalence of alpha-subunit hypersecretion in patients with pituitary tumors: clinically nonfunctioning and somatotroph adenomas. *J Clin Endocrinol Metab.* 1990;70:859–864.

87. Kourides IA, Weintraub BD, Rosen SW, Ridgway EC, Kliman B, Maloof F. Secretion of alpha subunit of glycoprotein hormones by pituitary adenomas. *J Clin Endocrinol Metab.* 1976;43:97–106.

88. Snyder PJ. Gonadotroph cell adenomas of the pituitary. *Endocr Rev.* 1985;6:552–563.

89. Ebersold MJ, Quast LM, Laws ER Jr, Scheithauer B, Randall RV. Long-term results in transsphenoidal removal of nonfunctioning pituitary adenomas. *J Neurosurg.* 1986;64:713–719.

90. Comi RJ, Gesundheit N, Murray L, Gorden P, Weintraub BD. Response of thyrotropin-secreting pituitary adenomas to a long-acting somatostatin analogue. *N Engl J Med.* 1987;317:12–17.

91. Burch W. Cushing's disease, a review. *Arch Intern Med.* 1985;145:1106–1111.

92. Burrow GN, Wortzman G, Rewcastle NB, et al. Microadenopmas of the pituitary and abnormal sellar tomograms in an unselected autopsy series. *N Engl J Med.* 1981;304:156–158.

93. Chandler WF, Schteingart DE, Lloyd RV, et al. Surgical treatment of Cushing's disease. *J Neurosurg.* 1987;66:204–212.

94. Fahlbusch R, Buchfelder M, Muller OA. Transsphenoidal surgery for Cushing's disease. *J R Soc Med.* 1986;79:262–269.

95. Guilhaume B, Bertagna X, Thomsen M, et al. Transsphenoidal pituitary surgery for the treatment of Cushing's disease: results in 64 patients and long term follow-up studies. *J Clin Endocrinol Metab.* 1988;66:1056–1064.

96. Hardy J. Cushing's disease: 50 years later. *Can J Neurol Sci.* 1982;2:375–380.

97. Mampalam TJ, Tyrell JB, Wilson CB. Transsphenoidal microsurgery for Cushing's disease. *Ann Intern Med.* 1988;109:487–493.

98. Nakane R, Kuwayama A, Watanabe M, et al. Long-term results of transsphenoidal adenomectomy in patients with Cushing's disease. *Neurosurgery.* 1987;21:218–222.

99. Saris SC, Patronas NJ, Doppman JL, et al. Cushing's syndrome: pituitary CT scanning. *Radiology.* 1987;162:775–777.

100. Dwyer AJ, Frank JA, Doppman JL, et al. Pituitary adenomas in patients with Cushing's disease: initial experience with Gd-DTPA-enhanced MR imaging. *Neuroradiology.* 1987;163:421–426.

101. Newton DR, Dillon WP, Normal D, et al. Gd-DTPA-enhanced MR imaging of pituitary adenomas. *AJNR.* 1989;10:949–954.

102. Orth DN. The old and the new in Cushing's syndrome. *N Engl J Med.* 1984;310:649–651.

103. Case Records of MGH. Case 53–1981. *N Engl J Med.* 1981;305:1637–1643.

104. Suda T, Kondo M, Totani R, et al. Ectopic adrenocorticotropin syndrome caused by lung cancer that responded to corticotropin-releasing hormone. *J Clin Endocrinol Metab.* 1986;63:1047–1051.

105. Case Records of the MGH. Case 52–1987. *N Engl J Med.* 1987;317:1648–1658.

106. Schteingart DE, Lloyd RV, Akil H, et al. Cushing's syndrome secondary to ectopic corticotropin-releasing hormone-adrenocorticotropin secretion. *J Clin Endocrinol Metab.* 1986;63:770–775.

107. Nieman LK, Chrousos GP, Oldfield EH, et al. The ovine corticotropin-releasing hormone stimulation test and the dexamethasone suppression test in the differential diagnosis of Cushing's syndrome. *Ann Intern Med.* 1986;105:862–867.

108. Lloyd RV, Chandler WF, McKeever PE, Schteingart DE. The spectrum of ACTH-producing pitu-

itary lesions. *Am J Surg Pathol.* 1986;10:618–626.

109. Post KD, Habas JE. Cushing's disease. In: Samii M, ed. *Surgery of the Sellar Region and Paranasal Sinuses.* Berlin: Springer-Verlag; 1991:294–301.

110. Reith P, Monnot EA, Bathija PJ. Prolonged suppression of a corticotropin-producing bronchial carcinoid by oral bromocriptine. *Ann Intern Med.* 1987;147:989–991.

111. Chrousos GP, Schulte HM, Oldfiefd EH, et al. The corticotropin-releasing factor stimulation test. *N Engl J Med.* 1984;310:622–626.

112. Chrousos GP, Schuermeyer TH, Doppman JL, et al. Clinical applications of corticotropin-releasing factor. *Ann Intern Med.* 1985;102:344–358.

113. Crapo L. Cushing's syndrome: a review of diagnostic tests. *Metabolism.* 1979;28:955–977.

114. Cunnah D, Jessop DS, Besser GM, Rees LH. Measurement of circulating corticotropin-releasing factor in man. *J Endocrinol.* 1987;113:123–131.

115. Findling JW, Aron DC, Tyrell JB, et al. Selective venous sampling for ACTH in Cushing's syndrome. *Ann Intern Med.* 1981;94:647–652.

116. Fukata J, Nakai Y, Imura H, et al. Human corticotropin-releasing hormone test in normal subjects and patients with hypothalamic, pituitary or adrenocortical disorders. *Endocrinol Jpn.* 1988; 35:491–502.

117. Hermus AR, Pieters GF, Pesman GJ, et al. The corticotropin-releasing hormone test versus the high dose dexamethasone test in the differential diagnosis of Cushing's syndrome. *Lancet.* 1986; 2:540–543.

118. Howlett TA, Drury PL, Perry L, et al. Diagnosis and management of ACTH-dependent Cushing's syndrome: comparison of the features in ectopic and pituitary ACTH production. *Clin Endocrinol (Oxf).* 1986;24:699–713.

119. Landolt AM, Valvanis A, Girard J, Eberle AN. Corticotropin-releasing factor test used with bilateral, simultaneous inferior petrosal sinus blood-sampling for the diagnosis of pituitary-dependent Cushing's disease. *Clin Endocrinol (Oxf).* 1986;25: 687–696.

120. Ludecke DK. Intraoperative measurement of adrenocorticotrophic hormone in peripituitary blood in Cushing's disease. *Neurosurgery.* 1989; 24:201–205.

121. Oldfield EH, Chrousos GP, Schulte HM, et al. Preoperative lateralization of ACTH-secreting pituitary microadenomas by bilateral and simultaneous inferior petrosal venous sinus sampling. *N Engl J Med.* 1985;312:98–103.

122. Schrell U, Fahlbusch R, Buchfelder M, et al. Corticotropin-releasing hormone stimulation test before and after transsphenoidal selective microadenomectomy in 30 patients with Cushing's disease. *J Clin Endocrinol Metab.* 1987;64: 1150–1159.

123. Zovickian J, Oldfield EH, Doppman JL, et al. Usefulness of inferior petrosal sinus venous endocrine markers in Cushing's disease. *J Neurosurg.* 1988; 68:205–210.

124. Findling JW, Tyrell JB. Occult ectopic secretion of corticotropin. *Am J Med.* 1986;146:929–933.

125. Carey RM, Varma SK, Drake CR, et al. Ectopic secretion of corticotropin-releasing factor as a cause of Cushing's syndrome. *N Engl J Med.* 1984; 311:13–20.

126. Boggan JE, Tyrell JB, Wilson CB. Transsphenoidal microsurgical management of Cushing's disease: a report of 100 cases. *J Neurosurg.* 1983; 59:195–200.

127. Tindall GT, Herring CJ, Clark RV, et al. Cushing's disease: results of transsphenoidal microsurgery with emphasis on surgical failures. *J Neurosurg.* 1990;72:363–369.

128. Krieger DT. Physiopathology of Cushing's disease. *Endocr Rev.* 1983;4:22–43.

129. Salassa RM, Laws ER, Carpenter PC. Cushing's disease—50 years later. *Trans Am Clin Climatol Assoc.* 1982;94:122–129.

130. Friedman RB, Oldfield EH, Nieman LK, et al. Repeat transsphenoidal surgery for Cushing's disease. *J Neurosurg.* 1989;71:520–527.

131. Fitzgerald PA, Aron DC, Findling JW, et al. Cushing's disease: transient secondary adrenal insufficiency after selective removal of pituitary microadenomas; evidence for a pituitary origin. *J Clin Endocrinol Metab.* 1982;54:413–422.

132. Derome PJ, Delalande O, Visot A, Jedynac CP, Dupuy M. In: Landolt AM, ed. *Progress in Pituitary Adenoma Research.* London: Pergamon Press; 1988:375–379.

133. Degerblad M, Rahn T, Bergstrand G, Thoren M. Long-term results of stereotactic radiosurgery to the pituitary gland in Cushing's disease. *Acta Endocrinol (Copenh).* 1986;112:310–314.

134. Sandler LM, Richards NT, Carr DH, et al. Long term follow-up of patients with Cushing's disease treated by interstitial irradiation. *J Clin Endocrinol Metab.* 1987;65:441–447.

135. Loli P, Berselli ME, Tagliaferri M. Use of ketoconazole in the treatment of Cushing's syndrome. *J Clin Endocrinol Metab.* 1986;63:1365–1371.

136. Sonino N. The use of ketoconazole as an inhibitor of steroid production. *N Engl J Med.* 1987;317: 812–818.

Craniopharyngiomas

Dachling Pang

Craniopharyngiomas are unique lesions in that they are histologically benign, but because of the technical difficulties and potential hazards involved in their radical excision, a surgical cure is seldom achieved except in expert hands. Their intimate adherence to the infundibular stalk and hypothalamus predisposes to a number of endocrinologic and neurobehavioral problems rarely seen in other brain tumors. They are slow-growing, but a mere fleck of residual tumor virtually guarantees a recurrence. With all these surgical idiosyncracies, microsurgery is still the mainstay of management, although recent advances in radiotherapy offer a number of nonsurgical options that could arguably be the treatments of choice in special circumstances. The treatment algorithm recommended in this chapter must therefore be regarded merely as the personal viewpoint of the author, not as the undisputed answer to this complex lesion. Neurosurgeons and oncologists must continue to modify their protocols along with advances in the frontiers of treatment for this tumor.

INCIDENCE

Craniopharyngiomas are relatively rare tumors, constituting between 2.5% and 4% of all intracranial tumors.[1,2] They are much more common among children, forming 9% of Matson's series of childhood brain tumors[3] and making up 54% of neoplasms in the sellar-chiasmal region in children. There is a bimodal age distribution, with the first peak at 5 to 10 years[4,5] and a second peak between 55 and 65 years,[6] but the tumor may become symptomatic at any age. Recent large series show equal sex distribution.[7,8]

EMBRYOLOGIC ORIGIN

For several decades, craniopharyngiomas were thought to arise exclusively from epithelial rests along the embryologic migration path of the anterior pituitary lobe. At the end of the third gestational week, the stomodeal ectoderm invaginates toward the diencephalon and eventually meets the downwardly projecting infundibular bud. As the sphenoid bone forms ventral to the diencephalon, the stomodeal cleft is pinched off from the pharyngeal epithelium to become a pouch (of Rathke), whose wall eventually thickens to form the various parts of the anterior pituitary lobe (Fig. 35.1). Ectoblastic cell rests have been found along this migration path (called the hypophysiopharyngeal duct), from

the partes tuberalis and distalis of the gland to the posterior pharyngeal mucosa (Fig. 35.2). The frequent occurrence of craniopharyngiomas around the infundibular stalk, their occasional occurrence within the sphenoid bone and pharynx, and the striking histologic resemblance between some craniopharyngiomas and tumors of known ectoblastic origin, such as adamantinomas, led Erdheim[9] and others[10–12] to implicate these embryonic ectoblastic remnants as the sole source of all craniopharyngiomas.

During the 1950s, the embryonic origin of craniopharyngioma was challenged when it was discovered that the pituitary squamous cell rests are rarely seen in children under 10 years but are found with increasing frequency in each succeeding decade of life, even though the peak incidence of craniopharyngiomas is between the ages of 5 and 10 years.[13] It was then postulated that the squamous cell rests from which craniopharyngiomas originate are products of metaplasia of the mature cells of the anterior pituitary gland, and not embryonic remnants.[10,13]

There is evidence to suggest that craniopharyngiomas may indeed have dual origins. The so-called childhood type, which occurs in all ages and contains palisading columnar cells that resemble the ameloblasts of fetal tooth buds, may be of embryonic origin.[14,15] The adult type, which occurs mostly in adults and consists mainly of mature stratified squamous cells, may be of metaplastic origin.

SURGICAL ANATOMY AND PATHOLOGY

Most craniopharyngiomas originate near the infundibular stalk and distort or completely obliterate the suprasellar cistern, depending on their size and direction of growth. Approximately one third of cases are retrochiasmatic (Fig. 35.3)—the tumor displaces the pituitary forward and the chiasm upward and forward towards the tuberculum so that both optic nerves appear shortened and acquire the false appearance of being prefixed (pseudoprefixity). Another one third of cases are subchiasmatic—the tumor displaces the stalk backwards and the chiasm directly upward so that the optic nerves are stretched. Both of these types are solid tumors and therefore have the hard consistency to indent and elevate the floor of the third ventricle all the way to the level of the foramen of Monro. The hypothalamic structures accommodate gradually by displacing to the sides, but generally maintain most of their normal functions, judging from the rarity of severe hypothalamic insuffi-

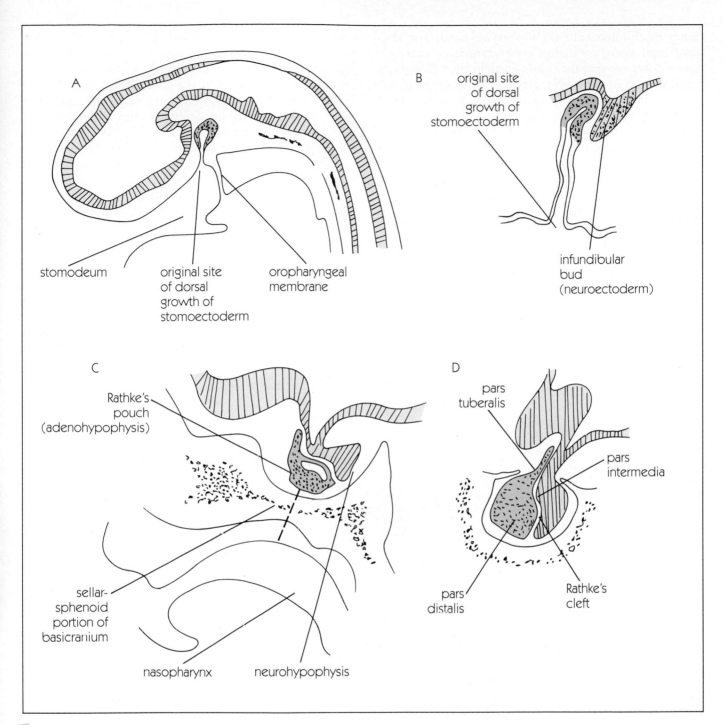

Figure 35.1 Embryogenesis of the pituitary gland. (A) Formation of Rathke's pouch from the stomodeal epithelium. (B) Fusion of stomodeal ectoderm with downgrowing infundibular bud, from neuroectoderm. (C) Interposition of mesoderm of basicranium to form the sella-sphenoid complex ventral to the pituitary gland, after Rathke's pouch has been pinched off from the stomodeum. S indicates original site of the dorsal growth of the stomoectoderm. Dotted line denotes the tract of the upgrowth, the hypophysiopharyngeal duct. (D) Final development of the adenohypophysis from thickening of Rathke's pouch wall. Stippled (red) area denotes Rathke's pouch epithelium and subsequent derivatives. Hatched (blue) area denotes infundibular bud from neuroectoderm and subsequent neurohypophysis.

ciency in children with craniopharyngiomas. The third ventricular floor, no matter how attenuated, keeps the tumor dome outside the third ventricle even though the CSF passage is often obstructed and the superior pole of the tumor appears on neuroimaging studies to be within the third ventricle (Fig. 35.4). True intraventricular craniopharyngiomas have been reported[16-18] and probably arise from dislocated tuberal ectoblastic cells, but they are exceedingly rare. For most craniopharyngiomas, the transventricular approach from above risks injuring the hypothalamus and is not recommended.

About 20% of craniopharyngiomas are prechiasmatic. These tumors are frequently cystic and, by burrowing under and expanding within the frontal lobes, may reach enormous sizes (Figs. 35.5, 35.6). The soft cystic component of the tumor may also extend out like fingers to the sylvian fissure laterally and over the dorsum sellae into the prepontine cistern posteriorly, be-

coming extensively multilobulated. This explains the occurrence of psychomotor seizures and cranial neuropathies in large rambling cystic tumors. Intrasellar craniopharyngiomas are the least common (10% to 15%),[19,20] but because they expand within the sella and cause pituitary insufficiencies early, they are often diagnosed when still relatively small (Fig. 35.7) and thus may be removed by the transsphenoidal route.

Craniopharyngiomas may be predominantly solid, predominantly cystic, or cystic with a large solid component that may in turn contain small cysts. The solid part is usually smooth, rubbery, firm, and pinkish gray, resembling fish flesh. The cyst wall may be diaphanous or a thick shell of solid tumor. The fluid is typically dark green with suspended birefringent cholesterol crystals.

Microscopically, the cyst lining is composed of simple stratified squamous epithelium supported by a collagenous basement membrane. Two histologic types

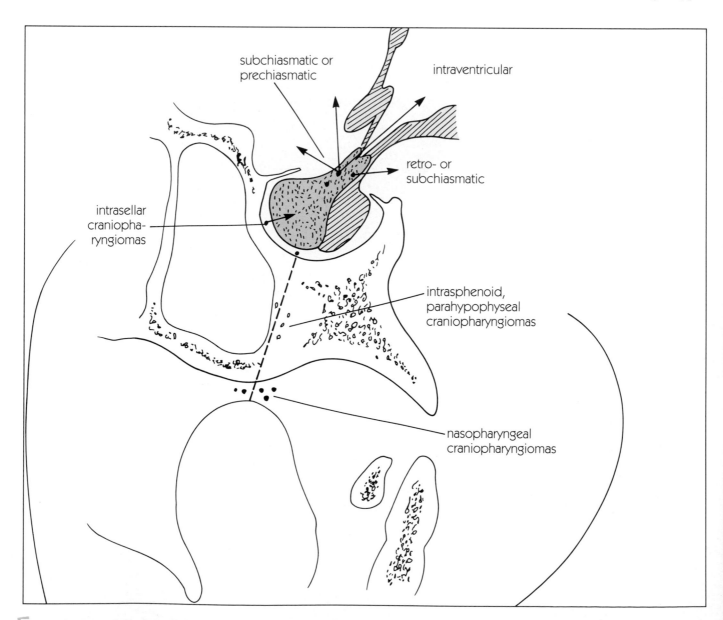

Figure 35.2 Possible sites of embryonic ectoblastic remnants and their relationship to subsequent locations of craniopharyngiomas. Dots indicate sites of ectoblastic remnants. Arrows indicate direction of growth and final location of tumors.

have been described in the solid parts. The more common *childhood* or *adamantinomatous* type is found in both children and adults.[14,15] It consists of epithelial trabeculae supported by a loose connective tissue stroma. These trabeculae are lined by palisading columnar cells

radially arranged around a central cord of round or polygonal cells with transparent cytoplasm and intercellular bridges (prickle cells). In other areas there are masses of dead cells that show whorled or laminated arrangements reminiscent of keratinization. It is this

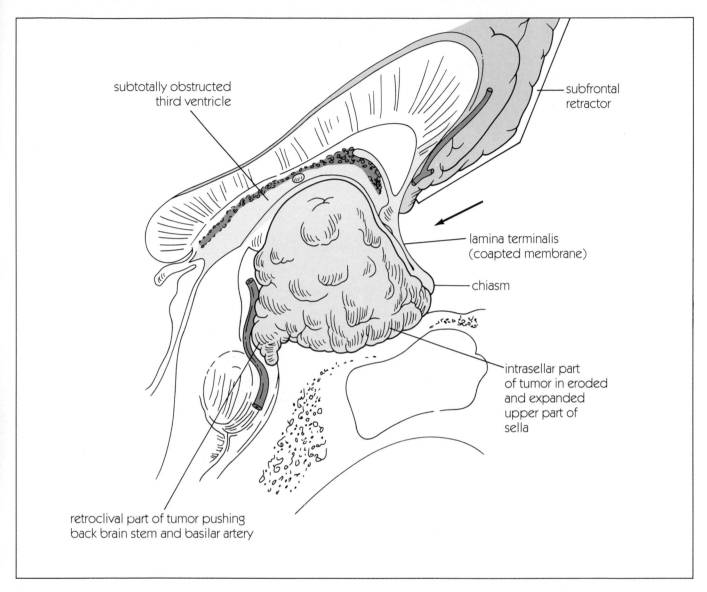

Figure 35.3 Schematic view of a large retrochiasmatic craniopharyngioma pushing the third ventricular floor upwards and coapting the attenuated midline basal hypothalamus with the lamina terminalis into a single membrane. Arrow indicates direction of the translamina terminalis approach.

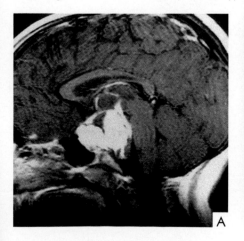
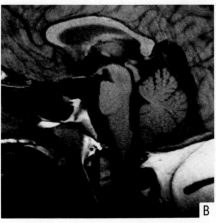

Figure 35.4 Postcontrast sagittal MRI of a large solid craniopharyngioma. **(A)** Note severe elevation of hypothalamus and third ventricular floor up to the level of foramen of Monro and distortion of the mamillary bodies. **(B)** After total resection of the tumor, the third ventricle resumes its normal location and its intact floor is again seen well. Note that the previously compressed mamillary body is now seen well.

combination of palisading columnar cells and central transparent cells that suggests a link with fetal tooth buds and other oral mucosal appendages (Fig. 35.8). The less common *adult* histologic type is found predominantly in adults[14,15] and consists of sheets of stratified squamous epithelium embedded in a matrix of vascular connective tissue. There are no laminellae or keratinization, and calcification is much less common (Fig. 35.9).

Either the solid part or the cyst wall, or both, may be calcified. Calcification marks the site of regressive changes in the epithelium and is therefore particularly prevalent within the laminated whorls of dead cells in the childhood type but not in the adult type. This explains why calcium is seen on CT in almost all childhood craniopharyngiomas but only in slightly over 50% of adult craniopharyngiomas.[4] Small calcium foci may

become confluent to form large stones, and actual bone formation has been reported.[14] It is important not to mistake a large stone as a sign of "burnt-out" tumor. Thin layers of *live* tumor cells are sandwiched between lamellae of calcium within the stone, which grows by further concretions being laid down after more live cells undergo regressive changes. In fact, reappearance of calcium or enlargement of a stone invariably means recurrence of an actively growing tumor.

The anterior, inferior, and lateral walls of the tumor capsule are normally separated from surrounding structures by a single layer of arachnoid. In contrast, the posterior wall is separated from the basilar artery and brain stem by the double-layered membrane of Liliequist. However, the dome of the tumor is almost always adherent to the infundibulum and basal hypothalamus due to an intense glial reaction in this region of the

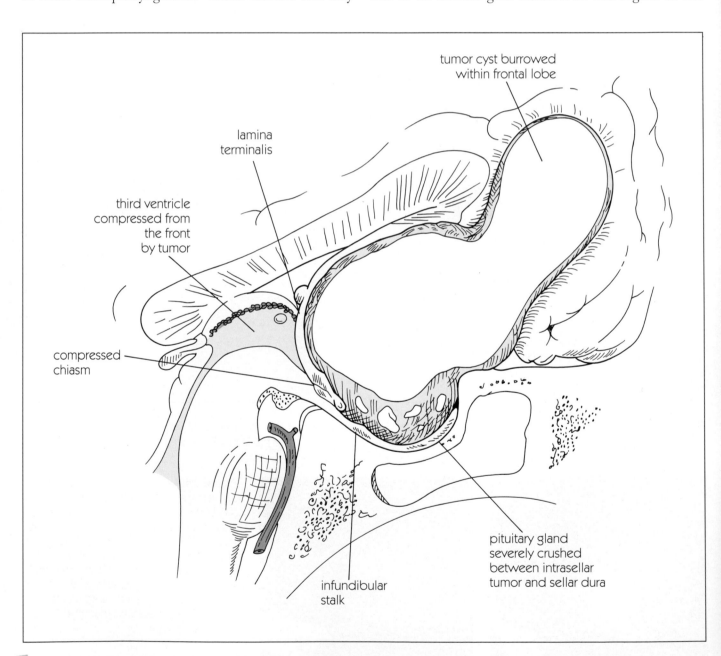

Figure 35.5 Prechiasmatic, predominantly cystic craniopharyngioma.

brain where most craniopharyngiomas arise. This tenacious glial sheath frequently contains pseudopods of tumor extending beyond the capsule. Occasionally, the inferior pole of the tumor expands within the sella and the capsule fuses tightly with the sellar dura and the medial walls of the cavernous sinus.

Having a common embryologic origin, craniopharyngiomas share the same blood supply as the anterior diencephalon (Fig. 35.10).[11,21,22] The anterior portion of the tumor thus receives arterial feeders from the anterior communicating artery and the A1 segment of the anterior cerebral arteries, and its lateral portion

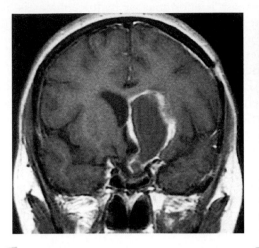

Figure 35.6 Postcontrast coronal MRI of a large, predominantly cystic craniopharyngioma that has expanded upwards and burrowed within the left frontal lobe.

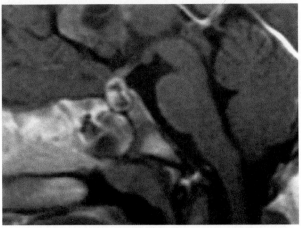

Figure 35.7 Postcontrast sagittal MRI of a mostly intrasellar craniopharyngioma. About two thirds of the tumor is intrasellar, and only one third is above the diaphragm.

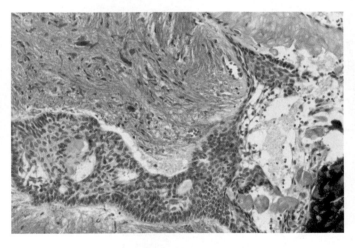

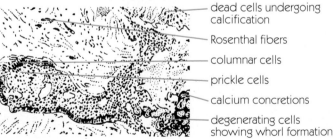

dead cells undergoing calcification
Rosenthal fibers
columnar cells
prickle cells
calcium concretions
degenerating cells showing whorl formation

Figure 35.8 Histology of the so-called juvenile-type or adamantinomatous craniopharyngioma, showing a pseudopod of tumor lined with palisading columnar cells surrounding central cells with transparent cytoplasm ("prickle cells"). Note intense gliosis of the brain around the tumor, with abundant Rosenthal fibers. (H & E; ×100)

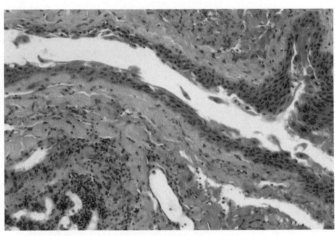

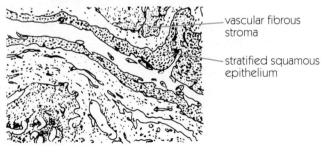

vascular fibrous stroma
stratified squamous epithelium

Figure 35.9 Histology of the so-called adult-type craniopharyngioma, showing stratified squamous epithelium overlying vascular fibrous stroma. Note absence of calcium and whorls (laminellae). (H & E; ×100)

receives branches from the posterior communicating artery. If the tumor involves the sella, it will also pick up arterial supply from the capsular and meningohypophyseal arteries. However, the tumor virtually never receives blood supply from the posterior cerebral or basilar artery, no matter how far posteriorly it extends,[11,23] since these vessels do not normally irrigate the anterior diencephalon. This fact is crucial to the safe removal of the retrosellar portion of the tumor.

CLINICAL FEATURES

The clinical presentation of craniopharyngiomas differs between children and adults (Fig. 35.11). Even though the optic chiasm and nerves are affected first by enlargement of the tumor, only 20% to 30% of children present with visual symptoms. This is because children tolerate progressive visual failure amazingly well, and they seldom complain until one eye is totally blind and the other barely can count fingers.[4,6,11,23] Subtle clues of progressive visual loss in young children include inex-

plicable deterioration in school performance, frequent stumbling, and an insistence on sitting very close to the television.

Other symptoms of an expanding intracranial mass such as headaches, personality changes, or even disturbance in orientation are likely to be overlooked in a young child. Diagnosis is therefore often delayed until the mass is enormous or hydrocephalus is already present due to third ventricular obstruction. Thus, 75% to 80% of children with craniopharyngiomas present with severe headache and vomiting without focal neurologic deficits.[4,6,11]

The two most frequent presenting endocrinopathies in children are short stature and delayed puberty (hypogonadism) in adolescents.[1,6] Diabetes insipidus (DI)[6,7] is less common and is usually only partial. Hypothyroidism and hypocortisolemia are unusual, although a blunter corticotropin response to provocative testing is common. Galactorrhea and hyperprolactinemia have been associated with craniopharyngiomas[21,24] and are thought to result from suppression of hypothalamic prolactin-inhibiting factor due to infundibular stalk compression.

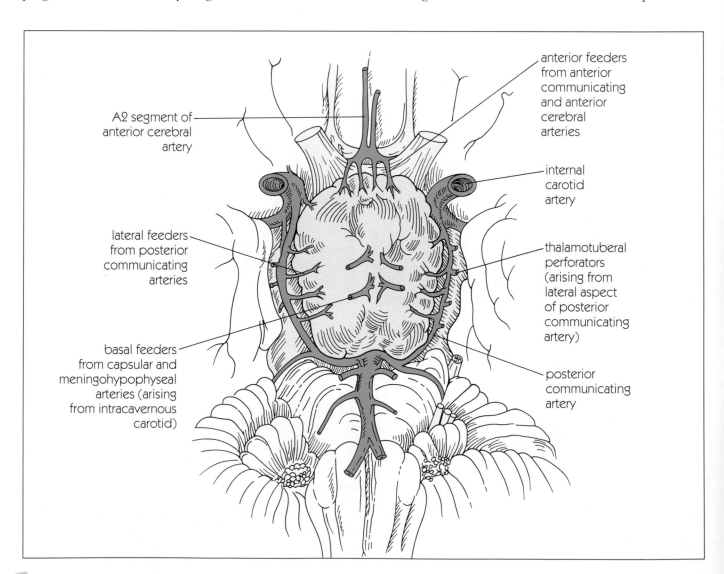

Figure 35.10 Blood supply of a craniopharyngioma.

The most common hypothalamic syndrome encountered in children is central hyperphagia and obesity, which is sometimes disproportionate to the food intake and may be partly due to metabolic derangement. An unusual disturbance of fat metabolism causing emaciation in spite of adequate food intake has been described by Northfield.[25] Precocious puberty has also been reported in four cases of craniopharyngiomas,[6,26–28] presumably because of compression of the arcuate nucleus luteinizing-hormone-releasing hormone (LH-RH) pacemaker. Flagrant disturbances of sleep and of thirst or temperature regulation are rarely seen in these children.

Neurobehavioral abnormalities occur in 20% of children with craniopharyngiomas.[1,4,6] In recent years, the author has repeatedly recognized signs of abulia minor in these children, such as psychomotor retardation, flattening of affect, and loss of enthusiasm toward the environment. Severely affected children also show significant recent memory deficits; the abulia and amnesia contribute most to the poor school performance. The amnesic syndrome has been attributed to compression of the hypothalamic component of the limbic memory circuit, such as the mamillary bodies. The abulia probably results from injury to the dopaminergic mesolimbic pathway, either within the medial forebrain bundle or at the medial septal region. This pathway is thought to be responsible for exploratory behaviors in animals and motivation in humans.[29–31] Thus, the typical child with a craniopharyngioma is short, obese, dull, and half-blind, and has a poor school record.

Unlike children, most adults are very sensitive to visual disturbance, and 80% of adults in Banna's series[32] presented with assorted patterns of field deficits, scotomas, and decreasing visual acuity. In contrast, less than one third of adults have signs of increased intracranial pressure (ICP). Nevertheless, neurobehavioral syndromes unrelated to raised ICP are also much more common in adults than children.[1,4,11] Bartlett estimated that 31.5% of patients older than 45 years had dementia,[33] and an even higher percentage had intermittent confusion and hypersomnia. A Korsakoff-like amnesia was found in 30% of adults,[34–36] and occasionally severe depression and apathy will complicate the intellectual deterioration.[33] The most common endocrinopathy in adults is gonadal failure (37%),[11] presenting as secondary amenorrhea in women and loss of libido in men.[11]

RADIOGRAPHIC DIAGNOSIS

Even though plain skull radiographs are seldom obtained for headache or visual symptoms today, craniopharyngioma is one of few intracranial tumors that can be accurately diagnosed with a skull film. Two thirds of adults and 95% of children with this tumor have an abnormal skull x-ray. The usual findings are erosion of the anterior clinoids and dorsum sellae, expansion of the upper sella, and suprasellar calcification (Fig. 35.12). Intrasellar extension of a craniopharyngioma may produce a "ballooned" sella that mimics a pituitary

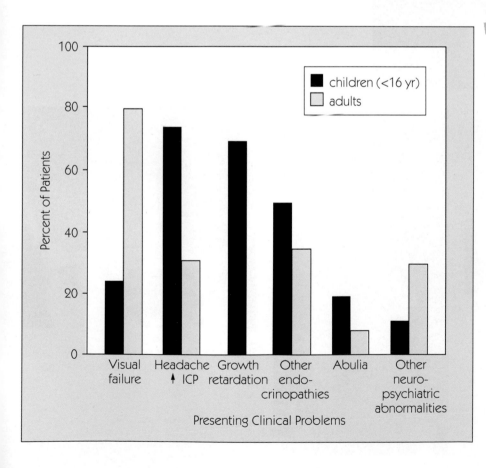

Figure 35.11 Presenting clinical problems of children and adults with craniopharyngiomas. Pooled data from references 11,12,17,23,36,61,63,64,66 and author's unpublished series.

adenoma, but the intrasellar calcium should exclude most adenomas.

CT and MRI are both important for craniopharyngiomas, for different reasons. CT is less ambiguous than MRI in distinguishing the solid from the cystic parts of the tumor. The MR signal intensity of the cyst fluid varies widely depending on protein, lipid, and methemoglobin contents, and may be confused with that of the solid part. The cyst fluid is always hypodense on CT and thus is easily distinguished from the solid or calcified tumor (Fig. 35.13). CT is therefore vital in classifying the tumor according to the solid/cyst ratio. A predominantly solid tumor is one that is at least 70% solid (Fig. 35.14), and a predominantly cystic tumor is less than 30% solid. This classification is important in choosing the optimal therapy.

Another important function of CT is to define the bony anatomy of the sphenoid sinus, tuberculum sellae, and sella in preparation for the frontobasal transsphenoidal approach to a low extension of the tumor (see below). The contiguous 3 to 5 mm coronal CT cuts using bone algorithms through the anterior skull base far surpass the old standard plain tomography. In addition, CT is much better than MRI in picking out small calcified parts of the tumor, particularly when these are close to the skull base.

On the other hand, MRI is better than CT in delineating the interface and relationship between tumor and brain in multiplane displays. The sagittal image, for instance, shows the distortion of the third ventricle and hypothalamic structures to great advantage and frequently will suggest whether a translamina terminalis approach to the dome of the tumor is necessary or feasible. Coronal images show the relationship of the lower pole of the tumor to the sella, sphenoid sinus, and cavernous sinus, and help determine whether the combined frontobasal transsphenoidal approach is necessary. Thus the MRI details enable the surgeon to select the surgical approach most likely to achieve total resection. Improving systems for MR angiography now completely re-

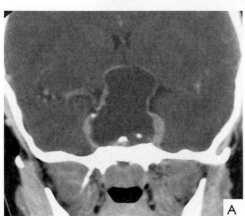

Figure 35.12 Lateral skull radiograph showing calcification within the sella and suprasellar regions in a child with a predominantly intrasellar craniopharyngioma.

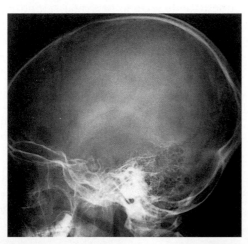

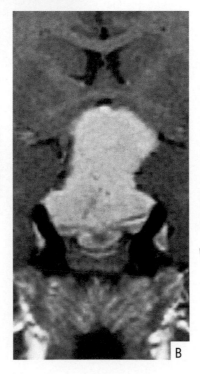

Figure 35.13 Predominantly cystic craniopharyngioma. **(A)** Postcontrast coronal CT shows clear distinction betwen cyst, cyst wall, basal solid part, and calcified part. **(B)** Postcontrast coronal T1-weighted MRI shows high-intensity cyst fluid and no distinction between solid, cyst, or calcium.

Figure 35.14 Postcontrast coronal CT of a predominantly solid craniopharyngioma.

place conventional angiography in defining the relationship of the tumor to the circle of Willis, except when an aneurysm of the cavernous carotid is strongly suspected.

MODALITIES AND OPTIONS OF TREATMENT

PRIMARY TUMOR, PREDOMINANTLY SOLID

Four treatment options are available for predominantly solid tumors diagnosed for the first time. The initial choice of therapy is guided by several factors: 1) the experience of the surgeon, 2) the availability of stereo-

tactic radiosurgery, 3) the age and medical condition of the patient, 4) the size and extent of the tumor on neuroimaging studies, and 5) the surgical anatomy, the degree of adherence, and the texture of the tumor capsule at surgery. A recommended treatment algorithm is summarized in Figure 35.15.

Total Resection

Total resection of craniopharyngiomas is feasible with low mortality and morbidity in skilled and experienced hands. Even though total resection is the starting objective for most craniopharyngiomas, the aggressiveness of tumor removal must be tempered by the degree of difficulty encountered at surgery. Resectability depends on the tumor size (tumors larger than 4 cm are

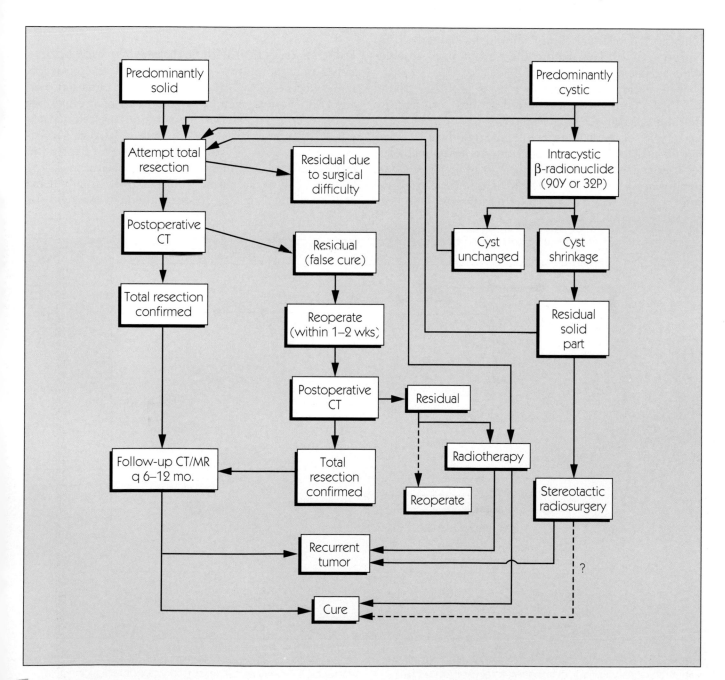

Figure 35.15 Recommended treatment algorithm for primary craniopharyngiomas in young and relatively healthy patients.

Planned partial resection and postoperative RT is recommended for elderly and medically infirm patients.

less likely to be totally resected), the degree of tumor adherence to the chiasm and great vessels, and the extent of rambling of the capsule within the basal cisterns and deep brain structures. Thus, the ratio of the number of cases in which total resection was accomplished (confirmed by postoperative neuroimaging) to the number in which total resection was attempted varies between 30% and 90%.[4,8,37–41] The realistic expectation for total resection is probably around 80% to 90%. CT with and without contrast should be performed within 24 hours after surgery to eliminate "false cure," i.e., to rule out residual tumor fragments in "blind spots" such as the underside of the chiasm, deep inside the sella, and behind the dorsum sellae in the prepontine cistern. MRI is not suitable for this purpose because of the exuberant contrast enhancement in the surgical bed within the first 2 postoperative months. Unexpected residual tumor should be reoperated on within 7 to 10 days, before the formation of troublesome adhesions in the surgical field.

The overall operative mortality is probably around 1% to 2%, and the best reported serious postoperative morbidity is below 10%.[7,8,38,39]

In spite of meticulous technique and diligent screening for false cures, a number of tumors will nonetheless recur after what has been deemed "complete" resection. Recurrences are usually detected within 5 years of the surgery,[4,39] but late recurrences after 20 years have been

reported.[7] A long-term review by Katz[37] of Matson's original series[42] reported recurrences in 25% of patients 4 to 19 years after "total" resection, and most other series recorded recurrence rates of 15% to 25%, with a mean of 20%.[7,8,38,39,41] Recent updating of results including the author's personal series (author's unpublished results) shows a 10-year recurrence rate of less than 15%. In any case, the 10-year survival rate of patients who have undergone total resection is well over 85% (Fig. 35.16). Thus, the overall results of total resection for solid craniopharyngiomas are excellent, and it is the treatment of choice in children and young adults. Obviously, the associated morbidity and, to an extent, the recurrence rate are dependent on the experience of the surgeon. Total resection should therefore be attempted only in centers where a large number of these tumors are managed.

Subtotal Resection With Postoperative Radiation

When only subtotal resection is achieved, the recurrence rate is unacceptably high if postoperative radiation therapy (RT) is not given. The combined recurrence rate from several large series for subtotal resection without RT is about 75%,[4,8,39,43–47] with a 10-year survival rate of only 25%. Postoperative RT significantly improves outcome and increases 10-year survival to 75% to 80%.[12,38,46] External beam radiotherapy is usually delivered by a three- or four-field technique over a field size

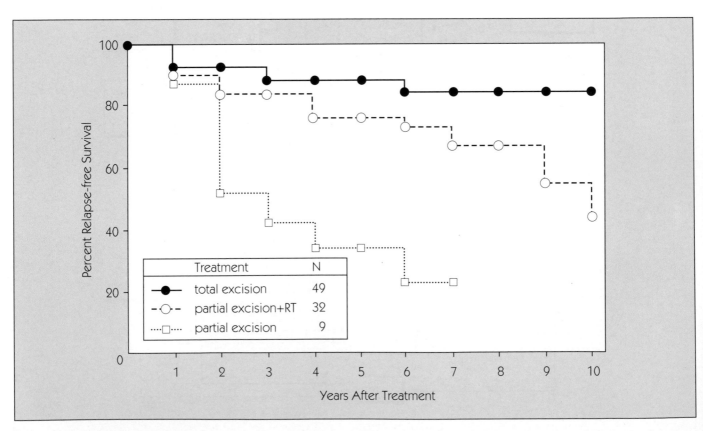

Figure 35.16 Actuarial relapse-free survival rates in patients with craniopharyngioma, comparing total excision (combined data from reference 67 and the author's unpublished series), subtotal or partial resection plus radiation (data from reference 17); and partial resection without radiation (data from reference 67). RT = radiation therapy.

of 6 × 7 cm, with a total dose of 50 to 60 Gy fractionated over 6 to 7 weeks, with the daily dose not exceeding 2 Gy.

Postoperative RT is an excellent adjunct after an attempt at total resection has proven unfeasible. Because of the good 10-year survival rate of subtotal resection and RT, and the sometimes unusually taxing nature of radical excision, some surgeons are adopting a planned incomplete resection combined with RT. However, conventional RT is not without hazard, especially in children. Visual failure, hypopituitarism, organic brain syndromes, dementia, and sensorimotor deficits have all been reported.[24,40,48–50] Frontal lobe dysfunction translating into severe learning disabilities is especially troublesome in children,[51] and RT has also been etiologically implicated in malignant mesenchymal tumors arising de novo in the radiated field.[52,53] Furthermore, recent long-term follow-up studies[1,54] are beginning to reveal that subtotal resection with RT delays but does not prevent eventual recurrence of the tumor. This treatment option is therefore not recommended as first choice for children and healthy young adults with potentially long life spans, but it is a wise alternative if total resection is found to be too risky at surgery, as when a piece of tumor is obstinately adherent to a great vessel. It is also a reasonable option for older patients with large tumors.

Biopsy and Radiation

Most workers now believe that simple tumor biopsy and postoperative RT are inferior to either total resection or subtotal resection and RT. Shapiro et al.[38] reported 5- and 10-year survival rates for biopsy and RT of only 62% and 50%, respectively. Sung et al.[55] and Manaka et al.[46] reported comparable figures. Thus, this option is only endorsed for the old, the infirm, or those patients refusing more radical approaches. Because the biologic effects of RT may take 6 to 9 months to occur, patients suffering from imminent optic compression or high ICP due to mass effect of the tumor will not benefit from this treatment method. If a cyst contributes significantly to the mass effect, an in-dwelling catheter connected to a subcutaneous reservoir may be implanted in the cyst to permit periodic percutaneous aspiration of fluid during the waiting period.

Stereotactic Radiosurgery

In several treatment centers in Europe and the United States, stereotactic radiosurgery using the gamma irradiation unit[56–59] and the linear accelerator has been used for the primary control of small solid craniopharyngiomas and solid recurrences following cyst aspiration. Radiosurgery is based on the principle that the biologic effects produced by a single radiation dose are greater than those produced by the same dose fractionated. Thus, if the single dose is delivered to sharply circumscribed and precisely targeted areas of tissue, tumor necrosis may be induced with comparatively low morbidity to the surrounding brain.[60] The gamma unit delivers 201 radially directed narrow beams of cobalt-60 gamma radiation towards a target region within a spherical sector (Fig. 35.17). The system of apertures for each individual beam and the spatial arrangements of the ^{60}Co sources are designed to give oval-shaped isodose fields with very steep dose gradients in the border zones of the lesions to minimize radiation damage to the adjacent optic pathways and hypothalamus. In order to adapt the irradiated volume to the shape of the target, a number of adjacent target points in a predetermined spatial pattern can be used.[56] For solid craniopharyngiomas, approximately

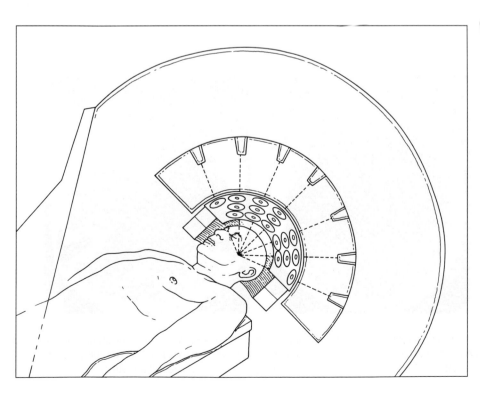

Figure 35.17 Schematic diagram of stereotactic radiosurgery using the gamma irradiation unit illustrating the principle of cross-firing with multiple beams stereotactically aimed at the target. The number of beams is underrepresented to preserve clarity. (Adapted with permission from Coffey RJ, Lunsford LD. Stereotactic radiosurgery using the 201 cobalt-60 source gamma knife. *Neurosurg Clin North Am.* 1990;1:955–990.)

Translamina Terminalis Approach

In patients with prefixed chiasm, the interoptic space is too small for the extensive maneuvers needed to extract a large craniopharyngioma. The lamina terminalis can then be traversed to gain access to the tumor dome (Fig. 35.23). Normally the lamina terminalis is a narrow structure that delimits the anterior third ventricle, but with large suprasellar tumors the tuberal portion of the basal hypothalamus, from the mamillary bodies to the chiasm, is stretched very thin and may actually be coapted with the lamina terminalis to form a single membrane (see Fig. 35.3). Both the infundibular and supraoptic recesses are obliterated, so that traversing this coapted membrane instantly gives access to the tumor without actually entering the third ventricle. In most large solid tumors, the lamina terminalis is widely expanded behind the chiasm, and the yellowish, gritty tumor can often be seen through the diaphanous coapted membrane in between the splayed-out optic tracts (Fig. 35.24). Opening this membrane carefully behind the crossing macular fibers of the chiasm (to avoid severe loss of acuity) will afford an excellent view of the tumor dome (Fig. 35.25). It appears likely that the basal hypothalamic nuclei are displaced laterally by

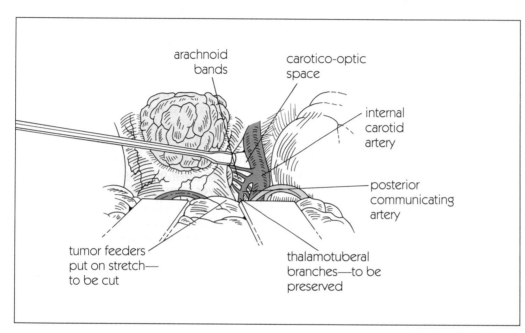

arachnoid bands

carotico-optic space

internal carotid artery

posterior communicating artery

thalamotuberal branches—to be preserved

tumor feeders put on stretch—to be cut

Figure 35.20 Right lateral dissection within carotico-optic space. The right lateral surface of the tumor capsule is pulled away from the internal carotid and posterior communicating arteries, putting the lateral feeders on stretch. The superiorly coursing thalamotuberal perforators to the hypothalamus and basal ganglia are preserved.

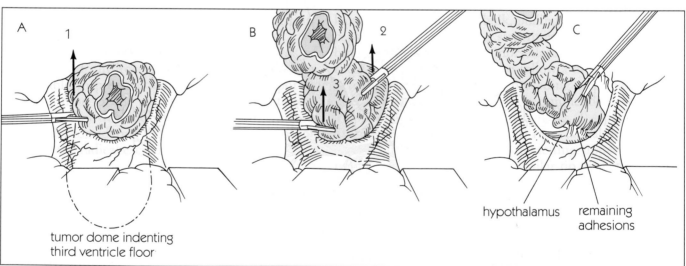

A 1

B 2 3

C

hypothalamus   remaining adhesions

tumor dome indenting third ventricle floor

Figure 35.21 Detaching the upper pole of the tumor from the hypothalamus. **(A)** After considerable reduction of tumor volume through interoptic debulking, the base of the upper tumor piece (indenting third ventricular floor) is firmly grasped by the left microforceps and pulled down towards the suprasellar cistern (grasp 1). **(B)** When more tumor appears in the interoptic space, it is, in turn, grasped by the right microforceps, which continues the downward pull (grasp 2), alternating with the left hand (grasp 3). **(C)** The upper pole is pulled down, and the previously severely elevated basal hypothalamus is now visible through the interoptic space.

the slow expansion of the tumor, since using the translamina terminalis route does not usually produce hypothalamic deficiency.

Subfrontal-Transsphenoidal Approach

If the preoperative MRI shows wide expansion of the sella by tumor or frank invasion of tumor into the sphenoid sinus, the inferior tumor capsule will almost certainly be densely fused with the sellar dura and walls of the cavernous sinus and cannot be extracted safely through the standard subfrontal approach (Fig. 35.26). In these situations, direct access to the intrasellar

tumor can be gained by drilling through the tuberculum sellae into the sphenoid sinus, sweeping aside the sphenoid mucosa, and then finally breaking open the anterior sellar wall (Fig. 35.27). A thin shell of pituitary gland is often sandwiched between the tumor capsule and the dura. If the pituitary stalk has already been cut, as with most of these tumors with large sellar extensions, there is no point in saving the gland. The sella is thus completely exenterated together with the tumor (Fig. 35.28). The circular and cavernous sinuses sometimes bleed profusely, but this type of venous bleeding can be readily controlled with tamponade.

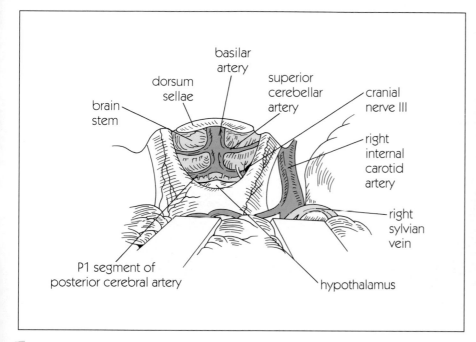

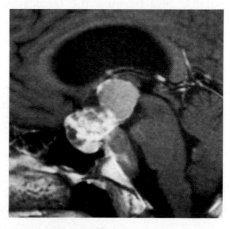

Figure 35.23 Postcontrast sagittal MR image of a partially solid craniopharyngioma with a large solid upper dome and a large retroclival part. Interoptic space is not adequate for removal of the upper part, nor does it afford the angle for the removal of the retroclival part.

Figure 35.22 View after total resection of tumor.

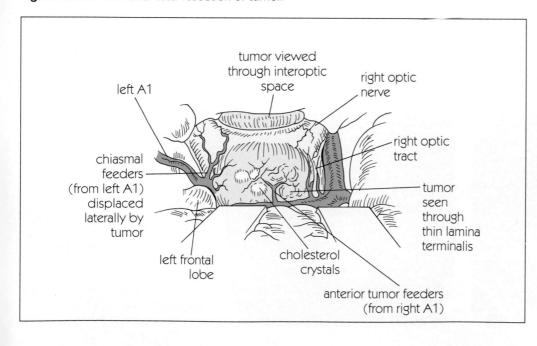

Figure 35.24 Large craniopharyngioma and prefixed chiasm. Only the most posterior segments of the optic nerves are seen. The small interoptic space is too small for tumor extraction. Tumor is seen bulging through the thin (coapted) lamina terminalis, splaying open the optic tracts. The chiasmal feeders from the anterior cerebral arteries are also displaced laterally by the tumor, and thus can be selectively preserved while the more medial feeders to the tumor are taken.

After complete tumor resection, the confluent sella-sphenoid cavity is packed with fat, and a piece of fascia lata is sutured to the edge of the tuberculum dural defect and laid over the sella (Figs. 35.29, 35.30). If the sphenoid mucosa is accidentally perforated, a lumbar drain may be needed to prevent postoperative CSF leak.

Staged Procedures

Lateral extension of tumor far into the choroidal fissure necessitates a second procedure using the subtemporal or pterional route. By itself the subtemporal route is not recommended as the primary approach, because of the high incidence of postoperative nerve III, IV, and VI palsies, and because the translamina terminalis and modified transsphenoidal options cannot be exercised from this angle.

Because most craniopharyngiomas do not actually penetrate the floor of the third ventricle no matter how high the hypothalamus has been lifted up by the tumor mass, using a primary transventricular approach from above has been associated with significant hypothalamic damage and poor results.[18,68] This approach is only used as a first procedure for the truly rare intraventricular craniopharyngiomas. It is also recommended as a second procedure if after the subfrontal operation a portion of the tumor is found to have penetrated far into the third ventricle and would not descend with suprasellar debulking.

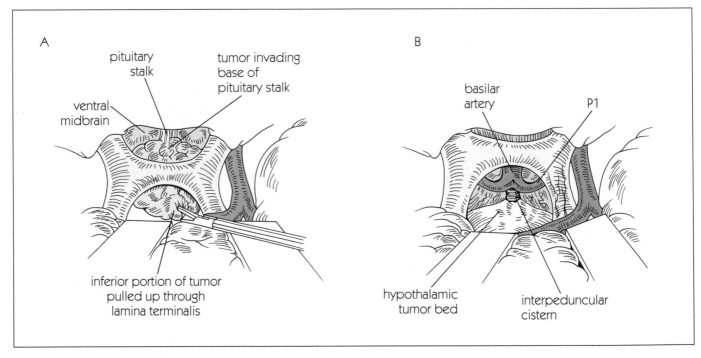

Figure 35.25 (A) Translamina terminalis resection of large craniopharyngioma. After debulking the main retrochiasmal portion of the tumor, the inferior pole is pulled up from the sella through the large opening in the lamina terminalis.

(B) After total resection of tumor, the tip of the basilar artery and the posterior cerebral arteries (P1), the midbrain, and the now "hanging" hypothalamic floor are seen through the lamina opening.

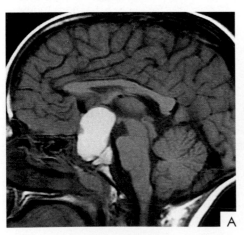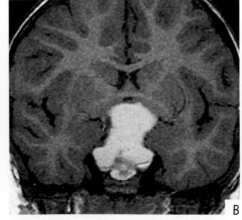

Figure 35.26 Precontrast MRI of a child with a partially cystic craniopharyngioma. (A) Sagittal image shows wide expansion of the sella and encroachment of the sphenoid sinus. Note level of the tumor dome almost at the level of the foramen of Monro and mamillary bodies just behind the tumor dome. (B) Coronal image shows wide lateral displacement of the cavernous sinuses, wide expansion of the sella, and a defect in the sella floor (arrows) through which the tumor extends into the sphenoid sinus.

Principles of Neurosurgery

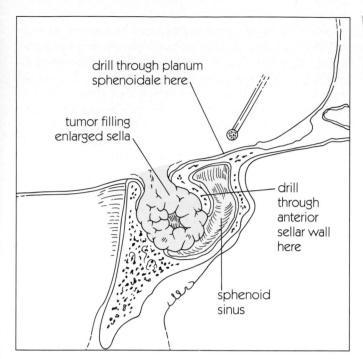

drill through planum
sphenoidale here

tumor filling
enlarged sella

drill
through
anterior
sellar wall
here

sphenoid
sinus

Figure 35.27 Subfrontal-transsphenoidal approach. Sagittal view shows large intrasellar and intrasphenoid tumor. Thick arrow shows direction of drilling through planum sphenoidale to gain entrance into sphenoid sinus, and access to the anterior sellar floor.

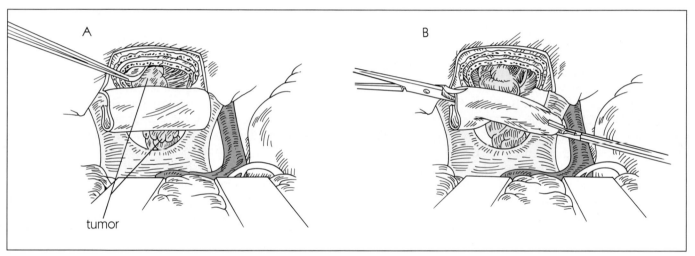

A

B

tumor

Figure 35.28 Subfrontal-transsphenoidal approach. (A) Exenteration of sella with microcurette scraping against bony sellar floor. (B) Intrasellar tumor is pushed into the interoptic space. If necessary, the remaining tuberculum sellae dura may be excised to improve exposure.

Figure 35.29 The sella-sphenoid confluent space is packed with free fat graft and overlaid with a fascial flap that is sutured to the anterior free dural edge.

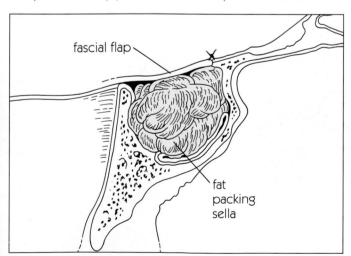

fascial flap

fat
packing
sella

MANAGEMENT OF POSTOPERATIVE COMPLICATIONS

Visual loss is the most common neurologic deficit after radical or subradical resection. The preoperative visual status is the most important determining factor for visual outcome.[17] Patients with total or near-total blindness do not regain useful vision, but those with scotomas and partial field cuts may well improve after surgery. Duration of preoperative visual loss is also an important prognostic factor: Visual impairment less than a year old has more than three times the chance of improvement that impairment longer than a year has.[69]

With the high likelihood of stalk sectioning or injury during tumor resection, postoperative DI is universal and frequently has a triphasic course. Excessive diuresis usually begins within the first 24 hours due to immediate cessation of normal intraaxonal transport of antidiuretic hormone (ADH). Degeneration of the hypothalamo-hypophyseal tract and necrosis of pitressin-neurophysin-laden axon terminals in the neurohypophysis then causes uncontrolled release of stored ADH 24 to 96 hours later to give paradoxic water retention.[4,70] This phase-2 response to stalk sectioning must be kept in mind when administering pitressin analogues in order to avoid causing water intoxication and lethal brain edema. The initial DI is best managed with small doses of intravenous DDAVP (desmopressin), which has a therapeutic effect lasting up to 18 hours. When the final, permanent diuretic phase of DI sets in, usually in a few days when the patient is more alert, DDAVP can be given by nasal spray. It is interesting that 10% to 15% of patients after stalk sectioning will resume partial production of ADH within 3 years, and their pitressin requirement may lessen. This is most likely due to formation of new neurovascular units in the magnocellular portion of the supraoptic and paraventricular nuclei of the hypothalamus.[71]

Stress doses of corticosteroid can be tapered to normal maintenance dosage in the form of oral cortisone acetate after the first 4 to 5 days. Dexamethasone used prophylactically for brain edema can also be tapered off completely according to the anticipated time course of postsurgical edema. Post-stalk-sectioning hypothyroidism requiring replacement occurs in 60% to 80% of patients. FSH and LH deficiencies are permanent. Children are begun on estrogen and testosterone replacement when the appropriate pubertal ages are reached, to impart secondary sexual characteristics. Testosterone is given to adult males to maintain libido. Ovulation in adult females can be induced by a costly process of priming ovarian follicular growth with human menopausal gonadotropins (Pergonal, containing FSH and LH) and then stimulating the follicles with a burst of human chorionic gonadotropin (possessing strong LH activity).[72] Patients with preserved pituitary stalk have been known to regain various endocrine functions, but recovery of the exquisitely sensitive LH-RH pacemaker function in the arcuate nucleus, vital to the induction of ovulation, has not been observed to date.

The growth rate of most children remains low after stalk section. Growth hormone (GH) therapy is usually started 6 to 9 months after surgery. Because estrogen and testosterone are known to accelerate closure of the epiphyseal plates of long bones in children, they are postponed until some growth has been made up by growth hormone therapy for several years, sometimes in spite of considerable psychosocial difficulties experienced by the hypogonadal adolescent patient. The initial 6 to 9 months wait before starting GH therapy is imposed to select out children who continue to grow normally despite the absence of GH.[73–78] In a few of these children, growth is attributed to hyperinsulinemia secondary to hyperphagia and weight gain,[73,74] but in

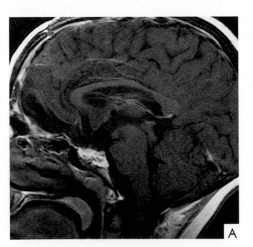 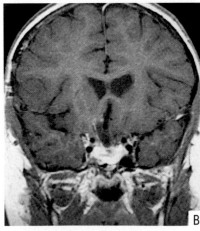

Figure 35.30 Postoperative MRI of the case shown in Figure 35.26, sagittal (**A**) and coronal (**B**) views. Note total excision of tumor by the subfrontal transsphenoidal route, loss of the tuberculum sellae "angle," and survival of fat graft within the sella-sphenoid space. Note resumption of air filling in the sphenoid sinus indicative of mucosal preservation.

others with normal insulin levels the growth is related to normal or supranormal levels of insulin-like growth factors (IGFs).[79] IGFs are probably stimulated by increased prolactin secretion from residual pituitary tissue caused by reduced prolactin-inhibiting factor output from the injured hypothalamus.

Serious hypothalamic syndromes such as loss of thirst sensation, dysthermia, and sleep disorders are now seldom seen in radical excisions. More likely are minor hypothalamic syndromes such as transient or mild recent memory deficits and appetite changes. In children and young adults it is especially common to see some degree of central hyperphagia 1 to 6 months after surgery.[23] The increased desire to eat is accompanied by weight gain. Severely affected children also have bizarre food-seeking behaviors and eating habits. Central hyperphagia has recently been postulated to result from injury to the serotoninergic eating inhibitory pathways originating from the anterior nucleus and preoptic area of the anterior hypothalamus. Weight gain usually stabilizes after hyperphagia subsides, but strict behavioral modification, stringent exercise programs, and psychologic counseling must be enforced to avoid morbid obesity.

Another interesting neurobehavioral syndrome, particularly following translamina terminalis resection of large tumors, is abulia minor, characterized by psychomotor retardation, flattening of affect, lack of enthusiasm and spontaneity of action and thoughts, loss of adventitious body motions and gesticulation, and reduction of exploratory behaviors.[80] Children thus affected are unmotivated in play and learning and consequently have extremely poor school performance. The neuropathologic basis for abulia is not known for certain, but it may be related to injury of the mesolimbic pathways projecting from the rostral midbrain to the medial septal nuclei, nucleus accumbens, and anterior cingulate gyrus[30,58,59,81] by way of the medial septal area, just underneath the deep subfrontal brain retractors.[80]

POSTOPERATIVE FOLLOW-UP

Postoperative CT with and without contrast should be obtained within 24 hours after surgery (when contrast enhancement of surgically traumatized brain is minimal) to detect residual tumor, hence to rule out false cure. Signal artifacts sometimes last as long as 10 weeks on the gadolinium-enhanced MRI, which makes MRI a less desirable test for this particular period. Presence of unsuspected residual tumor on the "next-day" CT should prompt a second-look operation within 1 to 2 weeks, i.e., before exuberant scarring makes reoperation difficult. If the "next-day" CT shows no residual tumor, or if the second attempt at total resection accomplishes its goal, the next CT and MRI can be obtained in 3 to 6 months. Thereafter, a yearly CT and MRI should be adequate.

Complete endocrine evaluation should be repeated 6 months after surgery to monitor thyroid and adrenocortical functions. Cortisone replacement is almost certainly permanent if stalk section was performed, but if the stalk was anatomically preserved, one may carefully withdraw cortisone in hospital and restudy the ACTH reserve to see if continued full replacement is necessary or whether the dose can be reduced. Excessive cortisone intake contributes potently to hyperphagia and must be categorically ruled out. Because of the recovery capacity of the magnocellular system of the supraoptic and paraventricular nuclei, the DDAVP requirement must also be re-evaluated 1 to 2 years after surgery even if total stalk section has been performed. At least 9 months should elapse before GH treatment is initiated, to determine whether adequate growth continues due to sustained IGF levels. A low postoperative GH level has no bearing on the growth curve after craniopharyngioma resection.[75,76,79]

Visual acuity and fields should be repeated twice yearly. This is most useful in cases of known residual or recurrent tumor, when a subtle change in vision may herald regrowth of a previously quiescent tumor before the increase in tumor size can be appreciated on imaging studies. At each clinical follow-up, the patient's neurobehavioral status is briefly evaluated as part of the routine. All growth indices are measured for children. The body weight and height are accurately documented since they remain the best indicators of abnormal eating behaviors, which are never truthfully reported by the patient and are often overlooked by the parents. Descriptions of the meal contents, timing, and patterns, as well as eating habits are best obtained from witnesses (siblings, friends), and are evaluated to distinguish between central hyperphagia, psychogenic polyphagia, and excessive corticosteroid intake. An abridged neuropsychologic minibattery should include verbal recall test, complex figure duplication and graphic recall to assess spatial orientation and nonlogic memory, respectively, object similarities and differences, and proverb interpretation. The patient's psychomotor activity level, mood, willingness to participate in work and recreation, and enthusiasm for social interaction are also recorded. A full neuropsychologic battery should be repeated on children 6 months to 1 year after surgery to plan school re-entry levels and long-term educational goals.

Reproductive Endocrinology: Physiology, Pathophysiology and Clinical Management. Philadelphia, Pa: WB Saunders Co; 1978:398–417.

73. Ayral D, Talot L, David M, Lecornu M, François R. Etude de la croissance paradoxale de certains enfants après chirurgie hypothalamo-hypophysaire en dépit de l'absence d'hormone de croissance. *Pediatrie.* 1980;35:389–401.

74. Costin G, Hogut MD, Philips LS, Daughaday WH. Craniopharyngioma: the rate of insulin in promoting postoperative growth. *J Clin Endocrinol Metab.* 1976;42:370–379.

75. Finkelstein JW, Kream J, Ludan A, Hellman L. Sulfaction factor (somatomedin): an explanation for continued growth in the absence of immunoassayable growth hormone in patients with hypothalamic tumor. *J Clin Endocrinol Metab.* 1972; 35:13–37.

76. Job JC, Lambertz J, Sizonenko PC, Rossier A. La croissance des enfants atteints de craniopharyngiome: vitesse de croissance et resultats des dosages d'hormone de croissance dans le plasma avant et après intervention chirurgicale. *Arch Fr Pediatr.* 1970;27:341–353.

77. Thomsen MJ, Conte FA, Kaplan SK, Grumbach MM. Endocrine and neurological outcome in childhood craniopharyngioma: a review of the effect of treatment in 42 patients. *J Pediatr.* 1980; 97:728–735.

78. Bucher H, Zapf J, Torresani T, Prader A, Froesch ER, Illig R. Insulin-like growth factors I & II, prolactin, and insulin in 19 growth hormone-deficient children with excessive, normal, and decreased longitudinal growth after operation for craniopharyngioma. *N Engl J Med.* 1983;309:1142–1146.

79. Pang D. Surgical management of craniopharyngioma. In: Sekhar LN, Janecka IP, eds. *Surgery of Cranial Base Tumors.* New York, NY: Raven Press; 1993:787–807.

80. Ungerstedt U. Stereotaxic mapping of the dopamine pathways in the rat brain. *Acta Physiol Scand.* 1971;367(suppl):1–48.

Chapter 36

Colloid Cysts
of the Third Ventricle

Arturo Camacho, Patrick J. Kelly

Colloid cysts of the third ventricle comprise 1% of CNS tumors.[1] When symptomatic, the outcome may be fatal if untreated. These lesions are benign. Complete removal will result in a cure. Although colloid cysts are virtually in the center of the brain, several excellent surgical options are available.

Colloid cysts afflict men and women with approximately equal frequency. In a recent study of 84 colloid cysts, 45 were in men and 39 in women.[2] Colloid cysts have been reported over a wide age range—from 7 to 82 years, with a case reported in a patient as young as 2 months—although they usually become symptomatic from the third to the sixth decades.[2]

The origin of colloid cysts has long been debated, and this in part is responsible for the various names associated with this lesion. The term *paraphysial cysts,* which indicates they originate in the paraphysis, was first proposed by Sjoval.[3] The term *paraphysis* was first used by Selenka[4] in 1890 to describe a vesicle evaginating from the roof of the telencephalon in sharks, reptiles, and marsupials. Kappers[5] studied the paraphysis in human embryos and found it to be a consistent structure comprised of a complex of short tubules. The structure was first present in embryos 17 mm in length, reached maximal development at about the tenth week, then degenerated such that by the 100 mm stage normally no trace of the organ remained. It is important to note that epithelium of the paraphysis as described by Kappers was devoid of cilia; therefore, cysts whose lining contains cilia and blepharoplasts are not of paraphyseal origin. It is perhaps more accurate to call these cysts *neuroepithelial cysts* as proposed by Stookey.[6] Hence, the term neuroepithelial cysts has also been used for with this lesion.[7,8]

More recently, scanning and electron microscope studies have found similarities to respiratory and enteric epithelium that suggest an endodermal rather than ectodermal origin.[9–11] Other possible cells of origin include the neuroepithelial ependymal lining, choroid, and tela choroidea.

In light of the failure to identify conclusively the cell type or structure of origin, it is more practical to refer to cystic lesions that appear to originate from the roof of the third ventricle at the level of the foramen of Monro as *colloid cysts.* The term colloid cyst is pathologically descriptive, thus avoiding the use of terms that may not accurately indicate the origin.

PATHOLOGY

Colloid cysts of the third ventricle are located anteriorly at the level of the foramen of Monro. Here the cysts may be attached to the roof of the third ventricle, the columns of the fornix, or the choroid plexus. The gross appearance is a characteristic blue or gray, and the cyst feels rubbery to gentle manipulation. The size may range from one centimeter to several centimeters (Fig. 36.1). Histologically, the cysts demonstrate either a single layer of pseudostratified columnar epithelium with or without cilia or cuboidal low columnar epithelium. Commonly present are mucous goblet cells with a mucin-positive mucicarmine on PAS staining. The epithelium and the fibrous capsule surrounding it together form the wall of the cyst (Fig. 36.2). The consistency of the contents varies among individual cysts. In 23 cases at the Mayo Clinic in which the content was described at the time of surgery 22 were either solid, semisolid, or viscous, and only one was liquid.[2] This fact may be important when considering surgical treatment. The amorphous material that makes up the content of the cyst is believed to be a result of cellular discharge of mucin and cellular desquamation.

PATHOPHYSIOLOGY

The signs and symptoms produced by these lesions are primarily related to increased intracranial pressure due

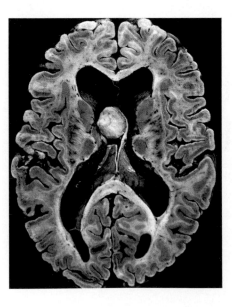

Figure 36.1 Gross transverse pathological specimen demonstrating a 2.5 cm colloid cyst in its characteristic position at the level of the foramen of Monro. Note the diffuse enlargement of lateral ventricles.

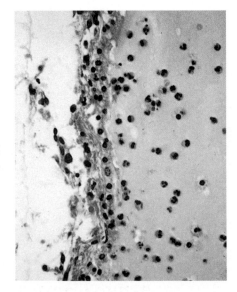

Figure 36.2 Photomicrograph of a colloid cyst demonstrating a fine fibrous capsule, epithelial layer, and amorphous contents. Sparse cellular debris is seen within the central portion.

to obstructive hydrocephalus. There are no pathognomonic signs. The most frequent findings in a recent series of surgically treated patients are summarized in Figure 36.3. As the cyst enlarges, it intermittently obstructs the flow of CSF at the level of the foramen of Monro. With continued growth, the obstruction becomes complete until surgical treatment or death (Fig. 36.4).

Other authors have speculated that even in the absence of hydrocephalus or increased intracranial pressure colloid cysts may become symptomatic as a result of local pressure on adjacent structures. In this regard Lobosky et al.[12] reported three cases in which, in the absence of hydrocephalus, patients presented with disturbances of memory, emotion, and personality. All three improved with surgical removal of the colloid cyst. The inference made was that direct pressure on diencephalic structures and fornix or vascular compromise of the same structures could explain the symptoms. Early reports regarding the presentation of symptoms emphasized a positional exacerbation of headaches. Sjovall[3] in 1909 first proposed that changes in head position could influence the position of the cyst, thereby intermittently obstructing the flow of CSF. Dandy[13] in 1933 and Stookey[6] in 1934, as well as other authors, attempted to explain the intermittent obstruction to flow in terms of a ball-valve effect caused by a moveable cyst at the foramen of Monro. Yenerman[14] in 1958 and more recent large series,[2,15,16] however, have not found this to be the case. Evidence against the ball-valve proposal consisted of autopsy findings in which the cyst was found below the foramen of Monro and the obstruction actually occurred at the anterior portion of the third ventricle. Furthermore, the colloid cyst appeared to be well fixed to the walls of the third ventricle. Of the 84 patients in our report, only two were affected by position; lying down worsened the headache in one patient but ameliorated the headache in the second patient.

Another aspect of the clinical course that perhaps has been overemphasized in the literature is the sudden death that can occur with these lesions.[17,18] If unattended death occurs, symptoms have usually been present for days to years; however, since the introduction of CT we have reported on 84 cases, and none of the deaths could be attributed directly to the colloid cyst save for one patient early in the series who did not have a CT scan. Ryder et al.[19] in 1986 reported on 55 patients with benign tumors of the third ventricle who suffered deterioration and death. The authors reported that most of the patients complained of symptoms for days to months, with only three showing courses of less than 24 hours.

We found that in 55 patients requiring surgical treatment the mean duration of symptoms was 29 months. The symptoms tended to be slowly progressive, only three having symptoms for less than 1 week. One patient had symptoms for 7 days, and the other two had symptoms for approximately 24 hours.

IMAGING STUDIES

Wallmann first described a colloid cyst in 1858,[20] but without accurate localization it remained an autopsy curiosity for over 60 years. The advancement of pneumoencephalography by Dandy cannot be overemphasized. Air pneumoencephalography—now only of historical interest—was fundamental to his work. He not only developed this diagnostic technique but used it to correctly identify, localize, and surgically remove the first colloid cyst in 1921.[13] One advantage of the air contrast study over more modern imaging studies is that it provides information about the presence or absence of communication between ventricles. The morbidity associated with the procedure, however, does not justify contem-

Figure 36.3 Signs and Symptoms of Colloid Cysts

Signs and Symptoms	Percentage of Patients
Headache	84
Change in mental status	36
Nausea and vomiting	26
Ataxia	20
Visual disturbance	14
Emotional lability/affect change	10
Depersonalization	6
Hypersomnolence	6

Modified from Camacho A, et al., 1989)

pory use. Nevertheless, knowledge of how each ventricle communicates with the remainder of the ventricular system is important in considering treatment (Fig. 36.5).

CT now forms the basis for diagnosing colloid cysts. It also provides important information regarding the presence or absence of hydrocephalus. On CT colloid cysts appear as round or oval lesions in the anterior and superior portion of the third ventricle at the level of the foramen of Monro. The attenuation relative to brain tissue may range from hypointense to hyperintense. Contrast enhancement is usually unimpressive (Figs. 36.6, 36.7). As CT scanning and modern imaging techniques become more widely used, the incidental finding of colloid cysts is becoming more frequent.

MRI may provide additional information and thus reduce the differential diagnosis prior to recommending treatment. Characteristically, colloid cysts appear as hyperintense round lesions on T1-weighted images (Fig. 36.8). Because multiplanar imaging is possible with MRI, the location and relationship of the lesion to surrounding anatomical structures is best ascertained with these studies.

On angiographic studies, colloid cysts appear as avascular lesions in the anterior-superior portion of the third ventricle. On the venous phase important information may be obtained regarding the deep venous system. The posterior segment of the septal vein will be displaced superolaterally. Additionally, evidence of hydrocephalus, such as elongation and stretching of the subependymal veins, may be present.

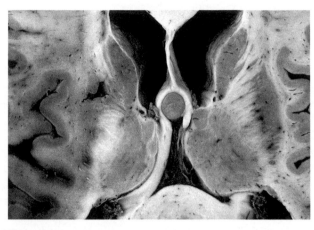

Figure 36.4 Gross coronal section of a pathological specimen demonstrating a small colloid cyst impacted between the foramen of Monro. The lateral ventricles are only mildly enlarged.

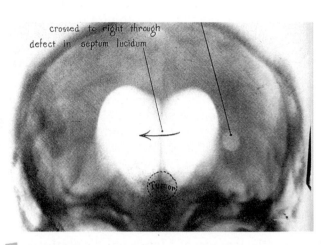

Figure 36.5 Anteroposterior pneumoencephalogram demonstrating outline of the colloid cyst and crossover of air contrast through a defect in the septum pellucidum. In such a case unilateral CSF diversion would decompress both lateral ventricles. (Reprinted with permission from Dandy WE, 1933)

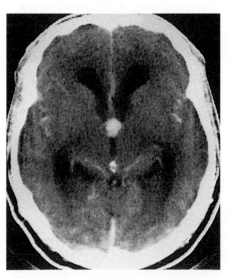

Figure 36.6 Axial CT scan showing a hyperintense colloid cyst at the level of the foramen of Monro, which is characteristic of this lesion. Note the temporal horns of the lateral ventricles are enlarged, indicating mild hydrocephalus.

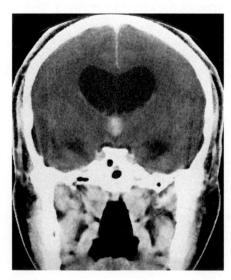

Figure 36.7 Coronal CT scan of a hyperdense colloid cyst producing symmetrical enlargement of the lateral ventricles including the temporal horns.

Principles of Neurosurgery

PATIENT MANAGEMENT

Since there are no pathognomonic signs and symptoms for colloid cysts, the correct diagnosis and treatment depends on the careful integration of history, neurologic exam, and imaging studies. A good medical history and detailed neurologic exam is imperative—signs of increased intracranial pressure, such as absent funduscopic venous pulsations, papilledema, change in mental status, etc., warrant close attention.

Not all patients in whom a colloid cyst is discovered require intervention. At our institution 24 patients with incidentally found colloid cysts are being followed closely. After a follow-up period of 19.3 months none have yet required surgery. Thus, in the patient without hydrocephalus whose symptoms cannot be attributed to the lesion in the anterior portion of the third ventricle, observation is a reasonable option. Taken into consideration, however, must be the patient's compliance, ready access to medical attention, and ability to deal with the knowledge and implications of the lesion's existence.

Which patients need urgent treatment and which patients have time to undergo work up must be decided. Some patients with elevated intracranial pressure and hydrocephalus note symptomatic relief following standard medical methods for reducing intracranial pressure. Chan and Thompson[17] reported on the use of hyperventilation, mannitol, and ventriculostomy to stabilize patients prior to definitive treatment of third ventricular colloid cysts. Unilateral ventriculostomy has been advocated to stabilize these patients, but caution should be exercised when employing this approach. An early air contrast ventriculogram from a patient of Dandy (Fig. 36.9) demonstrates that the lateral ventricle is entrapped without communication to the third ventricle or across the septum pellucidum. In such a patient, unilateral ventriculostomy may be insufficient and in fact may precipitate a shift of the midline structures. Thus, bilateral ventriculostomies may be required.

Once the patient is stabilized, definitive treatment at the earliest convenient time should be the goal.

SURGICAL TREATMENT

Transcortical Approach

Dandy performed the first successful removal of a colloid cyst in 1921. The surgical approach to the anterior third ventricle is still evolving. The approach first used by Dandy was a posterior transcallosal approach similar

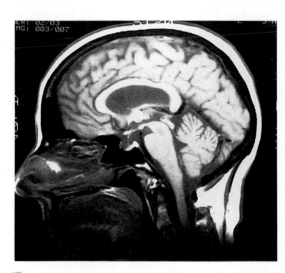

Figure 36.8 Sagittal T1-weighted MRI demonstrating increased T1 signal from a colloid cyst in the anterior third ventricle.

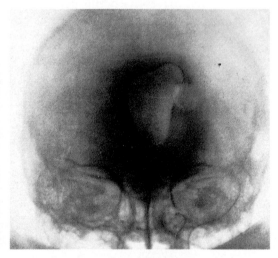

Figure 36.9 Anteroposterior pneumoencephalogram demonstrating the outline of a colloid cyst and entrapment of an enlarged left lateral ventricle. (Reprinted with permission from Dandy WE, 1933)

to that which had been used for tumors of the pineal region (Fig. 36.10). A pioneer and innovator, by 1930 Dandy modified his technique and used a frontal transcortical approach. In the absence of modern microsurgical methods, this required a somewhat extensive cortical resection (Fig. 36.11). This method was modified using a linear longitudinal transcortical incision[16,21,22] and, more recently, a transsulcal approach. This transfrontal-transcortical approach is best used when the ventricles are large, and in fact normal or small ventricles may contraindicate its use.

Transcallosal Approach

The next major step in the surgical removal of colloid cysts was by Greenwood[23] who in 1949 reported on the removal of four colloid cysts through an anterior transcallosal approach. The advantage of this approach is that it may be used when the ventricles are small, and since the cerebral cortex is not traversed there is less risk of postoperative seizures.[24] The relative disadvantages are that it is technically somewhat more demanding, and injury may occur to related vascular structures, that is, the superior sagittal sinus, parasagittal veins, and anterior cerebral arteries. One must also be careful not to confuse the cingulate gyrus with the corpus callosum and the callosomarginal artery with the pericallosal artery. In this regard, the white color of the corpus callosum may be helpful in its identification. The incision in the corpus callosum should be no more than 2 to 3 cm. In the anterior body of the corpus callosum this

does not produce a disconnection syndrome. Jeeves et al.[25] in 1979 after careful testing found impairment only in the transfer of tactile information. Once the corpus callosum has been divided, one of two trajectories may be taken. The first is to deviate to either side, enter the lateral ventricle, and then approach the colloid cyst through the foramen of Monro.[26] The second is to proceed in the midline and use the interforniceal entry.[27] The advantage to this latter method is that lesions too large to be delivered through the foramen of Monro may be removed. The disadvantage is that bilateral injury to fornix may occur. Sweet et al.[28] in 1959 were the first to document the recent memory deficit that is created by the bilateral section of the fornices.

Direct Removal of the Colloid Cyst

Following aspiration of its contents, the cyst ordinarily is removed through the foramen of Monro. The subchoroidal approach has been suggested for removal of partially calcified lesions or those with very viscous interiors that are too large to be delivered through an intact foramen of Monro. Alternatively, if the contralateral fornix is intact, the foramen of Monro may be enlarged anteriorly by section of the fornix anterior to the foramen of Monro. It should be noted that although this approach is usually well tolerated, it is not without some risk to memory.

Enlargement of the foramen of Monro posteriorly is more controversial, requiring division of the thalamostriate vein. Hirsch et al.[29] in 1979 described section of

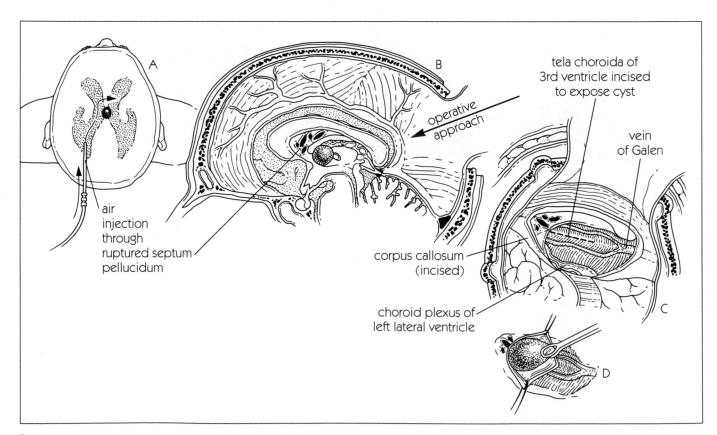

Figure 36.10 (A–D) Depiction of the earliest approach used by Walter Dandy to remove a third ventricle colloid cyst. An approach similar to that is used for pineal region tumors. (Reprinted with permission from Dandy WE, 1933)

the thalamostriate vein in the removal of third ventricular tumors without sequelae attributable to interruption of the venous drainage. Similar observations have been made by Lavyne and Patterson[30] using the subchoroidal transvelum interpositum approach. Hydrocephalus sometimes enlarges the foramen of Monro, facilitating work through it. In the best situation, however, the cyst can be aspirated to remove the fluid, and the remainder removed piecemeal, sparing the fornix and thalamostriate vein.

Percutaneous Aspiration Techniques
Several modalities have been reported in the aspiration of colloid cysts. The first report was by Gutierrez-Lara,[31] who in 1975 reported on the freehand aspiration of a colloid cyst. Bosch et al.[32] in 1978 reported on the successful application of stereotactic methods for colloid cyst aspiration. Powell et al.[33] in 1983 advocated ventriculoscopy for the aspiration of colloid cysts, especially in circumstances in which imaging studies were equivocal.

The simplicity of aspiration has a certain appeal.[30,34,35] However, there are also definite disadvantages. First, the content of colloid cysts is variable and, as mentioned above, of 23 colloid cysts that were systematically examined, 22 had contents that were solid, semisolid, or viscous. In such cases aspiration would fail. Second, in reported cases of aspiration, the aspiration is often incomplete; recurrences are documented.[36] Third, the spilled contents have been associated with ventriculitis and aqueductal stenosis.[6,15,37,38] Fourth, lesions other than colloid cysts can occupy the anterior third ventricle and may be difficult to differentiate on preoperative imaging studies.[39–44] In fact, the CT appearance of colloid cysts may be quite variable.[45–49] Finally, hemorrhage, impossible to control through a small biopsy cannula, may be devastating.

Stereotactic Resection of Colloid Cysts
Stereotactic resection of colloid cysts combines several advantages of the procedures described above. The procedure's technical aspects have been described in detail elsewhere[48–50]; also, see Chapter 49 for a discussion. Briefly, the procedure employs stereotactic CT and angiographic data bases. The CT margins of the lesion are digitized and interpolated into a target volume. A surgical trajectory is planned on a computer simulation system before the incision is made. Unlike nonstereotactic frontal transcortical approaches, where the bone flap is centered on the coronal suture, stereotactic resection employs a linear scalp incision at the patient's hairline and a 3 to 5 cm cranial trephine bone flap. In the stereotactic approach, the colloid cyst is approached from an anterior-superior direction as opposed to the superior approach employed in classical transcortical techniques. A more anterior trajectory enables the surgeon to establish the point where the cyst attaches to the roof of the third ventricle so it can be coagulated and removed with sharp dissection. After opening the dura, the superior frontal sulcus is split microsurgically. A 2 cm cylindrical retractor is advanced through the sulcus and the white

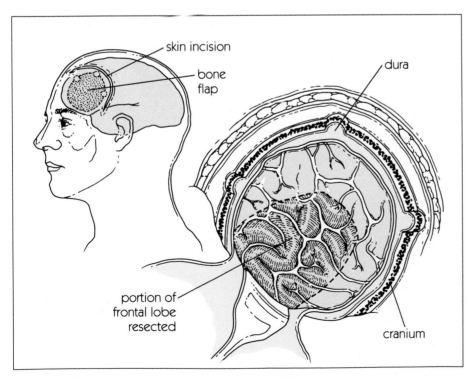

Figure 36.11 Outline of the scalp incision, craniotomy, and cortical resection for transfrontal transcortical removal of third ventricle colloid cyst as described by Dandy. (Reprinted with permission from Dandy WE, 1933)

skin incision

bone flap

dura

portion of frontal lobe resected

cranium

matter fibers are incised with the carbon dioxide laser until the lateral ventricle is reached (Fig. 36.12). Upon entering the ventricle, the retractor is rapidly advanced to the foramen of Monro. The design of the retractor makes it possible to spread the caudate head and septum pellucidum safely, which tends to dilate the foramen of Monro slightly. This facilitates direction of and removal of the cyst. Furthermore, this method can be used even when the ventricles are small, and important arteries and veins are avoided. At the Mayo Clinic stereotactic resection has been used in the removal of 19 colloid cysts. There have not yet been any postoperative seizures or other permanent surgical complications,[48–50] which contrasts with the 11% incidence of seizures associated with standard transcortical-transventricular approach.[2] The cyst is directly visible and the working area can be isolated from the lateral ventricle by the retractor, allowing total removal and minimizing spillage of the cyst contents into the lateral ventricle while protecting important anatomical structures.

SHUNTING PROCEDURES

The final surgical procedure that can be employed in patients with colloid cysts is CSF diversion. Although shunting procedures cannot be considered definitive treatment, they carry a relatively low risk. A shunt with fenestration of the septum pellucidum may be a reasonable option in elderly or medically unstable patients. In addition, like ventriculostomy, shunting procedures are used for stabilization until a definitive operation is performed. Shunt malfunctions and infections are frequent.[2]

CONCLUSION

The term colloid cyst should remain the preferred name for cystic lesions of the superior-anterior portion of the third ventricle until the structure of origin is better defined. With the aid of modern imaging techniques, early diagnosis of these lesions is now possible. Sudden death associated with colloid cysts should become less frequent. On the other hand, modern imaging methods have created a new dilemma: What should one do with incidentally discovered colloid cysts? The answer to this question is not straightforward, and one needs to tailor the recommendation to the individual patient, taking the surgeon's experience into account. In the symptomatic patient, surgical intervention is mandatory—total removal of the colloid cyst is the definitive treatment. Which surgical approach to use depends on the methods available to the surgeon and the advantages and disadvantages of each.

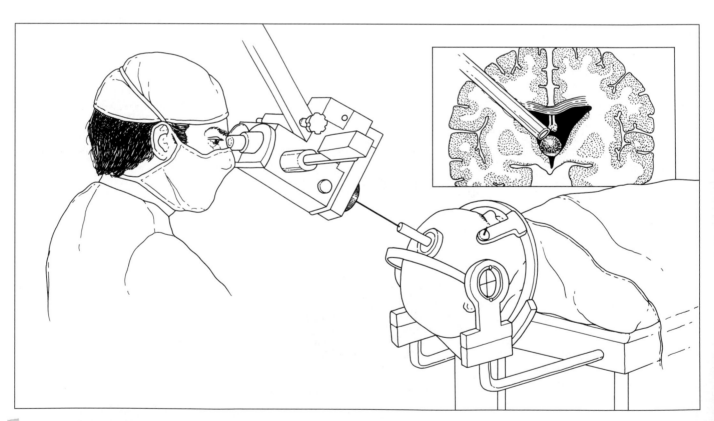

Figure 36.12 Computer assisted stereotactic microsurgical craniotomy technique for the treatment of colloid cysts of the third ventricle. Inset shows a coronal cross-sectional view of the cylindrical retractor and its relationship to structures in and around the third ventricle. (Adapted from Abernathey CD, et al., 1989)

REFERENCES

1. Rubenstein LJ. Tumors of the central nervous system. In: *Atlas of Tumor Pathology*. Washington, DC: Armed Forces Institute of Pathology; 1972.
2. Camacho A, Abernathey CD, Kelly PJ, et al. Colloid cysts: experience with the management of 84 cases since the introduction of computed tomography. *Neurosurgery*. 1989;24:693–700.
3. Sjovall E. Über eine Ependymcyste embryonalen Charakters (Paraphyse?) im dritten Hirnventrikel mit todlichem Ausgang. *Beitr z path Anat U.Z. allgem Path*. 1910;47:248–269.
4. Selenka E. Das Stirnorgan der Wirbeltiere. *Biol Centralbl*. 1890;10:323–326.
5. Kappers JA. The development of the paraphysis cerebri in man with comments on its relationship to the intercolumnar tubercle and its significance for the origin of cystic tumors in the third ventricle. *J Comp Neurol*. 1955;102:425–507.
6. Stookey B. Intermittent obstruction of the foramen of Monro by neuroepithelial cysts of the third ventricle: symptoms, diagnosis and treatment. *Bull Neurol Inst NY*. 1934;3:446–500.
7. Ciric I, Zivin I. Neuroepithelial (colloid) cysts of the septum pellucidum. *J Neurosurg*. 1975;43:69–73.
8. Shuangshoti S, Roberts MP, Netsky MG. Neuroepithelial (colloid) cysts: pathogenesis and relation to choroid plexus and ependyma. *Arch Pathol*. 1965; 80:214–224.
9. Leech RW, Freeman T, Johnson R. Colloid cyst of the third ventricle: a scanning and transmission electron microscopic study. *J Neurosurg*. 1982;57: 108–113.
10. Matsushima T, Fukui M, Kitamura K, et al. Mixed colloid cystxanthogranuloma of the third ventricle. A light and electron microscopic study. *Surg Neurol*. 1985;24:457–462.
11. Yagishita S, Itoh Y, Shiozawa T, et al. Ultrastructural observation on a colloid cyst of the third ventricle. *Acta Neuropathol (Berl)*. 1984;65:41–45.
12. Lobosky JM, Vangilder JC, Damasio AR. Behavioral manifestations of third ventricular colloid cysts. *J Neurol Neurosurg Psychiatry*. 1984;47: 1075–1080.
13. Dandy WE. *Benign Tumors of the Third Ventricle. Diagnosis and Treatment*. Springfield, Ill: Charles C Thomas Publisher; 1933.
14. Yenermen MH, Bowerman CI, Haymaker W. Colloid cyst of the third ventricle: a clinical study of 54 cases in the light of previous publications. *Acta Neuroveg*. 1958;17:211–277.
15. Brun A, Egund N. The pathogenesis of cerebral symptoms in colloid cysts of the third ventricle: a clinical and pathoanatomical study. *Acta Neurol Scand*. 1973;49:525–535.
16. Little JR, MacCarty CS. Colloid cysts of the third ventricle. *J Neurosurg*. 1974;40:230–235.
17. Chan RC, Thompson GB. Third ventricular colloid cysts presenting with acute neurological deterioration. *Surg Neurol*. 1983;19:358–362.
18. Weisz RR, Faxal M. Colloid cyst of the third ventricle: a neurological emergency. *Ann Emerg Med*. 1983;12:783–785.
19. Ryder JW, Kleinschmidt-DeMasters BK, Keller TS. Sudden deterioration and death in patients with benign tumors of the third ventricle area. *J Neurosurg*. 1986;64:216–223.
20. Wallman H. Eine Colloidcyste im dritten Hirnventrikel und ein Lipom im Plexus choroides. *Virchows Arch Path Anat*. 1858;11:385–388.
21. McKissock W. The surgical treatment of colloid cysts of the third ventricle. *Brain*. 1951;74:1–9.
22. Baker GS, Berke JJ. Colloid cysts of the brain. *Minn Med*. 1963;46:865–869.
23. Greenwood J. Paraphyseal cysts of the third ventricle. *J Neurosurg*. 1949;6:153–159.
24. Shucart WA, Stein BM. Transcallosal approach to the anterior ventricular system. *Neurosurgery*. 1978; 3:339–343.
25. Jeeves MA, Simpson DA, Geffen G. Functional consequences of the transcallosal removal of intraventricular tumours. *J Neurol Neurosurg Psychiatry*. 1979;42:134–142.
26. Ehni G, Ehni B. Consideration in transforaminal entry. In: Apuzzo MLJ, ed. *Surgery of the Third Ventricle*. Baltimore, Md: Williams & Wilkins; 1987: 326–353.
27. Apuzzo MLJ, Gianotta SL. Transcallosal interforniceal approach. In: Apuzzo MLJ, ed. *Surgery of the Third Ventricle*. Baltimore, Md: Williams & Wilkins; 1987:354–380.
28. Sweet WH, Talland GA, Ervin FR. Loss of recent memory following section of the fornix. *Trans Am Neurol Assoc*. 1959;84:76–82.
29. Hirsch JF, Zouaoui A, Renier D, et al. A new surgical approach to the third ventricle with interruption of the striothalamic vein. *Acta Neurochir*. 1979;47: 135–147.
30. Lavyne MH, Patterson RH. Subchoroidal transvelum interpositum approach to mid-third ventricular tumors. *Neurosurgery*. 1983;12:86–94.
31. Gutierrez-Lara F, Patino R, Hakim S. Treatment of tumors of the third ventricle: a new and simple technique. *Surg Neurol*. 1975;3:323–325.
32. Bosch DA, Rahn T, Backlund EO. Treatment of colloid cysts of third ventricle by stereotactic aspiration. *Surg Neurol*. 1978;9:15–18.
33. Powell MP, Torrens MJ, Thomson JLG, et al. Isodense colloid cysts of the third ventricle: a diagnostic and therapeutic problem resolved by ventriculoscopy. *Neurosurgery*. 1983;13:234–237.

34. Mohadjer M, Teshmar E, Mundinger F. CT-stereotaxic drainage of colloid cysts in the foramen of Monro and the third ventricle. *J Neurosurg.* 1987; 67:220–223.

35. Rivas JJ, Lobato RD. CT-assisted stereotaxic aspiration of colloid cysts of the third ventricle. *J Neurosurg.* 1985;62:238–242.

36. Donauer E, Moringlane JR, Ostertag CB. Colloid cysts of the third ventricle. *Acta Neurochir (Wien).* 1986;83:24–30.

37. Antunes JL, Louis KM, Ganti SR. Colloid cysts of the third ventricle. *Neurosurgery.* 1980;7:450–455.

38. Antunes JL, Kvam D, Ganti SR, et al. Mixed colloid cysts: xanthogranulomas of the third ventricle. *Surg Neurol.* 1981;16:256–261.

39. Gradin WC, Taylon C, Fruin AH. Choroid plexus papilloma of the third ventricle: case report and review of the literature. *Neurosurgery.* 1983;12:217–220.

40. Kendall B, Reider-Grosswasser I, Valentine A. Diagnosis of masses presenting with the ventricles on computed tomography. *Neuroradiology.* 1983;25:11–22.

41. Lanzieri CF, Sabato I, Sachear M. Third ventricular lymphoma: CT-findings. *J Comput Assist Tomogr.* 1984;8:645–647.

42. Loftus CM, Marquardt MD, Stein BM. Hemangioblastoma of the third ventricle. *Neurosurgery.* 1984;15:70–72.

43. Markwalder TM, Markwalder RV, Markwalder HM. Meningioma of the anterior part of the third ventricle. *J Neurosurg.* 1979;50:233–235.

44. Szper I, Oi S, Leestma J, et al. Xanthogranuloma of the third ventricle. *J Neurosurg.* 1979;51:565–568.

45. Bullard DE, Osborne D, Cook WA Jr. Colloid cyst of the third ventricle presenting as a ring-enhancing lesion on computed tomography. *Neurosurgery.* 1982;11:790–791.

46. Ganti SR, Antunes JL, Louis KM, et al. Computed tomography in the diagnosis of colloid cysts of the third ventricle. *Radiology.* 1981;138:385–391.

47. Zilka A. Computed tomography of colloid cysts of the third ventricle. *Clin Radiol.* 1981;32:397–401.

48. Abernathey CD, Kelly PJ, Davis DH. Treatment of colloid cysts of the third ventricle by stereotactic microsurgical laser craniotomy. *J Neurosurg.* 1989;70:525–529.

49. Kelly PJ. Nonglial mass lesions. In: *Tumor Stereotaxis.* Philadelphia, Pa: WB Saunders Co.; 1991.

50. Kelly PJ. Computer-assisted stereotaxic laser microsurgery. In: Apuzzo MLJ, ed. *Surgery of the Third Ventricle.* Baltimore, Md: Williams & Wilkins; 1987:811–828.

Chapter 37

Metastatic Tumors
of the Spine

Richard G. Perrin, R.J. McBroom

Metastatic tumors of the spine are an ominous complication of systemic cancer. The management of spinal metastases—establishing a diagnosis and determining and executing the optimal treatment—is a paradigm for the management of all spinal tumors.

Spinal metastases (and spinal tumors in general) are classified according to anatomic location.[1–3] The vast majority occur extradurally. Intradural extramedullary metastases are uncommon. Intramedullary spinal metastases are relatively rare (Fig. 37.1).

Metastatic tumors are the most frequently occurring tumors of the spinal column, and the spine is the most common site for skeletal metastases.[4] It is estimated that between 5% and 10% of cancer patients develop symptomatic spinal metastases.[5–8] Secondary spinal tumors most often originate from carcinomas of the breast, pros- tate, and lung, reflecting both the prevalence of these primary neoplasms and the propensity for carcinomas of the breast and prostate to metastasize to bone. Approximately 9% of patients with symptomatic spinal metastases present without known primary tumors.[9–11]

Postmortem studies have shown that secondary spinal tumors are distributed along the spinal column in approximate proportion to the bony bulk of the vertebrae. The lumbar region is the most common site, whereas the cervical spine is least often involved.[4] In clinical experience, however, *symptomatic* spinal metastases most frequently affect the thoracic segments, with particular predilection for the levels around T-4 and T-11.[10]

DIAGNOSIS

SYMPTOMS AND SIGNS

Symptomatic spinal metastases produce a characteristic clinical syndrome.[2,3,10–12] Pain is the earliest and most prominent feature in 90% of patients. Local back or neck pain may be associated with band-like radicular extension indicating nerve root involvement. Pain that is described as severe and burning or dysesthetic should raise suspicion of an intradural extramedullary tumor. Local back or neck pain that is aggravated by movement about the involved segment and relieved by immobilization indicates underlying mechanical instability. Palpation of the posterior spine usually elicits local tenderness at vertebrae involved with extradural metastases.

Local back or neck pain due to spinal metastases may be present for weeks or months and is often initially dismissed as arthritis, back strain, or disc disease. The correct diagnosis may not be established until more obvious manifestations of spinal cord or nerve root compromise appear.[13] It is axiomatic that *back or neck pain in a cancer patient heralds spinal metastasis until proven otherwise.*

Back or neck pain is eventually followed by weakness, numbness, and sphincter dysfunction. Once established, weakness progresses relentlessly to complete and irreversible paraplegia unless timely treatment is initiated.[9]

RADIOGRAPHIC STUDIES

Radiographic studies are essential for diagnosis, staging, surgical planning, and follow-up of patients with spinal metastases.

Figure 37.1 Relative Frequency of Spinal Metastases According to Anatomic Classification

Author	Patients	E (%)	ID/EM (%)	IM (%)
Rogers and Heard (1958)	17	94	6 (one case)	—
Barron et al (1959)	125	98	—	1.6
Edelson et al (1972)	175	97	—	3.4
Perrin et al (1981)	200	94	5	0.5

Plain Film

Plain x-ray studies of the spine provide a useful screening test, showing an abnormality in 90% of patients with secondary tumors of the spine. Evaluation of plain x-rays should include assessment of:

1. Qualitative bony alterations (i.e., lytic, blastic, or sclerotic abnormalities). The majority of spinal metastases produce osteolytic alteration. Osteoblastic or sclerotic changes most often occur with metastases arising from breast or prostate (Fig. 37.2).[14]
2. Site of involvement (i.e., posterior elements, pedicles, or vertebral body). It is uncommon for spinal metastases to involve only the posterior elements (spine and laminae). More often, the tumor focus is located in the vertebral body, causing compression of the dural sac and its contents from the front. Most often, however, spinal metastases evolve laterally, in the region of the pedicle, and extend anterolaterally or posterolaterally. Pedicle erosion is the earliest and most common abnormality seen on plain films of the spine in patients with spinal metastases. The AP radiograph of the spine normally resembles a "totem of owls" (Fig. 37.3A). Pedicle erosion produces a "winking owl" sign (Fig. 37.3B); bilateral pedicle erosion causes a "blinking owl" sign.[15]
3. Ancillary findings (i.e., paraspinal soft tissue shadow, vertebral collapse, pathologic fracture dislocation, and malalignment).[16] The region of pedicle erosion is often associated with paravertebral soft tissue shadow (Fig. 37.4). Loss of structural in-tegrity may lead to vertebral collapse with wedge compression (Fig. 37.5). Further destruction of the vertebral body can cause pathologic fracture dislocation (Fig. 37.6). Pathologic fracture dislocation is most often seen in the cervical region, where the wide range of neck movements, dependent position of the head, and lack of a rib cage supporting structure all jeopardize the structural integrity of the spinal column and the anatomic alignment of the spinal canal.

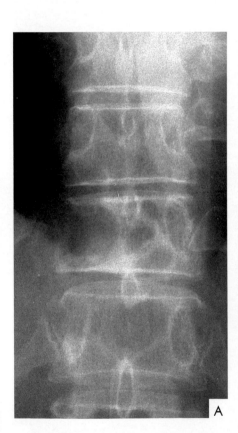
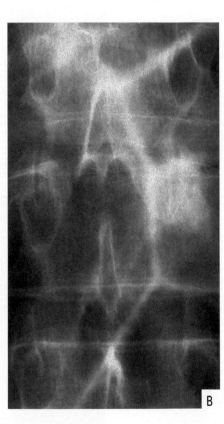

Figure 37.2 Osteolytic spinal metastases arising from the lung (**A**). Osteosclerotic spinal metastases arising from the prostate (**B**).

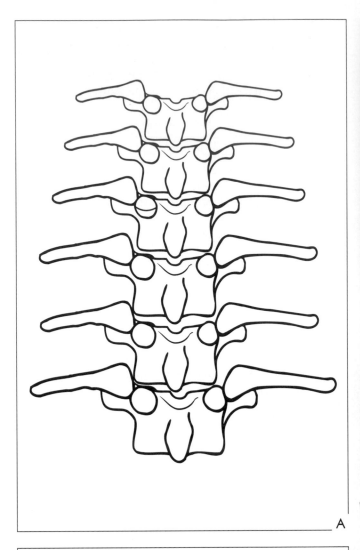

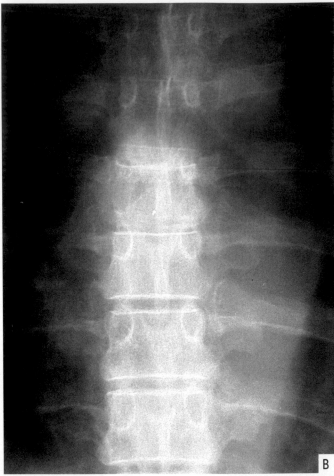

Figure 37.3 (A) "Winking owl" sign. (B) AP radiograph resembling a "totem of owls."

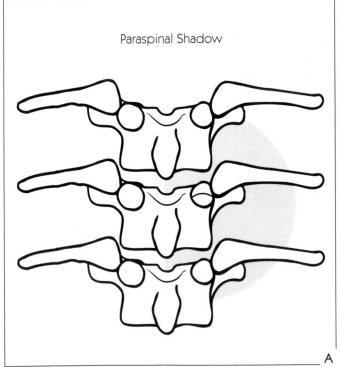

Paraspinal Shadow

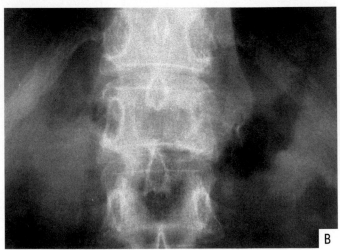

Figure 37.4 (A,B) Paraspinal soft tissue shadow at the site of symptomatic spinal metastasis.

Principles of Neurosurgery

Bone Scan

Radioisotope bone scan may show evidence of metastatic spinal tumor at an earlier stage than plain x-rays.[17–20] It has been estimated that 50% to 75% of the vertebral medullary space is replaced before radiographic changes are discernible.[21] However, bone scans are relatively nonspecific—degenerative changes and infection, as well as spinal tumors, cause positive uptake.[22]

Myelography

Myelography has been the standard method for identifying the location and level of spinal cord and nerve

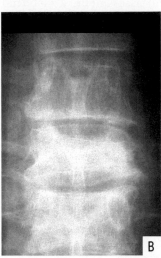

Figure 37.5 (A,B) Vertebral collapse due to spinal metastases.

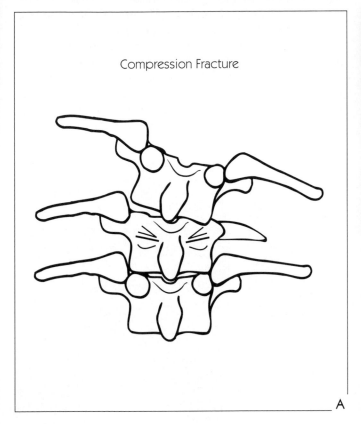

Compression Fracture

A

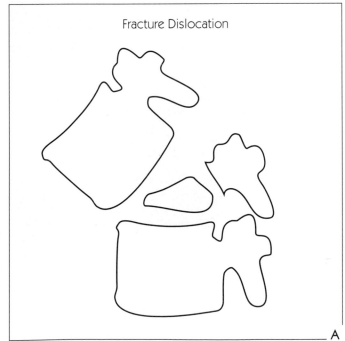

Fracture Dislocation

A

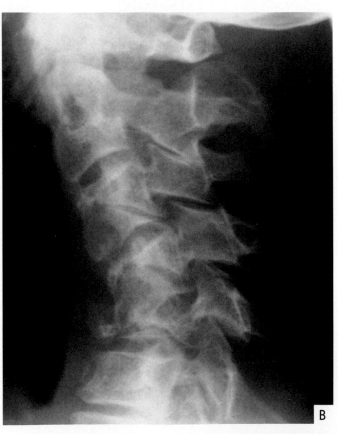

B

Figure 37.6 (A,B) Pathologic fracture-dislocation due to cervical spinal metastasis.

root compromise due to spinal tumors. Extradural, intradural extramedullary, and intramedullary spinal tumors are distinguished by characteristic myelographic patterns (Fig. 37.7A,B). Deviation of the dye column indicates the source (anterior, lateral, posterior) of the compression mass. When the level of a complete block identified by lumbar myelography is incongruent with the clinical assessment, a cisternal myelogram should be performed to determine the extent of a single lesion or to identify multiple levels of involvement (Fig. 37.7C).

Computerized Axial Tomography

Computerized axial tomography (CAT) scan is useful to demonstrate the distribution of spinal tumors, the displacement of the spinal cord and nerve roots, the degree of bony destruction, and paraspinal extension of the lesion in the horizontal plane (Fig. 37.8). CAT scan is also effective in distinguishing benign spinal degenerative disease from neoplastic lesions.[23,24]

Magnetic Resonance Imaging

MRI has become the imaging modality of choice for spinal tumors, including metastases.[25-28] MRI permits display of the entire spinal column in sagittal sections to confirm an isolated level of involvement, multiple levels of contiguous tumor spread, or disparate tumor foci at multiple levels (Fig. 37.9). Horizontal and coronal reconstructions provide important information concerning tumor geometry, useful in planning surgical decompression, as well as data about vertebral bony integrity, essential in executing the spinal reconstruction.

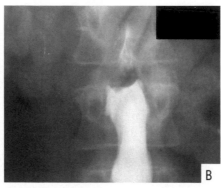

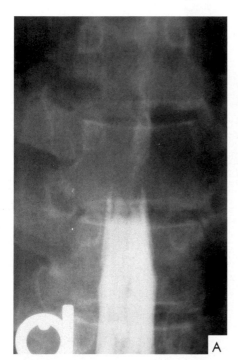

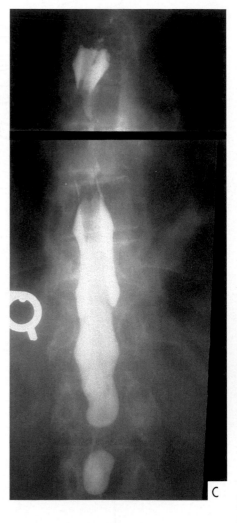

Figure 37.7 (A) Complete lumbar myelographic block at the site of extradural spinal metastasis. **(B)** Meniscus block due to intradural extramedullary spinal metastasis from a malignant melanoma. **(C)** Lumbar and cisternal myelograms delineate the extent of extradural spinal metastases.

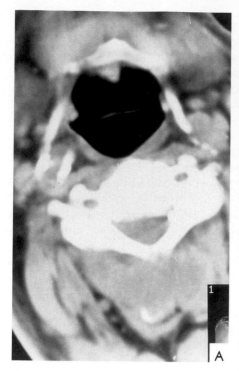

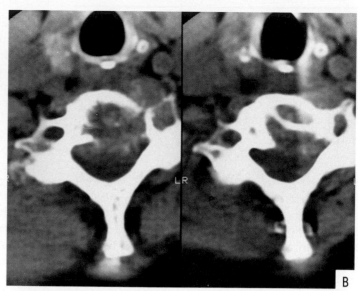

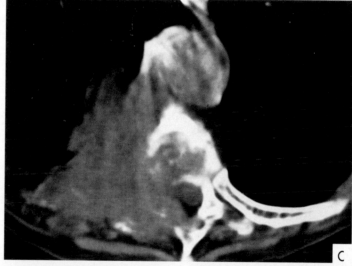

Figure 37.8 CAT scan of extradural spinal metastases located posteriorly (A), anteriorly (B), and laterally (C), and showing displacement of the dural sac and contents, bony destruction, and paraspinal extension.

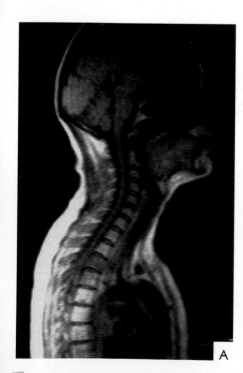

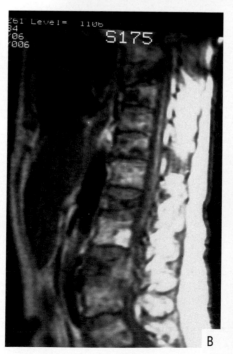

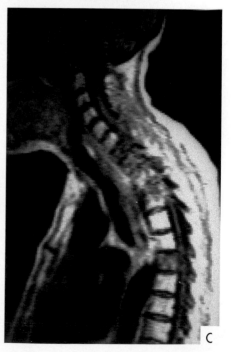

Figure 37.9 MRI demonstrating metastases at an isolated level (A), multiple levels of contiguous tumor spread (B), and disparate levels of tumor foci (C).

Metastatic Tumors of the Spine

MANAGEMENT

Treatment of patients with spinal metastases is designed to relieve pain and to preserve or restore neurologic function. The realistic objective is palliation. Nevertheless, relief from pain and preservation or restoration of neurologic function contribute immeasurably to the quality of remaining life for a cancer patient and reduce the burden of care.

RADIATION VERSUS SURGERY

The relative merits of therapeutic irradiation, surgery, or a combination of these treatment modalities for management of spinal metastases have been a matter of conjecture and continuing debate. Radiation therapy is usually considered the initial treatment of choice for the majority of patients with symptomatic secondary spinal tumors and is especially effective for lymphoreticular metastases.[9,29-32] Surgery is widely considered a treatment of last resort.[8] The generally accepted indications for surgical intervention are listed in Figure 37.10.[3,9,12,15,29,31,33]

Most patients referred for surgical management of spinal metastases have relapsed after radiation therapy. The majority have persistent or recurring tumor causing spinal cord and/or nerve root compromise after maximal tolerable therapeutic irradiation.

Surgery is indicated when the diagnosis is in doubt. Approximately 9% of patients with symptomatic spinal metastases present with no known primary tumor.[9-11] Surgical decompression may then be diagnostic as well as therapeutic. Surgery is also indicated when pathology other than metastatic tumor (e.g., disc protrusion, abscess, hematoma) is suspected of causing spinal cord or nerve root compromise in a cancer patient.[13]

Pathologic fracture dislocation of the spine produces neurologic compromise by a combination of factors, including distortion caused by spinal malalignment and compression produced by extradural tumor. Surgical intervention is then required to restore spinal alignment, eliminate the compressing tumor, and stabilize the spinal column.[12,34]

Urgent surgical decompression should be considered for patients with rapidly progressing or advanced paraplegia. Therapeutic irradiation can initially aggravate the neurologic compression syndrome[35]; therefore, complete and irreversible paraplegia may occur before any benefits of radiation therapy are manifest.

SURGICAL APPROACH

Surgery for spinal metastases must decompress the spinal cord and nerve roots and stabilize the spinal column.[10,12,16,36,37] The surgical approach can be primarily

---

Figure 37.10 Indications for Surgery in Spinal Metastasis

Failure of radiation therapy
Diagnosis unknown
Pathologic fracture-dislocation
Paraplegia, rapidly progressing/far advanced

Figure 37.11 Factors to Consider in Choosing an Approach to Spinal Metastases

Tumor location
Spinal level
Tumor extent
Bony integrity
Patient debility

---

anterior or posterior; each has its uses, and neither approach is always appropriate. The optimal avenue depends on a number of factors (Fig. 37.11).[38]

Intradural spinal metastases are usually best approached from behind.[2,3] The posterior approach permits craniocaudad exposure along the length of the spinal column and provides appropriate transdural access for intramedullary and intradural extramedullary metastases.

Extradural spinal metastases can be approached from the front or from behind.[38] Occasionally they involve only the posterior spine and laminae (see Fig. 37.8A), in which case decompression through a posterior approach (laminectomy) is appropriate. More often the compression mass is located in front of the dural sac (see Fig. 37.8B), calling for decompression through an anterior approach. Most extradural metastases, however, evolve laterally in the vertebral body, extending anterolaterally or posterolaterally (see Fig. 37.8C). Effective spinal decompression in these cases can be achieved through either an anterior or a posterior approach. Finally, extradural metastases often extend in napkin-ring fashion about the dural sac; in such cases the posterior approach permits more thorough circumferential decompression of the dural sac and nerve roots.

The anterior approach is awkward at the highest cervical (C-1 and C-2), high thoracic (T1-T3), and lowest lumbar (L-5 and sacrum) segments. A transoral approach and mandible-splitting maneuvers have been described for anterior access to the upper cervical spine. However, the technical challenge of such procedures and the difficulties for the patient, whose physical and emotional resources are already limited by systemic cancer, usually outweigh the palliative benefits. The highest thoracic segments can be reached from the front by splitting the manubrium and reflecting the first and second ribs laterally. More caudal exposure is limited by the heart and great vessels; furthermore, the natural thoracic kyphos restricts visualization during this approach for both decompression and instrumentation. Decompression at the lumbosacral junction from in front is relatively straightforward. However, spinal stabilization at this level is difficult. Thus, even if adequate decompression is achieved, anterior spinal reconstruction—particularly at the cephalad (C-1 and C-2) and caudad (L-5 and sacrum) extremes of the spinal column—poses enormous biomechanical problems.

Spinal stabilization is necessary after all anterior decompression (corpectomy) procedures and after most posterolateral decompression procedures.[15,16] Spinal stability after reconstruction depends on the integrity of the bony elements adjacent to the decompression site; they must be sufficient to accept, support, and maintain the fixation devices. The same structural factors that render the diseased cervical spine susceptible to pathologic fracture dislocation also jeopardize an anteriorly applied reconstruction prosthesis. Fixation of the prosthesis is also limited by the diminutive size of the cervical vertebral bodies. Consequently, an anterior stabilization construct in the cervical spine should be supplemented by a posterior stabilization construct or an external brace or appliance. Stabilization of the spine at any level is less likely to be achieved with an anterior fixation construct if the defect to be spanned encompasses two or more corpectomy segments, and it may be necessary in such cases to reinforce the anterior stabilization construct with a posteriorly applied device. Posterior stabilization can be achieved by sublaminar wiring fixed to rib grafts, steel rods, or methylmethacrylate struts at a minimum of two levels above and two levels below the decompression defect.

Patient debility, both local and systemic, plays an important role in selecting the surgical approach. Posterior spinal decompression and stabilization procedures performed through a radiation-saturated field carry a high risk of wound complications, including dehiscence with or without infection.[36,39,40] For this reason (other things being equal), previously irradiated thoracic and lumbar spinal metastases are best approached from the front. However, this does not apply to the cervical region, where radiation-induced soft tissue injury, scarring, and loss of anatomic planes increase the risk of vascular and esophageal injury along the anterior avenue of dissection. Finally, some patients may be unable to tolerate the more involved transthoracic or thoracoabdominal exposures because of systemic illness or concurrent conditions.

Embolization

Spinal metastases originating from thyroid or kidney are highly vascular. It is advisable to embolize such lesions before direct surgical intervention in an effort to minimize intraoperative blood loss (Fig. 37.12).

Posterior Decompression

Posterior decompression is performed with the patient in an appropriate prone position. In the face of existing or potential spinal instability, care must be taken to avoid exacerbation of spinal malalignment. When frank pathologic fracture dislocation affects the cervical seg-

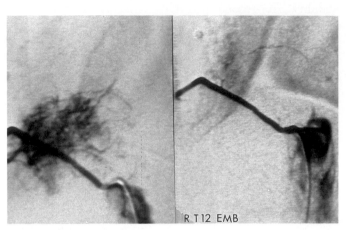

Figure 37.12 Spinal angiography before (left) and after (right) embolization of spinal metastasis originating from hypernephroma.

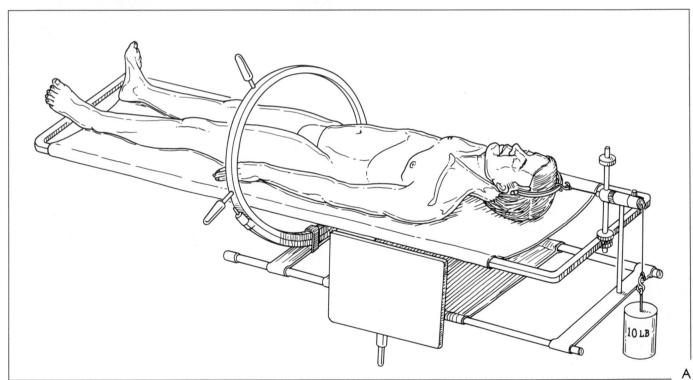

Figure 37.13 (A) Positioning for posterior decompression and stabilization with skeletal traction to restore and maintain spinal alignment.

ments, skeletal traction is applied to restore spinal alignment before surgery.

Manipulation of the diseased cervical spine during tracheal intubation may precipitate or aggravate a neurologic deficit; consequently, consideration should be given to intubating the awake patient with fiberoptic bronchoscopy.[41] Once the patient is intubated and anesthesized, skull tongs (if not already present) are applied for skeletal traction (10 pounds) during surgery (Fig. 37.13A). The surgical procedure is facilitated by use of a turning bed, such as a Stryker frame, so

that after induction of anesthesia, the patient can be repositioned from supine to prone with minimal risk of exacerbating spinal malalignment (Fig. 37.13B). If spinal instability is not a concern, the patient can be placed prone in the knee-chest position or on a suitable frame without thoracic or abdominal restriction (Fig. 37.13C).

The midline incision should be of sufficient length to permit decompression for at least half a segment above and half a segment below the area of spinal cord compromise. The paraspinal muscles are stripped sub-

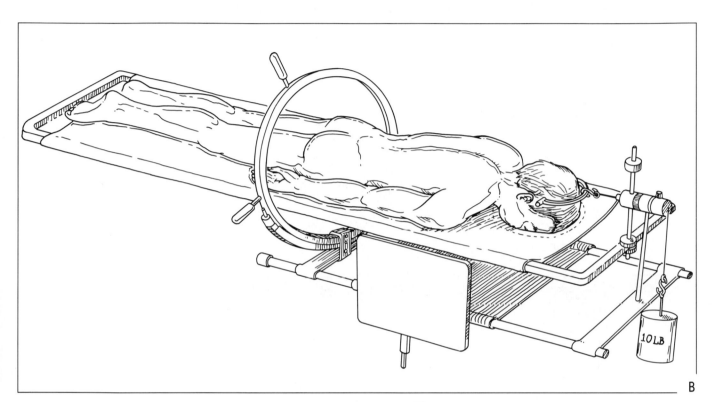

B

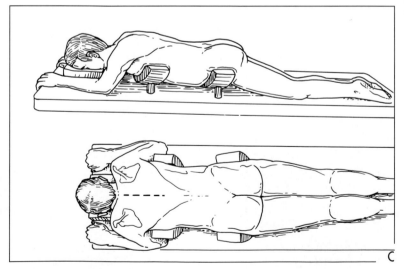

C

Figure 37.13, continued (B) Use of a turning bed (such as a Stryker frame) permits repositioning of the patient from supine to prone. (C) Positioning when spinal instability is not a concern.

periostially from the spines and laminae around the diseased area (Fig. 37.14). Care must be taken to avoid inadvertently plunging through the bony laminae, which may be destroyed by tumor. A wide laminectomy is performed that extends for a half segment above and a half segment below the area of spinal cord compression. In the uncommon event that the extradural tumor is restricted to the posterior elements (as, for example, in Figure 37.8A), laminectomy alone may provide adequate decompression.

In most cases, however, adequate decompression from a posterior approach requires posterolateral exposure for removal of tumor-destroyed lateral elements. This, in turn, provides anterior access into the vertebral body. Excavation of the tumor-involved vertebral body can be accomplished with angled cup curettes and pituitary forceps. A downward-angled cup curette can be used to decompress the dural sac anteriorly by displacing the compression mass into the hollowed vertebral body (Fig. 37.15). The tumor should be carefully peeled

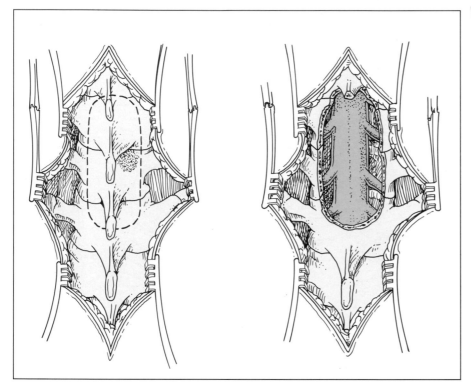

Figure 37.14 Posterior exposure is achieved by stripping muscles subperiosteally from the spines and laminae around the diseased area. Exposure must extend for at least a half segment above and a half segment below the area of cord compression.

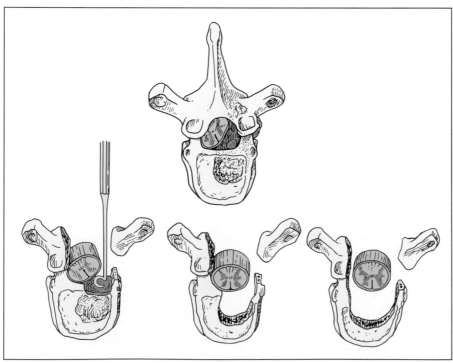

Figure 37.15 Adequate decompression from a posterior approach usually requires posterolateral exposure. Removal of tumor-destroyed elements provides access anteriorly into the vertebral body.

Principles of Neurosurgery

off the dural sac and root sleeves. Encased nerve roots in the thoracic segments can be intentionally crushed if radicular pain caused by involvement of these roots is present. This posterolateral decompression may be undertaken bilaterally to enable radical and circumferential decompression of the spinal cord and nerve roots (Fig. 37.16; see Fig. 37.15).

The posterior approach is based on standard laminectomy technique, is easily extended superiorly or inferiorly to include additional segments (as is often required), and is applicable along the length of the spinal column. Adequate posterolateral exposure provides access through the tumor-destroyed lateral elements into the vertebral body anterolaterally and permits removal of an anterior compression mass. Radical decompression circumferentially about the dural sac and root sleeves can thus be accomplished. Once adequate decompression has been achieved, the dural sac often pulsates.[12,15]

Brisk bleeding may occur during excavation of the vertebral body. This usually diminishes when the vertebral body has been gutted and can then be controlled by application of thrombin-soaked pledgets.

Posterior Stabilization

When spinal metastases involve only the posterior bony elements (spines and laminae) or occur exclusively within the spinal canal (without bony involvement), a laminectomy without spinal reconstruction may be adequate. However, in most cases an adequate posterior decompression procedure for spinal metastases (posterolateral decompression) precipitates or aggravates spinal instability and must therefore be followed by spinal stabilization.[36] Spinal instrumentation is used to secure and maintain normal spinal alignment with rigid internal fixation. The goal is to provide immediate spinal stability that will remain intact for the patient's lifetime.

Posteriorly applied spinal reconstruction involves laminar fixation to bone grafts, steel rods, or methylmethacrylate struts. Meticulous care must be taken with the sublaminar wiring to avoid dural laceration and spinal cord injury. Preoperative assessment of the spinal canal by radiograph and CAT scan helps to determine if there is adequate extradural space for the passage of sublaminar wires. Intraoperatively, the entry and exit points of each sublaminar wire trajectory are prepared by removing the overlapping inferior laminar

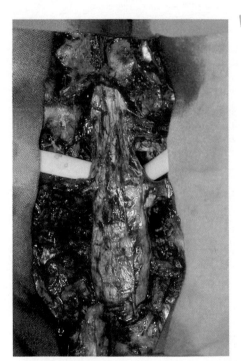

Figure 37.16 Operative photograph showing circumferential decompression of the dural sac and nerve roots through the posterolateral approach.

edge and associated ligamentum flavum (Fig. 37.17A). The doubled end of the stainless steel wire is curved to facilitate sublaminar passage; the leading tip is bent back somewhat to help one feel its location and to insure its proper emergence at the exit site. Intimate contact must be maintained between the sublaminar surface and the wire during its passage (Fig. 37.17B). The wire should be firmly twisted or cinched in place immediately after sublaminar passage so that it maintains snug and firm contact with the lamina, thus preventing displacement of the sublaminar loop against the dural sac and its contents (Fig. 37.17C). The firmly secured wires are then fixed to appropriately contoured bone, steel rod, or methylmethacrylate struts (Fig. 37.17D). Autogenous bone (e.g., rib, iliac crest, fibula) should be used for bony arthrodesis when the patient is expected to have prolonged survival. If bone struts are used, the contact surfaces between the bone graft and spinal elements (spines and laminae) should be roughened to promote fusion. Segmental instrumentation with steel rods or loops or methylmethacrylate struts is usually most appropriate when palliation is the realistic goal. If steel rods are used, the end of each rod should be bent at a right angle to prevent vertical migration of

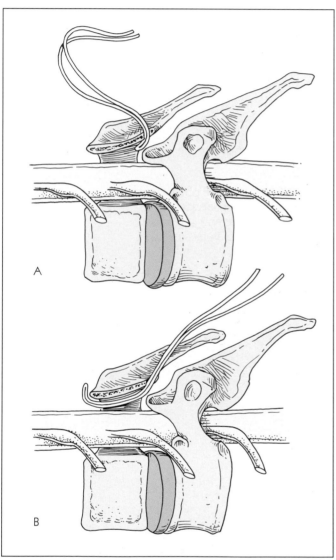

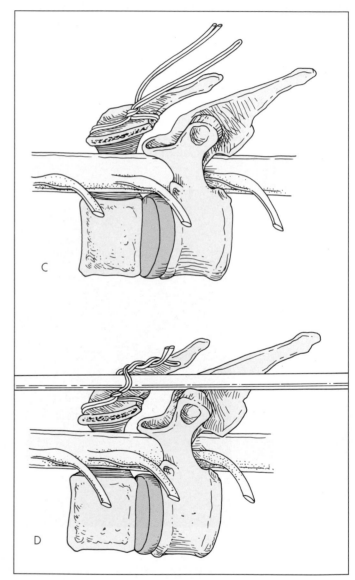

Figure 37.17 (A) Entry and exit points of each sublaminar wire trajectory. (B) Curving the doubled end of stainless steel wire facilitates sublaminar passage; the leading tip is bent back further to assist in its location and proper emergence at the exit site. Intimate contact must be maintained between the sublaminar surface and length of wire during and after its passage. (C) The wire should be firmly secured and placed by twisting or cinching to maintain snug and firm contact about the lamina to prevent displacement of the sublaminar loop. (D) The firmly secured wires are fixed to appropriately contoured stabilization constructs.

the struts. Use of a rectangular loop prevents both vertical and rotational displacement. If methylmethacrylate is used, the struts can be applied while malleable, thus enhancing the fit and providing intimate articulation with the spinal surface. Whatever supporting material is used (bone, steel, or methylmethacrylate), it is essential to secure multiple levels of fixation to the spine, and at a minimum of two levels above and two levels below the unstable segment (Fig. 37.18).

Anterior Decompression

Anterior decompression is performed with the patient in an appropriate supine position. The anterior approach used depends on the level of spinal involvement. Care must be taken, especially in the cervical region, to avoid exacerbation of spinal malalignment.

Cervical (C3–C7)

Spinal metastases affecting the cervical segments are most often associated with existing or potential spinal instability. Patients presenting with frank pathologic fracture dislocation are treated preoperatively with skeletal traction to restore spinal alignment. As with posterior decompressions, consideration should be given to intubating the awake patient with fiberoptic bronchoscopy,[4] followed by application of skull tongs

for intraoperative traction. When anterior and posterior procedures are performed under the same anesthetic, surgery is facilitated by use of a turning bed such as a Stryker frame (see Fig. 37.13A).

Neck dissection may be carried out from the right side or the left. The recurrent laryngeal nerve is at risk during a right-sided approach, and on the left side the long thoracic duct is in jeopardy. Preoperative evaluation of vocal cord function is essential when circumstances suggest that a patient's vocal cord function is already compromised and helps to determine the appropriate side for neck dissection.

A skin incision along the anterior border of the sternocleidomastoid muscle provides an approach to the anterior cervical spine (Fig. 37.19). The platysma is divided in line with the skin incision and the anterior border of the sternocleidomastoid is cleared. The cervical fascia is divided and a plane is developed between the carotid sheath and its contents laterally and the trachea and esophagus medially. It is often necessary to ligate and divide the superior thyroid artery and vein, and it may be necessary to divide the omohyoid muscle to achieve sufficient longitudinal exposure. Adequate access is thus gained to the vertebral bodies (and anterior spinal canal) from C-3 through C-7. The diseased vertebra is often identified by gross paraspinal tumor

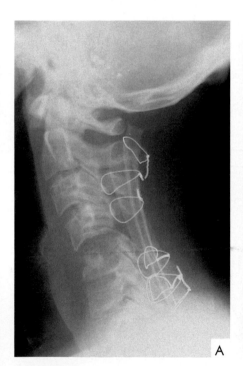
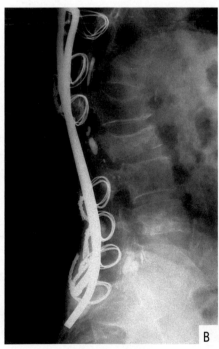
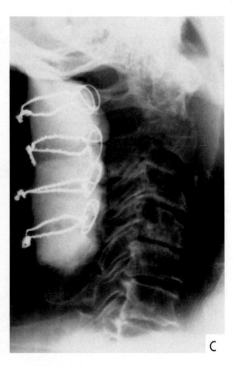

A   B   C

Figure 37.18 Postoperative radiographs showing segmental wiring to autogenous bone (rib struts) **(A)**, steel rod **(B)**, and methylmethacrylate strut **(C)**.

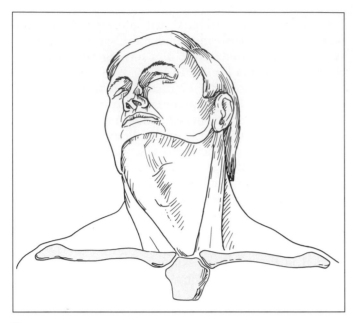

Figure 37.19 A skin incision along the anterior border of the sternocleidomastoid muscle is an appropriate approach to the anterior cervical spine.

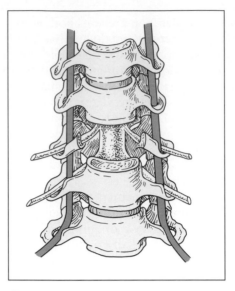

Figure 37.20 For resection of the vertebral body the intervertebral disc is excized above and below the affected segment, which is then removed with curettes, drill, and suction.

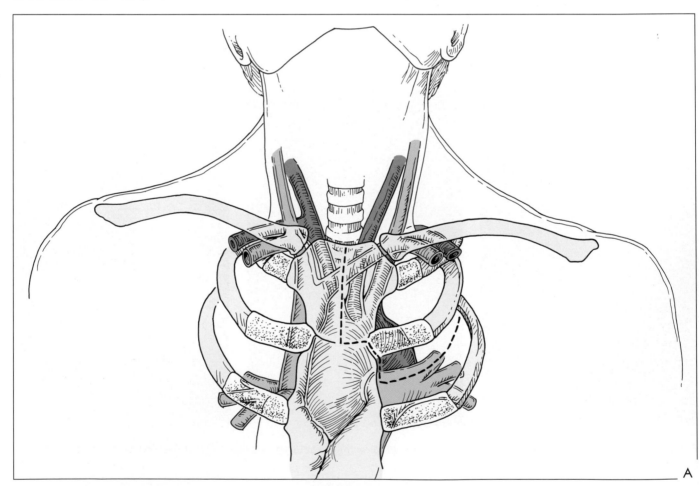

A

Figure 37.21 (A) Anterior exposure of the highest thoracic segments is achieved by extending the anterior neck approach inferiorly through a midline sternotomy.

Principles of Neurosurgery

extension, which causes discoloration and deformity of the anterior longitudinal ligament. Intraoperative x-ray is used to confirm the spinal level.

Further dissection should be performed, using the operating microscope to permit precise technique. The medial border of the longus coli muscle is detached across the area of the diseased vertebral body and adjacent disc spaces bilaterally. Resection of the vertebral body is facilitated by first excising the intervertebral disc above and below the diseased segment. The tumor-destroyed vertebral body is removed with the aid of curettes, drill, and suction (Fig. 37.20). Care must be taken to avoid injuring the vertebral arteries that may be buried in the tumor or tethered to lateral bone fragments. The posterior longitudinal ligament should be excised and the anterior dural sac cleared to insure complete removal of any epidural tumor extension.

Thoracic (T1–T3)
Anterior exposure of the highest thoracic segments is achieved through a midline sternotomy that extends through the second intercostal space (Fig. 31.21). The dissection begins with exposure of the lower cervical spine (as described above) and is carried inferiorly by dividing the omohyoid muscle. The manubrium sterni are divided in the midline and then to the second intercostal space with an oscillating saw. The soft tissues beneath the sternum are dissected and divided, with care taken to avoid injury to the internal mammary vessels and long thoracic duct (on the left side). A small sternal retractor assists in exposing the retrosternal space. The great vessels are identified down to the aortic arch and the dissection plane is established between the trachea and esophagus (medially) and the great vessels (laterally). Exposure of the upper thoracic segments is limited by the aortic arch and the oblique view of the upper thoracic spine coursing posteriorly to follow the natural kyphotic curve (Fig. 37.21B). The diseased vertebral body is removed as described above.

Thoracic (T4–T11)
Spinal metastases involving T-4 through T-11 can be approached anteriorly through the chest. The location of the major bony destruction or spinal cord compres-

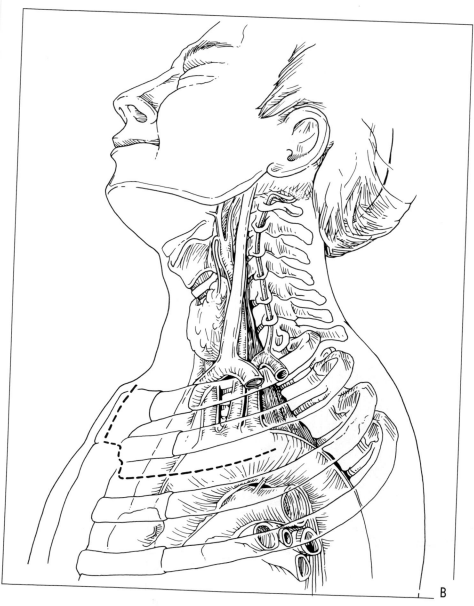

Figure 37.21, continued (B) The aortic view anteriorly and the oblique view of the upper thoracic spine posteriorly along the neutral kyphotic curve limit the exposure.

B

Metastatic Tumors of the Spine

tially ligated and divided. The segmental vessel at the level of the spinal tumor is frequently the most difficult to find. Once the segmental vessels are divided, the aorta and vena cava are gently retracted to expose the anterior and lateral surfaces of the vertebral bodies. Exposure of the vertebral bodies must extend for one intact vertebra above and below the diseased segment.

Adequate decompression of the dural sac and nerve roots involves removal of the tumor-destroyed vertebral body (corpectomy). The intervertebral discs above and below the diseased segment are excised, delineating the longitudinal extent of the surgical decompression. The affected bone is removed down to the posterior longitudinal ligament using curettes, drill, and suction. The posterior longitudinal ligament is excised and the dura is exposed to permit removal of extradural tumor extension (Fig. 37.23A). Careful removal of the pedicle (which is often destroyed by tumor) allows exposure of the inferiorly coursing segmental root sleeve (Fig. 37.23B). The dural root sleeves are rather delicate along the thoracic segments. If a sleeve is inadvertently torn, the defect should be repaired under magnification.

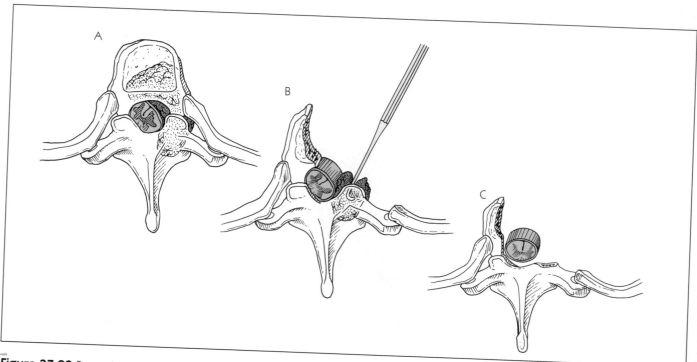

Figure 37.23 Resection of the vertebral body is facilitated by first excising the intervertebral disc above and below the diseased segment(s) and then removing the destroyed vertebral body. The posterior longitudinal ligament is excised and the dura exposed for removal of extradural tumor extension **(A)**. Removal of the pedicle exposes the inferiorly coursing segmental root sleeve **(B)**. Anterior thoracolumbar exposure permits decompression of the anterior and lateral spinal canal around approximately two thirds of the dural sac circumference **(C)**.

37.20

Oversewing the repaired defect with a muscle pledget helps to insure a water-tight closure.

The transthoracic approach permits decompression, under direct vision, of approximately two thirds of the dural sac circumference around the anterior and lateral spinal canal (Figs. 37.23C, 37.24). Nerve roots on the side opposite the surgical exposure are hidden from view. Attempts at blind circumferential decompression may result in dural laceration and nerve root injury.

Thoracolumbar (T12–L2)
The side on which to perform the thoracotomy is determined by the local spinal pathology. When the disease is symmetrical the left side is chosen, as the spleen is easier to mobilize than the liver. A double-lumen endotracheal tube or bronchial blocker is usually not necessary. The patient is placed in the lateral decubitus position and then rolled posteriorly 20° to facilitate visualization of the contralateral portion of the spinal canal. The operating table is extended with the apex at the level of the spinal pathology to facilitate the surgical exposure (Fig. 37.25A).

The skin incision is made along the course of the tenth rib. The incision crosses the costal cartilage anteromedially and proceeds along the lateral edge of the rectus sheath (Fig. 37.25B). Posterolaterally, the latissimus dorsi overlying the tenth rib is divided and the external oblique is separated in line with its fibers to expose the tenth rib (Fig. 37.25C). The tenth rib is separated from its cartilage attachment anteriorly and divided posterior to the angle of the rib (Fig. 37.25D). The parietal pleura is incised and the superior surface of the diaphragm visualized. The retroperitoneal space is identified by cutting the costal cartilage of the tenth rib. Once in the retroperitoneal space, the peritoneum is bluntly dissected from the posterior surface of the transversus abdominis. The muscles of the anterior abdominal wall can then be divided safely.

The diaphragm is exposed by bluntly dissecting the peritoneum from its inferior surface. The diaphragm is

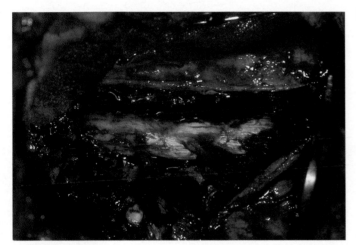

Figure 37.24 Intraoperative photograph showing anterolateral decompression of the dural sac and root sleeves.

then divided in a semicircular fashion near its peripheral attachment (see Fig. 37.25D). This incision should not stray into the center of the diaphragm because of the risk of denervating the muscle and the reduced healing capacity of the central tendon. Only a cuff of muscle (approximately 2 cm) is left attached to the rib to facilitate closure. The posterior portion of the diaphragm is divided medially to gain access to the psoas muscle so it can be retracted laterally to expose the vertebral body (Fig. 37.25E). The intervertebral discs are identified to facilitate isolation, ligation, and division of the segmental vessels. The aorta and vena cava are then retracted to expose the anterior and lateral surfaces of the vertebral bodies. The spinal level is confirmed by identifying the convergence of the twelfth rib and the first lumbar transverse process.

Decompression of the dural sac and nerve roots then proceeds with excision of the intervertebral disc above and below the diseased segment, removal of the tumor-destroyed vertebral body, excision of the posterior lon-

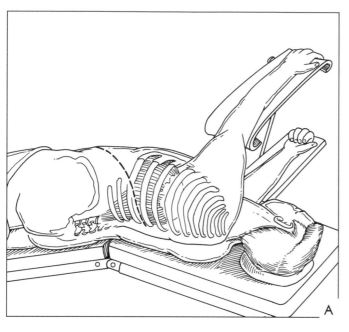

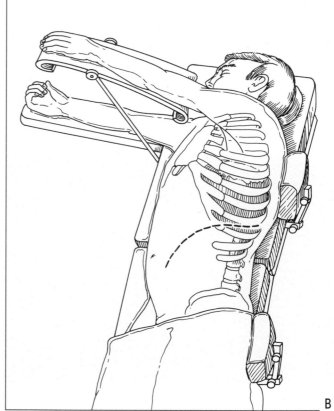

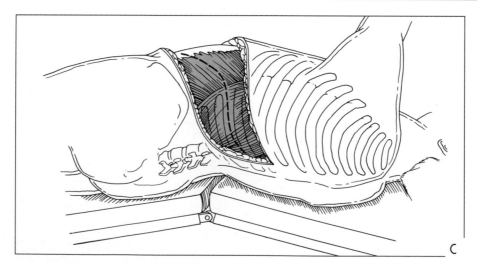

Figure 37.25 Positioning for thoracolumbar decompression. The operating table is extended with apex at the level of spinal pathology to facilitate the surgical exposure. The patient is placed in the lateral decubitus position and rolled posteriorly 20° (**A**) to aid in visualization of the contralateral portion of the spinal canal. (**B**) The skin incision is made along the course of the tenth rib, anteromedially crossing the costal cartilage and proceeding along the lateral edge of the rectus sheath. (**C**) The latissimus dorsi overlying the tenth rib is divided and the external oblique separated to expose the rib, which is separated (**D**) from its cartilage attachment anteriorly and divided posterior to the angle of the rib.

Principles of Neurosurgery

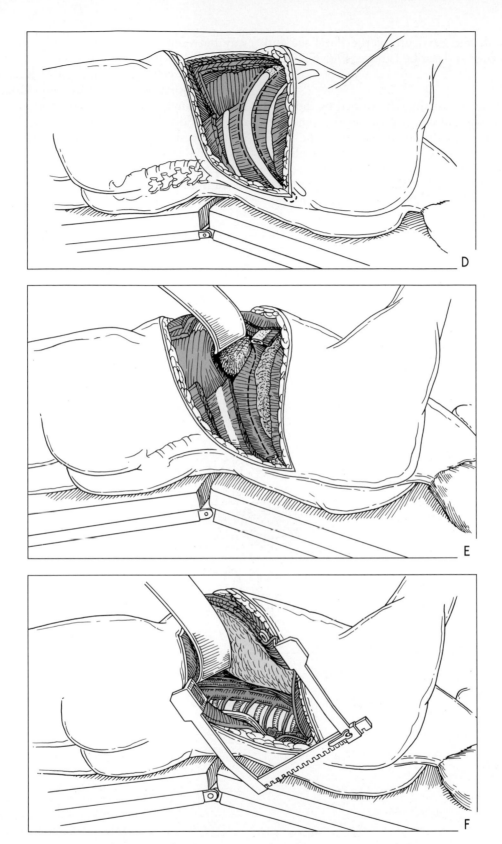

Figure 37.25, continued (E) The parietal pleura is incised to expose the superior surface of the diaphragm. The peritoneum is bluntly dissected from the posterior surface of the transversus abdominis so that the anterior abdominal wall muscles can be safely divided. (F) The posterior diaphragm is divided medially to gain access to the psoas muscle, which is retracted laterally to expose the spine. The diaphragm is exposed by bluntly dissecting the peritoneum from its inferior surface and is then divided near its peripheral attachment.

gitudinal ligament, and exposure of the dural sac and segmental root sleeve as described above (Fig. 37.26).

Lumbar (L3-L5)

The side of approach is usually determined by the local spinal pathology. The patient is positioned supine and then rolled up 30° to facilitate retraction of the peritoneal contents (Fig. 37.27). The operating table is extended at the level of the spinal pathology.

The skin incision is made obliquely across the anterior abdominal wall (Fig. 37.28). It extends from mid-way between the twelfth rib and superior iliac crest superiorly to just above the pubic rami at the lateral edge of the rectus sheath inferiorly. Each muscle layer of the abdominal wall is divided sequentially in line with the skin incision. Before the transversus abdominis muscle is divided the peritoneum must be bluntly dissected from its posterior surface to avoid inadvertent entry into the peritoneal cavity (Fig. 37.29). The retroperitoneal space is exposed by sweeping the peritoneum and fat off the inner surfaces of the ilium and psoas. Care must be taken not to extend the dissection

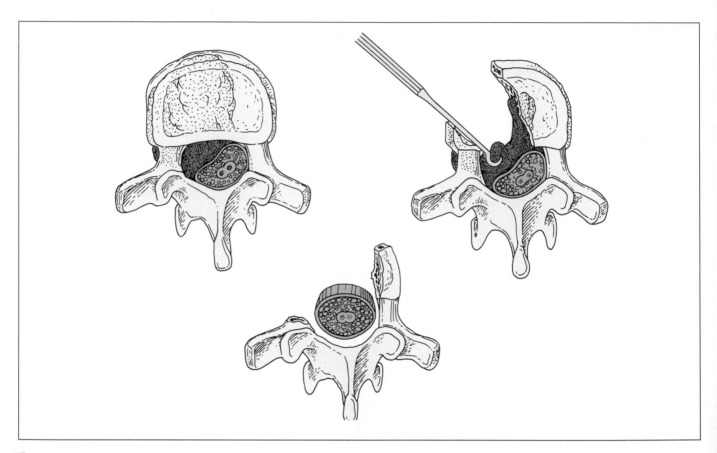

Figure 37.26 Decompression of the dural sac and nerve roots proceeds with excision of the intervertebral disc above and below the diseased segment, removal of the tumor-destroyed vertebral body, excision of the posterior longitudinal ligament, and exposure of the dural sac and segmental root sleeve.

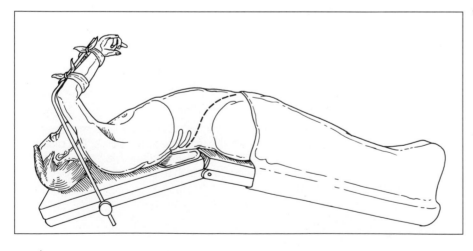

Figure 37.27 Position of the patient for transabdominal anterior approach to the spine. The operating table is extended with apex at the site of the spinal pathology. The patient is arranged supine and then rolled up 30° to aid in retraction of the peritoneal contents.

posterior to the psoas, as this would jeopardize the lumbosacral plexus. During exposure the ureter is retracted anteriorly and medially with the peritoneum. The spinal level is confirmed by identifying the prominence of the sacrum or by intraoperative radiography. The intervertebral discs are identified to facilitate localization and subsequent ligation and division of the segmental vessels. To expose L-5, the iliolumbar vein, which is usually a very large vessel that joins the poste-rior aspect of the common iliac vein, should be identified and ligated. Controlling this vessel is frequently the most difficult part of the dissection.

Decompression of the dural sac and nerve roots proceeds with excision of the intervertebral disc above and below the diseased segment. The tumor-destroyed vertebral body is removed, the posterior longitudinal ligament is excised, and the dural sac and nerve roots are exposed as described above. Since the approach for the

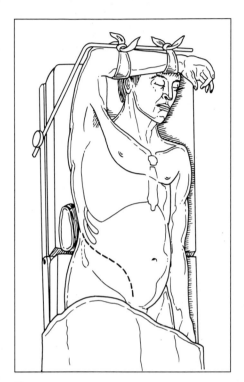

Figure 37.28 An oblique skin incision across the anterior abdominal wall extends (superiorly) from midway between the twelfth rib and superior iliac crest to (inferiorly) just above the pubic rami at the lateral edge of the rectus sheath.

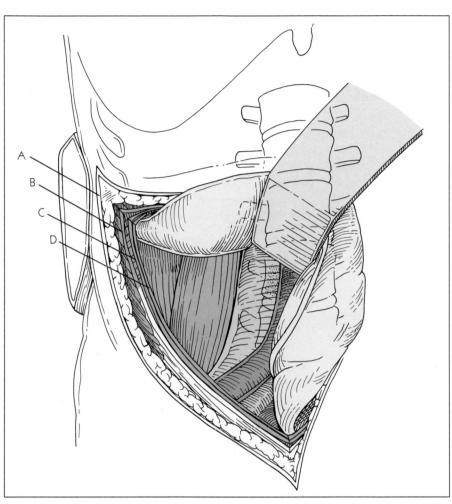

Figure 37.29 Each muscle layer of the abdominal wall is sequentially divided in line with the skin incision (**A**): external oblique (**B**), internal oblique (**C**), transverse (**D**). The peritoneum must be bluntly dissected from the posterior surface of the transversus abdominis before this muscle is divided to prevent inadvertent entry into the peritoneal cavity. The retroperitoneal space is exposed.

lumbar segments is more truly anterior, it is possible to expose and visualize the root sleeves bilaterally (Fig. 37.30).

Anterior Stabilization

Adequate procedures for anterior spinal decompression involve vertebral corpectomy at one or more levels and therefore *must* be followed by spinal stabilization. The variety of anterior spinal instrumentation devices and techniques that have been described suggests that there is no single outstanding method to secure and maintain normal spinal alignment for both immediate and long-term stability.

Autogenous bone should be used to secure bony arthrodesis if prolonged survival is anticipated. A tricorticate segment of iliac crest is usually an appropriate graft. After decompression of the dural sac and nerve roots and realignment of the spine, vertebral height is restored, using skeletal traction in the cervical segments and a vertebral spreader in the thoracic and lumbar spine. This tightens the lax and redundant soft tissues about the corpectomy segment and permits placement of the graft under compressive forces. The iliac crest strut is tailored to fit the corpectomy defect and is keyed into place, resting on the vertebral end plates above and below (Fig. 37.31). Obliquely oriented screws can be inserted through the graft and into the vertebral bodies

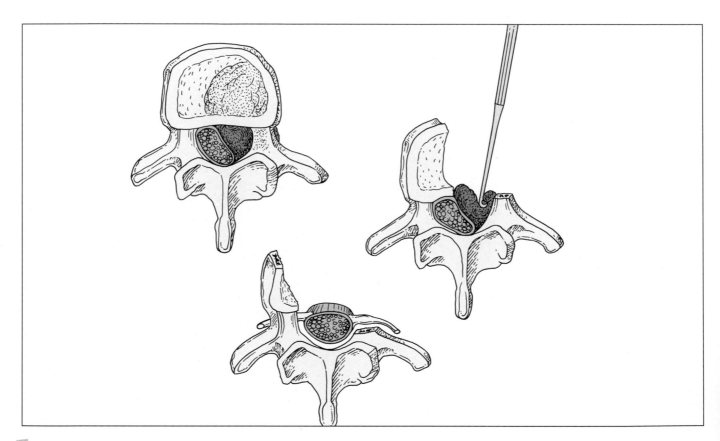

Figure 37.30 Decompression of the dural sac and nerve roots with excision of the intervertebral disc above and below the diseased vertebral body, its removal, excision of the posterior longitudinal ligament, and exposure of the dural sac and nerve roots.

above and below to increase the compression of the graft and its stability. Neutralization of the forces across the bone graft can be achieved by applying an anterior spinal plate to the vertebral bodies above and below the spanned segment and securing it with three or more screws. Postoperatively, an appropriate external brace is used for 3 months to protect the stabilization construct while bony arthrodesis occurs.

The use of bone graft is inappropriate for most pa-tients with symptomatic spinal metastases. Structurally intact autogenous bone is often not available, bone graft is incorporated slowly in a milieu characterized by residual tumor, osteoporosis, and changes caused by irradiation, and an external support is required for a minimum of 3 months. Consequently, it is usually more appropriate to use a synthetic construct, which can provide immediate spinal stabilization, thus eliminating the need for prolonged external orthotics.

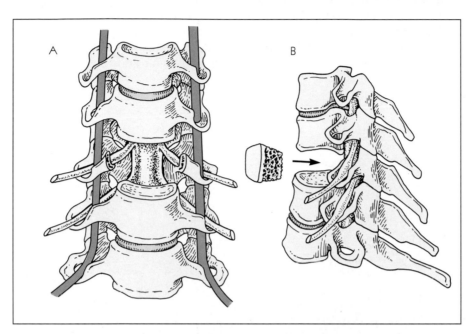

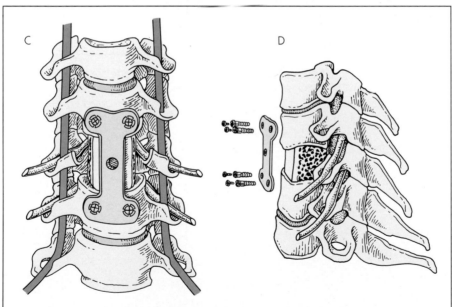

Figure 37.31 After decompression of realignment, restoration of vertebral height is achieved (in the cervical segments) with skeletal traction (**A**). An autogenous iliac crest strut is tailored to fit the defect and is keyed into place, resting on the vertebral end plates (**B**). Neutralization of forces across the bone graft can be achieved with an anterior spinal plate secured to the vertebral bodies above and below the spanned segment (**C,D**).

A simple and effective prosthetic fixation system is derived from a tailored AO construction plate and screws, augmented with methylmethacrylate (the Wellesley Wedge).[12] The stainless steel construction plate (3.5 mm wide for the cervical spine and 4.5 mm wide for the thoracic and lumbar spine) is contoured to size, with dimensions determined intraoperatively, to fit the decompression defect (Fig. 37.32). The U-shaped plate is secured to the vertebrae above and below with fully threaded cancellous screws. The plate can be extended for more than one vertebral segment above and below the decompression defect, depending on the local skeletal architecture. Each cervical vertebra can accommodate only one or two screws. In the upper thoracic spine two screws are inserted into each vertebral body. In the lower thoracic and lumbar spine fixation with three screws can be achieved (Fig. 37.33). Improved screw purchase can be obtained by preinjecting the holes with low-viscosity methylmethacrylate, provided the drill has not perforated the far cortex. Once the plate has been secured, methylmethacrylate in malleable form is used to fill the defect bracketed by the plate. The cement is inspissated through the empty screw holes and around the screw heads to prevent its dislodgement from the plate. During polymerization of the methylmethacrylate, the dura is protected by a fat graft and constant irrigation with cool normal saline. The fat graft is left in place to reduce postopera-

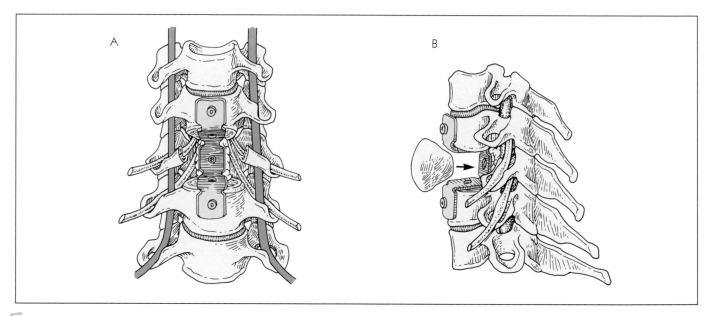

Figure 37.32 A simple and effective prosthetic fixation system is shown (the Wellesley Wedge). The stainless steel plate is contoured to size with dimensions determined intraoperatively to fit the decompression defect and the plate is secured to the vertebra above and below with fully threaded cancellous screws (**A**). Methylmethacrylate in malleable form fills the defect bracketed by the plate (**B**).

tive scar formation. The Wellesley Wedge provides a simple, safe, and effective means of spinal stabilization, particularly in the thoracic and lumbar regions (Fig. 37.34A,B).

Because the cervical vertebrae are smaller, the cervical spine poses a challenge in securing and preserving stability of the spinal column. Furthermore, the cervical spine's mobility makes stability difficult to maintain. Consequently, it is often advisable to supplement the anterior spinal instrumentation with a posterior stabi-

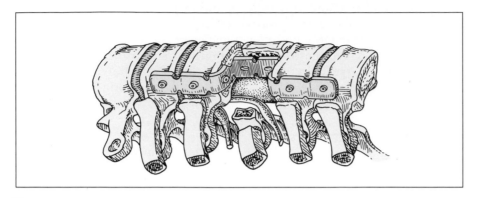

Figure 37.33 The Wellesley Wedge can be applied to replace the vertebral bodies of C3-L4. The tailored plate is inserted anteroposteriorly in the cervical segments, and is oriented laterally in the thoracic and lumbar levels.

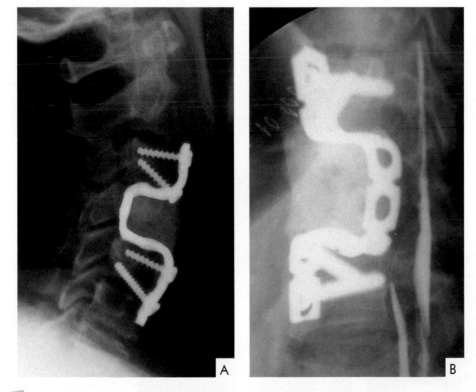

Figure 37.34 Postoperative radiographs showing an anterior fixation construct in place in the cervical spine (**A**) and thoracolumbar spine (**B**).

lization procedure (Fig. 37.35). Furthermore, when adequate anterior spinal decompression results in resection of two or more vertebral thoracic or lum-bar (corpectomy) levels, it is advisable to reinforce the anterior stabilization construct with a posteriorly applied device.

The fifth lumbar vertebra can be excised through an anterior approach. Spinal reconstruction with fixation to the sacrum is tenuous at best. Therefore, tumors involving L-5 are initially managed through a posterior approach. Once stable fixation is obtained (posteriorly), anterior spinal decompression (L-5 corpectomy) can be carried out at a second stage (see Fig. 37.35C).

RESULTS

The prognosis for patients with symptomatic spinal metastases is variable, given the heterogeneity of this patient population. The outcome of treatment depends on a number of factors.

Degree of Deficit
The degree of neurologic deficit at the time of treatment is the most reliable prognostic factor. Patients who are ambulatory do best, whereas patients with complete paralysis below the level of spinal cord compression do worst and have a poor chance of recovering useful motor function.

Duration of Symptoms
Recovery from spinal cord compression depends on the rate of onset and duration of symptoms. Long duration of symptoms and slowly evolving paraplegia are relatively favorable prognostic factors.

Tumor Type
The biologic properties of the culpable primary, including growth characteristics and radiation sensitivity, are factors that should determine method of management as well as the results of treatment and length of survival. Spinal metastases of reticuloendothelial origin have a relatively favorable outcome, whereas those arising from carcinoma of the lung carry a poor prognosis.

Tumor Location
Intradural spinal metastases are uncommon and carry a poor prognosis. Intradural extramedullary metastases, in particular, are associated with a virulent clinical syndrome and rapid deterioration to fatal outcome.

Advanced Disease
The degree of debility will determine the feasibility of surgery. Local and systemic factors influence the approach adopted and the surgical strategies employed.

Summary
A multidisciplinary approach with collaboration among neurosurgeon, oncologist, and orthopedic surgeon is advisable to achieve optimal outcome in the management of patients with symptomatic spinal metastases.

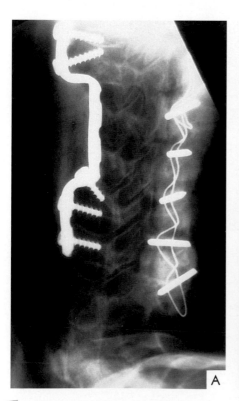
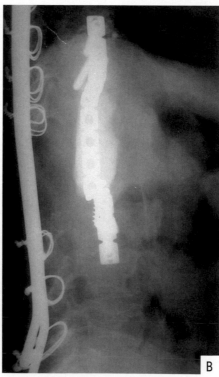
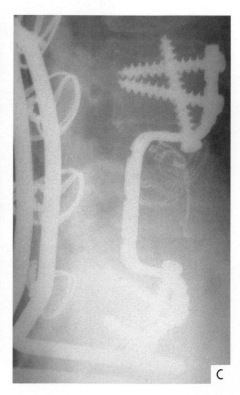

Figure 37.35 Combined anterior and posterior stabilization of the cervical spine (**A**) and thoracolumbar spine (**B**). Metastases involving the lumbar spine are initially approached posteriorly. Once fixation is obtained (posteriorly), anterior spinal decompression (L-5 corpectomy) can be carried out as a second stage (**C**).

REFERENCES

1. Chade HO. Metastatic tumors of the spine and spinal cord. In: Vinken PJ, Bruyn GW, eds. *Handbook of Clinical Neurology*. Amsterdam: North-Holland Publishing Co; 1976;20:415–433.
2. Murphy KC, Feld R, Evans WK, et al. Intramedullary spinal cord metastases from small cell carcinoma of the lung. *J Clin Oncol*. 1983;1:99–106.
3. Perrin RG, Livingston KE, Aarabi B. Intradural extramedullary spinal metastasis. *J Neurosurg*. 1982;56:835–837.
4. Willis RA. *The Spread of Tumors in the Human Body*. 3rd ed. London: Butterworths;
5. Barron KD, Hirano A, Araki S, Terry RD. Experiences with metastatic neoplasms involving the spinal cord. *Neurology* (Minneap). 1959;9:91–106.
6. Clarke E. Spinal cord involvement in multiple myelomatosis. *Brain*. 1986;79:332–348.
7. Galaski CSB. Skeletal metastases and mammary cancer. *Ann R Coll Surg Engl*. 1972;50:3–28.
8. Sundaresan N, Digiacinto GV, Hughes JEO, Cafferty M, Vallejo A. Treatment of neoplastic spinal cord compression: results of a prospective study. *Neurosurgery*. 1991;29:645–650.
9. Botterell EH, Fitzgerald GN. Spinal cord compression produced by extradural malignant tumors. *Can Med Assoc J*. 1959;80:791–796.
10. Livingston KE, Perrin RG. Neurosurgical management of spinal metastases. *J Neurosurg*. 1978;49:839–843.
11. Macdonald DR. Clinical manifestations. In: Sunderesan N, Schmidek H, Schiller A, Rosenthal A, eds. *Tumors of the Spine: Diagnosis and Clinical Management*. Philadelphia, Pa: WB Saunders Co; 1990;2:6–21.
12. Perrin RG, Livingston KE. Neurosurgical treatment of pathological fracture-dislocation of the spine. *J Neurosurg*. 1980;52:330–334.
13. Goodkin R, Carr BI, Perrin RG. Herniated lumbar disc disease in patients with malignancy. *J Clin Oncol*. 1987;5:667–671.
14. Shoskes DA, Perrin RG. The role of surgical management for symptomatic spinal cord compression in patients with metastatic prostate cancer. *J Urol*. 1989;142:337–339.
15. Perrin RG, McBroom RJ. Surgical treatment for spinal metastases: the posterolateral approach. In: Sundaresan N, Schmidek H, Schiller A, Rosenthal A, eds. *Tumors of the Spine: Diagnosis and Clinical Management*. Philadelphia, Pa: WB Saunders Co: 1990;30:305–315.
16. Perrin RG, McBroom RJ. Spinal fixation after anterior decompression for symptomatic spinal metastasis. *Neurosurgery*. 1988;22:324–327.
17. Belliveau RE, Spencer RP. Incidence and sites of bone lesions detected by ^{99m}Tc-polyphosphate scans in patients with tumors. *Cancer*. 1975;36:359–363.
18. Fletcher JW, Solaric-George E, Henry RE, et al. Radioisotope detection of osseous metastases. *Arch Intern Med*. 1975;135:553–557.
19. Low JC. The radionuclid scan in bone metastasis. In: Weiss L, Gilbert HA, eds. *Bone Metastasis*. Boston, Mass: GK Hall & Co; 1981;231–244.
20. McNeil BJ. Rationale for the use of bone scans in selected metastatic primary bone tumors. *Semin Nucl Med*. 1978;8:336–345.
21. Edelstyn GA, Gillespie PJ, Grebbell FS. The radiological demonstration of osseous metastases: experimental observations. *Clin Radiol*. 1967;18:158–162.
22. O'Mara RE. Bone scanning in osseous metastatic disease. *JAMA*. 1974;229:1915
23. O'Rourke T, George CB, Redmond J, et al. Spinal computed tomography and computed tomographic metrizamide myelography in the early diagnosis of metastatic disease. *J Clin Oncol*. 1986;4:576–583.
24. Redmond J, Spring DB, Munderloh SH, et al. Spinal computed tomography scanning in the evaluation of metastatic disease. *Cancer*. 1984;54:253–258.
25. Brunberg JA, Dipietro MA, Venes JL, et al. Intramedullary lesions of the pediatric spinal cord: correlation of findings from MR imaging, intraoperative sonography, surgery, and histologic study. *Radiology*. 1991;181:573–579.
26. Jaeckle KA. Neuroimaging for central nervous system tumors. *Semin Oncol*. 1991;18:150–157.
27. Lisbona R, Rosenthall L. Role of radionuclide imaging in osteoid osteoma. *Am J Roentgenol*. 1979;132:77–80.
28. Sze G. Magnetic resonance imaging in the evaluation of spinal tumors. *Cancer*. 1991;67:1229–1241.
29. Dunn RC Jr, Kelly WA, Wohns RN, Howe JF. Spinal epidural neoplasia: a 15-year review of the results of surgical therapy. *J Neurosurg*. 1980;52:47–51.
30. Friedman M, Kim TH, Panahon AM. Spinal cord compression in malignant lymphoma: treatment and results. *Cancer*. 1976;37:1485–1491.
31. Gilbert RW, Kim JH, Posner JB. Epidural spinal cord compression from metastatic tumor: diagnosis and treatment. *Ann Neurol*. 1978;3:40–51.
32. Maranzano E, Latini P, Checcaglini F, et al. Radiation therapy in metastatic spinal cord compression. *Cancer*. 1991;67:1311–1317.
33. Delaney TF, Oldfield EH. Spinal cord compression. In: DeVita VT, Hellman S, Rosenberg SA, eds. *Cancer: Principles and Practice of Oncology*. 3rd ed. New York, NY: JB Lippincott; 1989:1978–1985.
34. Perrin RG, Livingston KE. Pathological fracture-dislocation of the cervical spine. In: Tator CH, ed. *Early Management of Acute Spinal Cord Injury*. New York, NY: Raven Press; 1982;365–372.

35. Rogers L. Malignant spinal tumors and the epidural space. *Br J Surg.* 1958;45:416–422.

36. Heller M, McBroom RJ, MacNab T, Perrin RG. Treatment of metastatic disease of the spine with posterolateral decompression and Luque instrumentation. *Neuro-Orthopedics.* 1986;2:70–74.

37. Perrin RG, McBroom RJ, Perrin RG. Metastatic tumors of "the cervical spine. In: Block P, ed. *Clinical Neurosurgery.* Baltimore, Md: Williams & Wilkins; 1991;37:740–755.

38. Perrin RG, McBroom RJ. Anterior versus posterior decompression for symptomatic spinal metastasis. *Can J Neurol Sci.* 1987;14:75–80

39. Macedo N, Sundaresan N, Galicich JH. Decompressive laminectomy for metastatic cancer: what are the current indications? *Proc Am Soc Clin Oncol.* 1985;4:278.

40. Martenson JA, Evans RG, Lie MR, et al. Treatment outcome and complications in patients treated for malignant epidural spinal cord compression. *J Neurooncol.* 1985;3:77–84.

41. Tindall S, Perrin RG. Anesthesia for surgical management of spinal metastases. *Probl Anesth.* 1991; 5:80–90.

Spinal Intradural
Extramedullary Tumors

Chad D. Abernathey

Intradural extramedullary tumors of the spine constitute two thirds of all spinal neoplasms. Schwannomas (neurilemomas) and meningiomas make up approximately 90% of the total and occur in equal numbers.[1,2] The remaining 10% are divided amongst a host of clinical entities, including ependymoma (filum terminale), dermoid, epidermoid, angioma, lipoma, metastatic carcinoma, arachnoid cyst, ependymoma, chordoma, lymphoma, melanoma, myxoma, and sarcoma.[3-8]

Epidemiologic studies suggest that primary spinal tumors overall occur with an incidence of 2 per 100,000 population annually. Approximately 20% of all CNS tumors lie within the spinal canal. Rough estimates of location generally place 25% as extradural, 50% as intradural and extramedullary, and 25% as intramedullary.[9] Based upon this information, a neurosurgeon should anticipate an incidence of one intradural extramedullary tumor per 100,000 population per annum. Due to the fact that schwannomas and meningiomas make up approximately 90% of all intradural extramedullary tumors, the emphasis of this chapter will be devoted to the management of these two neoplasms. However, the diagnostic and treatment modalities discussed are applicable to all neoplasms that may occur in this location.

CLINICAL PRESENTATION

Most intradural extramedullary neoplasms present with progressive, slowly developing neurologic signs and symptoms. The clinical presentation of these tumors may be broken down into essentially two categories, mechanical and vascular. Compression of the spinal cord or nerve roots by a slowly growing mass will cause interruption of the normal physiologic and metabolic processes. As the mass effect increases, the resulting effect on the neural tissue will progress from irritative forces (pain and paresthesia) to destructive neurologic deficits (sensory loss, motor loss, and bladder and bowel dysfunction) or disinhibition of upper motor neuron pathways (hyperactive deep tendon reflexes and loss of autonomic control).

Pain is the primary symptom of intradural extramedullary tumors on initial presentation.[4,10,11] The pain is often radicular in nature but can occur in a diffuse, nondescript pattern. The pain is generally described as a dull, aching sensation with occasional sharp inflections. It is uncommon for patients to report burning or similar dysesthetic sensations, as in intramedullary neoplasms. Nocturnal pain may be prominent, as may recumbent exacerbation. This type of presentation is often relieved by an upright position. Paresthesias are also common, with descriptions of "numbness and tingling."

Weakness is the most readily identified objective finding. It typically follows the sensory symptoms but may, on occasion, occur as the primary complaint. Weakness universally is associated with hyperreflexia and spasticity in the afflicted extremities. Flexor spasms or muscle cramps will develop as weakness and spasticity increase. In addition to these upper motor neuron signs, lower motor neuron symptomatology can also be identified, including hyporeflexia, atrophy, and fasciculations along the innervation of the afflicted level. Specific segmental weakness also occurs.

Later symptoms and signs are associated with autonomic, bladder, and bowel disturbances. Urinary and fecal incontinence or retention are most common, while sexual dysfunction is infrequently identified. Rarely, clinicians will observe spinal deformities. It has become uncommon for these disturbances to develop due to early diagnosis by modern neuroimaging techniques, such as MRI and CT.

The clinical presentation is useful in determining the exact level and location of the lesion. A careful history may provide clues as to exact location of the lesion within the spinal canal; for example, lesions occurring in the posterior aspect of the spinal cord will produce posterior column dysfunction, such as joint position and vibratory sensation loss. Anterior lesions will spare the posterior column function while affecting weakness and sensation to the level of the abnormality. Anterior lesions may also affect the spinocerebellar tracts, resulting in uncoordinated and ataxic gait, unrelated to the degree of long tract dysfunction. Lesions lying at the anterolateral aspect of the spinal cord will demonstrate classic Brown-Séquard symptoms.

The speed with which neurologic deficits occur in spinal intradural extramedullary tumors is predictive of eventual outcome. Lesions that create sudden loss of function are due most commonly to immediate neurovascular compromise. The ischemia created by a vascular insult is almost always irreversible and function is poorly recoverable. If the symptoms are slowly progressive over weeks to months or even years, then they are most likely due to slow compressive effects on the neural elements themselves. In these cases, an excellent recovery after surgical decompression of the mass lesion heralds a very satisfying neurologic recovery. Often, severe neurologic injury will recover completely with surgical extirpation of the mass.

NEURODIAGNOSTIC INVESTIGATIONS

Plain spine roentgenograms have been overlooked in recent years as a source of valuable information in the assessment of spinal tumors. As lesions have been identified earlier in their course with MRI and CT myelography, plain spine roentgenography has become less useful. However, the classic descriptions of bony destruction warrant reiteration. Classically, approximately half of all neurogenic tumors and 10% of meningiomas would present with bony defects, including erosion of the pedicles, vertebral bodies, or neural arches. Widening of the neuroforamina and spinal canal may also be helpful in screening identification of these lesions. Calcification in long-standing tumors is common.

Lumbar puncture generally demonstrates elevation of protein levels in intradural extramedullary tumors. If the protein concentration is greater than 100 mg%, then the diagnosis of intraspinal neoplasm should be considered. Meningiomas commonly present with CSF protein levels of 300 to 500 mg%, neurofibromas with 600 to 800 mg%, and ependymomas with extremely high concentrations, as high as 3000 to 4000 mg%. Lumbar puncture is rarely performed alone without the introduction of contrast agents. CT myelography was considered the most useful diagnostic procedure for the demonstration of intradural extramedullary masses, before the development of MRI. Even today, if myelography is combined with poststudy CT imaging, additional information may be obtained that is not readily identifiable on an MRI (Fig. 38.1). Most experienced,

actively operating neurosurgeons continue to consider CT myelography to be the most definitive single procedure for the assessment of intradural extramedullary mass lesions, providing the most information: CSF studies, CSF flow dynamics around the tumor, specific localization in relation to the spinal cord, bony anatomy, and surgical considerations. The classic appearance of intradural extramedullary neoplasms is that of a compressive lesion, well outlined and defined by the contrast agent, resulting in concavity defects, inhibition of CSF flow, and partial or complete blockage.

Even though CT myelography still constitutes the definitive standard for imaging of the spinal canal, MRI has largely supplanted CT myelography as the initial diagnostic approach (Fig. 38.2).[12–14] Increasingly, MRI has become the primary diagnostic modality in the assessment of intradural extramedullary lesions.[15] At this time, less than 10% of patients proceed to CT

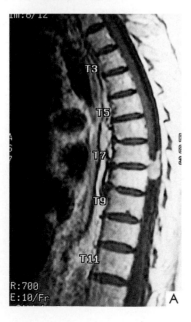

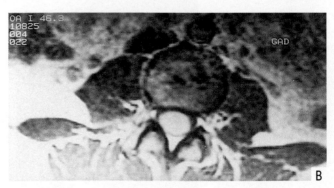

Figure 38.1 (A) Lumbar myelogram demonstrating complete blockage of subarachnoid contrast flow secondary to an L-5 intradural extramedullary ependymoma. (B) Postmyelographic CT showing a giant sacral schwanoma.

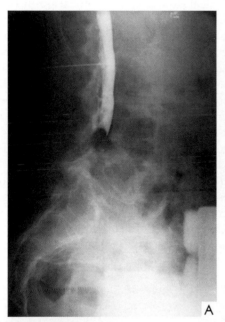

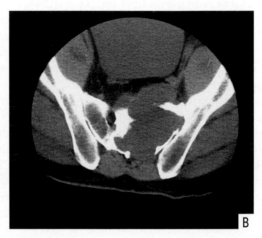

Figure 38.2 Gadolinium-enhanced MRI of a T7-T8 intradural extramedullary meningioma. (A) Sagittal view. (B) Axial view.

myelography after a definitive MRI study has been obtained at our institution. The development of motion-compensation imaging techniques, thin-section high-resolution imaging, and CSF flow dynamic protocols has been responsible for this change in diagnostic approach. The limitations of MRI are primarily related to partial volume averaging, motion artifact, blurring of tumor margins with peritumoral reaction, and simple limitations of scan fields (some lesions are simply missed because scan protocols of the spine may not overlap).

With the administration of paramagnetic contrast agents, many of the difficulties associated with MRI can be overcome. We currently use gadolinium diethylene-triamine pentaacetic acid (Gd-DTPA). Gd-DTPA administration has greatly enhanced the ability to distinguish the tumor margins from surrounding gliosis and reaction.[16–19] It also has allowed better interpretation of postsurgical results, with improved distinction between tumor and scar enhancement (Figs. 38.3, 38.4). The development of MRI myelography promises to replace the need for interventional CT myelography in the future.

Additional studies of occasional use include somatosensory evoked potentials, spinal electrograms, electromyography, and cistometrograms. These tests are purely diagnostic of the effects of the spinal cord tumor and do not aid greatly in the specific assessment from a diagnostic or therapeutic standpoint, although they can be helpful for localization of the lesion and quantification of the severity of injury. Additional procedures such as epidural venography, spinal angiography, ultrasound, thermography, and so on are rarely used in the modern preoperative assessment of intradural extramedullary lesions.

SURGICAL MANAGEMENT

The operative approach to intradural extramedullary tumors can largely be generalized throughout the spinal column. The following description represents the standard approach used at our institution.

The patient is brought to the operative suite after obtaining informed surgical consent and is placed under general endotracheal anesthesia. Electrophysiologic monitoring is employed and baseline electromyography and nerve conduction studies have been obtained prior to induction of anesthesia.[20] Evoked potentials, EMG, and NCV monitoring are continued throughout the procedure with a certified technician or specially trained neurologist present. The patient is then placed in a flexed crouch prone position and the skin overlying the surgical site is prepped and draped in the usual fashion.

An initial lateral radiograph is obtained with a marker placed on the skin surface to localize the incision more accurately. An attempt is made to limit the surgical exposure to the focal point of the tumor. Typically only two vertebral levels need to be exposed, as it is rare for these tumors to extend much beyond one or two vertebral segments. Dissection is carried sharply in a subperiosteal fashion, and the paraspinous musculature is swept laterally. A Miskimmon's or angled cerebellar retractor is used to hold the soft tissues laterally. If the tumor is laterally placed within the spinal canal and does not extend beyond the midline, only a unilateral hemilaminectomy is required. If the tumor is larger and extends across the midline, a complete laminectomy and removal of the spinous process is performed. The bony resection is achieved with assorted rongeurs. As bone removal progresses, a 4 mm diamond bur becomes increasingly useful to limit the potential for trauma to the thecal sac or neural elements. Once the bone is

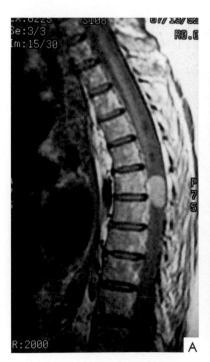
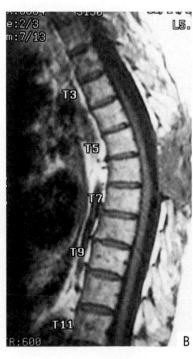

Figure 38.3 (A) Preoperative gadolinium-enhanced MRI showing a T6-T7 intradural extramedullary meningioma. (B) Postoperative gadolinium-enhanced MRI demonstrating complete resection of the meningioma. Note the operative scar tissue directly posterior to the thecal sac.

thinned, careful resection with orbital rongeurs is performed. The lamina is removed far enough laterally to expose the thecal sac and neoplasm adequately (Fig. 38.5). However, an attempt is made to limit the lateral resection, to aid in the prevention of postoperative instability.

If a dumbbell-type tumor projects through the neuroforamen, then resection of the heads of the ribs adjacent to the tumor may be required. The intercostal muscle bundle is divided to expose the pleura anteriorly. Hemostasis is achieved in the bony margins with bone wax, and the epidural veins are cauterized with bipolar cautery. Cottonoid pledgets are placed in the lateral gutters along the exposed dura mater after removal of the ligamentum flavum and epidural fat. The tumor can typically be identified prior to the opening of the dura mater. Often the tumor can be visualized directly or palpated with a fine ball-tip sounding probe. On occasion, ultrasound is useful in localizing the lesion. The dura mater is opened in a longitudinal fashion over the tumor along the midline. The margins of the dura

mater are held laterally with temporary tack sutures (Fig. 38.6). The tumor is visualized and the arachnoid is opened immediately over it. Depending on the location of the tumor, the spinal cord is protected from trauma by positioning cottonoid pledgets adjacent to the tumor. The tumor surface is cauterized with bipolar cautery to improve hemostasis as the resection proceeds. Cottonoid pledgets are placed at the superior and inferior aspects of the neoplasm to decrease the migration of hemorrhage into the subarachnoid space. Inevitably, some surgical hemorrhage will seep into the subarachnoid space and will require irrigation with normal saline solution to decrease the risk for postoperative aseptic arachnoiditis. The tumor is then entered and debulked with sharp and blunt dissection techniques. Typically, the tumor can be removed with simple microcup forceps dissection. However, the cavitronic ultrasonic aspiration device (CUSA) may be useful at low-power settings. If the tumor is significantly adherent to the spinal cord and surrounding dura mater, a CO_2 laser is quite helpful in the resection process. It is

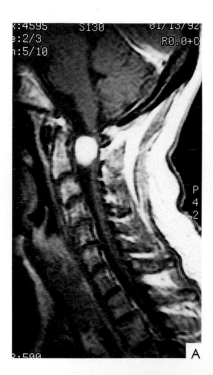
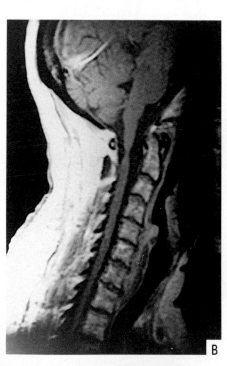

Figure 38.4 (A) Preoperative gadolinium-enhanced MRI showing a schwannoma in the foramen magnum region anterior to the upper cervical spinal cord and lower medulla. (B) Postoperative gadolinium-enhanced MRI demonstrating complete resection of the schwannoma.

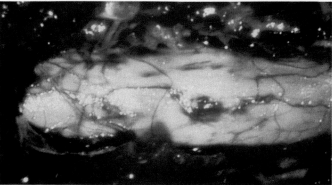
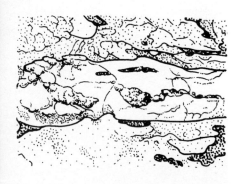

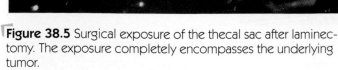

Figure 38.5 Surgical exposure of the thecal sac after laminectomy. The exposure completely encompasses the underlying tumor.

recommended that power be limited to 10 W in continous mode to decrease the risk for tissue spread of the imparted heat. The usefulness of the CUSA or laser is largely dependent on the degree of calcification within the tumor. For instance, in long-calcified meningiomas, it is often impossible to use these instruments with any significant efficacy.

The neoplasm is debulked in an intracapsular fashion. As the center of the tumor is removed, the capsule falls in upon itself and can be mobilized from the surrounding neural elements and dural margin (Fig. 38.7). Upon completion of the intracapsular resection, the capsule is carefully dissected free with bipolar and microscissor dissection. Any attachments to the dural margin are either cauterized with bipolar cautery or vaporized with the CO_2 laser.

Upon completion of the tumor removal, the spinal cord is often noted to return immediately to a more normal anatomic position (Fig. 38.8). However, with long-standing neoplasms, the spinal cord may be thinned to a ribbon-like shape and unable to regain its former bulk. The vascular supply to the tumor is inspected throughout the procedure to ensure that transient vessels that do not supply the tumor but in fact are feeding vessels to the spinal cord are not sacrificed. All vasculature relating to the spinal cord is preserved and protected. Once satisfied that a gross total resection of the tumor has been accomplished, immaculate hemostasis is obtained with bipolar cautery. The wound is irrigated with copious amounts of normal saline solution and the arachnoid is repositioned over the spinal cord and reapproximated with interrupted 6-0 nonabsorbable sutures. The dura mater is then closed in a watertight fashion with running 5-0 nonabsorbable suture such as Prolene (Fig. 38.9). Prior to the final suture placement, the thecal sac is re-expanded with normal saline solution to aid in the prevention of epidural hemorrhage. Significant hemostasis can be achieved with simple re-expansion of the thecal sac to tamponade the epidural venous channels. The paraspinous musculature and fascial tissues are then closed in anatomic layers with interrupted absorbable suture and the skin is closed with a running nonabsorbable suture (3-0 nylon) in a watertight fashion. An occlusive dressing is applied to the wound and the patient is subsequently transferred to the recovery room.

RESULTS

Short-term outcome in the surgical treatment of intradural extramedullary neoplasms is generally excellent, with very gratifying improvement of neurologic function the rule.[21] Depending on the severity of the initial pre-

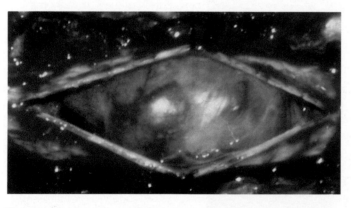
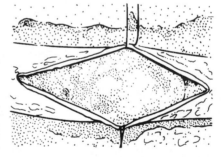

Figure 38.6 The intradural extramedullary schwannoma has been exposed by incision of the dura mater. The dural margins have been tacked to the paraspinous musculature.

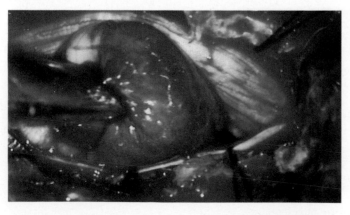
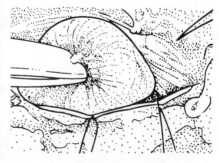

Figure 38.7 The tumor is mobilized from the surrounding neural elements using microdissection techniques.

sentation, if no evidence of vascular injury has occurred, excellent improvement in neurologic function can be anticipated. These patients will commonly return to normal or near normal status. Physical therapy and occupational therapy are considered standard postoperative treatment to optimize the neurologic recovery period. An initial surge of neurologic improvement is witnessed in the first 6 weeks following surgical intervention, and often dramatic results can occur. However, long-term recovery can continue for up to a year.

The risk of recurrence is estimated to be approximately 10% in gross total resections of benign intradural extramedullary tumors such as schwannomas and meningiomas. If a subtotal resection is accomplished, then a symptomatic recurrence rate of approximately 20% can be expected. Of note, filum terminale ependymomas tend to have a slightly higher recurrence rate and may require adjuvant radiation therapy. As a general rule, recurrences of most intradural extramedullary tumors are treated by repeat surgical intervention. Subsequent recurrences after repeat operation are then considered to be candidates for radiation therapy, as are tumors that extend beyond the bounds of reasonable surgical capabilities. At our institution, a follow-up MRI study of the tumor site is performed 1 year after surgery. If this study does not demonstrate obvious recurrence, a follow-up study is scheduled after 2 years. If this subsequent study does not demonstrate tumor recurrence, a follow-up study at 5 years is recommended.

Complications related to surgical intervention for intradural extramedullary tumors include standard risks, such as stroke, heart attack, death, infection, paralysis, DVT, PE, bladder or bowel dysfunction, sexual dysfunction, hemorrhage, tumor recurrence, CSF leakage, meningomyelocele, anesthetic complications, and drug reactions. The most significant and difficult complications to treat consist of initial new neurologic deficits which often do not return. Sensorimotor deficits are more likely to recover than bladder or bowel/autonomic dysfunction. These ultraoperative injuries are typically related to vascular insult of the spinal cord or manipulation of the neural elements. CSF fistula represents one of the more dreaded complications since treatment may be difficult. If CSF leakage occurs through the wound site, then standard treatment calls for lumbar drainage for approximately 48 hours at 10 to 15 mL per hour. If persistent leakage continues, then revision of the surgical wound is warranted. In dumbbell-type tumors that develop pleural or retroperitoneal CSF fistula, a trial with chest tube drainage is

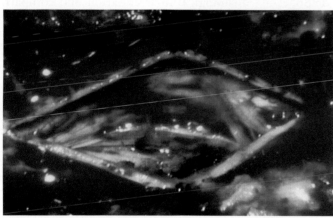
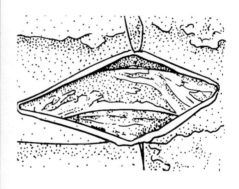

Figure 38.8 Following gross total resection of the neoplasm, the spinal cord is seen to resume a more normal position and appearance.

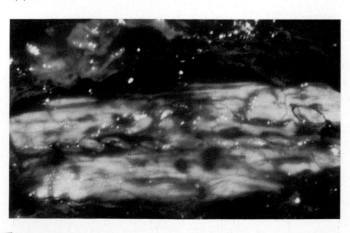
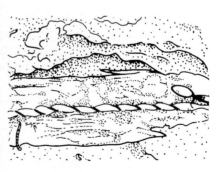

Figure 38.9 The dura mater has been closed in a watertight fashion with running 5-0 nonabsorbable suture.

performed. However, this maneuver is often unsuccessful and open repair is warranted.

CONCLUSION

The surgical management of spinal intradural extramedullary neoplasms has become simplified in the past 10 years. The excellent surgical outcomes obtained today are primarily related to the early diagnosis achieved with new neurodiagnostic studies and to improved surgical techniques. Surgical precision has made great advances with the advent of the operating microscope, cavitronic ultrasonic aspiration device, and laser technology. Additionally, intraoperative electrophysiologic monitoring has been exceedingly valuable in predicting, detecting, and preventing neurologic injury. In summary, neurosurgeons today can anticipate a very satisfying surgical result in the treatment of intradural extramedullary neoplasms.

REFERENCES

1. Levy W, Latchaw J, Hahn J, et al. Spinal neurofibromas: a report of 66 cases and a comparison with meningiomas. *Neurosurgery.* 1986;18:331–334.
2. Namer IJ, Pamir MN, Benli K, Saglam S, Erbengi A. Spinal meningiomas. *Neurochirurgia.* 1987; 30:11–15.
3. Abernathey CD, Onofrio BM. Foramen magnum meningiomas and schwannomas: operative approach. *Neurosurgical Operative Atlas.* AANS; 1991:387–396.
4. Abernathey CD, Onofrio BM, Schneithauer BW, Pairolero PC, Shives TC. Surgical management of giant sacral schwannomas. *J Neurosurg.* 1986; 65:286–295.
5. Dodge HW Jr, Love JG, Gottlieb CM. Benign tumors of the foramen magnum: surgical consideration. *J Neurosurg.* 1956;13:603–617.
6. Kernohan JW, Sayre GP. *Tumors of the Central Nervous System.* Washington, DC: Armed Forces Institute of Pathology; 1952:141. Atlas of Tumor Pathology, section 10, fascicles 35, 37.
7. Levy WJ Jr, Bay J, Dohn D. Spinal cord meningioma. *J Neurosurg.* 1982;57:804–812.
8. Paulus W, Jelinger K, Perneczky G. Intraspinal neurotherkoma (nerve sheath myxoma): a report of two cases. *Am J Clin Pathol.* 1991;95:511–516.
9. McCormick P, Post K, Stein B. Intradural extramedullary tumors in adults. *Neurosurg Clin North Am.* 1990;1:591–608.
10. Dodge HW Jr, Svien H, Camp J, Craig W. Tumors of the spinal cord without neurologic manifestations producing low back and sciatic pain. *Proc Staff Meet Mayo Clin.* 1951;26:88.
11. Horrax G, Poppen JL, Wu WQ, Weadon PR. Meningiomas and neurofibromas of the spinal cord: certain clinical features and end results. *Surg Clin North Am.* 1949;29:659–665.
12. Blews D, Wang H, Ashok J, et al. Intradural spinal metastases in pediatric patients with primary intracranial neoplasms: Gd-DTPA-enhanced MR vs CT myelography. *J Comput Assist Tomogr.* 1990;14:730–735.
13. Scotti G, Scialfa G, Colombo N, et al. MR imaging of intradural extramedullary tumors of the cervical spine. *J Comput Assist Tomogr.* 1985;9: 1037–1041.
14. Sze G. Magnetic resonance imaging in the evaluation of spinal tumors. *Cancer.* 1991;67:1229–1241.
15. Takemoto K, Matsumura Y, Hashimoto H, et al. MR imaging of intraspinal tumors—capability in histological differentiation and compartmentalization of extramedullary tumors. *Neuroradiology.* 1988;30:303–309.
16. Bronen R, Sze G. Magnetic resonance imaging contrast agents: theory and application to the central nervous system. *J Neurosurg.* 1990;73: 820–839.
17. Dillon W, Normal D, Newton T, et al. Intradural spinal cord lesions: Gd-DTPA-enhanced MR imaging. *AJNR.* 1989;170:229–237.
18. Parizel P, Baleriaux D, Rodesch G, et al. Gd-DTPA-enhanced MR imaging of spinal tumors. *AJR.* 1989;152:1087–1096.
19. Stimac G, Porter B, Olson D, et al. Gadolinium-DTPA-enhanced MR imaging of spinal neoplasms: preliminary investigation and comparison with unenhanced spin-echo and stir sequences. *AJR.* 1988;151:1185–1192.
20. Whittle I, Johnston I, Besser M. Recording of spinal somatosensory evoked potentials for intraoperative spinal cord monitoring. *J Neurosurg.* 1986;64:601–612.
21. Ciapetta P, Domenicucci M, Raco M. Spinal meningiomas: prognosis and recovery factors in 22 cases with severe motor deficits. *Acta Neurol Scand.* 1988;77:27–30.

Chapter 39

Intramedullary Tumors and Tumors of the Cauda Equina

Allan Friedman

Over the past 20 years, technological advances have aided the diagnosis and treatment of intramedullary cord tumors. MRI scanning has enhanced our ability to detect these lesions, and microsurgical techniques have better enabled us to resect some of these tumors surgically.

Intramedullary spinal cord tumors comprise 2% to 4% of all CNS tumors. They account for only 20% of adult intradural spinal tumors, but in children, in whom the incidence of meningiomas and neurofibromas is low, they account for 50% of intradural spinal tumors. Gliomas, particularly ependymomas and astrocytomas, are the most commonly encountered intramedullary spinal cord tumors (Fig. 39.1).[1] Ependymomas are slightly more common than astrocytomas in adults, but astrocytomas are more prevalent in children and adolescents. Anaplastic astrocytomas and glioblastomas account for approximately 10% of spinal cord gliomas. Hemangioblastomas account for 3% to 4% of intramedullary spinal cord tumors.

Tumors that rarely occur within the spinal cord include primary tumors such as gangliogliomas, oligodendrogliomas, and melanomas. Benign tumors such as lipomas, dermoids, epidermoids, cavernous angiomas, and schwannomas have been noted. Intramedullary mass lesions can result from inflammatory processes, such as sarcoidosis, infection, and multiple sclerosis and may be difficult to differentiate from intrinsic tumors[2,3] both clinically and radiologically.

INTRAMEDULLARY TUMORS

Ependymomas

Ependymomas are the most common intramedullary spinal cord tumors encountered in the adult population (Fig. 39.2). These tumors appear to be discrete with little invasive potential. The gray to purple tumor tissue readily separates from the adjacent white spinal cord. The tumor is frequently capped by a cyst over its cranial pole; less frequently there is a cyst below its caudal pole. Histologic examination most often reveals an epithelial ependymoma comprised of sheets of cells broken up by pseudorosettes (anuclear zones comprised of cytoplasmic processes surrounding blood vessels). True rosettes are rarely seen. The occasional tanocytic ependymoma contains free-standing anuclear areas of fibrillary processes reminiscent of an astrocytoma. In fact, this

---

Figure 39.1 Intramedullary Spinal Tumors

Most Common Tumors	Less Common Tumors	Expansile Nontumorous Lesions
Ependymoma	Oligodendroglioma	Multiple sclerosis
Astrocytoma	Ganglioglioma	Infection
Hemangioblastoma	Malignant glioma	Abscess
	Schwannoma	Sarcoidosis
	Melanoma	
	Metastatic tumors	
	Teratoma	
	Neuroenteric cyst	
	Dermoid tumor	
	Epidermoid tumor	
	Lipoma	
	Cavernous angiomas	

histology may lead to the erroneous diagnosis of an astrotoma. Myxopapillary ependymomas are virtually restricted to the cauda equina.

Intramedullary ependymomas occur anywhere along the spinal cord, although they have a slight propensity to appear in the cervical region. They are heralded by a slow, insidious clinical course, usually evolving for years prior to diagnosis. On MRI scan, the tumor appears as a well circumscribed gadolinium-enhancing mass capped by a nonenhancing cyst.

The primary treatment of intramedullary spinal cord ependymoma is surgical resection. A review of the literature reveals that approximately 80% of these lesions can be completely resected.[1,4–8] Although approximately 50% of patients develop new neurologic deficits immediately after surgery, the deficits are transient in all but 5% to 10% of patients. The patient's postoperative neurologic function is most strongly influenced by his or her preoperative state.[1] Marked neurologic improvement is only reported to occur in approximately 20% of patients. If the surgeon achieves gross total resection, the rate of recurrence is 5% to 10% over a 5 year follow-up period. Radiation therapy is reserved for patients in whom total gross resection cannot be achieved.[9] Even in this group, the efficacy of radiation therapy is suggested but not proven by the available literature.

Astrocytomas

Ninety percent of spinal cord astrocytomas are well differentiated. These "benign" lesions can be divided into two types: diffusely infiltrating and pilocytic. Infiltrating astrocytomas consist of cells that permeate a localized portion of the spinal cord, causing a restricted swelling. Although the heart of these tumors appears to consist of a pure population of tumor cells, these cells intermingle with the normal spinal cord around the tumor's periphery. Pilocytic astrocytomas are similar to their cranial counterparts (Fig. 39.3). They are relatively discrete lesions composed of compact fascicles of elongated cells separated by loose areas of stellate cells and microcysts. Pilocytic astrocytomas are frequently associated with large cysts that in extreme cases span the entire spinal cord. Ten percent of intramedullary astrocytomas are malignant.[4]

The progressive neurologic deficit produced by an intramedullary astrocytoma may unfold slowly.[10] One long-term follow-up study documenting the natural history of childhood spinal cord astrocytomas demonstrated an 80% 5-year survival rate and 55% 10-year survival rate. It should be noted that others have not reported such an optimistic prognosis.[11,12] In adult patients, the natural history of the disease varies greatly, with some tumors remaining quiescent and others pro-

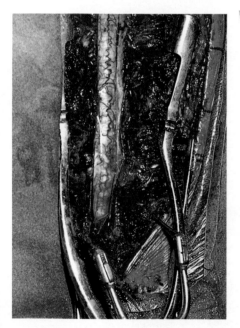

Figure 39.2 This 52-year-old female had a 3-year history of episodic radicular burning pain. Following laminectomies, her spinal cord was found to be enlarged by an ependymoma and its adjacent cyst. Note the stretched appearance of the vessels on the dorsum of the spinal cord.

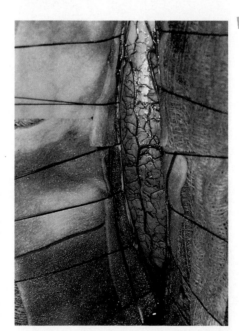

Figure 39.3 This 14-year-old presented with a 6-year history of scoliosis and 4 months of progressive leg numbness. At the time of surgery, his conus medullaris was found to be enlarged by an infiltrating astrocytoma.

gressing rapidly. Malignant astrocytomas are associated with a relentlessly progressive course.

On a myelogram an intramedullary spinal cord astrocytoma appears as a focal swelling of the spinal cord. Infiltrating fibrillary astrocytomas present as diffuse and nonenhancing masses when imaged on MRI (Fig. 39.4). The MRI scan may demonstrate cysts within the infiltrating tumor. Pilocytic astrocytomas enhance densely with gadolinium on MRI scan (Fig. 39.5). These tumors are usually associated with a large peritumoral cyst that is often several times as large as the tumor nodule.

The optimal therapy for intramedullary spinal cord tumors has yet to be determined. Surgical therapy is apparently not beneficial when treating malignant spinal cord astrocytomas.[13] Many childhood tumors appear to be amenable to surgical excision[11,14]; short-term follow up of surgical therapy for astrocytomas presenting during childhood and adolescence demonstrates good results, but long-term follow up remains to be published in detail.[15] The results of surgical therapy for low-grade spinal cord astrocytomas in adults are not as good[1,13,16,17]; surgery is associated with a significant incidence of neu-

rologic worsening and long-term follow up demonstrates a high incidence of tumor recurrence.[1] The available literature has failed to demonstrate a significant correlation between prognosis and degree of surgical resection.

Radiation therapy is difficult to assess for juveniles because these patients have such a variable long-term natural survival rate when untreated. Radiation therapy appears to be effective in impeding tumor growth in adults.[18,19] The role of chemotherapy has yet to be defined.

Metastatic Tumors

As patients with metastatic, systemic, malignant tumors are living longer, metastatic tumors of the spinal cord are becoming more common. Spinal cord symptoms produced by an intramedullary spinal metastasis must be differentiated from symptoms of metastasis to the vertebrae, radiation necrosis of the spinal cord, and paraneoplastic myelopathy. Spinal cord metastasis can produce symptoms without significantly enlarging the spinal cord, therefore notoriously difficult to detect by radiologic techniques.[20] Gadolinium-enhanced MRI appears to be the best method of detecting these lesions.[21,22]

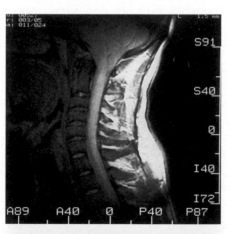

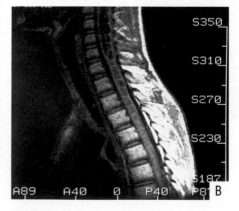

Figure 39.4 The MRI scan (TR 2000, TE 35) demonstrates a diffuse infiltrating astrocytoma of the cervical spinal cord. This lesion did not enhance with gadolinium.

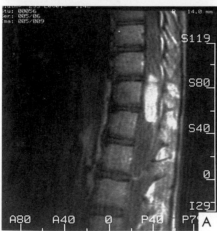

Figure 39.5 (A) MRI scan (TR 500, TE 20) contrasted with gadolinium demonstrating a well circumscribed

astrocytoma within the spinal cord. (B) The cyst associated with this tumor extends up into the cervical spinal cord.

Hemangioblastomas

Hemangioblastomas are slow-growing neoplasms that make up approximately 3% of intramedullary spinal cord tumors and usually present as slowly progressing masses or, rarely, subarachnoid hemorrhage.[23] These highly vascular tumors appear in the spinal cord either as a solid mass or as a nodule in a cyst (Fig. 39.6) and are comprised of clumps of yellow lipid-laden cells separated by pink vascular tissue (Fig. 39.7). In the cystic variety, it is usually the cyst that makes up the majority of the mass and causes the neurologic symptoms. The nodule within the cyst has a propensity to appear on the dorsum of the spinal cord and can be identified by the tortuous arteries and varices emerging from its surface. One quarter to one third of patients with intramedullary spinal cord hemangioblastomas have other manifestations of von Hippel-Lindau disease.[24]

Myelography demonstrates a nonspecific circumferential enlargement of the spinal cord that may extend beyond the borders of the tumor cyst.[25] The diagnosis of hemangioblastoma is suspected from the myelogram, if large dorsal varices are seen.

The tumor cyst shows a higher protein content than CSF on the MRI (Fig. 39.8). The elusive tumor nodule can be located on a gadolinium-enhanced MRI scan. If the tumor nodule is resected, the tumor can be cured. The gadolinium-enhanced MRI scan often demonstrates asymptomatic tumors in patients with von Hippel-Lindau disease.

Lipomas

Lipomas of the spinal cord are most often intimately related to the substance of the cord (Fig. 39.9). These lesions are usually not amenable to complete resection.

Schwannomas

Schwannomas may occur completely within the substance of the spinal cord.[26]

CLINICAL PRESENTATION

Early diagnosis of an intramedullary spinal cord tumor is a challenge for the clinical neurologist.[27] The earliest manifestations of an intraspinal mass are nonspecific and

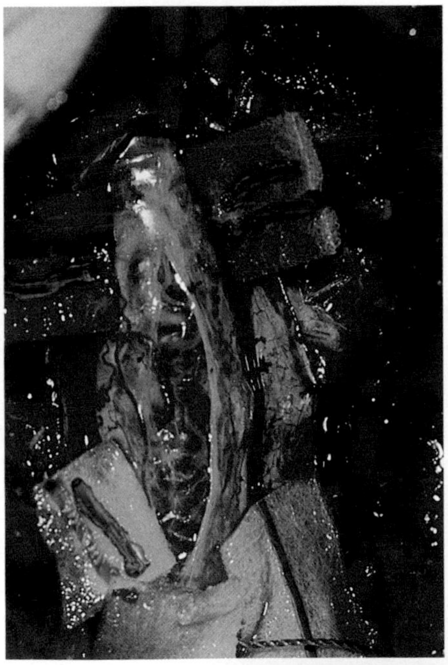

Figure 39.6 A 26-year-old presented with progressive leg numbness and weakness. This intraoperative photograph demonstrates venous varices emanating from the dorsum of an intramedullary solid spinal cord hemangioblatoma.

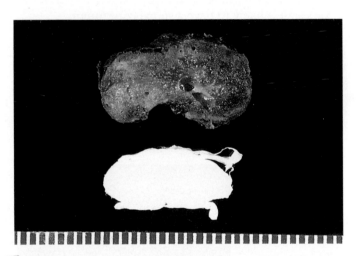

Figure 39.7 Following resection of this lesion, the patient had no new neurologic deficit. For comparison, an axial cross section of the resected tumor (top) is shown with a cross-section of a normal spinal cord obtained from an autopsy of a different patient.

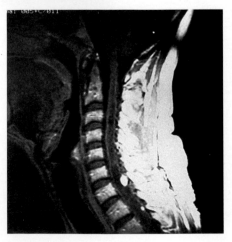

Figure 39.8 Gadolinium-enhanced MRI demonstrates the two tumor nodules and the extensive cyst of this spinal hemangioblastoma.

often masquerade as a more common and benign musculoskeletal disorder. The average reported time between the onset of symptoms and the establishment of the correct diagnosis is 31/2 years.

The most common initial symptom of an intramedullary spinal cord tumor is pain. Unfortunately, the pain that accompanies these lesions is usually not distinctive and cannot be classified. Most often the pain is initially a nonspecific deep, dull ache located adjacent to the affected spine. As time passes, the pain radiates either around the torso or into an extremity depending on the level of the tumor. The pain tends to be diffuse, eschewing dermatomal boundaries. Although the discomfort occasionally fluctuates in intensity, it almost always becomes more severe with time.

Occasionally the pain takes on characteristics that raise the suspicions of the examining physician.[28] When the pain is worse at night, awakening the patient from a sound sleep, the possibility of a spinal tumor must be considered. Unfortunately, only a minority of patients report nocturnal pain. A small group of patients report characteristic burning or intermittently lancinating pain. A patient with burning sciatic pain and a negative Lasègue's sign is likely to have a spinal cord tumor.

Some patients do not note radiating pain but report paresthesias in the dermatomes subserved by the compressed spinal cord. This zone of paresthesias tends to extend caudally with time.

Neurologic deficits may not appear until years after the onset of pain, but once present these deficits often accelerate rapidly.

A smaller group of patients present with weakness unaccompanied by numbness. This weakness may be only lower motor neuron weakness or a combination of upper and lower motor neuron weakness mimicking amyotrophic lateral sclerosis. Cervical spinal cord tumors may cause wasting confined to the patient's hands or, more rarely, the proximal musculature of the arms.

Sensory deficits are rarely an early manifestation of a spinal cord tumor, although such deficits appear as the clinical syndrome unfolds. The classic sensory deficit produced by a lesion intrinsic to the spinal cord is a dissociated, suspended sensory level that descends with time. Neurologic examination of adjacent dermatomes reveals loss of pain and temperature sensation, although touch, position, and vibratory sensation remain. Unfortunately this classic picture only occurs in approximately 20% of patients harboring intrinsic spinal cord tumors.

Incontinence is usually a late manifestation of cervical and thoracic tumors, but it occurs early in a patient who has a tumor of the conus medullaris.

Patients rarely present with sudden neurologic deficit secondary to a hemorrhage within the tumor.

_____IMAGING

Plain roentgenograms are a poor screening tool for intramedullary spinal cord tumors, but the observant physician may detect indirect evidence of an intraspinal mass on a routine exam. These indirect signs include scalloping of the posterior border of the vertebral body, erosion of the medial pedicles, and thinning of the lamina (Fig.

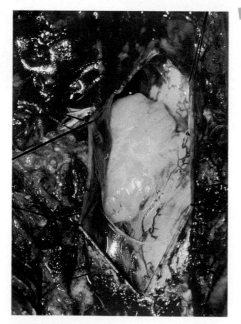

Figure 39.9 Intraoperative photograph demonstrating an exophytic lipoma infiltrating into the dorsum of the spinal cord. Although the exophytic component was resected, the intramedullary portion could only be incompletely removed.

39.10). More frequently, plain roentgenograms demonstrate the nonspecific finding of scoliosis.

An intramedullary tumor can be imaged by myelography and CT scanning. It appears on myelography as a nonspecific widening of the spinal cord shadow seen on coronal and sagittal views (Fig. 39.11A). This spinal cord enlargement is demonstrated on the postmyelogram CT scan (Fig. 39.11B). Unlike syringomyelia, the cystic cavity associated with an intramedullary spinal cord tumor only fills sporadically with contrast agent on a delayed postmyelogram CT scan. Although intramedullary tumors have occasionally been demonstrated on IV enhanced spinal CT scans, this technique is not widely used.

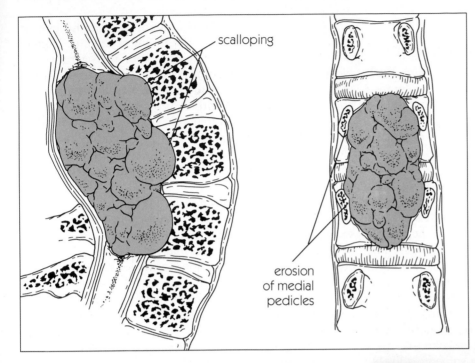

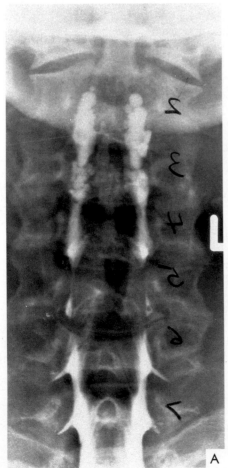

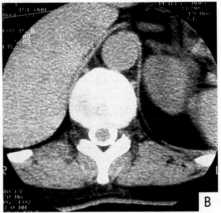

Figure 39.10 Although roentgenograms are a poor screening tool for the detection of an intramedullary tumor, the observant physician can sometimes note erosion of the medial lumina and scalloping of the posterior vertebral body, which betray the presence of an intraspinal mass.

Figure 39.11 (A) Cervical myelogram demonstrating a smooth widening of the spinal cord that reveals the location of the intramedullary spinal cord tumor. (B) This postthoracic myelogram x-ray CT scan better defines the enlarged spinal cord, which thins the subarachnoid space.

To date, contrast-enhanced MRI scans give the physician the most information concerning intramedullary spinal tumors.[21,29,30] The MRI scan allows the physician to see the extent of the tumor, and the gadolinium enhancement differentiates the tumor from an adjacent cyst (Fig. 39.12). In the past, spinal angiography has been used to seek out the vascular nodule associated with a cystic hemangioma. In most cases, the gadolinium-enhanced MRI scan obviates this study.

SURGICAL MANAGEMENT[31–33]

Most intramedullary spinal cord tumors are approached through an incision made between the posterior columns, although occasionally the best approach is through the dorsal root entry zone or even the anterior spinal cord.[34] The posterior aspect of the spinal cord is exposed by removing the overlying lamina. When cervical laminectomies are performed, special care is taken to maintain the integrity of the facets in order to maintain spinal stability. If feasible, the lamina are removed en bloc and wired or sutured back in place at the end of the case.[35]

If the tumor is wholly contained within the spinal cord, the spinal cord is opened between the posterior columns over the length of the solid portion of the tumor. The midline is usually easily discerned. Even in a distorted spinal cord, the midline is marked by the attachment of the posterior septum of arachnoid. The surgeon confirms this plane of dissection by noting the fine vessels that pass between the posterior columns.

If the tumor is an ependymoma, the surgeon is likely to encounter a gray to purple capsule that easily separates from the softer white spinal cord. Once the posterior portion of the tumor is separated from the spinal cord, the pia edges are gently retracted using 7-0 Prolene suture. The capsule is opened and a portion of the tumor's center is removed leaving 1 or 2 mm of tumor circumferentially. Overly vigorous gutting of the tumor will lead to

fragmentation of the friable tumor capsule. The circumferential dissection around the waist of the tumor is continuous using blunt dissection. Small feeding and draining vessels are cauterized and cut. Occasionally the plane separating the tumor from the spinal cord will be lost over a small portion of the capsule. Once the problem region has been flanked by a dissection above and below, the plane between the spinal cord and tumor in the problem area will become clearer.

Dissecting the poles of the tumor is more difficult. If a cyst is present, the end of the tumor is obvious. If there is no cyst, the tumor seems to taper into a root that blends into the spinal cord. As this cord of tumor tissue is pursued, histologic confirmation verifies that tumor and not gliotic spinal cord is being resected. Once one pole has been dissected free, it is gently retracted from its bed. Since the tumor's blood supply comes from the anterior spinal artery, vessels along the anterior aspect of the tumor are sought out, coagulated, and cut as the tumor is extracted.

If the spinal cord harbors an infiltrating astrocytoma, a tumor margin may be encountered, in which case dissection proceeds as outlined for ependymomas. One pole usually blends with the normal spinal cord. When the edge of the tumor is no longer obvious, the resection should stop. In cystic astrocytomas with a tumor nodule, the tumor is usually of a different consistency than the normal spinal cord, allowing the nodule to be grossly resected.

Hemangioblastomas have a propensity to occur at the dorsum of the spinal cord. When the lesion is associated with a large cyst, the edge of the pia around the tumor nodule is coagulated and the plaque of tumor is easily removed. When a larger solid tumor is encountered, the tumor capsule is gently coagulated with a bipolar cautery to diminish the tumor. The contracted tumor is then carefully dissected from the surrounding spinal cord; the feeding and draining vessels are coagulated and cut as

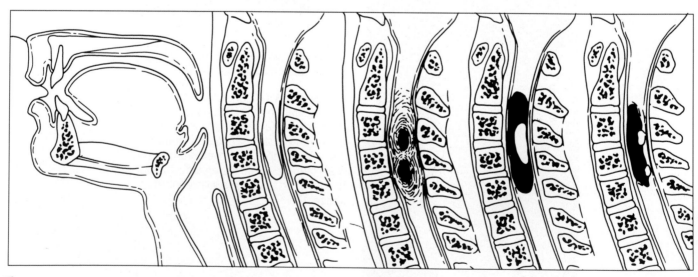

Figure 39.12 MRI scans are the best method for detecting intramedullary spinal tumors. These MRI scans demonstrate commonly seen intramedullary tumors: ependymoma (**A**), pilocytic astrocytoma (**B**), infiltrating astrocytoma (**C**), and hemangioblastoma (**D**).

they are encountered. Operating within the hemangioblastoma is treacherous, and gutting the tumor usually results in severe hemorrhage. Occasionally, a larger tumor is bisected to facilitate its removal.

TUMORS OF THE CAUDA EQUINA

Primary tumors of the cauda equina are listed in Figure 39.13. Ependymomas of the cauda equina have almost exclusively a myxopathic histology.[36] Some ependymomas are quite smooth, seemingly contained by the thinly stretched filum terminale (Fig. 39.15). Others are nodular, surrounding and incorporating the nerves of the cauda equina. On histologic examination, these tumors contain rings of ependymal cells that surround cores of blood vessels and mucin.

Epidermoid and dermoid tumors of the spine tend to occur along the cauda equina. Although these tumors are usually discrete, they may be bound to the surrounding nerve roots. Neurofibromas are well circumscribed lesions involving only a single nerve root until late in their courses (Fig. 39.14). Meningiomas rarely occur in the lumbar canal.

CLINICAL PRESENTATION

Pain is the most common presenting symptom of a tumor of the cauda equina and may precede any demonstrable neurologic deficits by several years (Fig. 39.16).[37] For approximately 50% of patients, the pain becomes more severe at night or when the patient assumes a

Figure 39.13 Tumors of the Cauda Equina	
Ependymoma	Lipoma
Schwannoma	Metastatic tumors
Meningioma	

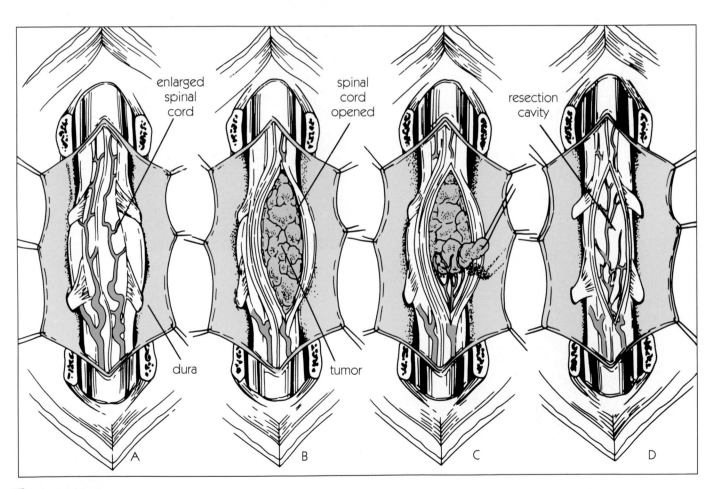

Figure 39.14 (A) The neurosurgeon first encounters a spinal cord that is swollen by the intramedullary mass. (B) A myelotomy is made between the dorsal columns. The gray tumor separates from the white matter of the spinal cord around the periphery. (C) The pole of the tumor is mobilized, and blood vessels emanating from the anterior spinal artery are coagulated and cut. (D) Following surgery, the resection cavity is lined by shaggy-looking thinned spinal cord that usually functions quite well.

recumbent position for any length of time. Unlike the more common musculoskeletal back pain, this pain is not relieved by shifting position while the patient remains recumbent.[38] The pain is only mitigated when the patient stands or sits up. Frequently the patient will report sleeping at night in the sitting position.

More rarely, patients with tumors of the cauda equina present with painless, progressive leg weakness. Patients with ependymomas occasionally present with subarachnoid hemorrhage or papilledema, presumably the result of an increase in spinal fluid protein.

IMAGING

Lumbar spine roentgenograms performed on a patient with a tumor of the cauda equina occasionally demonstrate widening of the intrapedicular distance, erosion of the posterior vertebral body, or enlargement of a neural foramen. Because of their subarachnoid location, these lesions are readily demonstrated by myelography or MRI.

SURGICAL MANAGEMENT

Surgery has been reported to be successful in removing approximately 50% of myxopapillary ependymomas. Urinary retention is the most common side effect of this procedure. It can only be assumed that newer imaging techniques that allow for earlier diagnosis and advances in microsurgical techniques will increase the number of tumors that can be completely removed. Neurofibromas usually remain discrete and can be completely removed surgically without adding to the patient's neurologic deficit.

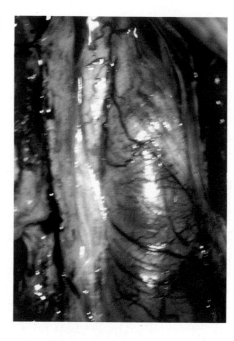

Figure 39.16 This patient presented with progressive radicular right leg pain. At the time of surgery, a large schwannoma was found to be compressing the conus medullaris and the nerve roots of the cauda equina.

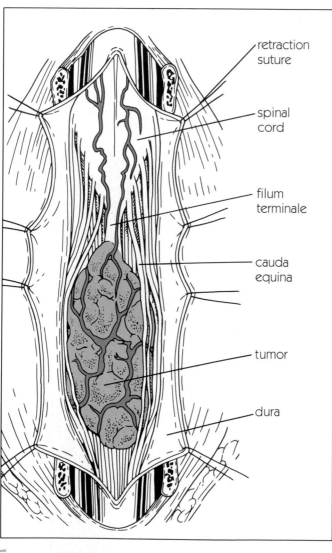

retraction suture

spinal cord

filum terminale

cauda equina

tumor

dura

Figure 39.15 Ependymomas of the lumbar spinal canal are tenuously contained within the filum terminale. Initially, they displace the nerve roots of the cauda equina, but as the tumor enlarges the roots become encased.

REFERENCES

1. Fornari M, Pluchino F, Solero CL, et al. Microsurgical treatment of intramedullary spinal cord tumours. *Acta Neurochir Suppl.* 1988;43:3–8.
2. Choksey MS, Powell M, Gibb WRG, et al. A conus tuberculoma mimicking an intramedullary tumour: a case report and review of the literature. *Br J Neurosurg.* 1989;3:117–122.
3. Lammoglia FJ, Short SR, Sweet DE, et al. Multiple sclerosis presenting as an intramedullary cervical cord tumor. *Kans Med.* 1989;90:219–221.
4. McCormick PC, Torres R, Post KD, et al. Intramedullary ependymoma of the spinal cord. *J Neurosurg.* 1990;72:523–532.
5. Yasui T, Hakuba A, Katsuyama J, et al. Microsurgical removal of intramedullary spinal cord tumours: report of 22 cases. *Acta Neurochir Suppl.* 1988;43:9–12.
6. Alvisi C, Cerisoli M, Guilioni M. Intramedullary spinal gliomas: long-term results of surgical treatments. *Acta Neurochir.* 1984;70:169–179.
7. Fischer G, Mansuy L. Total removal of intramedullary ependymomas: follow-up study of 16 cases. *Surg Neurol.* 1980;14:243–249.
8. Guidetti B, Mercuri S , Vagnozzi R. Long-term results of the surgical treatment of 129 intramedullary spinal gliomas. *J Neurosurg.* 1981;54:323–330.
9. Shaw EG, Evans RG, Scheithauer BW, et al. Radiotherapeutic management of adult intraspinal ependymomas. *Int J Radiat Oncol Biol Phys.* 1986;12:323–327.
10. Rossitch E Jr, Zeidman SM, Berger PC, et al. Clinical and pathological analysis of spinal cord astrocytomas in children. *Neurosurgery.* 1990;27:193–196.
11. Reimer R, Onofrio BM. Astrocytomas of the spinal cord in children and adolescents. *J Neurosurg.* 1985;63:669–675.
12. Hardison HH, Packer RJ, Rorke LB, et al. Outcome of children with primary intramedullary spinal cord tumors. *Childs Nerv Syst.* 1987;3:89–92.
13. Cohen AR, Wisoff JH, Allen JC, Epstein F. Malignant astrocytomas of the spinal cord. *J Neurosurg.* 1989;70:50–54.
14. Epstein F, Epstein N. Surgical treatment of spinal cord astrocytomas of childhood: a series of 19 patients. *J Neurosurg.* 1982;57:685–689.
15. Allen JC, Lassoff SJ. Outcome after surgery for intramedullary spinal cord tumors. *Neurosurgery.* 1980;26:1091. Letter.
16. Cooper PR. Outcome after operative treatment of intramedullary spinal cord tumors in adults: intermediate and long-term results in 51 patients. *Neurosurgery.* 1989;25:855–859.
17. Cooper PR, Epstein F. Radical resection of intramedullary spinal cord tumors in adults: recent experience in 29 patients. *J Neurosurg.* 1985;63:492–499.
18. Garcia DM. Primary spinal cord tumors treated with surgery and postoperative irradiation. *Int J Radiat Oncol Biol Phys.* 1985;11:1933–1939.
19. Schwade JG, Wara WM, Sheline GE, et al. Management of primary spinal cord tumors. *Int J Radiat Oncol Biol Phys.* 1978;4:389–393.
20. Winkelman MD, Adelstein DJ, Karlins NL. Intramedullary spinal cord metastasis. *Arch Neurol.* 1987;44:526–531.
21. Sze G, Krol G, Zimmerman RD, et al. Intramedullary disease of the spine: diagnosis using gadolinium-DTPA-enhanced MR imaging. *Am J Roentgenol.* 1988;151:1193–1204.
22. Post MJD, Quencer RM, Green BA, et al. Intramedullary spinal cord metastases, mainly of nonneurogenic origin. *Am J Roentgenol.* 1987;148:1015–1022.
23. Neumann HPH, Eggert HR, Weigel K, et al. Hemangioblastomas of the central nervous system: a 10-year study with special reference to von Hippel-Lindau syndrome. *J Neurosurg.* 1989;70:24–30.
24. Browne TR, Adams RD, Roberson GH. Hemangioblastoma of the spinal cord. *Arch Neurol.* 1976;33:435–441.
25. Solomon RA, Stein BM. Unusual spinal cord enlargement related to intramedullary hemangioblastoma. *J Neurosurg.* 1988;68:550–553.
26. Ross DA, Edwards MSB, Wilson CB. Intramedullary neurilemomas of the spinal cord: report of two cases and review of the literature. *Neurosurgery.* 1986;19:458–464.
27. Guidetti B, Fortuna A. Differential diagnosis of intramedullary and extramedullary tumours. In: Vinken PJ, Bruyn GW, eds. *Handbook of Clinical Neurology.* Amsterdam: North-Holland; 1975;19:51–75.
28. Austin GM. The significance and nature of pain in tumors of the spinal cord. *Surg Forum.* 1959;10:782–785.
29. Katz BH, Quencer RM, Hinks RS. Comparison of gradient recalled-echo and T2-weighted spin-echo pulse sequences in intramedullary spinal lesions. *AJNR.* 1989;10:815–822.
30. Scotti G, Scialfa G, Colombo N, et al. Magnetic resonance diagnosis of intramedullary tumors of the spinal cord. *Neuroradiology.* 1987;29:130–135.
31. Malis LI. Intramedullary spinal cord tumors. *Clin Neurosurg.* 1978;25:512–539.
32. McCormick PC, Stein BM. Intramedullary tu-

mors in adults. *Neurosurg Clin North Am.* 1990; 1:609–630.

33. Stein BM. Surgery of intramedullary spinal cord tumors. *Clin Neurosurg.* 1979;26:529–542.

34. Ahyai A, Woerner U, Markakis E. Surgical treatment of intramedullary tumors (spinal cord and medulla oblongata): analysis of 16 cases. *Neurosurg Rev.* 1990;13:45–52.

35. Zide BM, Wisoff JH, Epstein FJ. Closure of extensive and complicated laminectomy wounds. *J Neurosurg.* 1987;67:59–64.

36. Sonneland PRL, Scheithauer BW, Onofrio BM. Myxopapillary ependymoma: a clinicopathologic and immunocytochemical study of 77 cases. *Cancer.* 1985;56:883–893.

37. Fearnside MR, Adams CBT. Tumours of the cauda equina. *J Neurol Neurosurg Psychiatry.* 1978;41: 24–31.

38. Wiss DA. An unusual cause of sciatica and back pain: ependymoma of the cauda equina: case report. *J Bone Joint Surg.* 1982;64A:772–773.

Chapter 40

Tumors of the Cranial Base

Chandranath Sen

Tumors of the cranial base arise from or are in the vicinity of the bony structures at the base of the brain. The tumors may originate from the extracranial tissues, namely, the paranasal sinuses, pharynx, and connective tissues, secondarily invading the basal bones, meninges, and even the brain. Other tumors, such as osteosarcomas, chordomas, and chondrosarcomas, may arise from the basal bone and cartilage. Primarily intracranial tumors from the meninges, blood vessels, cranial nerves, and pituitary gland may arise from and encroach upon this region.

Despite their varied histology and biologic behavior, these tumors have a common feature—they are difficult to reach and involve critical structures. The base of the skull represents a transition area through which important blood vessels, like the internal carotid and vertebral arteries, enter and the cranial nerves exit. In addition, large venous sinuses draining blood from the brain aggregate at the skull base as they exit the cranial vault. They are difficult to reach because they are located ventral to the brain and posterior to the facial skeleton and aerodigestive system (Fig. 40.1).

Several advances in the last decade have significantly improved the surgical management of such tumors. These advances include a better understanding of microsurgical anatomy, refinements in neurodiagnostics and neuroanesthesia, and the development of microsurgical techniques using a variety of disciplines (neurosurgery, otolaryngology, and plastic surgery).

ANATOMY OF THE CRANIAL BASE

The cranial base is divided into three portions—anterior, middle, and posterior—that correspond to the respective cranial fossae. These are further divided into two segments—midline and lateral. Numerous surgical approaches to the cranial base have been described, and such subdivisions of this area greatly facilitate evaluation of radiographic studies and selection of the appropriate surgical procedure.

The anterior cranial base[1] is made up of the frontal, ethmoid, and sphenoid bones, which form the orbital roofs laterally and the cribriform plates and roofs of the ethmoidal and sphenoidal sinuses medially. Posteriorly it is limited by the tuberculum sellae and the lesser sphenoid wings. The optic canals (diverging caudolaterally), the superior orbital fissures, and the anterior genu of the cavernous internal carotid arteries (ICAs) form the posterior relations of the anterior fossa. About 44 olfactory fila exit the cribriform plate, each with their own arachnoidal and dural sheaths. The orbital roofs and the anterior clinoid processes can be pneumatized to a variable degree from extensions of the frontal, ethmoidal, and sphenoidal sinuses.

The middle cranial base[2] is made up of the body and greater wings of the sphenoid and petrous temporal bones (Fig. 40.2). Occupying a significant portion of this region, the cavernous sinus is situated between the temporal lobes and the pituitary gland (Fig. 40.3). It con-

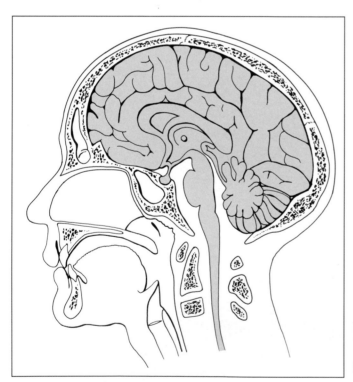

Figure 40.1 Midline sagittal section showing the anterior, middle, and posterior cranial bases and their relation to the brain and pharynx.

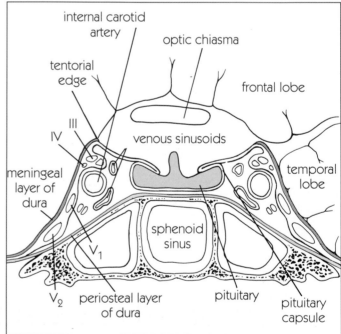

Figure 40.2 Coronal section of the parasellar region. The central portion of this region is occupied by the pituitary gland and the lateral portion is occupied by the temporal lobes. The dura of the middle cranial fossa consists of two layers, the outer periosteal and inner meningeal layers, which enclose the cavernous sinuses.

sists of a mixture of venous plexus and sinusoids within the dural leaves, through which the internal carotid artery and the abducens nerve travel. The oculomotor nerve pierces the roof posteriorly as it enters the cavernous sinus. Medially, the cavernous sinus is separated from the pituitary gland by a thin layer of periosteal dura (pituitary capsule). The floor is composed of dura, which rests on the lateral wall of the sphenoid sinus.

The petrous temporal bone houses the middle and inner ear structures and the petrous segment of the ICA. The petrous ICA is made up of an initial vertical segment and then a horizontal one before it enters the cavernous sinus. The genu of the petrous ICA is near the cochlea and the geniculate ganglion of the facial nerve.

The greater wing of sphenoid lies above the infratemporal and pterygopalatine fossae, which contain the masticatory and pharyngeal muscles, cranial nerves, internal and external carotid arteries, eustachian tube, and a venous plexus that communicates through the foramina at the skull base with the cavernous sinus above.

The posterior cranial base[3] is made up of the clivus in the middle and the posterior surface of the petrous temporal bones on either side. The upper portion of the clivus is formed by the sphenoid bone and the lower portion by the basiocciput. The posterior cranial base is related to the brain stem and cerebellum on its dorsal surface. Several cranial nerves exit the posterior cranial fossa: The abducens nerve leaves by piercing the meningeal layer of the dura on either side of the clivus to enter Dorello's canal, where it ascends, crosses the petrous apex, and enters the cavernous sinus. The facial and vestibulocochlear nerves enter the internal auditory canal (IAC). The jugular foramen is situated just caudal and lateral to the IAC and contains the jugular bulb and the glossopharyngeal, vagus, and accessory nerves. The hypoglossal canal is immediately medial and rostral to the occipital condyles. The articular surfaces of the occipital condyles face anterolaterally and the anterior ends point medially. The vertebral arteries exit the foramen transversarium of atlas, hug the joint capsule of the atlantooccipital joint closely, then enter the dura on the lateral aspect at the foramen magnum.

The venous plexus between the two layers of the clival dura is very well developed, and the superior and inferior petrosal sinuses travel between these layers to connect the cavernous sinuses to the jugular system. Ventrally, the posterior cranial base is situated over the nasopharynx, separated only by the mucosa and the constrictor.

TYPES OF TUMORS

Tumors in this region originate from three principal sources: intracranial tissues, cranial bones and cartilage, and extracranial tissues. Figure 40.4 lists the types of tumors encountered in our practice. Some of the more common types are described below.

MENINGIOMA[4]

Forty percent to 50% of meningiomas involve the skull base. The usual locations are the olfactory grooves, the sella and parasellar region, Meckel's cave, and the posterior fossa. These tumors often engulf cranial nerves and blood vessels and grow through the dura mater to

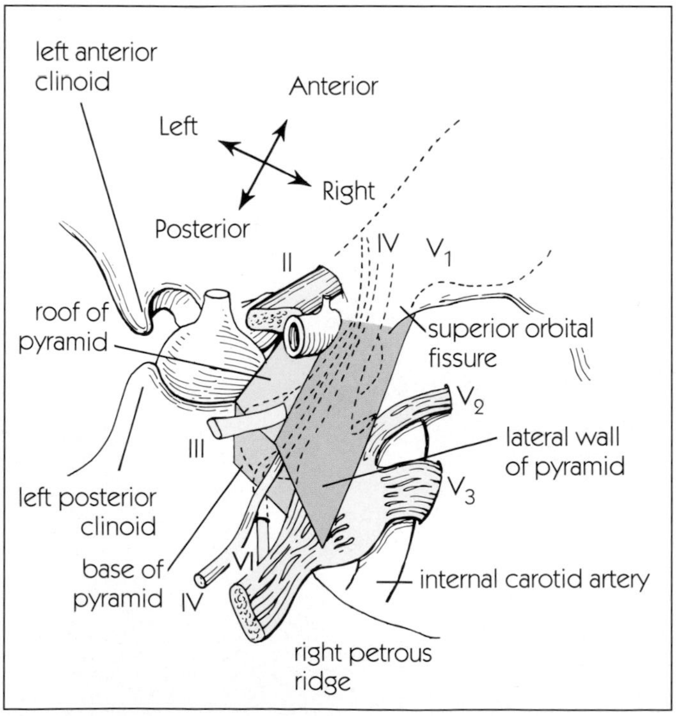

Figure 40.3 Diagram of the right cavernous sinus, demonstrating the pyramidal shape of the space (shaded) with its base towards the posterior fossa and the apex merging anteriorly with the orbital apex. The ICA exits the sinus anteriorly. Cranial nerves III, IV, and V occupy the lateral wall from above downwards, respectively, on their way to the superior orbital fissure.

invade the basal bony structures and enter the orbit, paranasal sinuses, and the muscles at the base of the skull (Fig. 40.5). Tumor touching bone causes a hyperostotic reaction; tumor cells are frequently found within such bone. Benign meningiomas usually displace rather than invade the brain. However, because they grow slowly, there may be extensive involvement of the basal structures at the time of presentation. Malignant meningiomas and those of the angioblastic type behave much more aggressively, tending to grow rapidly and metastasize to distant organs. The goals of surgery are to remove totally the tumor and involved tissues, to prevent recurrence, and to preserve neurovascular structures.

SCHWANNOMA

Schwannoma is a benign neoplasm arising from the cranial nerve sheaths. The vestibular nerve is the most fre-

Figure 40.4A Benign Lesions

Type of Tumor	Number of Operations**
Neurilemoma	30
V	18
IX, X	8
VII	4
Meningioma	156
Olfactory groove	3
Tuberculum sellae	4
Sphenoid ridge	10
Middle fossa	11
Cavernous sinus	65
Medial tentorial	7
Petrous ridge	13
Clivus	34
Foramen magnum	9
Epidermoid cyst/cholesterol granuloma	10
Craniopharyngioma	3
Juvenile angiofibroma	6
Invasive pituitary adenoma	8
Paraganglioma	12
Hemangioma of cavernous sinus	3
Brain stem cavernous angioma	2
Fibrous dysplasia	1
Ossifying fibroma	2
Chondroblastoma	1
Orbital osteoma	2
Metastatic cardiac myxoma to temporal bone	1
CSF leak*	9
Giant cell tumor of bone (middle fossa)	1
Vascular	
Cavernous ICA aneurysm	4
Petrous ICA aneurysm	2
Total	253

*Includes only patients referred here for management of CSF leaks

Figure 40.4B Malignant Lesions

Type of Tumor	Number of Operations**
Chordoma	35
Chondrosarcoma	18
Adenoid cystic carcinoma	17
Plasmacytoma	2
Esthesioneuroblastoma	7
Adenocarcinoma	4
Squamous cell carcinoma	26
Basal cell carcinoma	3
Osteogenic sarcoma	3
Melanoma	3
Rhabdomyosarcoma	3
Total	121

**The figures in Figures 40.4A and 40.4B indicate the number of operations. These are more than the number of patients since several patients had more than one operation.

quent site of origin. Less frequently, the trigeminal, facial, glossopharyngeal, vagus, and hypoglossal nerves are sites of origin. The tumor becomes symptomatic either from dysfunction of the parent or neighboring cranial nerves or from progressive distortion of the brain stem. The tumor does not invade tissue and tends to displace cranial nerves, blood vessels, and the brain. Tumors arising from nerve sheaths may occupy more than one compartment and extend extracranially along the course of the nerve (Fig. 40.6A). The tumor does not invade the bone; instead, smooth remodelling around the tumor, which is most remarkable in the region of the exit foramen of the cranial nerve, is a clue to the diagnosis (Fig. 40.6B). Multiple nerve sheath tumors that occur in patients with von Recklinghausen's disease behave more aggressively and are prone to malignant transformation.

ESTHESIONEUROBLASTOMA[5]

This is a malignant tumor arising from the olfactory epithelium on the nasal side under the cribriform plate. There are two peaks of incidence, at 30 and 60 years of age. It is slow-growing and has a 20% to 40% metastatic potential to the regional lymph nodes, bone, and lungs. Invasion of the anterior cranial base is common

by the time of presentation. Surgical resection entails en bloc removal of the tumor and surrounding tissues, including the bone of the cranial base, the dura, and the olfactory tracts. These tumors respond favorably to radiation, so surgery is followed by external beam irradiation. Large tumors can grow posteriorly, threatening the optic nerves and involving the middle cranial fossa (Fig. 40.7). When this occurs, only piecemeal removal is possible. Local recurrence is common, even years after surgical removal.

CHORDOMA[6]

This malignant tumor arises from the notochordal remnants that extend from the clivus to the sacrum. The average age at presentation is 40 years. About 35% of chordomas occur in the skull base, and the majority of the rest occur at the caudal end of the spine. These tumors are usually slow-growing and quite large at the time of presentation. They are grayish, lobulated masses without a distinct capsule, and they contain varying amounts of calcification. Bone destruction in an irregular manner is evident on the CT scan. The consistency of the tumor may vary from soft and gelatinous to rock hard. They are extradural in origin and tend to displace

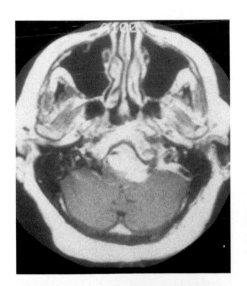
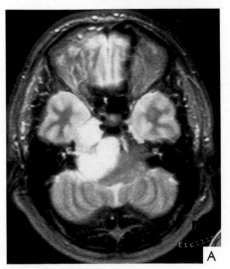
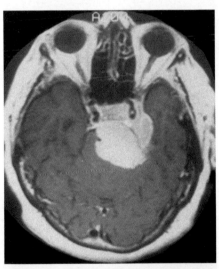
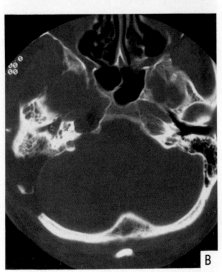

Figure 40.5 Extensive basal meningioma that involves the cavernous sinus, clivus, and sphenoid sinus and surrounds the left ICA and basilar artery.

Figure 40.6 (A) MRI scan shows a large trigeminal neurinoma in the middle and posterior fossa displacing the ICA and the basilar artery. (B) CT scan shows smooth remodeling of the bone in the region of Meckel's cave.

the dura. Large or recurrent tumors invade and penetrate the dura, and they may bury themselves inside the brain stem and surround important arteries and cranial nerves (Fig. 40.8). It is usually possible to establish a plane of dissection around the tumor and the neurovascular structures; however, because bone is infiltrated by the tumor, no such distinction can be made in the cranial bones. The local recurrence rate is quite high, and metastasis occurs in 10% to 40% of cases. Chordomas are relatively radioresistant, and aggressive surgical resection is the initial therapy of choice. There are no histologic indicators to predict the aggressiveness of a particular case.

CHONDROSARCOMA[6]

Like chordomas, these are slow-growing, malignant neoplasms. They are believed to originate in the primitive mesenchymal cell rests in the cartilaginous matrix at the skull base. Their gross appearance and biologic

behavior are similar to the chordoma, and they involve the middle, anterior, and posterior cranial base in decreasing order of frequency. The parasellar location is the most common (Fig. 40.9). These tumors are primarily extradural with dural invasion occuring at a later stage. They can be graded histologically to indicate their relative biologic aggressiveness. Radical surgical excision is the treatment of choice; however, this is done in a piecemeal fashion to preserve the important neurovascular structures. Local recurrence rate is high and is usually the ultimate cause of the patient's death.

ADENOID CYSTIC CARCINOMA[5]

This malignant neoplasm arises from the major and minor salivary glands and affects patients in their fourth to sixth decades. The natural course of the disease is relentless progression and local invasion. Its high propensity for perineural extension at distances from its gross location is a significant limiting factor in its surgi-

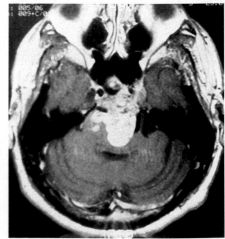

Figure 40.7 (A,B) MRI scan of a patient with a large esthesioneuroblastoma who presented with bilateral loss of vision.

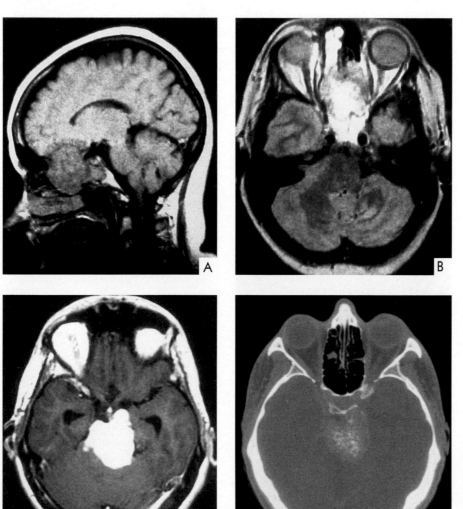

Figure 40.8 (A) MR scan with gadolinium in a 22-year-old patient with a large clivus chordoma. (B) CT scan with bone algorithms shows fine calcification within the tumor.

Figure 40.9 MRI scan of a young man with a large chondrosarcoma invaginating the clivus and extending into the sphenoid and cavernous sinus. Radiologically, a chondrosarcoma is indistinguishable from a chordoma.

Principles of Neurosurgery

cal treatment. The bones may be involved even if there is no radiographic evidence; however, usually irregular bone destruction is noted on the CT scans. Metastasis is a late finding in the disease. Because of its protracted course, follow up of more than 5 years is required for prognostication. Despite incomplete excision, long periods of survival are not uncommon. Multiple treatments for recurrent disease are justified to provide symptomatic relief.

NASOPHARYNGEAL CARCINOMA[7]

This type of tumor commonly occurs in Chinese people. The average age of the patient at presentation is 45 years, and males are more frequently affected. There is a high incidence of invasion of the skull base, and spread into the cervical lymph nodes occurs early in the course of the disease. Three histologic types exist, whose biologic behavior and prognosis vary. The nonkeratinizing and undifferentiated types, which are strongly associated with exposure to the Epstein-Barr virus, carry a better prognosis than the squamous cell variety, which is not radiosensitive and has a 5-year survival rate of 20%. Radiation is the initial treatment for the nonkeratinizing and undifferentiated types, with surgery reserved for recurrent disease. Surgery plays a greater role, however, in the treatment of the squamous cell carcinoma.

PARAGANGLIOMAS[5]

These tumors arise from the paraganglia of the head and neck. Of this group the glomus jugulare and tympanicum are of interest to the cranial base surgeon. These tumors are multicentric in 10% of cases and appear at different times in the patient's life. They are extremely vascular and their response to radiation is variable. The average age at the time of presentation is 45 years, and females are more frequently affected. These tumors are generally regarded as benign and slow-growing, progressively involving critical structures in the temporal bone. The initial presentation is pulsatile tinnitus, which progresses to conductive hearing loss and cranial neuropathies of nerves VII through XII as the tumor grows. Intracranial extension occurs in larger tumors. The tumor also extends for distances inside the lumen of the sigmoid and transverse sinus and internal jugular vein. Involvement of the internal carotid artery and the caudal cranial nerves is the major cause of surgical morbidity. Surgical excision is the primary treatment.

RADIOGRAPHIC EVALUATION

Current progress in treating tumors at the cranial base is partly attributable to advances in imaging techniques. Radiographic imaging is essential for diagnosing the tumor and, more importantly, estimating accurately the extent of the disease to facilitate surgical planning. Polytomography has been completely replaced by high-resolution CT and MRI. The goals of radiographic evaluation of skull base lesions are 1) to screen for base of the skull involvement, 2) to determine the extent of bony involvement, 3) to determine the relationship of the soft tissue structures in the region of the tumor (i.e., whether there is invasion or displacement of the brain, pituitary, arteries, and extracranial soft tissues), and 4) to determine the vascular anatomy in the vicinity of the tumor and, in case of involvement of major vessels by the tumor, to determine the collateral channels and the circulatory reserve. It is also possible to predict the histology of the lesion based on characteristic changes produced by the lesion.

COMPUTED TOMOGRAPHY

A high-resolution CT scanner is essental for minute details. The area of the tumor is scanned in 1.5 to 3 mm slices parallel to the planum sphenoidale. To obtain an overview of the region and identify associated abnormalities like hydrocephalus, the remainder of the head is scanned in 10 mm slices. Axial scans are always supplemented with coronal scans of the same thickness; these are performed with the gantry and head angled to provide a true coronal view, which is preferable to a computer reformatted study. The scanning is carried out before and after intravenous contrast medium has been administered and uses bone and soft-tissue algorithms. This provides an accurate estimate of the bone and shows to a degree the relation of soft tissue to the tumor. Thus the study of the lesion in two planes gives a three-dimensional evaluation. Software for three-dimensional reconstruction is currently available and is helpful in some cases. The CT scan is the most sensitive way of detecting minute amounts of calcification in the tumor (see Fig. 40.8B). It provides the best possible view of the type of bony involvement—e.g., irregular bone destruction as in a malignant tumor (Fig. 40.10), smooth remodeling of bone as in a neurilemoma (see Fig. 40.6B), or hyperostosis (Fig. 40.11)—and its extent and relation to the various foramina, paranasal sinuses, and the labyrinth, which is important for planning surgical resection. The major drawback of the CT scan is its inability to depict the vascular relations of the tumor.

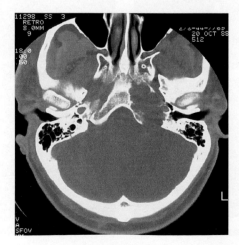

Figure 40.10 CT scan of a patient with a chondrosarcoma shows irregular bone destruction in the region of the petroclival synchondrosis. The scalloping of the bone margins is typical of this tumor.

Currently, MRI is the best technique available for studying the relation of the tumor to soft tissue. It has excellent contrast resolution, and a magnet of a high field strength yields high quality images. Like CT, MRI is performed in thin slices in the axial, coronal, and sometimes sagittal planes. Intravenous gadolinium further enhances the contrast of the lesion. MRI enables the tumor to be distinguished from the neurovascular structures, fat, and extracranial soft tissues. It allows the surgeon to determine whether a distinct plane exists between the tumor and the brain or if the tumor has invaded the brain or soft tissues. When an important blood vessel like the ICA or the vertebrobasilar system is in close proximity to the tumor, the status of the parent vessel or its major branches (i.e., whether they are completely surrounded by the tumor) is best determined by MRI (Fig. 40.12). A similar assessment of the venous sinuses can also be made. The limitation of MRI seems to be its inability to differentiate specks of calcification from flowing blood in tumor vessels; thus a densely calcified tumor may appear to be very vascular. Consequently, CT and MRI provide complementary information.

Although MRI has limited its use, arteriography is still important for investigating tumors at the cranial base. Arteriography is better able to define the relationship of the major arteries and their branches to the tumor. When there is encasement, arteriography enables the length of involvement, the caliber of the lumen, and the status of the vessel wall to be evaluated. It is also used to determine a tumor's vascularity and the angioarchitecture, which can sometimes indicate the type of tumor in question, e.g., juvenile angiofibroma (Fig. 40.13), meningioma, glomus tumor, etc. Simple displacement, as opposed to constriction with irregularity of the vessel wall in a particular segment, can indicate whether the vessel will separate from the tumor without injury. Because of the heavy bony overlay in the region of the skull base, subtraction technique is essential when studying the angiograms. Important drainage veins and their patency should be known preoperatively so they will not be compromised. This is especially important with tumors in the vicinity of the sigmoid sinus and jugular bulb, in which case dominance of the jugular bulb and adequacy of communication between

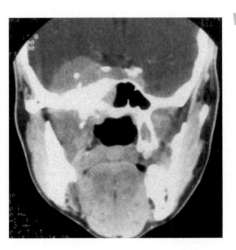

Figure 40.11 Coronal CT scan of a patient with an extensive meningioma of the middle fossa and extracranial region shows severe hyperostotic bone involvement.

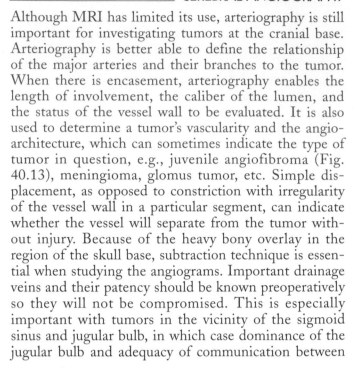

Figure 40.12 MRI scan of a patient with a chondrosarcoma surrounding the ICA without compromise of the lumen on arteriography.

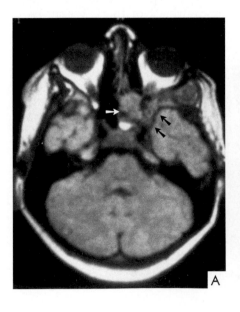
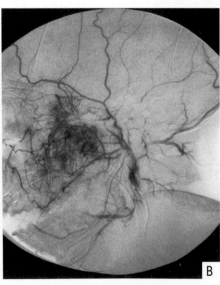

A
B

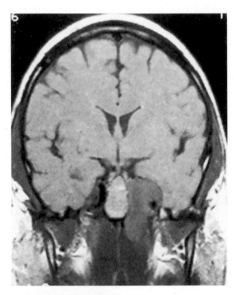

Figure 40.13 (A) MRI scan of a patient with a juvenile angiofibroma occupying the nasopharynx and extending into the sphenoid sinus, superior orbital fissure, and the anterior cavernous sinus (arrows) (B) External carotid arteriogram showing typical hypervascularity of the tumor.

the transverse sinuses must be assessed (Fig. 40.14). Free communication between the various sinuses at the torcula exists in 57% of patients, while the remainder have some type of anomaly.[8]

The collateral arterial circulation can be estimated by observing the presence and size of the anterior and posterior communicating arteries and the pattern of flow with cross compression of the ICA. An accurate knowledge of the cerebral circulatory reserve is extremely important because the ICA is frequently involved in the skull base by the tumor. In certain cases the vessel may need to be sacrificed, if there is a malignant tumor or the tumor and vessel are inseparable (with a meningioma). In other instances the artery may be injured and need to be occluded temporarily for repair. The consequences of such a course of action must be predetermined. The balloon test occlusion is used for this purpose at our institution and forms a part of the arteriographic examination.[9] A balloon catheter is floated into the ICA in question and clinical evaluation of the patient is carried out with the artery occluded (Fig. 40.15). About 8% to 10% of the patients show a neurologic deficit on this test. If the patient passes the test, a stable xenon cerebral blood flow examination is performed, with the artery both occluded and patent. About 15% of patients show a significant reduction in their flows during this test (Fig. 40.16). Thus, patients who fail the clinical test and those who show critical reduction in blood flow need some type of vascular reconstructive procedure to maintain their cerebrovascular reserve in case of injury to or sacrifice of the artery. This revascularization is usually carried out under barbiturate and hypothermic brain protection. In patients with adequate collaterals, the artery may be ligated in such a way that there is no blind stump to act as an embolic source.

Knowledge of the extent and source of the blood supply to the tumor is also important. In addition to its diagnostic importance, it is helpful to perform superselective catheterization of the feeding vessels preoperatively and embolize them to reduce intraoperative blood loss and facilitate surgical removal. Despite significant

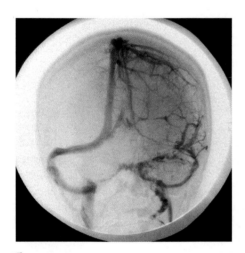

Figure 40.14 Venous phase of an arteriogram showing lack of communication between the transverse sinuses on either side with the superior sagittal sinus draining into the right transverse sinus.

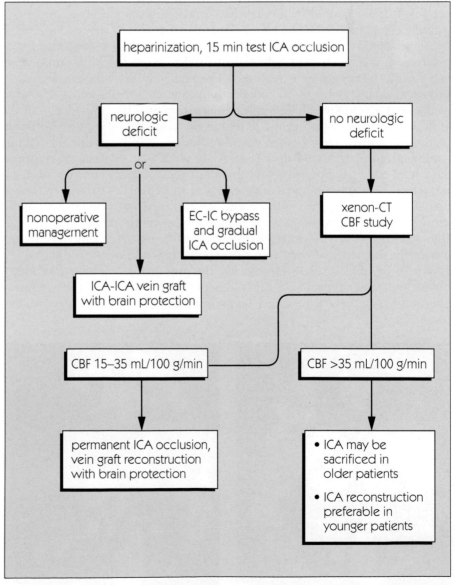

Figure 40.15 Balloon test occlusion.

advances in this field, certain vessels cannot be safely embolized, especially if they are small and arise directly from the ICA or the vertebrobasilar system.

SURGICAL MANAGEMENT

ANESTHESIA AND MONITORING

The length and complexity of the operative procedures require constant communication between the surgeon and anesthetist and the use of sophisticated anesthetic techniques, including intracranial hypertension management, brain relaxation, brain protection during vascular occlusion and reconstruction, intraoperative electrophysiologic monitoring of brain and cranial nerve function, and finally, after the long operation, a smooth and rapid emergence from anesthesia to allow neurologic evaluation. Because the surgeon needs to work beneath the brain, brain retraction is a major cause of morbidity. Several techniques of brain relaxation are used, including hyperventilation, osmotic diuretics, and CSF drainage. CSF drainage through a spinal subarachnoid drain is used in the absence of a significant intradural mass or distortion of the brain. The drain is usually inserted by the anesthetist after induction and intubation, and gradual withdrawal of fluid is carried out during the operation as required. The brain can be protected against ischemia by sodium thiopental or etomidate for electroencephalographic burst suppression and concomitant hypothermia.[10] These measures are instituted immediately before vascular clamping and continued until the blood flow is re-established. Standard methods of monitoring vital functions include an intraarterial catheter and a central venous or right atrial catheter to measure the volume and protect against venous air embolism. Sequential pneumatic compression stockings over the lower extremities are used to reduce the incidence of deep vein thrombosis. It is necessary to be able to estimate closely the amount of blood lost, and appropriate replacement during the operation is necessary to avoid hemodilution-related coagulopathy, which can be a significant problem. Fresh frozen plasma and platelet replacement is based on coagulation profile tests performed at regular intervals.

To some extent the type of intraoperative electrophysiologic monitoring dictates the anesthetic technique. Brain stem auditory evoked responses and somatosensory evoked responses (SER) are frequently monitored so that important brain stem functions can be assessed constantly.[11] Retraction or direct injury by manipulations made in the vicinity can cause problems in these areas, and changes can be made according to the evoked responses to prevent serious sequelae. When cranial nerve manipulation is anticipated, the spontaneous and evoked activity of the nerves is monitored to facilitate positive identification and reduce the operative trauma. Motor nerves are best suited for such monitoring, and the anesthetist must refrain from using longacting paralytic agents and rely on inhalation agents like isoflurane, although these can interfere with SER monitoring. Thus, a concerted effort by the surgeon, the anesthetist, and the neurophysiologist is essential to execute the operation safely.

SURGICAL PRINCIPLES

Adequate Exposure
Many innovative operative exposures for approaching these lesions have been devised. Each provides exposure of a specific region of the skull base. Thorough knowledge of the surgical anatomy is essential to maximize the benefits of a particular approach while reducing complications. The surgeon may use more than one approach simultaneously to obtain multiple viewing angles. This is necessary not only because of the restrictive nature of many of the approaches, but because a combination of approaches, at one or more than one sitting, permits more thorough removal, especially of larger tumors.

Control of Important Neural and Vascular Structures
The procedure may involve separation of the tumor from major neurovascular structures, or these structures

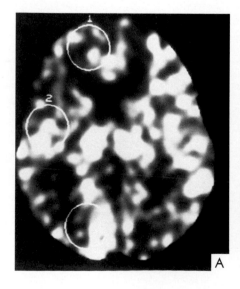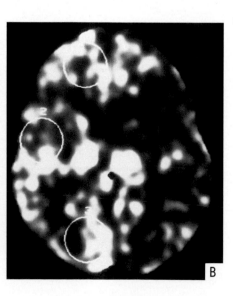

Figure 40.16 Stable xenon CT showing preocclusion cerebral blood flow (A) and the drop in flow in the left middle cerebral artery territory during occlusion of the left ICA (B).

may be encountered during surgical exposure. The surgeon must establish proximal and distal control of major vessels during these maneuvers so inadvertent injury can be satisfactorily managed. Such control is a prerequisite during arterial grafting when an involved segment of the ICA is resected.

Staging of Operations for Radical Surgical Excision

Radical tumor removal, which includes the involved margins, is the goal of surgery. Staging may be required for several reasons. Intra- and extradural tumors may need to be removed in stages to reduce the risks of CSF leakage. Large tumors requiring tedious and lengthy dissections may need more than one operative approach. These may be tackled in stages to reduce the surgeon's fatigue and thus increase the effectiveness of the operation. In some instances residual tumor may be seen on postoperative imaging studies and a second operation may be undertaken to remove the remaining tumor.

Strategies to Reduce or Eliminate Brain Retraction

Major morbidity in these operations arises from prolonged and excessive brain retraction. One of the most effective ways of reducing this is by judicial resection of nonessential bony structures or temporary displacement of the facial skeleton to improve exposure and access to a particular region. Other means of brain relaxation are also used.

Adequate Reconstruction After Tumor Removal

The purpose of this is to prevent infection, CSF leakage, and disfigurement. Complete separation of the CSF, brain, and major arteries from the contaminated regions of the paranasal sinuses and pharynx must be restored at the end of the operation. Vascularized tissue is the mainstay of reconstruction, along with pieces of fat, muscle, or bone. The vascularized flaps may be local tissue, such as the galeal pericraneal flap, temporalis and sternomastoid muscle transfers, or vascularized free flaps (rectus abdominis, greater omentum, etc.).

SURGICAL APPROACHES

Figure 40.17 lists the commonly used approaches for cranial base tumors, which are broadly divided into anterior and lateral. Some of these approaches are described below.

Figure 40.17 Surgical Approaches to the Cranial Base

Approach	Principal Region Exposed
Intradural	
Retrosigmoid	Cerebellopontine angle
Posterior subtemporal-presigmoid-transpetrous	Petrous ridge, upper and middle clivus
Frontotemporal transsylvian	Parasellar
Transsylvian-anterior subtemporal-transcavernous	Tentorial notch, upper clivus
Anterior subtemporal-preauricular infratemporal	Upper and middle clivus
Extreme lateral transcondyle	Ventral craniocervical junction
Extradural Anterior	
Transbasal	Anterior cranial base, sphenoid sinus,
Extended subfrontal (with orbital osteotomy)	middle clivus, medial to petrous ICA
Transethmoidal	Sphenoid, ethmoid sinus, middle clivus
Transsphenoidal	
Transoral (and extensions)	Midclivus, craniocervical junction
Bilateral maxillotomy	Maxillary sinus, pterygopalatine fossa,
Unilateral maxillotomy	craniocervical junction
Transcervical	Craniocervical junction
Lateral	
Subtemporal-preauricular infratemporal	Infratemporal fossa, petrous apex,
Postauricular-infratemporal	middle clivus
Transcochlear	Middle clivus
Total petrosectomy	Middle and lower clivus
Extreme lateral transcondyle	Anterior craniocervical junction

Anterior Approaches

These are used for pathology involving the anterior cranial base as far posterior as the optic foramina. These approaches may also be used for the sella turcica, clivus, and craniocervical junction. When these approaches are used posteriorly to the optic foramina, they are restricted to the median and paramedian areas, limited laterally by the exit foramina of cranial nerves VI through XII, the cavernous sinuses, and the internal carotid arteries, and caudally by the jugular bulbs and occipital condyles. Additionally, the surgeon may not have proximal control of the ICA and the vertebral arteries and thus will be unable to deal with intraoperative vascular problems. Another limitation of the anterior approaches is the paucity of reconstructive options. This can be a serious handicap if a large defect created in the skull base causes free communication between the intradural space or the great vessels with the contaminated spaces of the pharynx and paranasal sinuses. Complications like infections and CSF fistulae can have disastrous consequences. Nevertheless, the anterior approaches are ideal for certain lesions confined to this particular anatomic region.

Extended Subfrontal Approach
With Supraorbital Osteotomies[12]

A bicoronal incision is made from zygoma to zygoma at or behind the coronal suture to create a long pericranial flap for reconstruction. The pericranium is elevated with the scalp and reflected down to the lateral walls of the orbits. The periorbita is stripped from the roof and lateral wall of the orbit after the supraorbital nerves and vessels are freed

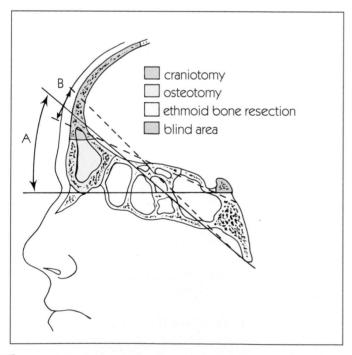

□ craniotomy
□ osteotomy
□ ethmoid bone resection
□ blind area

Figure 40.18 Additional room can be obtained underneath the frontal lobes by performing a supraorbital and ethmoidal osteotomy. However, a superficially wide exposure is required for access to the deeper areas of the clivus, and the posterior clinoids are in a blind area with this approach.

from the foramen. A bifrontal craniotomy is performed, following which the supraorbital rims, along with the anterior portions of the orbital roofs, are removed with a reciprocating saw. Removal of the supraorbital rims permits an additional 2.5 to 3 cm of room underneath the frontal lobes, thus reducing the degree of brain retraction. The brain can be further slackened by withdrawing spinal fluid through a lumbar subarachnoid drain inserted before positioning the patient. The olfactory nerves are divided, and the frontal lobes are elevated extradurally. Limited access to the anterior fossa through the frontal sinus has been described and is suitable for smaller and anteriorly located pathology. The entire anterior fossa is exposed, while only the midline portion of the middle and posterior cranial base down to the foramen magnum is accessible by the extended subfrontal approach. The major advantage of this approach is that it allows wide exposure of the pathology with minimal brain retraction (Fig. 40.18), and the basal defect can be satisfactorily reconstructed with a galeal or pericraneal flap (Fig. 40.19). This approach is useful for both intra- and extradural tumors of the anterior base and predominantly extradural tumors of the middle and posterior cranial base. The wide exposure is particularly important when treating deep lesions. The extended subfrontal approach has been used either singly or in combination with a transfascial or lateral approach for esthesioneuroblastomas, meningiomas of the anterior cranial base that have extended inferiorly in the sinuses and bony structures, sinonasal carcinomas, orbital tumors, and chordomas and chondrosarcomas of the middle and posterior cranial base, and for repair of CSF leaks through the anterior fossa and the sphenoid sinus.

Transoral Approach

This approach provides access to the clivus and anterior craniocervical junction through the oropharynx (Fig. 40.20).[13] It is used predominantly for extradural lesions, but in specific instances it can be used for intradural lesions.[14] It is most commonly used for basilar invagination from a variety of causes and cervicomedullary compression in rheumatoid arthritis. A special mouth gag is inserted to depress the tongue while the soft palate is retracted upward. The posterior pharyngeal wall is incised in the midline, and the prevertebral muscles are stripped and retracted laterally. The anterior tubercle of the atlas is the most important landmark to the midline, and the lateral limits of the exposure are formed by the occipital condyles and the jugular and hypoglossal foramina, which are about 18 mm to either side of the midline. The bone of the clivus, the anterior arch of C-1, and the vertebral bodies are removed with a high-speed drill as needed.

After removal of the lesion the prevertebral muscles and pharyngeal mucosa are reapproximated in layers. On occasion a bone strut from the iliac crest may be left in the bony defect to "fill out" the space, preventing postoperative velopharyngeal insufficiency. Thus the approach is extensive in a longitudinal direction but

Principles of Neurosurgery

quite limited laterally. Another limitation of the approach is its depth from the surface (about 10 cm from the level of the incisors in the adult). Adequate reconstruction of the operative area is severely restricted, and this limitation should be seriously considered in the preoperative planning. The major advantage of the procedure is direct access to the ventral aspect of the craniocervical junction without need for brain retraction. Modifications like the Le Fort maxillotomy, mandibulotomy, and glossotomy along with division of the soft and hard palate can be added to the standard transoral approach depending on the particular lesion in question. These additions increase the longitudinal limits of the exposure, but the lateral restrictions remain.

Lateral Approaches

Understanding the three-dimensional anatomy of the temporal bone is essential for the proper selection and optimal use of the lateral approaches to the skull base (Fig. 40.21). The major structures in consideration here are the petrous ICA, cochlea, labyrinth, facial nerve, and the jugular bulb and foramen. The preoperative radiographs of the patient need to be analyzed in relation to these landmarks and the appropriate surgical approach selected accordingly. The approach is determined by the location and extent of the tumor, whether or not there is extradural extension of the tumor, status of hearing, and existing cranial nerve dysfunction. Tumors in the cavernous sinus are approached through the transsylvian and subtemporal routes. Intradural clival lesions are approached through the subtemporal, presigmoid subtemporal, transtemporal, preauricular infratemporal, or extreme lateral transcondylar routes. Lateral approaches are also indicated for lesions lateral to or surrounding the ICA and for extradural tumors involving the temporal bone, infratemporal, and pterygoid regions. Figure 40.22 indicates the areas of the clivus exposed by the various approaches. The advantages of the lateral approaches are several: the ipsilateral internal carotid and vertebral arteries, the internal jugular vein, and the cranial nerves can be controlled; a wider exposure reduces the working depth; the plane between the brain and the tumor is better defined; contaminated spaces are usually not traversed; and the options for reconstruction are numerous.

Subtemporal and Preauricular Infratemporal Approach

This approach is used for extradural lesions that are predominantly unilateral, involve the middle and posterior cranial base, and may extend across the midline up to the opposite petrous apex.[15] Certain intradural tumors can also be managed by this approach,[16] including meningiomas that have extended into the infratemporal fossa. In the case of large tumors, the intra- and extradural portions may be removed at separate stages to reduce the chances of CSF leakage. An important reason this approach is preferable to a transtemporal approach is that it preserves hearing, since the approach

path stays anterior to the critical portion of the temporal bone and there is no need to displace the facial nerve.

A frontotemporal craniotomy is made and the supraorbital rims and zygomatic arch are removed (Fig. 40.23). The mandibular condyle is excised after dislocating it from the joint. The greater sphenoid wing is rongeured down to unroof the foramina ovale and rotundum to allow access to the base of the pterygoid

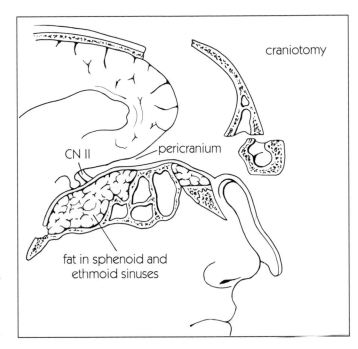

Figure 40.19 Reconstruction of the floor is performed by exenterating the sphenoidal, ethmoidal, and frontal sinuses, filling them with fat, and laying a long pericranial flap.

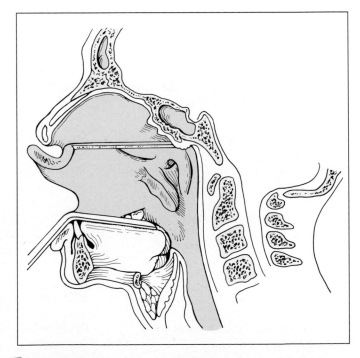

Figure 40.20 The exposure obtained by adding a bilateral maxillectomy to a standard transoral approach.

plate (Fig. 40.24). The petrous ICA is completely unroofed from its entry into the skull base up to the cavernous sinus and displaced laterally after establishing control in the neck. The bone medial to the petrous ICA is part of the clivus and can be drilled away after completely displacing the ICA from the bony canal to expose the clival dura. The sphenoid sinus can also be entered by removing the bone between V_2 and V_3. The eustachian tube situated immediately lateral to the petrous ICA is transected during this approach and

must be obliterated adequately to avoid a CSF fistula. Surgical exposure extends from the foramen rotundum in front to the hypoglossal foramen (Fig. 40.25). Only the middle portion of the clivus from the level of the trigeminal root to the hypoglossal foramen is exposed. The upper clivus can be exposed only through an intradural transsylvian or subtemporal route by traversing the posterior cavernous sinus.

Following removal of the tumor the clival defect can be filled with fat while the area around the petrous ICA

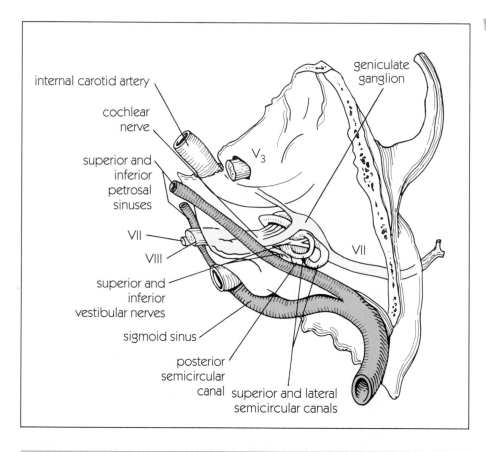

Figure 40.21 Superior view of the contents of the temporal bone. The surgical approaches to the clivus go through these structures or in front of or behind them, depending on the status of hearing and size of the tumor.

Figure 40.22 Areas of the Clivus Exposed by Surgical Approaches

Area of Clivus Exposed	Surgical Approach
Superior clivus (above V root) and posterior clinoid	Transsylvian Subtemporal
Middle clivus (between V root and jugular bulb)	Presigmoid-subtemporal Preauricular infratemporal Transoral transpalatal or with Le Fort maxillotomy Retrosigmoid Total petrosectomy
Lower clivus (jugular bulb to foramen magnum)	Extreme lateral transcondylar Transoral

Principles of Neurosurgery

is covered by transposing the temporalis muscle pedicled on the coronoid process. If a large defect is produced, as with malignant tumors, a vascularized free flap of the rectus abdominis or latissimus dorsi is used, deriving its blood supply from the external carotid artery or one of its branches. The orbitozygomatic segment and craniotomy bone flap are replaced (Fig. 40.26). Disadvantages of this approach include excision of the mandibular condyle with resultant jaw deviation

(with proper care this is not a significant disability) and destruction of the eustachian tube with conductive hearing loss (managed with a tympanostomy tube).

Total Petrosectomy
In contrast to the previous operation this approach involves removal of the entire petrous temporal bone, providing wider access to the intradural clivus and cerebellopontine angle. It is usually used for large petrocli-

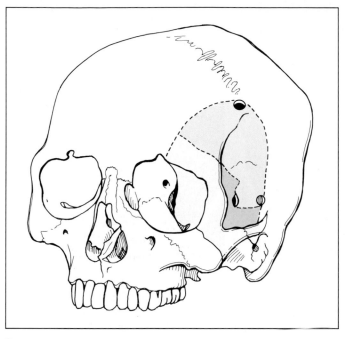

Figure 40.23 The incision, craniotomy, and orbitozygomatic bone flap are shown. The major vessels are controlled in the neck, while the needle electrodes are used for intraoperative neurophysiologic monitoring.

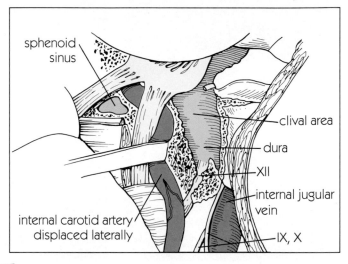

Figure 40.24 The greater sphenoid wing and the anterior portion of the petrous bone are rongeured to unroof the maxillary and mandibular nerves and the petrous ICA is completely exposed, dividing the eustachian tube. The ICA at its entry into the skull base is surrounded by a dense fibrous ring that is continuous with the periosteum; this has to be divided to mobilize the artery fully out of the bone. Removal of bone between V_2 and V_3 leads into the sphenoid sinus while drilling the bone medial to the ICA exposes the clival dura.

Figure 40.25 Diagram showing the area of the skull base exposed by the subtemporal and preauricular infratemporal approach.

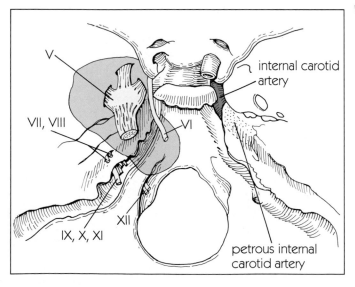

val meningiomas, glomus jugulare tumors, and temporal bone carcinomas, particularly in patients with hearing loss. The surgical incision is usually a postauricular one and the external ear canal is divided and closed as a blind pouch. The ICA is uncovered as in the previous procedure, and the temporal bone is drilled down between the sigmoid sinus and the ICA. The facial nerve is com-

pletely lifted out of the temporal bone and rerouted anteriorly or posteriorly as required (Fig. 40.27). The jugular bulb and the sigmoid sinus can be obliterated, if adequate communication with the opposite transverse sinus is demonstrated angiographically. When this approach is used for malignant tumors of the temporal bone, an en bloc resection that includes the cranial

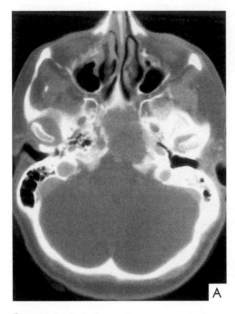
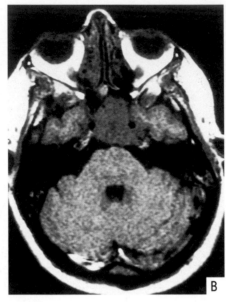
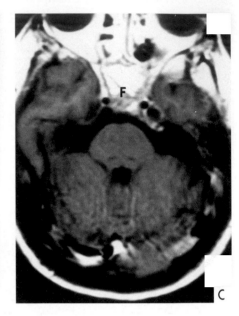

Figure 40.26 Preoperative CT (**A**) and MRI (**B**) scans showing the tumor in the clivus and left petrous apex with irregular bone destruction. The first operation was carried out through a bifrontal craniotomy and an extended subfrontal extradural approach. The tumor, which was found to be an adenoid cystic carcinoma, was very fibrous and tenacious and was only partially removed. The floor was reconstructed with a galeal pericraneal flap. Two weeks after the first operation the

remaining tumor around the left petrous ICA and the clivus was removed through a left subtemporal and preauricular infratemporal approach, after a left temporal craniotomy and orbitozygomatic osteotomy and resection of the mandibular condyle. The petrous ICA was completely exposed and mobilized and a gross total excision of tumor was achieved. Postoperative MRI (**C**) showing the area of tumor removal filled with fat and pericranial flap F (high-intensity signal).

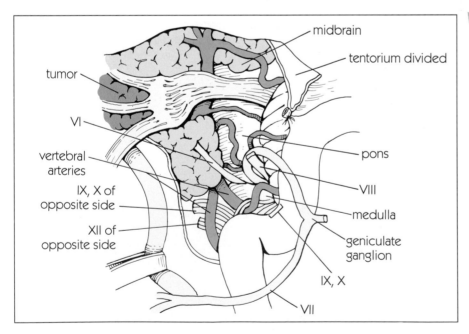

Figure 40.27 Petrosectomy approach used for a large intradural clival tumor. Note the removal of the temporal bone from the sigmoid sinus to the ICA and from the trigeminal root above to the jugular bulb below, allowing mobilization of the facial nerve. This approach provides a wide access to these extensive tumors.

nerves is preferred. However, when the approach is used for benign tumors or to provide access to an intradural tumor, the bone is removed piecemeal, usually with a high-speed drill, preserving the cranial nerves anatomically. When this approach is used to gain access to a large intradural clival tumor, the tumor removal is performed at a separate stage.

Reconstruction involves a thorough dural closure with a graft and a temporalis or sternomastoid flap to fill the defect. If the facial nerve has been transected it is also reconstructed with a greater auricular or sural nerve graft.

Presigmoid Subtemporal Approach

This approach is used primarily to treat intradural clival tumors (e.g., meningiomas and neurilemomas) in patients who have intact hearing.[17] The skin incision begins in the postauricular area and curves anteriorly in the temporal region. Following a temporal craniotomy and craniectomy in the posterior fossa retrosigmoid area, the sigmoid sinus and the lateral portion of the transverse sinus are completely unroofed with a high-speed drill. This bone removal is carried up to the mastoid segment of the facial nerve and the semicircular canals, which are not disturbed. The dura is opened in front of the sigmoid sinus and in the temporal area (Fig. 40.28). The superior petrosal sinus is ligated and divided, the incision extending medially toward the tentorial notch posterior to the entry of the trochlear nerve. The temporal lobe is elevated, protecting the vein of Labbé, while the cerebellum is retracted posteriorly along with the sigmoid sinus to expose the tumor. The advantage of this approach over a standard retrosigmoid approach is that the labyrinth is preserved while enough bone is removed in the petrous temporal

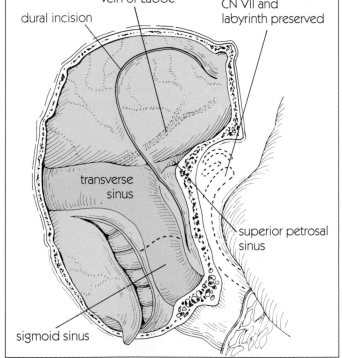

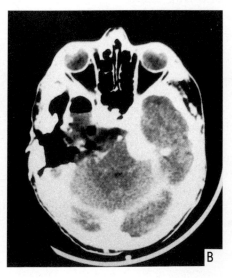

Figure 40.28 Exposure provided by the presigmoid subtemporal approach, used to reach petroclival tumors.

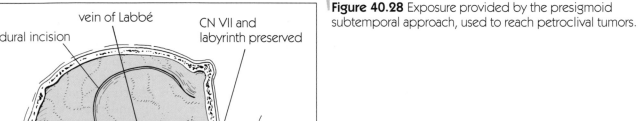

Figure 40.29 (A) Axial MRI showing a patient with bilateral medial tentorial meningiomas distorting the brain stem. The arrowhead points to the fetal origin of the posterior cerebral artery within the tumor. (B) The patient underwent a frontotemporal craniotomy, orbitozygomatic osteotomy, and removal of the supratentorial portion of the tumor. Two months later the remaining tumor, including its extension into the posterior cavernous sinus, was removed by a presigmoid subtemporal approach. A postoperative CT scan shows satisfactory tumor removal on the right.

region to bring the surgeon closer and more lateral to the tumor (Fig. 40.29). Following tumor removal the dura is closed in a watertight fashion, using a graft if necessary. The bone fragments are replaced and the remaining defect is filled with fat harvested from the abdomen or thigh. In patients with no hearing the approach can be further extended anteriorly into the labyrinth to provide a combined translabyrinthine and subtemporal access to the tumor.

Extreme Lateral Transcondylar Approach

This approach is used for intra- and extradural tumors at the lower clivus or foramen magnum, and those at C-1 and C-2 that are situated ventrally and ventrolaterally to the neuroaxis.[18,19] The incision is similar to the presigmoid approach without the temporal extension. Bone is removed by a partial mastoidectomy that does not disturb the labyrinth and facial nerve, and the sigmoid sinus is unroofed down to the jugular bulb. Craniectomy is extended in the retrosigmoid area to include the foramen magnum (C-1 and C-2 hemilamina and articular facets can be included when lower access is desired). The vertebral artery is isolated from the C-2 or C-1 foramen transversarium up to its dural entry, and part or all of the occipital condyle is drilled away. Removal of the occipital condyle and isolation of the extradural vertebral artery permits a true lateral perspective of this area. The vertebral artery is also completely released at its dural entry point to allow full mobilization and thus safe dissection from the tumor. The area of access is indicated in Figure 40.30. This approach provides access to the ventral craniocervical junction without brain retraction, and it enables the surgeon to remove all involved bone in the region of the occipital condyle, hypoglossal and jugular foramina, and the ventral clivus below the level of the jugular bulbs. If the tumor extends into the jugular foramen and the jugular bulb is either occluded or nondominant and has adequate cross-communication with its counterpart, the caudal cranial nerves can be completely skeletonized. The sigmoid sinus and the jugular vein can then be ligated and the tumor within the jugular foramen can be thoroughly removed (Fig. 40.31). Following tumor removal the dura is closed with a graft, and fat or a temporalis flap is used to obliterate the defect.

POSTOPERATIVE CARE AND COMPLICATIONS

Postoperative problems are usually related to fluid and electrolyte balance, brain swelling, delayed vascular occlusion, CSF leaks, and, most frequently, difficulties arising as a consequence of cranial nerve palsies. Serious and irreversible complications may result if these problems are not anticipated or detected and treated early. Although cranial base surgery is a team effort, most of the life-threatening complications are neurologic or vascular, and thus the neurosurgeon must exercise special vigilance to prevent them.

Initial postoperative management, provided in the intensive care unit, can extend several days. Close monitoring of the fluid balance and serum electrolytes reveals imbalances early. A CT scan is performed on the first postoperative day to obtain a "baseline study," which reveals the presence of intracranial air, brain swelling, and hematomas as well as ventricle size, and can be compared to subsequent studies. In addition, this study allows the degree of tumor resection to be assessed. CSF leakage is a relatively common problem after these operations because of entry, deliberate or otherwise, into the paranasal sinuses, temporal air cells, or eustachian tube. Early detection helps prevent meningitis. Thorough reconstruction with vascularized tissue is a key step in preventing this problem. When the leak is small, it can usually be managed with a temporary spinal fluid drain; however, larger leaks require accurate determination of the fistula site and surgical repair. Occult hydrocephalus caused by a fistula can be rectified by a simple shunting procedure.

Following tumor resection the major intracranial arteries must be carefully protected from the contaminated spaces of the sinuses and the nasopharynx by vascularized tissue (e.g., temporalis muscle flap or galeal-pericranial flap) or a vascularized tissue transfer. Secondary infection with erosion of one ICA and one vertebral artery, resulting in death, can occur. Postoperative angiography is recommended when the integrity of a particular vessel is in question. Occlusion of the vessel or formation of a psuedoaneurysm may thus be detected, and revascularization or obliteration of the vessel by neuroradiologic intervention may be undertaken before a catastrophic event develops.

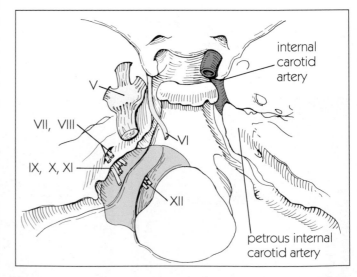

Figure 40.30 Area of access and bone removal by the extreme lateral transcondylar approach.

Principles of Neurosurgery

Cranial nerve dysfunction occurs frequently and can cause secondary problems. When the trigeminal or the facial nerve is impaired, protection of the ipsilateral eye must involve shielding and adequately lubricating it. An eyelid augmentation is necessary if prolonged difficulty is anticipated. When the temporomandibular joint or the masticatory muscles have been disrupted, early jaw exercises can prevent trismus and limited jaw excursion. Dysfunction of the glossopharyngeal, vagus, or hypoglossal nerves affects swallowing and airway protection. Under such circumstances, tracheostomy and feeding gastrostomy or jejunostomy are performed early—preventing aspiration, and facilitating adequate nutrition and a smooth postoperative course—and can be reversed when these functions are recovered. Although nerve dysfunction is usually temporary, secondary disability is great if the nerves are affected jointly rather than individually and grave if they are bilaterally impaired.

Fortunately, infection is infrequent considering the nature and duration of these operations. Infection can present as meningitis and intradural or extradural abscess. Its presence is heralded by fever and changes in the patient's mental status or local wound appearance. Spinal fluid examination and contrast enhanced CT scan provide the diagnosis. Treatment involves prolonged intravenous antibiotics and debridement of the abscess if present. Removal of the bone flaps may also be necessary. Because the operations and confinement to bed are prolonged, deep venous thrombosis and pulmonary thromboembolism are risks. Pneumatic compression stockings and subcutaneous heparin are continued until the patient is ambulatory. Deep venous thrombosis should be detected early and anticoagulation therapy instituted if indicated. If this is contraindicated, insertion of a vena caval filter should be considered.

CONCLUSION

Tremendous progress has been made in the field of cranial base surgery, especially in the last decade. It continues to be a challenging multidisciplinary collaboration. Constant refinement and critical evaluation of the results are necessary to define the role of such treatment. Adjunctive treatment modalities need to be explored so the efficacy and safety of the management of lesions in these areas can be enhanced and supplemented.

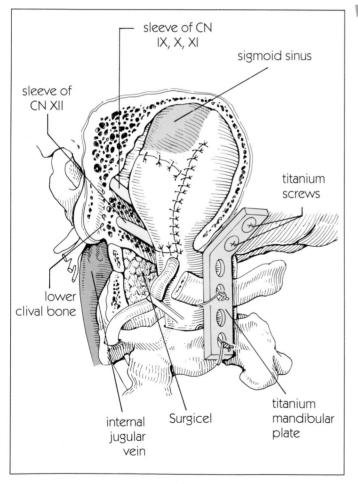

Figure 40.31 Bony removal includes unroofing of the sigmoid sinus, partial or total condylectomy, and complete isolation of the vertebral artery up to its dural entry. The extradural portions of the nerves of the jugular and hypoglossal foramina have been skeletonized and the condyle has been completely resected. The sigmoid sinus has been ligated to skeletonize the jugular foramen and an occipito-cervical fusion has also been performed.

REFERENCES

1. Lang J. Anterior cranial base anatomy. In: Sekhar LN, Schramm VL Jr, eds. *Tumors of the Cranial Base: Diagnosis and Treatment.* Mt. Kisco, NY: Futura Publishing Co; 1987:247–264.
2. Lang J. Middle cranial base anatomy. In: Sekhar LN, Schramm VL Jr, eds. *Tumors of the Cranial Base: Diagnosis and Treatment.* Mt. Kisco, NY: Futura Publishing Co; 1987:313–334.
3. Lang J. Posterior cranial base anatomy. In: Sekhar LN, Schramm VL Jr, eds. *Tumors of the Cranial Base: Diagnosis and Treatment.* Mt. Kisco, NY: Futura Publishing Co; 1987:441–460.
4. Chou SM, Miles JM. The pathology of meningiomas. In: Al-Mefty O, ed. *Meningiomas.* New York, NY: Raven Press; 1991:37–57.
5. Batsakis JG. *Tumors of the Head and Neck—Clinical and Pathological Considerations.* 2nd ed. Baltimore, Md: Williams & Wilkins; 1979.
6. Sen CN, Sekhar LN, Schramm VL, Janecka IP. Chordomas and chondrosarcomas of the cranial base. *Neurosurgery.* 1989;25:931–941.
7. Weiland LH. Nasopharyngeal carcinomas. In: Barnes L, ed. *Surgical Pathology of the Head and Neck.* New York, NY: Marcel Dekker; 1985:453–466.
8. Osborn AG. *Introduction to Cerebral Angiography.* Hagerstown, Md: Harper & Row; 1980:331.
9. Erba SM, Horton JA, Latshaw RB, et al. Balloon test occlusion of the internal carotid artery with stable xenon/CT cerebral blood flow imaging. *AJNR.* 1988;9:533–538.
10. Batjer HH, Frankfurt AI, Purdy PD, Smith SS, Samson DS. Use of etomidate, temporary arterial occlusion, and intraoperative arteriography in surgical treatment of large and giant cerebral aneurysms. *J Neurosurg.* 1988;68:234–240.
11. Moller AR. *Evoked Potentials in Intraoperative Monitoring.* Baltimore, Md: Williams & Wilkins; 1988.
12. Sekhar LN, Sen CN. An extended frontal approach to tumors involving the skull base. In: Wilkins R, Rengachary S, eds. *Neurosurgery Update I.* New York, NY: McGraw-Hill; 1990:292–301.
13. Menezes AH, VanGilder JC. Transoral transpharyngeal approach to the anterior craniocervical junction. *J Neurosurg.* 1988;69:895–903.
14. Crockard HA, Sen CN. The transoral approach for the management intradural lesions at the craniovertebral junction. *Neurosurgery.* 1991;28:88–98.
15. Sekhar LN, Schramm VL, Jones NF. Subtemporal-preauricular infratemporal fossa approach to large lateral and posterior cranial base neoplasms. *J Neurosurg.* 1987;67:488–499.
16. Sen CN, Sekhar LN. The subtemporal and preauricular infratemporal approach to intradural structures ventral to the brain stem. *J Neurosurg.* 1990; 73:345–354.
17. Al-Mefty O, Fox JL, Smith RR. Petrosal approach for petroclival meningiomas. *Neurosurgery.* 1988; 22:510–517.
18. Sen CN, Sekhar LN. An extreme lateral approach to intradural lesions of the cervical spine and foramen magnum. *Neurosurgery.* 1990;27:197–204.
19. Sen CN, Sekhar LN. Surgical management of anteriorly placed lesions of the craniocervical junction—an alternative approach. *Acta Neurochir.* 1991;122:108.

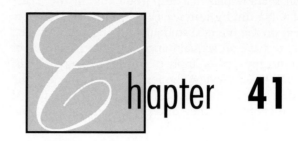

Chapter **41**

Radiation Therapy for
Central Nervous System Tumors

Edward C. Halperin, Mitchell S. Anscher

Radiation therapy plays an important role in the treatment of CNS malignancies (Figs. 41.1, 41.2). It is incumbent on the medical student studying neurosurgery, therefore, to have an acquaintance with the principles of radiation therapy as they apply to neuro-oncology. To this end, we will briefly review the forms of radiotherapy, the clinical decision-making process involved in the use of radiation therapy, and the concepts underlying radiation injury of the CNS.

THE FORMS OF RADIATION THERAPY

The most commonly used form of radiation therapy for CNS tumors is *teletherapy*. Teletherapy refers to the projection through space of x-rays or gamma rays aimed at a target (Figs. 41.3, 41.4). The standard machines for administering teletherapy are the *linear accelerator* and the *cobalt-60 machine*. The linear accelerator consists of an electron gun, an accelerator tube, a bending magnet, and a target. Linear accelerators may be used to generate therapeutic x-rays or electrons. Commercially available linear accelerators will produce x-rays from 4 to 35 million electron volts. Careful radiation therapy field design and custom lead alloy blocking are used to obtain a precise arrangement of beams for the treatment of intracranial or spinal malignancies. The cobalt-60 machine relies on the radioactive decay of cobalt for the production of gamma rays. Employing a system of field-shaping devices and custom designed blocks, the cobalt machine can also be used to obtain shaped fields for precision treatment.

Another form of radiation therapy used in the treatment of CNS malignancies is *brachytherapy*. Brachytherapy refers to continuous low-dose-rate irradiation such as that generated from radioisotopes. These radioisotopes may be implanted directly into a tumor, either temporar-

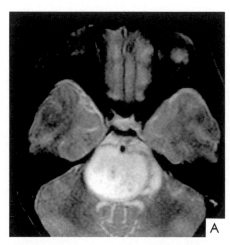 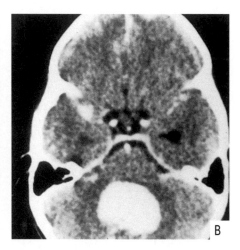

Figure 41.1 Among the more common CNS malignancies of adults are glioblastoma multiforme and anaplastic astrocytoma—the supratentorial high-grade gliomas. Surgery, local field radiotherapy, and chemotherapy clearly affect the survival of patients with these tumors (see Fig. 41.2). The cure rate for anaplastic astrocytoma is about 20% and for glioblastoma multiforme is less than 3%—clearly there is much room for improvement. Similarly, childhood pontine glioma (**A**), in spite of radiotherapy once or twice daily, has a 3-year survival rate of only 10% to 20%. Medulloblastoma (**B**) is a tumor of the posterior fossa in children that is almost never cured by resection alone. Postoperative craniospinal irradiation (CSI) addresses the risk of local tumor recurrence as well as the possibility of neuroaxis tumor dissemination. This form of therapy cures 60% to 80% of patients with this malignancy. CSI is a complex technique that calls for a highly skilled radiotherapy team and modern equipment.

ily or permanently. The most common form of CNS brachytherapy is the interstitial implantation of radioactive iodine-125 or iridium-192 as a component of the treatment of supratentorial malignant gliomas.

A third form of radiation therapy is *radiosurgery*. Radiosurgery may be performed with a specially designed cobalt-60 machine referred to as a "gamma knife," an adapted linear accelerator, or a machine that can produce protons, helium ions, pions, or heavy ions. Radiosurgery refers to the use of an extremely precise and well-delineated beam of radiation that generates lesions within the brain. Such lesions might be used to obliterate small intracranial metastases, arteriovenous malformations, or gliomas.

THE CLINICAL REASONING PROCESS OF THE RADIATION ONCOLOGIST

When faced with a patient with a CNS malignancy, the radiation oncologist's clinical reasoning typically moves through several steps. First the physician ascertains the *intent of treatment.* By this we mean the specific goal of the therapeutic intervention. Goals are most commonly

Figure 41.2 Results of Three Phase III Trials of the Brain Tumor Study Group Evaluating Postoperative Therapy for Malignant Supratentorial Gliomas of Adults

Treatment	Number of Patients	Median Survival Time in Weeks
Trial 6091	222	
Support only		14
BCNU		19
Radiotherapy		36*
Radiotherapy + BCNU		35*
Trial 7201	358	
Methyl-CCNU		24
Radiotherapy		36*
Radiotherapy + methyl-CCNU		42*
Radiotherapy + BCNU		51*
Trial 7501	527	
Radiotherapy + Medrol		40
Radiotherapy + procarbazine		47*
Radiotherapy + BCNU		50*
Radiotherapy + BCNU + Medrol		41

*Significantly better than first arm of respective study.

Adapted from Shapiro WR. Therapy of adult malignant brain tumors: what have clinical trials taught us? *Semin Oncol.* 1986;13:38–45.

divided into *curative* and *palliative* (Fig. 41.5). For patients treated with curative intent, the physician and the patient are willing to accept some degree of risk in return for a reasonable probability of permanent eradication of the malignancy. For example, in the postoperative treatment of medulloblastoma, a brain tumor of childhood, the patient, the patient's family, and the physician might be willing to accept risks of radiation injury to cognition, a diminution of bone growth, or other toxicities of irradiation in return for a 60% to 80% probability of cure.

An alternative intent of treatment is palliative. In palliative radiotherapy the physician is specifically attempting to ameliorate a symptom for a patient who is incurable. In this situation, there is little reason to risk treatment-induced toxicities. For example, a patient with breast carcinoma with metastases involving lung, liver, and brain might merit palliative whole brain irradiation intended to forestall further growth of brain metastases and consequent morbidity. However, the course of radiation would be short to avoid consuming much of the patient's remaining life span, and the dosage should be low to avoid radiation-induced CNS toxicity.

After determining the intent of treatment, the radiotherapist selects the appropriate *dose, volume,* and *technique.* Doses of radiation are typically prescribed in cGy (centiGray). The cGy, a unit of absorbed dose in tissue, became the standard dose unit of radiation in 1980 when it replaced the term *rad* (radiation absorbed dose). There are two factors that help the radiation oncologist select the appropriate dose of radiation. One is the known radiation tolerance of the surrounding normal CNS tissue. The second factor is the data concerning the dose-

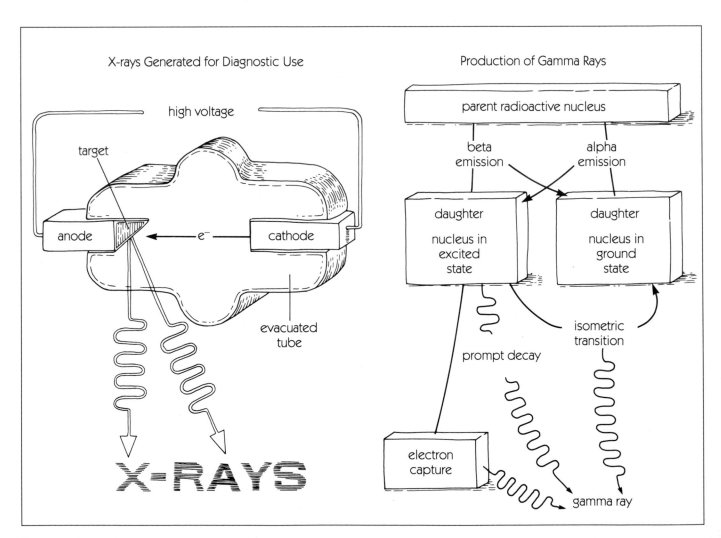

Figure 41.3 *Radiation oncology* is a clinical and scientific endeavor devoted to the diagnosis and treatment of humans with malignant and benign neoplasms. The radiation oncologist is familiar with the principles of cancer management, including pathology, diagnostic imaging, chemotherapy, surgery, and pain management, but is particularly skilled in the use of therapeutic ionizing and nonionizing radiation. Two forms of ionizing radiation are commonly used: *x-rays* are photons produced by the acceleration of electrons in an electric field, *gamma rays* are photons emitted as the result of transition of a nucleus from a higher to a lower energy level. (Adapted from Selman J. *The Basic Physics of Radiation Therapy.* 2nd ed. Springfield, Mass: Charles C Thomas Publishers; 1976:64, and Perez CA, Brady LW, eds. *Principles and Practice of Radiation Oncology.* Philadelphia, Pa: JB Lippincott Co; 1987:137)

response of the histologic type of tumor to radiation. Such dose-response data have been compiled and are extremely helpful in selecting the dose most likely to obtain local tumor control of any given malignancy.

Having selected a dose, the physician next selects an appropriate volume for irradiation. This refers to the amount of tissue that needs to be encompassed in the radiation beam. For example, while it is known that medulloblastoma most commonly arises in the posterior fossa, it is also known that it is a malignancy with a proclivity to seed to the spinal axis. Therefore, the volume of irradiation must encompass the entire craniospinal axis. In contrast, pediatric brain stem gliomas tend to grow and relapse only at the local site of disease. Therefore, the appropriate radiotherapy field need only encompass the tumor, as ascertained by appropriate imaging

studies, with a margin. A sound understanding of the patterns of spread of each tumor type is necessary to establish the appropriate treatment volume.

Finally, having determined the appropriate dose and volume for treatment, the oncologist must choose the necessary technique. A common technique for radiation of lesions in the brain is parallel opposed lateral beams directed at the brain. Other techniques include parallel opposed lateral fields and a vertex field, arc treatment, or single beams. In the treatment of spinal malignancies, one may treat with either a single posterior field, parallel opposed anterior and posterior fields, or various angled fields. To determine the optimum field configuration in any given case most radiation oncologists perform a computer reconstruction of the radiation dose distribution—a process referred to as *computerized dosimetry*.

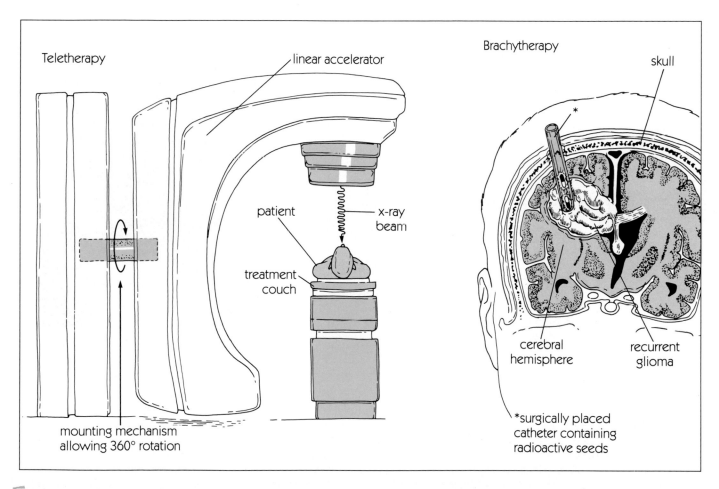

Figure 41.4 Radiation therapy for CNS neoplasms is most commonly administered with *teletherapy*. Teletherapy refers to the projection of photon and/or electron beams through space using, most frequently, a high-energy linear accelerator or a cobalt-60 machine. Teletherapy is administered in multiple daily fractions (i.e., 2 Gy per fraction, 5 fractions per week for 6 weeks = 60 Gy; 1 Gy = 1 J/kg = 100 cGy = 100 rad; Gy is an abbreviation for "Gray"). Another form of radiation therapy is *brachytherapy*. This is continuous low-dose-rate irradiation such as that generated from implanted radioisotopes.

RADIATION INJURY TO THE CENTRAL NERVOUS SYSTEM

The Mechanism of Normal Tissue Injury

The dose of irradiation that can be delivered to the tumor is often limited by the tolerance to radiation of the surrounding normal tissues (Figs. 41.6, 41.7). This is true in the CNS as well as in other regions of the body. The development of a normal tissue injury depends on the interaction of a number of factors, including the ability of irradiated cells to repair damage to their DNA, the total dose of radiation, the daily dose of radiation, the ability of tissues to regenerate after radiation injury, and the effect of intercurrent insults such as chemotherapy, surgery, trauma, or infections. The complex interaction between these various factors is diagrammed in Figure 41.8.

Radiation oncologists have learned that by adjusting the total dose and the dose per fraction one can minimize the risk of normal tissue injury while maximizing the chances of achieving tumor control. In general, the use of daily doses above 2 Gy will require that the total dose be lowered in order to avoid late normal tissue injury.

Clinical Aspects

Radiation injury to the CNS is divided into acute, subacute, and late forms, depending on the interval between irradiation and the onset of injury. Acute radiation injury

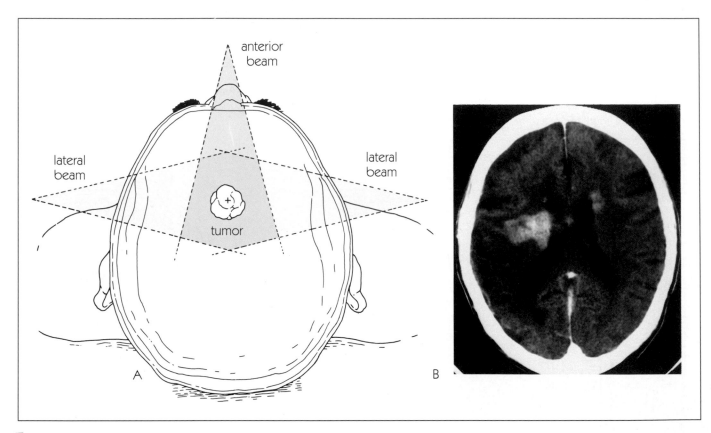

Figure 41.5 Radiation therapy plays a central role in the treatment of many CNS neoplasms. Each case may be classified as either *curative* or *palliative*. In a curative case, the patient and the physician are willing to run a risk of long-term side effects in return for a reasonable chance of cure. For example, the young adult with a pituitary adenoma might be willing to run the risk of visual or neuroendocrine injury following subtotal resection and 45 to 50 Gy with three convergent fields in return for a high chance of arrest of tumor growth (**A**). In a palliative case, on the other hand, one seeks to ameliorate certain symptoms without any significant chance of cure. The risk of side effects should be small insofar as improved quality of life is of great importance. For example, 30 Gy in 2 weeks is unlikely to eradicate brain metastases from breast carcinoma definitively. The noxious effects of cerebral metastases may be reduced for a reasonable period of time by such a dose—without a high risk of radiation injury to the brain. Such treatment would generally be deemed worthwhile (**B**). (A: Reproduced with permission from Halperin EC, Burger PC. Conventional external beam radiotherapy for central nervous systems malignancies. *Neurol Clin.* 1985;3:867–882)

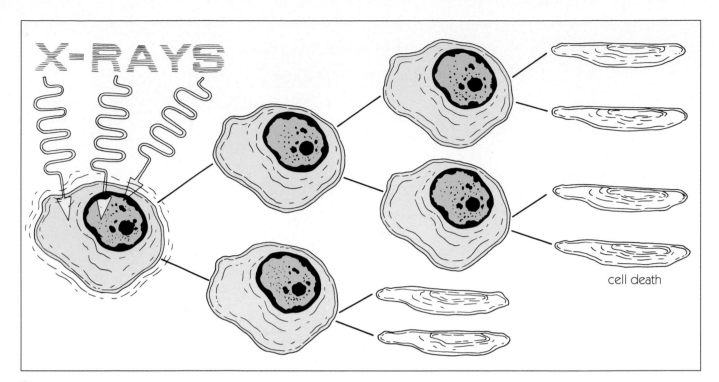

Figure 41.6 The causes and consequences of the lethal effect of ionizing radiation on normal and tumor cells are of great interest to the clinician. The loss of cell viability means a loss of capacity for sustained proliferation of the tumor with its attendant local compression/infiltration, metabolic demands on the host, and risk of tumor dissemination. The target for the cytotoxic effects of radiation is DNA. Cell death is most commonly the result of nonrepaired double-strand breaks in the double helix. Death is manifested by an inability to carry out cell division successfully—a *clonogenic death*. As this cell pedigree shows, a cell may go through one or several divisions before death occurs.

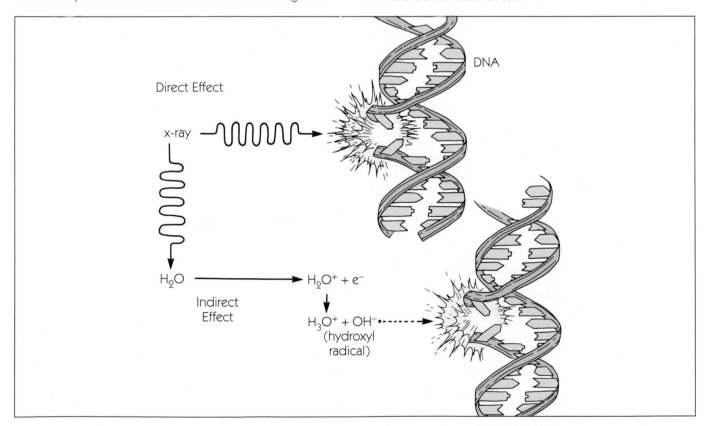

Figure 41.7 Ionizing radiation may damage DNA following ionization of purine or pyrimidine bases via a direct interaction of photons with the DNA—radiation's *direct effect*. The effects of radiation may be secondary to biochemical intermediates such as those produced by the interaction of radiation with water—radiation's *indirect effect*. The most important of the biochemical intermediates generated by radiation are hydroxyl radicals. These highly reactive compounds have an unpaired electron in the outer shell. The chemical changes wrought by free radicals produce the biologic damage leading to clonogenic death. Most radiation biologic damage is caused by the indirect effect.

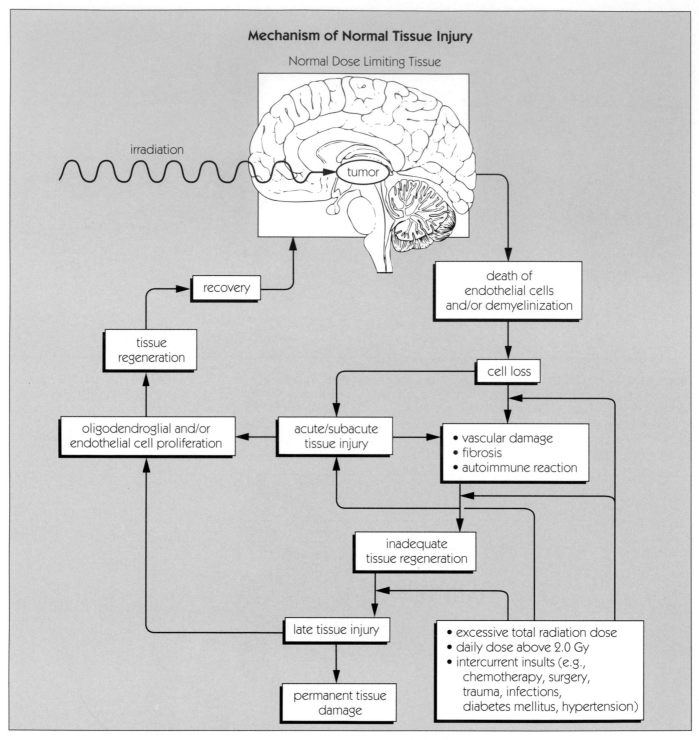

Figure 41.8 The dose of radiation delivered to a tumor is often limited by the surrounding normal tissues' tolerance to irradiation. This normal tissue injury may be divided into acute, subacute, or late forms of injury depending on the interval between irradiation and the onset of injury (see Figs. 41.9–41.11). Acute injury occurs during the course of irradiation or within 4 weeks following its completion. Subacute injury occurs from 1 to 6 months after the completion of radiation therapy. Late injury occurs more than 6 months after radiation treatments have ceased. The patient generally recovers from the acute effects of irradiation, but under certain circumstances, such as in the setting of mechanical trauma, acute injury may progress to late injury. It is also possible for patients to develop late injury without ever developing clinical signs of acute injury. This most often occurs in the setting of intercurrent insults, such as surgery, or following treatments using daily doses above 2 Gy. Late radiation injury may be reversible, but it is more likely to be irreversible than acute injury.

generally begins hours to days after the initiation of radiation treatments. This form of injury generally occurs during a course of radiation treatment and is usually reversible. The development of acute injury does not necessarily predispose a patient to the development of subacute or late radiation injury. The acute forms of radiation injury to the CNS are summarized in Figure 41.9.

Subacute forms of radiation injury generally begin 1 to 6 months after the completion of a course of irradiation. Like acute forms of radiation injury, the subacute forms are generally reversible and do not necessarily progress to late forms of radiation injury. The subacute forms of radiation injury are summarized in Figure 41.10.

The late forms of radiation injury are the most feared complications of CNS irradiation. The clinical manifestations of late radiation injury vary depending on the region of the CNS that has been irradiated. Most forms of late radiation injury are irreversible. The notable

Figure 41.9 Acute Forms of Radiation Injury to the Central Nervous System[7]

Onset After Irradiation	Dose	Clinical Presentation	Clinical Course
Hours–days	≥100 Gy in 1 dose to whole brain	Nausea, vomiting, diarrhea, disorientation, loss of muscle control, respiratory distress, seizures, coma, death	Always fatal; seen, for example, in the setting of nuclear accidents
<24 hours	≤3 Gy in 1 fraction to brain or spinal cord	Headache, nausea, vomiting, worsening of pre-existing neurologic symptoms due to increasing peritumoral edema	Reversible with steroids; preventable by premedication with steroids prior to initiating radiation therapy

Figure 41.10 Subacute Forms of Radiation Injury to the CNS[8–10]

Onset After Irradiation	Dose	Clinical Presentation	Clinical Course
1–3 months	30 Gy to spinal cord	Lhermitte's sign (tingling paresthesias induced by neck flexion)	Reversible over 1–9 months
4–8 weeks	18 Gy to brain	Somnolence syndrome (somnolence, anorexia, fever, apathy, headache, dizziness, nausea, occasional vomiting)	Reversible over 4–14 days
6–13 weeks	*Not known	Rapidly progressive ataxia, focal motor signs, cranial nerve palsies, nystagmus	May be reversible over 6–8 weeks or progress to death

*This syndrome is very rare. It has been reported to occur after 50 Gy in 4 weeks to the brain.

Subacute forms of radiation injury, the result of transient demyelinization,[11] are usually mild and reversible.

exceptions to this rule are the endocrine manifestations of hypothalamic/pituitary irradiation that can be treated medically. The clinical manifestations of late radiation injury to the CNS are summarized in Figure 41.11. Treatment of late radiation injury to the CNS is summarized in Figures 41.11 and 41.12.

An additional form of late radiation injury is the development of second malignancies within the irradiated field. The criteria for establishing that a second malignancy is radiation-induced are as follows: 1) the tumor must arise within the previously irradiated region; 2) the tumor must be of a different histologic type than

Figure 41.11 Late Forms of Radiation Injury to the CNS[12-16]

Onset After Irradiation	Dose	Clinical Presentation	Clinical Course
Brain			
>6 months	≥60 Gy to whole brain ≥70 Gy to ≤25% of brain	Loss of motor function, sensory deficits, cortical blindness, seizures, headache, speech impairment, gait and/or balance disturbances	May be reversible with surgery, corticosteroids
Spinal Cord			
>6 months	>45 Gy to spinal cord	Acute complete paraplegia/quadriplegia developing over several hours	Irreversible
		Lower motor neuron syndrome (muscle atrophy, loss of deep tendon reflexes, fasciculations) developing over weeks–months	Irreversible
		Chronic progressive myelitis (gradual loss of all spinal cord functions)	Irreversible
Retina/Optic Nerve/Optic Chiasm			
1.5–6 years	≥50 Gy to retina	Painless progressive visual loss	Irreversible
2–4 years	≥50 Gy to optic nerve head	Painless progressive visual loss (ischemic optic neuropathy)	Usually irreversible; may respond to hyperbaric oxygen if instituted within 72 hours of visual loss
1–9 years	≥50 Gy to proximal optic nerve	Sudden partial or complete visual loss; may be painful	Irreversible

the original malignancy; and 3) there must be a sufficient time interval (generally at least 4 years) between the completion of irradiation and the development of the second malignancy.

In order to avoid late radiation injury to the CNS, radiation oncologists have developed guidelines regarding the maximum doses that can be safely delivered to normal tissues and organs. These dosing guidelines are adhered to by most radiation oncologists and are exceeded only under exceptional circumstances. Tolerance of the various CNS tissues to irradiation doses is outlined in Figure 41.13.

Figure 41.11 Late Forms of Radiation Injury to the CNS (continued)[12–16]

Onset After Irradiation	Dose	Clinical Presentation	Clinical Course
Intellectual Functioning			
>6 months	Varies with age (younger children are more easily affected)	Memory deficits, decline in IQ	Variable; may progress or stabilize
Hypothalamic/Pituitary Axis			
>6 months	≥24 Gy	Growth hormone deficiency causing decreased growth rate, reduced growth hormone response to stimulation (children)	Treatable with growth hormone
	≥55 Gy	Signs of hypothyroidism, elevated TSH, decreased thyroxine	Treatable with thyroid replacement
	≥55 Gy	Amenorrhea, diminished libido due to hyperprolactinemia	Treatable with bromocriptine
	≥55 Gy	Failure to enter puberty, loss of secondary sexual characteristics, infertility due to gonadotropin deficiency	Treatable with hormone replacement
	≥55 Gy	All of above plus diabetes insipidus and glucocorticoid deficiency due to panhypopituitarism	Treat as above, plus D-amino-D-arginine-vasopressin, corticosteroids

The late syndromes are usually severe, progressive, and irreversible and result from irreversible vascular damage and demyelinization.[17,18]

Figure 41.12 Treatment of Late Radiation Injury[20–22]

Injury	Treatment
Brain necrosis	Surgical resection (treatment of choice)
	Corticosteroids (dexamethasone 12 to 16 mg per day for 4 to 6 weeks, then taper slowly over 4 months)
	Heparin followed by warfarin (if surgery and/or steroids fail)
Brain necrosis or spinal cord injury	Hyperbaric oxygen

The treatment of late radiation injury to the brain is generally more successful than treatment of late radiation injury to the spinal cord. Surgical resection of a brain lesion may result in marked or complete recovery if the lesion is focal and in a favorable location or if symptomatic increased intracranial pressure is present.[20] Surgery is the treatment of choice for resectable lesions. In lesions not amenable to surgery, corticosteroids may be an effective alternative.[21]

Therapy of radiation myelitis is generally ineffective. Hyperbaric oxygen has been reported to be helpful on occasion.[23]

Figure 41.13 Tissue Tolerance Doses of the Nervous System to Radiation Therapy[19]

Organ	Injury	TTD 5/5 (Gy)	TTD 50/5 (Gy)
Brain	Necrosis Infarction	60	70
Spinal cord	Necrosis Infarction	45	55
Peripheral nerves	Demyelinization Fibrosis Vascular damage	60	100
Eye 　Retina	Blindness	55	70
Optic nerve/chiasm	Blindness	50	—
Hypothalamus/pituitary	Hypopituitarism	45	200–300

The concept of minimum and maximum tissue tolerance dose (TTD) was developed in an attempt to provide practical guidelines for normal tissue and organ tolerance to irradiation.[19] The minimum tissue tolerance dose (TTD 5/5) is defined as that dose associated with a 5% rate of complications occurring within 5 years of treatment. The maximum tissue tolerance dose (TTD 50/5) is the dose associated with a 50% complication rate in the same time span.[12] The goal of clinical practice is to achieve cure or palliation while minimizing complications. The TTD 5/5 and TTD 50/5 dose limits are commonly used as guidelines for dose prescriptions. The values given assume a standard set of treatment conditions: 1) megavoltage irradiation, i.e., a cobalt-60 machine or a linear accelerator; 2) a dose delivery schedule of 2.0 Gy/d, 5 days per week with 2-day rest intervals, and 3) completion of treatment in 6 to 8 weeks.

Pathologic Aspects

The gross pathology of radiation injury is characterized in the brain by a shrinking and shriveling of the cortex, indicating a cavitation of the underlying white matter. Telangiectasias and focal hemorrhage may be found. In the spinal cord, radiation necrosis is characterized by a narrowing of the cord. On cross-section the gray columns have a washed-out appearance and the white tracts are reduced in size.

Histopathologically, radiation necrosis is characterized by areas of confluent coagulative necrosis of the white matter and deepest layers of the cortex, atypia or absence of endothelial cells of the vessels, vascular thickening, telangiectasia formation, and vascular proliferation.

Radiation necrosis must often be distinguished from necrosis of tumor or spontaneous necrosis of the brain. If the lesions of radiation necrosis are distant from an intracranial tumor and the appropriate histologic findings are present, the identity of radiation necrosis is readily accepted. Frequently, however, the lesions of radionecrosis occur adjacent to a neoplasm. In this setting delayed radionecrosis may be difficult to distinguish from the entities mentioned above. Representative examples of radiation necrosis are given in Figure 41.14.

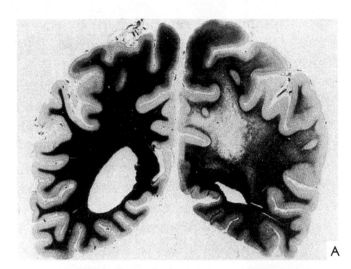

A

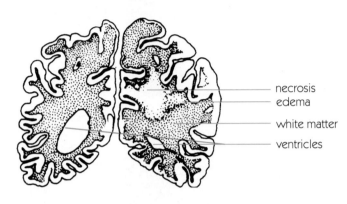

necrosis
edema
white matter
ventricles

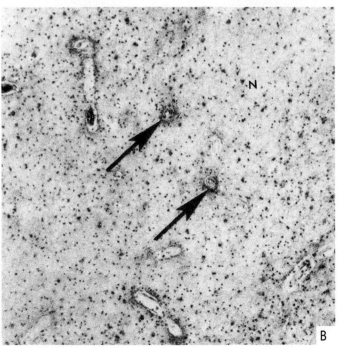

B

Figure 41.14 This patient was a 65-year-old with bronchogenic carcinoma and brain metastases. Radiation therapy consisting of 3600 cGy in 300 cGy fractions, 5 days per week, over 2 1/2 weeks was given. Five months later another 2000 cGy using 200 cGy fractions, 5 days per week, over 2 weeks were given. The patient died 5 months after the second dose. **(A)** At autopsy, a granular necrotic area was noted in the parieto-occipital region posterior to a small metastatic carcinoma (not shown). The granular region is characteristic of radiation necrosis. As is also common, there is edema of the more distant white matter surrounding the focus of radiation necrosis and compressing the ventricle. There is sparing of the subcortical myelinated fibers. **(B)** A section taken from the edge of the lesion in A shows a discrete focus of parenchymal necrosis (N), not associated with neoplasm. Several vessels with fibrinoid necrosis are seen (arrows). (Reproduced with permission from Halperin EC, Burger PC, 1985)

Radiologic Aspects

There are no radiographic changes that are pathogno-monic of radionecrosis of the CNS. If the lesions seen radiographically occur in the same location as the original tumor, it may be impossible to distinguish recurrent tumor from radionecrosis without histologic confirma-tion. Radiographic changes occurring distant from the site of the tumor but within the radiation field may be stronger evidence of radionecrosis. However, histologic confirmation should be obtained whenever possible. Examples of radiographic changes that herald radiation necrosis of the brain are given in Figure 41.15.

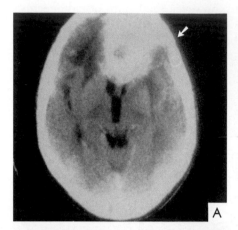

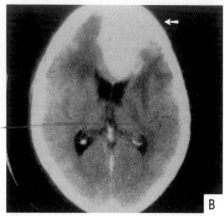

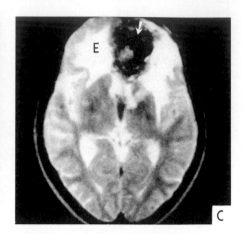

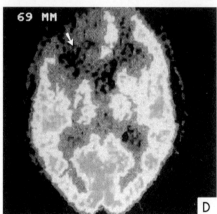

Figure 41.15 Changes due to radionecrosis appear on CT scanning of the brain as either regions of low density without mass effect or contrast enhancement, a localized low density contrast-enhancing mass, or diffuse lesions of varying density without mass effect but with occasional enhancement. **(A,B)** These postcontrast CT scans show marked bifrontal enhancement surrounded by hypodense halo (arrows). Postradiation changes on MRI due to increased water content of the brain, appear as periventricular hyperintensity of varying degrees of severity. Changes on MRI may correspond geographically with those seen on CT, but neither modality can rule out tumor recurrence and histologic confirmation of radionecrosis should be obtained whenever possible.[2] **(C)** This MRI study shows mixed intensity signal (arrow) from the area corresponding to the enhancement area on CT scan **A** and **B** and high-intensity signal from surrounding edema *(E)*. PET may be able to distinguish tumor recurrence from necrosis in selected situations. Radiation necrosis usually appears as an area of relatively less metabolic activity compared to the surrounding tissues. This feature may be useful in distinguishing radionecrosis from high-grade gliomas or metastases that appear hypermetabolic.[3] However, low-grade gliomas usually appear hypometabolic, so PET may not be useful in distinguishing radionecrosis from recurrent low-grade glioma.[4] **(D)** This PET scan shows marked hypometabolism (arrow) in both prefrontal areas, larger on the left. Radiation myelopathy may appear on CT as a widening of the spinal cord that returns to normal size after several months.[6] (D: Reproduced with permission from DiChiro G, Oldfield E, Wright DC, et al., 1988)

Principles of Neurosurgery

REFERENCES

1. Halperin EC, Burger PC. Conventional external beam radiotherapy for central nervous system malignancies. *Neurol Clin North Am.* 1985;3: 867–882.

2. Dooms GC, Hecht S, Brant-Zawadzki M, et al. Brain radiation lesions: MR imaging. *Radiology.* 1986;158:149–155.

3. Doyle WK, Budinger TF, Valk PE, et al. Differentiation of cerebral radiation necrosis from tumor necrosis by (^{18}F)FDG and ^{82}Rb positron emission tomography. *J Comput Assist Tomogr.* 1987;11: 563–570.

4. DiChiro G, DeLaPaz RL, Brooks RA, et al. Glucose utilization of cerebral gliomas measured by (^{18}F) fluorodeoxyglucose and positron emission tomography. *Neurology.* 1982;32:1323–1329.

5. DiChiro G, Oldfield E, Wright DC, et al. Cerebral necrosis after radiotherapy and/or intraarterial chemotherapy for brain tumors: PET and neuropathologic studies. *AJR.* 1988;150:189–197.

6. Tugendhaft P, Baleriaux D, Gerard JM, et al. Sequential CT scanning in radiation myelopathy. *J Neurooncol.* 1984;2:249–252.

7. Hall E. *Radiobiology for the Radiologist.* 3rd ed. Philadelphia, Pa: JB Lippincott; 1988;367–368.

8. Jones A. Transient radiation myelopathy: with reference to Lhermitte's sign of electrical paresthesias. *Br J Radiol.* 1964;37:727–744.

9. Littman P, Rosenstock J, Gale G, et al. The somnolence syndrome in leukemic children following reduced daily dose fractions of cranial radiation. *Int J Radiat Oncol Biol Phys.* 1984;10:1851–1853.

10. Lampert PW, Davis RL. Delayed effects of radiation on the human central nervous system. *Neurology.* 1964;14:912–917.

11. Boldry E, Sheline G. Delayed transitory clinical manifestations after radiation treatment of intracranial tumors. *Acta Radiol (Ther).* 1966;5:5–10.

12. Rubin P, Cooper RA Jr, Phillips TL. The dose limiting organs in radiation oncology. In: Cooper RA Jr, Phillips TL, eds. *Radiation Biology and Radiation Pathology Syllabus.* Chicago, Ill: American College of Radiology; 1975.

13. Reagan TL, Thomas GE, Colby MY. Chronic progressive radiation myelopathy: its clinical aspects and differential diagnosis. *JAMA.* 1968;203:128–132.

14. Lambert PM. Radiation myelopathy of the thoracic spinal cord in long-term survivors treated with radical radiotherapy using conventional fractionation. *Cancer.* 1978;41:1751–1760.

15. Parsons JT, Fitzgerald CR, Hood CI, et al. The effects of irradiation on the eye and optic nerve. *Int J Radiat Oncol Biol Phys.* 1983;9:609–622.

16. Guy J, Schatz NJ. Hyperbaric oxygen in the treatment of radiation induced optic neuropathy. *Ophthalmology.* 1986;93:1083–1088.

17. Zeman W, Samorajaski. Effects of irradiation on the central nervous system. In: Berdjis CC, ed. *Pathology of Irradiation.* Baltimore, Md: Williams & Wilkins; 1971:213–277.

18. Lyman RS, Kupalov PS, Scholz W. Effects of roentgen rays on the central nervous system: results of large doses on the brains of adult dogs. *Arch Neurol Psychiatry.* 1933;29:56–87.

19. Rubin P, Casarett G. A direction for clinical radiation pathology: a tolerance dose. *Front Radiat Ther Oncol.* 1972;6:1–15.

20. Leibel SA, Sheline GE. Tolerance of the central and peripheral nervous system to therapeutic irradiation. In: Lett JT, Altman KI, eds. *Advances in Radiation Biology: Relative Radiation Sensitivities of the Human Organ Systems.* Orlando, Fla: Academic Press; 1987;12:257–288.

21. Lee AW, Ng SH, Ho JHC, et al. Clinical diagnosis of late temporal lobe necrosis following radiation therapy for nasopharyngeal carcinoma. *Cancer.* 1988;61:1535–1542.

22. Rizzoli HV, Pagnanelli DM. Treatment of delayed radiation necrosis of the brain: a clinical observation. *J Neurosurg.* 1984;60:589–594.

23. Hart GB, Mainous EG. The treatment of radiation necrosis with hyperbaric oxygen (OHP). *Cancer.* 1976;37:2580–2585.

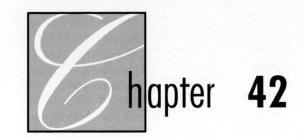

Stereotactic Radiosurgery and Focused Beam Irradiation

Robert J. Coffey

In 1951 Lars Leksell, a visionary Swedish neurosurgeon, introduced "stereotactic radiosurgery...a technique for noninvasive destruction of intracranial tissues or lesions that may be inaccessible or unsuitable for open surgery."[1] Leksell's technique involved the delivery of a large, single-fraction "dose of ionizing radiation to a...stereotactically localized intracranial volume...."[2,3] Open stereotactic operations using a variety of devices had been performed experimentally on human patients and animals during the late 19th and early 20th centuries; multifractionated, multiport external beam orthovoltage irradiation techniques had been applied to intracranial targets in patients before Leksell developed his first stereotactic instrument in 1949.[4,5] However, Leksell was the first to employ an image-guided stereotactic instrument that had the target coordinates set at the center of a semicircular arc to crossfire multiple narrow radiation beams through the intact skull. Early on, he explored the use of 280 kV x-rays to treat obsessive-compulsive states and trigeminal neuralgia.[1,6] By fixing the x-ray tube to an instrument carrier on the arc, and by altering the arc angle or position of the tube along the arc, many stationary entry portals could be used.

Leksell also explored the technical and clinical utility of linear accelerators (linac) and entry plateau (non-Bragg-peak) proton beams for radiosurgery (Fig. 42.1).[2,3,7,8] While other investigators subsequently refined stereotactic linac and particle-beam irradiation techniques, Leksell, his colleagues, and his successors developed several generations of the cobalt-60 gamma unit (currently called the "gamma knife") (Fig. 42.2).

Until the 1980s, only a few centers in the world performed radiosurgical operations. The recent increased interest in stereotaxis in general and radiosurgery in particular is in large measure due to the revolution in neuroimaging brought about by the introduction of CT and MRI. Additionally, the growing power and shrinking size (and price) of modern computers has made the integration of imaging and physics dosimetry data—a necessary component of radiosurgery—accessible and affordable for a large number of medical centers. Currently, the total number of each type of radiosurgical instrument in operation worldwide is inversely related to cost. Thus, more linac-based instruments than gamma units are being used, and only a handful of cyclotron-based particle beam radiosurgical centers are available.

RADIOSURGERY VERSUS RADIOTHERAPY

The goal of radiosurgery is to obliterate a relatively small intracranial target with a high, single-fraction irradiation dose while sparing adjacent and distant tissues. In contrast to conventional fractionated radiation therapy, radiosurgery does not rely on the supposed differential radiation sensitivity of the target compared to the normal brain. Rather, radiosurgical treatment relies on the relatively steep fall-off of the dose delivered outside the target, thereby preventing complications.[4] Stereotactic imaging and target localization using CT, MRI, and/or angiography must be fully integrated with the radiation

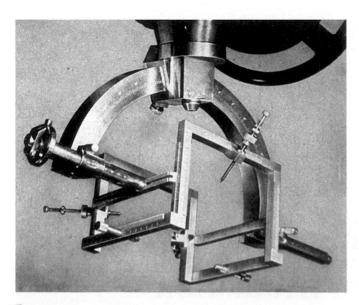

Figure 42.1 Leksell's stereotactic device, circa 1953, adapted to radiosurgery using a 300 kV x-ray tube, and later adapted to proton beam radiosurgery at the Gustaf Werner Institute, Uppsala, Sweden. The heavy-duty arc and instrument carrier supported the final beam collimator during irradiation of the target through 21 beam-entry portals.

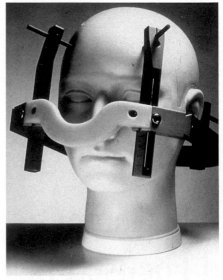

Figure 42.2 The current Leksell (Model-G) stereotactic instrument, compatible with computed tomographic, magnetic resonance, and angiographic localization for radiosurgery and/or open stereotaxis.

Principles of Neurosurgery

delivery device for maximal effect. The irradiation isocenter must accurately and repeatedly coincide with the desired target. Different radiosurgical systems satisfy these essential criteria by using various technical solutions. Similarly, a variety of computer-based approaches to radiosurgical dose planning provide a three-dimensional representation of isodose contours superimposed on the stereotactic images of the target and surrounding intracranial structures.

RADIOSURGICAL INSTRUMENTATION AND TECHNIQUES

THE ⁶⁰Co GAMMA UNIT

Leksell and Larsson designed the first 179-source ⁶⁰Co gamma unit as a "practical, precise and simple tool which could be handled by the surgeon himself."[2] Gamma Unit I was installed at the Sophiahemmet Hospital in Stockholm in 1968. Its disk-shaped irradiation fields were best suited to create lesions in fiber tracts or thalamic nuclei to treat functional disorders or involuntary movements. As the number of functional neurosurgical operations waned, and as promising results were obtained in the treatment of a few small arteriovenous malformations and tumors, a second gamma unit was constructed to produce nearly spherical irradiation fields. Gamma Unit II was used at the Karolinska Hospital in Stockholm between 1974 and 1988. Later generations of the Leksell Gamma Unit were installed during the 1980s in Argentina, England, the United States, Norway, Sweden, and Japan. While some of the European and Asian units differ from each other in source number and array, all of the instruments in the United States are identical (Fig. 42.3).[11] The 18 metric ton central body contains the 201 ⁶⁰Co sources, each having an average initial activity of 30 curies; the total initial activity loaded into a gamma unit is approximately 6000 curies. The Nuclear Regulatory Commission closely monitors the on-site loading and ongoing quality assurance testing of all gamma units. The nearly hemispheral array of sources forms an anteroposterior arc of 96° and a transverse arc of 160° in relation to the patient's head (±48° and ±80°, respectively, in relation to the central beam). The size and shape of the irradiated volume is controlled by the use of four inner collimator helmets, each having 201 beam channels of either 4, 8,

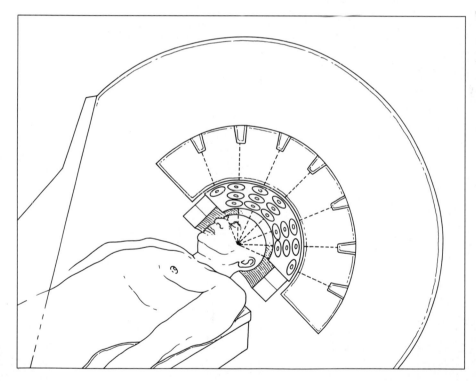

Figure 42.3 Cross-sectional diagram of the 201-source gamma knife (United States model) with the patient in position during irradiation. The cobalt-60 sources are focused at a central point. CT, MR, or angiographic guidance is used to place the desired target at the focal point. (Adapted from Coffey RJ, Lunsford LD, 1990)

14, or 18 mm in diameter. One or more collimator helmets is used alone or in combination for each radiosurgical procedure. The isodose distributions in the axial, coronal, and sagittal planes for each collimator are illustrated in Figure 42.4. The dosimetry for multiple iso-center irradiations and selected beam-channel plugging patterns has also been verified (Fig. 42.5).

The selection of the radiation target(s) in each case, as well as the calculation of target coordinates, is based upon stereotactic cerebral angiography, CT, and/or MR

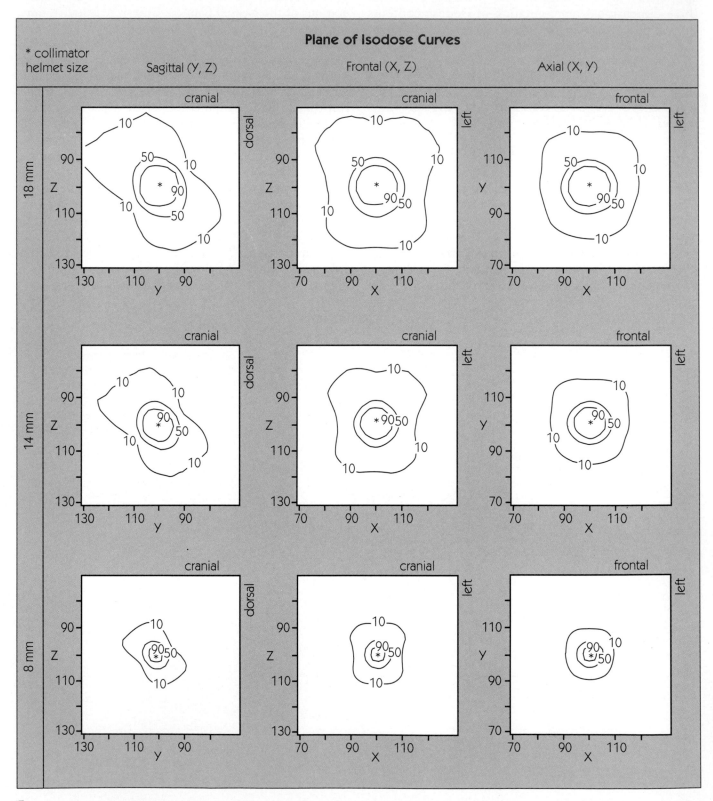

Figure 42.4 Isodose distributions for the 201 cobalt-60 source gamma knife in the sagittal, frontal, and axial planes using the 18, 14, and 8 mm collimator helmets. The 90%, 50%, and 10% isodose lines are shown (4 mm collimator not illustrated). The 50% isodose shell of the 18 mm collimator covers a volume 22 x 21 x 25 mm in diameter in the X, Y, Z planes, respectively (approximately 6100 mm³).

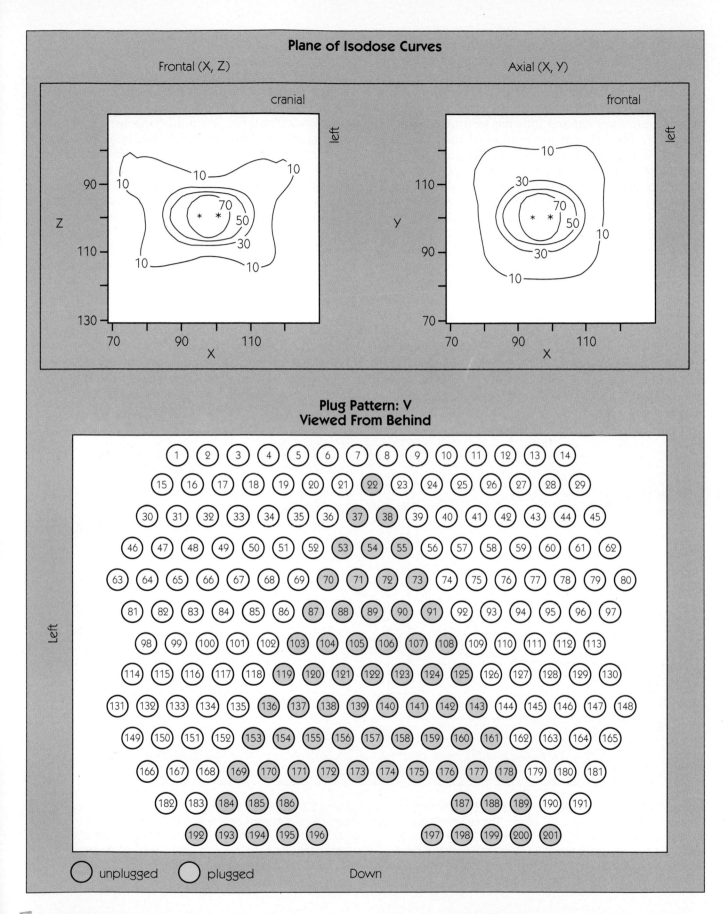

Figure 42.5 Gamma knife multiple-isocenter isodose distributions showing two shots with the 14 mm collimator, separated by 7 mm in the X-axis. The 70%, 50%, 30%, and 10% isodose lines are illustrated in the frontal and axial planes. Selective beam-channel plugging in a "V" pattern has been employed to flatten the dose distribution in the vertical (Z) axis. This type of dose plan is especially useful to treat pituitary adenomas or other anterior skull-base lesions as the dose to the optic chiasm, lying superiorly in the frontal plane, is minimized. Diameters of the 50% isodose shell are 22 x 16 x 14 mm, respectively, along the X, Y, and Z axes.

images. Other data necessary for computer dose planning are measurements of the patient's head shape and the angle of the stereotactic frame to the central beam with the patient fixed in the collimator helmet. The coordinates, collimator size, and relative weighting of each isocenter are entered into the treatment-planning computer. The current generation of institutionally developed and commercially available dose-planning systems provides an interactive video display of multiplanar isodose contours superimposed on the stereotactic images, plus a three-dimensional analysis of isodose volumes in relation to adjacent intracranial structures. During the planning process, isocenters can be moved or modified both graphically (on screen) and manually (by entering new coordinate or collimator data).

Since the gamma unit employs fixed sources with a constant relation to the collimator helmet and stereotactic frame, "isocenter verification films" or "port films" are unnecessary. The radiosurgical team, consisting of the surgeon, radiation oncologist, and radiation physicist, determine the dose to be delivered to the target. Almost all targets are enclosed within the 50% or higher isodose shell.

The use of accelerated charged particle beams to ablate intracranial targets in humans began in the early 1950s. The first target was the normal pituitary gland in cases of advanced, metastatic, hormone-responsive carcinomas and diabetic retinopathy.[4,12] Later, large numbers of pituitary adenomas and vascular malformations were treated.[12–16] In several thousand patients, especially those treated before the CT and MRI era, target selection was based on plain skull film anatomy compared to preoperative angiograms or air studies rather than on any fixed stereotactic coordinate system.[18,19] Thus, only since the 1980s have publications describing the techniques and results of charged-particle-beam intracranial irradiation employed the terms *stereotactic*, *stereotaxic*, or *radiosurgery*.

The overwhelming number of patients treated with charged-particle beams have been irradiated with either protons (hydrogen nuclei) or helium ions. Attractive features of particle beams for radiosurgery include minimal beam scatter and phenomena related to the Bragg-peak effect—increased dose at the depth rather than at the

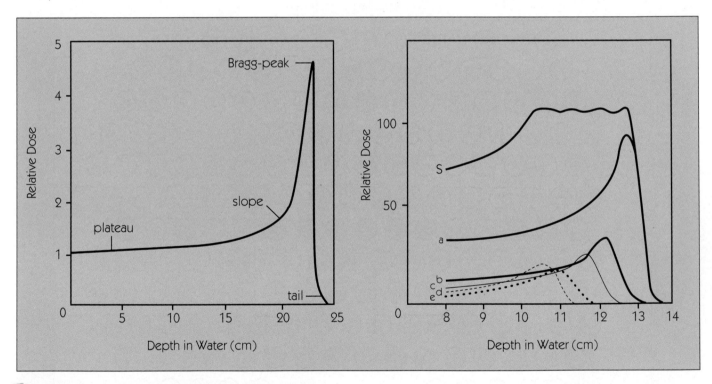

Figure 42.6 (A) Depth-dose curve for a 187 MeV proton beam showing the Bragg peak effect. The relatively low entry dose (plateau) rapidly increases at depth (rising slope) to reach a maximum dose (Bragg peak) after which the dose rapidly drops off to zero (Tail). (B) The effect of adding several modulated particle beams (S=sum of B, C, D, and E) to cover a 2.8 cm target volume versus a single unmodulated beam (A) that covers only a few millimeters. While the entry plateau dose of beam A represents less than half of the maximum dose, the entry dose in case S represents over 70% of the maximum dose. (Adapted from Hall EJ, 1988)

surface of tissue, and finite range in tissue (Fig. 42.6A). Since the size of the unmodulated Bragg peak of proton or helium ion beams is only a few millimeters—much smaller than the usual intracranial lesion being treated—the peaks of various entering beams must be "spread out" to encompass the lesion volume (Fig. 42.6B).[17] Telescoping or variable length water absorbers, fixed absorbers, and variable thickness rotating modulators within the beam path have been used in various combinations to match the dose distribution to the size and shape of the lesion being treated.[15,19] Some centers have refined the beam shape further by using custom-formed collimator apertures that correspond to the geometry of the target lesion in a particular imaging projection. Additional calculations are necessary to determine the depth or range of the Bragg peak in tissues of variable density and thickness (scalp, bone, brain) to insure appropriate beam modulation. Currently, this is accomplished most accurately by computerized analysis of beam paths through bone and soft tissue based on x-ray absorption data from CT scans.

Due to the complexity of particle beam treatment planning and the fact that treatment is usually performed in a physics laboratory, remote from hospital facilities, imaging is performed one or more days before treatment. Investigators at the Lawrence Berkeley Laboratory have performed stereotactic imaging studies with a modified Leksell frame mated to a vacuum-formed polystyrene mask molded to each patient's face and head (Fig. 42.7). During treatment, reapplication of the mask accurately reproduces the patient's head position in stereotactic space in relation to the helium

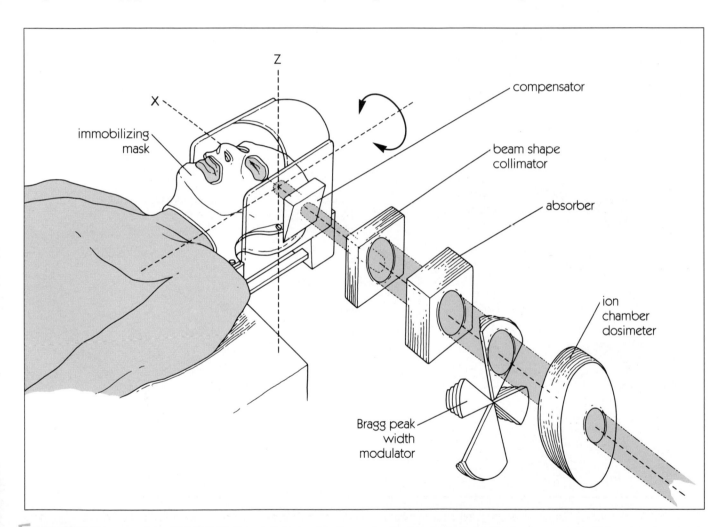

Figure 42.7 Diagram of the 230 MeV helium-ion-beam irradiation system at the Lawrence Berkeley Laboratory, University of California. The custom-formed mask for each patient reproduces stereotactic localization coordinates for the target from pretreatment imaging studies. The final beam shape, range in tissue, and width of the Bragg ionization peak are determined by the beam shape collimator, range modifying absorber, and Bragg peak width modulator, respectively. A tissue-equivalent compensator mounted close to the patient's head adjusts for skull curvature. (Adapted from Levy RP, Fabrikart JF, Frankel KA, et al., 1989)

ion beam.[12,15] Other particle-beam irradiation facilities have not employed stereotactic imaging techniques. Despite head fixation with a coordinate frame during treatment, the coordinates for irradiation targets were derived from intraoperative comparision of x-ray port films with nonstereotactic diagnostic imaging studies (Fig. 42.8).

At Berkeley, patients are treated during one or two sessions using three or more irradiation portals per session. Five to 10 portals are routine when treating vascular malformations, while up to 12 portals have been used for pituitary disorders. The lesion is often enclosed within the 90% isodose shell. Given the high linear energy transfer of helium ions compared to photon or gamma ray beams, a relative biological effectiveness "quality factor" of 1.3 has been calculated to compare dosimetry using the 230 MeV/amu helium ion beam with x-rays or gamma rays.

The theoretical biophysical advantages of particle beam irradiation have led some investigators to treat larger lesions at higher doses than employed by others using gamma unit or linac-based radiosurgery.[16,20] However, the possibility of delayed complications due to finite dose-volume tolerances of brain tissue may limit the safe treatment of large intracranial lesions with high (single-fraction) radiosurgical doses, regardless of the modality employed.

LINEAR ACCELERATOR RADIOSURGERY

Linear accelerators are room-sized devices that accelerate a stream of electrons at nearly the speed of light to hit a metal target, producing a beam of photons (x-rays) with energies in the megavoltage (MeV) range. Linac-produced photon beams of 4 to 18 MeV have energies roughly equivalent to the gamma radiation emitted by ^{60}Co sources in the gamma units.[4,21,22]

All linacs can rotate along a fixed axis parallel to the floor and perpendicular to the beam axis. Irradiation can be performed through a series of stationary portals or, more commonly for radiosurgery, via a series of noncoplanar intersecting arcs. Depending on the system used for head support and patient orientation, the irradiation arcs can be arrayed at various angles to the right and left of the sagittal skull axis or, alternatively, at various angles anterior or posterior to the coronal skull axis. Each arc is produced by a partial (less than 360°) rotation of the linac gantry. The series of arcs is generated

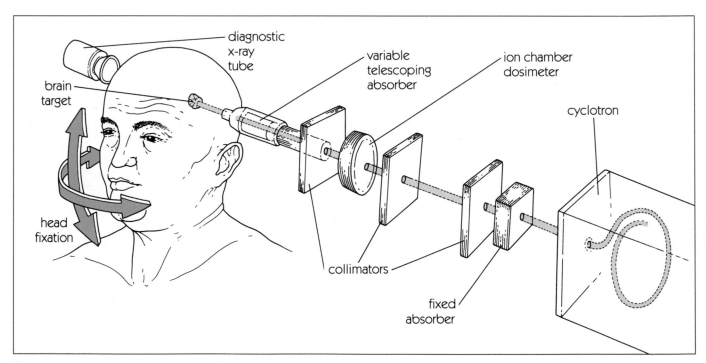

Figure 42.8 Schematic diagram of Bragg peak proton beam therapy at the 160 MeV Harvard Cyclotron (circa 1961–present). The telescoping water-filled absorber corrected for unevenness in the skull surface and depth to target in order to place the Bragg peak at the desired target. An on-axis (beam's-eye-view) x-ray tube was employed to align the head fixation instrument with the desired target according to comparisons with pretreatment diagnostic imaging studies. (Adapted from Kjellberg RN, Koehler AM, Preston WM, et al., 1962)

by orienting the patient at a slightly different angle to the axis of gantry rotation by using different stations of the treatment chair or couch. A stereotactic frame fixes the imaging-defined radiosurgical target at the common isocenter of all the arc rotations. One linac system employs simultaneous movement of both the gantry and the patient, producing a unique beam-entry geometry. In essence, many of the geometric features of linac radiosurgery are based upon refinements of Leksell's original arc-radius principle.

Although linear accelerators have been used by radiation therapists since the 1950s, the development of linac-based radiosurgical systems began in the 1980s.[22] Betti and colleagues adapted the Talairach stereotactic frame to a treatment chair mounted on curved rails (Fig. 42.9).[23,24] A 10 MeV linac was rotated through a series of seven to 17 isocentric, paracoronal arcs determined by various stationary chair positions (Fig. 42.9, inset). Submillimeter isocentric accuracy was claimed, and collimators 5 to 20 mm in diameter were employed.

Colombo adapted his own arc-radius stereotactic frame for radiosurgery using a 4 MeV linac.[25,26] He did not add any final beam collimation but used the variable internal collimators of the linac beam head to pro-

duce 5 to 35 mm square or rectangular fields. With the patient supine on the treatment couch, a series of stationary positions allowed the delivery of 9 to 17 irradiation arcs along either side of the sagittal skull axis. Subsequently, this "football seam" arc arrangement has become the most popular beam geometry for linac radiosurgical systems. Later, Colombo modified his technique to treat complex or nonspherical targets.[27] The treatment couch rotates at a constant velocity, with the linac gantry set at predetermined angles above and below a horizontal axis through the target. A series of such paired irradiation sequences produces conical irradiation fields with their vertices at the target. This modified technique yields semicircular beam entry paths anterior and posterior to the coronal skull plane.

Hartmann, Sturm, and colleagues developed a 15 MeV linac radiosurgical system based upon a modified Reichert-Mundinger stereotactic apparatus.[28] Sophisticated dose-planning software, 6 to 54 mm collimators, and an 11-arc (sagittal axis) technique were used. Later modifications of the system at other centers included an improved head frame support system, and an in-vivo port-film method to check final isocenter accuracy.

Winston and Lutz pioneered the use of linac radio-

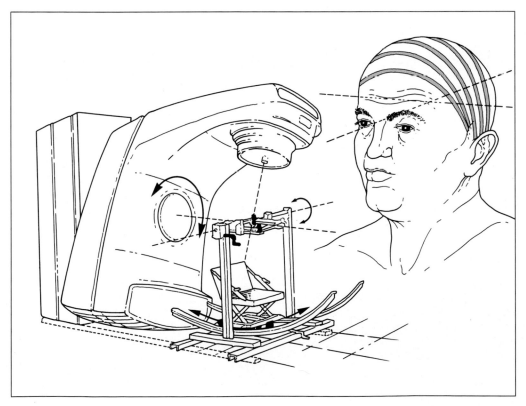

Figure 42.9 Schematic diagram of the stereotactic linear accelerator system introduced by Betti and colleagues. Talairach's stereotactic frame is mounted to upright supports attached to the center of tandem, floor-mounted arcs. The patient treatment chair moves to various stations along the arcs. Since the linear accelerator rotates perpendicular to the anteroposterior axis of the head, a series of coronal arcs, intersecting at the target, is produced (inset). (Adapted from Betti OO, Derechinsky VE, 1984)

surgery in the United States.[29] Their original system, currently employed with various modifications in several centers, included a Brown-Roberts-Wells stereotactic head frame, floor-stand, and a 6 MeV linac (Fig. 42.10). Four or more sagittally-oriented irradiation arcs were delivered using 12.5 to 30 mm circular collimators. They also introduced a phantom-target film technique to detect any mechanical inaccuracy in system alignment for every treatment arc.

Friedman and Bova further refined linac-based radiosurgical techniques by adding a high precision attachment to control movements of the patient's head and the tertiary collimators (5 to 35 mm diameter) independently of potential variations in gantry or treatment couch alignment.[21,30] They also used a 6 MeV linac and the same stereotactic system as the Boston group. A number of centers in the United States and Europe have purchased the commercial version of this system.

Podgorsak, Olivier and colleagues developed a novel "dynamic" radiosurgery system in which the 10 MeV linac gantry and patient couch move simultaneously.[31] Thus, instead of several intersecting arcs, the beam entry geometry resembles a continuous seam (Fig. 42.11). The actual irradiation treatment time may be shorter with this method than with multiple arc techniques.

STEREOTACTIC RADIATION THERAPY

In contrast to high, single-fraction irradiation doses delivered to the target volume during radiosurgery, some investigators have applied stereotactic techniques to increase the precision and safety of multifraction radiation therapy. While a number of particle-beam and linac-radiosurgery centers have administered irradiation through multiple portals over 2 days, stereotactic radiation therapy is administered over a period of weeks. Image-guided target localization and image-integrated dose planning are as essential in stereotactic radiation therapy as in radiosurgery. An added technical consideration is precise, repeatable head fixation during as many as 30 or more dose fractions.

In 1985 and 1986 Van Buren, Landy, Houdek, and colleagues reported that a plastic halo ring applied to the skull could provide repeatable fixation for stereotactic imaging and fractionated radiation therapy using a 10 MeV linac.[32,33] They found the technique especially applicable to large, moderately radiosensitive neoplasms in the parasellar region (pituitary adenoma, craniopharyngioma, hypothalamic glioma). Daily dose fractions of 2 to 3 Gy were administered to the tumor margins for total doses of 36 to 62.5 Gy. In the first 11 patients, tumors were controlled for up to 3 years. Two

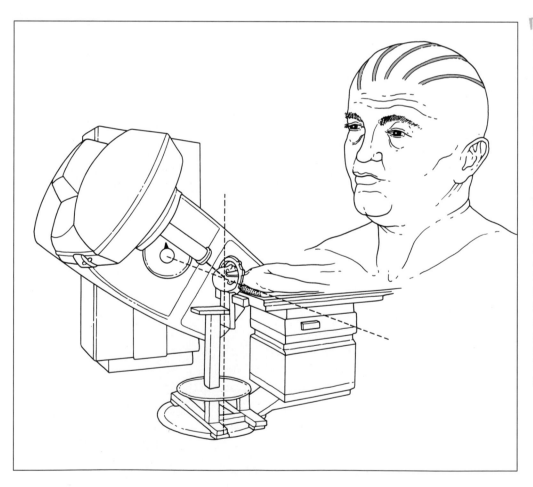

Figure 42.10 The "Boston" radiosurgical system designed by Winston and Lutz. The principle is similar to most linear accelerator-based systems. Rotation of the patient (fixed horizontally within a stereotactic frame and floor or table-mounted support system) to various couch angles, causes the photon beam to enter the skull through multiple, noncoplanar, sagittally oriented arcs (inset). The final beam collimator, having inserts of various sizes, is brought relatively close to the patient's head to minimize the radiation penumbra and to optimize beam alignment. (Adapted from Winston KR, Lutz W, 1988 and Columbo F, Benedetti A, Pozza F, et al., 1985)

patients experienced visual complications. Vision was recovered after tumor removal (pituitary adenoma) in one patient; visual loss persisted in another patient, who had a hypothalamic glioma.

Austin-Seymour and a multidisciplinary group of collaborators have reported the results of fractionated proton-beam irradiation for low-grade malignant skull base tumors.[18] They performed three-dimensional dose planning based on CT and MR imaging. A thermoplastic mesh face mask similar to the one illustrated in Figure 42.7 immobilized the patient during treatment in the supine or seated position, depending on the entry portal for each fraction. Beam's-eye-view port films assured target accuracy within 2 mm. Daily dose fractions of 1.8 to 2.1 cobalt Gy equivalent units were administered (CGE based on a relative biological effectiveness for protons of 1.1 compared to cobalt-60) to a median tumor dose of 69 CGE (range = 56.9 to 75.6 CGE). Actuarial 5 year and predicted 10 year local control rates for chordomas and chondrosarcomas were 82% and 58%, respectively. Treatment-related complications included visual loss in three patients (two unilateral, one bilateral), hypopituitarism in nine patients (treatable with hormone replacement), and seizures in one of the patients, who also experienced unilateral

visual loss. For recurrent or residual skull base tumors that are too large for single-fraction radiosurgery, even after surgical debulking, fractionated stereotactic radiation therapy may be the therapy of choice.

CLINICAL RESULTS OF RADIOSURGERY

INDICATIONS

Current interest in radiosurgery is primarily concerned with the treatment of vascular malformations and tumors. Patient selection criteria usually include some or all of the following: deeply seated, high risk, or inoperable lesion; failure of previous surgical, irradiation, or other treatments to eliminate the lesion; advanced patient age or poor medical condition precluding anesthesia and open surgery; or refusal of open surgery by a patient with a lesion otherwise appropriate for radiosurgical treatment. Among the various radiosurgical centers, patient selection, and hence clinical reports, have reflected the interests and referral patterns of the investigators involved. Also, especially at centers employing new or recently designed systems, a larger proportion of patients with intraparenchymal lesions

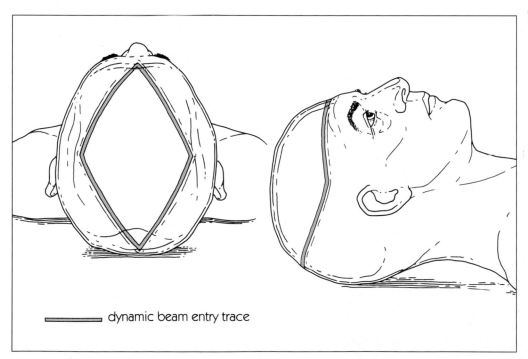

dynamic beam entry trace

Figure 42.11 Diagram of the dynamic radiosurgery beam-entry trace from the system developed by Podgorsak and colleagues. In this unique system the linear accelerator gantry and patient treatment couch rotate simultaneously, producing the illustrated pattern centered at the stereotactically defined target. The entry and exit beams never coincide. (Modified from Podgorsak EB, Olivier A, Pla M, et al., 1987)

(metastases, primary brain tumors, vascular malformations) have been reported compared to histologically benign extraaxial neoplasms.[21,25,26,28] The available reports of specific indications for radiosurgical treatment with various irradiation modalities are summarized in Figure 42.12.

The gamma unit has been employed to treat a broad spectrum of radiosurgical indications in over 6000 patients with results reported over the past 2 decades. In addition to vascular malformations, pituitary disorders, and malignant brain tumors, several series of acoustic neuromas, meningiomas, and functional procedures for

---

Figure 42.12 Summary of Reported Radiosurgical Treatment Indications

Gamma Unit	Particle Beam	Linear Accelerator
Vascular malformations*	Vascular malformations*	Vascular malformations*

Pituitary adenoma
  Pituitary ablation
	Pituitary adenoma
	  Pituitary ablation	

Craniopharyngioma	Benign tumors[†]	Craniopharyngioma[†]
Acoustic neuroma	Malignant tumors[†]	Acoustic neuroma[†]
Meningioma		Meningioma[†]
Metastases		Metastases
Primary brain neoplasms		Primary brain neoplasms
Functional neurosurgery	Functional neurosurgery[†]	Functional neurosurgery[†]

*Arteriovenous malformations and angiographically occult vascular malformations.
[†]Few, isolated reports or detailed data and results not available.

Figure 42.13 Summary of Results: Radiosurgical Treatment of Arteriovenous Malformations

	Gamma Unit	Particle Beam	Linear Accelerator
Total obliteration (%)			
1 year	40	NA	38–52
2 years	80–86	up to 80*	67–75
Rehemorrhage (nonfatal/fatal) (%)	2–4/0.9	10/4	3–4/3
Radiation-induced complications (%) (temporary/permanent)	3–4.4/2.2–3	2–12/10	3–12.5[†]
Death (%)	0	2–3	0

NA = Data not available
*Lawrence Berkeley Laboratory series; arteriovenous malformation obliteration rate after proton beam therapy not available.
[†]Permanent versus temporary complications not always specified.

pain and psychiatric illness have also been reported.[3,6,11,34–51] Over a somewhat longer time span, nearly 12,000 patients have been treated at particle beam facilities in the United States and Soviet Union using stereotactic or semistereotactic techniques.[12] However, in virtually all of these patients, the indication for treatment was either a vascular malformation, pituitary tumor, or the need to suppress a normally functioning pituitary gland.[21,23–26,28,52–54] Most reports describing the results of linac-based radiosurgery have involved vascular malformations and malignant intraaxial tumors. The results of radiosurgical treatment for a variety of intracranial lesions are summarized in Figures 42.13 to 42.16.

Figure 42.14 Summary of Results: Radiosurgical Treatment of Angiographically Occult Vascular Malformations

	Gamma Unit	Particle Beam
Clinical status (%)		
Stable or improved	79	80
Worse	21	14
Dead	0	6
Rehemorrhage	4	20
Radiation-induced complications (%) (temporary/permanent)	12.5/8	5.7/3
Open surgery posttreatment (%)	0	9

Figure 42.15 Summary of Results: Radiosurgical Treatment of Metastases

	Gamma Unit	Linear Accelerator
Tumor size (%)		
Smaller or stable	94	94–95
Increased	6	5–6
Clinical status (%)		
Stable or improved	93	84–100
Worse	7	0–8
Survival		
Median (months)	10	NA
One year (%)	33	NA
Radiation-induced complications (%)	0	3–22
Open surgery posttreatment (%)	6	11

In patients with small AVMs, radiosurgery can achieve a complete obliteration rate of up to 86% in 2 years (Fig. 42.17).[11,14–16,24,34,38,39,46,48] For deep, high-risk AVMs, the complication rate of radiosurgery compares favorably with the best current microsurgical series (Fig. 42.18). Rebleeding during the latency period before obliteration has occurred at a rate of 2% to 3% per year in most centers. Most rehemorrhages have been nonfatal and did not lessen the likelihood of eventual nidus obliteration. Angiographically occult vascular malformations have remained a more controversial and problematic entity to treat, either by radiosurgery or open methods. The natural history of these lesions has yet to be defined for long time periods, and many AOVMs represent incidental or multiple imaging findings of equivocal relationship to the patient's symptoms. Furthermore, no imaging modality can determine when or if the lesion has been obliterated by radiosurgery. The author currently reserves radiosurgical treatment for deep, inoperable AOVMs that clearly have caused repeated or progressive neurologic symptoms due to multiple bleeding episodes.[44]

Acoustic neuromas, pituitary adenomas, and meningiomas constitute the majority of histologically benign neoplasms treated by various radiosurgical techniques. To date, the largest experience with acoustic neuromas and meningiomas has been at centers using the gamma knife (Fig. 42.19).[38,39,43] Long-term clinical and radiographic tumor control rates of 75% to 90% and 86% to 98%, respectively, have been reported with little permanent neurologic morbidity. Although 18% to 25% of patients with acoustic neuromas larger than 10 mm may experience the delayed onset of facial or trigeminal nerve deficits, such deficits have resolved completely or partially in almost all cases. The few exceptions have been patients who underwent open operation after the onset of facial weakness and probably sustained anatomic disruption of the facial nerve during surgery.

Excellent results have also been obtained in the gamma knife radiosurgical and heavy-charged-particle treatment of endocrinologically active pituitary adenomas, especially those associated with acromegaly or Cushing's disease.[13,50,55] Tumor control and endocrinological remission have been achieved in over 90% of

Figure 42.16 Summary of Results: Radiosurgical Treatment of Histologically Benign Extraaxial Tumors Using the ^{60}Co Gamma Unit

	Tumor Size (%)		Clinical Status (%)	
	Decreased or Stable	Increased	Improved	Worse
Acoustic neuroma*	86–98	2–14	75–82	18–25**
Pituitary adenoma	92	8	92	8
Meningioma	96	4	90	6†

*Karolinska Hospital and University of Pittsburgh experience.
**Cranial neuropathy of trigeminal or facial nerves improved at a median time of 13 or 8 months, respectively, after delayed onset.
†Two patients died due to seizure (n=1) or glomerulonephritis (n=1).

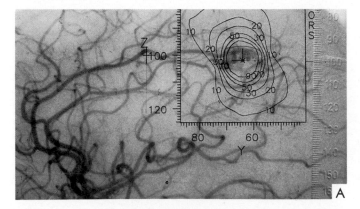
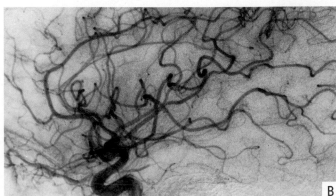

Figure 42.17 (A) Stereotactic right carotid angiogram film during gamma knife radiosurgical treatment of an interhemispheric AVM that had bled 3 weeks earlier in a 13-year-old boy. Radiosurgical dosimetry: single isocenter, 14 mm-collimator, 25 Gy to margin of nidus (70% isodose line), 35.7 Gy maximum central dose. (B) Follow-up angiogram film 1 year after treatment showing complete obliteration of the AVM nidus. The patient remains neurologically normal.

patients in some series, with minimal morbidity. The development of hormone-blocking drugs may herald the expansion of radiosurgery to treat patients with potentially life-threatening endocrinopathy. In such a situation, the drug could suppress the hypersecretion syndrome during the latency period before radiosurgically induced tumor necrosis.

Several reports have been published describing the results of radiosurgery in lieu of open surgery for recurrent or newly diagnosed brain metastases.[40,41,51–55] Both linac and gamma knife techniques appear comparable in terms of tumor shrinkage and clinical response (Figs. 42.20, 42.21). The higher complication and secondary open surgery rates in some linac-based series are

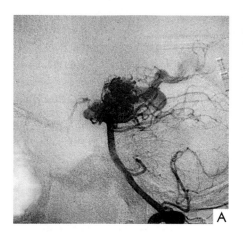
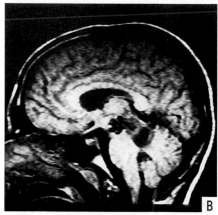
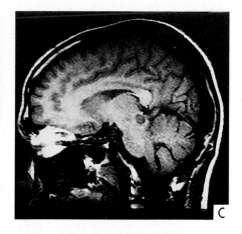

Figure 42.18 (A) Vertebral angiogram film, lateral view, before gamma knife radiosurgical treatment of a midbrain AVM in a 14-year-old boy. A ventriculoperitoneal shunt had been placed to relieve hydrocephalus secondary to intraventricular hemorrhage and brain stem distortion from the engorged deep venous drainage of the nidus. Radiosurgical dosimetry: single isocenter, 14 mm collimator, 20 Gy to margin of nidus (50%i sodose line), 40 Gy maximum central dose. (B) Pretreatment sagittal T1-weighted MRI scan showing the AVM nidus in the brain stem and dilated veins draining into the Galenic system. (C) Follow-up T1-weighted MRI scan 16 months after treatment showing obliteration of the AVM nidus (proven by subsequent angiography) and return of the deep cerebral veins to normal caliber.

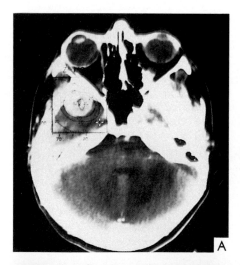
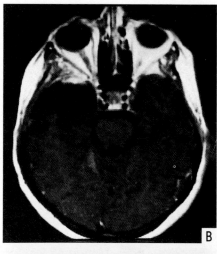

Figure 42.19 (A) Stereotactic contrast enhanced CT scan during gamma knife radiosurgical treatment of a recurrent sphenoid wing meningioma in a 42-year-old woman. Radiosurgical dosimetry: 2 isocenters, 18 mm-collimator, 20 Gy to tumor margin (50% isodose line), 40 Gy maximum central tumor dose. (B) Follow-up T1-weighted MRI scan with gadolinium enhancement in the same axial plane as the previous figure 1 year after treatment. The tumor had decreased in size dramatically. The patient's imaging studies and clinical follow up 2.5 years after radiosurgery have revealed no evidence of tumor recurrence.

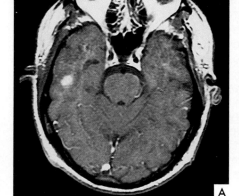
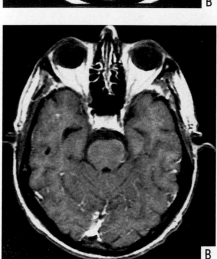

Figure 42.20 (A) Gadolinium-enhanced MRI scan showing a small metastasis from malignant melanoma in the right temporal lobe after 30 Gy fractionated whole brain irradiation. Radiosurgical dosimetry: single isocenter, 8 mm collimator, 18 Gy to margin (50% isodose line), 36 Gy maximum central dose. (B) Gadolinium-enhanced MRI scan in the same axial plane 3 months after radiosurgery using the gamma knife. The tumor had disappeared, leaving a small cleft in the right temporal lobe.

more likely related to tumor size than any other factor. Since nearly all patients with brain metastases receive conventional fractionated irradiation, the timing, volume, and dose of boost radiosurgery must be carefully orchestrated to maximize tumor control and minimize radiation-induced side effects. The available data suggest that boost radiosurgery plus whole-brain radiation therapy is as effective as open surgery plus whole-brain irradiation for solitary metastases less than 3 cm in diameter, regardless of prior therapy, tumor histology, or so-called radioresistance.

The treatment of highly selected patients with apparently well-circumscribed primary glial neoplasms also has been explored. Dramatic tumor shrinkage or stabilization of growth was observed in 56% of patients in the author's early experience (Fig. 42.22).[42] Several patients with persistent or recurrent malignant tumors in the basal ganglia (one glioblastoma), third ventricle (one anaplastic astrocytoma, one ependymoma) or fourth ventricle (ependymoma) have survived longer than 24 months after treatment, well beyond similar patients treated with other available modalities (Fig. 42.23).

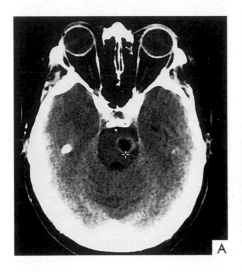
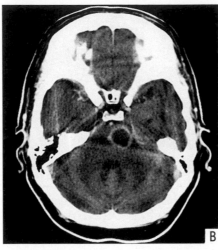

Figure 42.21 (A) Stereotactic contrast-enhanced CT scan during gamma knife radiosurgical treatment of a pontine metastasis (lung primary). Whole brain radiation therapy, 20 Gy in five fractions, had been administered 1 year earlier after resection of a left parietal lobe metastasis. Radiosurgical dosimetry: single isocenter, 14 mm collimator; 16 Gy to the margin (60% isodose line), 26.7 Gy maximum central dose. (B) Follow-up contrast-enhanced CT scan 8 months after radiosurgery at a slightly different gantry angle. The tumor size had not changed appreciably. The patient remained stable clinically and the tumor had not progressed on imaging studies 13 months after treatment.

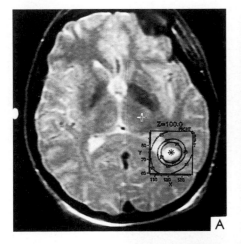
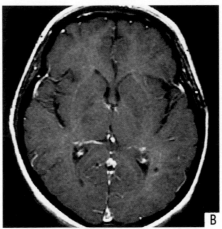

Figure 42.22 (A) Stereotactic T2-weighted MRI scan during radiosurgical treatment of a biopsy-proven left parietal lobe astrocytoma after 45 Gy fractionated external beam irradiation. Radiosurgical dosimetry: 1 isocenter, 14 mm collimator, 18 Gy to the margin (70% isodose line), 25.7 Gy maximum central dose. (B) Follow-up MRI scan with gadolinium enhancement 24 months after gamma knife radiosurgery shows no evidence of tumor. The stereotactic biopsy site can be seen just lateral to the trigone of the left lateral ventricle. The patient remained neurologically normal.

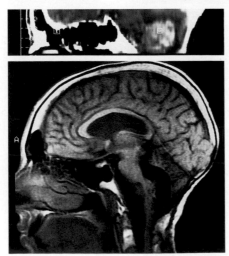

Figure 42.23 (Top) Stereotactic contrast-enhanced CT image sagittal reformation, during gamma knife radiosurgical treatment of a recurrent fourth ventricle ependymoma in a 20-year-old man after open surgery, conventional irradiation, and intraarterial chemotherapy. Radiosurgical dosimetry: incomplete coverage, 2 isocenters, 18 mm collimator, margin dose ≤16 Gy (50% isodose), 32 Gy maximum central dose. (Bottom) Sagittal T1-weighted MRI scan 15 months after radiosurgery showing progressive tumor shrinkage. The patient's pretreatment neurologic progression had been arrested.

REFERENCES

1. Leksell L. The stereotactic method and radiosurgery of the brain. *Acta Chir Scand.* 1951;102:316–319.
2. Leksell DG. Stereotactic radiosurgery: present status and future trends. *Neurol Research.* 1987;9:60–67.
3. Leksell L. Stereotactic radiosurgery. *J Neurol Neurosurg Psychiatry.* 1983;46:797–803.
4. Larson DA. Radiosurgery. Refresher Course at the American Society for Therapeutic Radiology and Oncology; October 15–19, 1990; Miami Beach, Fl.
5. Leksell L. A stereotaxic apparatus for intracerebral surgery. *Acta Chir Scand.* 1949;99:229–233.
6. Leksell L. Stereotactic radiosurgery in trigeminal neuralgia. *Acta Chir Scand.* 1971;137:311–314.
7. Larsson B, Leksell L, Rexed B, et al. The high-energy proton beam as a neurosurgical tool. *Nature.* 1953;182:1222–1223.
8. Larsson B, Leksell L, Rexed B. The use of high energy protons for cerebral surgery in man. *Acta Chir Scand.* 1963;125:1–7.
9. Leksell L, Lindquist C, Adler JR, et al. A new fixation device for the Leksell stereotaxic system. *J Neurosurg.* 1987;66:626–629.
10. Barcia-Salorio JL, Hernandez G, Broseta J, et al. Radiosurgical treatment of carotid-cavernous fistula. *Appl Neurophysiol.* 1982;45:520–522.
11. Lunsford LD, Coffey RJ, Flickinger JC. Stereotactic gamma knife radiosurgery: initial North American experience in 207 patients. *Arch Neurol.* 1990;47:169–175.
12. Levy RP, Fabrikant JI, Frankel KA, et al. Charged-particle radiosurgery of the brain. In: Friedman WA, ed. *Stereotactic Neurosurgery. Neurosurg Clin North Am.* Philadelphia, Pa: WB Saunders Co; 1990;1:955–990.
13. Kjellberg RN, Shintani A, Frantz A, et al. Proton-beam therapy in acromegaly. *N Engl J Med.* 1968;278:689–695.
14. Kjellberg RN, Hanamura T, Davis KR, et al. Bragg-peak proton beam therapy for arteriovenous malformations of the brain. *N Engl J Med.* 1983;309:269–274.
15. Levy RP, Fabrikant JI, Frankel KA, et al. Stereotactic heavy-charged-particle Bragg peak radiosurgery for the treatment of intracranial arteriovenous malformations in childhood and adolescence. *Neurosurgery.* 1989;24:841–852.
16. Steinberg GK, Fabrikant JI, Marks MP, et al. Stereotactic heavy-charged-particle Bragg-peak radiation for intracranial arteriovenous malformations. *N Engl J Med.* 1990;323:96–101.
17. Hall EJ. *Radiobiology for the Radiologist.* Philadelphia, Pa: JB Lippincott; 1988:261–291.
18. Austin-Seymour M, Munzenrider J, Goitein M, et al. Fractionated proton radiation therapy of chordoma and low-grade chondrosarcoma of the base of the skull. *J Neurosurg.* 1989;70:13–17.
19. Kjellberg RN, Koehler AM, Preston WM, et al. Stereotaxic instrument for use with the Bragg peak of a proton beam. *Confin Neurol.* 1962;22:183–189.
20. Hosobuchi Y, Fabrikant J, Lyman J. Stereotactic heavy-particle irradiation of intracranial arteriovenous malformations. *Appl Neurophysiol.* 1987;50:248–252.
21. Friedman WA. LINAC radiosurgery. In: Friedman WA, ed. *Stereotactic Neurosurgery. Neurosurg Clin North Am.* Philadelphia, Pa: WB Saunders Co; 1990;1:991–1008.
22. Heifetz MD, Wexler M, Thompson R. Single-beam radiotherapy knife: a practical theoretical model. *Journal Neurosurg.* 1984;60:814–818.
23. Betti OO, Derechinsky VE. Hyperselective encephalic irradiation with linear accelerator. *Acta Neurochir.* 1984;33(suppl):385–390.
24. Betti OO, Munari C, Rosler R. Stereotactic radiosurgery with the linear accelerator: treatment of arteriovenous malformations. *Neurosurgery.* 1989;24:311–321.
25. Colombo F, Benedetti A, Pozza F, et al. External stereotactic irradiation by linear accelerator. *Neurosurgery.* 1985;16:154–160.
26. Colombo F, Benedetti A, Pozza F, et al. Linear accelerator radiosurgery of cerebral arteriovenous malformations. *Neurosurgery.* 1989;24:833–840.
27. Colombo F, Benedetti A, Pozza F, et al. Linear accelerator radiosurgery of three-dimensional irregular targets. *Stereotact Funct Neurosurg.* 1990;54,55:541–546.
28. Hartmann G, Schlegel W, Sturm V, et al. Cerebral radiation surgery using moving field irradiation at a linear accelerator facility. *Int J Radiat Oncol Biol Phys.* 1985;11:1185–1192.
29. Winston KR, Lutz W. Linear accelerator as a neurosurgical tool for stereotactic radiosurgery. *Neurosurgery.* 1988;22:454–464.
30. Friedman WA, Bova FJ. The University of Florida radiosurgery system. *Surg Neurol.* 1989;32:334–342.
31. Podgorsak E, Olivier A, Pla M, et al. Physical aspects of dynamic stereotactic radiosurgery. *Appl Neurophysiol.* 1987;50:263–268.
32. Houdek PV, Fayos JV, Van Buren JM, et al. Stereotactic radiotherapy technique for small intracranial lesions. *Med Phys.* 1985;12:469–472.
33. Van Buren JM, Landy HJ, Houdek PV, et al. CT-directed stereotactic fractionated rotational radiotherapy by linear accelerator. *Neurosurgery.* 1986;19:149. Abstract.
34. Altschuler EM, Lunsford LD, Coffey RJ, et al. Gamma knife radiosurgery for intracranial arteriovenous malformations in childhood and adolescence. *Pediatr Neurosci.* 1989;15:33–61.
35. Backlund EO, Johansson L, Sarby B. Studies on craniopharyngiomas, II: treatment by stereotaxis and radiosurgery. *Acta Chir Scand.* 1972;138:749–759.
36. Backlund EO, Rahn T, Sarby B, et al. Closed stereotaxic hypophysectomy by means of ^{60}Co gamma

radiation. *Acta Radiologica (Therapy, Physics Biol).* 1972;11:545–555.

37. Backlund EO, Rahn T, Sarby B. Treatment of pinealomas by stereotaxic radiation surgery. *Acta Radiol (Stockholm).* 1974;13:368–376.

38. Coffey RJ, Lunsford LD, Bissonette D, et al. Stereotactic gamma radiosurgery for intracranial vascular malformations and tumors: report of the initial North American experience in 331 patients. *Stereotact Funct Neurosurg.* 1990;54,55:535–540.

39. Coffey RJ, Lunsford LD. Stereotactic radiosurgery using the 201 cobalt-60 source gamma knife. In: Friedman WA, ed. *Neurosurg Clin North Am.* Philadelphia, Pa: WB Saunders Co; 1990;1:955–990.

40. Coffey RJ, Flickinger JC, Lunsford LD. Radiosurgery for brain metastases using the cobalt-60 gamma unit: methods and results in 24 patients. *Int J Radiat Oncol Biol Phys.* 1991;20:1287–1295.

41. Coffey RJ, Flickinger JC, Lunsford LD, et al. Solitary brain metastasis: radiosurgery in lieu of microsurgery in 32 patients. *Acta Neurochirurgica.* 1991; (suppl 52). In press.

42. Coffey RJ, Flickinger JC, Bissonette DB, et al. The role of radiosurgery in the treatment of malignant brain tumors. In: Lunsford LD, ed. *Radiosurgery. Neurosurg Clin North Am.* Philadelphia, Pa: WB Saunders Co; 1991;2.

43. Flickinger JC, Lunsford LD, Coffey RJ, et al. Radiosurgery of acoustic neuromas. *Cancer.* 1991;67:345–353.

44. Kondziolka D, Lunsford LD, Coffey RJ, et al. Stereotactic radiosurgery of angiographically occult vascular malformations: indications and preliminary experience. *Neurosurgery.* 1990;27:892–900.

45. Kondziola D, Lunsford LD, Coffey RJ, et al. Stereotactic radiosurgery of meningiomas. *J Neurosurg.* 1991;74:552–559.

46. Lunsford LD, Kondziolka D, Flickinger JC, et al. Stereotactic radiosurgery for arteriovenous malformations. *J Neurosurgery.* 1991;512–524.

47. Noren G, Arndt J, Hindmarsh T. Stereotactic radiosurgery in cases of acoustic neurinoma: further experiences. *Neurosurgery.* 1983;13:12–22.

48. Steiner L. Radiosurgery in cerebral arteriovenous malformations. In: Flamm E, Fein J, eds. *Textbook of Cerebrovascular Surgery.* New York, NY: Springer-Verlag; 1986;4:1161–1215.

49. Steiner L, Forster D, Leksell L, et al. Gamma thalamotomy in intractable pain. *Acta Neurochir (Wien).* 1980;52:173–184.

50. Stephanian E, Lunsford LD, Coffey RJ, et al. Gamma knife radiosurgery for pituitary adenomas. *Int J Radiat Oncol Biol Phys.* 1990;19(suppl 1):228. Abstract.

51. Thompson BG, Coffey RJ, Flickinger JC, et al. Stereotactic radiosurgery of small intracranial tumors: neuropathological correlation in three patients. *Surg Neurol.* 1990;33:96–104.

52. Engenhart R, Kimmig B, Sturm V. Stereotactically guided convergent beam irradiation of solitary brain metastases and cerebral arteriovenous malformations. In: Dyck P, Bouzaqlou A, eds. *Brachytherapy of Brain Tumors and Related Stereotactic Treatment.* Philadelphia, Pa: Hanley and Belfus; 1989:119–132.

53. Loeffler JS, Kooy AM, Wen PY, et al. The treatment of recurrent brain metastases with stereotactic radiosurgery. *J Clin Oncol.* 1990;8:576–582.

54. Sturm V, Kober B, Hover K-H, et al. Stereotactic percutaneous single dose irradiation of brain metastases with a linear accelerator. *Int J Radiat Oncol Biol Phys.* 1987;13:279–282.

55. Degerblad M, Rahn T, Bergstrand G, et al. Long-term results of stereotactic radiosurgery to the pituitary gland in Cushing's disease. *Acta Endocrinol (Copenh).* 1986;112:310–314.

Chapter 43

Chemotherapy of Central Nervous System Tumors

S. Clifford Schold, Jr.

Cytotoxic drugs have had a significant impact on the natural history of many forms of cancer in the last 40 years. Acute lymphocytic leukemia in children and testicular cancer have become curable diseases because of the introduction of chemotherapy. Many other forms of leukemia, most forms of lymphoma, and several solid tumors, including breast cancer and small cell lung cancer, are sensitive to conventional doses of currently available agents. On the other hand, numerous common forms of cancer have been only minimally responsive to chemotherapy. Examples include non-small cell lung cancer, melanoma, pancreatic cancer, and renal cell carcinoma. Unfortunately, the most common forms of primary brain tumor also belong in this unresponsive category (Fig. 43.1). There have been many instances of unequivocal responses to chemotherapy among patients with anaplastic gliomas, and other forms of CNS tumors are clearly sensitive to chemotherapy. Nevertheless, the impact of chemotherapy on the most common and malignant forms of brain tumor has been slight.

Discovery of new forms of chemotherapy remains a major area of emphasis in cancer research. This will undoubtedly lead to new treatments for CNS tumors in the near future. In this chapter, I will review and discuss the process of evaluation of new chemotherapeutic agents, the agents themselves, the current status of chemotherapy of CNS tumors, and some special problems with respect to the chemotherapy of brain tumors.

CLINICAL TRIALS

Formal clinical trials are both expensive and complicated. Before embarking on a trial, there should be a reasonable and answerable question of sufficient interest to justify application of the necessary resources. It is also extremely important that the precise objectives of a trial be specified and that there be in-depth statistical input into the design of the trial. This increases the likelihood of the study resulting in a new or deeper understanding of a disease process or its treatment. There is no doubt that too many poorly designed and inconclusive studies have been conducted and published on the chemotherapy of CNS tumors. This both clutters the literature and confuses the reader who is not intimately involved in the field.

There is a standardized sequence for evaluating new cancer chemotherapeutic agents in people, which allows progressive and continuous assessment of toxicity and efficacy. These stages are referred to as phase I, II, III trials (Fig. 43.2).

PHASE I

Phase I trials are designed to identify the qualitative toxicity of new chemotherapeutic agents and to determine the maximum tolerated dose in humans. These are the first trials done in people with a new drug, and they are generally conducted with patients whose disease is considered refractory to standard forms of therapy. It is unusual for standard phase I trials to be done in patients with CNS tumors because the confounding variable of intracranial disease would make identification of neurologic toxicity difficult. However, in specialized situations, such as intracarotid drug administration and other targeted routes of delivery, it is important to conduct the phase I trials in patients being treated for CNS disease to identify toxicity associated with a particular route or drug formulation.

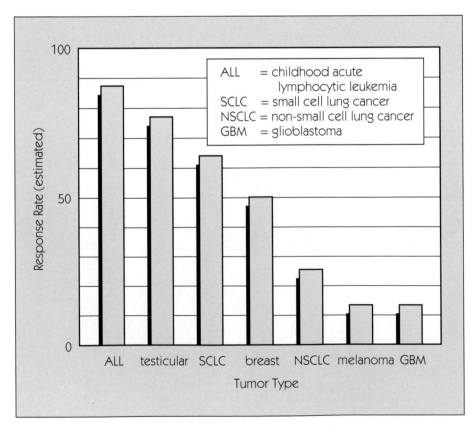

Figure 43.1 Estimated response rates to conventional chemotherapy of a variety of common forms of cancer.

PHASE II

Phase II trials are the initial tests of a drug's activity against specific forms of cancer. The doses and schedules are determined by the experience in the phase I trial, and the treated population is made as homogeneous as possible. Consequently, with an adequate number of patients, such a trial allows one to estimate the response rate of a specific form of cancer to a specific drug using a particular dose and schedule.

PHASE III

Phase III trials are the definitive tests of a drug's efficacy. They are generally randomized trials in which the new agent is compared against a treatment of known activity in a disease. A much larger number of patients is required for phase III trials than for phase II trials because of the statistical comparison to a control arm, but the phase III trial is virtually the only way to be certain of a new drug's role in the treatment of a disease.

Objectives, Statistics, Expense

An important question in the conduct of these trials is what level of activity in a phase II trial justifies advancing the treatment to a phase III trial, a much longer and more expensive enterprise. This decision rests primarily on the activity of the control or standard drug in a phase II setting in a disease. If the phase II level of activity of the new drug is comparable to or exceeds that of the historic results with a standard drug, it is reasonable to proceed with the phase III trial. Clearly, this level of activity in a phase II setting varies widely with the disease under consideration, and it emphasizes the importance of selecting the appropriate population for the phase II trial.

DRUGS IN USE

NITROSOUREAS AND RELATED ALKYLATING DRUGS

The most common and effective drugs in the treatment of gliomas are the nitrosoureas (Fig. 43.3). These com-

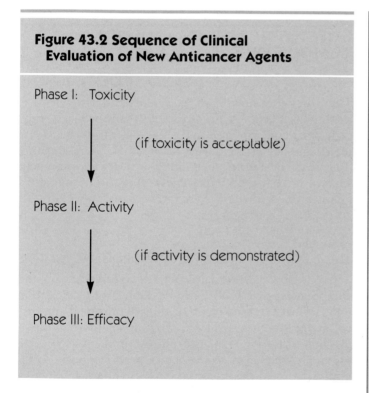

Figure 43.2 Sequence of Clinical Evaluation of New Anticancer Agents

Phase I: Toxicity

(if toxicity is acceptable)

Phase II: Activity

(if activity is demonstrated)

Phase III: Efficacy

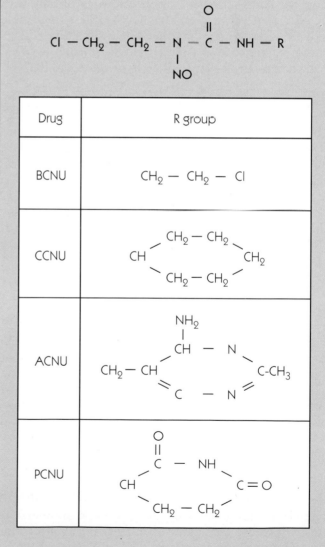

Figure 43.3 Structures of nitrosoureas in common use.

pounds act by alkylating tumor DNA at the O-6 position of guanine, thereby interfering with DNA replication. The alkyl group produced by many nitrosoureas is chloroethylguanine, but similar alkylation at the O-6 position of guanine is produced by related methylating agents, such as procarbazine, streptozocin, and DTIC. The most common drugs in this class for the treatment of gliomas are BCNU (carmustine), CCNU (lomustine), and procarbazine. A number of other nitrosoureas have been introduced into clinical trial, including PCNU, ACNU, and methyl-CCNU, but none has shown clear superiority to the widely available agents.

In the widely quoted trial of therapy for adults with anaplastic gliomas conducted by the Brain Tumor Study Group in the 1970s,[1] BCNU increased the percentage of survivors at 18 months after diagnosis in comparison to patients treated with radiotherapy alone. This study has defined BCNU as the standard against which newer forms of therapy are compared, although the results were modest at best. Procarbazine was shown in a later study by the BTSG not to be significantly different from BCNU, and therefore it also is presumed to have some efficacy in the treatment of this group of diseases.[2] Interestingly, CCNU has never been compared directly with BCNU, so it is not clear that CCNU has comparable activity. However, its pharmacologic similarity and its ease of administration (since it is taken orally) have led many neuro-oncologists to use it in preference to BCNU.

MUSTARD DERIVATIVES

The other major class of alkylating drugs is the mustard derivatives, the most common examples of which are cyclophosphamide and L-phenylalanine mustard (melphalan). These drugs also alkylate DNA, but they do so at a different site and hence their spectrum of activity is different from that of the nitrosoureas. Cyclophosphamide has shown activity against recurrent gliomas at high doses,[3] and melphalan appears to have activity against oligodendroglial tumors and neuronal tumors, such as medulloblastoma and pineoblastoma.

CISPLATIN

Cis-diaminedichloroplatinum II (cisplatin) is a DNA-intercalating agent that has shown impressive antitumor activity in a number of human cancers, including germ cell tumors, head and neck tumors, and small cell lung tumors. Cisplatin, at least when given by the intraarterial route, has activity against both recurrent glioma and newly diagnosed anaplastic glioma.[4] It is also effective against intracranial germ cell tumors.

ANTIMETABOLITES

The classic antineoplastic agents are the antimetabolites, which are analogues of normal metabolites that function by serving as artificial and imperfect substrates for natural metabolic reactions. The most widely used of these agents are methotrexate, a folic acid antagonist,

5-fluorouracil, 6-mercaptopurine, and cytosine arabinoside (ara-C). The antimetabolites as a class are relatively inactive against CNS tumors, at least when used as single agents. They are cell-cycle-specific agents that are most effective against tumors with a high growth fraction.

NATURAL PRODUCTS

There are several natural product drugs that have been used in the treatment of brain tumors and other forms of cancer. These include the vinca alkaloids (vincristine and vinblastine), the topoisomerase II inhibitors etoposide (VP-16) and veniposide (VM-26), the antitumor antibiotics such as adriamycin and actinomycin D, and the recently introduced novel agent, taxol. These drugs are usually large, complex molecules that penetrate the blood-brain barrier poorly. They have been of interest recently because the multidrug resistant (MDR) phenotype appears to produce cross-resistance to many of these natural product anticancer drugs.

CHEMOTHERAPY OF INDIVIDUAL TUMOR TYPES

ASTROCYTIC TUMORS

The drugs that have been used most extensively in the treatment of astrocytic tumors are the nitrosoureas, procarbazine, cisplatin, and to a lesser extent other alkylating drugs such as cyclophosphamide. BCNU is the only drug that has shown unequivocal efficacy in improving survival of patients with newly diagnosed anaplastic gliomas. It is usually given intravenously at a dose of $200 \ mg/m^2$ every 6 weeks.

OLIGODENDROGLIAL TUMORS

There is now substantial reported experience with the combination of CCNU, procarbazine, and vincristine ("PCV") in the treatment of oligodendroglial tumors, and it appears that this form of glioma is more sensitive to chemotherapy than the more common astrocytic tumors.[5] Melphalan has also produced responses in an impressive percentage of patients. Standard practice is evolving toward the use of chemotherapy in preference to radiotherapy in the treatment of these tumors.

MEDULLOBLASTOMAS

Two large cooperative trials in medulloblastoma used CCNU and vincristine (with or without prednisone) in the adjuvant treatment of patients with newly diagnosed disease and compared outcome in patients receiving combination therapy with that in patients treated with radiotherapy alone. There was a marginal benefit from chemotherapy in both trials.[6,7] Treatment of recurrent medulloblastoma, however, suggests that cyclophosphamide and cisplatin may be more active agents. This has not yet been confirmed in a phase III setting. Packer and colleagues have also shown that a combination of cisplatin, vincristine, and CCNU has substantially delayed recurrence in children with high-risk medulloblastoma.[8]

PRIMARY CNS LYMPHOMAS

Primary CNS lymphomas are generally highly sensitive to corticosteroids and radiotherapy, but despite this therapeutic sensitivity, the prognosis for patients with this disease is quite poor. Consequently, there has been substantial interest in using chemotherapeutic agents, and it appears that recurrent CNS lymphoma will respond to the same drugs that are effective in systemic lymphoma: cyclophosphamide, adriamycin, vincristine, and prednisone (CHOP) and subsequent derivatives of this combination.[9] It remains to be seen whether inclusion of these active regimens in the treatment of newly diagnosed patients will materially affect survival.

OTHER TUMORS

Germ Cell Tumors

The most common germ cell tumor of the CNS is the pure germinoma. This is a highly radiosensitive tumor that generally does not require chemotherapy. However, other cellular elements in a germ cell tumor, such as endodermal sinus tumor, teratoma, or choriocarcinoma, are associated with a worse prognosis, and these are often treated with a combination of radiotherapy and chemotherapy. Cisplatin and its derivatives are the most active agents in the treatment of intracranial germ cell tumors, as they are in the treatment of germ cell tumors that appear elsewhere in the body.

Ependymal Tumors

It also appears that ependymal tumors in the brain and spinal cord respond to conventionally administered cisplatin or carboplatin, but again it is not clear whether the addition of chemotherapy at the time of diagnosis will materially affect the outcome.

MENINGIOMAS, CHORDOMAS, NEUROMAS

There are several relatively common extraaxial intracranial tumors for which chemotherapy is employed when surgery (and occasionally radiotherapy) has failed. Unfortunately, there is very little evidence of any activity of standard drugs in this setting.

SPECIAL PROBLEMS

PREDICTING RESPONSE

A major problem in the treatment of human cancer is that it has not been possible to predict reliably the response of an individual patient to a particular treatment. One can make general statements about the probability of response based on the histologic type of tumor, the extent of disease, and certain demographic features, such as the age of the patient. However, with few exceptions it has not been possible to assay an individual tumor in some sense and select the most appropriate therapy, as is done in microbiology. Consequently, for example, a small percentage of children with acute lymphoblastic leukemia do not respond to conventional chemotherapy, just as a small percentage of patients with anaplastic glial tumors respond dramatically to standard systemic chemotherapy at conventional doses. A reliable method to make these determinations in advance would have a profound impact on the treatment of patients suffering from these diseases.

There are several possibilities. One is simply growing the tumor in culture or in an animal and doing some kind of sensitivity test. The limitation of this approach has been the low percentage of tumor cells that are clonogenic, i.e., that form colonies in culture or masses in animals over time. Since the percentage of clonogenic cells is low (probably less than 1% of neoplastic cells in a glioma, for example), one can ask whether they are truly representative of the parent tumor. Nevertheless, there has been some progress in using soft agar cloning techniques to identify cells that are resistant to certain drugs, and this resistance pattern appears to correlate with the lack of clinical response.[10] Another approach can be used if the primary mechanism of action of a chemotherapeutic agent is known, the mechanisms of resistance to this action have been determined, and it is possible to assay a tumor or a portion of a tumor for mechanisms of resistance. For example, it is thought that the primary biochemical mechanism of resistance to the nitrosoureas is an enzyme (O6-alkylguanine-DNA alkyltransferase) that removes the alkyl adduct formed by the drug on the guanine base of the tumor DNA. If this repair enzyme is present in high levels, tumors are relatively resistant to the nitrosoureas, but if the tumor is transferase-deficient the tumor is very sensitive to the cytotoxic effects of these alkylating drugs.[11] An assay of this type might be performed on resected tissue to guide the choice of therapeutic agent to be used.

DRUG DELIVERY

A unique aspect of the chemotherapy of tumors in the brain is the physiologic blood-brain barrier. Generally speaking, chemotherapy is ineffective in the treatment of CNS tumors. To what extent is this failure a result of inadequate drug delivery to the brain and spinal cord because of this barrier? On the one hand, lipid-soluble agents, i.e., those that are able to penetrate the barrier, are the most effective drugs in the treatment of CNS tumors. On the other hand, the barrier is clearly disrupted in many of these tumors, at least as measured by contrast enhancement on CT or MR scanning. The question is important because its resolution will herald the strategy of new therapeutic developments by emphasizing either new methods of delivery or totally new agents.

It appears that the answer will not be simple. There is experimental and clinical evidence that there is considerable variability in capillary permeability among primary CNS tumors,[12] and it is likely that the biochemical sensitivity of these tumors is similarly variable. To the extent that capillary permeability, blood flow, and biochemical sensitivity of individual tumors can be measured, it will become possible to select treatment rationally on the basis of measurable traits.

EVALUATING RESPONSE

Another peculiar and difficult problem in the treatment of CNS tumors is the determination of response to therapy. This was accomplished largely on clinical grounds in the early cooperative trials, and more recently assessment of treatment response has been based on a combination of clinical factors and imaging data from CT or MRI. Unfortunately, there are complexities even with the sophisticated imaging equipment available. First, these tumors are often irregular and highly infiltrative with indistinct margins, so attempts to determine tumor volume are subject to considerable measurement error. Second, contrast enhancement on CT or MRI lacks specificity, so in the setting of recurrent disease after primary treatment it is not always possible to distinguish active disease from gliosis or necrosis. This of course makes precise determination of a change in tumor volume after treatment nearly impossible. Third, the clinical neurologic status of a patient may not be reflected in the change on the imaging study. Patients can be considerably worse despite little change on CT or MRI, particularly those with very large tumors. On the other hand, tumors in relatively silent areas of the brain can show considerable change without any effect on the neurologic examination. Furthermore, established neurologic deficits tend to remain fixed despite reversal of the pathologic process, so it is usually not reasonable to require improvement in the neurologic exam in the definition of response. Finally, all of these things can be profoundly affected by a change in the dose of corticosteroids being administered to the patient.

Because of the uncertainty surrounding the assessment of response in CNS tumors, study design and reports of clinical trials must include precise definitions. The variability in reported response rates in different trials probably largely reflects different definitions of response to therapy.

REFERENCES

1. Walker MD, Alexander E III, Hunt WE, et al. Evaluation of BCNU and/or radiotherapy in the treatment of anaplastic gliomas. *J Neurosurg.* 1978;49:333–343.
2. Green SB, Byar DP, Walker MD, et al. Comparisons of carmustine, procarbazine, and high-dose methylprednisolone as additions to surgery and radiotherapy for the treatment of malignant glioma. *Cancer Treat Rep.* 1983;67:1–12.
3. Longee DC, Friedman HS, Albright RE Jr, et al. Treatment of patients with recurrent gliomas with cyclophosphamide and vincristine. *J Neurosurg.* 1990;72:583–588.
4. Dropcho EJ, Rosenfeld SS, Morawetz RB, et al. Pre-radiation intracarotid cisplatin treatment of newly diagnosed anaplastic gliomas. *J Clin Oncol.* In press.
5. Cairncross JG, Macdonald DR. Successful chemotherapy for recurrent malignant oligodendroglioma. *Ann Neurol.* 1988;23:360–364.
6. Evans AE, Jenkin RDT, Sposto R, et al. The treatment of medulloblastoma: results of a prospective randomized trial of radiation therapy with and without CCNU, vincristine, and prednisone. *J Neurosurg.* 1990;72:572–582.
7. Tait DM, Thornton-Jones H, Bloom HJG, et al. Adjuvant chemotherapy for medulloblastoma: the first multi-centre control trial of the International Society of Pediatric Oncology (SIOP I). *Eur J Cancer.* 1990;26:464–469.
8. Packer RJ, Diegel KR, Sutton LN, et al. Efficacy of adjuvant chemotherapy for patients with poor-risk medulloblastoma: a preliminary report. *Ann Neurol.* 1988;24:503–508.
9. Hochberg FH, Loeffler JS, Prados M. The therapy of primary brain lymphoma. *J Neurooncol.* 1991; 10:191–201.
10. Von Hoff DD, Clark GM, Stogdill BJ, et al. Prospective clinical trial of a human tumor cloning system. *Cancer Res.* 1983;43:1926–1931.
11. Schold SC Jr, Brent TP, von Hofe E, et al. O6-alkylguanine-DNA alkyltransferase and sensitivity to procarbazine in human brain tumor xenografts. *J Neurosurg.* 1989;70:563–577.
12. Groothuis DR, Vriesendorp FJ, Kupfer B, et al. Quantitative measurements of capillary transport in human brain tumors by computed tomography. *Ann Neurol.* 1991;30:581–588.

Chapter 44

Cervical Disc Disease
and Spondylosis

Eric S. Nussbaum, Setti S. Rengachary

CERVICAL DISC DISEASE

Mixter and Barr are generally credited with introducing the concept of disc herniation as a source of nerve root compression.[1] In 1934, they reported the first removal of a preoperatively diagnosed ruptured lumbar intervertebral disc. Three years earlier, however, Dandy had removed "chondroid material" from two patients with sciatica and realized that it was normal disc tissue rather than neoplasm.[2] Since these early reports, surgical treatment of intervertebral disc disease has become an area of major interest for neurosurgeons. Tremendous attention has been focused on the cervical spine; it is estimated that cervical spine disorders now account for up to 2% of all admissions to large hospital centers.

ANATOMY

The axial skeleton, including the cervical spine, must bear both the weight of the body and externally applied axial forces, and still maintain a considerable degree of mobility. The spine therefore has seemingly opposing functional attributes: serving as a rigid structural support while concurrently allowing functional mobility. This dual purpose is achieved by the segmented structure of the spine, much like a goose-neck lamp, with the links being the vertebrae and the intervertebral discs allowing motion while maintaining stability.

The relative amounts of structural support and functional mobility vary among regions of the spine. The cervical spine exhibits a great deal of mobility but little weight-bearing function, whereas for the lumbar spine the reverse is true. The intervertebral discs serve as mechanical buffers that absorb axial loading, bending, and shear forces. As a result of the evolution of bipedal posture in hominoids, the intervertebral discs have become further stressed, which accounts for the high incidence of degenerative disc disorders in humans.

The intervertebral disc consists of two distinct components: a soft central portion, the nucleus pulposus, and a tough, round peripheral component, the annulus fibrosus (Fig. 44.1).

The nucleus pulposus is composed of a three-dimensional meshwork of collagen fibers (Fig. 44.2). Filling the interstices between the collagen fibers is a matrix composed primarily of proteoglycan molecular aggregates. The structure of the aggregate is best understood by examining the organization of one of its monomeric subcomponents. This consists of a central protein with side-chain glycosaminoglycans. Glycosaminoglycans (mucopolysaccharides) are proteins conjugated with sugar polymers. Two major types of glycosaminoglycans are commonly found in the nucleus pulposus: keratin and chondroitin sulfate. The former is recognizable by its shorter length. Proteoglycan monomers are attached to long chains of hyaluronic acid by a link protein to form the proteoglycan aggregate.

The annulus fibrosus consists of concentric layers of collagen fibers which run in a diagonal fashion and attach to the hyaline cartilaginous endplates. The fibers pass in opposite directions in alternating layers, much like the layers of steel-belted radial tires (see Fig. 44.1). The superficial fibers of the annulus that attach to the body are known as Sharpey's fibers. Anomalous excessive motion induces calcification at the origin of Sharpey's fibers, so-called traction spurs of Macnab.

In childhood 80% of the nucleus pulposus is water, osmotically bound to the proteoglycan matrix. With

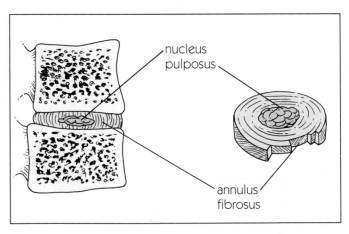

nucleus pulposus

annulus fibrosus

Figure 44.1 Structure of the intervertebral disc. The *annulus fibrosus* consists of concentric layers of collagen fibers in a diagonal array that attach to hyaline cartilaginous endplates. The fibers pass in opposite directions in alternating layers, much like the layers of steel-belted radial tires. The soft central portion is the *nucleus pulposus*.

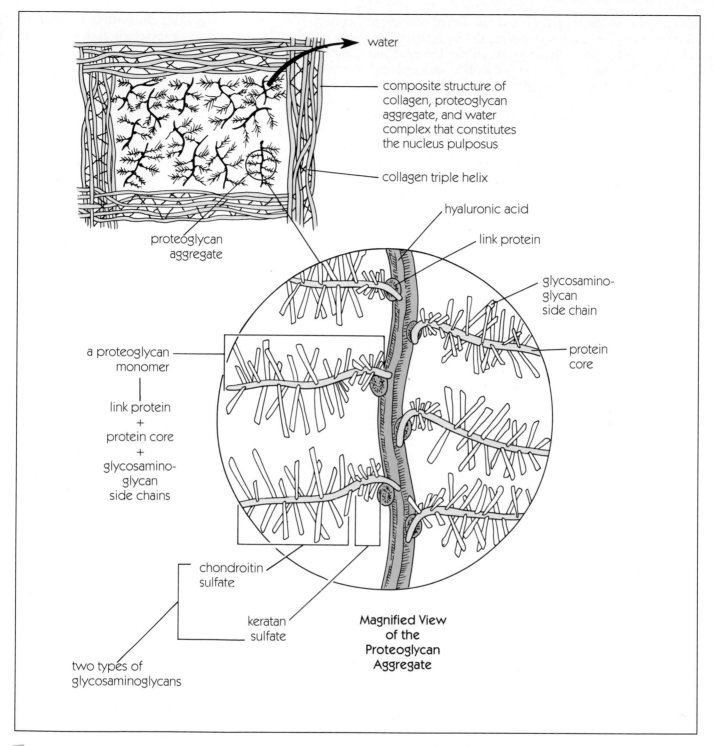

water

composite structure of collagen, proteoglycan aggregate, and water complex that constitutes the nucleus pulposus

collagen triple helix

proteoglycan aggregate

hyaluronic acid

link protein

glycosamino-glycan side chain

protein core

a proteoglycan monomer

link protein
+
protein core
+
glycosamino-glycan side chains

chondroitin sulfate

keratan sulfate

two types of glycosaminoglycans

Magnified View of the Proteoglycan Aggregate

Figure 44.2 Molecular structure of the nucleus pulposus. The nucleus pulposus is a three-dimensional network of collagen fibers. The interstices of the matrix are filled with proteoglycan molecular aggregrates and water. The proteoglycan molecular aggregate consists of a central core of hyaluronic acid to which proteoglycan monomers are attached through link proteins (see magnified view). Each proteoglycan monomer consists of a central core protein to which glycosaminoglycans (mucopolysaccharides) are attached.

aging, both the proteoglycan and the intradiscal water content decrease. Dessication results in lack of disc turgor, causing poor distribution of the biomechanical load. The negatively charged sulfate and carboxyl groups in the glycosaminoglycan chains confer a net negative charge to the disc matrix with respect to plasma. Because osmotic pressure results from the relative difference in the concentration of charged particles between the disc and the plasma, there is a high osmotic pressure within the disc caused by a higher density of charged particles (Gibbs-Donnan equilibrium).

An important support that prevents spontaneous disc herniation is afforded by the posterior longitudinal ligament. This structure is a flat, ribbon-like band of collagenous fibers running along the posterior surface of the vertebral bodies and the intervertebral discs. At the level of the disc space, the ligament has thin, pointed extensions bilaterally, giving an overall dentate configuration to the ligament (Fig. 44.3). The central portions of the discs are therefore well reinforced by the tough posterior ligament, but the lateral portions are relatively unsupported. This, in part, accounts for the higher frequency of lateral as opposed to medial disc herniations.

The spine as a whole is divided into alternating mobile and fixed segments (Fig. 44.4). The transitional zones between the mobile and fixed regions undergo the greatest amount of stress during motion. Therefore, in humans the lower cervical and lumbar intervertebral

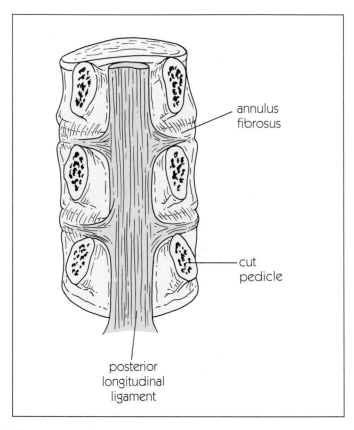

Figure 44.3 The posterior longitudinal ligament is a flat, ribbon-like band of collagenous fibers running along the posterior surface of the vertebral bodies and the intervertebral discs. At the level of the disc space the ligament has thin, pointed extensions bilaterally, giving the ligament a dentate configuration overall.

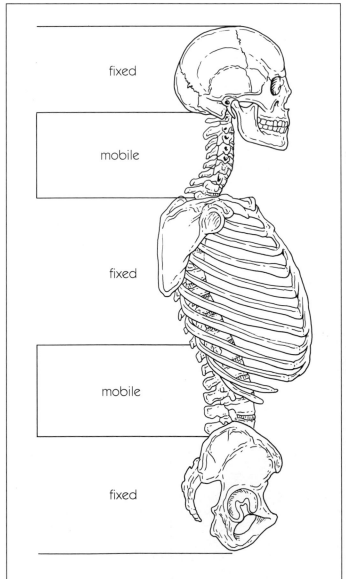

Figure 44.4 The spine as a whole is divided into alternating mobile and fixed segments. The transitional zones between the fixed and mobile regions undergo the most stress during motion.

Principles of Neurosurgery

discs are most frequently affected by degenerative changes. Not surprisingly, 60% of cervical disc herniations occur at the C6-7 level and another 25% at C5-6.[3]

PATHOLOGY

Cervical disc rupture can occur after an acute traumatic injury to a previously normal disc or, more commonly, after repetitive wear and tear that causes progressive degenerative injury. Early degenerative changes lead to radial fissuring of the annulus (Fig. 44.5). The nucleus pulposus then escapes through these fissures, extending to the margin of the annulus: this stage is designated a *contained disc rupture;* it can usually be managed without surgery.

With further degenerative injury, the nucleus pulposus, still contained within the confines of the greatly thinned annulus and posterior longitudinal ligament,

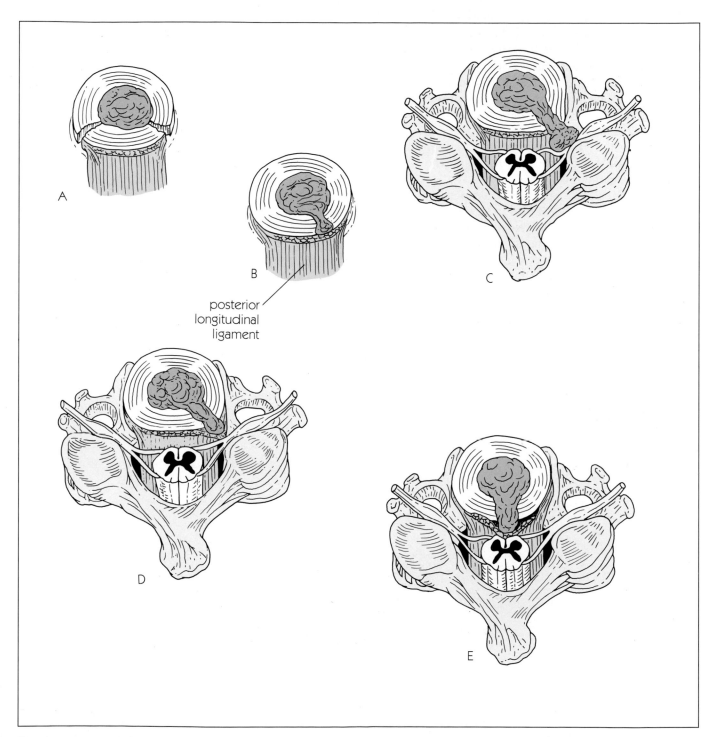

posterior
longitudinal
ligament

Figure 44.5 (A) Radial fissures in annulus. (B) "Contained" ruptured disc. (C) Extruded "soft" disc (tear in the annulus and the posterior longitudinal ligament; free fragments of nucleus pulposus in the epidural space impinging against the root). (D) Protruded "soft" disc causing radiculopathy (Posterior longitudinal ligament intact). (E) Centrally herniated disc.

protrudes beyond the perimeter of the disc space. It extends into the epidural space, where it may impinge on a nerve root, resulting in radiculopathy. In extreme stages there is a complete rent in the annulus and the posterior ligament, allowing an extruded fragment of the nucleus pulposus to impinge on the nerve root. Less frequently, the disc may rupture centrally and cause direct compression of the spinal cord (see Fig. 44.5).

CLINICAL SYNDROME

The patient with a cervical disc herniation may present with radiculopathy, myelopathy, or a combination of these. Soft disc herniations with root compression usually manifest acutely. Myelopathic signs and symptoms are more insidious in onset and present later in the course of disease. The incidence of cervical disc herniation peaks in the third or fourth decade of life; it typically occurs in a paracentral unilateral location where the annulus fibrosus is weakest and the posterior longitudinal ligament is thin.

After cervical disc rupture, most patients present with neck, shoulder, and/or arm pain, which may follow a well-demarcated radicular distribution. The pain can be sharp but is more commonly described as a constant dull ache exacerbated by neck motion. This is typically associated with paresthesias, numbness, and tingling in a similar distribution. Many patients describe parascapular aching pain, which is thought to be referred pain (Fig. 44.6). Sensory complaints often extend fur-

ther down the upper extremity to involve the fingers, providing an important clue to the level of the lesion.

Other symptoms may include headache, upper extremity weakness, or frank atrophy with muscle wasting. Neck extension closes the facets over the nerve root, thus increasing compression and sometimes inciting symptoms. Patients with central disc herniation may describe neckache, loss of dexterity, diffuse upper extremity weakness, clumsiness or instability of gait, and bowel or bladder dysfunction.

Physical findings will depend on the level and location of disc herniation. Lateral disc herniation causes nerve root compression with specific motor group weakness, reflex changes, and objective sensory loss in a radicular pattern. More centrally located herniations can cause spinal cord compression with hyperreflexia below the level of the lesion, clumsiness and ataxia of the lower extremities, gait disturbance, and bowel or bladder dysfunction.

Specific examples of neurologic signs and symptoms associated with compression of a given nerve root are summarized in Figure 44.7. C-4 root injury causes pain along the side of the neck to the point of the shoulder. C-5 root involvement results in neck pain to the shoulder and the upper anterior arm, with paresis of the supraspinatus, infraspinatus, deltoid, and elbow flexors. There may be some decrease in the biceps jerk and sensory changes over the deltoid region.

C-6 lesions cause pain radiating to the lateral arm and dorsum of the forearm, with marked elbow flexor

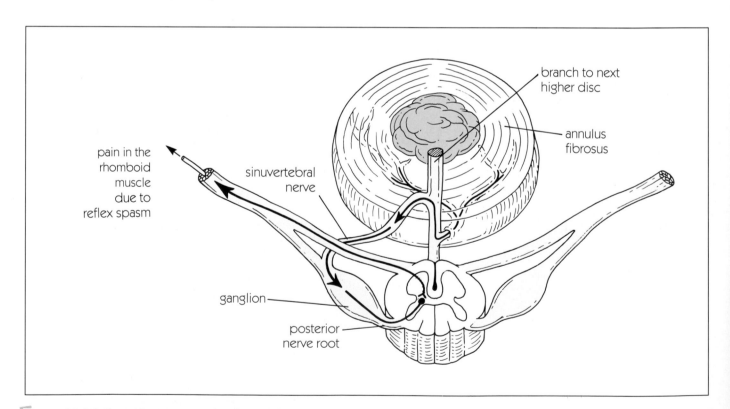

Figure 44.6 Pathway for parascapular discogenic pain.

weakness. The biceps jerk is diminished or absent. Paresthesias typically involve the thumb. C-7 lesions result in pain to the dorsal forearm, with weakness of the triceps, supinator, and pronator and wrist and finger extension. The triceps jerk is diminished. Sensory changes involve the index and middle fingers. C-8 root involvement causes pain in the medial aspect of the arm and forearm, with intrinsic hand muscle weakness.

Uncommonly, patients with acute central cervical disc herniation present with frank spinal cord injury (Fig. 44.8). With severe cord compression the lesion may be "complete," with functional cord transection and loss of all function below the level of the lesion. More commonly an "incomplete" injury is present and the patient may demonstrate one of a number of classic syndromes.

Central cord syndrome refers to the acute development of painless weakness, involving predominantly the upper extremities, distal more than proximal. The sensory changes are less dramatic. The *Brown–Séquard syndrome* is characterized by a functional hemisection of the cord, with loss of pain and temperature sensation

Figure 44.7 Cervical Roots Syndrome

Level of cervical disc rupture	C3-4	C4-5	C5-6	C6-7	C7-T1
Root compressed	C4	C5	C6	C7	C8
Distribution of pain and paresthesia	Side of neck to the top of the	Around shoulder and arm	Forearm index finger thumb	Forearm and ring finger	Forearm little finger
Motor Weakness Sensory loss (dermatome)	Diaphragm	Deltoid	Biceps	Triceps extensors of wrist and fingers	Intrinsic muscles of hand
Reflex Impairment	----	Biceps	Biceps	Triceps	----

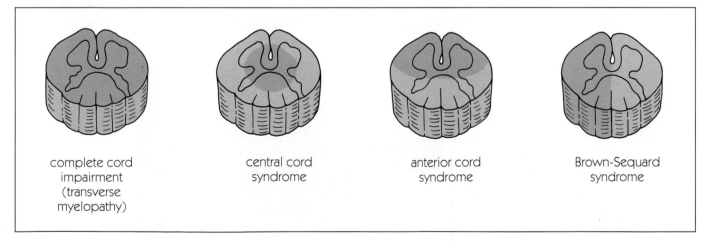

complete cord impairment (transverse myelopathy)   central cord syndrome   anterior cord syndrome   Brown-Sequard syndrome

Figure 44.8 Cervical cord syndromes.

contralateral to the lesion and with ipsilateral weakness and posterior column involvement. *Anterior cord syndrome* involves the anterior two thirds of the cord, with sparing of only the posterior columns. This syndrome can be caused by anterior spinal artery thrombosis.

DIFFERENTIAL DIAGNOSIS

The differential diagnosis of cervical disc rupture includes lesions that may mimic radicular findings, with or without associated spinal cord compression. Tumors, most notably schwannomas or meningiomas, can produce a cervical radicular syndrome. Syringomyelia can be identified by the suspended, dissociated sensory loss associated with bilateral dysesthetic pain. Brachial plexus lesions can be difficult to localize, presenting a diagnostic challenge. Involvement of more than one root should raise the suspicion, and electromyography should confirm the diagnosis, of such an injury.

Pancoast's syndrome may mimic a C-8 or T-1 lesion, with intrinsic hand weakness and Horner's syndrome. Chest radiography or tomography of the apices of the lungs should identify a lesion in this situation. Peripheral entrapment syndromes can also be confused with disc herniation. Carpal tunnel syndrome, for example, may cause pain and paresthesias involving the entire arm. The clinical pattern of symptoms typically suggests the correct diagnosis in such cases.

DIAGNOSTIC STUDIES

Patients who undergo evaluation for cervical disc herniation are first studied with plain radiographs of the cervical spine, including anteroposterior, lateral, and odontoid views. This allows assessment of vertebral body alignment and integrity, disc space height, neural foramen encroachment, advanced osteophytic changes, and ossification of the posterior longitudinal ligament. Oblique views may demonstrate foraminal spurs nicely.

Myelography with subsequent CT scanning remains the standard for evaluation of degenerative disease of the cervical spine. CT provides excellent delineation of the cross-sectional detail of the bony elements. The spinal cord and proximal nerve roots can be seen against the dense contrast background, allowing easy assessment of cord or root compression (Fig. 44.9). CT scanning is also an excellent study for diagnosis of neural foraminal stenosis.

MRI is less invasive and has recently gained great popularity as a tool for studying the cervical spine. Although the soft tissue anatomy is clearly visualized, MRI provides poor osseous detail, requires a long acquisition time, and yields variable image quality. However, it is useful to demonstrate soft disc herniations (Fig. 44.10).

NONOPERATIVE TREATMENT

Nonoperative or conservative treatment typically consists of bed rest, avoidance of heavy lifting, physical therapy, application of heat, neck massage, analgesics, muscle relaxants, and cervical traction. In many cases these maneuvers obviate the need for surgical intervention. Presumably, as the disc dessicates and shrinks, nerve root compression should resolve and the symptoms improve. A reasonable trial period for such treatment should be decided on the basis of the severity of symptoms and the presence or absence of neurologic deficit.

INDICATIONS FOR SURGERY

A central disc herniation causing spinal cord compression, as heralded by myelopathy, deserves surgical consideration. Which patients with isolated radiculopathy should undergo surgery, however, remains controversial. In general, the best indication for surgery in a patient with a standard posterolateral disc herniation and radiculopathy is failure of conservative management. This includes patients who have intractable pain or a progressive neurologic deficit.

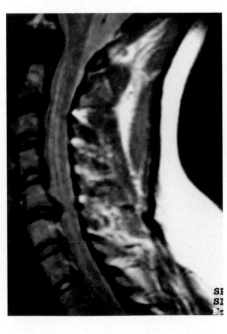

Figure 44.10 MR image of the cervical spine, sagittal section showing ruptured disc at C5-6 level.

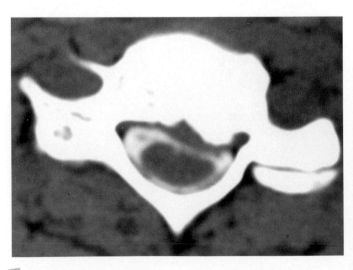

Figure 44.9 CT scan, axial view with intrathecal contrast. There is distortion of nerve root and thecal sac by a herniated disc and an osteophyte.

Posterior Approach for Excision of a "Soft" Lateral Cervical Disc

A posterior midline incision is centered on the desired level. A lateral radiograph is taken, with a metallic marker to confirm the pathologic interspace. A "keyhole" foraminolaminotomy is performed that includes the inferior border of the lamina above, the superior border of the lamina below, and the medial half of the facet joint. The ligamentum flavum is excised. The cervical root is retracted cephalad and the extruded disc fragments are removed (Fig. 44.11).

Anterior Approach for Excision of Cervical Disc and Removal of Osteophyte

A horizontal incision is made in the anterior neck, centered over the desired interspace. After soft-tissue dissection in a plane medial to the carotid artery, the prevertebral space is entered. The disc material is removed from the interspace and the osteophytes are drilled out (Fig. 44.12). A "bread-loaf" tricortical bone graft is harvested from the patient's iliac crest; alternatively, bone-bank allograft can be used. The graft is impacted under distraction (Fig. 44.13). Fusion usually occurs within 3 months.

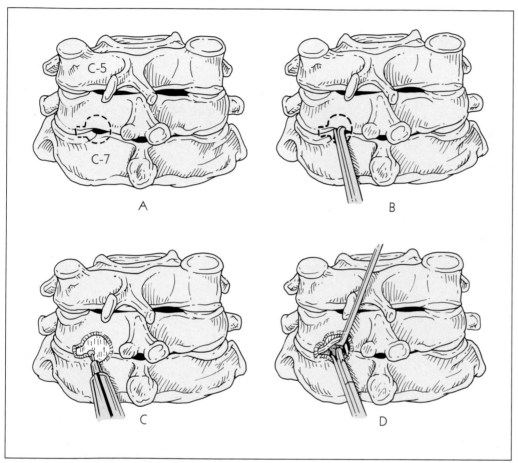

Figure 44.11 Technique of excision of "soft" lateral cervical disc.

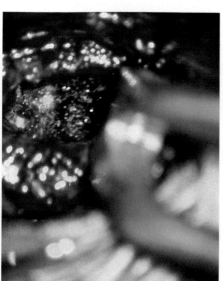

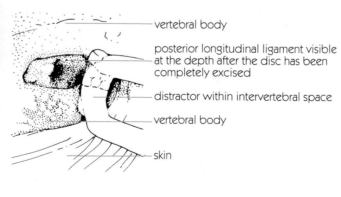

Figure 44.12 Excision of intervertebral disc through the anterior approach.

— vertebral body

— posterior longitudinal ligament visible at the depth after the disc has been completely excised

— distractor within intervertebral space

— vertebral body

— skin

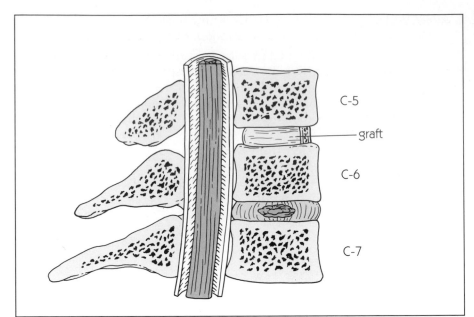

Figure 44.13 Application of interbody graft.

C-5

graft

C-6

C-7

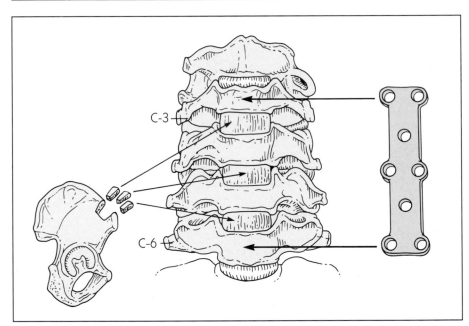

Figure 44.14 Multilevel discectomy, osteophytectomy, fusion, and internal stabilization.

C-3

C-6

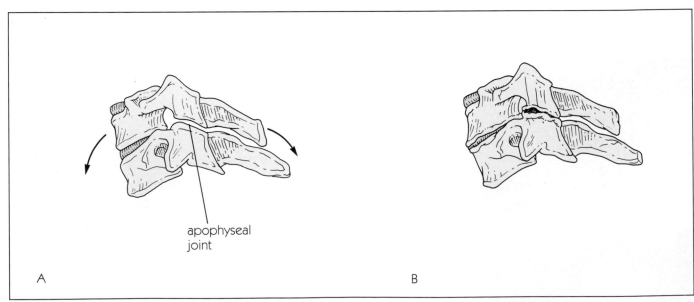

apophyseal joint

A

B

Figure 44.15 (A) Normal intervertebral disc and apophyseal joint. (B) Narrowing of intervertebral disc space and formation of osteophytes in intervertebral and apophyseal joint spaces in cervical spondylosis.

Multilevel Discectomy, Osteophytectomy, Fusion, and Internal Stabilization

This procedure is usually indicated in patients who have osteophytes at multiple levels causing myelopathy or myeloradiculopathy, but no associated congenital spinal stenosis. The technique is quite similar to that of single-level discectomy and osteophytectomy. However, at the completion of discectomy and interbody fusion, internal stabilization is achieved with a plate-and-screw system. This acts as an internal splint, improves the chances of solid fusion, and minimizes the possibility of delayed kyphotic deformity caused by collapse of the graft (Fig. 44.14).

CERVICAL SPONDYLOSIS

In 1838, Key described a firm bony ridge crossing the cervical disc space and encroaching on the spinal cord. Later, Horsley successfully operated on such a lesion, demonstrating that spinal cord compression caused by bony stenosis can be amenable to surgical treatment. Since that time our understanding of the pathophysiology and the natural history of cervical spondylosis has grown, allowing earlier recognition and more effective treatment of this disorder.[4]

PATHOPHYSIOLOGY

The primary event that leads to spondylotic degeneration is reduction in disc height. This occurs as part of the aging process and is caused by a decrease in the water content of the nucleus pulposus. In younger individuals, because of optimal disc height, adjacent vertebral bodies never contact each other, even in extremes of flexion and extension. The normal intervertebral disc thus acts as a spacer between the vertebral bodies.

In older individuals, loss of disc height allows the anterior and posterior edges of adjacent vertebral bodies to touch during flexion and extension, inducing osteophyte formation. Degenerative changes in the apophyseal joints (facet joints) also induce formation of osteophytes that encroach on the neural foramina (Fig. 44.15).

The uncovertebral joints also deserve a brief description. The superior surfaces of the cervical vertebrae are not flat—the superolateral edges curve upwards into hook-like uncinate processes. These processes allow interlocking of vertebral bodies and appear to confer some degree of lateral stability. Early anatomists found cleft-like spaces in the lateral edges of the intervertebral discs near the uncinate processes. These clefts were mistaken for synovium-lined joint spaces and were named uncovertebral joints (joints of Luschka) (Fig. 44.16). On the basis of current understanding, we know that these are not true joints but are actually degenerative clefts within the discs near the uncinate process. The practical significance is that osteophytes are prone to occur in this area, and because of their proximity to the intervertebral foramen they may encroach on the foramen and cause root compression (Fig. 44.17).

Certain additional factors can lead to spinal cord compression in spondylosis (Fig. 44.18). Congenital narrowing of the spinal canal predisposes to cord compression. The presence and degree of stenosis can be judged on lateral radiographs of the cervical spine. Normally, the anteroposterior diameter of the spinal canal should be at least 80% of the sagittal diameter of the midvertebral body (Pavlov's ratio); lesser ratios can be assumed to indicate spinal stenosis.

Hypertrophy and infolding of the ligamentum flavum resulting from loss of elastic tissue in the ligament further compromise the already limited space within the spinal canal. Chronic subluxation caused by laxity of ligaments causes repetitive microtrauma to the spinal cord during normal motion of the cervical spine. In particular, hyperextension of the neck, which further narrows the canal by causing inward buckling of the ligamentum flavum, traps the spinal cord between impinging ventral and dorsal forces.

From the foregoing discussion of the pathogenesis of spinal cord compression in cervical spondylosis, it is apparent that any surgical procedure designed to alleviate the symptoms of myelopathy should aim at both decompression and stabilization of the affected area. Satisfying only one of these goals is likely to yield suboptimal results.

CLINICAL SYNDROME

Much like cervical disc herniation, cervical spondylosis may lead to radiculopathy, myelopathy, or myeloradiculopathy. Nerve root compression caused by spondylotic osteophytes develops either insidiously or acutely, especially after minor trauma. There is usually a history of chronic neckache with intermittent, recurring pain and paresthesias. Clinically, root compression results in some combination of motor weakness, sensory loss, reflex changes, and neck and arm pain.

Myelopathy caused by cervical spondylosis typically develops insidiously and is accompanied by a history of chronic, intermittent symptoms. The presentation can include any of the myelopathic syndromes described above for central disc herniation, including the central cord syndrome, Brown-Séquard syndrome, anterior cord syndrome, or transverse myelopathy. Rarely, "myelopathy hand," akin to the weak, wasted hand of amyotrophic lateral sclerosis may result from cervical spondylosis. Lhermitte's sign is a sudden, brief sensation resembling an electric shock that radiates down the spine and/or into the extremities, associated with neck movement. This finding further suggests impingement by the narrowed canal on the spinal cord.

Cervical spondylosis may cause difficulties unrelated to direct nerve root compression. Vertebral artery compression caused by impingement of osteophytes on the vertebrarterial foramina may lead to intermittent ischemic symptoms associated with changes in neck

Figure 44.16 Anatomy of uncovertebral joint and intervertebral foramen.

intervertebral disc

uncovertebral joint (joint of Luschka)

uncinate process of vertebral body

Front View

uncovertebral joint

inferior articular process

root

apophyseal (facet) joint

transverse process

superior articular process

Side View

inferior articular process

facet joint capsule (capsule of apophyseal joint)

superior articular process

uncinate process of vertebral body

Oblique View

Figure 44.17 Impingement on nerve root in the intervertebral foramen by uncovertebral and apophyseal osteophytes.

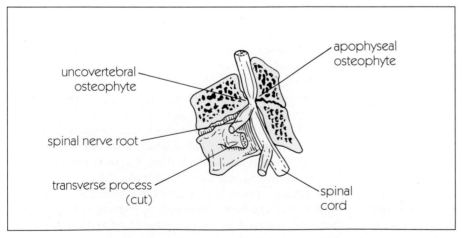

uncovertebral osteophyte

apophyseal osteophyte

spinal nerve root

transverse process (cut)

spinal cord

position. *Forestier disease* is characterized by dysphagia resulting from compression by a large anterior osteophyte on the esophagus.

IMAGING

Some degree of cervical spondylosis can be identified on radiographic examination in 25% to 50% of the population over the age of 50 years and in 75% of the population over the age of 75 years.[5] Obviously, radiologic evidence of cervical spondylosis may not correlate with physical findings. Plain radiographs demonstrate osteophytes at the disc space level, foraminal spurs, loss of disc height, narrowing of the spinal canal, and bony ridging across the disc space.

Myelography with postmyelogram CT scanning still provides the best delineation of bony detail, allowing assessment of neural impingement (Fig. 44.19). A C1-2 puncture usually provides the best images, although a lumbar puncture can be used instead. MRI can reveal

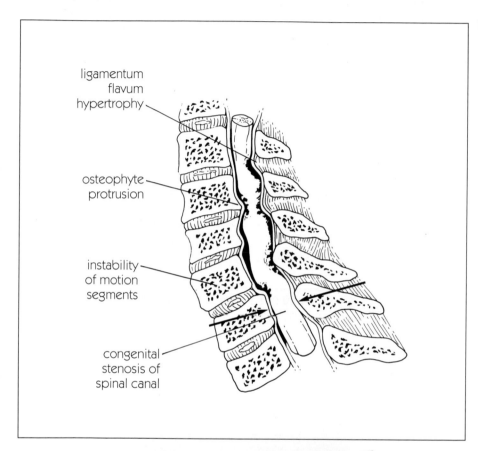

Figure 44.18 Factors leading to cervical spondylotic myelopathy.

ligamentum flavum hypertrophy

osteophyte protrusion

instability of motion segments

congenital stenosis of spinal canal

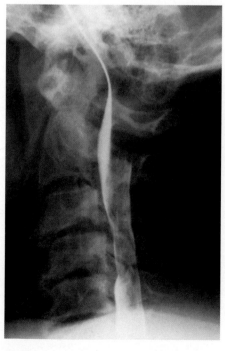

Figure 44.19 Cervical myelogram in a patient with multilevel spondylotic disease.

osteophytic spurring and narrowing of the spinal canal, and can also demonstrate associated changes in signal intensity within the spinal cord caused by repetitive microtrauma from opposing osteophytes. Neural foraminal stenosis is less well visualized than on myelography.

_____ NONOPERATIVE TREATMENT

Nonoperative treatment is similar to that for simple disc herniation. Bedrest with heat application, massage, physical therapy, and intermittent cervical traction may be helpful. A rigid cervical collar may also markedly improve the symptoms. The patient who is treated in this fashion must be followed for progression of neurologic deficit.

_____ SURGICAL OPTIONS

Partial Median Corpectomy With Strut Grafting

In patients with congenital spinal stenosis associated with cervical spondylosis and myelopathy, partial median corpectomy is the procedure of choice (Fig. 44.20). Through the standard anterolateral approach, the cervical spine is exposed. The vertebral bodies, the intervening discs, and the posterior longitudinal ligament are removed. The gap is filled with a strut graft, which is impacted under distraction. Creating a trough in the inferior surface of the vertebra above and the superior surface of the vertebra below allows stable seating of the graft. Internal stabilization can be carried out with plate and screws.

Cervical Decompressive Laminectomy With Luque Loop/Flexible Cable Stabilization

This procedure (Fig. 44.21) represents an alternative approach for patients with cervical myelopathy associated with spinal stenosis and multilevel spondylosis. Instead of dealing directly with the compressive pathologic process, which is situated anteriorly, additional room is provided for the spinal cord to expand by removing the laminae and spinous processes in the involved segments. The spinal cord then migrates back.

Laminectomy by itself does not provide optimal results—stabilization is required. This can be accomplished by anchoring a Luque loop or using flexible multistrand cables. The intervening facet joints are excised and filled with cancellous bone chips.

OSSIFICATION OF THE POSTERIOR LONGITUDINAL LIGAMENT

Rarely, the posterior longitudinal ligament itself becomes ossified (OPLL) (Fig. 44.22). This ossification is

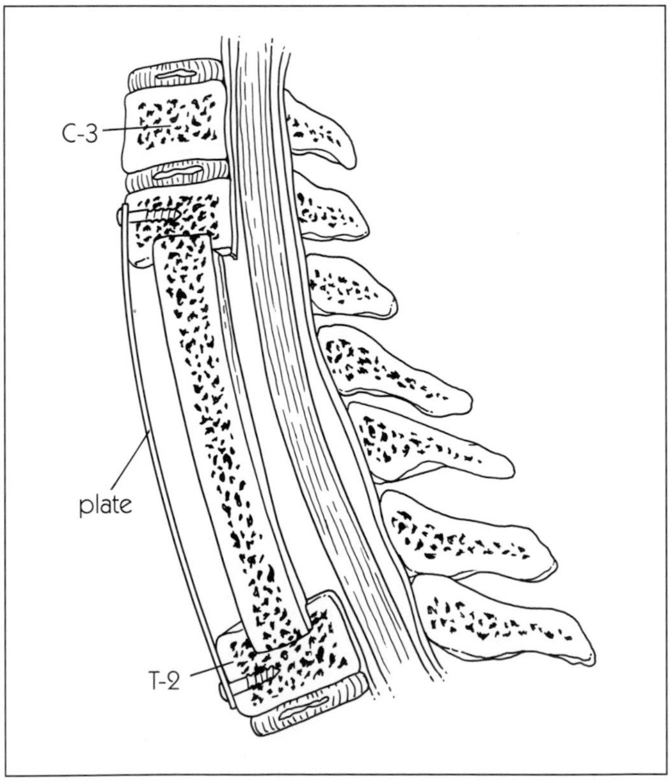

Figure 44.20 Partial median corpectomy with strut grafting.

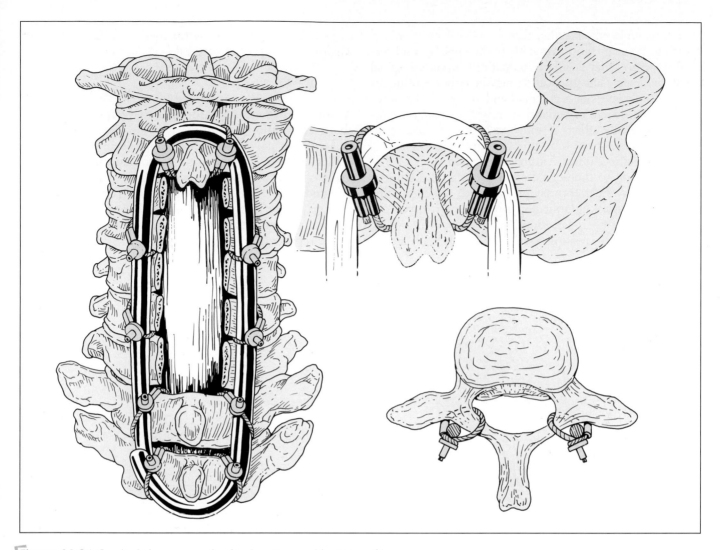

Figure 44.21 Cervical decompressive laminectomy with strut grafting.

Figure 44.22 Ossification of posterior longitudinal ligament.

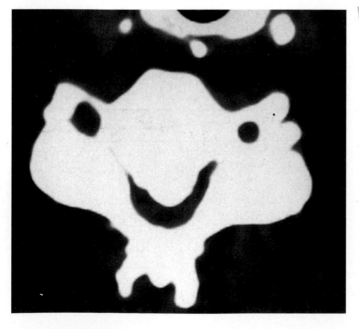

true bone replacement rather than simple calcification and spurring. It occurs most frequently in the upper to mid cervical spine and may encroach dramatically upon the spinal canal diameter.[6] The ossification may be either continuous over multiple levels or segmented and appears to be unrelated to the degree of cervical spondylotic changes. This condition usually afflicts in individuals over the age of 40 years and appears to be most prevalent in Japan.

The specific clinical features associated with OPLL vary according to the degree of root and cord compression. Again, the patient may present with radiculopathy, myelopathy, or myeloradiculopathy, although myelopathy appears to be most common in this setting. The diagnosis of OPLL can be established with plain lateral cervical spine films and confirmed with CT scanning. Treatment is typically surgical.

SURGICAL OPTIONS

Available surgical techniques include those described above. In addition, laminoplasty is sometimes an option.

Laminoplasty is indicated primarily in patients with OPLL. Instead of removing the laminae entirely, a lamina is opened on one side over a hinge on the opposite side and is anchored in that position (Fig. 44.23). This operation has not gained as much popularity as the anterior procedures because of the wide range of outcomes reported.

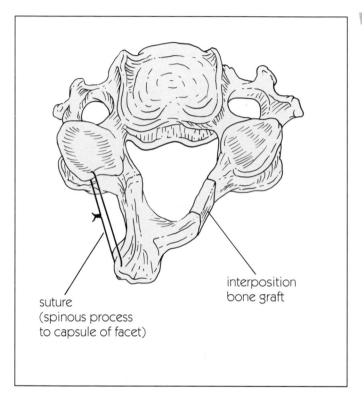

suture
(spinous process
to capsule of facet)

interposition
bone graft

Figure 44.23 Technique of laminoplasty.

REFERENCES

1. Mixter WJ, Barr JS. Rupture of the intervertebral disc with involvement of the spinal canal. *N Engl J Med.* 1934;211:210–215.
2. Dandy WE. Loose cartilage from the intervertebral disk simulating tumor of the spinal cord. *Arch Surg.* 1929;19:660–672.
3. Vanderburgh DF, Kelly WM. Radiographic assessment of discogenic disease of the spine. *Neurosurg Clin North Am.* 1993;4:13–33.
4. Wilkinson M. Historical introduction. In: *Cervical Spondylosis.* Philadelphia, Pa: WB Saunders Co; 1971.
5. Pallis C, Jones AM, Spillane JD. Cervical spondylosis: Incidence and complications. *Brain.* 1954; 274–289.
6. Bakay L, Cares HL, Smith RJ, Ossification in the region of the posterior longitudinal ligament as a cause of cervical myelopathy. *J Neurol Neurosurg Psychiatry.* 1970;33:263–268.

Chapter 45

Lumbar Intervertebral Disc Herniation

Robert H. Wilkins

NORMAL ANATOMY OF THE LUMBAR SPINE

An intervertebral disc is composed of three parts: the annulus fibrosus, the nucleus pulposus, and the cartilaginous plates (Fig. 45.1).[1-3] The annulus fibrosus is a tough outer ring composed of 10 to 12 concentric layers of fibrous tissue and fibrocartilage (Figs. 45.1, 45.2). It is reinforced anteriorly by the anterior longitudinal ligament and posteriorly by the posterior longitudinal ligament (Figs. 45.1–45.3). The nucleus pulposus, contained within this outer ring and slightly eccentric in a posterior direction (Figs. 45.1, 45.2), is a remnant of the notochord composed of a softer form of cartilage. In the child, the nucleus pulposus is semiliquid, but it becomes more solid and fibrous with age. Each lumbar intervertebral disc is bonded to the vertebral body above it by a thin plate of hyaline cartilage, and to the vertebral body below it by a similar thin plate of hyaline cartilage (Fig. 45.1). Each of these cartilaginous plates is an unossified segment of the vertebral body.

The bony arch that encircles the spinal canal posteriorly is formed by the two pedicles, two laminae, and the spinous process (see Fig. 45.2). The laminal arches of adjacent vertebrae are connected by an elastic yellow ligament, the ligamentum flavum (Fig. 45.1). The caudal end of the spinal cord, the conus medullaris, extends down to about the level of the L-1 vertebra. It is continuous inferiorly with a thin band called the filum terminale. The spinal canal in the lumbar area also contains the lumbar and sacral sensory and motor nerve rootlets, which in the aggregate are referred to as the cauda equina (Fig. 45.2). These nerve roots lie within a cylindrical sac of dura mater and arachnoid and are bathed by the CSF contained within the lumbar subarachnoid cistern.

At each spinal level, on each side, a nerve root containing both motor and sensory components exits from the dural sac. It then lies adjacent to the dural sac laterally for an inch or so before it turns further laterally to exit from the bony spinal canal one vertebral level below where it exited the dural sac. Therefore, the left L-5

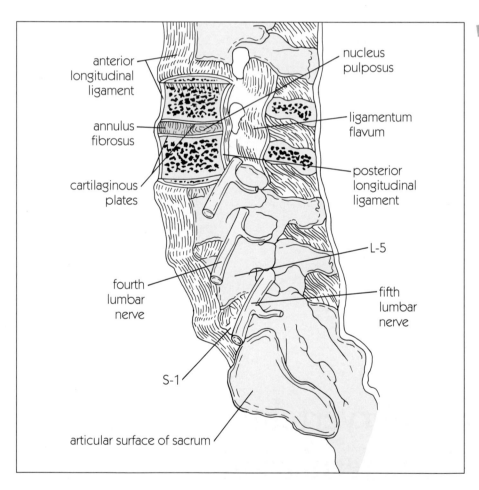

anterior longitudinal ligament

annulus fibrosus

cartilaginous plates

fourth lumbar nerve

S-1

articular surface of sacrum

nucleus pulposus

ligamentum flavum

posterior longitudinal ligament

L-5

fifth lumbar nerve

Figure 45.1 Sagittal view of the lumbar spine, with some components removed to better demonstrated the anatomy. (Modified from Keim HA, 1973)

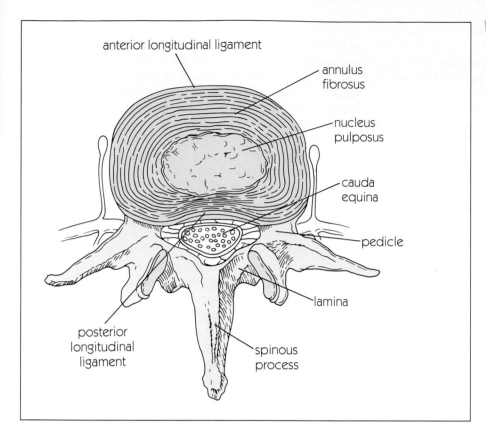

anterior longitudinal ligament

annulus fibrosus

nucleus pulposus

cauda equina

pedicle

lamina

posterior longitudinal ligament

spinous process

Figure 45.2 Axial view of the lumbar spine, showing an intervertebral disc, the contents of the spinal canal, and the elements of the posterior bony arch.

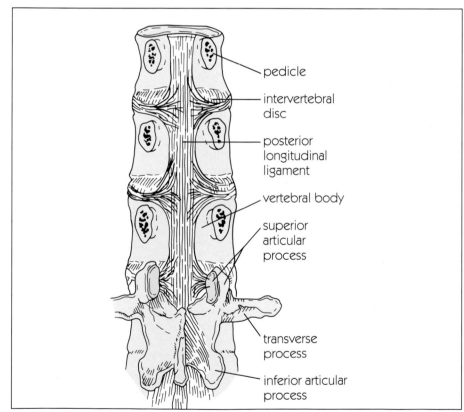

pedicle

intervertebral disc

posterior longitudinal ligament

vertebral body

superior articular process

transverse process

inferior articular process

Figure 45.3 Posterior view of the lumbar spine, with some components removed to show the posterior surface of the vertebral bodies and intervertebral discs, reinforced by the posterior longitudinal ligament. (Modified from Keim HA, 1973)

nerve root, which exits from the bony spinal canal through the left L5-S1 intervertebral foramen (just caudal to the left L-5 pedicle), actually leaves the dural sac at about the level of the L4-5 intervertebral disc (Fig. 45.5).

PATHOPHYSIOLOGY OF LUMBAR DISC HERNIATION

The nucleus pulposus may herniate in any direction out of its normal confines. If it herniates superiorly or inferiorly through the cartilaginous plate into the adjacent vertebral body, it is referred to as a Schmorl's nodule. Generally these are incidental findings noted radiographically or at autopsy.

Probably because the nucleus pulposus is situated somewhat posteriorly, and because the posterior longitudinal ligament reinforces the annulus fibrosus in the midline posteriorly, the majority of clinically significant disc herniations occur in a posterolateral direction. This process has been called by several names such as ruptured annulus fibrosus, herniated nucleus pulposus, ruptured disc, herniated disc, and slipped disc.[3-7]

The nucleus pulposus first herniates into tears in the concentric rings of the annulus fibrosus (Fig. 45.4A), even-

tually causing the remaining outer rings to bulge focally (disc protrusion) (Fig. 45.4B). If the process continues, the nuclear material may then escape from the disc (disc extrusion) to lie just anterior to the posterior longitudinal ligament (subligamentous disc herniation), or to lie free in the spinal canal (free fragment disc herniation) (Fig. 45.4C).

The usual posterolateral disc protrusion or disc extrusion ordinarily compresses the ipsilateral nerve root at its exit from the dural sac (e.g., a left L4-5 disc herniation compresses the left L-5 nerve root and a left L5-S1 disc herniation compresses the left S-1 nerve root) (Fig. 45.5). Such nerve root compression causes radicular symptoms and signs in the distribution of that specific nerve (Fig. 45.6). However, a centrally located disc herniation of significant size may involve several elements of the cauda equina on both sides of the midline, causing bilateral radiculopathy and even, at times, sphincteric disturbances such as urinary retention (Fig. 45.6).

In the lumbar area, approximately 95% of disc herniations occur at the L5-S1 or L4-5 level. Approximately 4% occur at the L3-4 level, and only about 1% at the L2-3 and L1-2 levels. Therefore, the physician evaluating a patient with a suspected lumbar disc rupture doesn't have many choices to consider in localizing the level of the lesion (Fig. 45.6).

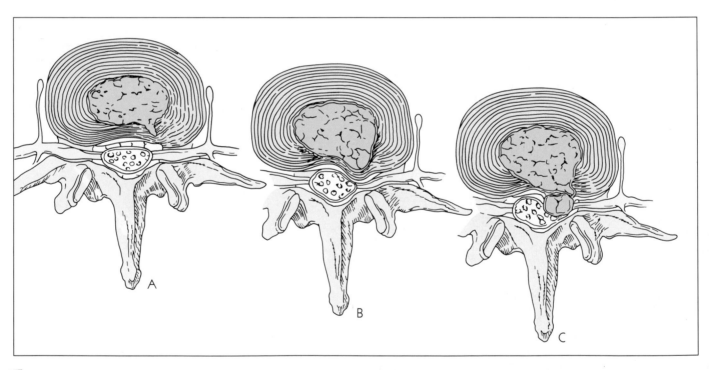

Figure 45.4 Stages in the herniation of an intervertebral disc. **(A)** Tearing of the rings of the annulus fibrosus. **(B)** Protrusion of the disc against the nerve root. **(C)** Extrusion of part of the nucleus pulposus, with further nerve root compression.

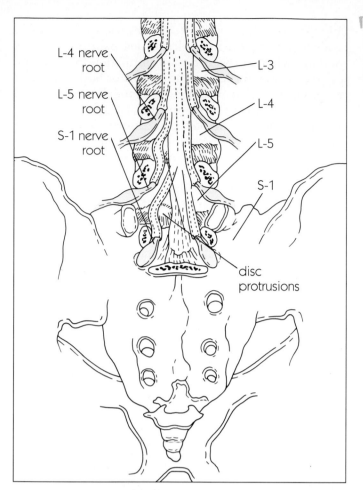

L-4 nerve root
L-5 nerve root
S-1 nerve root
L-3
L-4
L-5
S-1
disc protrusions

Figure 45.5 Posterior view of the lower lumbar spine. A disc protrusion at L4-5 on the left results in compression of the L-5 nerve root where it leaves the dural sac, but before it exits from the spinal canal. (Modified from Keim HA, 1973)

Figure 45.6 Typical Clinical Features of Unilateral Lumbar Herniated Nucleus Pulposus

Disc	Nerve Root	Pain	Paresthesias, Numbness	Weakness	Reflexes
L3-4	L-4	Lower back, buttock, lateral/anterior thigh, anterior leg	Anterior thigh, anterior leg	Quadriceps femoris	Knee jerk diminished or absent
L4-5	L-5	Lower back, buttock, lateral thigh, anterolateral calf, occasionally groin	Anterolateral calf to great toe	Dorsiflexion of foot, extension of great toe	Usually no changes
L5-S1	S-1	Lower back, buttock, lateral thigh and calf	Lateral calf to small toe	Plantarflexion of foot	Ankle jerk diminished or absent

SYMPTOMS AND SIGNS

The typical patient with a posterolateral lumbar disc rupture will have intermittent low back pain for a period varying from several weeks to several years and then also pain in the distribution of one sciatic nerve (sciatica). This pain is usually aggravated by movement of the back, by coughing or straining, or by standing or sitting for long periods. It tends to improve with bed rest. The patient may also notice tingling paresthesias or numbness and perhaps weakness in the distribution of the involved nerve (Fig. 45.6).

On physical examination, the patient usually demonstrates one or more of the following mechanical signs (Fig. 45.7): lumbar paravertebral muscle spasm, lumbar scoliosis, limitation by back and leg pain of low back motion such as forward flexion, limitation by back and leg pain of straight leg raising on one or both sides, and the production of pain along the sciatic distribution into the back by ipsilateral popliteal compression. The straight leg raising and popliteal compression tests cause pain by stretching the sciatic nerve, thereby pulling the involved nerve root in the lumbar spine more tightly against the herniated disc.

The patient may also have evidence of neurologic deficits in the distribution of the affected nerve root (Figs. 45.6, 45.7). There may be a reduction or loss of the ankle

---

Figure 45.7 Examination of Patient

Standing
Body build, posture
Deformities, pelvic obliquity,
   spine alignment
Paravertebral muscle spasm,
   spinal tenderness
Spinal column movements:
   flexion, extension, lateral
   bending, and rotation
Posterior sensation
Walking on toes
   (tests plantarflexion of feet)
Walking on heels
   (tests dorsiflexion of feet
   and extension of great toes)
Stepping onto step

Sitting on Table
Straight leg raising
Popliteal compression test
Knee jerks, ankle jerks
Anterior sensation
Strength of hip flexion,
   knee extension and flexion,
   foot dorsiflexion, great
   toe extension, and foot
   plantarflexion

Lying on Table
Supine
Straight leg raising:
1. Flex hip with knee extended
   (sciatic nerve stretch)
2. Flex hip with knee flexed

Prone
Spine extension
Hip extension

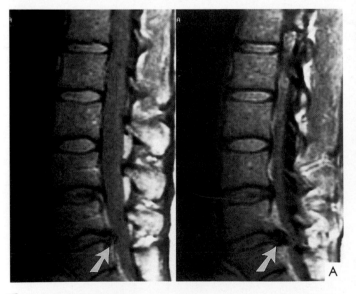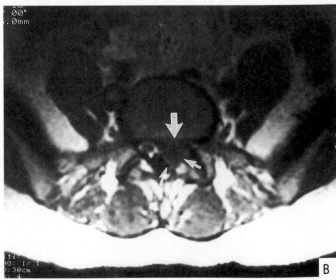

Figure 45.8 Two sagittal views (A) and one axial view (B) from an MRI study, showing a left posterolateral herniation of the L5-S1 intervertebral disc (arrows).

jerk or knee jerk, a reduction or loss of sensation to touch or pin-prick in a dermatomal distribution, or a reduction or loss of strength in certain muscle groups. The distribution of such neurologic deficits may permit the clinical localization of the disc rupture (Fig. 45.6).

DIAGNOSTIC STUDIES

Plain x-ray films of the lumbosacral spine and pelvis are obtained to rule out other causes of pain in the back and leg such as spondylolisthesis, a metastatic or primary neoplasm, a pyogenic or tuberculous infection, etc. If the back and leg symptoms continue despite conservative therapy, and surgical treatment is contem-

plated, the process can be delineated with an MRI study of the lumbar spine (Fig. 45.8) or a lumbar myelogram with a delayed CT scan (Fig. 45.9).

TREATMENT

Initially, most patients are treated conservatively for at least 2 weeks because the symptoms and signs will often resolve with this form of management. This is probably due to a reduction in the degree of disc protrusion and healing of the tears in the annulus fibrosus.

Such conservative therapy consists mainly of rest—ideally bed rest on a flat, firm mattress. Administration of an analgesic and a muscle relaxant may also help to

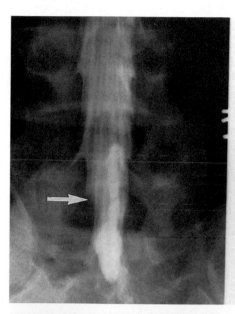
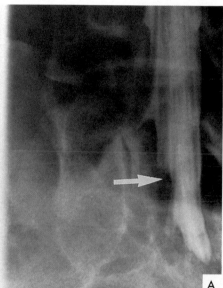
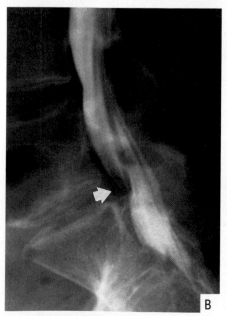
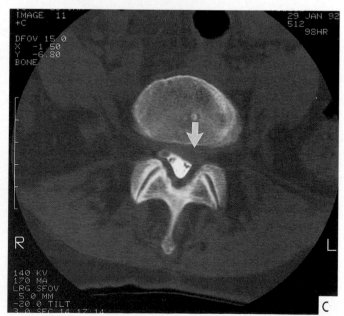

Figure 45.9 Anteroposterior (left) and oblique (right) (**A**) and lateral (**B**) views of a lumbar myelogram, showing a left posterolateral herniation of the L5-S1 intervertebral disc, impinging on the S-1 nerve root (arrows). (**C**) Axial view from the postmyelogram CT study, showing that a portion of a left posterolateral L5-S1 disc herniation has migrated superiorly behind the L-5 vertebral body (arrow).

reduce the discomfort, as may the application of a heating pad to the painful area. When the patient is again out of bed, the use of a lumbosacral corset for a few days or weeks may provide additional pain relief. After the period of pain has passed, lumbosacral exercises and attention to body mechanics (correct posture; use of preferred methods of lifting, sitting, and standing; etc.) may help prevent a recurrence.

If conservative measures do not provide sufficient relief, if significant weakness develops, or if urinary hesitancy or retention occurs, surgical treatment should be considered. At that point, an MRI scan or myelogram/CT scan is ordinarily obtained to provide information that is important in surgical decision-making, especially regarding whether to operate and the specifics of such an operation. Patients with a focal disc protrusion or a disc extrusion can usually be helped by a discectomy, but those with disc degeneration without focal protrusion or extrusion ordinarily cannot. In the circumstance of a diffusely bulging disc, the surgeon needs to decide whether there is sufficient nerve root compression to justify an attempt at operative relief.

The standard surgical treatment of a posterolateral lumbar disc herniation consists of a partial hemilaminectomy at the involved interspace on the appropriate side, with removal of the herniated disc material, removal of loose cartilage from within the disc, and decompression of the affected nerve root (Fig. 45.10).[2-9] For an unusually large disc herniation, a free fragment that has migrated, or a central disc herniation, a full bilateral laminectomy may be required to provide the necessary exposure. The patient usually recovers sufficiently to leave the hospital within 5 days after the operation and ordinarily is ready to return to work 4 to 6 weeks later.

In recent years, the operating microscope and microsurgical instruments have permitted a partial hemilaminectomy and discectomy to be performed through a smaller incision, with less tissue dissection and a somewhat more rapid recovery.[10,11] This procedure is referred to as a microsurgical lumbar discectomy. More recently, an approach has been introduced to permit the removal of lumbar disc tissue through a long metal cylinder of small diameter that is inserted into the disc through the

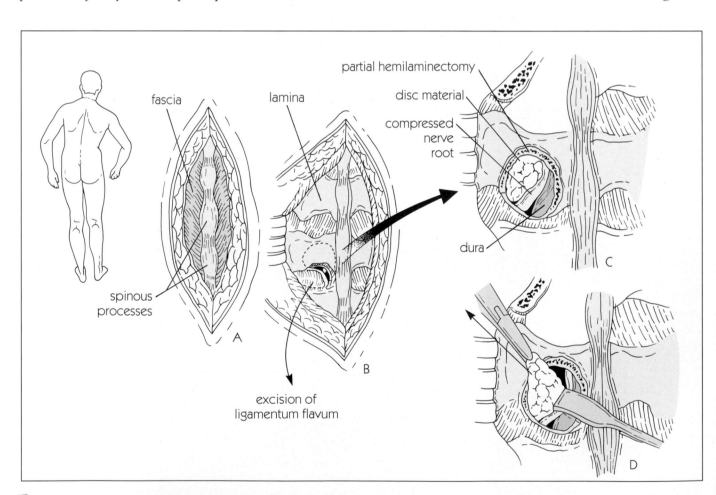

Figure 45.10 Posterior surgical approach to a lateral lumbar disc herniation. **(A)** This procedure ordinarily can be performed through a much shorter incision than that shown, with only unilateral exposure. **(B)** Portions of the adjacent laminae are removed, as is the ligamentum flavum. **(C,D)** The exposed nerve root is retracted medially and the herniated disc material is removed from its location anterior to the nerve root. (Modified from Netter FH, 1986)

Principles of Neurosurgery

skin of the back and the paravertebral muscles.[10] The value of this procedure, referred to as percutaneous lumbar discectomy, is still being assessed.[12]

For the ordinary lumbar disc herniation, a spinal fusion or a spinal stabilization procedure is not used. Such operations are considerably larger, with a longer incision, bilateral exposure, more tissue dissection, and a longer recovery time. Blood transfusion is commonly required during these procedures but is rarely needed during the standard or microsurgical lumbar discectomy.

About 85% to 95% of patients treated for a lumbar disc herniation by a partial hemilaminectomy and discectomy will have excellent or good relief. As a general rule, patients treated for a large disc extrusion fare better than those treated for a small disc protrusion, and those treated for a diffusely bulging disc are less likely to be helped than those with a disc extrusion or protrusion. Overall, about 15% of patients with a lumbar disc herniation will later have another disc herniation, either at the same location or at a different spinal level.

REFERENCES

1. Coventry MB, Ghormley RK, Kernohan JW. The intervertebral disc: its microscopic anatomy and pathology. *J Bone Joint Surg.* 1945;27:105–112, 233–247, 460–474.

2. DePalma AF, Rothman RH. *The Intervertebral Disc.* Philadelphia, Pa: WB Saunders Co; 1970.

3. Spurling RG. *Lesions of the Lumbar Intervertebral Disc With Special Reference to Rupture of the Annulus Fibrosus With Herniation of the Nucleus Pulposus.* Springfield, Ill: Charles C Thomas Publisher; 1953.

4. Hardy RW Jr. *Lumbar Disc Disease.* New York, NY: Raven Press; 1982.

5. Semmes RE. *Ruptures of the Lumbar Intervertebral Disc.* Springfield, Ill: Charles C Thomas Publisher; 1964.

6. Simeone FA. Lumbar disc disease. In: Wilkins RH, Rengachary SS, eds. *Neurosurgery.* New York, NY: McGraw-Hill; 1985:2250–2259.

7. Weinstein JN, Wiesel SW. *The Lumbar Spine.* Philadelphia, Pa: WB Saunders Co; 1990.

8. Cauthen JC. *Lumbar Spine Surgery: Indications, Techniques, Failures, and Alternatives.* 2nd ed. Baltimore, Md: Williams & Wilkins; 1988.

9. White AH, Rothman RH, Ray CD. *Lumbar Spine Surgery: Techniques & Complications.* St. Louis, Mo: CV Mosby Co; 1987.

10. Dunsker SB. Alternatives in the surgical treatment of herniated lumbar disks. *Clin Neurosurg.* 1989; 35:459–473.

11. Williams RW, McCulloch JA, Young PH. *Microsurgery of the Lumbar Spine.* Rockville, Md: Aspen Publishers; 1990.

12. Diagnostic and Therapeutic Technology Assessment (DATTA). Percutaneous lumbar diskectomy for herniated disks. *JAMA.* 1989;261:105–109.

13. Keim HA. Low back pain. *Clin Symp.* 1973; 25(3):1–32.

14. Netter FH. *Nervous System, Part II: Neurologic and Neuromuscular Disorders.* West Caldwell, NJ: CIBA Pharmaceutical Co; 1986:197. The CIBA Collection of Medical Illustrations, Volume I.

Lumbar Spinal Stenosis and Lateral Recess Syndrome

Philip R. Weinstein, Samuel F. Ciricillo

Patients suffering from lumbar spinal stenosis develop pain, paresthesias, numbness, and weakness in the back and legs due to entrapment of lumbosacral nerve roots in the constricted neural canal and foramina.[1] The symptoms and signs of central canal stenosis may mimic cauda equina syndrome due to tumor or fracture, while lateral recess stenosis may cause a unilateral or bilateral radiculopathy suggestive of a herniated disc syndrome.[2,3]

Lumbar spinal stenosis bears little or no relationship to physique or stature; it is a developmental variation that results in the formation of a neural arch smaller than normal in diameter and triangular rather than round (Fig. 46.1A,B).[4] The normal dimensions of the neural canal and its pathologic variations have been established from anatomic, radiologic, and surgical observations (Fig. 46.1C).[5–7] Acquired changes, including lumbar disc degeneration, ligamentous hypertrophy, and articular spondylosis, may be superimposed on the developmentally small neural canal and foramina, usually in later life (Fig. 46.2). Developmental stenosis is the sole cause of clinically significant radiculopathy in only 2% of patients with sciatica, but it is a predisposing factor that contributes to the effects of disc herniation or spondylosis in 30% of such patients.[8]

Congenital stenosis is most often due to diffuse skeletal dysplasias, such as achondroplastic dwarfism[9] or spondyloepiphyseal dysplasia. The neurologic complications of lumbar stenosis were first described by Sarpyener[10] in children born with dysraphic abnormalities. The surgical treatment of combined congenital and acquired lumbar stenosis in adults was first reported by Verbiest.[11]

PATHOGENESIS

Factors contributing to lumbar stenosis are listed in Figure 46.3. Embryogenesis of the lumbar vertebra begins after the seventh week of gestation. Two sets of paired chondrification centers form the vertebral body and neural arch (Fig. 46.4).[12] Fusion and ossification of growth centers in the vertebral body and pedicles are completed several years after birth. Theoretically, in

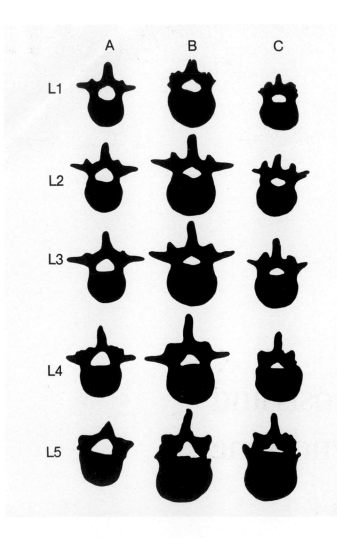

A

Figure 46.1 (A) Three sets of lumbar vertebrae from photographs of cadaver spinal preparations showing normal *A*, borderline *B*, and stenotic *C*, neural canals. Stenosis is most severe in L-4 and L-5 segments. In set *C*, the L-5 canal is triangular because the pedicles and laminae are shortened, which reduces the anteroposterior diameters of the midline canal and lateral recesses.

cases of developmental spinal stenosis or dwarfism, stenosis may result from premature cessation of growth or fusion at these sites. While symptomatic lumbar stenosis and cervical stenosis may occur together in up to 50% of patients with myelopathy,[13] thoracic spinal stenosis not associated with dwarfism is rare.[14]

Developmental lumbar stenosis requiring surgical treatment is three times more prevalent in females.[2] Although most cases are sporadic, familial cases of stenosis not associated with dwarfism have been re-ported,[15] which suggests that genetic factors may be involved. Relatively low prevalence rates were reported for lumbar stenosis before the era of CT and MRI.[16] Now that more accurate methods of diagnosis are available, the prevalence rates need to be updated.

In patients with lumbar stenosis, the pedicles and laminae are short and thick, and therefore the facets extend downward almost to the floor of the canal and inward almost to the midline (see Fig. 46.2). The anteroposterior diameter of the canal may be less than 12

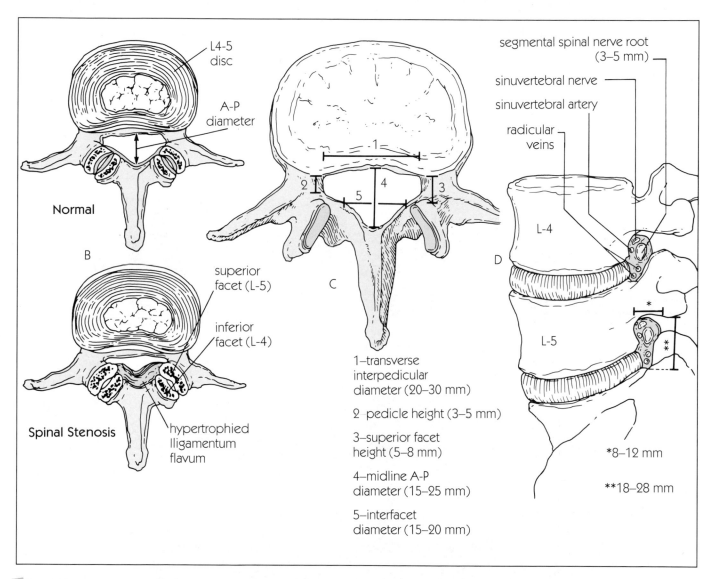

Figure 46.1 *continued* (B) Detailed diagrams of axial sections at the L4-5 level of normal and stenotic neural canals illustrate the anatomical features of both developmental and acquired factors that contribute to entrapment radiculopathy due to lumbar stenosis. Note the almost complete obliteration by stenosis of the subarachnoid space, which normally occupied approximately 80% of the cross-sectional area of the thecal sac. Axial section (C) and lateral view (D) of vertebrae at L4-5 showing measurements of normal and stenotic lumbar vertebral canal and foramina. Although these measurements may vary depending to a certain extent on the CT or MR scan technique and settings used, they are useful guidelines for diagnostic purposes, especially in borderline cases. (A: Reproduced with permission from Weinstein, 1982; C,D: Adapted with permission from Wilson CB, ed. *Neurosurgical Procedures: Personal Approaches to Classic Operations.* Baltimore: Williams & Wilkins, 1992: ch. 20)

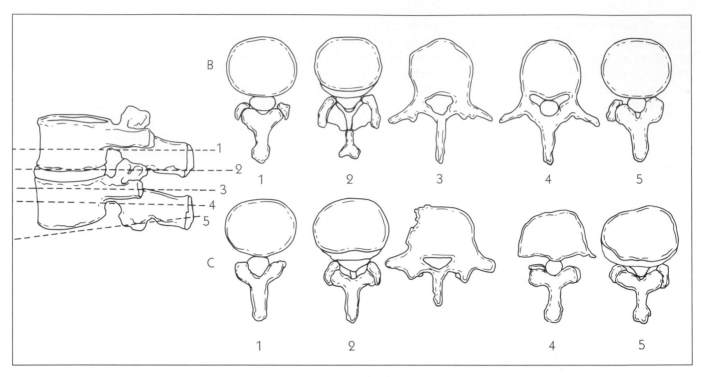

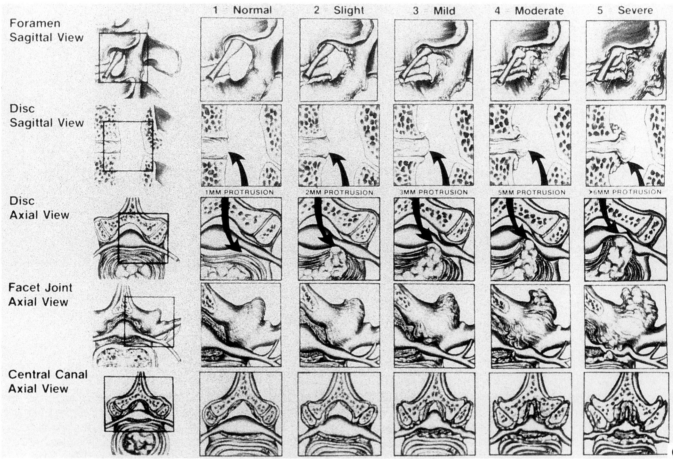

	1 Normal	2 Slight	3 Mild	4 Moderate	5 Severe
Foramen Sagittal View					
Disc Sagittal View	1MM PROTRUSION	2MM PROTRUSION	3MM PROTRUSION	5MM PROTRUSION	>6MM PROTRUSION
Disc Axial View					
Facet Joint Axial View					
Central Canal Axial View					

Figure 46.2 Serial axial sections at L4-5 with localization diagrams illustrate **(A)** a case of severe developmental lumbar stenosis without significant degenerative changes at the midbody level or at the level of disc and facets and **(B)** a case of severe acquired ligamentous hypertrophy with disc and facet osteophytes superimposed upon mild developmental narrowing without significant stenosis at the midbody level. **(C)** A grading system for assessing the relative severity of factors contributing to stenosis on CT scans or MR images. (B: Adapted with permission from Schonstrum NS, Boldender NF, Spengler DM, 1985; C: Reproduced with permission from Kerber CW, Glenn WV Jr, Rothman SLG. Lumbar computed tomography/multiplanar reformations: a reading primer. In: Post MJ, ed. *Computed Tomography of the Spine.* Baltimore, Md: Williams & Wilkins; 1984:164)

mm centrally and less than 4 mm in the lateral recesses and foramina. The transverse interpedicular diameter may be less than 25 mm (see Fig. 46.1C). Disc protrusion anteriorly and massive hypertrophy of the ligamentum flavum posteriorly may encroach further upon the space available for nerve roots,[17] substantially reducing the circumferential area of the thecal sac and eliminating the cushion of CSF surrounding the cauda equina.[18]

The pathogenesis of spondylosis, which originates with aging and degeneration of the intervertebral disc, has been described in detail.[17] In younger patients, acute lumbosacral radiculopathy in the sciatic, or less often femoral, nerve distribution is most often due to primary disc injury and displacement. In elderly patients, chronic radicular symptoms are more likely to be associated with spondylostenosis (Fig. 46.5A). Char-

Figure 46.3 Pathogenesis of Lumbar Spinal Stenosis

A. Congenital/Developmental
1. Idiopathic
2. Achondroplasia/hypochondroplasia
3. Hypophosphatemic vitamin D-resistant rickets (spondyloepiphyseal dysplasia)
4. Morquio's mucopolysaccharidosis
5. Spinal dysraphism (lipoma, myelomeningocele)

B. Acquired
1. Degenerative
   a. Spondylosis
   b. Spondylolisthesis
   c. Scoliosis
   d. Ossification of the posterior longitudinal ligament
   e. Ossification of the ligamentum flavum
   f. Intraspinal synovial cysts
2. Postoperative
   a. Laminectomy
   b. Fusion
   c. Fibrosis

3. Traumatic
   a. Laminectomy
   b. Kyphosis/scoliosis
   c. Burst fracture
4. Metabolic/endocrine
   a. Epidural lipomatosis (Cushing's disease)
   b. Osteoporosis (pathologic fractures)
   c. Acromegaly
   d. Pseudogout (calcium pyrophosphate dihydrate deposition disease)
   e. Renal osteodystrophy
   f. Hypoparathyroidism
5. Skeletal
   a. Paget's disease of bone
   b. Ankylosing spondylitis
   c. Rheumatoid arthritis
   d. Diffuse idiopathic skeletal hyperostosis (DISH)

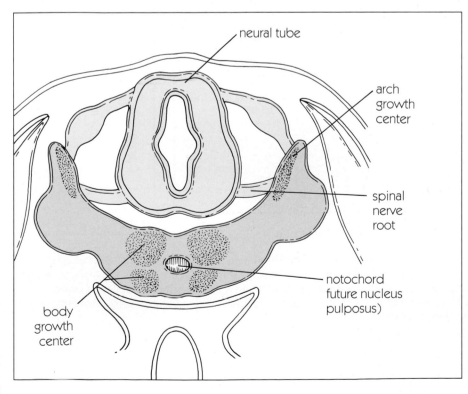

Figure 46.4 Developing lumbar vertebra shows bilateral paired vertebral body growth centers that join after 9 weeks' gestation to form a single chondrification site. Premature cessation of growth in the neural arch could result in short pedicles and laminae and reduce the size of the neural canal, resulting in developmental lumbar stenosis.

acteristic alterations of normal articular anatomy include cartilaginous degeneration and osteophyte proliferation at sites of attachment of the annulus, facet capsule, and ligamentum flavum (Fig. 46.5B). Chronic discogenic osteophyte protrusion is virtually ubiquitous, but it may not be the most important compressive element.

Degenerative spondylolisthesis (pseudospondylolisthesis) is a relatively common complication of lumbar spondylosis that results in anterior subluxation of the upper vertebra not associated with spondylolysis (Fig. 46.5C).[19] Although the malaligned intervertebral joint is usually stable, severe nerve root entrapment may ensue, especially beneath the hypertrophic ligamentum flavum and anteriorly displaced inferior facet in the lateral recess at the level of or just below the affected disc.

Other spinal disorders that may cause lumbar stenosis (see Fig. 46.3) are disc space infection, osteomyelitis, Pott's disease, and postsurgical or posttraumatic deformities.[20,21] Systemic skeletal disorders, including Paget's disease, rheumatoid or ankylosing spondylitis, and diffuse idiopathic skeletal hyperostosis, may also cause or contribute to caudal radiculopathy. Metabolic and endocrine abnormalities, such as acromegaly, pseudogout, hypoparathyroidism, renal osteodystrophy, and Cushing's disease with epidural lipomatosis, may also be associated with lumbar stenosis.

CLINICAL PRESENTATION

The most characteristic feature of the syndrome of lumbar spinal stenosis is back and leg pain caused by standing, aggravated by walking, and relieved by rest in a flexed or seated position (Fig. 46.6).[2] The symptom patterns and neurologic signs vary among patients and in the same patient. For example, the pain may be sharp and lancinating in a neurologically localized lower extremity distribution, or it may be dull, aching, and of gradual onset in the sacroiliac and posterolateral thigh areas.[22] In cases of central canal stenosis, the pain may be bilateral, although not necessarily symmetric; in cases where the lateral recess is the most prominent site of nerve root entrapment, it may describe a pattern that suggests a unilateral monoradiculopathy.[3,23,24] Symptoms of sensory and motor dysfunction, often in the same anatomic distribution as the radicular pain, may also be present.

Lumbar stenosis is usually a chronic condition, often beginning with many years of low-back pain punctuated with acute but temporary episodes of incapacitating lumbago with or without sciatica (see Fig. 46.5A). Initial or recurrent symptoms are associated in some cases with trauma or unusual physical stress. Often the history includes a satisfactory response to medical therapy after a previous diagnosis of acute sprain, disc herniation, or even fracture. Many patients with recurrent

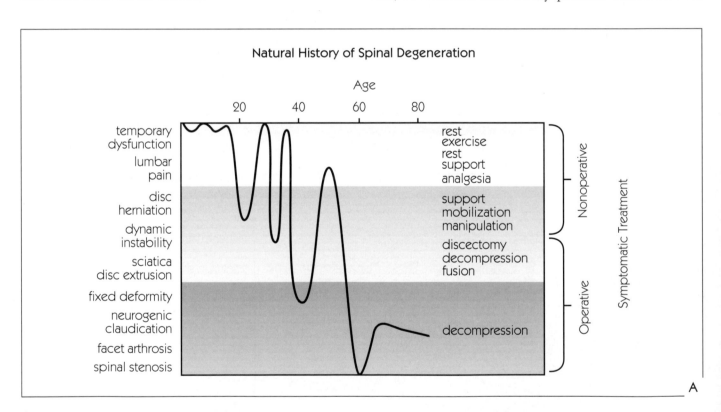

Figure 46.5 (A) The natural history of symptomatic degenerative lumbar disc disease and spondylosis, showing the progression from temporary symptoms of low back pain to those of acute sciatic radiculopathy and ultimately to a pattern of chronic neurogenic claudication as initial disc degeneration leads to herniation, which results in spondylosis that aggravates the underlying stenosis. Treatment is initially medical and includes physiotherapy, but recurrent disability or lack of recovery from a flare-up may necessitate surgical treatment.

symptoms have already undergone discectomy or laminectomy and sometimes fusion as well. In fact, residual or recurrent stenosis is a frequent cause of relapse or persistence of radiculopathy after failed lumbar spinal decompression.[25]

The age at presentation varies inversely with the severity of the developmental component of the stenosis. Thus, in cases of dwarfism or severe primary stenosis, the acute onset of excruciating sciatica, sometimes associated with paralytic lumbosacral radiculopathy, may occur at 20 to 30 years of age. Acute paraplegia may be due to a relatively mild disc protrusion that obliterates an already constricted subarachnoid space (Fig. 46.7). More common is presentation in the seventh, eighth, or even ninth decade, with progressive loss of the capacity to stand and walk because of leg pain or paresthesias with or without mild motor and reflex deficits (Fig. 46.8). In very elderly patients, the medical risks of surgical decompression for spondylotic lumbar radiculopathy may be justified to avoid lost independence and restriction to bed or wheelchair.

The symptoms that help to distinguish lumbar stenosis from other causes of caudal radiculopathy are the neurogenic claudication, postural aggravation, and cauda equina syndromes (see Fig. 46.1).[26] Neurogenic claudication consists of the progressive onset of radicular pain, paresthesias, numbness, and eventually, in some cases, weakness initiated or aggravated by walking. The order of onset and the severity of these symptoms may vary. In fact, numbness, fatigue, or weakness

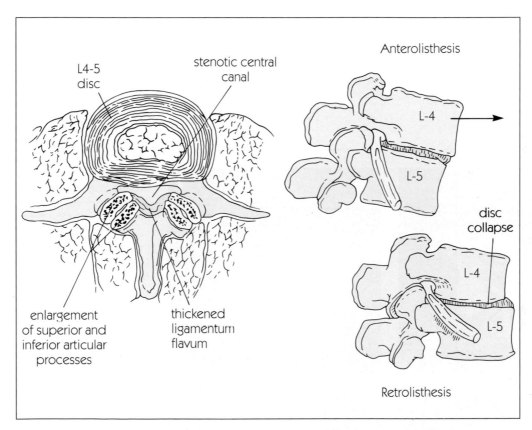

Figure 46.5 *continued* (B) Lumbar intervertebral joint showing degenerative changes at bone attachment sites on the annulus of a collapsing disc, thickening of the ligamentum flavum, and the ossifying hypertrophic facet capsule. These structural alterations, which contribute to nerve root compression in acquired lumbar stenosis, result from the excessive biomechanical stresses and relative hypermobility of the motion segment that follow desiccation and loss of functional competence of the disc. (C) Drawing of the L4-5 intervertebral joint showing the stenotic deformity resulting from degenerative spondylolisthesis, which may cause compression of either the L-5 roots (anterolisthesis) or the L-4 roots (retrolisthesis). Subluxation also results from degenerative collapse of the disc and from incompetence of the facet joints, whose articular surfaces may be oriented in a more vertical than oblique plane. (A: Adapted with permission from Hing KY, Kirkaldy-Willis WH, Shannon R, Wedge JH. Anatomy, pathology and pathogenesis of lateral spinal stenosis. In: Lin PM, ed. *Posterior Lumbar Interbody Fusion.* Springfield, Ill: Charles C Thomas Publisher; 1982:174)

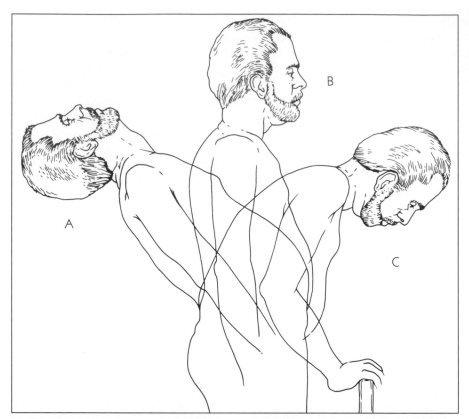

Figure 46.6 Postures that initiate, aggravate, and relieve symptoms of lumbosacral radiculopathy in cases of spinal claudication syndrome. (A) Extended posture (reaching overhead or backward) causes acute or gradual onset of radiculopathy. (B) Erect posture causes pain similar to that in the extended posture, and the patient cannot remain standing. (C) Flexed posture relieves pain produced by A or B and may be the only position in which the patient may walk comfortably. Some patients may get relief by leaning forward on a counter or by ambulating with a walker. In severe cases, the lateral recumbent knee-chest position may be the only pain-free posture.

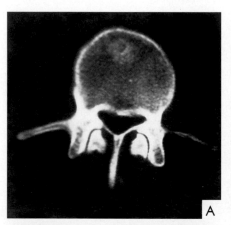
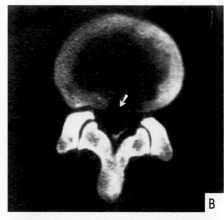
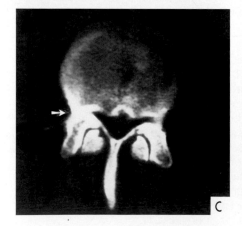
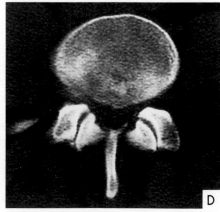

Figure 46.7 CT scan obtained in a mentally retarded 28-year-old laborer with short stature who had subacute back and leg pain followed by the acute onset of paraparesis, urinary retention, incontinence, and an L-3 sensory level shows midline disc herniation at L3-4 and L4-5 with severe developmental stenosis. Axial images were obtained at the L-3 pedicles (A), the bulging L3-4 disc (arrow) (B), the shortened L-4 pedicles (arrow) (C), and L4-5 (D). Bulging discs aggravate severe congenital stenosis in B and C. A sharp-pointed triangular (trefoil) canal configuration typical of lumbar stenosis is apparent in C; stenosis is slightly less severe in D. The anteroposterior canal diameter was 8 mm at the L-3 midbody level. Recovery was only partial after wide decompressive laminectomy and foraminotomies without discectomy. After decompression the thecal sac dilated to more than twice its preoperative circumference.

to the extent of footdrop or knee-buckling may occur without or before the appearance of pain. Incapacitating sensory dysesthesias may also occur without pain or weakness. These symptoms are characteristically relieved within minutes by sitting, but not by merely standing, as is often the case with claudication due to iliofemoral arterial stenosis.[27] Other features that distinguish neurogenic from vascular claudication relate to differences between the effects of nerve and muscle ischemia (Fig. 46.9).

In cases of neurogenic claudication, patients can often walk farther without rest during shopping while

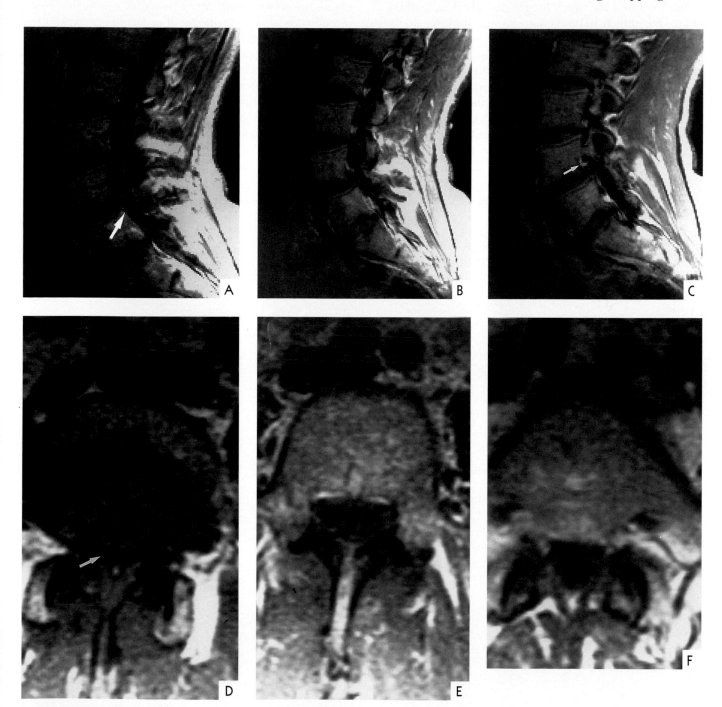

Figure 46.8 MRI scans of a 72-year-old man with postural aggravation of leg pain, neurogenic claudication, and bilateral footdrop demonstrable only after walking two blocks. Midline sagittal (A), near lateral (B), and far lateral sagittal (C) images show severe central canal (arrow) (A) and lateral recess (B) but not foraminal stenosis (arrow) (C) that is focal at L3-4 and L4-5. Axial images show severe thecal sac constriction (arrow) at the L4-5 disc level (D) and subarticular nerve root compression in the lateral recesses. The patency of the foramina and the absence of canal stenosis are confirmed by images of L-4 (E) and L-5 (F) obtained at the midbody levels above and below the site of focal stenosis.

leaning forward on a market basket than they can while standing erect to cross the parking lot. Similarly, a tennis player may be able to finish a set played in a relatively crouched position and then be unable to walk less than a block back to the car. Bicycling, especially with the handle bars lowered to allow lumbar flexion, is often tolerated for much longer periods than walking.[27] Thus, for elderly patients with lumbar stenosis, an exercise bike may be the only way to engage in aerobic activity required for weight reduction or cardiac rehabilitation. The ability to perform a bicycling exercise in the supine position can be used to distinguish neurogenic from vascular claudication syndromes.

The pathogenesis of radiculopathy during neurogenic claudication remains speculative.[27] Paresthesias, pain, and weakness are thought to result from relative nerve root ischemia due to physiologic activation during walking in the presence of compression of the radicular microcirculation by stenosis.[28,29] During experimental limb tourniquet compression in one study, the nerve fibers first became hyperexcitable, and spontaneous volleys of afferent impulses were recorded; later a reversible conduction block was observed.[30] This sequence of events might explain the occurrence of paresthesias and pain followed by numbness and weakness in cases of neurogenic claudication. When an ambulation-induced increase in the metabolic rate of the nerve root cannot induce a compensatory increase in blood flow and substrate availability, the resulting microvascular insufficiency is thought to result in the ischemic radiculopathy of neurogenic claudication.[28]

Figure 46.9 Differential Diagnosis of Arteriovascular and Neurospinal Claudication Syndromes

| | Iliofemoral Arterial Insufficiency | Lumbosacral Nerve Root Entrapment | |
		Ischemic	Mechanical
Pain	characteristic (cramping)	present or absent (radicular)	present or absent (radicular)
Induced by	muscular contraction (muscle ischemia)	axonal activation	lordotic posture (axonal compression)
Location	exercised muscles	lumbosacral (sciatic)	lumbosacral (sciatic)
Spread	absent	up or down	usually down
Character	usually cramping, dull	varies, often dysesthetic	varies, often lancinating
Relieved by	rest (standing)	rest (standing)	flexion posture or sitting
Motor deficit	rare; during walking, exercised muscles cramp and spasm	mild, variable; aggravated by any leg activity	mild, variable; aggravated by walking but not by bicycling
Sensory deficit	rare	mild, variable	mild, variable
Lasègue's sign	normal	frequently normal	normal
Pulse	femoral or distal pulse decreased	normal	normal
Arterial bruit	iliofemoral	absent	absent
Lumbar radiographs and ultrasound	arterial calcification	abnormal lumbar spine (osteophytes, short pedicles)	abnormal lumbar spine (osteophytes, short pedicles)
Aortography	diagnostic	normal	normal
Myelogram, CT, MRI	normal	diagnostic	diagnostic

The syndrome of postural aggravation of radiculopathy, or spinal claudication, consists of the immediate onset of back and leg pain upon standing in an erect or hyperextended position. The pain is rapidly relieved by sitting or bending forward (Fig. 46.10). Thus, patients may have greater difficulty walking uphill or upstairs than downhill or downstairs.

Postural aggravation of radiculopathy is more readily understood than neurogenic claudication, as lumbar lordosis and extension are known to aggravate stenosis of the neural canal and foramina (see Fig. 46.10).[1] In the extended position, disc protrusion may increase if spondylotic ossification has not already stabilized the annulus or fused the joint. The interlaminar space is reduced, and "shingling," or overlapping, of the rostral edge of the lower lamina under the caudal edge of the upper lamina occurs. The ligamentum flavum relaxes and buckles inward, increasing its dorsolateral mass effect. Rostral and anterior migration of the superior facets further constricts the foramina, while caudal movement of the inferior facets may further narrow the lateral recesses. Thus, the postural aggravation of radiculopathy may be explained by intermittent direct neural compression, which stimulates or inhibits nerve root function, as the patient moves into the erect or extended position.

The cauda equina syndrome includes intermittent or progressive symptoms of urinary or fecal incontinence, impotence, and sensory loss in the "saddle" distribution. In lumbar stenosis, in contrast to acute disc extrusion or chronic tumor progression, the onset of sacral paresthesias, incontinence, and paraparesis may be related to standing and walking. Bladder control may be lost only if ambulation continues after the onset of pain, paresthesias, and weakness because rest is impossible. Severe compromise of the neural canal that causes sacral nerve root compression, usually at L3-4 or L4-5 in the midline, is responsible for the impairment of sphincter control and perineal sensation.

In our earlier series, patients with cauda equina syndrome often had a complete myelographic block; however, the prognosis for recovery was quite good.[2]

Neurologic deficits may be absent or intermittent in patients with lumbar stenosis, being temporarily detectable only after ambulation and not at rest. Because involvement of the midlumbar segments is most common, sensory and motor deficits and reflex changes may herald L-4 and L-5 rather than S-1 root involvement. However, correlation of observed deficits with the anatomic sites of root entrapment demonstrated radiographically may be complex. For example, absence of the patellar reflex may result from L-4 root compression due to canal stenosis at L2-3 or L3-4, disc protrusion and inferior facet or ligamentous osteophyte at L3-4, lateral recess stenosis at L3-4, or far lateral disc and superior facet encroachment in the foramen at L4-5 (Fig. 46.11). Often, bilateral stenosis is associated with only unilateral symptoms. Pain and deficit patterns that implicate only one root pair may be associated with radiographic abnormalities at more than one level. Finally, the stenosis may be unilateral and asymmetric or discontinuous with a skipped level in between. A narrow central canal may be associated with a normal lateral recess and foramina, or the midline anteroposterior canal diameter may be normal and the lateral recess severely stenotic.

Surprisingly, the straight leg-raising test is most often negative in patients with lumbar stenosis.[2] This finding may help to differentiate spondylotic radiculopathy from that due to disc herniation, where nerve root displacement and inflammation may lower the threshold to stretch-induced, mechanical stimulation of the nerve root. In fact, the straight leg-raising maneuver may relieve the root compression by reducing the baseline lumbar lordosis that is present in the supine position or even by flexing the lower spine as the hip is flexed and the pelvis tilts backward.[26]

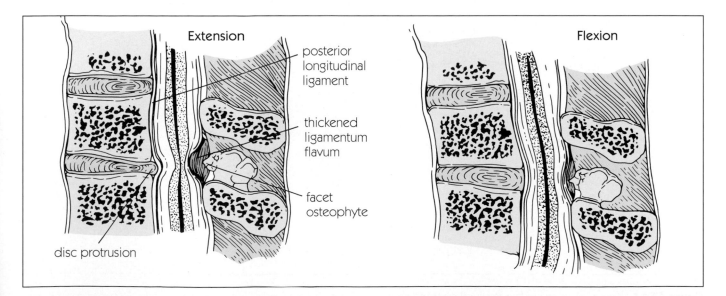

Figure 46.10 Effects of extension and flexion on the lumbar spine. Diagrams of a lumbar motion segment in the lateral view illustrate aggravation of stenosis by disc protrusion anteriorly and folding of the ligamentum flavum posteriorly during extension; this is relieved by flexion. Similar effects in the lateral recesses have been observed by CT scanning during extension and flexion.

DIAGNOSIS

The clinical history often distinguishes lumbar stenosis from other causes of radiculopathy. The level, side, and severity of involvement may be identified by the neurologic examination, including tests of anal sphincter tone and strength, sacral sensation, and, when a history of dysuria or incontinence is obtained, urodynamic studies of bladder function. Electromyography and sensory conduction studies may also help to localize the site(s) of involvement.[22] Electrophysiologic studies may be normal at rest but abnormal after ambulation induces symptoms of neurogenic claudication.

Spinal radiographs are needed to demonstrate degenerative changes in the discs and facet joints as well as evidence of instability, traumatic deformity, spondylolisthesis, or scoliosis. Skeletal disorders, such as osteoporosis, Paget's disease, and dwarfism, may be identified. Lumbar stenosis may be diagnosed in some cases by measuring the anteroposterior diameter of the neural canal and foramina on lateral radiographs. Accurate localization of lumbar lesions also requires radiographic identification of anatomic variations in the number of lumbar vertebra due to such anomalies as lumbarization of S-1 or sacralization of L-5.

Definitive diagnostic information is most readily obtained from lumbar spinal MR images or CT scans with sagittal reconstructions. These studies clearly show the size, shape, and anatomic relationships of spinal and neural elements (see Fig. 46.7) and can demonstrate the relative contribution of developmental stenosis, as well as disc, facet, and ligamentous elements of nerve root compression. MRI, when available, is the preferred initial scanning procedure.[31] The conus medullaris and cauda equina, as well as the individual nerve roots, can be seen without intrathecal injection of myelographic contrast material by lateral cervical or lumbar puncture often required to demonstrate the neural structures with CT (see Fig. 46.8). Direct multiplanar MR image construction provides more precise anatomic detail on sagittal images than CT. However, CT remains the best choice for detailed imaging and analysis of osseous anatomy and pathology.

For postoperative studies, intravenous administration of a paramagnetic contrast agent is an invaluable aid in differentiating peridural scar from recurrent disc herniation or stenosis on MRI. For postoperative studies or when MRI is not available, intrathecal administration of contrast material before CT scanning is advis-

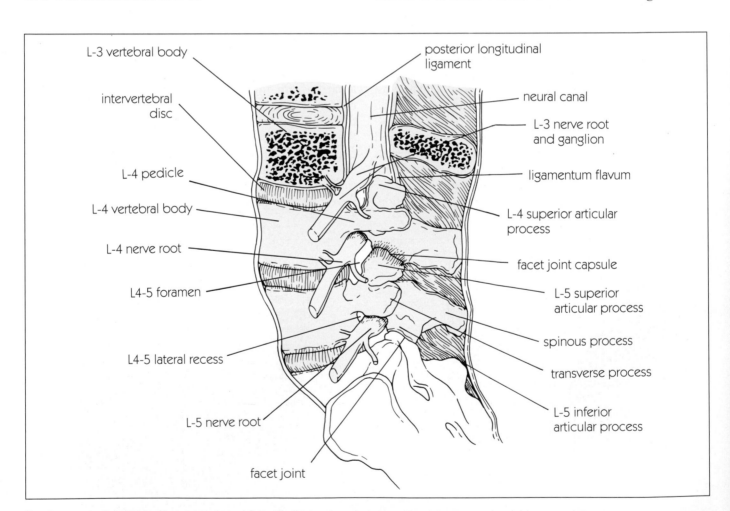

Figure 46.11 Normal anatomy of the midlumbar spine showing sites of potential compression of an individual nerve root (L-4 or L-5) in spinal stenosis: neural canal L3-4 (disc L-3, inferior articular process L-4), lateral recess L4-5 (superior articular process L-4), foramen L4-5 (superior articular process L-5, disc L-4).

Principles of Neurosurgery

able to demonstrate the subarachnoid space and neural elements.[32]

Myelography is now rarely, if ever, required to diagnose lumbar stenosis. However, it does provide a remarkable demonstration of the pathophysiology of the postural effects that produce spinal claudication. A severe "hourglass" constriction or complete obstruction of the subarachnoid space seen in the prone (extended) position is usually partially or completely relieved in the flexed knee-chest or sitting position (see Fig. 46.10).

TREATMENT

Medical management begins with rest and analgesic, antispasmodic, and, when tolerated, nonsteroidal antiinflammatory medications. Some patients may benefit from a brief (3 to 5 day) course of systemic corticosteroid administration or a series of three epidural steroid injections above the stenotic levels every 2 weeks. The aim is to reduce inflammation, which may contribute to nerve root compression by aggravating swelling due to edema. Use of a lumbar corset or flexion orthosis may relieve pain

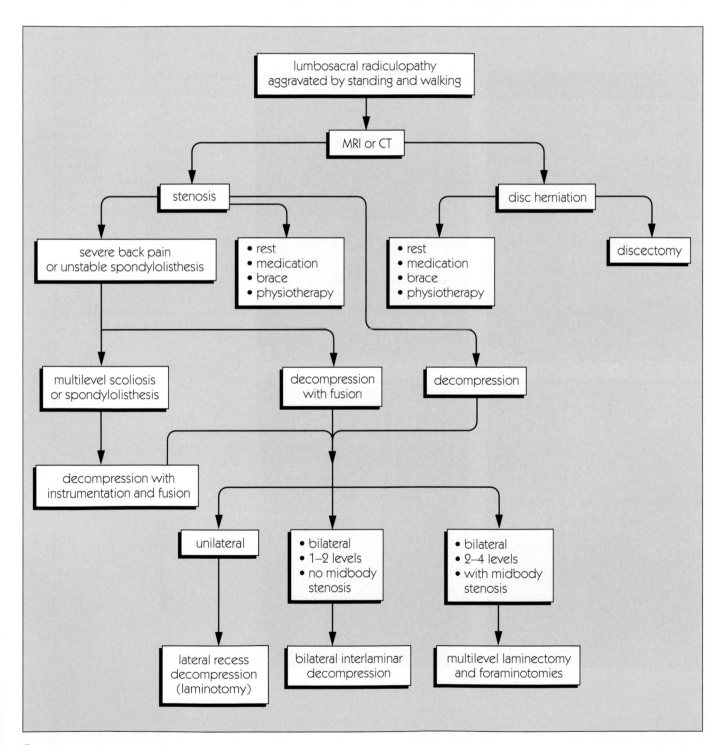

Figure 46.12 Protocol for the management of lumbar stenosis and lateral recess syndrome.

and facilitate ambulation. A walker may provide support for walking while the lower back remains flexed. Physiotherapy may help to alleviate pain, improve mobility and posture, and strengthen the abdominal and paravertebral musculature. Although these nonsurgical therapies may provide temporary relief, painful radiculopathy may recur upon resumption of normal activity.

Surgical treatment is indicated in the rare cases of progressive radicular neurologic deficit and cauda equina syndrome that do not respond to medical therapy. However, in patients without neurologic deficit, the most common indication for surgery is recurrent intolerable pain that restricts or prevents activities of daily living.

Selecting the most effective surgical procedure requires detailed analysis of the clinical and radiographic data (Fig. 46.12).[3] The goals of surgery are to decompress fully the thecal sac and exiting nerve roots and to minimize the risk of resulting spinal instability. Decompression of the stenotic lumbar spine is a technically difficult operation (Fig. 46.13). The initial muscle dissection for vertebral exposure demands meticulous hemostasis to avoid excessive blood loss. Intraoperative radiographic localization of the involved levels is essential. Removal of hypertrophic bone and osteophytes requires the use of heavy bone-cutting instruments and a power drill. The final ligament removal, dural exposure, and nerve root

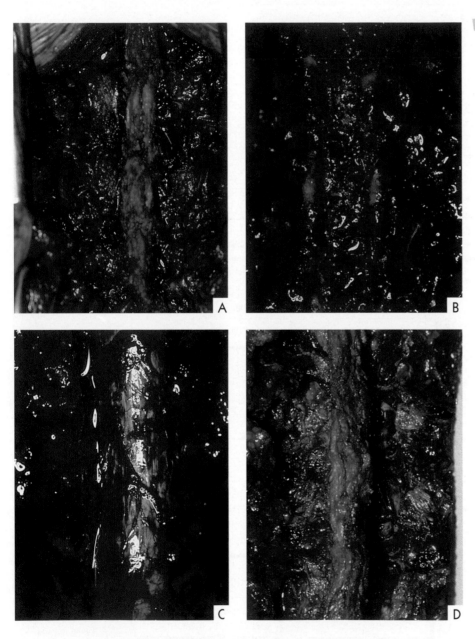

Figure 46.13 Surgical photographs showing the anatomy and operative procedures for decompression of lumbar stenosis or lateral recess syndrome. (A) Incision of lumbar fascia and retraction of detached dorsal paravertebral muscles. (B) Resection of spinous processes and creation of trenches at the junction of lamina and facets. (C) Completion of laminectomy and medial facet resection sufficient to explore the nerve roots and decompress the foramina by undercutting. (D) Interlaminar decompression without laminectomy as shown here on the right preserves the spinous processes and supraspinous ligaments as well as a central strut of the lamina.

Principles of Neurosurgery

decompression are delicate dissections that require powerful illumination and microsurgical technique. The normal epidural fat layer may be atrophic; adhesions between ligamentum flavum and dura may increase the risk of dural laceration and nerve root injury. Repair within the narrow spinal canal may be difficult because the surgical exposure is also limited by increased venous bleeding that follows drainage of CSF. To avoid further injuring compressed nerve roots, care must be taken not to place large instruments, such as curettes or rongeurs, within the stenotic neural canal or foramina.

The standard surgical approach for the relief of lumbar stenosis is a wide laminectomy with bilateral foraminotomies (Fig. 46.14A,B). The number of levels to be operated on and the lateral extent of decompression are determined by inspecting and measuring the canal on MR images or CT scans. This procedure is required in all patients with developmental stenosis severe enough to reduce the midbody anteroposterior canal diameter as demonstrated on axial sections just below the level of the pedicles (see Fig. 46.2). In such cases, the entire lamina as well as the medial facet must be removed to insure an adequate decompression.

When relative stenosis is primarily due to spondylosis, interlaminar decompression by bilateral laminotomies and foraminotomies may be performed at one or more levels to unroof the neural canal and lateral recesses without sacrificing the laminae, spinous processes, and supraspinous ligaments (Fig. 46.14C–F).[33] Although this procedure is somewhat more difficult and lengthy than the standard laminectomy approach, especially if performed at multiple levels, it has two major advantages: It preserves the neural arch, which protects the dura and nerve roots from epidural scarring, and it provides a site for paravertebral muscles and ligaments to reattach. This less destructive operation is thought to assist in maintaining spinal stability, especially in patients with degenerative spondylolisthesis or scoliosis.

In patients with lateral recess syndrome due to focal lumbar spondylosis and stenosis causing unilateral radiculopathy at a single level, simple interlaminar laminotomy and foraminotomy on the affected side should relieve symptoms. However, as in a full laminectomy procedure, substantial surfaces of the superior and inferior facets are required for an adequate decompression that completely unroofs the lateral recess and exposes the medial surface of the pedicle (see Fig. 46.14). Care must be exercised to preserve the pars interarticularis so as to prevent inadvertent inferior facetectomy. Undercutting techniques are used to remove the ligamentum flavum entirely and to resect the rostral portion

of each superior facet that contributes to foraminal stenosis. A malleable probe or angled dissector is used to verify that the foraminotomies are adequate.

Discectomy or removal of ventral osteophytes is rarely if ever required for adequate decompression of lumbar stenosis. Unless an extruded soft disc is encountered, the disc should be left intact to preserve the stability of the degenerated and partially resected intervertebral joint postoperatively. Because instability occurs after laminectomy in only 2% to 15% of patients over 35 years of age,[34,35] spinal fusion is usually not indicated as a part of the initial decompressive procedure. However, in patients with severe back pain or preoperative instability due to degenerative spondylolisthesis demonstrated on lateral flexion-extension radiographs, and in advanced cases of rotoscoliosis requiring complete bilateral facetectomy, fusion and internal fixation may be indicated as part of the primary procedure.[36] Secondary fusion is rarely necessary in patients over 50 years of age.

After surgical treatment, good or excellent results and return to premorbid activity levels have been reported in 80% to 85% of cases.[22,37,38] However, some patients may not be able to resume work requiring heavy physical labor. Patients with advanced chronic radicular neurologic deficits associated with muscle atrophy are unlikely to recover fully. Low back pain in the paravertebral area, which may be due to underlying degenerative arthritis rather than to an entrapment radiculopathy, is the least likely symptom to be relieved by decompressive surgery[39,40]; however, in many patients surgery eliminates the preoperative claudication-like low back and sacroiliac pain aggravated by ambulation. Perhaps such pain is triggered by ischemic activation of the posterior ramus, the dorsal root ganglia, or the nerve fibers that innervate the articular facets and paraspinous musculature.

CONCLUSION

Lumbar stenosis is an important cause of painful and incapacitating radiculopathy that has been diagnosed more frequently as the population has aged and as improved spinal imaging methods, such as MRI and CT, have become available. Surgical decompression is indicated when back and leg pain initiated and aggravated by standing and walking becomes disabling or intolerable or when progressive neurologic deficit develops. The results of wide laminectomy or more limited interlaminar lateral recess decompression are gratifying when normal ambulation and activity are restored.

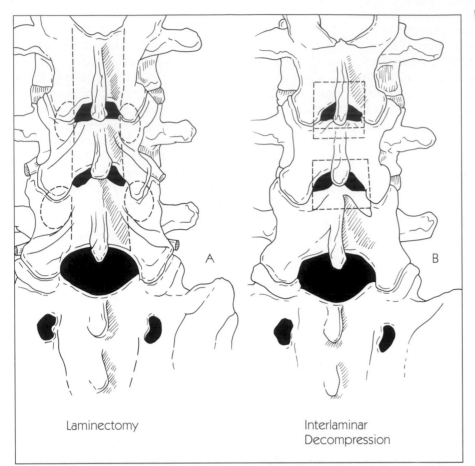

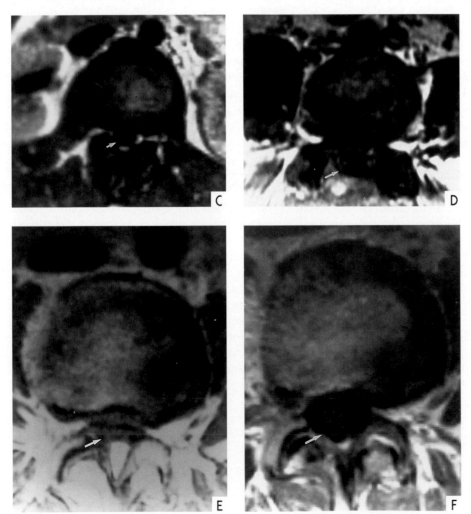

Laminectomy

Interlaminar
Decompression

Figure 46.14 Landmarks for adequate extent and prudent limits of bone resection (dotted lines) during laminectomy (**A**) and interlaminar decompression (**B**). Preoperative (**C**) and postoperative (**D**) axial MR images at L4-5 after laminectomy as well as before (**E**) and after (**F**) interlaminar decompression for stenosis at the L3-4 intervertebral disc level. These figures illustrate the preoperative constriction (arrows) and postoperative expansion (arrows) of the thecal sac in the cases presented in Figures 46.6 and 46.7, respectively.

Principles of Neurosurgery

REFERENCES

1. Weinstein PR. Diagnosis and management of lumbar spinal stenosis. *Clin Neurosurg*. 1983;30 677–697.
2. Weinstein PR. Lumbar stenosis. In: Hardy RW, ed. *Lumbar Disc Disease*. New York, NY: Raven Press; 1982:257–276.
3. Lee CK, Rauschning W, Glenn W. Lateral lumbar spinal canal stenosis: classification, pathologic anatomy and surgical decompression. *Spine*. 1988;13: 313–320.
4. Epstein BS, Epstein JA, Lavine L. The effect of anatomic variations in the lumbar vertebrae and spinal canal on cauda equina nerve root syndromes. *Am J Roentgenol Radium Ther Nucl Med*. 1964;91:1055–1063.
5. Kirkaldy-Willis W, Heithoff KB, Tchang S, et al. Lumbar spondylosis and stenosis: correlation of pathological anatomy with high-resolution computed tomographic scanning. In: Post MJ, ed. *Computed Tomography of the Spine*. Baltimore, Md: Williams & Wilkins; 1984:546–569.
6. Schonstrom NS, Bolender NF, Spengler DM. The pathomorphology of spinal stenosis as seen on CT scans of the lumbar spine. *Spine*. 1985;10:806–811.
7. Eisenstein S. Lumbar vertebral canal morphometry for computerized tomography in spinal stenosis. *Spine*. 1983;8:187–191.
8. Paine K, Haung P. Lumbar disc syndrome. *J Neurosurg*. 1972;37:75–82.
9. Epstein JA, Malis LI. Compression of spinal cord and cauda equina in achondroplastic dwarfs. *Neurology*. 1955;5:875–881.
10. Sarpyener MA. Congenital stricture of the spinal canal. *J Bone Joint Surg*. 1945;27:70–79.
11. Verbiest H. A radicular syndrome from developmental narrowing of the lumbar vertebral canal. *J Bone Joint Surg*. 1954;36B:230–237.
12. Angevine JB. Clinically relevant embryology of the vertebral column and spinal cord. *Clin Neurosurg*. 1973;20:95–113.
13. Epstein NE, Epstein JA, Carras R, et al. Coexisting cervical and lumbar spinal stenosis: diagnosis and management. *Neurosurgery*. 1984;15:489–496.
14. Barnett GH, Hardy RW Jr, Little JR, et al. Thoracic spinal canal stenosis. *J Neurosurg*. 1987;66:338–344.
15. Postacchini F, Massobrio M, Ferro L. Familial lumbar stenosis: case report of three siblings. *J Bone Joint Surg*. 1985;67A:321–323.
16. Teng P, Papatheodorou C. Lumbar spondylosis with compression of cauda equina. *Arch Neurol*. 1963;8:221–228.
17. Kirkaldy-Willis WH. Pathology and pathogenesis of lumbar spondylosis and stenosis. *Spine*. 1978;3: 319–328.
18. Weinstein PR. The application of anatomy and pathophysiology in the management of lumbar spine disease. *Clin Neurosurg*. 1980;27:517–540.
19. Ehni G. Surgical treatment of spondylotic caudal radiculopathy. In: Weinstein PR, Ehni G, Wilson CB, eds. *Lumbar Spondylosis: Diagnosis, Management and Surgical Treatment*. Chicago, Ill: Year Book Medical Publishers; 1977: 146–183.
20. Moreland LW, Lopez-Mendez A, Alarcon GS. Spinal stenosis: a comprehensive review of the literature. *Semin Arthritis Rheum*. 1989;19:127–149.
21. Weisz GM. Post-traumatic spinal stenosis. *Arch Orthop Trauma Surg*. 1986;106:57–60.
22. Hall S, Bartleson JD, Onofrio MB, et al. Lumbar spinal stenosis. *Ann Intern Med*. 1985;103:271–275.
23. Epstein JA, Epstein BS, Rosenthal AD, et al. Sciatica caused by nerve root entrapment in the lateral recess: the superior facet syndrome. *J Neurosurg*. 1972;36:584–589.
24. Reynolds AF, Weinstein PW, Wachter RD. Lumbar monoradiculopathy due to unilateral facet hypertrophy. *Neurosurgery*. 1982;10:480–486.
25. Quencer RM, Murtagh FR, Post JD, et al. Postoperative bony stenosis of the lumbar spinal canal: evaluation of 164 symptomatic patients with axial radiography. *AJR*. 1978;131:1059–1064.
26. Dyck P, Pheasant IIC, Doyle JB, et al. Intermittent cauda equina compression syndrome: its recognition and treatment. *Spine*. 1977;2:75–81.
27. Wilson CB. Significance of the small lumbar spinal canal: cauda equina compression syndromes due to spondylosis. *J Neurosurg*. 1969;31:499–505.
28. Watanabe R, Parke WW. Vascular and neural pathology of lumbosacral spinal stenosis. *J Neurosurg*. 1986;64:64–70.
29. Evans JG. Neurologic intermittent claudication. *Br Med J*. 1964;2:985–987.
30. Denny-Brown D, Brenner C. Paralysis of nerve induced by direct pressure and by tourniquet. *Arch Neurol Psychiatry*. 1944;51:1–26.
31. Schnebel B, Kingston S, Watkins R, et al. Comparison of MRI to CT in the diagnosis of spinal stenosis. *Spine*. 1989;14:332–337.
32. Bolender NF, Schonstrom NSR, Spengler DM. Role of computerized tomography and myelography in the diagnosis of central spinal stenosis. *J Bone Joint Surg*. 1985;67A:240–245.
33. Lin PM. Internal decompression for multiple levels of lumbar spinal stenosis: a technical note. *Neurosurgery*. 1982;11:546–549.
34. White AH, Wiltse LL. Postoperative spondylolisthesis. In: Weinstein PR, Ehni G, Wilson CB, eds. *Lumbar Spondylosis: Diagnosis, Management and Surgical Treatment*. Chicago, Ill: Year Book Medical Publishers; 1974:184–194.
35. Shenkin HA, Hash CJ. Spondylolisthesis after multiple bilateral laminectomies and facetectomies for lumbar spondylosis. *J Neurosurg*. 1979;50:45–47.
36. Epstein JA, Epstein BS, Lavine LS. Surgical

treatment of nerve root compression caused by scoliosis of the lumbar spine. *J Neurosurg.* 1974; 41:449–454.

37. Verbiest H. Results of surgical treatment of idiopathic developmental stenosis of the lumbar vertebral canal. A review of twenty-seven years' experience. *J Bone Joint Surg.* 1977;59B:181–188.

38. Russin LA, Sheldon J. Spinal stenosis: report of series and long term follow-up. *Clin Orthop.* 1976; 155:101–103.

39. Grabias S. The treatment of spinal stenosis. *J Bone Joint Surg.* 1980;62A:308–313.

40. Johnsson KE, Uden A, Rosen I. The effect of decompression on the natural course of spinal stenosis: a comparison of surgically treated and untreated patients. *Spine.* 1991;16:615–619.

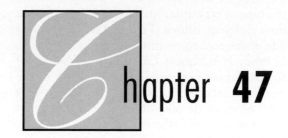

Trigeminal Neuralgia

Robert H. Wilkins

Trigeminal neuralgia, also known as tic douloureux, is a characteristic type of repetitious unilateral facial pain that can arise from different causes (Fig. 47.1).[1-4] It involves the right side of the face more often than the left side in about a 3:2 ratio. It is almost exclusively a disorder of adults, with the commonest time of onset being in the sixth and seventh decades. Less than 10% of patients experience the onset of tic douloureux before the age of 40. Women are more often affected than men in a ratio that has varied from 2:1 to 4:3 in reported series.

ETIOLOGY AND PATHOGENESIS

Tic douloureux can be caused by any of a number of conditions affecting the ipsilateral trigeminal system (Fig. 47.2).[4] In the majority, the etiology seems to be compression of the trigeminal nerve at its exit from the pons by an adjacent artery that has elongated with time to become wedged against the nerve. In about 5% to 8% of cases, the pain results from a benign tumor in the cerebellopontine angle such as a meningioma, epidermoid tumor, or acoustic neuroma. And about 2% to 3% of cases arise from multiple sclerosis. A variety of other rare etiologic associations have been reported, but all of these together probably do not account for more than a few percent of cases. Finally, in a significant number of patients the etiology of the tic douloureux is not apparent.

Various theories have been proposed to explain how the conditions just enumerated actually cause tic douloureux.

For example, some authors have postulated that demyelination resulting from neural compression by a blood vessel or tumor or resulting from multiple sclerosis is an important feature, perhaps permitting ephaptic transmission between adjacent axons. However, as attractive as such ideas are, no theory has yet been postulated that explains all aspects of tic douloureux such as the pain-free periods, which may last months early in the course of the condition.

CLINICAL FEATURES

Tic douloureux is diagnosed on the basis of the patient's history (see Fig. 47.1). Typically, the pain is sudden in onset, severe in degree, and short in duration, with each paroxysm usually lasting less than a minute. Although it is ordinarily spontaneous in onset, it can frequently be triggered by a nonpainful stimulus such as touching the skin on that side of the face, chewing, or talking. It has been described as lancinating, lightning-like, or electrical in quality, and has been likened to the pain experienced when a dentist drills into the unanesthetized pulp of a tooth. The patient may wince in response to the pain, hence the name tic douloureux. The pain is confined to some part of the distribution of one trigeminal nerve (see Fig. 47.2) and more commonly affects the lower part of the face than the upper.

The pain of untreated tic douloureux occurs unpredictably. Often the patient experiences many paroxysms

---

Figure 47.1 Characteristics of Trigeminal Neuralgia (Tic Douloureux)

Confined to an area within the distribution of one trigeminal nerve, most often within the lower two thirds of the face

Sudden, lancinating, severe, brief pain

Repetitious, but with significant pain-free intervals

Can be triggered by a nonpainful stimulus

Ordinarily prevented or reduced by carbamazepine

Almost exclusively a disorder of adults

Involves the right side of the face more often than the left (about a 3:2 ratio)

Affects women more often than men (about a 2:1 to 4:3 ratio)

Has various causes

---

of pain within a single hour, and such bouts may go on for days, with some fluctuation in frequency from hour to hour and day to day. Then a spontaneous remission may occur. Early in the course of the syndrome, pain-free periods lasting months are common, but as time goes on these natural remissions tend to become less frequent and less prolonged.

Often the patient who develops tic douloureux sees the dentist first, because lancinating lower facial pain seems to be arising from a certain tooth or teeth. Such teeth may be pulled or other dental procedures performed without providing relief. The patient may consult more than one physician before the correct diagnosis is made.

DIAGNOSIS

As already indicated, the diagnosis of tic douloureux is based on the history. The neurologic examination is ordinarily normal, with the exception that those few patients with multiple sclerosis or a large structural lesion such as a tumor in the cerebellopontine angle usually have altered trigeminal sensation and other evidence that heralds the underlying disorder. Likewise, diagnostic radiologic studies such as CT or MRI are normal in the usual patient with tic douloureux, but they are performed to identify the exceptional patient with a recognizable etiologic condition such as those just mentioned.

TREATMENT

Many effective treatments have been developed for tic douloureux, but none is successful in all cases. Furthermore, the individual patient frequently requires more than one form of treatment during the course of the disease.

In those few patients with an abnormality along the path of the trigeminal nerve that can be detected radiologically, such as a neoplasm in the cerebellopontine angle, the treatment is directed against the lesion that

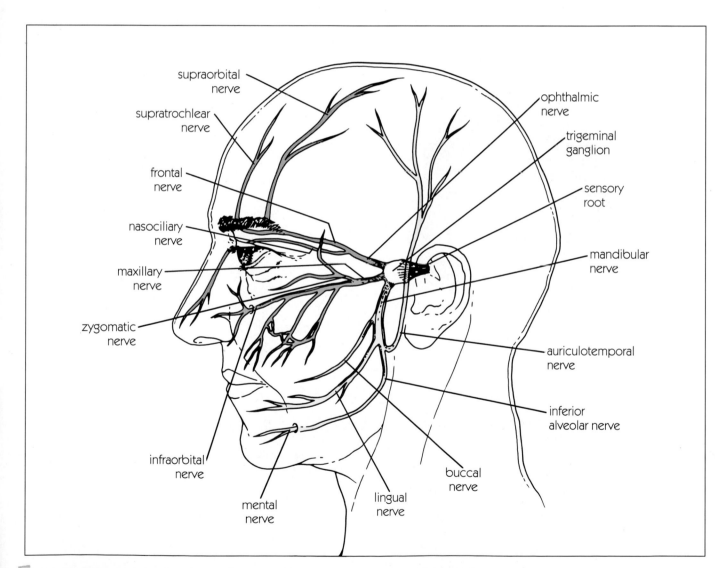

Figure 47.2 The peripheral and central aspects of the trigeminal nerve and its branches.

has been demonstrated. This approach ordinarily will also relieve the tic douloureux. However, most patients do not fall into this category and must be treated in other ways.

MEDICATION

The anticonvulsants carbamazepine and phenytoin have been found to reduce or control the pain of tic douloureux. Likewise, baclofen may have a beneficial effect.

Carbamazepine is ordinarily begun at a dosage of 200 mg/d and is increased as tolerated to 200 mg three or four times a day, or more. The goal is to reach the smallest dose that provides adequate pain relief. At high doses the patient may experience the side effects of lethargy, sluggish thinking, and imbalance. Carbamazepine may also interfere with the production of blood elements and may alter hepatic function. Therefore, a patient being treated with carbamazepine should have periodic complete blood counts and hepatic function studies.

Phenytoin is ordinarily begun at a dosage of 100 mg three times a day, and baclofen at a dosage of 5 or 10 mg three times a day. These also can cause side effects and need to be monitored from that standpoint.

Any of these three medicines is used alone at first, and is increased as needed to control the facial pain. With time, a patient may need progressively larger dosages to provide the same degree of relief. The development of toxicity may necessitate a reduction in the dosage, and the occurrence of some other significant side effect may require cessation of the medication altogether. In this case, a second drug may be added to or substituted for the first. At times, it may be necessary to use all three.

PERIPHERAL BRANCH INJECTION OR AVULSION

One of the peripheral branches of the trigeminal nerve may be injected with a neurolytic agent such as alcohol, or it may be surgically divided or avulsed. This approach provides pain relief at the expense of sensation. If a peripheral branch is injected, numbness of the face in its distribution will result. However, with time the nerve branch regenerates and both sensation and pain return. A somewhat more prolonged effect can be achieved by dividing or avulsing the nerve branch. For example, injection of the infraorbital nerve can be expected to give relief for about 1 year, whereas avulsion of the infra-

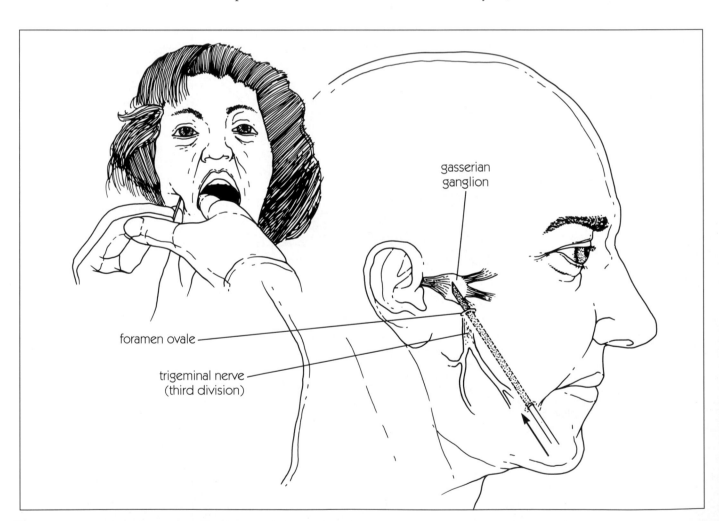

Figure 47.3 Percutaneous trigeminal/gasserian rhizolysis. The needle is inserted through the cheek into the third division of the trigeminal nerve at the foramen ovale and is advanced into the gasserian ganglion and sensory root.

orbital nerve will ordinarily provide pain relief for 2 to 3 years.[3,4]

TRIGEMINAL OR GASSERIAN RHIZOLYSIS

In these procedures, the gasserian ganglion and adjacent sensory root of the trigeminal nerve are injured, with the expectation that a more permanent effect can be achieved because neural regeneration is less likely to occur in these areas than in the peripheral trigeminal branches. In the past, anterior trigeminal rhizotomy was performed by exposing and dividing or otherwise injuring part or all of the main trigeminal sensory root adjacent to the gasserian ganglion.[2,3]

At present, this procedure is ordinarily done by inserting a needle through the cheek into the third division of the trigeminal nerve at the foramen ovale, and then advancing the needle into the gasserian ganglion and sensory root (Fig. 47.3).[1,5–7] The neural destruction is produced by injecting a neurolytic agent such as glycerol, by using a radiofrequency current to create a thermal lesion, or by inflating a small balloon to compress the neural tissue. In general, patients are relieved for a longer period than they are by the injection or avulsion of a peripheral branch. However, some degree of facial hypesthesia is expected with this form of treatment as well.

With radiofrequency lesioning, more than 60% of patients will have excellent pain relief and another 25% or so will have good relief.[7] Approximately 5% to 10% will not obtain relief initially or will have an early recurrence of pain; during the 5 years after the procedure, about 25% will experience recurrence.[5,6] With glycerol gasserian rhizolysis, the results are not quite as good: there is a 5% to 15% incidence of early failure and about a 20% to 30% incidence of later failure.[5,6]

MICROVASCULAR DECOMPRESSION OR POSTERIOR TRIGEMINAL RHIZOTOMY

Because it seems that vascular compression of the trigeminal nerve at its entrance into the pons is a common etiologic factor in trigeminal neuralgia, an operation has been devised to move the offending vessel(s) away from the nerve. This procedure is referred to as microvascular decompression because it involves an operating microscope and microsurgical technique. The area is exposed through a lateral posterior fossa craniectomy (retromastoid craniectomy), and after the vessel or vessels are separated from the nerve, a material such as a synthetic sponge is inserted to maintain the separation (Fig. 47.4). This procedure ordinarily provides pain relief without any facial sensory loss.

If no significant vascular compression is identified at operation, the main sensory root of the trigeminal nerve can be partially divided adjacent to the pons (posterior trigeminal rhizotomy). This has a similar probability of pro-

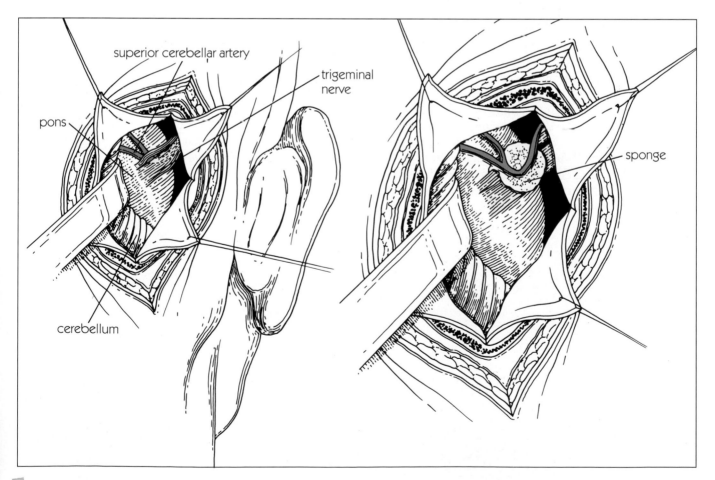

Figure 47.4 Retromastoid craniectomy with microvascular decompression of the trigeminal nerve.

viding pain relief, but will usually cause some degree of facial hypesthesia.

The results of microvascular decompression are good if arterial compression is identified. Among 68 personal patients followed an average of 54 months, 72% had excellent pain relief and 6% had good relief.[8] The initial failure rate for microvascular decompression is in the 5% to 10% range.[5,6,8] Subsequently, the rate of pain recurrence averages about 3.5% per year.[9] Similar detailed data about the results of modern posterior trigeminal rhizotomy have not been published. In a personal series of 22 patients followed for an average of 21 months, 86% obtained excellent pain relief.[8]

one of the surgical approaches should then be considered, with the selection based on the location of the pain, the patient's age and health, and the experience and preference of the surgeon. For example, for an elderly or infirm patient with pain in the cheek despite medication, an alcohol injection or surgical avulsion of the infraorbital nerve should be considered. If relief is obtained for a reasonable length of time and the pain subsequently recurs, medication should be given another try before a decision is made about repeating the injection or avulsion or trying a different approach such as a gasserian glycerol rhizolysis.

The patient with trigeminal neuralgia may need different forms of treatment during his or her life. The physician should be aware of the options, selecting the one most likely to help at that particular time, with the least risk.

CONCLUSION

A patient with trigeminal neuralgia who has no discernable mass along the trigeminal pathways should first receive a trial of appropriate medical therapy. If this fails,

REFERENCES

1. Rovit RL, Murali R, Jannetta PJ. *Trigeminal Neuralgia*. Baltimore, Md: Williams & Wilkins; 1990.
2. Stookey B, Ransohoff J. *Trigeminal Neuralgia: Its History and Treatment.* Springfield, Ill: Charles C Thomas Publisher; 1959.
3. White JC, Sweet WH. *Pain and the Neurosurgeon: A Forty-Year Experience.* Springfield, Ill: Charles C Thomas; 1969.
4. Wilkins RH. Trigeminal neuralgia: introduction. In: Wilkins RH, Rengachary SS, eds. *Neurosurgery.* New York, NY: McGraw-Hill; 1985:2337–2344.
5. Gybels JM, Sweet WH. *Neurosurgical Treatment of Persistent Pain: Physiological and Pathological Mechanisms of Human Pain.* Basel: Karger; 1989.
6. Sweet WH. Trigeminal neuralgia: problems as to cause and consequent conclusions regarding treatment. In: Wilkins RH, Rengachary SS, eds. *Neurosurgery Update II: Vascular, Spinal, Pediatric, and Functional Neurosurgery.* 1991:366–372.
7. Nugent GR. Trigeminal neuralgia: treatment by percutaneous electrocoagulation. In: Wilkins RH, Rengachary SS, eds. *Neurosurgery.* New York, NY: McGraw-Hill; 1985:2345–2350.
8. Piatt JH Jr, Wilkins RH. Treatment of tic douloureux and hemifacial spasm by posterior fossa exploration: therapeutic implications of various neurovascular relationships. *Neurosurgery.* 1984:14:462–471.
9. Burchiel KJ, Clarke H, Haglund M, et al. Longterm efficacy of microvascular decompression in trigeminal neuralgia. *J Neurosurg.* 1988:69:35–38.

Chapter **48**

Chronic Pain

Bennett Blumenkopf

All individuals at some time feel pain; undoubtedly, it is the most common presenting complaint. Whether one has a headache from a brain tumor, angina from coronary artery disease, or postprandial right upper quadrant colic from cholecystitis, the common denominator is pain. The experience of pain generally provides "protective usefulness" to an organism, although after this use has been served pain is debilitating.

The cause and duration of the pain experience often have a significant impact on its medical management. *Etiologically,* there are two broad categories of pain, *benign* and *malignant.* Benign pain may have a multitude of causes, while malignant pain is associated with cancer, generally widespread metastatic disease. *Physiologically,* pain is categorized as *somatic,* due to ongoing tissue injury and the resultant release of a variety of neurohumoral agents, and *neurogenic* or *deafferentation,* the result of injury to either the peripheral or central nervous system. *Temporally,* pain is considered *acute* if it is relatively short-lived, and its resolution is expected imminently. *Chronic* pain, however, is persistent and there is no foreseeable resolution.

Neurosurgeons are intimately involved with pain management. The neurosurgical approach may directly ad-

dress the underlying mechanism of pain, as in the case of diskectomy for radicular syndrome caused by a ruptured lumbar disc, but often the pain can only be palliated. This discussion reviews the neurosurgical approach to chronic pain management. First, a review of the basic anatomy and physiology involved in pain transmission is presented. Second, using these concepts, several neurosurgical procedures to alleviate chronic pain are offered. Finally, an interesting subclass of pain—deafferentation pain—will be discussed. This type of pain is less understood scientifically and certainly more difficult to manage clinically than other types of pain, and a new neurosurgical approach to it will be presented.

NEUROANATOMY AND NEUROPHYSIOLOGY OF PAIN

An appreciation of the anatomy and physiology of pain transmission is required to understand not only the many causes of pain but also the procedures employed to alleviate it (Fig. 48.1).[1-3] In pain transmission the peripheral nerves convey important sensory information about the organism to the central centers—the spinal

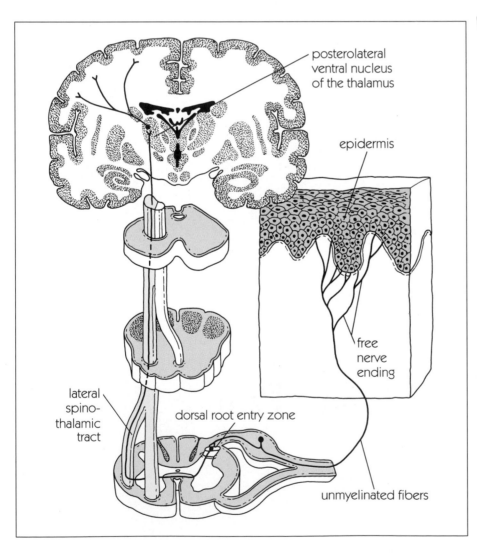

Figure 48.1 The nervous system pathway for nociception (pain) begins with the free nerve endings as receptors, which are present in the skin, mucous membranes, and periosteum. The nociceptive afferent fibers, represented by the unmyelinated C fibers and the thinly myelinated A-delta fibers with their cell bodies in the dorsal root ganglia, enter the dorsal root entry zone and synapse in the dorsal horn. Here, the first integration of pain occurs. The secondary nociceptive afferents decussate (cross) and then traverse the lateral spinothalamic tract to the rostral centers. Ultimately, pain is perceived at the cortical level.

posterolateral ventral nucleus of the thalamus

epidermis

free nerve ending

lateral spino-thalamic tract

dorsal root entry zone

unmyelinated fibers

cord, brain stem, and the brain itself—where pain is perceived at the cortical level.

The skin, mucous membranes, and periosteum can be considered the most peripheral parts of the nervous system since these structures contain the sensory receptors. Some receptors are specific for a single modality, while others are polymodal. Free nerve endings are generally believed to be the pain receptors. The impulses generated by these free nerve endings are conveyed to the central centers by the peripheral nerves. Two of the various subtypes of peripheral nerve fibers, the non-myelinated C fibers and the thinly myelinated A-delta fibers, are more likely to be involved in nociceptive transmission and seem to subserve different types of pain experience. The A-delta fibers conduct rapidly and convey a sharp, localized pain, while the unmyelinated C fibers conduct more slowly and convey a poorly localized dull, burning, or aching sensation.

The cell bodies or neurons of all the nociceptive afferent fibers are located within the dorsal root ganglia of the spinal roots or the gasserian ganglia of the trigeminal roots. These neurons are bipolar, and their central connections are in the spinal cord or brain stem. The central fibers of the primary nociceptive afferents—the A-delta and C fibers—terminate in the superficial regions of the dorsal aspect of the spinal cord, specifically laminae I, II, III of Rexed. In this region, the dorsal root entry zone (DREZ), the first integration of pain information occurs.

The neurons in the DREZ project their fibers—the secondary nociceptive afferents—to the thalamus. These fibers constitute the spinothalamic tract. The spinothalamic tract decussates within a segment or two of its segmental level and traverses the anterolateral column of the spinal cord. An additional pathway of secondary afferents projects to the brain stem reticular formation. Both the direct spinothalamic tract and the indirect spinoreticulothalamic tract terminate in the thalamus, particularly in the ventrobasal complex. From the thalamus, tertiary projections lead to the cerebral cortex, specifically the primary and secondary somatosensory areas.

Additional neural systems exist that modify pain (Fig. 48.2). In the peripheral nerves, the large myelinated A-alpha and A-beta fibers have an inhibitory effect on the spinothalamic neurons. This effect is probably mediated by inhibitory interneurons locally at each level of the dorsal horn laminae II, III. Also, the dorsal column

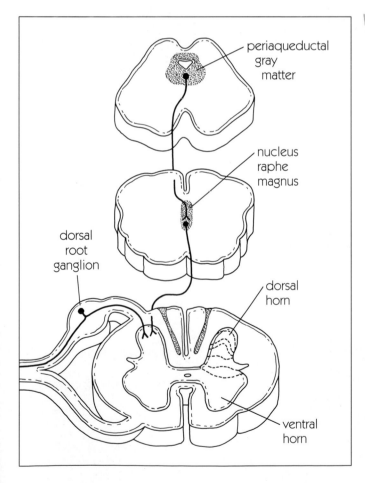

Figure 48.2 Neural pathways exist that inhibit pain at the dorsal horn level. These include brain stem pathways originating in the periaqueductal gray via the nucleus raphe magnus and peripheral nerve pathways involving the large A-alpha and A-beta fibers.

periaqueductal gray matter

nucleus raphe magnus

dorsal root ganglion

dorsal horn

ventral horn

nuclei and other brain stem locations project caudally to lamina I or laminae IV, V and with direct stimulation they inhibit the activity in the nociceptive thalamic cells (Fig. 48.3).

NEUROSURGICAL PAIN PROCEDURES

PERIPHERAL PROCEDURES

A variety of neurosurgical procedures based on this knowledge can alleviate pain (Fig. 48.4). Most peripherally, the peripheral nerves carrying the pain can be addressed. One might suppose that cutting a nerve (*peripheral neurectomy*) would eliminate pain impulses conveyed from the periphery, thereby abolishing pain.

However, a number of problems limit the applicability of this approach. There is significant overlap among the peripheral nerves in the distribution of innervation. Thus, pain is rarely limited to the zone of a single peripheral nerve. Furthermore, most peripheral nerves have both motor and sensory functions. A peripheral neurectomy could, therefore, cause an unacceptable neurologic deficit. Finally, development of deafferentation pain (discussed below) is a major complication of peripheral nerve section. Accordingly, this procedure is rarely performed to alleviate pain. An exception would be neurectomy performed for pain following injury to the superficial radial nerve.[4,5] In contrast, *peripheral nerve stimulation* is frequently used in the management of chronic pain, particularly that following nerve injury. With this approach, the large myelinated fibers that inhibit the

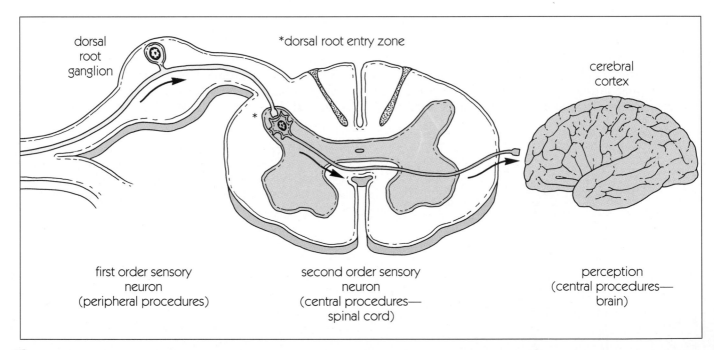

Figure 48.3 The sensory neural pathway beginning with the first-order neuron in the dorsal root ganglion, continuing with the second-order neuron in the dorsal root entry zone of the dorsal horn, and ultimately extending to the cortex where pain is perceived. Conceptually, palliative procedures for pain can be divided according to the level of the pathway approached.

Figure 48.4 Neurosurgical Pain Procedures

Peripheral	Central—Spinal Cord	Central—Brain
Peripheral neurectomy[4,5]	Cordotomy[11]	Mesencephalotomy[16]
Rhizotomy[6,7,8]	Midline myelotomy[12]	Brain stimulator[17,18]
Selective posterior rhizotomy[9]	Spinal stimulator[13]	Hypophysectomy[19]
Ganglionectomy[10]	Intraspinal narcotic analgesia[14,15]	
	Dorsal root entry zone (DREZ) lesion[21]	

nociceptive pathway at the level of the dorsal horn are selectively stimulated with either a transcutaneous or an implanted device.

The next most proximal approach involves sectioning the sensory fibers that make up the peripheral nerves (Fig. 48.5). This procedure (*rhizotomy*[6-8]) may be performed extra- or intradurally. Extradurally, the entire dorsal root is sectioned, while intradurally the multiple rootlets that make up the dorsal root are cut. *Selective posterior rhizotomy*[9] has also been described; this procedure is limited to the ventrolateral aspect of the rootlet, where the small fibers are organized. Rhizotomy has proven useful in the management of pain caused by malignant involvement of the brachial plexus (Pancoast syndrome), the chest wall, and occasionally the pelvis; its usefulness is limited in benign processes due to the frequent development of a deafferentation pain syndrome (postrhizotomy dysesthesiae).

Excision of the sensory ganglia (*ganglionectomy*[10]) has also been proposed for segmentally restricted pain, generally of malignant origin. This procedure removes the dorsal root ganglia at multiple levels. Ganglionectomy may be preferred over sensory rhizotomy because up to 20% of the nociceptive afferents traverse the *ventral* root.

CENTRAL PROCEDURES

Spinal Cord

A number of procedures, both ablation and stimulation, can be performed on the spinal cord itself in an attempt to palliate chronic pain. Included among these are procedures designed to destroy the spinothalamic tract—*cordotomy*[11]—through a formal hemilaminectomy with sectioning of the ventral spinothalamic tract or, more recently, through a percutaneous approach using a radiofrequency electrode. This results in contralateral analgesia below the level of the procedure and is remarkably effective in alleviating malignant pain, which is predominately one sided. Bilateral cordotomies are generally not performed because they can create respiratory complications. Furthermore, deafferentation pain syndrome (postcordotomy dysesthesia) severely limits its usefulness in benign pain syndromes.

Procedures that simultaneously divide the decussating nociceptive fibers from both sides of the body at the level of the anterior commissure—*midline commissurotomy* or *myelotomy*[12]—have been used in cases of midline perineal, pelvic, and rectal pain of malignant etiology. Bilateral effects are produced through a single cord incision as long as the site of the pain is limited. This procedure does, however, have a significant morbidity risk and is not popular.

Stimulation of the spinal cord, particularly the dorsal columns—*dorsal column stimulator* or *spinal cord stimulator*[13]—has been used for chronic benign pain, particularly the failed back syndrome following a ruptured intervertebral disk. The stimulation current is thought to provide pain relief by activating the descending inhibitory pathways. Paresthesiae, which have the same distribution as the pain, are perceived upon stimulation.

A spinal approach to pain relief that takes advantage of the basic neurochemistry of pain—*intraspinal narcotic analgesia*[14,15]—has gained popularity. Small doses of morphine instilled directly into the cerebrospinal

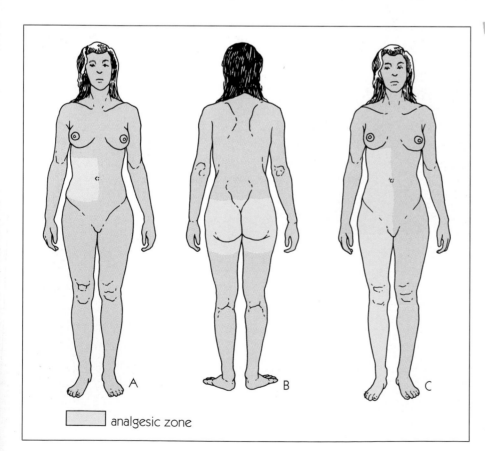

Figure 48.5 The effects of a variety of pain procedures on the sensory system can be described as: (**A**) *unilateral, segmental*, the result of a rhizotomy or ganglionectomy, creating a zone of analgesia useful for regional and lateralized pain in the thoracoabdominal area; (**B**) *bilateral, segmental*, the result of a midline myelotomy, providing a bilateral zone of analgesia particularly appropriate for lower pelvic pains; (**C**) *contralateral*, the result of an anterolateral cordotomy, creating a spinal level of analgesia that provides relief in diffuse, lateralized pains.

analgesic zone

fluid or into the epidural space provide profound and prolonged analgesia in a number of circumstances. ISNA is usually employed in metastatic malignancies, although recently it has been used for benign pain. A variety of pump devices have been designed for chronic therapy. Tolerance to the opiate is a long-term concern.

Brain

As is the case at the spinal cord level, both stimulation and ablation procedures for pain have been described. Stereotactic techniques are used on regions in the mesencephalon and diencephalon. *Stereotactic mesencephalotomy*[16] is indicated for cephalobrachial pain due to carcinoma and for thalamic syndrome pain. Interestingly, not only the pain but also the suffering are relieved by this procedure. Stimulation of areas in the midbrain and thalamus—*deep brain stimulation*[17,18]—has been used in cases of chronic benign pain and malignant pain (Fig. 48.6). The analgesia following midbrain stimulation appears to be opiate-mediated, while that following thalamic stimulation does not.

A central procedure that is particularly effective in palliating the pain of metastatic cancer (especially osseous metastases) is hypophysectomy (Fig. 48.7).[19] The pituitary gland may be surgically excised by the transsphenoidal route or chemically ablated using absolute ethanol injections. In cases of hormone-responsive malignancies (e.g., in the breast or prostate) long-lasting

pain relief is often achieved. The mechanisms responsible for this remarkable effect are not understood.

DEAFFERENTATION PAIN

A conceptually different and probably less familiar type of pain is *deafferentation pain*.[20] Deafferentation pain involves the perception of painful sensations (burning, tearing, throbbing, etc.) in a region of the body that is partially or totally deprived of sensation; that is, some or all of the peripheral nociceptors are physically disconnected from the central centers. As mentioned above, a number of deafferentation pain syndromes develop after ablative neurosurgical procedures; however, because these syndromes often do not develop for 12 to 18 months, these procedures are useful in cases of malignant pain with a limited life expectancy.

The prevalence of deafferentation pain is surprisingly high in amputation, root avulsion, peripheral nerve injury, quadriplegia and paraplegia, and postherpetic neuralgia. Fifty to 90% of amputees, 80% to 90% of brachial plexus avulsions, and 10% to 20% of paraplegics suffer some sort of deafferentation pain. The cause of these pains remains unclear. It has been suggested that deafferentation not only results in the loss of sensory input from the periphery but that the disconnected central spinal sensory neurons may also behave pathologically. This abnormal neu-

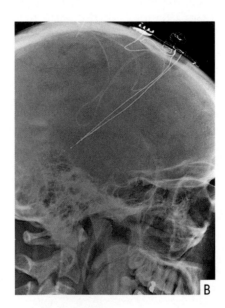
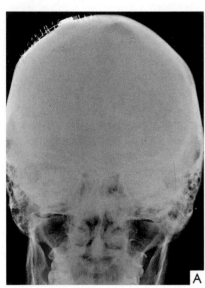
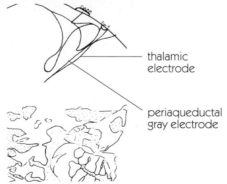
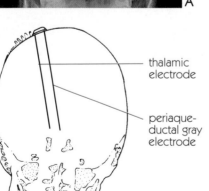

thalamic electrode

periaqueductal gray electrode

thalamic electrode

periaqueductal gray electrode

Figure 48.6 Anteroposterior (A) and lateral (B) skull radiographs show the placement of depth electrodes in the brain for stimulation-produced analgesia. The electrodes are placed either in the thalamus or the periventricular gray region.

ronal activity is perceived as pain. The neurophysiologic explanations for this activity include 1) hypersensitivity of the disconnected central neuron—an epileptic-like pain phenomenon, 2) release from the influences of powerful central inhibitory systems, and 3) change in the local concentrations of some of the classic neurotransmitters or recently described peptide neuromodulators.

The often disabling pain syndromes that develop after brachial plexus avulsion, amputation, quadriplegia, and paraplegia may involve these mechanisms. The conventional procedures detailed above have been ineffective. Knowledge of dorsal horn region anatomy and neurophysiology, especially nociceptive transmission and pain, led Nashold to believe that a nonfunctional or destroyed pathologic central neuron was better than a sick one. Thus, he developed the DREZ (dorsal root entry zone) operation (Fig. 48.8),[21] in which lesions made in the dorsal root entry zone convert partially injured (i.e.,

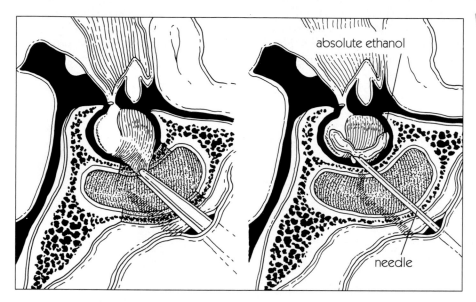

Figure 48.7 Transsphenoidal removal of the pituitary gland (hypophysectomy) provides excellent pain relief in cases of osseous metastases from endocrine-sensitive cancers (e.g., breast and prostate). The pituitary gland can also be chemically ablated with an injection of absolute alcohol through a needle placed within the sella turcica.

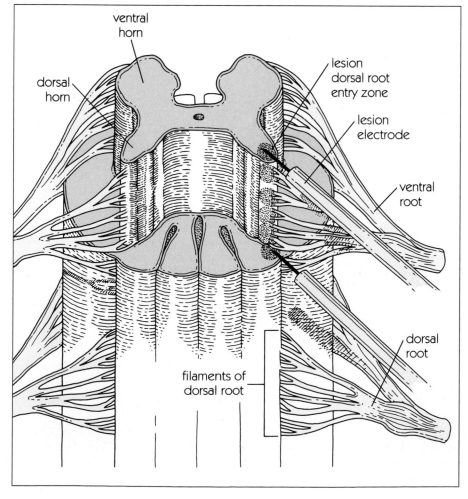

Figure 48.8 The DREZ procedure is designed to treat deafferentation pain by destroying the abnormally active dorsal horn neurons in the spinal cord at each segmental level of the pain. A small electrode is advanced into the spinal cord and radiofrequency lesions approximately 1 mm in diameter are created in a serial fashion.

"hyperactive") central neurons into quiescent scars at each segmental level of pain. This is accomplished by advancing a small electrode into the spinal cord, creating radiofrequency lesions approximately 1 mm in diameter in a serial fashion.

The DREZ procedure was initially performed in a group of patients with brachial plexus avulsion pain.[21] Long-term relief (5 years) has been described in 66% of those cases. Subsequently, it was recognized that there also exist cases of sacral plexus avulsion associated with pelvic trauma. Spinal cord injury and pain (quadriplegic or paraplegic), postherpetic pain, and postamputation phantom pain are types of deafferentation pain also considered appropriate for the DREZ procedure. Recently, a second group of patients with intractable pain of peripheral origin, including postamputation stump pain, postthoracotomy pain, and reflex sympathetic dystrophy syndrome have been treated with the procedure (Fig. 48.9). In addition, a *trigeminal nucleus caudalis DREZ* procedure has been developed for patients with pain after herpes zoster ophthalmicus and carcinoma of the orbit; however, the results are only preliminary.

One question to consider: why does the DREZ operation not create a deafferentation situation more distal in the circuitry? Perhaps because it limits the damage to nerve cells rather than fiber tracts. Nevertheless, deafferentation is a concern, and continued follow up is required. For the moment, an encouraging new procedure exists for these difficult pain problems.

Figure 48.9 Dorsal Root Entry Zone (DREZ) Procedure

Brachial/lumbar plexus avulsion pain

Paraplegic/quadriplegic pain

Amputation phantom pain

Postherpetic neuralgia

Amputation stump pain

Postthoracotomy pain

Reflex sympathetic dystrophy pain

REFERENCES

1. Albe-Fessard D, Berkley KJ, Kruger L, Ralston HJ III, Willis WD Jr. Diencephalic mechanisms of pain sensation. *Brain Res Rev.* 1985;9:217–296.
2. Basbaum AI, Fields HL. Endogenous pain control systems: brainstem spinal pathways and endorphin circuitry. *Annu Rev Neurosci.* 1984; 7:309–338.
3. Fields HL, Heinricher MM. Anatomy and physiology of a nociceptive modulatory system. *Phil Trans R Soc Lond.* 1985;B308:361–374.
4. Dellon AL, Mackinnon SE. Susceptibility of the superficial sensory branch of the radial nerve to form painful neuromas. *J Hand Surg.* 1984;9B: 42–45.
5. Dellon AL, Mackinnon SE. Treatment of the painful neuroma by neuroma resection and muscle implantation. *Plast Reconstr Surg.* 1986;77:427–435.
6. Esposito S, Bruni P, Delitala A, Canova A, Hernandez R, Callovini GM. Therapeutic approach to the Pancoast pain syndrome. *Appl Neurophysiol.* 1985; 48:262–266.
7. Loeser JD. Dorsal rhizotomy for the relief of chronic pain. *J Neurosurg.* 1972;36:745–750.
8. Onofrio BM, Campa HK. Evaluation of rhizotomy. *J Neurosurg.* 1972;36:751–755.
9. Sindou M, Goutelle A. Surgical posterior rhizotomies for the treatment of pain. In: Krayenbuhl H, ed. *Advances and Technical Standards in Neurosurgery.* Wien: Springer-Verlag; 1983;10:147–185.
10. Smith FP. Trans-spinal ganglionectomy for relief of intercostal pain. *J Neurosurg.* 1970;32:574–577.
11. Spiller WG, Martin E. The treatment of persistent pain of organic origin in the lower part of the body by division of the anterolateral column of the spinal cord. *JAMA.* 1912;58:1489–1490.
12. Sindou M, Daher A. Spinal cord ablation procedures for pain. In: Dubner R, Gebhart GF, Bond MR, eds. *Proceedings of the Vth World Congress on Pain.* New York, NY: Elsevier Science; 1988: 477–495.
13. De La Porte C, Siegfried J. Lumbosacral spinal

fibrosis (spinal arachnoiditis): its diagnosis and treatment by spinal cord stimulation. *Spine.* 1983; 8:593–603.

14. Auld AW, Maki-Jokela A, Murdoch DM. Intraspinal narcotic analgesia in the treatment of chronic pain. *Spine.* 1985;10:777–781.

15. Penn RD, Paice JA, Gottschalk W, Ivankovich AD. Cancer pain relief using chronic morphine infusion. *J Neurosurg.* 1984;61:302–306.

16. Nashold BS Jr. Brainstem stereotaxic procedures. In: Schaltenbrand G, Walker AE, eds. *Stereotaxy of the Human Brain*, New York, NY: Georg Thieme Verlag; 1982:475–483.

17. Adams JE, Hosobuchi Y, Fields HL. Stimulation of internal capsule for relief of chronic pain. *J Neurosurg.* 1974;41:740–744.

18. Hosobuchi Y. Subcortical electrical stimulation for control of intractable pain in humans. *J Neurosurg.* 1986;64:543–553.

19. Levin AB, Katz J, Benson RC, Jones AG. Treatment of pain of diffuse metastatic cancer by stereotactic chemical hypophysectomy: long term results and observations on mechanism of action. *Neurosurgery.* 1980;6:258–262.

20. Nashold BS Jr. Deafferentation pain in man and animals as it relates to the DREZ operation. *Can J Neurosci.* 1988;15:5–9.

21. Nashold BS Jr, Ostdahl RH. Dorsal root entry zone lesions for pain relief. *J Neurosurg.* 1979;51:59–69.

Chapter 49

Stereotactic Surgery

Ronald R. Tasker, Mark Bernstein

Stereotactic surgery is performed using a geometric guidance instrument fixed to the head that is capable of directing a probe or energy beam to an unseen target. Thus it is the interdigitation of four disciplines—surgery, some type of imaging since the surgeon cannot actually see the target, mathematical principles to determine the route from the surface of the body to the target, and computer technology for the many, sometimes complex calculations that must be made along the way. The term itself, adopted by the World Society for Stereotactic and Functional Neurosurgery in 1973,[1] is derived from the Greek word *stereos,* which implies three dimensions, and the Latin verb *tangere,* meaning to touch. This replaces the previously used term "stereotaxic," which is derived from *stereos* and the Greek word *taxis,* which implies a system or order.

Long before the concept was used in the operating room it was employed routinely in the animal laboratory by Horsley and Clarke.[2] In 1908 they built a sophisticated frame (Fig. 49.1) that they attached to the skull of an experimental animal in order to guide a probe into its brain with reference to a brain atlas constructed from serial brain sections of the species under study. Superimposed upon this was a three-dimensional scale, measuring in millimeters.

The stereotactic principle had been applied to humans before 1908 with the encephalometer designed by Zernov (Fig. 49.2). (The encephalometer was first used in 1891, to locate the central sulcus in order to drain an abscess at that site.[3]) The first subcortical human stereotactic procedures on record were performed by Spiegel and Wycis of Philadelphia[4,5] in 1948 using a stereotactic frame they designed (Fig. 49.3). Human stereotactic surgery required a strategy different from that used in the laboratory since skull landmarks were not usually accurate enough to guide a probe safely to the intended target. Instead, Spiegel and Wycis hit upon the idea of using internal brain landmarks, which they first pictured using air and later positive contrast media. Initially the foramen of Monro-pineal line, then the foramen of Monro-posterior commissure line along with the midsagittal plane were used in supratentorial procedures, and subsequently the anterior-posterior commissure line (Fig. 49.4). Human atlases were constructed with three-dimensional scaling based on these ventricular landmarks (Fig. 49.5).

The early impetus for stereotactic surgery came from the demonstration that pallidotomy was able to control the tremor of Parkinson's disease without producing paralysis,[6] a procedure ideally suited to the stereotactic method. Although the advent of L-dopa reduced the

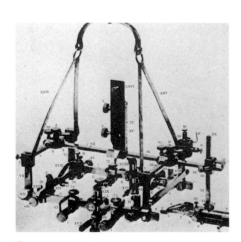

Figure 49.1 Stereotactic frame used by Horsley and Clarke. (Reprinted with permission from Krieg WJS. *Stereotaxy.* Evanston, Ill: Brain Books; 1975)

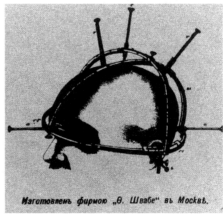

Figure 49.2 The encephalometer used by Zernov. (Reprinted with permission from Kandel EI, 1989)

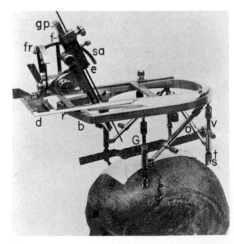

Figure 49.3 An early stereotactic frame designed by Spiegel and Wycis (Stereo-encephalotome V). (Reprinted with permission from Nashold B. Stereotactic instrumentation: a round table discussion. *J Neurosurg.* 1966;24(suppl):465)

Principles of Neurosurgery

number of procedures required to treat Parkinson's disease, the stereotactic technique still has a wide range of other applications today. First, procedures were developed to treat various movement disorders, intractable pain, and psychiatric illness. For these applications a wide variety of stereotactic frames appeared throughout the world, leading to procedures to modify functional diseases by destructive lesions, chronic stimulation, or instillation of specific neuroactive substances, including living cells. Then procedures for biopsy or treatment of deep, relatively inaccessible brain lesions, particularly tumors, were developed. This led to techniques for the destruction of deep lesions, using probes of various types, including radioactive sources (brachytherapy) and stereotactically directed energy beams from external sources, such as those derived from the linear accelerator, collimated radioactive cobalt sources, or proton beams. Finally, stereotactic techniques have been used for open craniotomies including the use of robotics; even maneuvers such as the clipping of aneurysms have been accomplished stereotactically.

GENERAL PRINCIPLES

A stereotactic procedure requires some or all of the following:

- Suitable stereotactic instrument
- Appropriate imaging of the target area
- The means to cross-correlate coordinates of the imaged target with those of the stereotactic instrument
- A brain atlas containing a coordinate system transferable to the stereotactic instrument and based on the coordinates of identifiable brain landmarks
- Appropriate probes or beams for the manipulation of the target
- When the stereotactic target can be directly identified by imaging, manipulation can be performed at once; otherwise its location must be extrapolated from brain landmarks and an atlas and its identification corroborated by physiologic techniques.
- Computer assistance, though not indispensable, greatly facilitates most stages of a stereotactic operation.

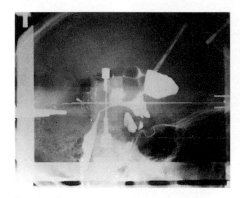

Figure 49.4 Anterior and posterior commissures identified with positive contrast media. (Reprinted with permission from Wilkins RH, Rengachary SS, eds. *Neurosurgery.* New York, NY: McGraw-Hill; 1985)

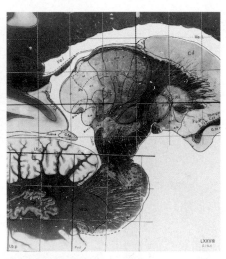

Figure 49.5 Sagittal diagram 14.5 mm from the midline of a human brain, ruled in a centimeter grid based on the intercommissural line for supratentorial structures. (Reprinted with permission from Schaltenbrand G, Wahren W, eds. *Atlas for Stereotaxy of the Human Brain.* Stuttgart: Georg Thieme Verlag; 1977)

Stereotactic frames in common use today include the Leksell (Fig. 49.6), CRW (Fig. 49.7), BRW (Fig. 49.8), Kelly (Compass System) (Fig. 49.9), McGill, Narabayashi (Fig. 49.10), Talairach, Sugita (Fig. 49.11), Hitchcock, Riechert-Mundinger, Laitinen (Fig. 49.12), and Patil. They all accomplish similar tasks in different ways. Some function purely on rectilinear principles, like the original Horsley-Clarke frame, using a translational system. The target is located in terms of millimeters anterior, posterior, right, left, dorsal, and medial to a given reference point on the frame (Fig. 49.13). These measurements are set on the three scales of the frame, the electrode carriage is slid back and forth to match, and the probe is directed into the brain. Other frames use polar coordinates based on arcs. The three-dimensional coordi-

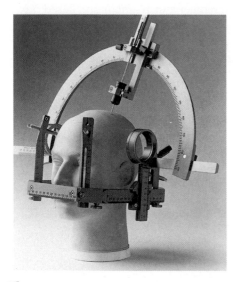

Figure 49.6 The "G" Leksell frame. (Courtesy of Elekta Instruments, Atlanta, Ga)

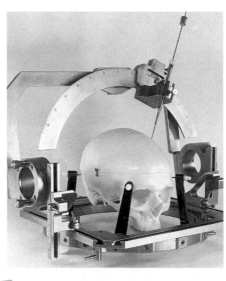

Figure 49.7 The CRW frame. (Courtesy of Radionics, Burlington, Mass)

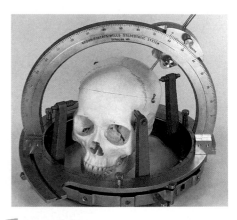

Figure 49.8 The BRW frame. (Courtesy of Radionics, Burlington, Mass)

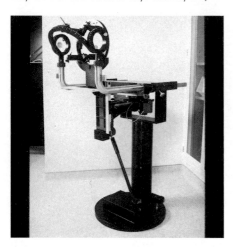

Figure 49.9 The Compass Stereotactic System. (Courtesy of PJ Kelly, Mayo Clinic, Rochester, Minn)

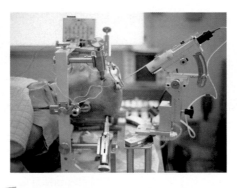

Figure 49.10 The Narabayashi frame. (Courtesy of Professor H Narabayashi, Tokyo, Japan)

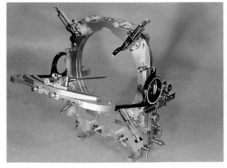

Figure 49.11 The Sugita frame. (Courtesy of DR Sugita, Nagoya, Japan)

Figure 49.12 (A) The Laitinen Stereotactic System. **(B)** The Laitinen Stereoadapter. (Courtesy of L Laitinen, Stockholm, Sweden)

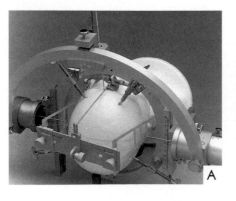

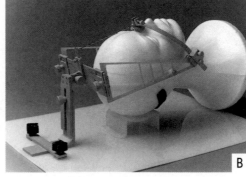

nates of the target are determined as they are for rectilinear frames, but the probe is introduced along the radius of the sphere described by revolving an arc fixed to the frame so that its center is the intended target (Fig. 49.14). Still other instruments consist of probe guides fixed to the skull—often to the burr hole itself—that can aim the probe into the brain, using angles determined by the imaging (see Fig. 49.12).

_____ IMAGING

Human stereotactic surgery requiring internal brain landmarks originally used ventriculography with either air or positive contrast media (see Fig. 49.4). This simple, effective technique is gradually being replaced by CT and MRI, techniques that have many advantages:
  • They are noninvasive.
  • They eliminate the need to introduce contrast media into the ventricles.
  • They prevent CSF loss and the resultant headache, nausea, vomiting, and brain shift.
  • MRI in particular depicts a variety of brain structures, sometimes even the target.
  • Computer graphics technology incorporated into the scanners usually allows simple computation of target sites.
  • Computers make possible the superposition of various types of images, including CT, MRI, and angiography, on frame coordinates, even incorporating physiologic data.
  • They are at least as precise as ventriculography and pneumoencephalography.[7,8]

Either MRI or CT can be used as the sole imaging technique for stereotactic procedures. With the Leksell frame, for example, the frame is fixed to the patient's head and to the gantry with a specially designed clamp; the imaging cuts are made parallel to one plane of the stereotactic frame—often the base—producing axial

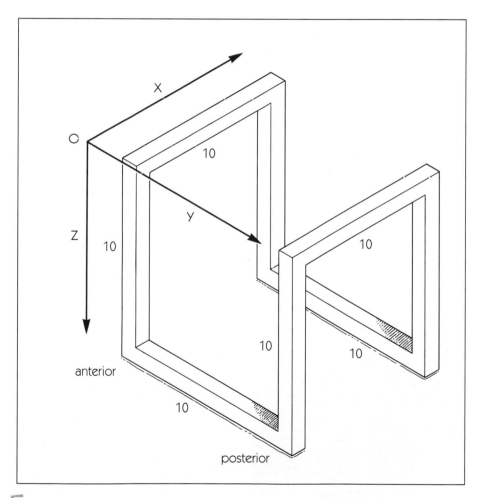

Figure 49.13 The three rectilinear planes in which a stereotactic frame measures. (Courtesy of E Dolan, Billings, Mont)

cuts. A special set of reference plates attached to one face of the frame contains a "picket fence" arrangement of fiducial bars (Fig. 49.15) that are visible in the overall image. Their positions along the periphery of the overall image allow precise identification of, first, the level of a cut in terms of stereotactic coordinates (Fig. 49.16) and,

second, the other two coordinates of the target structure (Fig. 49.17). With other frames, the BRW for example, imaging cuts are made with the head and frame placed at any position within the gantry, though they must remain still during the imaging. A computer program is then used to calculate target coordinates.

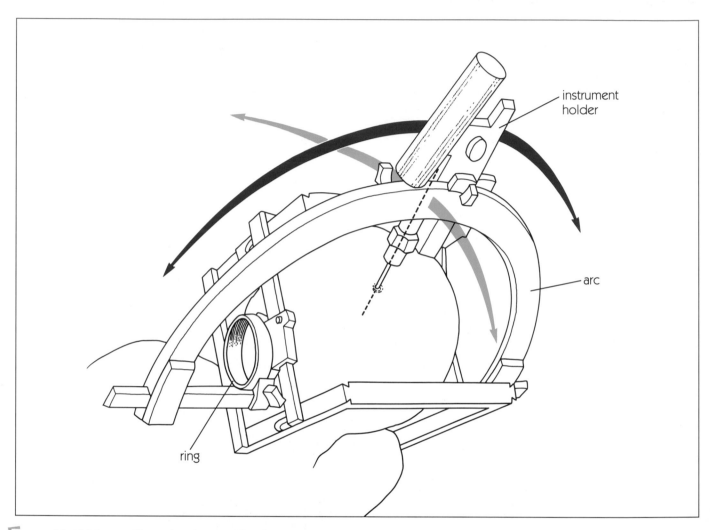

instrument holder

arc

ring

Figure 49.14 Diagram illustrating the use of polar coordinates with the Leksell frame. (Courtesy of E Dolan, Billings, Mont)

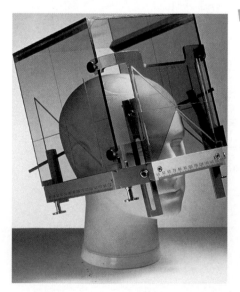

Figure 49.15 Leksell frame, illustrating guide plates with "picket fence" fiducial bars attached. (Courtesy of Elekta Instruments, Atlanta, Ga)

Whether to use CT or MRI depends on several factors in addition to the availability of the imaging system and compatible stereotactic frames. MRI depicts a much wider variety of potential brain structures than CT, but on the other hand, MRI must be repeatedly calibrated to prevent distortion and targets must be kept near the center of the image. The most accurate results have been obtained with MRI in functional stereotaxis when the coordinates of anterior and posterior commissures are first approximated in the midsagittal plane, and their coordinates are determined from either axial or coronal cuts that bracket their locations.

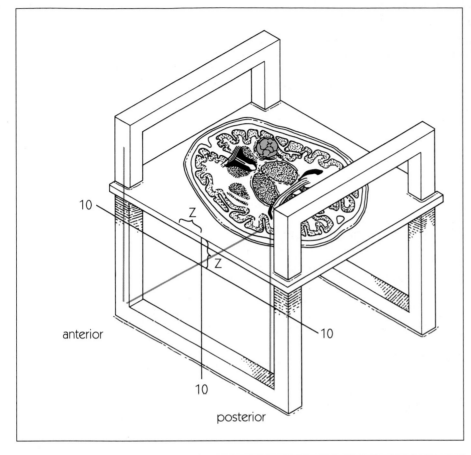

Figure 49.16 The position of the oblique fiducial bars, shown in Figure 49.15, in the axial image of the brain identifies which axial cut is being examined. For the Leksell frame they bear a 45° angle with the vertical bars so that the distance z of their images from the midpoint between the vertical bars is also the distance above or below the middle of the vertical bars. (Courtesy of E Dolan, Billings, Mont)

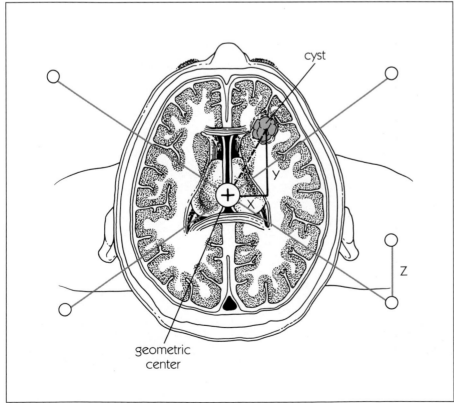

Figure 49.17 The anteroposterior and mediolateral coordinates of a target can be measured directly. (Courtesy of E Dolan, Billings, Mont)

For functional stereotactic procedures, an atlas of the brain is usually essential (see Fig. 49.5). Some of those in common use are listed in the references.[9–19] The desired target, located in millimeters from the midsagittal plane and landmark structures such as anterior and posterior commissures, is visualized first in the atlas and if possible on the imaging. Otherwise its location must be extrapolated on the imaging from the location of structures that can be visualized. Infratentorial procedures require imaging of features of the fourth ventricle along with the midsagittal plane for reference.

PROBES AND OTHER MEANS OF TARGET MANIPULATION

A wide variety of probes for the various types of stereotactic procedures are available (Fig. 49.18).

Physiologic Probes

Physiologic probes are used to verify that the site the surgeon has reached is, in fact, the one being sought, particularly when it is not directly identifiable from imaging. The two methods most frequently used are electrical stimulation and microelectrode recording, although evoked potentials and EEG recordings can also be made.

Stimulation is the simplest method since it is usually performed with a macroelectrode (Fig. 49.19), which requires no highly specialized equipment. Moreover, due to volume conduction, it activates structures at least 2 mm away, so in the course of most exploratory trajectories information is obtained from a wide variety of brain structures.[19]

Microelectrodes (Figs. 49.20, 49.21), on the other hand, require specialized equipment and "see" only for a very short distance, so unless the electrode tip is very close to a neuron or axon, nothing is recorded and no

---

Figure 49.18 Probes and Other Means of Target Manipulation

Physiologic Exploration	Lesion-Making	Biopsy
1. Macrostimulation (Fig. 49.19)	1. Injection of necrotizing substances	1. Simple aspiration (Fig.49.27)
2. Microstimulation (Figs. 49.20, 49.21)	2. Cryoprobes	2. "Corkscrew" coring (Fig. 49.27)
3. Microelectrode recording (Figs. 49.20, 49.21)	3. Radiofrequency probes[22] (Fig. 49.23)	3. Biting (Fig. 49.26)
4. Evoked potential recording[20]	4. Mechanical leukotomes[23]	4. Side-cutting aspiration to produce a core (Fig. 49.27)
5. EEG recording		5. Hematoma aspiration, Archimedes screw
6. Impedance recording		

Brachytherapy, Clipping Aneurysms and Other Special Purposes, Chronic Stimulating Electrodes (Fig. 49.28), Focused External Radiation—protons, x-rays, and gamma rays (Fig. 49.37)—Beams

localizing information is gleaned.[23-27] The same applies if the microelectrode is used for stimulation, as in our practice, in which we alternate recording and stimulation up to 100 μA. In contrast to macrostimulation, only a few types of neurons can be identified with microelectrode recording: tactile, some nociceptive, kinesthetic, dentatothalamic, motor, and auditory. Range limitations are also advantageous: If a neuron with a tactile receptive field is recorded, for example, one can be certain that it is very close to the microelectrode tip, whereas if a macroelectrode induces paresthesiae, the responsible structure may be 2 mm or more away.

Impedance monitoring is particularly useful combined with stereotactic biopsy. It readily distinguishes the low impedance of ventricles and many lesions from that of normal brain (Fig. 49.22).[28]

Stereotactically implanted electrodes are frequently used to record depth EEG for the surgical treatment of epilepsy.

Probes for Making Lesions

Brain lesions are usually made with radiofrequency current (Fig. 49.23). The size of the lesion depends on the geometry of the bare electrode tip, the duration and level of current flow, and the temperature to which the tip is

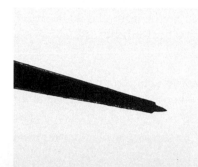

Figure 49.19 "Tasker" concentric bipolar macrostimulation electrode 1.1 mm in diameter with 0.5 mm pole and 0.5 mm pole separation. (Courtesy of Diros Technology, Toronto, Ontario)

Figure 49.20 Microelectrode used at the Toronto Hospital with a 30 μm tip. (Courtesy of JO Dostrovsky, Department of Physiology, University of Toronto, Toronto, Ontario)

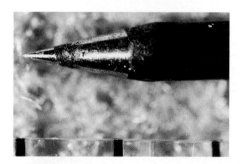

Figure 49.21 Semimicroelectrode used by H. Narabayashi. (Courtesy of Professor H Narabayashi, Tokyo, Japan)

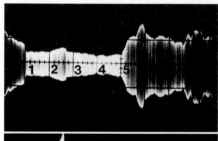

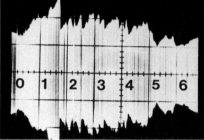

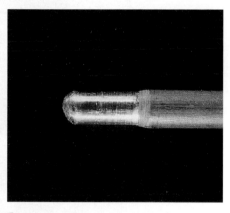

Figure 49.23 Radiofrequency lesion-making electrode with 3 mm bare tip with 1.1 mm diameter. (Courtesy of Diros Technology, Toronto, Ontario)

Figure 49.22 Impedance "profile" of the human brain showing (above) a fall in impedance at a depth of about 1 cm as the impedance probe was stereotactically advanced out of the brain into a glioblastoma multiforme, its rise again at about 5 cm as it emerges from tumor, and (below) its rise at a depth of about 0.4 cm as it enters a tough meningioma, falling again at about 5.2 cm as it emerges. (Reproduced with permission from Tasker RR. Physiological monitoring of stereotactic biopsy. *Appl Neurophysiol.* 1985;48:444–447)

raised.[29] Lesions are made by a backup electronic system such as the OWL (Diros Technology, Toronto, Ontario) (Fig. 49.24) or Radionics (Radionics, Burlington, Mass) (Fig. 49.25). This equipment also provides impedance recording, stimulation at a variety of parameters, and temperature recording. Radiofrequency is particularly convenient to use since lesions of varying sizes can be easily made, and lesion-making can be coupled with physiologic studies. It appears fraught with fewer risks than other techniques: Specially constructed small leukotomes, though providing directionally tailored lesions, must be carefully handled to avoid hemorrhage. Cryoprobes, often based on liquid nitrogen, have the advantage of elegantly making temporary lesions, but they require a ponderous backup, and the probe must not be disturbed while frozen to the brain to avoid inducing hemorrhage.

Probes for Biopsy

Personal preference of biopsy equipment varies widely. Three devices are commonly used. Our preference is for the Sedan design (Fig. 49.26), which consists of two hollow tubes that fit snugly inside one another with a stilette for introduction. Each tube has a distally placed side window, 1 cm long, arranged so that as the inner tube rotates within the outer, the two windows alternately coincide and become occluded. The device is introduced to the desired biopsy site, the tubes are rotated so both side windows are open to the brain; gentle suction is then applied with a syringe at the proximal end to draw tissue into the window and is maintained while the tubes are rotated to amputate the specimen. A rubber O-ring insures that suction is maintained. Thus a series of longitudinal cores—like those obtained by geologists—can be made, starting at the brain-lesion boundary and progressing in stages through the lesion itself.

Also commonly used is the Backlund biopsy kit (Elekta Instruments, Atlanta, Ga) (Fig. 49.27). The probes contain a variety of aspiration tubes, and one probe contains a terminal corkscrew 1 cm long. To use the latter, an introductory cannula and stilette are ad-

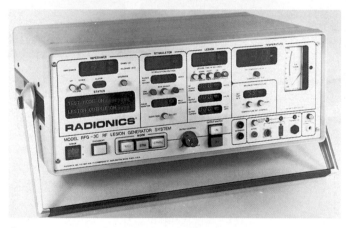

Figure 49.24 Electronic backup manufactured by Diros Technology for functional neurosurgical procedures provides electrical stimulation at a variety of parameters, measures electrical impedance, makes radiofrequency lesions at a variety of parameters, and monitors the temperature of lesions. (Courtesy of Diros Technology, Toronto, Ontario)

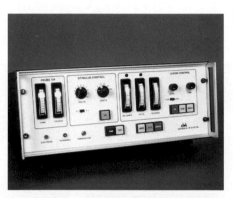

Figure 49.25 Similar equipment provided by Radionics Corp. (Courtesy of Radionics, Burlington, Mass)

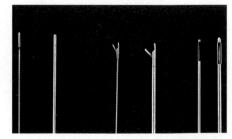

Figure 49.26 Instruments available to sample tissue during stereotactic biopsy. (Left) Obturator and outer cannula for introduction. (Middle) Small and large biting biopsy forceps. (Right) Inner and outer cannulae of side-window cutting biopsy needle of the Sedan type.

vanced to the biopsy site, the stilette is replaced by the corkscrew probe, and as the corkscrew probe is extruded 1 cm beyond the tip of the introductory probe, it is rotated. The introductory tube is then advanced over the extruded corkscrew to amputate tissue gripped by the corkscrew, the equipment is removed, and the specimen collected.

Some surgeons prefer microbiting devices (see Fig. 49.26) introduced through a hollow tube, and sharp and dull aspirating devices of various sizes can be used for small and large, thin- and thick-walled lesions whose contents vary in consistency. A suction-driven Archimedes screw device is available for the aspiration of hematomas.

CHRONIC STIMULATING ELECTRODES

To control chronic pain or movement disorders, electrodes are stereotactically inserted at various physiologically verified brain sites and anchored in place (Fig. 49.28). Temporary transcutaneous test stimulation is usually carried out over several days to determine: 1) if the electrode remains in the intended position, 2) if stimulation is beneficial, and 3) what the optimal parameters are. If unsuccessful, the electrodes are removed; otherwise they are joined to a device that enables chronic stimula-

tion to proceed. The simplest type is radiofrequency coupled, activated by a radio transmitter and antenna, with the implanted electrode connected to a subcutaneous receiver, usually placed in the chest wall below the clavicle. More sophisticated devices are totally implantable, battery-powered, and capable of being programmed externally (Figs. 49.29, 49.30).

COMPUTERS

While not essential for stereotactic surgery, computers facilitate the surgeon's work, a matter addressed in a volume edited by Kelly and Kall.[30] Computers assist in the arithmetic used to determine the three-dimensional stereotactic coordinates of the target or reference landmarks identified with imaging, and by placing cursors on the images of these structures and those of the "picket fence" fiducials (see Fig. 49.15), the computer can calculate XYZ stereotactic coordinates directly.

Once these coordinates are determined, the computer provides a second service. In functional stereotactic operations it is usually impossible to image the target directly. Rather, the location is established with reference to landmarks such as anterior and posterior commissures. The

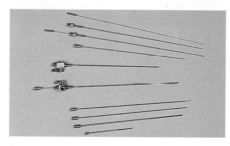

Figure 49.27 Backlund biopsy kit includes various aspiration devices, and second, third, and fourth from bottom: cannula, obturator, and "corkscrew" biopsy device. (Courtesy of Elekta Instruments, Atlanta, Ga)

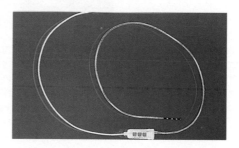

Figure 49.28 Tripole chronic stimulation electrode for implantation into brain. (Courtesy of Neuromed, Ft. Lauderdale, Fla)

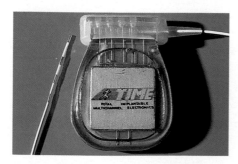

Figure 49.29 Totally implantable and programmable battery-powered stimulating device (TIME) manufactured by Neuromed, also capable of radiofrequency coupling. (Courtesy of Neuromed, Ft. Lauderdale, Fla)

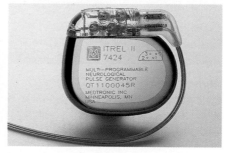

Figure 49.30 Totally implantable and programmable battery powered stimulating device (ITREL II) manufactured by Medtronic Corp. (Courtesy of Medtronic, Minneapolis, Minn)

computer facilitates this process by drawing a whole set of brain atlas diagrams; they are stretched or shrunk to match the particular dimensions of the patient's brain and the coordinates of the stereotactic frame as placed (Fig. 49.31). This type of computer graphics can be incorporated into an interactive system that superimposes physiologic data and MRI, CT, or angiographic images (Figs. 49.32–49.34). If such data are stored, a computer graphics technique can be used to search the database for data of a particular type in all patients studied and to plot them on computerized diagrams (Fig. 49.35).

Finally, computers can be used to direct the whole stereotactic procedure, whether it is performed by a human or robotic neurosurgeon (Fig. 49.36).[31–36]

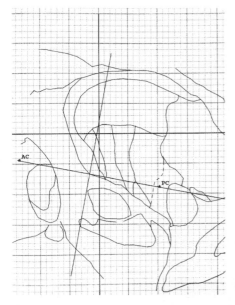

Figure 49.31 Computer-generated sagittal atlas diagram redrawn to conform to the patient's intercommissural distance and reading in terms of stereotactic coordinates according to the placement of the frame on the patient's head.

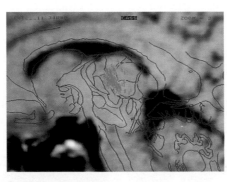

Figure 49.32 10.5 mm lateral sagittal MRI of the brain with superimposed outline from an atlas by Schaltenbrand and Wahren, upon which are marked in blue the locations of nonevoked tremor cells using the CASS system. (Courtesy of Tyrone Hardy, Lovelace Medical Center, Albuquerque, NM)

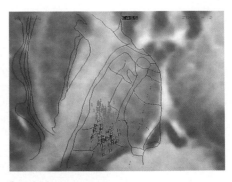

Figure 49.33 Similar horizontal illustration 6.5 mm above the intercommissural line, showing nonevoked tremor cells in green and facial tactile cells in red. (Courtesy of Tyrone Hardy, Lovelace Medical Center, Albuquerque, NM)

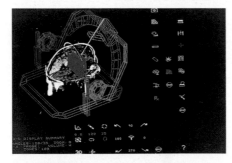

Figure 49.34 Computer-generated three-dimensional MR image showing in yellow a stereotactic probe being directed towards the thalamus; motor strips are red. (Courtesy of Tyrone Hardy, Lovelace Medical Center, Albuquerque, NM)

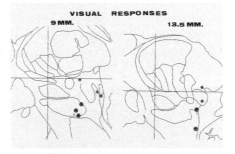

Figure 49.35 Computer-generated 9 mm and 13.5 mm sagittal brain diagrams that plot all macrostimulation-induced visual responses in patients studied. Small circles indicate sites where stimulation induced a sense of movement in the visual fields; large circles indicate where visual fields were obscured.

APPLICATIONS OF STEREOTACTIC SURGERY

FUNCTIONAL STEREOTACTIC SURGERY

Movement Disorders Including Spasticity

Destructive stereotactic lesions in the thalamus, subthalamus, globus pallidus, internal capsule, and dentate nucleus, as well as chronic stimulation of the thalamus and dentate nucleus, have been used to treat a variety of movement disorders. There has been much recent publicity about implanting living tissue, either from the patient's own adrenal glands or fetal mesencephalic tissue, to treat Parkinson's disease.[40–47]

Chronic Pain

Some authors consider percutaneous procedures performed on the spinal cord, such as cordotomy, commissurotomy, and trigeminal nucleotomy and tractotomy,[48–58] to be stereotactic procedures, but the term is usually reserved for operations in which the brain is manipulated. Destructive lesions are usually made in the spinoreticulothalamic tract. This has been accomplished in the pons[59–62] and mesencephalon, involving at the latter site both its somatotopographically organized lateral component and its nonsomatotopographically organized medial component. In addition, lesions have been made in Hassler's parvicellular ventrocaudal nucleus, thought to be the specific relay for the spinothalamic tract, and even in the ventrocaudal nucleus itself. Another popular lesion site is the medial thalamus in a variety of structures (centrum medianum, parafascicular nucleus, internal thalamic lamina), thought to represent the thalamic relay of the medially distributed, nonsomatotopographically organized portion of the spinoreticulothalamic tract. Lesions have also been made in pulvinar and hypothalamus.[63–70] Chronic stimulation, however, has been performed mainly in the ventrocaudal nucleus, medial lemniscus, and sensory capsule and in the periventricular or periaqueductal gray, although stimulation has also been used in the hypothalamus.

Psychiatric Illness

Although the earliest stereotactic operation was a psychosurgical procedure[71] with the lesion made in the dorsomedian nucleus, psychosurgery is rarely performed now. Cingulumotomy, anterior internal capsulotomy, and, possibly, hypothalamotomy are done most often.[72–77]

Epilepsy

Two types of stereotactic procedures have been used to treat epilepsy—deep EEG recording electrodes can be stereotactically inserted to guide future ablative surgery, or stereotactic surgery itself can control epilepsy. Though both stimulation and destructive procedures have been performed, these are rarely used today. The destructive procedures were undertaken for two different purposes: Lesions in the medial temporal lobes were meant to destroy epileptic foci, while procedures such as stereotactic subthalamotomies were meant to sever major pathways, thus limiting the spread of epileptic discharges.[78–83]

MORPHOLOGIC STEREOTACTIC SURGERY

The stereotactic approach has many morphologic applications. The stereotactic procedure most frequently performed, however, is the stereotactic biopsy.

Stereotactic Biopsy

Stereotactic biopsy enhances neurosurgery in a number of ways. First, it offers a relatively simple, safe technique for diagnosing a lesion so therapy can be more accurately planned. This is particularly applicable in deep, relatively inaccessible or multifocal lesions or when the patient's general condition makes radical surgery risky.

Therapeutic Aspiration

The philosophy of biopsy can be applied to certain cystic lesions such as abscesses, hematomas, colloid cysts, or craniopharyngiomas, which can be aspirated and possibly cured.

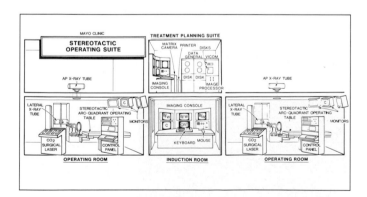

Figure 49.36 Kelly's stereotactic operating room. (Courtesy of PJ Kelly, Mayo Clinic, Rochester, Minn)

Brachytherapy

Stereotactic insertion of radioactive sources into a deep lesion is an alternative method of treating certain types of tumors.

Stereotactic Open Craniotomy

When a lesion is located deeply, particularly in sensitive structures, the impact of open surgery can be minimized by using stereotactic guidance.

Stereotactically Guided External Radiation

A new development in the treatment of neoplasms and arteriovenous malformations is stereotactically guided external radiation, to deliver a maximum dose of destructive energy to the lesion with minimal damage to surrounding normal structures. This has been accomplished using three different strategies: The stereotactically directed proton beam, whose site of impact is determined by the Bragg peak of proton absorption, was the earliest form[84-86]; more recent alternatives are a stereotactically directed x-ray beam from a linear accelerator[87,88] or collimated gamma emission from a cobalt-60 source (Fig. 49.37).[89-92]

Miscellaneous

Stereotactic techniques can be used to access small ventricles in order to place an Ommaya reservoir for intrathecal antineoplastic therapy in a cancer patient with positive cerebrospinal fluid. In the case of hydrocephalus, stereotactic surgery has been used to treat symptoms in a number of ways, for example, third ventriculostomy[93] and reconstruction of the aqueduct of Sylvius.[94] Significant experience has been acquired in the stereotactic clipping of aneurysms and arteriovenous malformations,[95-98] but this modality is not currently employed in most neurosurgical centers. Stereotactic aspiration of spontaneous intracerebral hematoma with and without instillation of clot-lysing compounds has been studied clinically,[99,100] but conclusive statements regarding the efficacy cannot be made. In one series of 175 putaminal hemorrhages drained stereotactically more than 6 hours after the ictus, level of consciousness and motor function were improved in approximately one third.[99] Further interest in this technique may evolve since effective evacuation of a deeply sit-uated clot can be achieved relatively easily and with minimal trauma to overlying functional tissue. Stereotaxis is also well-suited for the removal of foreign bodies.[101]

Stereotactic Endoscopy

Stereotactic endoscopy combines the best of both possible worlds—the accuracy of stereotactic guidance and the ability to see the brain.[102]

SELECTED STEREOTACTIC PROCEDURES IN CURRENT USE

THALAMOTOMY FOR MOVEMENT DISORDERS

Dyskinesias were originally treated by severing the "final common path" in the brain or spinal cord, thus accepting partial paralysis in exchange for relief from an exhausting dyskinesia. Meyers,[6,103,104] however, demonstrated that excision of the globus pallidus accomplishes the same thing without producing paralysis. Because the morbidity of the procedure was significant it never would have gained wide acceptance except for the introduction of human stereotactic surgery about that time. Stereotactic pallidotomy suddenly became a common procedure. As time passed, it was realized that since the globus pallidus projects to the thalamus, the thalamus should also be an appropriate target for relief of movement disorders. Cooper and Bravo[105] and Riechert and Hassler[106] showed that thalamotomy is superior to pallidotomy for the relief of dyskinesias, and to date thalamotomy has remained the principal stereotactic procedure for that purpose. However, a number of alternate targets (e.g., the subthalamus, dentate nucleus, internal capsule) have been used, and interest in pallidotomy is being revived because of possible relief of bradykinesia[46]; dentatectomy has proven most useful for the relief of spasticity.[107-126] Though most surgeons attempt to treat movement disorders by making lesions, it is also possible to suppress them using chronic stimulation, thus avoiding the risk of lesions.[127-134]

An entirely new chapter in the treatment of movement disorders was written when Backlund first transplanted cells from a patient's adrenal medulla to the caudate

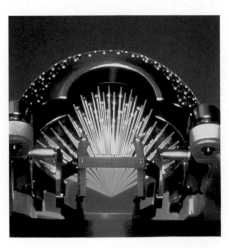

Figure 49.37 Diagrammatic illustration of collimated gamma rays delivered by the Leksell Gamma Knife. (Courtesy of Elekta Instruments, Atlanta, Ga)

nucleus in order to exploit the laboratory observation that such cells might survive, grow, and exude dopamine into surrounding tissue. Subsequent observations have shown that such treatment is on the one hand not dramatic and on the other somewhat enigmatic, since it appears not to cause the same effects in humans as had been expected from animal studies. Attempts to transplant human fetal mesencephalic multipotential cells destined to form substantia nigra into the corpus striatum have been designed to reproduce observations made in nonhuman primates that such cells survive, establish synaptic connections with striatal cells, and produce dopamine.[135–138] These types of therapy must await more extensive evaluation before they can be placed in proper perspective. Though often performed as open procedures, such surgery in sick, disabled patients carries a high risk and is more conveniently and safely accomplished by stereotactic means. These strategies are the first examples of what will probably become a major type of therapy. Whereas currently radiofrequency lesions indiscriminately kill all the tissue at a target site, and electrical stimulation indiscriminately activates all adjacent cells, in the future it will be possible to introduce specific neuroactive substances capable of destroying selected types of neurons either anterograde or retrograde. Instead of using stimulation, neuroactive substances will be available to activate or inhibit particular neurons. The only current clinical example of this strategy is the infusion of morphine into either the third ventricle or the spinal theca.

Although thalamotomy is most often performed for the relief of tremor, particularly that of Parkinson's disease, essentially the same lesion is made to relieve other types of tremor and dyskinesia. A somewhat larger lesion extending more rostral may be necessary in nontremorous disorders. Surgical treatment is indicated for dyskinesias that do not respond appropriately to medical therapy, are disabling, and particularly affect distal limb joints, such as the tremor of Parkinson's disease, essential tremor, and cerebellar tract lesions (of which only the tremor, not the ataxia, and in particular the distal rather than proximal tremor, responds) and dystonia affecting in particular the distal limbs (not, in our experience, the trunk or neck).

The CT-compatible stereotactic frame is attached to the patient's head under local anesthesia, usually in the ward or the CT suite, and axial cuts are made. The three-dimensional frame coordinates for the anterior and posterior commissures are determined. With the Leksell frame this is done as follows: Axial cuts are made every 1.5 mm with the GE 9800 scanner extending from the upper midbrain (Fig. 49.38), where the thickness of the collicular plate is seen, to the foramen of Monro's "rabbit ears" (Fig. 49.39). The posterior commissure lies in the posterior wall of the third ventricle in the first 1.5 mm cut above the tectal plate, where it narrows down to a thin membrane (Fig. 49.40). Though calcification in the pineal may be visible in this cut, its maximum dimension is usually seen in the next higher cut (Fig. 49.41). The

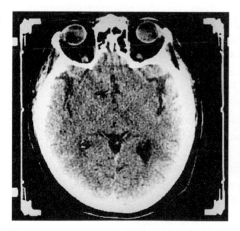
Figure 49.38 Axial stereotactic CT cut through upper midbrain using Leksell frame.

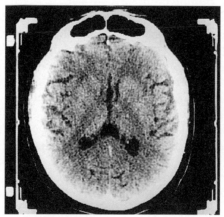
Figure 49.39 Axial cut as in Figure 49.38 showing "rabbit ears" appearance of the foramen of Monro region.

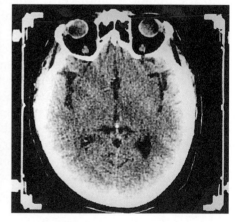
Figure 49.40 Axial cut 1.5 mm above Figure 49.38 showing posterior commissure.

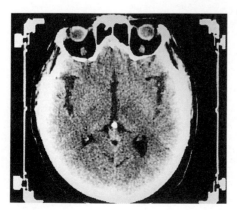
Figure 49.41 Axial cut 1.5 mm above Figure 49.40 showing pineal calcification at its fullest.

anterior commissure may be difficult to see, but since stereotactic targets lie close to the posterior commissure, even an error of several millimeters has little effect on their eventual localization. The commissure is sought on the anterior wall of the third ventricle, where it sometimes appears as a solid bar (Fig. 49.42); otherwise it can be assumed to lie about 3 mm below the "rabbit ears" of the foramen of Monro. It is now convenient to use a PC program to construct a series of sagittal brain diagrams based on one of the standard atlases (see Fig. 49.31). These diagrams, digitized in the computer's memory, are stretched or shrunk so their intercommissural distance conforms to that of the patient under study. At the same time the program applies to these reconstructed diagrams a millimeter grid that reads in terms of the particular patient's stereotactic frame coordinates.

The appropriate target is selected, and its coordinates are read off and set on the frame for probe introduction. A 5/16-inch twist drill hole is made anterior to the coronal suture in the same sagittal plane as the intended target. This size of hole allows a wide variety of trajectories to be made without the bony edges bending the probe. The hole is made in the same plane as the target so that all electrode trajectories traverse a single sagittal plane; this facilitates the mapping and comprehending of physiologic data (Fig. 49.43).

Though it is not entirely certain what structure or structures need to be destroyed to stop tremor, the usual strategy is to select a site with neurons firing in time with the tremor (tremor cells), where tremor is most effectively suppressed (or in some conditions driven) by electrical stimulation at the lowest possible threshold.[139-154] This is accomplished as follows: The tactile representation of the contralateral fingers is located in the 15 mm sagittal plane, and its position corroborated either by stimulation-induced paresthesiae at minimum threshold in the fingers or by identifying the tactile neurons with receptive fields in those digits. Should the first electrode trajectory reveal responses in either the face or the proximal upper extremity, trunk, or lower extremity, a second trajectory is made, laterally or medially respectively, based on the known medial-to-lateral somatotopographic organization of the tactile nucleus. Immediately rostral to these tactile cells microelectrodes locate neurons that respond to passive joint bending or muscle perturbation in the upper extremity, presumably in the lemniscal kinesthetic or spindle pathways. Further rostrally will be "voluntary" neurons firing in advance of a particular contralateral voluntary movement, presumably in the dentatothalamic tract destined for motor cortex. Stimulation of kinesthetic cells usually induces paresthesiae in a related part of the limb; rarely, it induces the sensation that a movement has taken place in the limb, although no movement is apparent. Stimulation of the "voluntary" cells often induces contraction in corresponding muscles at the onset of a stimulus train but not tetanization. The more rostrally the electrode is moved, the higher the threshold for inducing paresthesiae. In patients with tremor, microelectrodes demonstrate that kinesthetic and voluntary cells are also "tremor cells." Other tremor cells cannot be characterized. The degree of synchrony with EMG and tremor varies. Patients with dystonia have "dystonia cells" with similar firing patterns. Acute electrical stimulation, particularly at 300 Hz, is now applied, searching for sites where involuntary movement is arrested or driven most effectively at the lowest current. Such sites are chosen as targets.

Having located the target, a radiofrequency lesion is made, coagulating the largest possible volume in which dyskinesia cells and stimulation effects on the dyskinesia are observed. This requires a lesion or collection of lesions 5 mm or more in diameter, achieved by heating a lesion-making electrode with a 1 X 3 mm bare tip for at least 30 seconds with a current of 45 to 65 mA (Fig. 49.44). It is unclear how far the lesion must extend medially and laterally to achieve the best results.

Such surgery for Parkinson's disease arrests contralateral tremor, usually completely, at the time of surgery, though some degree of recurrence can take place up to 2 to 3 months postoperatively in perhaps 10% to 20% of patients; tremor seldom recurs later. Relief of contralateral rigidity is usually achieved in part at least, though this is not usually pursued since it requires a larger lesion and increases risk, and rigidity itself is seldom a major disability. Bradykinesia, manifested by impoverished facial expression, speech disturbance, loss of manual dexterity, and interference with gait, is never improved by thalamotomy; however, Delong and his group[155] recently observed that subthalamic nucleus lesions improve bradykinesia in monkeys made parkinsonian with MPTP,

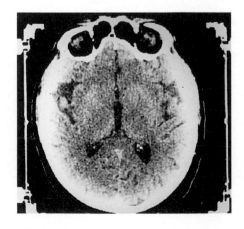

Figure 49.42 Axial cut showing anterior commissure.

and there is evidence that lesions in the globus pallidus (receiving the main outflow of subthalamic nucleus) ameliorate bradykinesia and akinesia. These intriguing points require further study.

The primary risks of thalamotomy are worsening dysarthria, ataxia of the hand, and disturbance of gait. They are seen in 3% or 4% of patients. Very rarely, intracerebral hemorrhage occurs. Whereas chronic stimulation to treat movement disorders obviates most of these risks, it demands further study.

Destructive Surgery

Destructive stereotactic procedures for pain relief were much more commonly employed in the past, but they have largely been supplanted by either chronic brain stimulation or chronic morphine instillation. The earliest stereotactic attempts at pain relief were destructive lesions in the spinothalamic tract in the mesencephalon and in the medial and lateral thalamus. Mesencephalic tractotomy continues to be widely used, its efficacy apparently

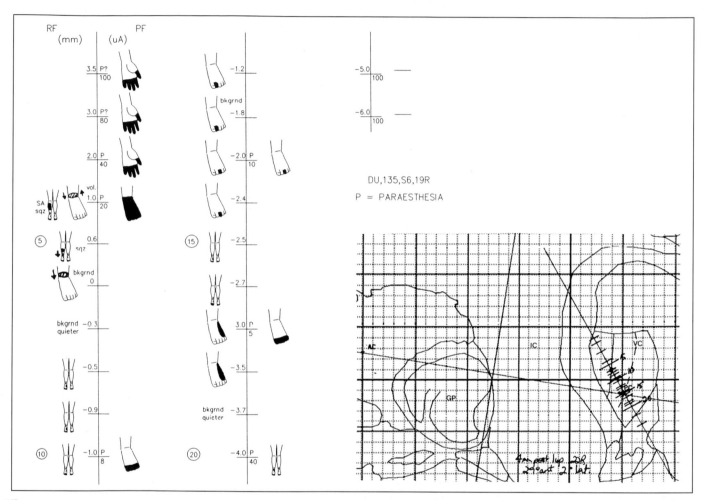

Figure 49.43 Computer-generated 19 mm sagittal brain diagram illustrating the course of a microelectrode trajectory through the lateral portion of the ventrocaudal nucleus (lower right) on which recording sites (illustrated to the left) are indicated. GP = globus pallidus; IC = internal capsule; VC = ventrocaudal nucleus; RF = contralateral receptive fields of neurons studied; PF = contralateral body part to which microstimulation-induced response was referred. Data to the left of trajectory line (numbers indicate distance in millimeters above target) indicate RFs; circled numbers refer to similarly numbered sites on the sagittal diagram. SA = slowly adapting; Sqz = squeeze; arrows indicate direction of passive movement evoking response. For PFs to right of midline, P = paresthesiae; numbers, threshold in µA. Thus neurons recorded from +1.0 to 0 are kinesthetic, all others are tactile, evoked by touching the parts indicated.

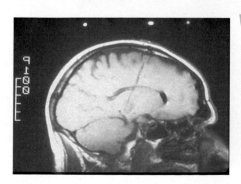

Figure 49.44 Sagittal MR image of patient with parkinsonism showing thalamotomy lesion and needle tract on the second postoperative day.

enhanced by including both somatotopographically organized fibers destined for parvicellular ventrocaudal nucleus and nonsomatotopographically organized fibers destined for medial thalamus.[19,22,71,156-209] The original practice of creating a lesion in the main lemniscal relay in the ventrocaudal nucleus, which was thought also to contain the spinothalamic relay, proved less effective and more likely to cause dysesthesia than creating a lesion in the medial thalamus, which has gradually supplanted it.[210-214] Medial thalamotomy and mesencephalic tractotomy (Fig. 49.45) continue to be the principal destructive procedures for pain relief; medial thalamotomy has a lower morbidity (chiefly transient cognitive disorders) but also a lower efficacy. Creating a lesion in the specific spinothalamic relay in Hassler's parvicellular ventrocaudal nucleus also appears to be a very effective procedure, although not often used.[63,64] Such procedures are most useful for treating cancer pain and the intermittent attacks of neuralgic and lancinating pain, not the constant burning dysesthetic discomfort associated with central and deafferentation pain.

As in thalamotomy, the likely locations—the spinothalamic tract in the upper midbrain and the parafascicular nucleus or the internal thalamic lamina—are selected from the position of the anterior-posterior commissure line. The medial lemniscus is distinguished from spinothalamic tract with macrostimulation: the former is recognized by the induction of somatotopographically organized contralateral paresthesiae, the latter by induction of somatotopographically organized contralateral warm or cold sensations. The medial lemniscus generally extends 10 to 12 mm and the spinothalamic tract 6 to 9 mm from the midline. The reticulothalamic fibers, which are usually insensitive to stimulation, lie medial to the spinothalamic tract. A lesion is planned, using the same equipment as for thalamotomy, that interrupts the spino-reticulothalamic fibers but spares the medial lemniscus, inducing dissociated sensory loss in the contralateral half of the body, in the area corresponding to that in which sensory effects were induced (see Fig. 49.45).

The site for medial thalamotomy must usually be identified by extrapolation. Whereas the tactile relay in ventrocaudal nucleus is readily identified with stimulation by inducing paresthesiae in the corresponding part of the contralateral body, stimulation in the parafascicular nucleus

or the internal thalamic lamina usually produces only volume conduction to the nearby sensory thalamus. Their location must be determined using the brain atlas from the proven position of the tactile relay (see Fig. 49.45). Pain relief from medial thalamotomy is less likely and more temporary than that from mesencephalic tractotomy, but it is rarely associated with mortality, usually exposing the patient only to the risk of transient cognitive disturbance. Mesencephalic tractotomy on the other hand carries a mortality of 5% to 10% and a 5% risk of dysesthetic phenomena and oculomotor disturbances.

Chronic Stimulation

Chronic stimulation of the brain has been employed for decades,[215-217] but Mazars[218-220] and Hosobuchi[221] appear to have been the first to popularize its use in the lemniscal relay in the ventrocaudal nucleus as a rostral extension of chronic stimulation of peripheral nerves and dorsal columns. The concept of using chronic stimulation to control pain by inducing paresthesiae in the area of pain came out of the gate theory of pain,[222] which suggested that activation of large fibers would suppress activity in small fibers (presumably pain conducting). Such stimulation was at first used indiscriminately to treat various types of pain; however, it is more effective for controlling pain caused by damage to the nervous system (central and deafferentation pain) than for nociceptive pain. The pathophysiology of central and deafferentation pain is poorly understood. Presumably chronic stimulation suppresses deranged central neuronal activity induced by the neural injury, which is in some way responsible for sending false messages into consciousness that are interpreted as pain. The nature of the deranged central neural activity is unknown, as is the reason why not every patient with a particular lesion develops pain.

The choice of chronic stimulation of the brain, rather than the spinal cord or peripheral nerve, is based on the following considerations: Patients with central pain caused by brain lesions (usually stroke) commonly respond only to stimulation of the lemniscal path in the brain. Similarly, brain stimulation may be the only useful technique available for central pain caused by cord lesions (usually from trauma) because patients with severe cord injuries have atrophied dorsal columns up to the dorsal column nuclei, leaving no site at which cord

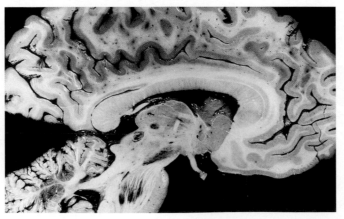

Figure 49.45 Sagittal section of the brain of a patient with carcinoma of the gingiva who underwent stereotactic mesencephalic tractotomy and medial thalamotomy for intractable pain in the head and neck 4 months before he died of the disease.

stimulation can be effected; or the epidural space may be inaccessible because of previous spinal surgery. Brain stimulation may also be considered in desperate patients for whom peripheral nerve or cord stimulation has failed.

Lemniscal Pathway Stimulation
As with peripheral nerve or dorsal column stimulation, brain stimulation in the lemniscal pathway is intended to produce paresthesiae in the part of the body affected by pain. This is accomplished by placing a stimulating electrode in either the tactile relay in the ventrocaudal nucleus of the thalamus, the medial lemniscus, or the sensory capsule; usually it is placed in the tactile relay (Fig. 49.46). The technique is performed in a similar way to thalamotomy for parkinsonian tremor except that the physiologic exploration is focused on the lemniscal relay. Microelectrodes are used to locate somatosensory tactile cells with receptive fields in the area of the patient's pain, or else sites are sought where micro- or macrostimulation produces paresthesiae in the area of the patient's pain.

When the optimum site is found, a chronic stimulating electrode is inserted, locked in place, and tunnelled under the scalp to the side of the head where a transcutaneous lead is attached for trial stimulation. The patient is then stimulated for 2 hours on and 1 hour off with a battery-powered TENS unit and records where the paresthesiae are felt, what effect they have on the pain, and any untoward experiences. If successful, the electrode is internalized to either a radiofrequency-coupled or battery-powered self-contained unit as mentioned above (see Figs. 49.28–49.30). Only half of the apparently suitable candidates actually derive relief from this stimulation,[218–221,223–228] and there is up to a 4% infection rate and a 10% incidence of transient neurologic effects. Perhaps one patient in five develops some technical problem with the device, such as electrode migration or lead breakage.

Periventricular–Periaqueductal Gray Stimulation
A second site commonly used for chronic brain stimulation is the periventricular or periaqueductal gray in the medial midbrain or thalamus. The use of this site evolved from the work of Reynolds,[229] who showed that analgesia could be induced there in animals, leading Richardson

and Akil to apply the technique in humans.[230,231] This stimulation may activate the patient's opiate and endorphin receptors, setting in action a serotonin-mediated descending pathway through the nucleus raphae magnus that in turn inhibits entry of impulses into the spinothalamic tract. While such stimulation would be expected to affect only nociceptive pain and other noxious mechanisms that depend on traffic in the spinothalamic tract, there is no consensus in the matter. Possibly, multiple medial descending pathways exist.

The choice between periventricular and periaqueductal gray depends not so much on efficacy—stimulation at both sites can suppress pain—but on the ancillary effects. Some patients stimulated in periventricular gray may perceive no effect, except through volume conduction to nearby sensitive structures; however, in other patients it may induce a feeling of generalized warmth, pleasure, and satiety in addition to pain relief. Stimulation in periaqueductal gray, on the other hand, may induce a sense of anxiety, unexplainable psychic discomfort, nystagmus, and diplopia, when using the site is impractical.

The procedure is done as above, except that no method for physiologically identifying the appropriate stimulation site exists. Therefore, it is usually chosen directly from the CT scan, 2 mm lateral to the wall of the third ventricle and 2 to 5 mm in front of the posterior commissure on the anterior-posterior commissure line, which is likely to be in the medial parafascicular nucleus (see Fig. 49.46). When using microelectrodes, the presence of neuronal discharge guarantees that the electrode has not inadvertently entered the nearby third ventricle. Neurons firing in bursts, common in dorsomedian nucleus, may cease abruptly at the border of the parafascicular nucleus. If acute stimulation induces a feeling of warmth or satiety plus pain relief, that site is a desirable one for a trial of chronic stimulation. If none of these localizing features are found, additional trajectories may be explored until the best possible site is found. Whatever the method of target selection, a chronic stimulating electrode is implanted for testing exactly as for the lateral thalamus. Chronic stimulation at this site is useful in patients who have nociceptive pain or who have central pain with a major element of allodynia (experiencing a normally non-noxious stimulus as painful) or hyperpathia (experiencing a noxious stimulus such as a pin prick as excessively unpleasant).

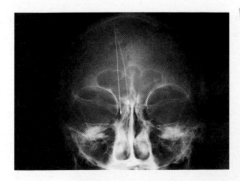

Figure 49.46 AP radiograph of the head showing chronic brain-stimulating electrodes in the lemniscal relay nucleus (lateral) and in the periventricular gray (medial).

PSYCHOSURGERY: CINGULUMOTOMY

It is perhaps not widely appreciated how useful cingulumotomy can be in treating severe, disabling monopolar depression. It is less useful for treating obsessive-compulsive patients who have not responded to more conventional therapy. Ballantyne's series at Massachusetts General Hospital have established its effectiveness and safety. The procedure can be performed more readily than most other functional stereotactic procedures because the cingulum itself can be directly visualized in MRI scans (Fig. 49.47), and its stereotactic coordinates can be read off directly as in a stereotactic biopsy. Radiofrequency lesions are usually made without physiologic corroboration, though techniques for it have been described.

STEREOTACTIC BIOPSY

One of the most common and important applications of stereotactic surgery is biopsy of intracranial mass lesions, an essential and everyday procedure in virtually all neurosurgical units. It ascertains the histologic or microbiologic nature of a brain lesion with high accuracy and relatively low risk. Targets within the lesion in question are selected by neurodiagnostic imaging (i.e., CT or MRI) performed with the patient wearing the stereotactic frame. A sample of tissue is obtained by aspiration of liquid lesions, or by using one of a number of tissue-cutting tools for solid tumors (see Figs. 49.26, 49.27). In most cases (except for young children) the procedure is done under local anesthesia and light sedation.

The technique of stereotactic biopsy and selection of the frame and sampling tool are relatively straightforward. The challenge is selecting the appropriate patient for stereotactic biopsy as opposed to standard craniotomy or nonsurgical therapy. Improved neurodiagnostic imaging has obviated the need for tissue diagnosis of numerous types of lesions, such as cavernous angiomas, which have a relatively distinctive appearance on MRI. However, one can never be certain of the diagnosis of a brain lesion until tissue is examined; the incidence of "unexpected" diagnosis was 12% in one recent biopsy series.[232] Once the clinician has concluded that the patient requires a tissue diagnosis, how is the stereotactic approach selected over craniotomy?

To answer this question, characteristics of both the lesion and the patient must be considered. The ideal lesion for stereotactic biopsy is too small and too deep for a safe approach by open craniotomy. Multiple lesions and diffuse, ill-defined lesions are also well suited for stereotactic biopsy. Furthermore, patients too old or ill to tolerate a craniotomy under general anesthesia usually tolerate a stereotactic biopsy uneventfully. If the patient is well and neurologically intact, one may not wish to subject him or her to the higher risk of neurologic morbidity associated with craniotomy as opposed to biopsy, assuming that cytoreductive surgery is not necessary or can wait.

When stereotactic biopsy is used, the diagnosis should be achieved more than 90% of the time; this number approaches 99% to 100% in the case of neoplasia.[233] Tumor cases usually do not pose a problem for the pathologist if the lesion is properly sampled. However, sampling only the central low-density portion of a ring-enhancing CT lesion may well supply only nondiagnostic necrotic tissue, whereas a sample from the enhancing edge may reveal the true nature of the lesion (for example, a malignant astrocytoma or the edge of a resolving hematoma). The rate of positive specific diagnosis is lower for inflammatory lesions, such as viral cerebritis or toxoplasmosis, but thorough laboratory investigation of patients suspected of harboring such lesions has obviated the need for tissue sampling in a significant number of cases.

The complication rate of stereotactic biopsy varies in the literature from 0% up to 10% in some series.[233] The most common and devastating complication is intracerebral hemorrhage, which is more likely to occur after biopsy of malignant neoplasms (e.g., malignant astrocytoma, lymphoma) as opposed to low-grade gliomas. In our experience, the rate of significant hemorrhage following stereotactic biopsy is about 5%. The rate of this complication can be reduced by proper planning, which in some situations requires preoperative angiography and/or MRI to demonstrate a safe trajectory through the brain, although most hemorrhages result from disruption of small tumor microvasculature not visible on imaging. Epidural, subdural, and subarachnoid hemorrhage may also complicate stereotactic biopsy.[233]

Case History

A 48-year-old heterosexual lumberjack presented with a 3 week history of headache, diplopia, and left hemipare-

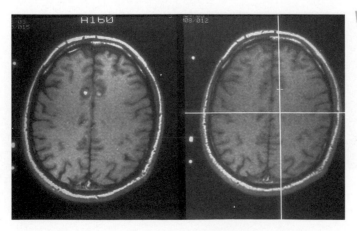

Figure 49.47 Axial MRI scan showing bilateral cingulumotomy lesions.

sis. On examination he had bilateral papilledema, pyramidal weakness of the left face, arm, and leg, and bilateral third and sixth cranial nerve pareses. CT showed a densely enhancing lesion in the posterior right thalamus and upper brain stem without significant mass effect (Fig. 49.48). CT-guided stereotactic biopsy confirmed the diagnosis of lymphoma (Fig. 49.49). The patient was treated with cranial radiation (50 Gy in 25 fractions via parallel opposed regional fields) and 2 months later was neurologically intact with no evidence of tumor on CT (Fig. 49.50).

Case History

A 33-year-old Vietnamese male presented with a short history of progressive limb weakness, diplopia, and fever. On examination he was cachectic, febrile, and appeared moribund. He groaned incomprehensibly, had bilateral intranuclear ophthalmoplegia, and was quadriparetic. Enhanced CT demonstrated a ring-enhancing lesion in the dorsal pons and midbrain (Fig. 49.51). Stereotactic aspiration of 3 mL of green pus resulted in immediate neurologic improvement. Subsequent culture grew mixed flora including anaerobic Gram-positive cocci, and fur-

ther treatment consisted of 6 weeks of intravenous antimicrobial therapy and two more stereotactic abscess drainages. Two months after admission he had a normal CT and was markedly improved with a moderate right hemiparesis and persistent diplopia. He was transferred to a rehabilitation facility.

STEREOTACTIC CRANIOTOMY AND TUMOR RESECTION

Stereotactic technique can be used to do more than biopsy a lesion—it can be used as a surgical adjunct in a number of ways. First, it can help the surgeon accurately plan a craniotomy flap and find a small lesion. For small cortical or subcortical lesions, the lesion is targeted on CT or MRI with the frame in place, and an entry point on the scalp is selected. The trajectory described will show where the craniotomy flap overlies the lesion. For subcortical lesions that do not present to the surface of the brain, the biopsy probe is simply inserted to its target (i.e., the lesion), and the surgeon follows the probe to the lesion, which is removed using standard microneurosurgical techniques.[234] Stereotactic endoscopy has been

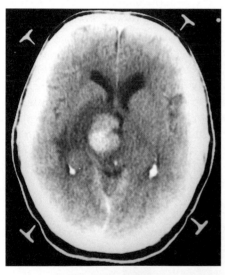

Figure 49.48 Enhanced CT scan showing lesion in diencephalon and upper brain stem.

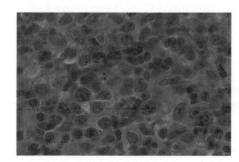

Figure 49.49 Light micrograph of biopsy specimen from lesion demonstrating lymphoma. Hematoxylin, phloxine, saffron stain of B5-fixed tissue. (X 242).

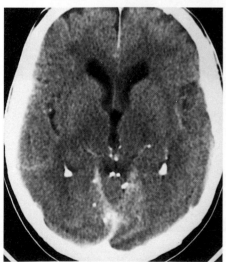

Figure 49.50 Enhanced CT scan 2 months following biopsy and radiation. No enhancing lesion is visible.

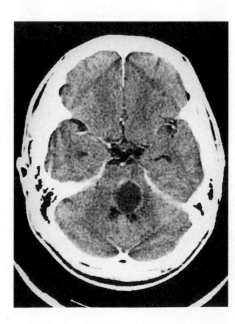

Figure 49.51 Enhanced CT scan showing ring-enhancing lesion in pons and midbrain. Abscess.

used to locate and remove intraventricular lesions, particularly within the third ventricle.[233]

Another way the stereotactic technique provides a surgical adjunct is by electrically and mechanically coupling a surgical tool (such as a laser) to a stereotactic system to effect a computer-assisted volumetric stereotactic resection. As areas on images of the lesion sliced perpendicular to the line of sight are targeted, the laser can be directed to the corresponding areas of the tumor in vivo and the lesion sequentially removed. Therefore, whatever is identified as tumor on the CT or MRI slices can be totally extirpated, resulting in postoperative images devoid of visible lesion. To date, this technique has been used mainly for deep, thalamic vascular malformations[235] and gliomas,[236] and while it is an exciting technical innovation, the inherent oncologic value of "gross total resection" of supratentorial glioma remains to be elucidated.[237] The limiting factor in the surgical ablation of brain tumors is that the tumor margin outlined on CT or even MRI may not accurately reflect the true tumor borders.

Stereotactic surgery has also made use of technological advances by combining neuroimaging, stereotactic technique, and robotic equipment to create the "neurosurgical robot."[238] Potential applications of neurosurgical robots include biopsy, interstitial brachytherapy, and surgical resection of lesions.

STEREOTACTIC CYST ASPIRATION

A number of neoplastic and nonneoplastic cysts can be effectively treated by stereotactic drainage in isolation or as the first stage of other therapies. A small but interesting experience with stereotactic aspiration of colloid cyst of the third ventricle has been reported.[239] Treatment is effective with low morbidity, in over half the cases, but a significant proportion of failures occur in hyperdense cysts on unenhanced CT, which are more likely to contain viscous fluid. Sequential aspiration and antibiotic therapy for brain abscesses appear to be a very effective treatment for this disease, as mentioned above.[240] Stereotactic aspiration of glioma cysts at the time of biopsy not only provides the diagnosis but in selected cases affords excellent symptomatic improvement until cranial radiation is completed.

Case History

A 65-year-old male presented with a 1 week history of progressive right hemiparesis and global dysphasia. CT demonstrated a cystic lesion in the left hemisphere with an enhancing nodule (Fig. 49.52). Stereotactic biopsy and aspiration of 50 mL of yellow fluid was performed, demonstrating a malignant astrocytoma with necrosis. Twenty-four hours later he had marked improvement of his hemiparesis and dysphasia, and CT showed significant diminution in the size of the cyst and mass effect (Fig. 49.53). He was transferred to another hospital for cranial radiation.

STEREOTACTIC BRACHYTHERAPY AND INTRACAVITARY RADIATION

The word brachytherapy, derived from the Greek root for short *(brachys)*, refers to treatment from a short distance. Brachytherapy is a radiation modality in which radioactive sources are placed directly into a tumor to irradiate it from the inside out. The approach is predicated on the assumption that it is desirable to deliver as high a radiation dose as possible to achieve better local control of a malignant tumor. While this has been demonstrated to be true in laboratory in vivo and in vitro models,[241] human data sup-

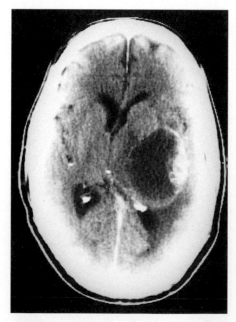

Figure 49.52 Enhanced CT scan showing cystic lesion in left hemisphere with peripheral (lateral) enhancement.

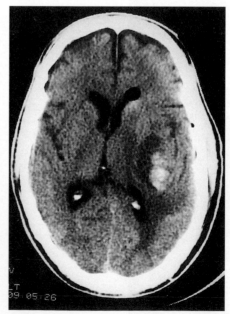

Figure 49.53 CT scan 24 hours after biopsy and cyst drainage. Malignant astrocytoma.

porting this hypothesis are sparse. The amount of radiation that can be delivered safely to a brain tumor by conventional teletherapy is limited by the unacceptable damage to normal brain that results from large doses. Brachytherapy provides the opportunity to administer very large doses of radiation to a tumor with relative sparing of surrounding brain, due to rapid fall-off of dose with distance determined by the inverse-square law and tissue attenuation.[241] Furthermore, the radiobiologic characteristics of continuous low-dose-rate radiation favor damage to neoplastic tissue over normal tissue because normal cells are better able to repair sublethal damage than tumor cells.[241]

In brachytherapy, after dosimetry for the lesion has been planned, plastic catheters are placed in the desired position and then after-loaded with line sources of radia-

tion seeds (Fig. 49.54). The most commonly used isotopes for brain brachytherapy are iodine-125 and iridium-192. After the desired minimum tumor dose has been delivered (usually 4 to 7 days) the catheters are removed. In most brachytherapy protocols, dosimetry is planned by multiplanar two-dimensional isodose distribution generation or computerized three-dimensional reconstruction models. Near-perfect accuracy of planning and actual catheter insertion is possible because of the stereotactic technique (Fig. 49.55).

Most experience with brachytherapy has been in the treatment of patients with recurrent malignant astrocytoma, specifically tumors that are reasonably small and well circumscribed on imaging, do not abut the midline and have not seriously compromised the patient's func-

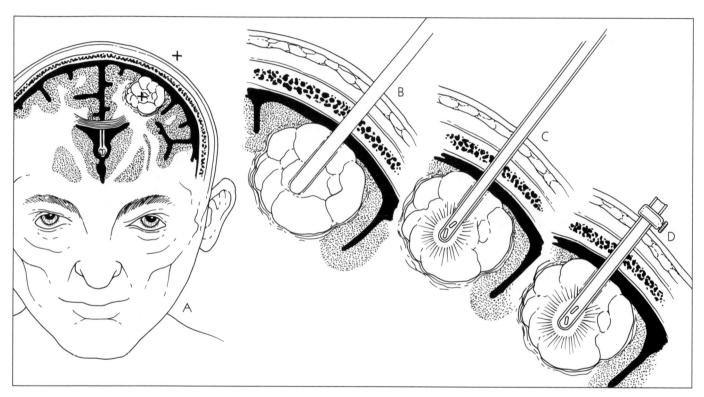

Figure 49.54 The technique of brachytherapy. **(A)** Tumor identified on imaging and the end point and trajectory of the catheter(s) chosen. **(B)** Outer catheter introduced stereotactically via twist drill hole. **(C)** Inner catheter housing radioactive seeds afterloaded into outer catheter. **(D)** Inner and outer catheters fixed to scalp with plastic flange.

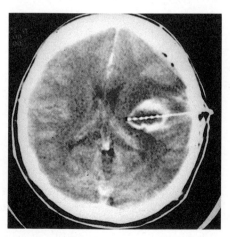

Figure 49.55 Postimplant CT scan demonstrating accurate placement of a single iodine-125 seed catheter in a malignant astrocytoma in a 35-year-old female. The patient was participating in the University of Toronto randomized brachytherapy trial examining the role of brachytherapy as part of initial management of patients with malignant astrocytoma.

tional performance.[242] In this group of well-selected patients, additional median survivals of approximately 1 year over those without brachytherapy have been obtained in most series.[242,243] The role of brachytherapy in the initial therapy of patients with malignant astrocytoma is not yet defined but is the subject of a handful of ongoing randomized studies.[242] Patients eligible for such studies are selected by tumor size and performance status and represent only about 30% of all patients with this tumor.[242,243] There is also increasing interest in and experience with patients who have a single recurrent brain metastasis refractory to surgery and external radiation, among whom a very small number of highly selected patients may well benefit.[244] There has been limited experience with brachytherapy for histologically benign and malignant skull base tumors (e.g., meningioma, chordoma) refractory to other modalities.[245,246]

The stereotactic technique also allows interstitial brachytherapy to be combined with hyperthermia,[247] which is not only cytotoxic when used alone but also a potent radiation sensitizer. Difficulty with adequate heating (42° to 45°C) of all portions of the tumor have thus far limited progress in achieving the desired effect with hyperthermia, particularly with brain tumors. Stereotactically directed radiation by multiple external radiation sources or a linear accelerator produces finely focussed radiation or "external brachytherapy" and is discussed in Chapters 41 and 42.

Lesions that recur after brachytherapy appear to be particularly circumscribed and produce mass effect, so that reoperation because of recurrent tumor plus radiation necrosis is required for palliation in 25% to 50% of patients undergoing brachytherapy.[242,243] The complications of brachytherapy include infection (i.e., scalp infection or brain abscess) and acute and chronic mass effect with increased intracranial pressure.[242,243]

Intracavitary irradiation involves the stereotactic placement of radioactive colloidal suspension of a beta-emitting isotope (e.g., yttrium-90, phosphorus-32) into a predominantly cystic neoplasm, such as certain gliomas and craniopharyngiomas, either at initial therapy or at recurrence.[248,249] Since beta particles do not penetrate deeply into tissue, lesions with significant solid components are not appropriate for such intracavitary treatment. Complications of this approach are few, and efficacy has been demonstrated in providing palliation in patients with recurrent glioma cysts.[249] For cystic craniopharyngiomas, this modality of treatment is effective in improving visual and endocrine function and has been suggested as a possible first-line treatment for predominantly cystic tumors.[248]

THE FUTURE

If the current exploitation of the stereotactic technique for such a variety of purposes seems impressive, future directions have inestimable scope. More widespread use of computer technology is heralded in morphologic stereotactic surgery, providing stereotactic imaging guidance for open craniotomy in the manner pioneered by Kelly, while in functional stereotactic surgery a wide range of neuroactive substances capable of being introduced into a spectrum of specific brain sites will revolutionize current endeavors.

REFERENCES

1. Gildenberg PL. General concepts of stereotactic surgery. In: Lunsford LD, ed. *Modern Stereotactic Neurosurgery*. Boston, Mass: Martinus Nijhoff; 1988:3–11.
2. Horsley V, Clarke RH. The structure and functions of the cerebellum examined by a new method. *Brain*. 1908;31:45–124.
3. Kandel EI; Watts G, trans. *Functional and Stereotactic Neurosurgery*. New York, NY: Plenum Publishing Corp; 1989:69.
4. Spiegel EA, Wycis HT, Marks M, et al. Stereotaxic apparatus for operations on the human brain. *Science*. 1947;106:349–350.
5. Spiegel EA, Wycis HT. Pallidothalamotomy in chorea. Presented at the Philadelphia Neurological Society; April 22, 1949.
6. Meyers HR. Surgical procedures for postencephalitic tremor with notes on the physiology of premotor fibers. *Arch Neurol Psychiatry*. 1940;44:453–459.
7. Tasker RR. Computerized tomography (CT) is just as accurate as ventriculography for functional stereotactic thalamotomy. *Stereotact Funct Neurosurg*. 1991;57:157–166.
8. Kondziolka D, Dolan EJ, Tasker RR. Functional stereotactic surgery and stereotactic biopsy using a magnetic resonance imaging directed system: results and comparisons to CT guidance. *Stereotact Funct Neurosurg*. 1990;249:54–55.
9. Afshar F, Watkins ES, Yap JC. *Stereotactic Atlas of the Human Brainstem and Cerebellar Nuclei*. New York, NY: Raven Press; 1978.
10. Andrew J, Watkins ES. *A Stereotactic Atlas of the Human Thalamus and Adjacent Structures: A Variability Study*. Baltimore, Md: Williams & Wilkins; 1969.
11. Hassler R, Mundinger F, Riechert T. *Stereotaxis in Parkinson Syndrome, with an Atlas of the Basal Ganglia in Parkinsonism by R. Hassler*. Berlin: Springer-Verlag; 1979.
12. Schaltenbrand G, Bailey P. *Introduction to Stereotaxis with an Atlas of the Human Brain*. Stuttgart: Georg Thieme Verlag; 1959.
13. Schaltenbrand G, Wahren W. *Atlas for Stereotaxy of the Human Brain*, rev. ed. Stuttgart: Georg Thieme Verlag; 1977.
14. Spiegel EA, Wycis HT. *Stereoencephalotomy (Thal-*

amotomy and Related Procedures), Part 1: Methods and Stereotaxic Atlas of the Human Brain. New York, NY: Grune & Stratton; 1952.

15. Szikla G, Bouvier G, Hari T, Petrov T. *Angiography of the Human Brain Cortex: Atlas of Vascular Patterns and Stereotactic Cortical Localization.* Berlin: Springer-Verlag; 1977.

16. Talairach J, David M, Tournoux P, Corredor H, Kvasina T. *Atlas d'anatomie stéréotaxique.* Paris: Masson; 1957.

17. Talairach J, Szikla G. *Atlas d'anatomie stéréotaxique du télencéphale.* Paris: Masson; 1967.

18. Van Buren JM, Bourke RC. *Nuclei and Cerebral Connections of the Human Thalamus, I. Variations of the Human Diencephalon, II.* Berlin: Springer-Verlag; 1972.

19. Tasker RR, Organ LW, Hawrylyshyn PA. *The Thalamus and Midbrain of Man. A Physiological Atlas Using Electrical Stimulation.* Springfield, Ill: Charles C Thomas Publisher; 1982.

20. Fukushima T, Mayanagi Y, Bouchard G. Thalamic evoked potentials to somatosensory stimulation in man. *Electroencephalogr Clin Neurophysiol.* 1976; 40:481–490.

21. Cooper IS, Lee ASJ. Cryostatic congelation: a system for providing a limited, controlled region of cooling or freezing of biologic tissues. *J Nerv Ment Dis.* 1961;133:259–263.

22. Sweet WH, Mark VII, Hamlin H. Radiofrequency lesions in the central nervous system of man and cat: including case reports of eight bulbar pain-tract interruptions. *J Neurosurg.* 1960;17:213–225.

23. Bertrand C, Martinez SN, Hardy J, et al. Stereotactic surgery for parkinsonism: microelectrode recording, stimulation and oriented sections with a leucotome. *Prog Neurol Surg.* 1973;5:79–112.

24. Guiot G, Hardy J, Albe-Fessard D. Délimitation précise des structures sous-corticales et identification de noyaux thalamiques chez l'homme par l'éléctrophysiologie stéréotaxique. *Neurochirurgie.* 1962;5:1–18.

25. Jasper HH, Bertrand G. Thalamic units involved in somatic sensation and voluntary and involuntary movements in man. In: Purpura D, Yahr M, eds. *The Thalamus.* New York, NY: Columbia University Press; 1966:365–390.

26. Ohye C. Depth microelectrode studies. In: Walker AE, Schaltenbrand G, eds. *Stereotaxy of the Human Brain.* Stuttgart: Georg Thieme Verlag; 1982: 372–389.

27. Tasker RR, Yamashiro K, Lenz F, Dostrovsky JO. Thalamotomy for Parkinson's disease: microelectrode technique. In: Lunsford LD, ed. *Modern Stereotactic Neurosurgery.* Boston, Mass: Martinus Nijhoff; 1988:297–314.

28. Organ LW, Tasker RR, Moody NF. The impedance profile of the human brain as a localization technique in stereoencephalotomy. *Confin Neurol.* 1967;29:192–196.

29. Alberts WW, Wright EWJ, Feinstein B, von Bonin G. Experimental radiofrequency brain lesion size as a function of physical parameters. *J Neurosurg.* 1966;25:421–423.

30. Kelly PJ, Kall BA, eds. *Computers in Stereotactic Neurosurgery.* Boston, Mass: Blackwell Scientific Publications; 1992. Contemporary Issues in Neurological Surgery.

31. Bertrand G, Olivier A, Thompson CJ. Computer display of stereotactic brain maps and probe tracts. *Acta Neurochir.* 1974;(suppl 21):235–243.

32. Bertrand G, Olivier A, Thompson CJ. The computer brain atlas: its use in stereotactic surgery. *Confin Neurol.* 1975;36:312–313.

33. Hardy TL, Koch L, Lassiter A. Computer graphics with computerized tomography for functional neurosurgery. *Appl Neurophysiol.* 1983;46:217–226.

34. Hardy TL. Stereotactic CT atlases. In: Lunsford LD, ed. *Modern Stereotactic Neurosurgery.* Boston, Mass: Martinus Nijhoff; 1988:425–430.

35. Hawrylyshyn P, Rowe IH, Tasker RR, Organ LW. A computer system for stereotaxic neurosurgery. *Comput Biol Med.* 1976;6:87–97.

36. Kelly PJ. Volumetric stereotaxis and computer-assisted stereotactic resection of subcortical lesions. In: Lunsford LD, ed. *Modern Stereotactic Neurosurgery.* Boston, Mass: Martinus Nijhoff; 1988: 169–184.

37. Peluso F, Gybels J. Computer calculation of the position of the side-protruding electrode tip during penetration in human brain. *Confin Neurol.* 1972; 34:94–100.

38. Tasker RR, Hawrylyshyn P, Organ LW. Computerized graphic display of physiological data collected during human stereotactic surgery. *Appl Neurophysiol.* 1978;41:183–187.

39. Vries JK, McLinden S, Banks G, Latchaw RE. Computerized three-dimensional stereotactic atlases. In: Lunsford LD, ed. *Modern Stereotactic Neurosurgery.* Boston, Mass: Martinus Nijhoff; 1988:441–459.

40. Adams JE, Rutkin BB. Lesions of the centrum medianum in the treatment of movement disorders. *Confin Neurol.* 1965;26:231–236.

41. Andy OJ, Jurko MF, Sias FR Jr. Subthalamotomy in the treatment of Parkinsonian tremor. *J Neurosurg.* 1963;20:860–870.

42. Burzaco J. Stereotactic pallidotomy in extrapyramidal disorders. *Appl Neurophysiol.* 1985;48:283–287.

43. Gildenberg PL. Survey of stereotactic and functional neurosurgery in the United States and Canada. *Appl Neurophysiol.* 1975;38:31–37.

44. Krayenbühl H, Wyss OAM, Yasargil MG. Bilateral thalamotomy and pallidotomy as treatment for bilateral Parkinsonism. *J Neurosurg.* 1961;18:429–444.

45. Laitinen L. Thalamic targets in the stereotaxic treatment of Parkinson's disease. *J Neurosurg.* 1966; 24:82–85.

46. Laitinen L, Bergenheim AT, Hariz MI. Leksell's

posteromedial pallidotomy in the treatment of Parkinson's disease. *J Neurosurg.* 1992;76:53–61.

47. Spiegel EA, Wycis HT. Pallidothalamotomy in chorea. *Arch Neurol Psychiatry.* 1950;64:295–296.

48. Crue BL Jr, Todd EM, Carregal EJA, Kilham O. Percutaneous trigeminal tractotomy: case report utilizing stereotactic radiofrequency lesion. *Bull Los Angeles Neurol Soc.* 1967;32:86–92.

49. Crue BL Jr, Todd EM, Carregal EJ. Percutaneous radiofrequency stereotactic trigeminal tractotomy. In: Crue BL, ed. *Pain and Suffering.* Springfield, Mass: Charles C Thomas Publisher; 1970:69–79.

50. Fox JL. Delineation of the obex by contrast radiography during percutaneous trigeminal tractotomy: technical note. *J Neurosurg.* 1972;36:107–112.

51. Fox JL. Percutaneous trigeminal tractotomy: variations in delineation of the obex using emulsified pantopaque. *Confin Neurol.* 1974;36:97–100.

52. Hitchcock ER. Stereotactic spinal surgery: a preliminary report. *J Neurosurg.* 1969;31:386–399.

53. Hitchcock ER. Stereotactic cervical myelotomy. *J Neurol Neurosurg Psychiatry.* 1970;33:224–230.

54. Hitchcock ER. Stereotactic trigeminal tractotomy. *Ann Clin Res.* 1970;2:131–135.

55. Hitchcock ER, Schvarcz JR. Stereotaxic trigeminal tractotomy for post-herpetic facial pain. *J Neurosurg.* 1972;37:412–417.

56. Schvarcz JR. Spinal cord stereotactic techniques re trigeminal nucleotomy and extralemniscal myelotomy. *Appl Neurophysiol.* 1978;41:99–112.

57. Schvarcz JR. Stereotactic spinal trigeminal nucleotomy for dysesthetic facial pain. In: Bonica JJ, Liebeskind JC, Albe-Fessard DG, eds. *Advances in Pain Research and Therapy.* New York, NY: Raven Press; 1979;3:331–336.

58. Schvarcz JR. Stereotactic high cervical extralemniscal myelotomy for pelvic cancer pain. *Acta Neurochir Suppl.* 1984;33:431–435.

59. Barbera J, Barcia-Salorio JL, Broseta J. Stereotaxic pontine spinothalamic tractotomy. *Surg Neurol.* 1979;11:111–114.

60. Hitchcock ER. Stereotaxic pontine spinothalamic tractotomy. *J Neurosurg.* 1973;39:746–752.

61. Hitchcock ER, Kim MC, Sotelo M. Further experience in stereotactic pontine tractotomy. *Appl Neurophysiol.* 1985;48:242–246.

62. Hitchcock ER, Sotelo M, Kim MC. Analgesic levels and technical method in stereotactic pontine spinothalamic tractotomy. *Acta Neurochir.* 1985;77:29–36.

63. Hassler R. The division of pain conduction into systems of pain sensation and pain awareness. In: Janzen R, Keidel WD, Herz A, Steichele C, eds. *Pain: Basic Principles-Pharmacology-Therapy.* Stuttgart: Georg Thieme Verlag; 1972:98–112.

64. Hitchcock ER, Teixeira MJ. A comparison of results from center-median and basal thalamotomies for pain. *Surg Neurol.* 1981;15:341–351.

65. Fraioli B, Guidetti B. Effect of stereotactic lesions of the pulvinar and lateralis posterior nucleus on intractable pain and dyskinetic syndromes of man. *Appl Neurophysiol.* 1975;38:23–30.

66. Laitinen L. Anterior pulvinotomy in the treatment of intractable pain. *Acta Neurochir Suppl.* 1977;24:223–225.

67. Siegfried J. Stereotactic pulvinarotomy in the treatment of intractable pain. In: Krayenbühl H, Maspes PE, Sweet WH, eds. *Progress in Neurological Surgery.* Basel: Karger; 1977;8:104–113.

68. Yoshii N, Mizokami T, Ushikubo T, et al. Long-term followup study after pulvinotomy for intractable pain. *Appl Neurophysiol.* 1980;43:128–132.

69. Mayanagi Y, Sano K, Suzuki I, et al. Stimulation and coagulation of the posteromedial hypothalamus for intractable pain, with reference to β-endorphins. *Appl Neurophysiol.* 1982;45:136–142.

70. Sano K, Mayanagi Y, Sekino H, Ogashiwa M, Ishijima B. Results of stimulation and destruction of the posterior hypothalamus in man. *J Neurosurg.* 1970;33:689–707.

71. Spiegel EA, Wycis HT. *Stereoencephalotomy, II. Clinical and Physiological Applications.* New York, NY: Grune & Stratton; 1962.

72. Ballantine HT Jr, Cassidy WL, Flanagan NB, et al. Stereotaxic anterior cingulotomy for neuropsychiatric illness and intractable pain. *J Neurosurg.* 1967;26:488–495.

73. Bertrand C, Martinez N, Hardy. Frontothalamic section for intractable pain. In: Knighton RS, Dumke PR, eds. *Henry Ford Hospital International Symposium.* Boston, Mass: Little, Brown & Co; 1966:531–533.

74. Mayanagi Y, Sano K. Posteromedial hypothalamotomy for behavioural disturbances and intractable pain. In: Lunsford LD, ed. *Modern Stereotactic Neurosurgery.* Boston, Mass: Martinus Nijhoff; 1988:377–388.

75. Meyerson BA, Mindus P. The role of anterior internal capsulotomy in psychiatric surgery. In: Lunsford LD, ed. *Modern Stereotactic Neurosurgery.* Boston, Mass: Martinus Nijhoff; 1988:353–364.

76. Narabayashi H, Nagao T, Saito Y, et al. Stereotaxic amygdalotomy for behaviour disorders. *Arch Neurol.* 1963;9:1–25.

77. Turnbull IM. Bilateral cingulumotomy combined with thalamotomy or mesencephalic tractotomy for pain. *Surg Gynecol Obstet.* 1972;134:958–962.

78. Hassler R, Riechert T. Über einen Fall von doppelseitiger Fornicotomie bei sogenannter temporalen Epilepsie. *Acta Neurochir (Wien).* 1957;5:330–340.

79. Jelsma RK, Bertrand CM, Martinez SN, Molina-Negro P. Stereotaxic treatment of frontal lobe and centrencephalic epilepsy. *J Neurosurg.* 1973;39:42–51.

80. Jinnai D. Clinical results and the significance of Forel-H-tomy in the treatment of epilepsy. *Confin Neurol.* 1966;27:129–136.

81. Kalyanaraman S, Ramamurthi B. Stereotaxic surgery for generalized epilepsy. *Neurol India.* 1970;18 (suppl 1):34–41.

82. Li CL, Van Buren JM. Micro-electrode recordings in the brain of man with particular reference to epilepsy and dyskinesia. In: Somjen GG, ed. *Neurophysiology Studied in Man*. Amsterdam: Exc Med; 1972:49–63.

83. Spiegel EA, Wycis HT, Baird HW III. Pallidotomy and pallidoamygdalotomy in certain types of convulsive disorders. *Arch Neurol Psychiatry*. 1958; 80:714–728.

84. Kjellberg RN, Kliman B. Treatment of acromegaly by proton hypophysectomy. In: Morley TP, ed. *Current Controversies in Neurosurgery*. Philadelphia, Pa: WB Saunders Co; 1976:392–405.

85. Kjellberg RN, Abe M. Stereotactic Bragg peak proton beam therapy. In: Lunsford LD, ed. *Modern Stereotactic Neurosurgery*. Boston, Mass: Martinus Nijhoff; 1988:471–480.

86. Levy RP, Fabrikant I, Frankel KA, Phillips MH, Lyman JT. Charged-particle radiosurgery of the brain. In: Lunsford LD, ed. *Modern Stereotactic Neurosurgery*. Boston, Mass: Martinus Nijhoff; 1988:955–990.

87. Friedman WA. LINAC radiosurgery. In: Lunsford LD, ed. *Modern Stereotactic Neurosurgery*. Boston, Mass: Martinus Nijhoff; 1988:991–1005.

88. Hitchcock E, Kitchen G, Datton E, Pape B. Stereotactic LINAC radiosurgery. *Br J Neurosurg*. 1989;3:305–312.

89. Coffey RJ, Lunsford LD. Stereotactic radiosurgery using the 201 cobalt-60 source gamma knife. In: Friedman WA, guest ed; Winn HR, Mayberg MR, eds. Stereotactic Neurosurgery. *Neurosurg Clin North Am*. Philadelphia, Pa: WB Saunders Co; 1990:933–954.

90. Forster DMC, Leksell L, Meyerson BA, et al. Gammathalamotomy in intractable pain. In: Janzen R, Keidel WD, Herz A, Steichele C, eds. *Pain: Basic Principles-Pharmacology-Therapy*. Stuttgart: Georg Thieme Verlag; 1972:194–198.

91. Leksell L, Meyerson BA, Forster DMC. Radiosurgical thalamotomy for intractable pain. *Confin Neurol*. 1972:34:264.

92. Steiner L, Forster D, Leksell L, et al. Gammathalamotomy in intractable pain. *Acta Neurochir (Wien)*. 1980;52:173–184.

93. Jack CR, Kelly PJ. Stereotactic third ventriculostomy: assessment of patency with MR imaging. *AJNR*. 1989;10:515–522.

94. Backlund EO, Grepe A, Lunsford LD. Stereotactic reconstruction of the aqueduct of Sylvius. *J Neurosurg*. 1981;55:800–810.

95. Kandel EI, Peresedov W. Stereotaxic clipping of arterial aneurysms and arteriovenous malformations. *J Neurosurg*. 1977;46:12–23.

96. Mullan S. Experiences with surgical thrombosis of intracranial berry aneurysms and carotid cavernous fistulas. *J Neurosurg*. 1974;41:657–670.

97. Rand RW. Stereotaxy for vascular anomalies. In: Schaltenbrand G, Walker AE, eds. *Stereotaxy of the Human Brain: Anatomical, Physiological and Clinical Applications*. Stuttgart: Georg Thieme Verlag; 1982: 674–685.

98. Riechert T, Mundinger F. Combined stereotaxic operation for treatment of deep-seated angiomas and aneurysms. *J Neurosurg*. 1964;21:358–363.

99. Niizuma H, Shimizu Y, Yonemitsu T, et al. Results of stereotactic aspiration in 175 cases of putaminal hemorrhage. *Neurosurgery*. 1989;24:814–819.

100. Mohajder M, Eggert R, May J, et al. CT-guided stereotactic fibrinolysis of spontaneous cerebellar hemorrhage: long-term results. *J Neurosurg*. 1990; 73:217–222.

101. Hitchcock E, Cowie R. Stereotactic removal of intracranial foreign bodies: review and case report. *Injury*. 1982;14:471–475.

102. Hellwig D, Eggers F, Bauer BL, Likoyiannis A. Endoscopic stereotaxis preliminary results. *Stereotact Funct Neurosurg*. 1990;418:54–55.

103. Meyers R. The modification of alternating tremors, rigidity and festination by surgery of the basal ganglia. *Res Publ Assoc Res Nerv Ment Dis*. 1942;21: 602–665.

104. Meyers R. Surgical interruption of the pallidofugal fibers, its effect on the syndrome of paralysis agitans and technical consideration in its application. *NY State J Med*. 1942;42:317–325.

105. Cooper IS, Bravo CJ. Implications of a five-year study of 700 basal ganglia operations. *Neurology*. 1958;8:701–707.

106. Hassler R, Riechert T. Über die Symptomatik und operative Behandlung der extrapyramidalen Bewegungsstörungen. *Med Klin*. 1958;53:817–824.

107. Andrew J, Fowler CJ, Harrison MVG. Stereotaxic thalamotomy in 55 cases of dystonia. *Brain*. 1983;106:981–1000.

108. Bullard DE, Nashold BS Jr. Stereotaxic thalamotomy for treatment of post-traumatic movement disorders. *J Neurosurg*. 1984;61:316–321.

109. Cooper IS. *Involuntary Movement Disorders*. New York, NY: Hoeber-Harper Row; 1969.

110. Gros C, Frerebeau PH, Perez-Dominguez E, et al. Long-term results of stereotaxic surgery for infantile dystonia and dyskinesia. *Neurochirurgie*. 1976; 19:171–178.

111. Jokura H, Otsuki T, Niizuma H, et al. Long-term results of VIM-thalamotomy for post-apoplectic tremor. *Stereotact Funct Neurosurg*. 1990;54+55:216.

112. Kandel EI. Treatment of hemihyperkinesis by stereotactic operations on basal ganglia. *Appl Neurophysiol*. 1982;45:225–229.

113. Kandel EI. Long-term follow up results after stereotactic surgery of Parkinsonism. Presented at the tenth meeting of the WSSFN; Maebashi, Japan; 1989.

114. Kelly PJ, Gillingham FJ. The long-term results of stereotactic surgery and L-dopa therapy in patients with Parkinson's disease. *J Neurosurg*. 1980;53: 332–337.

115. Matsumoto K, Shichijo F, Fukami T. Long-term followup review of cases of Parkinson's disease after

unilateral or bilateral thalamotomy. *J Neurosurg.* 1984;60:1033–1034.

116. Miyamoto T, Bekku H, Moriyama E, Tsuchida S. Present role of stereotactic thalamotomy for Parkinsonism: retrospective analysis of operative results and thalamic lesions in computed tomograms. *Appl Neurophysiol.* 1985;48:294–304.

117. Mohadjer M, Goerke H, Milios E, Eton A, Mundinger F. Long-term results of stereotaxy in the treatment of essential tremor. *Stereotact Funct Neurosurg.* 1990;54+55:125–129.

118. Mundinger F, Kuhn I. Postoperative and long-term results after stereotactic operations for action myoclonia in cases of encephalomyelitis disseminata. *Appl Neurophysiol.* 1982;45:299–305.

119. Mundinger F. Postoperative and long-term results of 1,561 stereotactic operations in Parkinsonism. *Appl Neurophysiol.* 1985;48:293.

120. Nagaseki Y, Shibazaki T, Hirai T, et al. Long-term followup results of selective VIM-thalamotomy. *J Neurosurg.* 1986;65:296–302.

121. Narabayashi H. Choreoathetosis and spasticity. In: Schaltenbrand G, Walker AE, eds. *Stereotaxy of the Human Brain.* Stuttgart: Georg Thieme Verlag; 1982:532–543.

122. Narabayashi H, Maeda T, Yokochi F. Long-term followup study of nucleus ventralis intermedius and ventrolateralis thalamotomy using a microelectrode technique in parkinsonism. *Appl Neurophysiol.* 1987;50:330–337.

123. Ohye C, Hirai T, Miyazaki M, et al. VIM-thalamotomy for the treatment of various kinds of tremor. *Appl Neurophysiol.* 1982;45:275–280.

124. Taira T, Hitchcock E. Stereotactic thalamotomy for patients with dystonia. *Stereotact Funct Neurosurg.* 1990;54+55:215–216.

125. Tasker RR, Siqueira J, Hawrylyshyn P, Organ LW. What happened to VIM-thalamotomy for Parkinson's disease? *Appl Neurophysiol.* 1983;46:68–83.

126. Tasker RR, Doorly T, Yamashiro K. Thalamotomy in generalized dystonia. In: Fahn S, et al, eds. *Advances in Neurology, 50: Dystonia 2.* New York, NY: Raven Press; 1988:615–631.

127. Andy OJ. Thalamic stimulation for control of movement disorders. *Appl Neurophysiol.* 1983;46:107–123.

128. Benabid AL, Pollak P, Louveau A, et al. Combined (thalamotomy and stimulation) surgery of the VIM thalamic nucleus for bilateral Parkinson's disease. *Appl Neurophysiol.* 1987;50:344–346.

129. Brice J, McLellan L. Suppression of intention tremor by contingent deep-brain stimulation. *Lancet.* June 7, 1980;1221–1222.

130. Cooper IS, Upton ARM, Amin I. Chronic cerebellar stimulation (CCS) and deep brain stimulation (DBS) in involuntary movement disorders. *Appl Neurophysiol.* 1982;45:209–217.

131. Mazars G, Merienne L, Cioloca G. Control of dyskinesia due to sensory deafferentation by means of thalamic stimulation. *Acta Neurochir Suppl.* 1980;30:239–243.

132. Mundinger R, Neumuller H. Programmed stimulation for control of chronic pain and motor diseases. *Appl Neurophysiol.* 1982;45:102–111.

133. Schvarcz JR, Sica RS, Morita E, et al. Electrophysiological changes induced by chronic stimulation of the dentate nuclei for cerebral palsy. *Appl Neurophysiol.* 1982;45:55–61.

134. Siegfried J, Rea GL. Deep brain stimulation for the treatment of motor disorders. In: Lunsford LD, ed. *Modern Stereotactic Neurosurgery.* Boston, Mass: Martinus Nijhoff; 1988:409–412.

135. Backlund EO, Granberg PO, Hamberger B, et al. Transplantation of adrenal medullary tissue to striatum in parkinsonism: first clinical trials. *J Neurosurg.* 1985;62:164–173.

136. Backlund EO. Transplantation to the brain. In: Lunsford LD, ed. *Modern Stereotactic Neurosurgery.* Boston, Mass: Martinus Nijhoff; 1988:389–393.

137. Bakay RAE. Transplantation into the central nervous system: a therapy of the future. In: Friedman WA, guest ed; Winn HR, Mayberg MR, eds. Stereotactic Neurosurgery. *Neurosurg Clin North Am.* Philadelphia, Pa: WB Saunders Co. 1990:881–895.

138. Hitchcock ER, Kenny BG, Clough CG, Hughes RC, Henderson BTH, Detta A. Stereotactic implantation of foetal mesencephalon (STIM): the UK experience. In: Dunnett SB, Richards SJ, eds. *Progress in Brain Research.* Amsterdam: Elsevier Science Publishing Co; 1990;82:723–728.

139. Albe-Fessard D. Electrophysiological methods for the identification of thalamic nuclei. *Z Neurol.* 1973;205:15–28.

140. Alberts WW, Libet B, Wright EW, Feinstein B. Physiological mechanisms of tremor and rigidity in Parkinsonism. *Confin Neurol.* 1965;26:318–327.

141. Bertrand G, Jasper H, Wong A. Microelectrode study of the human thalamus: functional organization in the ventrobasal complex. *Confin Neurol.* 1967;29:81–86.

142. Guiot G, Derome P, Arfel G, Walter S. Electrophysiological recordings in stereotaxic thalamotomy for Parkinsonism. *Prog Neurol Surg.* 1973;5:189–221.

143. Jones MW, Tasker RR. The relationship of documented destruction of specific cell types to complications and effectiveness in thalamotomy for tremor in Parkinson's disease. *Stereotact Funct Neurosurg.* 1990;54+55:207–211.

144. Lenz FA, Dostrovsky JO, Kwan HC, et al. Methods for microstimulation and recording of single neurons and evoked potentials in the human central nervous system. *J Neurosurg.* 1988;68:630–634.

145. Lenz FA, Dostrovsky JO, Tasker RR, et al. Single-unit analyses of the human ventral thalamic nuclear group: somatosensory responses. *J Neurophysiol.* 1988;59:299–316.

146. Lenz FA, Schnider S, Tasker RR, et al. The role of feedback in the tremor frequency activity of tremor cells in the ventral nuclear group of human thalamus. *Acta Neurochir Suppl.* 1987;39:54–56.

147. Lenz FA, Tasker RR, Kwan HC, et al. Functional classes of "tremor cells" in the ventral tier of lateral thalamic nuclei of patients with Parkinsonian tremor. In: Brock M, ed. *Modern Neurosurgery.* Berlin: Springer-Verlag; 1991.

148. Lenz FA, Tasker RR, Kwan HC, et al. Single unit analysis of the human ventral thalamic nuclear group: correlation of thalamic 'tremor cells' with the 3–6 Hz component of Parkinsonian tremor. *J Neurosci.* 1988;8:754–764.

149. Matsumura M, Hirato M, Wada H, et al. Electrophysiological study of the thalamic ventralis intermedius nucleus in cases with central pain. *Appl Neurophysiol.* 1986;49:297.

150. Narabayashi H. Tremor mechanisms. In: Schaltenbrand G, Walker AE, eds. *Stereotaxy of the Human Brain.* Stuttgart: Georg Thieme Verlag; 1982:510–514.

151. Ohye C, Fukamachi A, Narabayashi H. Spontaneous and evoked activity of sensory neurons and their organization in the human thalamus. *Z Neurol.* 1972; 203:219–234.

152. Ohye C, Narabayashi H. Activity of thalamic neurons and their receptive fields in different functional states in man. In: Somjen GG, ed. *Neurophysiology Studied in Man.* Amsterdam: Exc Med; 1972:79–84.

153. Ohye C, Narabayashi H. Physiological study of presumed ventralis intermedius neurons in the human thalamus. *J Neurosurg.* 1979;50:290–297.

154. Strüppler A, Lücking CH, Erbel F. Neurophysiological findings during stereotactic operation in thalamus and subthalamus. *Confin Neurol.* 1972;34:70–73.

155. Bergman H, Wickmanso T, DeLong MR. Reversal of experimental parkinsonism by lesions of the subthalamic nucleus. *Science.* 1990;249:1436–1438.

156. Amano K, Iseki H, Notani M, et al. Rostral mesencephalic reticulotomy for pain relief with reference to electrode trajectory and clinical results. *Appl Neurophysiol.* 1979;42:316.

157. Amano K, Kawamura H, Tanikawa T, et al. Long-term follow-up study of rostral mesencephalic reticulotomy for pain relief—report of 34 cases. *Appl Neurophysiol.* 1986;49:105–111.

158. Askenasy HM, Levinger M. Stereoencephalotomy for relief of pain. *Harefuah.* 1968;74:85–89.

159. Bettag W, Yoshida T. Über stereotaktische Schmerzoperationen. *Acta Neurochirurgica.* 1960;8:299–317.

160. Cassinari V, Pagni CA. *Central Pain: A Neurosurgical Survey.* Cambridge, Mass: Harvard University Press; 1969.

161. Frank F, Tognetti F, Gaist G, Frank G, Galassi E, Sturiale C. Stereotaxic rostral mesencephalotomy in treatment of malignant faciothoracobrachial pain syndromes. *J Neurosurg.* 1982;56:807–811.

162. Frank F, Fabrizi AP, Gaist G, et al. Stereotactic mesencephalotomy versus multiple thalamotomies in the treatment of chronic cancer pain syndromes. *Appl Neurophysiol.* 1987;50;314–318.

163. Hageman R, DeGrood MPAM. Experiences with stereotactic treatment of intractable pain. *Psychiatr Neurol Neurosurg.* 1970;73:113–134.

164. Hassler R, Riechert T. Klinische and anatomische Befunde bei stereotaktischen Schmerzoperationen im Thalamus. *Arch Psychiatr z Gesamte Neurol.* 1959;200:93–122.

165. Hécaen H, Talairach J, David M, Dell MB. Coagulations limitées du thalamus dans les algies du syndrome thalamique. *Rev Neurol (Paris).* 1949;81: 917–931.

166. Helfant MH, Leksell L, Strang RR. Experiences with intractable pain treated by stereotaxic mesencephalotomy. *Acta Chir Scand.* 1965;129:573–580.

167. Kudo T, Yoshii N, Shimizu S. Stereotaxic surgery for pain relief. *J Exp Med.* 1968;96:219–234.

168. Mayanagi Y, Bouchard G. Evaluation of stereotactic thalamotomies for pain relief with reference to pulvinar intervention. *Appl Neurophysiol.* 1977;39:154–157.

169. Monnier M, Fischer R. Localisation, stimulation et coagulation du thalamus chez l'homme. *J Physiol.* 1951;43:818.

170. de Montreuil CB, Lajat Y, Resche R, et al. Apport de la neurochirurgie stéréotaxique dans le traitment dcs algies des cancers cervico-faciaux. *Ann Otol Laryngol (Paris).* 1983;100:181–186.

171. Mundinger F. Stereotaktische Operationen gegen anderweitig unbehandelbar schwere Schmerzzustande. *Z Allg Med.* 1975;50:860–864.

172. Nashold BS Jr. Brainstem stereotaxic procedures. In: Schaltenbrand G, Walker AE, eds. *Stereotaxy of the Human Brain. Anatomical, Physiological and Clinical Applications.* Stuttgart: Georg Thieme Verlag; 1982:475–483.

173. Nashold BS, Slaughter DG, Wilson WP, Zorub D. Stereotactic mesencephalotomy. In: Krayenbühl H, Maspes PE, Sweet WH, eds. *Progress in Neurological Surgery.* Basel: Karger; 1977;8:35–49.

174. Nashold BS, Wilson WP, Slaughter DG. Stereotaxic midbrain lesions for central dysesthesia and phantom pain. *J Neurosurg.* 1969;30:116–126.

175. Niizuma H, Kwak R, Ikeda S, et al. Follow-up results of centromedian thalamotomy for central pain. *Appl Neurophysiol.* 1982;45:324–325.

176. Niizuma H, Kwak R, Saso S, et al. Follow-up results of center median thalamotomy for central pain. *App Neurophysiol.* 1980;43:336.

177. Orthner H, Roeder F. Further clinical and anatomical experiences with stereotactic operations for relief of pain. *Confin Neurol.* 1966;27:418–430.

178. Pagni CA. Place of stereotactic technique in surgery for pain. In: Bonica JJ, ed. *Advances in Neurology.* New York, NY: Raven Press; 1974;4:699–706.

179. Pagni CA. Central pain and painful anesthesia. In:

Krayenbühl H, Maspes PE, Sweet WH, eds. *Progress in Neurological Surgery*. Basel: Karger; 1977;8:132–257.

180. Pagni CA, Maspes PE. The relief of intractable pain in malignant disease of the head and neck by stereotactic thalamotomy or sensory root lesions. In: Janzen R, Keidel WD, Herz A, Steichele C, eds. *Pain: Basic Principles-Pharmacology-Therapy*. Stuttgart: Georg Thieme Verlag; 1972:202–204.

181. Richardson DE. Thalamotomy for intractable pain. *Confin Neurol*. 1967;29:139–145.

182. Richardson DE. Recent advances in the neurosurgical control of pain. *South Med J*. 1967;60:9–12.

183. Richardson DE. Thalamotomy for control of chronic pain. *Acta Neurochir Suppl*. 1974;21:77–88.

184. Riechert T. Das stereotaktische Operationsverfahren bei der Schmerzbekämpfung. *Dtsch Med Wochenschr*. 1963;87:1177–1179.

185. Riechert T. Die chirurgische Behandlung der zentralen Schermerzzustande; einschliesslich der stereotaktischen Operation am Thalamus und Mesencephalon. *Acta Neurochir*. 1960;8:136–152.

186. Sano K. Intralaminar thalamotomy (thalamolaminotomy) and postero-medial hypothalamotomy in the treatment of intractable pain. In: Krayenbühl H, Maspes PE, Sweet WH, eds. *Prog Neurol Surg*. 1977;8:50–103.

187. Sano K. Stereotaxic thalamolaminotomy and posteromedial hypothalamotomy for the relief of pain. In: Bonica JJ, Ventafridda V, eds. *Advances in Pain Research and Therapy*. New York, NY: Raven Press; 1979;2:475–485.

188. Sano K, Yoshioka M, Ogashiwa N, et al. Thalamolaminotomy: a new operation for relief of intractable pain. *Confin Neurol*. 1966;27:63–66.

189. Sano K, Yoshioka M, Sekino H, et al. Functional organization of the internal medullary lamina in man. *Confin Neurol*. 1970;32:374–380.

190. Siegfried J, Krayenbühl H. Clinical experience in the treatment of intractable pain. In: Janzen R, Keidel WD, Herz A, Steichele C, eds. *Pain: Basic Principles-Pharmacology-Therapy*. Stuttgart: Georg Thieme Verlag; 1972:202–204.

191. Spiegel EA, Wycis HT. Mesencephalotomy in treatment of "intractable" facial pain. *Arch Neurol Psychiatry*. 1953;69:1–13.

192. Speigel EA, Wycis HT. Mesencephalotomy for the relief of pain. In: *Stereoencephalotomy, II: Clinical and Physiological Applications*. New York, NY: Grune & Stratton; 1962:206.

193. Sugita K, Mutsuga N, Takaoka Y, Doi T. Results of stereotaxic thalamotomy for pain. *Confin Neurol*. 1972;34:265–274.

194. Takaku A, Kwak R, Sakamoto T, Okudaira Y. Stereotactic thalamotomy for postherpetic central pain and muscular hypertonicity. *Tohoku J Exp Med*. 1973;85:87–92.

195. Talairach J, Tournoux P, Bancaud J. Chirurgie pariétale de la douleur. *Acta Neurochir*. 1960;8:153–250.

196. Tasker RR. Thalamotomy for pain: lesion localization by detailed thalamic mapping. *Can J Surg*. 1969;12:62–74.

197. Tasker RR. Neurosurgical concepts of pain management in head and neck cancer. *Can J Otolaryngol*. 1975;4:480–484.

198. Tasker RR. Thalamic stereotaxic procedures. In: Schaltenbrand G, Walker AE, eds. *Stereotaxy of the Human Brain*. Stuttgart: Georg Thieme Verlag; 1982:484–497.

199. Tasker RR. Stereotactic surgery. In: Wall PD, Melzack R, eds. *Textbook of Pain*. Edinburgh: Churchill-Livingstone; 1984:639–655.

200. Tasker RR. Stereotactic surgery. In: Wall PD, Melzack R, eds. *Textbook of Pain*. 2nd ed. Edinburgh: Churchill-Livingstone; 1989:840–855.

201. Tsubokawa T, Moriyasu N. Follow-up results of centre median thalamotomy for relief of intractable pain. *Confin Neurol*. 1975;37:280–284.

202. Uematsu S, Konigsmark B, Walker AE. Thalamotomy for alleviation of intractable pain. *Confin Neurol*. 1974;36:88–96.

203. Urabe M, Tsubokawa T. Stereotaxic thalamotomy for the relief of intractable pain. *Tohoku J Exp Med*. 1965;85:286–300.

204. Von Roeder F, Orthner H. Erfabrungen mit stereotaktischen Eingriffen, III. Mitteilung. *Confin Neurol*. 1961;21:51–97.

205. Voris HC, Whisler WW. Results of stereotaxic surgery for intractable pain. *Confin Neurol*. 1975;37:86–96.

206. Whisler WW, Voris HC. Mesencephalotomy for intractable pain due to malignant disease. *Appl Neurophysiol*. 1978;47:52–56.

207. Wycis HT, Spiegel EA. Long-range results in the treatment of intractable pain by stereotaxic midbrain surgery. *J Neurosurg*. 1962;19:101–107.

208. Mazars GL, Pansini A, Chiarelli J. Coagulation du faisceau spinothalamique et du faisceau quintothalamique par stéréotaxie. Indications-resultats. *Acta Neurochir*. 1960;8:324–326.

209. Mazars GL, Roge R, Pansini A. Stereotactic coagulation of the spinothalamic tract for intractable trigeminal pain. *J Neurol Neurosurg Psychiatry*. 1960; 23:352.

210. Ervin FR, Mark VH. Stereotactic thalamotomy in the human, II: physiologic observations on the human thalamus. *Arch Neurol*. 1960;3:368–380.

211. Mark VH, Ervin FR, Hackett TP. Clinical aspects of stereotactic thalamotomy in the human, I: the treatment of chronic severe pain. *Arch Neurol*. 1960; 3:351–367.

212. Mark VH, Ervin FR. Role of thalamotomy in treatment of chronic severe pain. *Postgrad Med*. 1965;37:563–571.

213. Mark VH, Ervin FR, Yakovlev PI. Correlation of pain relief, sensory loss and anatomical lesion sites in pain patients treated by stereotactic thalamotomy. *Trans Am Neurol Assoc*. 1961;86:86–90.

214. Mark VH, Ervin FR, Yakovlev P. Stereotactic thalamotomy, III: the verification of anatomical lesion sites in the human thalamus. *Arch Neurol.* 1963;8: 78–88.

215. Heath RG, Mickle WA. Evaluation of seven years' experience with depth electrode studies in human patients. In: Ramey ER, O'Doherty DS, eds. *Electrical Studies on the Unanaesthetized Brain.* New York, NY: PB Hoeber; 1960:214–247.

216. Pool JL. Psychosurgery in older people. *J Am Geriatr Soc.* 1954;2:456–466.

217. Pool JL, Clark WK, Hudson P, Lombardo M. Hypothalamic–hypophyseal dysfunction in man: laboratory and clinical assessment. In: Fields WS, Guillemin R, Carton CA, eds. *Hypothalamic–Hypophyseal Interrelationships.* Springfield, Ill: Charles C Thomas Publisher; 1956:114–124.

218. Mazars GL. Intermittent stimulation of nucleus ventralis posterolateralis for intractable pain. *Surg Neurol.* 1975;4:493–495.

219. Mazars GL, Merienne L, Ciolocca C. Stimulations thalamiques intermittentes antalgiques: note préliminaire. *Rev Neurol (Paris).* 1973;128:273–279.

220. Mazars GL, Merienne L, Ciolocca C. Treatment of certain types of pain by implantable thalamic stimulators. *Neurochirurgie.* 1974;29:117–124.

221. Hosobuchi Y, Adams JE, Rutkin B. Chronic thalamic stimulation for the control of facial anesthesia dolorosa. *Arch Neurol.* 1973;29:158–161.

222. Melzack R, Wall PD. Pain mechanisms: a new theory *Science.* 1965;150:971–979.

223. Adams JE, Hosobuchi Y, Fields HL. Stimulation of internal capsule for relief of chronic pain. *J Neurosurg.* 1974;41:740–744.

224. Hosobuchi Y, Adams JE, Fields HL. Chronic thalamic and internal capsular stimulation for the control of anesthesia dolorosa and dysesthesia of thalamic syndrome. In: Bonica JJ, ed. *Advances in Neurology, 4: International Symposium on Pain.* New York, NY: Raven Press; 1974:783–787.

225. Hosobuchi Y, Adams JE, Linchitz R. Pain relief by electrical stimulation of the central gray matter in humans and its reversal by naloxone. *Science.* 1977; 197:183–197.

226. Levy RM, Lamb S, Adams JE. Deep brain stimulation for chronic pain: long-term results and complications. In: Lunsford LD, ed. *Modern Stereotactic Neurosurgery.* Boston, Mass: Martinus Nijhoff; 1988: 395–407.

227. Sweet WH. Intracranial electrical stimulation for relief of chronic intractable pain. In: Krayenbühl H, Maspes PE, Sweet WH, eds. *Progress in Neurological Surgery.* Basel: Karger; 1977;8:258–269.

228. Young RF. Brain stimulation. In: Friedman WA, guest ed; Winn HR, Mayberg MR, eds. Stereotactic Neurosurgery. *Neurosurg Clin North Am.* Philadelphia, Pa: WB Saunders Co; 1990: 865–879.

229. Reynolds DV. Surgery in the rat during electrical analgesia induced by focal brain stimulation. *Science.* 1969;164:444–445.

230. Richardson DE, Akil H. Pain reduction by electrical brain stimulation in man, I: acute administration in periaqueductal and periventricular sites. *J Neurosurg.* 1977;47:178–183.

231. Richardson DE, Akil H. Pain reduction by electrical brain stimulation in man, II: chronic self-administration in the periventricular grey matter. *J Neurosurg.* 1977;47:184–194.

232. Friedman WA, Sceats DJ, Nestok BR, et al. The incidence of unexpected pathological findings in an image-guided biopsy series: a review of 100 consecutive cases. *Neurosurgery.* 1989;25:180–184.

233. Apuzzo MLJ, Chandrasoma PT, Cohen D, et al. Computed imaging stereotaxy: experience and perspective related to 500 procedures applied to brain masses. *Neurosurgery.* 1987;20:930–937.

234. Moore MR, Black PM, Ellenbogen R, et al. Stereotactic craniotomy: methods and results using the Brown-Roberts-Wells stereotactic frame. *Neurosurgery.* 1989;25:572–578.

235. Davis DH, Kelly PJ. Stereotactic resection of occult vascular malformations. *J Neurosurg.* 1990; 72:698–702.

236. Kelly PJ. Stereotactic biopsy and resection of thalamic astrocytomas. *Neurosurgery.* 1989;25:185–195.

237. Nazzaro JM, Newwelt EA. The role of surgery in the management of supratentorial intermediate and high-grade astrocytomas in adults. *J Neurosurg.* 1990;73:331–344.

238. Drake J, Joy M, Goldenberg A, et al. Computer and robotic assisted resection of thalamic astrocytomas in children. *Neurosurgery.* 1991;29:27–31.

239. Kondziolka D, Lunsford LD. Stereotactic management of colloid cysts: factors predicting success. *J Neurosurg.* 1991;75:45–51.

240. Dyste GN, Hitchon PW, Menezes AH, et al. Stereotaxic surgery in the treatment of multiple brain abscesses. *J Neurosurg.* 1988;69:188–194.

241. Bernstein M, Gutin PH. Interstitial irradiation of brain tumors: a review. *Neurosurgery.* 1981;9: 741–750.

242. Bernstein M, Laperriere N, Leung P, et al. Interstitial brachytherapy for malignant brain tumors: preliminary results. *Neurosurgery.* 1990;26:371–380.

243. Leibel SA, Gutin PH, Wara WM, et al. Survival and quality of life after interstitial implantation of removable high-activity iodine-125 sources for the treatment of patients with recurrent malignant gliomas. *Int J Radiat Oncol Biol Phys.* 1989;17: 1129–1139.

244. Prados M, Leibel S, Barnett CM, et al. Interstitial brachytherapy for metastatic brain tumors. *Cancer.* 1989;63:657–660.

245. Bernstein M, Gutin PH. Interstitial irradiation of skull base tumors. *Can J Neurol Sci.* 1985;12: 366–370.

246. Kumar PP, Good RR, Leibrock LG, et al. High-

activity iodine-125 endocurietherapy for recurrent skull base tumors. *Cancer.* 1988;61:1518–1527.

247. Sneed PK, Stauffer PR, Gutin PH, et al. Interstitial irradiation and hyperthermia for the treatment of recurrent malignant brain tumors. *Neurosurgery.* 1991;28:206–215.

248. Pollack IF, Lunsford LD, Slamovits TL, et al. Stereotaxic intracavitary irradiation for cystic craniopharyngiomas. *J Neurosurg.* 1988;68:227–233.

249. Hood TW, McKeever PE. Stereotactic management of cystic gliomas of the brainstem. *Neurosurgery.* 1989;24:373–378.

Chapter 50

Medical and Surgical Treatment of Epilepsy

Allen R. Wyler

A *seizure* is an attack of cerebral origin that affects a person in apparent good health or suddenly aggravates a chronic pathologic state. These sudden and transitory abnormal motor, sensory, autonomic, or psychic phenomena result from transient dysfunction of part or all of the brain. *Epilepsy* is a chronic brain disorder characterized by spontaneous recurrent seizures. The characteristics of a seizure depend on the regions of the brain involved during the beginning and the duration of the seizure.

DIAGNOSIS

When diagnosing epilepsy two determinations must be made. First, *seizure type* must be diagnosed, which requires a knowledge of epileptic seizure classifications. Second, *etiology* must be determined. After these two steps have been completed, a rational treatment plan can be devised and implemented. Recently, emphasis has been placed on diagnosing the epileptic *syndrome* because it can help the physician make a significantly more accurate long-term prognosis.

SEIZURE HISTORY

The diagnosis of epilepsy is primarily clinical; laboratory data is secondary. The clinical history generates an accurate diagnosis approximately 80% of the time.[1] However, if treatment fails, it is often wise to reconsider the original diagnosis. To correctly diagnose epilepsy, the patient may need to undergo long-term EEG/video monitoring. As with any clinical problem, a history is necessary and should start with a description of the attacks. Because the seizure may impair memory of the event, the patient is often unable to provide a complete description. Additional information should be obtained from a parent or other significant person who has seen the seizures. Any information that helps diagnose the seizure should be obtained. It is useful to ask:

1. Does the patient have a *prodrome* (i.e., a symptom that occurs hours or minutes before the seizure)? For example, some patients complain of a dull headache for a day prior to the seizure.
2. Does the patient have a recognizable *aura* (i.e., a feeling or experience during the initial moments of the seizure)? It is thought that this first portion of the seizure reaches consciousness as a subjective feeling, manifesting the neuronal circuits through which the seizure is spreading. For example, if the seizure were beginning in the hand portion of the primary sensory cortex, the seizure's aura might be a tingling sensation in the hand. It is important to determine if an aura exists because it strongly suggests that the seizure can be classified as partial. In addition, the aura may help localize the *epileptogenic focus,* the region of the cortex intrinsically responsible for generation of the seizures. Theoretically, if the epileptogenic focus is removed, the seizures will cease.
3. What is the first signal to an observer that a seizure is beginning? For example, does the seizure begin with a motionless stare or tonic extension of the arms? If the initial event is immediate tonic extension of the arms, it is likely that the seizure is primarily generalized. On the other hand, if the seizure begins with a motionless stare, it is likely that the seizure is complex partial.
4. Does the seizure end with convulsive motor movements (i.e., clonic activity)?
5. Are there circumstances that increase the likelihood of a seizure? For example, many women find that seizures occur a few days preceding their menses.

Figure 50.1 is a table showing a classification of seizures.

Partial seizures had been called *focal* seizures because they originate from confined, focal regions of cortex. The EEG often has epileptiform discharges confined to focal regions of the scalp, such as the temporal area. In contrast, *generalized* seizures do not originate from focal cortical regions, although it is unclear from where within the brain they arise. The EEG is often characterized by bilaterally synchronous epileptiform (spike) discharges, suggesting that they arise from diencephalic or deep midline structures. Furthermore, a generalized seizure will frequently begin with bilateral symmetrical body movements, such as tonic extension of both arms (frequently seen with tonic seizures). Complex partial seizures often begin with an arrest of movement, a vacant facial expression, and, after several seconds, progress to repetitive, semipurposeful movements known as *automatisms.* In *simple* partial seizures consciousness is not lost, whereas in *complex* partial seizures consciousness is lost. For example, a simple partial seizure that involves the visual cortex may be manifested by flashing phosphenes in the contralateral visual field. The person is fully alert and can notify an observer of the seizure. At the start of a complex partial seizure the patient may verbalize, but if asked to respond, will be unable to do so. Partial seizures may *secondarily generalize,* which means they may progress into a tonic-clonic convulsion. When this occurs, they should be called complex partial seizures with secondary generalization rather than tonic-clonic seizures. The term *tonic-clonic* seizure should be reserved for the specific form of *primarily generalized* seizure that begins with tonic posturing rather than one that begins as a complex partial seizure.

Absence seizures are very similar to short complex partial seizures in that they may be brief and consist only of an arrest of movement and unresponsiveness. The longer an absence seizure lasts, the more it may resemble a complex partial seizure. Generally, absence seizures are not followed by postictal confusion. Following an absence seizure the person may continue with whatever activity preceded the seizure. Mistaking an absence seizure for a complex partial seizure is a common diagnostic error. Because the therapy and prognosis of these two seizure types are entirely different a correct diagnosis is important. Often discrimination between the two will depend on the EEG findings. Absence seizures have a characteristic pattern of 3/sec spike-and-wave discharges. With appropriate drug treatment these spike-and-wave discharges disappear from the EEG.

Myoclonic seizures are characterized by brief jerks that occur alone or in pairs. Often a series of jerks will progress into a clonic seizure. *Atonic* seizures are spells in which axial body tone is abruptly lost and the patient may fall to the ground. These seizures can cause bodily damage, especially to the face and head.

ETIOLOGY

Chronic seizures develop from damaged cortex. More specifically, epilepsy results from damage to neurons, not axons. Thus, epilepsy is a problem of gray matter rather than white matter. This is most obvious for partial epilepsy because, if the epileptogenic focus is removed surgically, routine pathologic examination will usually show focal neuronal damage and gliosis. For primary generalized epilepsy, focal pathology is not demonstrable. When taking the history one must ask questions that enable an etiologic diagnosis. For example, has the person had a significant head injury, febrile seizures, subarachnoid hemorrhage, or CNS infection? Does the person have a syndrome, like tuberous sclerosis, that affects the CNS? As a rule, the age of seizure onset can help guide the history. For example, seizure disorders that begin in infancy are more likely due to severe perinatal injuries, while seizures that begin in adulthood are more likely due to brain tumors or alcoholism. Remember that seizures are a symptom of a malfunctioning or damaged nervous system and are not specific to the agent.

Genetic factors are important in both inherited and acquired epilepsy. The best example of an inherited epilepsy is juvenile myoclonic epilepsy, which shows linkage with the BF and HLA loci on human chromosome 6.[2] On the other hand, partial epilepsy has a genetic component but its occurrence is also explained by other factors. If 100 people have identical head injuries, only a percentage will subsequently develop recurrent seizures. Those who develop posttraumatic epilepsy are more likely to have a positive maternal family history of seizures. Genetics explains why some children develop febrile seizures and other children with the same illness do not, and why only a small number of those children with febrile seizures develop chronic seizures. Everyone has a threshold. A person deprived of sleep long enough will have convulsions. When these convulsions occur, however, depends on the individual's threshold, a function of genetically determined excitatory and inhibitory neurotransmitter

Figure 50.1 Classification of Seizures

I. Generalized seizures (convulsive or nonconvulsive)
A. 1. Absence seizures
    a. Impairment of consciousness only
    b. With mild clonic components
    c. With atonic components
    d. With tonic components
    e. With automatisms
    f. With autonomic components
  2. Atypical absence
B. Myoclonic seizures
C. Clonic seizures
D. Tonic seizures
E. Tonic-clonic seizures
F. Atonic seizures

II. Partial seizures
A. Simple partial seizures
  1. With motor signs
  2. With autonomic symptoms or signs
  3. With sensory symptoms
  4. With psychic symptoms
B. Complex partial seizures with the same changes seen in II.A.1–4
C. Partial seizures with secondary generalization

III. Unclassified epileptic seizures

mechanisms, which are RNA influenced. Therefore, family history is relevant when evaluating a person with suspected epilepsy.

LABORATORY CONFIRMATION

Once the clinical history is taken, the physician should have an opinion about the presence of epilepsy and the etiology of the seizures. It is helpful to obtain an EEG to confirm the diagnosis. But, it should be emphasized that, for various reasons, many patients with epilepsy have a normal EEG. First, a routine EEG samples only 20 to 30 minutes, which is a relatively small time period. Epilepsy is paroxysmal, and 30 minutes may not be enough time to catch episodic discharges in the EEG. Second, vast amounts of brain are not adjacent to the skull or do not reflect EEG activity to the scalp. For example, the scalp EEG often will not show epileptiform activity that is occurring within the basal temporal and hippocampal regions of the temporal lobe. In a study of 1824 EEGs in over 300 epileptic patients, definite interictal epileptiform discharges were seen in 60% of EEG records and in 83% of patients,[3] but it took an average of six EEG recordings per patient to reach this yield. Only 56% of the initial EEG tracings showed epileptiform discharges. Clearly, then, *an initial normal EEG does not disprove the diagnosis of epilepsy*. If the clinical history supports the diagnosis of epilepsy, the patient should be treated in spite of a normal EEG. If the seizures are not brought under control with appropriate therapy, repeat EEGs or long-term EEG/video monitoring should be considered.

Routine EEGs should be performed with the International 10-20 electrode placement system, which uses a set number of electrodes affixed to the scalp at proportional intervals that are relatively consistent from patient to patient. An initial routine EEG study should include periods when the patient is awake and asleep. Usually one needs to request a sleep EEG specifically. Sleep can be induced by either sleep deprivation or chloral hydrate (from 1 to 3 g depending on patient size). Slow-wave sleep activates interictal epileptiform spike activity in some patients and therefore enhances the diagnostic yield of the procedure. Both hyperventilation and photic stimulation also enhance the incidence of spike activity in some forms of epilepsy and should be included in the initial EEG studies.

Unless there is a specific reason to analyze the CSF, a lumbar puncture is unnecessary in the initial evaluation of epilepsy.

IMAGING STUDIES

Every patient who is diagnosed with epilepsy should have an MRI scan to determine if a structural lesion is present. MRI is preferred to CT because causal lesions are significantly more likely to be identified with MRI.[4,5] It is sometimes thought that if a patient has had seizures for many years that began at a young age, a tumor is unlikely. This is not true—many such patients have benign tumors. Thus, regardless of the patient's age at seizure onset or duration of epilepsy, MRI should be used to diagnose tumors. Skull films are unnecessary because they do not image the brain.

SYNDROME DIAGNOSIS AND PROGNOSIS

With the above information, often the syndrome can be diagnosed and a prognosis made. For example, a young patient who has only true absence seizures clinically, is of normal intelligence, has no structural lesion on the MRI scan, and has an uncomplicated EEG showing classical 3/sec spike-and-wave discharges fits a syndrome with a modestly good prognosis if treated with appropriate drugs. In contrast, another patient of the same age who suffers atypical absence seizures, has evidence of frontal lobe damage on MRI, is mentally retarded, and has a complicated EEG tracing with evidence of encephalopathic slowing and slow spike-wave discharges, has a very poor long-term prognosis. There is much debate over what should be included in the syndrome classification, and a discussion of this issue is beyond the scope of this chapter. Attempts should be made to determine if seizures are symptomatic of an underlying brain abnormality that belongs within a known neurologic syndrome.

MEDICAL THERAPY

Epilepsy treatment depends on correct seizure diagnosis. Different types of seizures respond better to some anticonvulsant medications than to others. Related diagnoses (e.g., mental retardation and depression) often modify the drug choice. For example, barbiturate anticonvulsants should be avoided in patients prone to de-

Figure 50.2 Antiepileptic Drugs

Generic Name	Brand Name
phenytoin	Dilantin
carbamazepine	Tegretol
phenobarbital	phenobarbital
valproic acid	Depakote
ethosuximide	Zarontin
primidone	Mysoline
clonazepam	Clonopin

pression. There are seven effective drugs available for treating epilepsy (Fig. 50.2). Some epileptologists consider there to be six primary anticonvulsants because primidone (Mysoline) is metabolized to phenobarbital, which provides primidone's major drug effect. Clonazepam has very limited use and is reserved for either true absence seizures (refractory to ethosuximide or valproic acid) or myoclonic seizures. Benzodiazepine drugs (Valium, Tranxene, and Ativan) should not be used habitually and are not considered primary anticonvulsants.

First, it should be determined whether the patient's seizure is primarily generalized or partial, because each type requires different medications. For example, valproic acid or phenobarbital is generally more effective for primarily generalized epilepsy than partial epilepsy, and ethosuximide is indicated only for true absence seizures. Either carbamazepine or phenytoin is the drug of choice for partial epilepsy. A large 5-year multicenter drug study compared the efficacy and toxicity of carbamazepine, phenobarbital, phenytoin, and primidone in treating partial and generalized tonic-clonic seizures. The results showed that each of the four drugs used as monotherapy were similarly effective in the treatment of generalized tonic-clonic seizures, but carbamazepine was more effective in treating partial seizures.[6]

For true absence seizures ethosuximide or valproic acid is the drug of choice. Ethosuximide is not indicated for partial seizure disorders.

TREATMENT STRATEGY

When initiating drug therapy, one should always start with a single antiepileptic drug, an approach termed *monotherapy*. The reasons are that 1) toxic side effects are more managable when caused by one drug, 2) it is easier to judge drug efficacy, 3) patients are more likely to comply with treatment, 4) there are no effects from drug interactions, and 5) therapeutic serum levels are more easily maintained.

Unless there is an overriding clinical reason to treat the patient with a loading dose, the drug is initiated at a low dose and slowly increased until the patient's drug serum level is within the suggested therapeutic range. The drug is maintained within therapeutic levels (unless that level causes toxic side effects) until seizures recur. If seizures are controlled, the therapeutic goal has been achieved. If seizures persist, the dosage is slowly increased until either toxic side effects occur, at which point the dosage should be lowered, or the seizures are brought under control. Therapeutic serum drug levels indicate what is therapeutic for the majority of patients. If a patient's seizures are controlled at a level that is below the therapeutic range, an increased dose is unnecessary. Likewise, if seizure control is obtained with a serum level slightly above the therapeutic range and the patient has no symptoms of drug toxicity, there is no need to reduce the level.

If the initial drug fails to control the seizures, a second drug should be substituted for the first. Only after all reasonable attempts at control with monotherapy have failed should a second drug be tried in combination (co-therapy). There is seldom a need to prescribe more than two anticonvulsant drugs in combination.

DOSING SCHEDULE

The aim of anticonvulsant treatment is to control seizures by maintaining a constant drug serum level. Serum levels depend largely on the drug's half life (the time required for half of the drug to be eliminated from the body), which varies from patient to patient (Figs. 50.3,

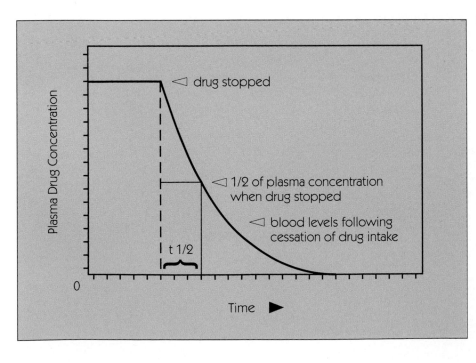

Figure 50.3 Graphic representation of a drug's half life. The drug's plasma concentration is kept constant and then stopped (arrow), at which time the plasma concentration begins to drop toward zero. The time it takes for the plasma concentration to become half of what it was when the drug was stopped is the half life ($T_{1/2}$).

50.4). Thus, if the serum level of a drug is 100 mg/mL and it takes 6 hours for the level to drop to 50 mg/mL, the drug's half life is 6 hours.

Each dose of drug is ingested and absorbed. During absorption the serum level rises (Fig. 50.5). Meanwhile, the drug is being eliminated. When absorption stops and elimination continues, the serum level falls. The physician should aim for a dosage that maintains the serum level within the therapeutic range. Thus, a drug with a very long half life, such as phenobarbital, can be given once a day and a stable serum level will be maintained. On the other hand, a drug like carbamazepine may need to be given four times per day. Because drug serum levels fluctuate following a drug dose, the relationship between dosage and serum sample must be kept in mind. For example, the serum level one hour after a dose is the *peak* level, whereas a serum level in the early morning before any drug has been given is the *trough* level (see Fig. 50.5). The point at which to obtain a serum level is dictated by the clinical question. To establish that symptoms indicate drug toxicity, a drug level should be obtained while the patient is symptomatic. To establish that seizures are refractory to a drug, a serum level should be obtained immediately after a seizure. Peak and trough levels should be obtained to determine the patient's metabolism of a drug.

When initiating drug treatment, remember that a drug's steady-state is not reached until after approximately five half lives (see Fig. 50.5). Thus, if a drug's half life is 24 hours, and the drug's first dose is given Monday morning, the steady state will not be reached until after Friday. It is also true that if the same drug is stopped on Monday, it will take several days for the blood levels to become insignificant.

The most common reason for patient noncompliance with medication schedules is toxic side effects. These can be minimized by advising patients to take the drugs after meals, when adsorption may be slower, and at bedtime.

GENERIC DRUGS

Because many newer anticonvulsant drugs are costly, prescribing generic drugs to minimize patient expense is appealing. However, in recent years it has become evident that using generic anticonvulsant medications may be problematic. Some patients require fairly specific serum levels, which are easily maintained when working with one drug made by one company. But the bioavailability of the drug, (carbamazepine, for example) may be markedly different when produced by different companies. At times there have been as many as six different companies supplying generic carbamazepine. Because pharmacies often buy generic drugs in bulk and bid for the lowest price, the patient may receive a different preparation each time the prescription is refilled. Thus, even if the patient maintains the same dose, the bioavailability of the active drug will vary, causing the patient's serum level to vary, perhaps considerably, after each refill. If the patient buys the brand name drug (Tegretol), the drug bioavailability remains constant with prescription refills.

TREATMENT FAILURES

The most common reason for treatment failure is poor compliance, that is, the patient is not taking the drug or not taking it as prescribed. The reasons for poor compliance include but are not limited to toxic side effects,

Figure 50.4 Antiepileptic Drug Plasma Half Life

Drug	Half Life	Time to Steady State
phenytoin	24 h	5 d
carbamazepine	12 h	3 d
phenobarbital	4 d	3 wk
valproic acid	12 h	3 d
ethosuximide	2 d	10 d
primidone	12 h	3 d

(From Porter RJ, 1984)

depression, poor memory, boredom with a habitual task, and denial of the disorder. Noncompliance, then, may be due to factors other than a willful attempt by the patient to sabotage the treatment plan.

The second most common reason for continued seizures is an incorrect seizure diagnosis. Many events may be misdiagnosed as seizures, including cardiac arrhythmia, hypoglycemia, sleep disorders, tics, and pseudoseizures. To insure that a correct diagnosis has been made, long-term EEG/video monitoring may be indicated. This type of monitoring is done in specialized facilities that are part of comprehensive epilepsy centers. A patient is constantly observed by trained personnel while undergoing EEG and videotape recordings. These recordings are maintained 24 hours per day until several of the patient's typical seizures are recorded. By analyzing the recorded events several issues can be settled. Has the wrong seizure diagnosis been made? Absence seizures may be mistaken for complex partial seizures and be treated ineffectively with phenytoin when ethosuximide is a more appropriate drug. Are the events epileptic?

Pseudoseizures, also termed nonepileptic seizures, are events that may resemble seizures but are not epileptic. Whether this represents a hysterical event, true malingering, or a somatic exaggeration to mild simple partial seizures that are not recorded with scalp EEG electrodes is often unclear. The differential diagnosis between true epileptic seizures and pseudoseizures may be difficult to determine. A diagnosis of pseudoseizures has serious implications, and it should be based on positive findings and not solely on the interictal EEG.

A modest number of patients take the correct medications in therapeutic doses and continue to have seizures. These patients are considered refractory to anticonvulsant medication and should be surgically evaluated if seizures persist.

Status epilepticus is either a seizure that continues for longer than 20 minutes or repetitive seizures where the patient is unconsciousness between seizures. Status epilepticus with convulsive seizures is a medical emergency, because it has a significant mortality rate if not controlled expeditiously.[7] As with any medical emergency treatment, first establish control of the airway; no object should be placed in the patient's mouth. The patient should be turned on his or her side so any secretions or vomitus can drain from the oral pharynx. Only after the seizures have stopped should an oral airway or endotracheal tube be inserted. Oxygen can be administered by nasal cannula.

The next step is to establish a route for intravenous administration of medication using at least an 18-gauge intracath. If the patient's history is unknown, 50 mL of blood should be removed and 20 mL sent for a complete blood count, a toxic drug screen and serum electrolyte, blood sugar, magnesium, and calcium levels. The remaining 30 mL should be frozen in case additional tests are needed later. An IV drip of 5% dextrose in lactated Ringer's solution should be started.

Efforts should then be directed at stopping the seizures. Opinions differ as to which drugs are best used to treat status epilepticus,[8,9] but it is recommended that a combination of phenytoin and lorazepam be used routinely. The one exception to this treatment is a patient suspected of being in acute withdrawal from phenobarbital (or primidone), in which case the initial treatment should be IV phenobarbital. Otherwise, phenytoin should be given as a long-acting anticonvulsant and lorazepam as a short-acting immediate anticonvulsant. For a normal sized adult 1 g of phenytoin is given intravenously. Because parenteral phenytoin is extremely

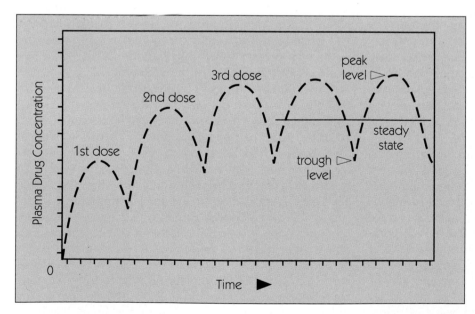

Figure 50.5 Graphic representation of a drug reaching steady state. An individual's serum level for a drug is zero before administration of the drug. After the first dose the drug serum level increases until all of the drug is absorbed. The highest serum level reached after the dose is absorbed is the drug's peak level. Elimination causes the plasma level to drop. Before the serum level falls to zero a second dose is given. This causes the drug's peak level to become higher than it was after the first dose. This process continues during a regular drug dosing schedule until the peak and trough drug levels remain constant. This is steady state.

alkaline (pH=11), it must be infused at a rate *no greater than 50 mg/min*. Simultaneously, lorazepam can be given rapidly in repetitive 2 mg doses until seizure control is achieved. The lorazepam doses can be repeated every 2 minutes. If status epilepticus has not been stopped after 1 g of phenytoin and a cumulative lorazepam dose of 50 mg, one should consider phenobarbital and/or general anesthesia administered by an anesthesiologist. Once the seizures have been stopped, appropriate medical care should be administered, taking into account how much the medication and seizures have sedated the patient. Then a cause for the status epilepticus should be sought.

SURGICAL TREATMENT

If a patient's seizures are refractory to anticonvulsant medication, surgery should be considered. There is no formula for determining just how many seizures the patient must have or how frequently they must occur before surgery should be considered. A consideration more important than seizure frequency is how seizures affect the person's social and economic potentials. If seizures keep a person from driving an automobile, they may restrict normal social development and vocational opportunities. One seizure a year would be a disaster to an airline pilot, while two seizures a day may have no consequence for a mentally retarded, institutionalized patient. How seizures affect a person's life is a personal issue and is best determined by the patient, not the physician.

Epilepsy surgery requires a multidisciplinary approach to a complex and chronic problem. Surgically removing a seizure focus in a person who may have long-standing psychological, social, and vocational sequelae as a result of this chronic disorder is not sufficient treatment. Therefore, epilepsy surgery should be done only within specialized comprehensive epilepsy centers staffed to treat patients and their rehabilitation holistically.

Surgical evaluation begins with the assumption that the patient is refractory to a reasonable trial of anticonvulsant medication. This does not mean that every known drug must be tried in every conceivable combination. At the very least phenytoin, carbamazepine, and phenobarbital must have been tried alone or in combination with each other. Whether valproic acid needs to be tried prior to surgical evaluation is debatable.

The surgical work-up can be divided into phases, with the least invasive tests being done initially. The first phase begins with a review of recent structural studies (less than 1 year old) in case a causal structural lesion can be identified. A current MRI scan that includes coronal sections is necessary. Long-term EEG/video monitoring should be done. An accurate seizure diagnosis is essential because the rest of the work-up largely depends on it. A neuropsychological evaluation should also be performed. A psychological test battery can help localize the seizure focus, determine if memory is sufficient to proceed with surgery, and aid in postoperative vocational rehabilitation planning.

An *intracarotid sodium amytal test* (known as the Wada test) determines which side of the brain is dominant for speech and is performed concomitantly with a retrograde carotid arteriogram. The carotid arteries are studied sequentially. The patient is supine with both arms extended (to test for subsequent paresis) and the carotid artery is injected with approximately 100 mg of sodium amytal. The patient undertakes a series of tasks designed to test for aphasia and, sometimes, memory. The object of the test is to produce a hemiparesis contralateral to the side of the injected artery, thereby confirming that a sufficient drug dose was delivered to the hemisphere, and then determine if speech is abolished. For example, if a left carotid artery injection causes a right hemiparesis with aphasia and a similar subsequent injection of the right carotid causes only left hemiparesis, one can assume the left hemisphere is dominant for speech. Depending on the specific test protocol, memory can also be assessed, but this is controversial.

If long-term EEG/video monitoring has found that the patient has complex partial seizures, it can be assumed that the patient has an epileptogenic focus somewhere within the brain. On the other hand, if the patient has an obvious form of primarily generalized seizures and no structural lesion, it can be assumed that the patient does not have a focal epileptogenic focus. Thus, if the patient has been found to have idiopathic primarily generalized seizures, there is no need for further investigation to find an epileptogenic focus; the patient may be considered for corpus callosotomy. If the patient has complex partial seizures, it is assumed that he or she has an epileptogenic focus, and attention is turned to lateralizing and localizing the focus. The most accurate method of locating the focus is MRI. A solitary *cortical lesion* that correlates with the EEG findings is almost assuredly the epileptogenic focus.

If the MRI scan does not provide localization, invasive long-term EEG/video monitoring should be considered (Fig. 50.6). There is considerable debate about when to use only noninvasive studies to plan surgery and when to resort to invasive monitoring.[10] Some surgeons plan surgery based solely on interictal EEG data, while others first identify the epileptogenic focus with invasive *ictal* recordings. The advantage of ictal invasive monitoring is that it not only provides more precise localization than scalp EEG recordings, but it also can be more accurate in identifying patients who are not surgical candidates.[11,12] Invasive recordings localize and lateralize seizure foci, and localize seizure foci in relation to functional cortex. The techniques for obtaining these goals vary. Localization can be done by implanting either subdural strip electrodes or depth electrodes. There are pros and cons to both methods; in some centers both types of electrodes are used to maximize results. The second goal (to localize seizure foci in relation to functional cortex) is best met by implanting a large multiple contact grid electrode. The grid is implanted via craniotomy only after the general location of the focus has been determined.[13] With the grid in place, chronic ictal recordings are made to localize the epileptogenic focus. Electrical stimulation at electrodes over different cortical sites "map" cortical function.[14,15] If electrical stimulation at a particular electrode blocks speech production, it is assumed that the underlying cortex is involved in speech. Mapping is commonly used for cases in which structural lesions, such as tumors, are near the speech cortex.

Other less invasive tests can be used to localize epileptogenic foci. The positron emission tomogram (PET) scan has been useful in some centers, since interictally many foci will show up as zones of glucose hypometabolism.[16,17] PET scans are not available in all surgical epilepsy centers, however, and are still considered a research tool by many surgeons. Their accuracy in local-

izing epileptogenic foci is not sufficient to justify their use over invasive ictal monitoring. Likewise, single photon emission computed tomographic scans (SPECT) have been thought useful for localizing foci, but they are currently less reliable than PET scans and thus not acceptable to many neurosurgeons.

Epilepsy surgery can be divided into two major types: *focal resections* and *commissurotomy*. Focal resection removes the epileptogenic focus from the brain, potentially ridding patients of all their seizures. This operation is indicated for treatment of complex partial seizures (with or without secondary generalization) that

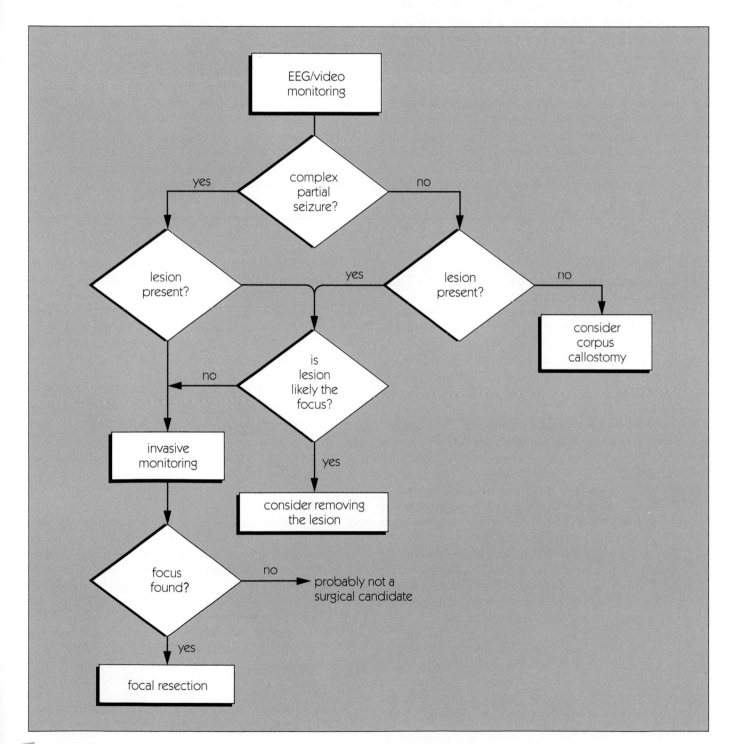

Figure 50.6 This diagram outlines when EEG/video monitoring is indicated.

originate within surgically accessible cortex. Because the majority of patients with complex partial seizures have seizure foci within the temporal lobe, the most common focal resection is anterior temporal lobectomy. The techniques for performing anterior temporal lobectomy range from selective amygdalohippocampectomy (where only the amygdala and hippocampus are removed by a microsurgical approach) to large temporal lobe resections guided by acute intraoperative electrocorticography.

The results of focal resection depend on the region of brain resected and the presence of a lesion. For nonlesional complex partial seizures, best results follow anterior temporal lobectomy with 70% to 90% of patients either seizure-free or significantly improved (only a few seizures annually). After a frontal lobectomy, however, only 50% of patients are seizure-free or significantly improved. Focal resection of other lobes is far less common and produces mixed results. For all regions of cortex the odds of a good result are improved if the epilepsy is associated with a MRI lesion that can be completely removed. Thus, resection of a frontal lobe with a lesion in the frontal pole is likely to generate a better outcome than a resection of a nonlesioned frontal lobe.

Commissurotomy refers to surgery that divides all or some of the midline commissures.[18-20] In the last few years only the corpus callosum has been divided by most surgeons. Hence, the surgery is termed *corpus callosotomy*. This surgery is reserved for epilepsy that is not confined to one discrete cortical location. The operation disrupts the interhemispheral pathways thought to be used in seizure generalization. The surgery does not remove the epileptogenic tissue that causes seizures. Consequently, the majority of patients continue to have some seizures. Only approximately 10% of patients undergoing callosotomy are seizure-free. A typical result is a 65% reduction in total seizure frequency. Because of these rather poor results some surgeons reserve this operation for those who suffer severe physical injury from atonic seizures.

Hemispherectomy is sometimes considered a separate form of epilepsy surgery because it has associated complications different from those of the standard focal resections. However, it is basically just a large focal resection reserved for those few cases in which the entire hemisphere has been damaged. Such damage is often associated with infantile hemiplegia due to massive cortical infarction. In those cases, the entire hemisphere can be removed without physical or psychological damage.

REFERENCES

1. King DW, Gallagher BB, Murvin AJ, et al. Pseudoseizures: diagnostic evaluation. *Neurology.* 1982; 32:18–23.
2. Delgado Escueta AV, Greenberg DA, Treiman L, et al. Mapping the gene for juvenile myoclonic epilepsy. *Epilepsia.* 1989;30:S8–18.
3. Marsan CA, Zivin LS. Factors related to the occurrence of typical paroxysmal abnormalities in the EEG records of epileptic patients. *Epilepsia.* 1970;11:361–381.
4. Brooks BS, King DW, el Gammal T, et al. MR imaging in patients with intractable complex partial epileptic seizures. *Am J Roentgenol.* 1990;154: 577–583.
5. Sperling MR, Wilson G, Engel J Jr, Babb TL, Phelps M, Bradley W. Magnetic resonance imaging in intractable partial epilepsy: correlative studies. *Ann Neurol.* 1986;20:57–62.
6. Smith DB, Mattson RH, Cramer JA, Collins JF, Novelly RA, Craft B. Results of a nationwide Veterans Administration Cooperative Study comparing the efficacy and toxicity of carbamazepine, phenobarbital, phenytoin, and primidone. *Epilepsia.* 1987;28:S50–58.
7. Porter RJ. *Epilepsy: 100 Elementary Principles.* Philadelphia, Pa: WB Saunders Co; 1984:1–162.
8. Delgado Escueta AV, Wasterlain C, Treiman DM and Porter RJ. Current concepts in neurology: management of status epilepticus. *N Engl J Med.* 1982;306:1337–1340.
9. Gabor AJ. Lorazepam versus phenobarbital: candidates for drug of choice for treatment of status epilepticus. *J Epilepsy.* 1990;3:3–6.
10. Ojemann GA. Surgical therapy for medically intractable epilepsy. *J Neurosurg.* 1987;66:489–499.
11. Spencer SS. Depth electroencephalography in selection of refractory epilepsy for surgery. *Ann Neurol.* 1981;9:207–214.
12. Wyler AR, Richey ET, Hermann BP. Comparison of scalp to subdural recordings for localizing epileptogenic foci. *J Epilepsy.* 1989;2:91–96.
13. Goldring S, Gregorie EM. Surgical management of epilepsy using epidural electrodes to localize the seizure focus: review of 100 cases. *J Neurosurg.* 1984;60:457–466.
14. Lesser RP, Luders H, Klem G, et al. Extraoperative cortical functional localization in patients with epilepsy. *J Clin Neurophysiol.* 1987;4:27–53.
15. Luders H, Hahn JF, Lesser RP, et al. Basal temporal subdural electrodes in the evaluation of patients with intractable epilepsy. *Epilepsia.* 1989;30: 131–142.
16. Engel J Jr, Brown WJ, Kuhl DE, Phelps ME, Mazziotta JC, Crandall PH. Pathological findings underlying focal temporal lobe hypometabolism in partial epilepsy. *Ann Neurol.* 1982;12:518–528.
17. Laster DW, Penry JK, Moody DM, Ball MR, Witcofski RL, Riela AR. Chronic seizure disorders: contribution of MR imaging when CT is normal. *AJNR.* 1985;6:177–180.

18. Wilson DH, Culver CM, Waddington M, Gazzaniga M. Disconnection of the cerebral hemispheres. *Neurology.* 1975;25:1149–1153.

19. Wilson DH, Reeves AG, Gazzaniga MS. "Central" commissurotomy for intractable generalized epilepsy: series two. *Neurology.* 1982;32:687–697.

20. Wyler AR. Corpus callosotomy in the treatment of epilepsy. *Contemp Neurosurg.* 1990;17:1–5.

Chapter 51

Intracranial Arachnoid Cysts

Samuel F. Ciricillo, Michael S.B. Edwards

Arachnoid cysts are intraarachnoid collections of CSF that produce neurologic symptoms either by compressing adjacent neural tissue or by obstructing CSF flow.[1] Most of these cysts are congenital; consequently, about 75% of those causing symptoms are diagnosed in young children.[2-5] They constitute 1% of all intracranial mass lesions not resulting from trauma.[6]

The previous use of such terms as "external hydrocephalus," "chronic cystic arachnoiditis," "meningitis serosa circumscripta," "leptomeningeal cyst," "relapsing juvenile subdural hematoma," and "temporal lobe agenesis syndrome" to describe these lesions has led to confusion regarding their pathology, pathogenesis, diagnosis, and treatment. Recent studies have shown that arachnoid cysts arise from the accumulation of CSF within a split or duplicated arachnoid membrane.[1,7] The accumulated CSF, either secreted by arachnoid cells lining the cyst[8] or trapped as a result of unidirectional flow into the cyst, progressively increases in volume. The resulting expansion of the cyst compresses surrounding brain or obstructs intraventricular or extraventricular CSF pathways, resulting in clinical symptoms. A thorough understanding of the pathogenesis and the altered CSF flow dynamics in patients with these lesions is necessary for successful treatment.

PATHOLOGY

More than 150 years ago, Bright suggested that arachnoid cysts form between the layers of the arachnoid membrane.[1] He emphasized that their chronic nature was evident from the tendency of superficial cysts to erode the bone above them and to compress the brain below them. In 1971, Robinson[6] maintained that arachnoid cysts in the middle cranial fossa are a secondary anomaly of mesenchymal differentiation resulting from agenesis of the temporal lobe. However, the normal histologic structure of compressed brain,[1,8] the identical weight of affected and contralateral hemispheres,[9] and the re-expansion of compressed brain after successful treatment[2-4,10-13] suggest that cyst formation and expansion, rather than temporal lobe agenesis, is the primary abnormality.[14]

Histologic studies of autopsy specimens in 1958 by Starkman et al.[15] confirmed that arachnoid cysts result from a developmental aberration involving splitting or duplication of the arachnoid membrane (Fig. 51.1). Subsequent analysis of the cyst wall by electron microscopy has shown that the arachnoid membrane splits into an inner and outer layer at the margin of the cyst.[8] The cysts ordinarily contain clear CSF with a normal cellular and biochemical content. A mildly increased protein content may suggest relative isolation from the CSF pathways or, when combined with xanthochromia, previous intracystic hemorrhage. A markedly elevated protein level or pleocytosis in the cyst cavity, however, suggests the possibility of a cystic neoplasm instead of an arachnoid cyst.

The pathogenesis of arachnoid cysts is best understood in terms of the development of the arachnoid. Loose mesenchymal tissue, the so-called perimedullary mesh, surrounds the embryonic brain and is the precursor of both the pia and the arachnoid.[1,7] The pulsatile force exerted by the choroid plexus propels CSF through this rarefied embryonic tissue, dissecting it into inner pia and outer arachnoid components. Alterations in the flow of CSF during these early stages of leptomeningeal differentiation may cause the arachnoid to separate into two distinct layers. Arachnoid cysts result from enlargement of these arachnoid diverticula.

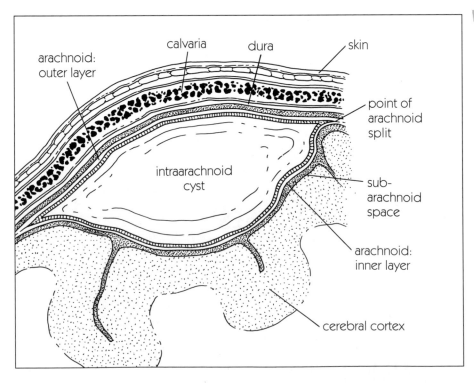

Figure 51.1 Arachnoid cyst and its relation to the meninges and the subarachnoid space.

Unlike leptomeningeal cysts caused by trauma or infection, in which loculated CSF is surrounded by scarred arachnoid,[8,11] true arachnoid cysts are lined by cells that contain specialized membranes and lining cells capable of secretion.[8] Thus, arachnoid cysts may expand either by accumulation of CSF secreted by these inner lining cells, or by unidirectional (ball-valve) CSF flow.[16] Progressive expansion of the cyst compresses the underlying brain but usually allows preservation of its cytoarchitecture; chronic compression, however, may cause gliosis. Hydrocephalus may result from intraventricular blockage of CSF flow or from extraventricular obstruction of the pathways through which CSF normally flows or is absorbed.[1,7,8,17] Arachnoid cysts can arise in any part of the central nervous system where arachnoid is found (Fig. 51.2).

CLINICAL PRESENTATION

The clinical manifestations of arachnoid cysts are often mild even in patients with large lesions.[17–19] Some neurologic signs and symptoms are common to all patients, whereas others are specific for patients with cysts in particular anatomic locations.[2,4,20] Headache and craniomegaly caused by cyst expansion or hydrocephalus occur in patients with cysts in any location. Seizures, in contrast,

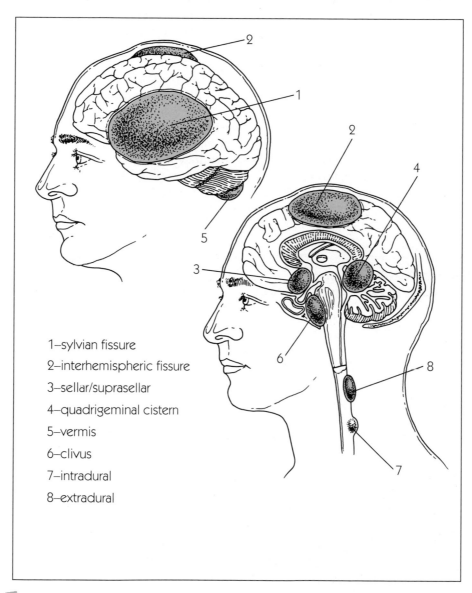

1–sylvian fissure
2–interhemispheric fissure
3–sellar/suprasellar
4–quadrigeminal cistern
5–vermis
6–clivus
7–intradural
8–extradural

Figure 51.2 Anatomic distribution of arachnoid cysts along the craniospinal axis.

herald a supratentorial location. Clinical syndromes associated with cysts in the most common locations (see Fig. 51.2) are discussed in the following sections.

SYLVIAN FISSURE CYSTS

One half of all arachnoid cysts involve the sylvian fissure[4,7,10] (Fig. 51.3); male patients have cysts in this location over four times as frequently as female patients,[1] and these patients are usually younger than 20 years old at presentation. Headache is their most common presenting symptom.[1] Focal motor, generalized, or complex partial seizures also occur frequently (Fig. 51.4).[4,10] A focal bulge in the temporal bone or unilateral proptosis may be present as a result of gradual cyst expansion. Subdural hematoma, either intracystic or superficial to the cyst, can occur spontaneously or after minor head trauma.[21] The risk of this well-recognized complication has prompted some authors to recommend surgical intervention in all patients with arachnoid cysts.

POSTERIOR FOSSA CYSTS

Cysts in the posterior fossa, many of which arise near the midline, can cause obstructive hydrocephalus resulting in symptoms of intracranial hypertension, craniomegaly, and developmental retardation.[16,22,23] Cysts arising at the cerebellopontine angle may, in addition, cause symptoms and signs referable to dysfunction of the brain stem or cranial nerves. Arachnoid cysts in the posterior fossa must be distinguished from other collections of CSF, such as an enlarged cisterna magna or the Dandy-Walker malformation.[4]

SUPRASELLAR CYSTS

Arachnoid cysts can also arise in the suprachiasmatic cistern.[5,24] If large, they may erode the sella turcica, compress the pituitary stalk, optic chiasm, and hypothalamus, or obliterate the anterior third ventricle or foramen of Monro.[5] Obstructive hydrocephalus, the most common cause of initial symptoms, occurs in almost 90% of patients with suprasellar arachnoid cysts (Fig. 51.5). Other common symptoms include visual and endocrine dysfunction.[24] The bobble-head doll syndrome, an unusual movement disorder characterized by a to-and-fro bobbing and nodding of the head and torso, was first described in two patients with suprasellar arachnoid cysts.[25] Noncommunicating suprasellar arachnoid cysts must be distinguished from other mass lesions in this location, including pituitary adenomas, craniopharyngiomas, meningiomas, and aneurysms of the internal carotid artery.[4]

QUADRIGEMINAL CISTERN CYSTS

Cysts in the quadrigeminal cistern are thought to arise from arachnoid overlying the quadrigeminal plate and tentorial notch.[1,26] The relative immobility of midbrain structures and the close approximation of many cranial nerve nuclei, fiber tracts, and CSF pathways may lead to significant symptoms even in patients with small cysts in this location. Obstruction of the aqueduct of Sylvius results in headaches, nausea, vomiting, and papilledema.[4] Parinaud's syndrome occurs in approximately 25% of these patients. Other lesions causing similar clinical features include pinealomas, dermoid cysts, tentorial meningiomas, and vein of Galen malformations. Pineal cysts, the result of focal degeneration of the pineal parenchyma, are often seen on MR images but rarely grow large enough to cause symptoms and thus do not require treatment.

DIAGNOSIS

Before the introduction of modern computer-assisted imaging modalities, the diagnostic work-up of patients thought to have arachnoid cysts relied on plain roentgenograms and cerebral angiograms. Skull radiographs of patients with cysts in the middle cranial fossa usually show evidence of a slowly expanding temporal mass. In these cases, the lesser wing of the sphenoid is elevated, and the squamous portion of the temporal bone is eroded and outwardly displaced. Angiograms, which show an avascular mass displacing normal vessels, may help differentiate arachnoid cysts from the occasional subacute sub-

Figure 51.3. Anatomic Distribution of Arachnoid Cysts Along the Cerebrospinal Axis

Intracranial cysts

Supratentorial
  Sylvian fissure (1)
  Cerebral convexity
  Interhemispheric fissure (2)
  Sellar/suprasellar (3)
  Quadrigeminal cistern (4)

Infratentorial
  Cerebellopontine angle
  Posterior midline
  Vermis (5)
  Clivus (6)

Intraspinal cysts

Intradural (7)
Extradural (8)

Numbers in parentheses refer to Figure 51.2.

Adapted with permission from di Rocco C. Arachnoid cysts. In: Youmans JR, ed. *Neurological Surgery*. Philadelphia, Pa: WB Saunders Co; 1990:1300.

dural hematoma or suprasellar aneurysm. Now that CT and MRI are available, the invasive techniques of angiography and pneumoencephalography are rarely needed.

A definitive diagnosis can often be made using CT alone.[2,4,5,23] An arachnoid cyst appears on CT scans as a noncalcified, low-density, extraaxial mass with regular borders that do not enhance with the administration of contrast media.[2,3] In cysts that communicate with the subarachnoid space, metrizamide CT cisternography and ventriculography show delayed homogeneous uptake of contrast. Other findings on CT scans include compression of adjacent brain and the lateral ventricle, gyral effacement, and midline shift. If CSF pathways are obstructed, ventricular enlargement also occurs. CT usually allows arachnoid cysts to be differentiated from low-grade gliomas, infarcts, and chronic subdural hygromas;[2] it is less reliable, however, in differentiating arachnoid cysts from cysts associated with isodense tumors, such as gangliogliomas, cerebellar hemangioblastomas, and cystic astrocytomas.[4] Radioisotopic or metrizamide CT cisternograms or ventriculograms may be necessary to differentiate arachnoid cysts from other abnormal collections of CSF,[3,5,24] such as porencephalic cysts or the posterior fossa cyst of a Dandy-Walker malformation, or from an enlarged cisterna magna.[4]

MRI has become the radiographic study of choice in patients in whom an arachnoid cyst is suspected.[27,28] Multiplanar imaging allows better visualization of the underlying pathology of the cyst and its anatomic relationship to surrounding neural structures. The contents of arachnoid cysts have the same signal characteristics as CSF on both T1-weighted and T2-weighted images.[28] MRI readily discriminates between the CSF of true arachnoid cysts and the high-protein fluid of neoplastic cysts,[8] and it often shows cyst walls separating encysted fluid from the surrounding ventricular or subarachnoid fluid. New MRI techniques that assess pulsatile motion of CSF show reduced signal intensity within these lesions, indicating fluid motion; it appears, however, that this signal loss is secondary to arterial systolic pulsations transmitted from the surrounding brain tissue rather than bulk CSF flow through the cyst.[29] Thus, metrizamide CT cisternography and ventriculography remain the only reliable techniques for confirming communication of the cyst with the subarachnoid space.

TREATMENT

PATIENT SELECTION

Not all arachnoid cysts require surgical intervention. Patients with asymptomatic cysts discovered during radiographic imaging for an unrelated complaint and those with cysts producing minor skull defects should be followed clinically with annual CT or MRI and neuropsychiatric testing.[4,10] Surgical intervention should be considered if symptoms develop, if the patient's school performance deteriorates, or if other evidence of cognitive impairment is seen.[10] Treatment is certainly required for patients with symptoms of intracranial hypertension, intractable seizures, or focal neurologic deficits.[4,5,10,11,24,30] Children with arachnoid cysts that compress the brain directly or indirectly should be treated as well,[3,4,8,10,13] despite the risks of operative intervention. In children, these risks are outweighed by the potential for impaired development

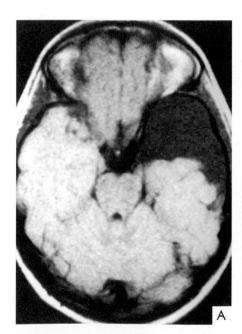 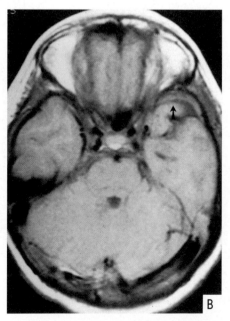 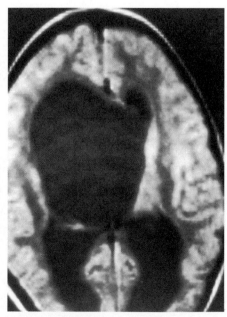

Figure 51.4 (A) Preoperative T1-weighted MR image in a 14-year-old girl with complex partial seizures shows a large cyst in the left middle temporal fossa, displacing the temporal lobe posteriorly (TR = 600, TE = 20). (B) Follow-up MR image 1 year after cystperitoneal shunting shows complete re-expansion of the temporal lobe. The shunt tubing is visible in the middle cranial fossa (arrow).

Figure 51.5 T1-weighted MR image in a 7-year-old boy with precocious puberty shows a large suprasellar arachnoid cyst obstructing the foramen of Monro with resulting hydrocephalus.

and function of brain tissue[8] or for rapid neurologic deterioration caused by intracystic or subdural hemorrhage.[3,4,6,12,21]

GOALS OF THERAPY

GOALS OF THERAPY

The goals of therapy are to relieve the brain of compression and to relieve the CSF pathways from obstruction. Surgical options include needle aspiration; craniotomy for partial or complete cystectomy or for fenestration into the subarachnoid space, basilar cisterns, or ventricle; and cyst-peritoneal shunting. The choice of surgical therapy depends on the age and health of the patient, the size and location of the cyst, and the presence or absence of hydrocephalus.[10] Needle aspiration by transcranial puncture in infants or through a burr hole in older children or adults results in only temporary benefit because cyst fluid reaccumulates and symptoms recur;[2,31] thus, needle aspiration is no longer considered a reasonable option.[4]

CYST FENESTRATION

Craniotomy has been the most common method of treatment.[2,5,6,20,32,33] Advantages of this approach include direct inspection and excision of the cyst,[2,5,20] confirmation of the diagnosis by biopsy,[34] and coagulation of the fragile arachnoidal blood vessels under direct inspection.[12] Craniotomy sometimes averts the complications that can occur in a shunt-dependent patient.[32,34,35]

Recent experience, however, suggests that for most types of arachnoid cysts, the presumed advantages of craniotomy are insignificant or outweighed by attendant complications.[4,10,13,18,30,31,33] Arachnoid cysts frequently recur after craniotomy for drainage or fenestration.[2,12,13] Recurrence may result from reclosure of the cyst wall after partial resection, from fenestration of the cyst into the subdural space with the inner arachnoidal membrane left intact, or from inadequate flow of CSF through the subarachnoid space into which the cyst is opened.[16] In addition, the communicating or noncommunicating hydrocephalus that accompanies some cysts is not always relieved by fenestration or excision of the cyst. When hydrocephalus persists, a subsequent CSF shunting procedure is necessary.[5,30] Finally, craniotomy for excision of arachnoid cysts is not a benign procedure: its complications include aseptic meningitis, severe neurologic deficits, delayed hemorrhage, and infrequently, death.[2,12,17,22]

Despite these risks, craniotomy is the preferred surgical approach for quadrigeminal[26] and suprasellar arachnoid cysts.[4,5,11,20,24] Because of their proximity to the brain stem, small lesions in these locations are more safely approached under direct visualization. Suprasellar arachnoid cysts can be excised through a standard subfrontal,[20,36] transventricular, or transcallosal approach.[5,24] We prefer the transcallosal approach, especially in patients with hydrocephalus, because it minimizes frontal lobe retraction and avoids interruption of frontal white matter tracts (Fig. 51.6). After a standard horseshoe-shaped scalp

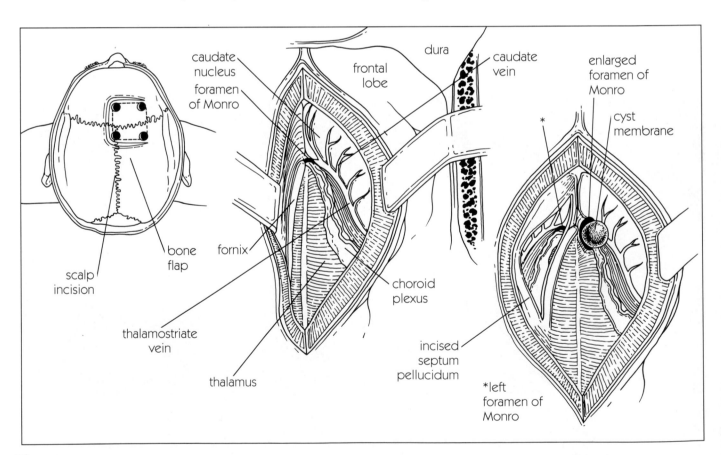

Figure 51.6 Anterior transcallosal approach to a suprasellar arachnoid cyst. The cyst can be seen obstructing the foramen of Monro. The cyst is fenestrated into the ventricle, and a catheter is used to shunt the ventricle to the peritoneal cavity.

incision, a four-hole free bone flap is constructed with the medial holes over the sagittal sinus. The bone flap is positioned so that it is transected by the coronal suture approximately two thirds of the way from the anterior margin of the flap. A U-shaped dural opening is made and the dura reflected along the sagittal sinus. The retractor blades are carefully deepened to avoid damage to the pericallosal arteries, until the corpus callosum is identified. The callosal fibers are separated in the anterior-posterior direction, and the lateral ventricle is entered. The dome of the cyst can then be seen through the thinned, tented floor of the lateral ventricle (Fig. 51.7). It is not necessary to excise the cyst wall down to the floor of the third ventricle; in fact, wide excision may damage the hypothalamus unnecessarily and lead to endocrine dysfunction.[24] After communication is established between the cyst interior and the ventricle

(Fig. 51.8), a silastic tube is placed into the cyst bed, and its distal end is placed into the peritoneal cavity to prevent cyst recurrence (Fig. 51.9).

In patients with suprasellar cysts without hydrocephalus, a subfrontal approach may be equally successful.[5,36] When this approach is used, manipulations are limited to the arachnoid membranes, the optic nerves are released from arachnoid adhesions, and the basal CSF circulation is restored.

Cysts in the quadrigeminal cistern can be safely fenestrated with a supracerebellar approach.[26] The patient is placed prone in the concord position and a standard midline craniectomy is performed in the posterior fossa. The dura is incised and reflected superiorly, and the supracerebellar bridging veins are coagulated and divided. The cerebellar hemispheres are then gently retracted inferiorly

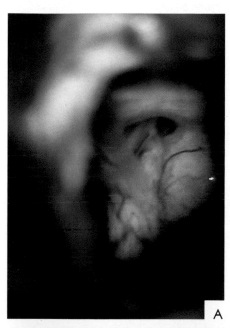

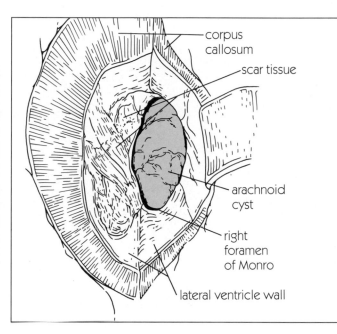

Figure 51.7 Intraoperative photograph of the trans-callosal approach to a suprasellar arachnoid cyst. The thin lining of the cyst is seen bulging through the right foramen of Monro.

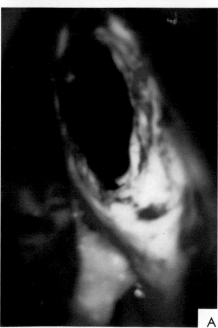

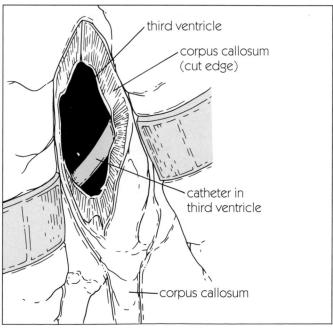

Figure 51.8 Intraoperative photograph of the suprasellar cyst shown in Figure 51.7 after wide fenestration into the right lateral ventricle.

until the tentorial notch and cyst are exposed. The cyst wall may then be excised safely (Fig. 51.10).

For patients with cysts in the middle cranial fossa, some authors advocate cyst fenestration as the initial treatment. Galassi et al.[12] reported only one death, caused by bacterial meningitis, and two major postoperative complications (one extradural and one intracystic hematoma) in their series of 77 adult and pediatric patients with cysts in the middle cranial fossa that were initially treated by fenestration. The vast majority (95%) of these patients showed clinical or radiographic improvement after fenestration. These good results may reflect the fact that adults generally suffer fewer complications and that cysts in the middle cranial fossa are among the least difficult to treat. If fenestration is performed, wide excision of the outer arachnoid membrane is necessary, along with fenestration of the inner arachnoid membrane into the chiasmatic and interpeduncular cisterns.[11–13]

Poorer results are seen in studies that involve only children and in those that include patients with cysts outside the middle cranial fossa. Raffel and McComb[32] reported that 11 (73%) of 15 patients without hydrocephalus had cysts successfully fenestrated and remain shunt-independent. Lange and Oeckler[37] reported a series in which 13 (68%) of 19 patients treated by craniotomy showed significant clinical improvement. Four of the six patients whose condition did not improve after craniotomy required subsequent shunting procedures. In 10 of our 15 patients, with cysts in various locations, fenestration failed to cause clinical or radiographic improvement.[10]

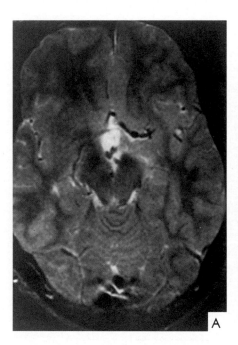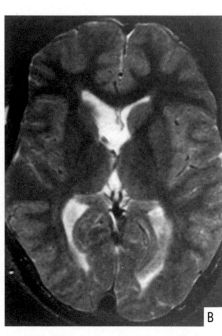

A   B

Figure 51.9 Follow-up MR images of the suprasellar arachnoid cyst shown in Figure 51.5, 1 year after cyst fenestration and shunting. The large obstructing lesion has completely resolved.

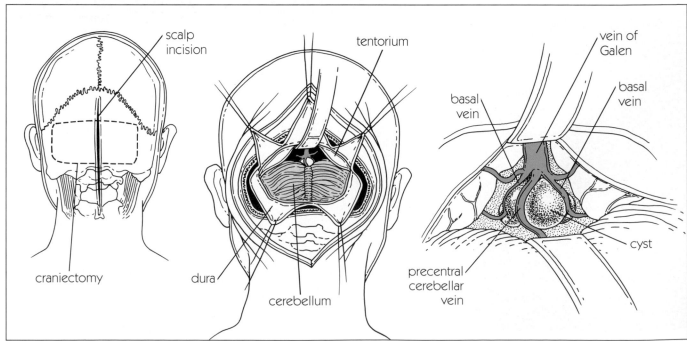

Figure 51.10 Supracerebellar approach to an arachnoid cyst of the quadrigeminal cistern.

Principles of Neurosurgery

Cyst-peritoneal shunting, in combination with ventriculoperitoneal (VP) shunting if hydrocephalus is present, is the procedure of choice for the treatment of most arachnoid cysts.[4,10,13,18,31,38] Fenestration alone rarely allows ventricular decompression in patients with hydrocephalus; therefore, most of these patients later require VP shunting for relief of hydrocephalus[4,5,16,20] or cyst-peritoneal shunting to treat recurrent cysts.[12,13] In our series, only one of nine patients with hydrocephalus was successfully treated with fenestration alone.[10] VP shunting is frequently necessary in patients with hydrocephalus, and an additional shunt from the cyst to the peritoneal tubing does not substantially increase the risk of the procedure. A cyst-VP shunt therefore appears to be a more prudent surgical option than fenestration in these patients.

For arachnoid cysts that recur after fenestration, shunting is effective as a secondary treatment to decompress the cyst.[2,4,5,30,39] Shunting is also necessary when a cyst is successfully treated by fenestration, but an obstructive or communicating hydrocephalus persists.[16]

The major complications of cyst shunting—malfunction and infection—occur infrequently.[4,31,33] If the arachnoidal leaves are reapproximated after shunting, fluid may not reaccumulate between them, even if the shunt is later occluded. Symptoms of nausea and headache, which sometimes occur after shunting, are not dangerous and invariably diminish with time.[10] Intracystic or subdural hematomas precipitated by excessively rapid cyst decompression[17] are rare in our experience. A drawback of shunting is that the shunt must usually remain in place throughout the patient's life. Despite its permanence, however, shunting seems to cause few complications and to impose few limitations on patients.

The technique used in cyst-peritoneal shunting of cysts in the middle cranial fossa is similar to that used in VP shunting. Shunt design and the method of insertion can be adapted to meet the specific needs of each patient, but a simple shunt from the cyst to the peritoneum suffices for most middle cranial fossa cysts.[4] The patient is placed supine on the operating table, and the head is rotated into the lateral position on a doughnut headholder. A curvilinear incision is then made over the temporal region (Fig. 51.11). The temporalis fascia and muscle are incised in the direction of the muscle fibers and the underlying bone exposed. A burr hole is then made, and the dura, which often appears blue-gray because of the underlying collection of CSF, is coagulated. The peritoneum is then

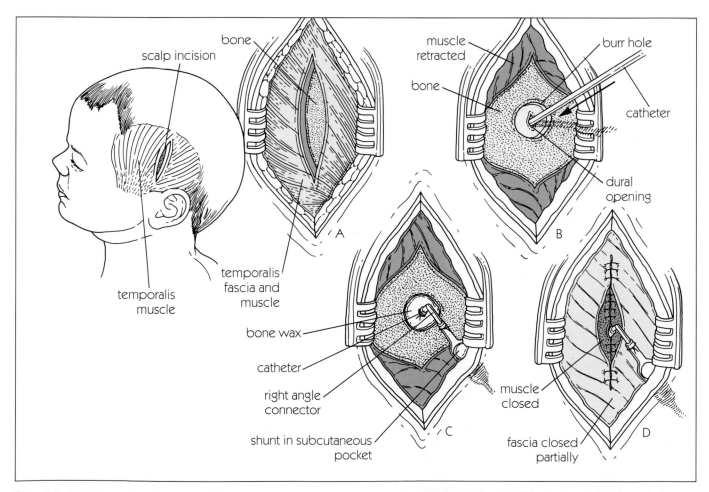

Figure 51.11 Cyst-peritoneal shunting technique. (A) A linear incision is made in the temporalis fascia and muscle, and a burr hole is drilled over the cyst. (B) The dura is perforated just large enough to permit passage of the catheter. Bone wax is used to seal the burr hole. (C) The reservoir is placed in a subcutaneous pocket away from the burr hole and connected to the cyst catheter via a right angle connector. (D) The temporalis muscle and fascia are then closed in layers around the catheter tubing to prevent formation of a pseudomeningocele.

exposed and the shunt tunneled subcutaneously. An incision just large enough to permit passage of the shunt tubing is then made in the dura, and the tubing is advanced into the cyst cavity. After confirmation of distal flow, the peritoneal end is placed into the abdominal cavity and secured. Bone wax may be placed in the burr hole to limit the leakage of subcutaneous fluid. The temporalis muscle and fascia are then closed in layers to minimize tracking around the catheter. The patient can usually leave the hospital after 48 to 72 hours.

Patients with cysts in the posterior fossa can also be treated successfully by cyst shunting. In these patients, a single burr hole is drilled over the posterior fossa. The overlying cervical muscles are closed to reduce the likelihood of pseudomeningocele formation. Cyst location appears to influence the success of shunt therapy. Among patients in our series[10] with cysts in the middle cranial fossa, shunting resulted in clinical improvement for all of seven children with cysts treated initially by shunting and four with temporal cysts shunted after unsuccessful fenestration. In contrast, cyst shunting was successful in only about half of the children with cysts in the posterior fossa, whether shunting was used as the first mode of treatment (five of nine patients) or after failed fenestration or shunting (three of five patients). Cysts in both locations, however, were more successfully treated by shunting than by fenestration.

All patients should undergo postoperative CT or MRI to assess the size of the cyst and to confirm catheter placement. Patients whose follow-up scans show no improvement require close clinical and radiographic observation and may warrant radionuclide evaluation to rule out shunt malfunction.[4] Periodic radiographic evaluation is also prudent after successful shunting and is imperative if clinical symptoms recur or if symptoms of shunt malfunction or infection develop.

REFERENCES

1. Rengachary SS, Watanabe I, Brackett CE. Pathogenesis of intracranial arachnoid cysts. *Surg Neurol.* 1978;9:139–144.
2. Anderson FM, Segal HD, Caton WL. Use of computerized tomography scanning in supratentorial arachnoid cysts: a report on 20 children and four adults. *J Neurosurg.* 1979;50:333–338.
3. Galassi E, Piazza G, Gaist G, et al. Arachnoid cysts of the middle cranial fossa: a clinical and radiological study of 25 cases treated surgically. *Surg Neurol.* 1980;14:211–219.
4. Harsh GR IV, Edwards MSB, Wilson CB. Intracranial arachnoid cysts in children. *J Neurosurg.* 1986;64:835–842.
5. Hoffman HJ, Hendrick EB, Humphreys RP, et al. Investigation and management of suprasellar arachnoid cysts. *J Neurosurg.* 1982;57:597–602.
6. Robinson RG. Congenital cysts of the brain: arachnoid malformations. *Prog Neurol Surg.* 1971;4:133–174.
7. Rengachary SS, Watanabe I. Ultrastructure and pathogenesis of intracranial arachnoid cysts. *J Neuropathol Exp Neurol.* 1981;40:61–83.
8. Go KG, Houthoff H-J, Blaauw EH, et al. Arachnoid cysts of the sylvian fissure: evidence of fluid secretion. *J Neurosurg.* 1984;60:803–813.
9. Shaw C-M. "Arachnoid cysts" of the sylvian fissure versus "temporal lobe agenesis" syndrome. *Ann Neurol.* 1979;5:483–485.
10. Ciricillo SF, Cogen PH, Harsh GR, et al. Intracranial arachnoid cysts in children: a comparison of the effects of fenestration and shunting. *J Neurosurg.* 1991;74:230-235.
11. Dyck P, Gruskin P. Supratentorial arachnoid cysts in adults: a discussion of two cases from a pathophysiologic and surgical perspective. *Arch Neurol.* 1977;34:276–279.
12. Galassi E, Gaist G, Giuliani G, et al. Arachnoid cysts of the middle cranial fossa: experience with 77 cases treated surgically. *Acta Neurochir Suppl (Wien).* 1988;42:201–204.
13. Geissinger JD, Kohler WC, Robinson BW, et al. Arachnoid cysts of the middle cranial fossa: surgical considerations. *Surg Neurol.* 1978;10:27–33.
14. von Wild K, Gullotta F. Arachnoid cyst of the middle cranial fossa—aplasia of temporal lobe? *Childs Nerv Syst.* 1987;3:232–234.
15. Starkman SP, Brown TE, Linell EA. Cerebral arachnoid cysts. *J Neuropathol Exp Neurol.* 1958;17:484–500.
16. di Rocco D, Caldarelli M, di Trapani G. Infratentorial arachnoid cysts in children. *Childs Brain.* 1981;8:119-133.
17. Aicardi J, Bauman F. Supratentorial extracerebral cysts in infants and children. *J Neurol Neurosurg Psychiatry.* 1975;38:57–68.
18. McCullough DC, Harbert JC, Manz HJ. Large arachnoid cysts at the cranial base. *Neurosurgery.* 1980;6:76–81.
19. Menezes AH, Bell WE, Perret GE. Arachnoid cysts in children. *Arch Neurol.* 1980;37:168–172.
20. Raimondi AJ, Shimoji T, Gutierrez FA. Suprasellar cysts: surgical treatment and results. *Childs Brain.* 1980;7:57–72.
21. Page AC, Mohan D, Paxton RM. Arachnoid cysts of the middle fossa predispose to subdural haematoma formation: fact or fiction: *Acta Neurochir Suppl (Wien).* 1988;42:210–215.
22. Little JR, Gomez MR, MacCarth CS. Infratentorial arachnoid cysts. *J Neurosurg.* 1973;39:380–386.

23. Vaquero J, Carrillo R, Cabezudo JM, et al. Arachnoid cysts of the posterior fossa. *Surg Neurol.* 1981;16:117–121.
24. Murali R, Epstein F. Diagnosis and treatment of suprasellar arachnoid cyst: report of three cases. *J Neurosurg.* 1979;50:515–518.
25. Benton JW, Nellhaus G, Huttenlocher PR, et al. The bobble-head doll syndrome: report of a unique truncal tremor associated with third ventricular cyst and hydrocephalus in children. *Neurology.* 1966;16: 725–729.
26. Yanaka K, Enomoto T, Nose T, et al. Postinflammatory arachnoid cyst of the quadrigeminal cistern: observation of development of the cyst. *Childs Nerv Syst.* 1988;4:302–305.
27. Gandy SE, Heier LA. Clinical and magnetic resonance features of primary intracranial arachnoid cysts. *Ann Neurol.* 1987;21:342–348.
28. Weiner SN, Pearlstein AE, Eiber A. MR imaging of intracranial arachnoid cysts. *J Comput Assist Tomogr.* 1987;11:236–241.
29. Brooks ML, Jolesz FA, Patz S. MRI of pulsatile CSF motion within arachnoid cysts. *Magn Reson Imaging.* 1988;6:575–584.
30. Stein SC. Intracranial developmental cysts in children: treatment by cystoperitoneal shunting. *Neurosurgery.* 1981;8:647–650.
31. Kaplan BJ, Mickle JP, Parkhurst R. Cystoperitoneal shunting for congenital arachnoid cysts. *Childs Brain.* 1984;11:304–311.
32. Raffel C, McComb JG. To shunt or to fenestrate: which is the best surgical treatment for arachnoid cysts in pediatric patients? *Neurosurgery.* 1988;23: 338–342.
33. Locatelli D, Bonfanti N, Sfogliarini R, et al. Arachnoid cysts: diagnosis and treatment. *Childs Nerv Syst.* 1987;3:121–124.
34. Anderson FM. Arachnoid cysts. *J Neurosurg.* 1979; 51:132. Letter.
35. Garcia-Bach M, Isamat F, Vila F. Intracranial arachnoid cysts in adults. *Acta Neurochir Suppl (Wien).* 1988;42:205–209.
36. Marinov M, Undjian S, Wetzka P. An evaluation of the surgical treatment of intracranial arachnoid cysts in children. *Childs Nerv Syst.* 1989;5:177–183.
37. Lange M, Oeckler R. Results of surgical treatment in patients with arachnoid cysts. *Acta Neurochir (Wien).* 1987;87:99–104.
38. Pomeranz S, Wald U, Amir N, et al. Arachnoid cysts: unusual aspects and management. *Neurochirurgia.* 1988;31:25–28.
39. Cilluffo JM, Onofrio BM, Miller RH. The diagnosis and surgical treatment of intracranial arachnoid cysts. *Acta Neurochir (Wien).* 1983;67:215–229.

INDEX

Note: Numbers in **bold** type refer to figures.

in meningioma, 28.7–28.8, **28.12**
Angioplasty, 14.2
　in atheromatous arterial stenosis, 14.20–14.21
　in cerebral arterial vasospasm, 14.20, 14.24, 14.25, **14.26–14.27**
　　decision tree for, 14.23, **14.25**
Annulus fibrosus, **44.1**, 44.2, **45.1–45.2**, 45.2, 45.3
Antibiotics in brain abscess, 24.4
Anticoagulants in stroke prevention, 10.12
Anticonvulsant drugs, **50.2**, 50.4
　in head injuries, 16.17
Antidiuretic hormone, 32.32–32.36
　deficiency of, **32.34–32.35**, 32.34–32.36
　inappropriate secretion of, **32.33**, 32.33–32.34
　plasma osmolality affecting, **32.32**, 32.33
　regulation of, **32.31**, 32.32
Antifibrinolytic therapy in intracranial aneurysms, 11.7
Antimetabolite therapy, 43.4
Antisepsis, history of, 1.17
Antishock garment, pneumatic, in multiple injuries, 15.5–15.6, **15.6**
Apneustic breathing, 3.8, 3.9, **3.9**
Apoplexy, pituitary, 33.2, 33.3, **33.6**
Ara-C therapy, 43.4
Arabic medicine, **1.3–1.4**, 1.4–1.6
Arachnoid cysts, 51.2–51.10
　anatomic distribution of, **51.2–51.3**, 51.3, 51.4
　clinical features of, 51.3–51.4
　diagnosis of, 51.4–51.5
　hydrocephalus in, 6.4, **6.4**, 6.5, 6.17
　middle cranial fossa, 51.8
　pathology of, **51.1**, 51.2
　posterior fossa, 51.4
　quadrigeminal cistern, 51.4
　　supracerebellar approach in, 51.7–51.8, **51.10**
　shunting procedures in, 51.9–51.10, **51.11**
　suprasellar, 51.4, 51.5, **51.5**
　　transcallosal approach in, 51.6–51.7, **51.6–51.9**, 51.8
　sylvian fissure, 51.4, **51.4**, 51.5
　treatment of, 51.5–51.10
　　goals in, 51.5–51.6
　　patient selection in, 51.5-51.6
Arachnoid granulations, hydrocephalus in, 6.7–6.8, **6.10**
Arteriovenous fistula of spinal dura, embolization therapy in, 14.9, **14.11**
Arteriovenous malformations, 12.4–12.5, **12.8–12.11**, 13.4, 13.5–13.6
　angiographic appearance of, 12.8, 12.10, **12.14**, **12.19**
　embolization therapy in, **14.2–14.10**, 14.3–14.9
　　in brain, **14.2–14.9**, 14.3–14.7
　　dural, 14.18–14.20, 14.21, 14.22, **14.22–14.24**
　　in spinal cord, 14.7–14.9, **14.10**
　intraoperative appearance of, 12.8, **12.15**
　radiosurgery results in, 42.12, **42.13**, 42.14, 42.15, **42.17–42.18**
Aspiration procedures

percutaneous, in colloid cysts of third ventricle, 36.7
　stereotactic, 49.13, 49.22, **49.52–49.53**
Aspirin in stroke prevention, 10.12
Astrocytomas, 26.7–26.11
　age distribution of, **26.3**, 26.6
　anaplastic, 26.7–26.8, 26.11
　　clinical features of, **26.8**, 26.12–26.13
　brain stem, 31.16, **31.18**
　　magnetic resonance features of, **31.1**, 31.3
　cerebellar, **31.2–31.3**, 31.4, 31.10–31.11, **31.12**
　chemotherapy in, 43.4
　chiasmal-hypothalamic, hydrocephalus in, 6.5
　chromosomal loss in, 25.14–25.15, **25.14–25.15**
　classification of, **26.2**, 26.2–26.3, 26.4–26.5
　clinical features of, **26.7**, 26.10–26.11
　intramedullary, 39.3–39.4, **39.3–39.5**, 39.8
　medulla oblongata, 31.18, 31.19, **31.20–31.22**
　parietal lobe, radiosurgery results in, 42.16, **42.22**
　periaqueductal, hydrocephalus in, 6.6, **6.7**
　pilocytic, 26.7
　　cerebellar, 31.10, **31.12**
　　cerebral, **26.5**, 26.7, 26.9
　　in chiasm and hypothalamus, **26.6**, 26.7, 26.10
　　clinical features of, **26.4**, 26.8–26.9
　　magnetic resonance imaging in, **31.1**, 31.3
Ataxic breathing, 3.8, 3.9, **3.9**
Atherosclerosis
　aneurysms in, 13.5
　angioplasty of arterial stenosis in, 14.20–14.21
　cerebrovascular, 10.6
Atlantooccipital dislocation, 20.3, **20.6**
　treatment of, 20.8, **20.21**
Atlas fractures, 20.4, **20.7**
　treatment of, 20.8–20.9
Avicenna, **1.4**, 1.4–1.5
Axis fractures, 20.4–20.5, **20.8–20.11**
　treatment of, 20.9–20.10, **20.22–20.24**
Axonal injury, diffuse, 16.6–16.7
Axonotemesis, 22.3

Baclofen in trigeminal neuralgia, 47.4
Ballistic studies in gunshot wounds of head, 17.4–17.7, **17.6–17.9**, 17.8
Balloon occlusion
　in carotid-cavernous fistula, 14.14–14.16, **14.17–14.18**
　in cerebral aneurysms, 14.9–14.14
　　decision tree for, 14.10, **14.12**
　　intrasaccular occlusion in, 14.11–14.14, **14.15**
　　parent vessel occlusion in, 14.9–14.11, 14.12, **14.14**
　in cerebral arteriovenous fistula, 14.18, **14.20**
　detachable balloons in, 14.2
　test occlusion in cranial base tumors, 40.9, **40.15–40.16**
　two systems for, 14.11, **14.13**
　in vertebral artery fistula, 14.16–14.18, **14.19**

Vertebral artery fistula, embolization therapy in, 14.16–14.18, **14.19**

Vertebrobasilar ischemia, 10.16–10.17
    vertebral artery transposition in, **10.14**, 10.16–10.17

Vesalius, Andreas, 1.10, **1.15**

Vinca alkaloids, 43.4

Viruses, oncogenicity of, 25.18

Visual acuity tests
    in craniopharyngiomas, 35.8
    in pituitary adenomas, 33.2, **33.4**, 34.4

von Hippel-Lindau disease, 25.9, **25.10**, 25.12
    cerebellar hemangioblastoma in, 31.14

Warfarin in stroke prevention, 10.12

Water deprivation test in diabetes insipidus, 32.34–32.35

William of Saliceto, 1.7

Willis, Thomas, 1.11, 1.12, **1.17–1.18**

Wound healing, postoperative, 4.8, 4.9, **4.9**

Yonge, James, 1.12

Zygoma fractures, 18.27, 18.28, 18.29, **18.41–18.43**